BLOOD TRANSFUSION IN
CLINICAL MEDICINE

BLOOD TRANSFUSION IN CLINICAL MEDICINE

P.L. MOLLISON
CBE, MD, FRCP, FRCPath, FRCOG, FRS
Emeritus Professor of Haematology in the University of London
Formerly Director, MRC Experimental Haematology Unit
St Mary's Hospital Medical School, London

C.P. ENGELFRIET
MD
Professor of Immunohaematology in the University of Amsterdam
Head of Department of Immunohaematology
Central Laboratory of The Netherlands
Red Cross Blood Transfusion Service

MARCELA CONTRERAS
BSc, MD, MRCPath, FRCP(Edin)
Director, North London Blood Transfusion Centre
Honorary Senior Lecturer, Department of Haematology
St Mary's Hospital Medical School, London

The chapter on Transfusion in Oligaemia
revised by
JENNIFER JONES
BSc, FRCP, FFARCS
Consultant Anaesthetist and
Consultant in Charge of the Intensive Care Unit
St Mary's Hospital, London

NINTH EDITION

OXFORD
BLACKWELL SCIENTIFIC PUBLICATIONS
LONDON EDINBURGH BOSTON
MELBOURNE PARIS BERLIN VIENNA

© 1961, 1967, 1972, 1979, 1983, 1987, 1993 by
Blackwell Scientific Publications
Editorial Offices:
Osney Mead, Oxford OX2 0EL
25 John Street, London WC1N 2BL
23 Ainslie Place, Edinburgh EH3 6AJ
238 Main Street, Cambridge
  Massachusetts 02142, USA
54 University Street, Carlton
  Victoria 3053, Australia

Other Editorial Offices:
Librairie Arnette SA
2, rue Casimir-Delavigne
75006 Paris
France

Blackwell Wissenschaft-Verlag
Meinekestrasse 4
D-1000 Berlin 15
Germany

Blackwell MZV
Feldgasse 13
A-1238 Wien
Austria

First published 1951
Spanish translation of first edition 1955
Spanish translation of seventh edition 1987
Italian translation of seventh edition 1987
Second edition 1956
Third edition 1961
Reprinted 1963, 1964
Fourth edition 1967
Reprinted 1967
Fifth edition 1972
Reprinted 1974
Sixth edition 1979
Seventh edition 1983
Eighth edition 1987
Reprinted 1988
Ninth edition 1993

Set by Semantic Graphics, Singapore
Printed and bound in the United States
of America by Hamiltons, New York

DISTRIBUTORS

Marston Book Services Ltd
PO Box 87
Oxford OX2 0DT
(*Orders*: Tel: 0865 791155
        Fax: 0865 791927
        Telex: 837515)

USA
  Blackwell Scientific Publications, Inc.
  238 Main street
  Cambridge, MA 02142
  (*Orders*: Tel: 800 759-6102
          617 876-7000)

Canada
  Times Mirror Professional Publishing Ltd
  5240 Finch Avenue East
  Scarborough, Ontario M1S 5A2
  (*Orders*: Tel: 800 268-4178
          416 298-1588)

Australia
  Blackwell Scientific Publications
  (Australia) Pty Ltd
  54 University Street
  Carlton, Victoria 3053
  (*Orders*: Tel: 03 347-0300)

A catalogue record for this title is
available from the British Library

ISBN 0-632-02584-0

CONTENTS

CHAPTER 1
The Withdrawal of Blood

FIGURES

CHAPTER 2
Transfusion in Oligaemia

TABLES

CHAPTER 3
Immunology of Red Cells

FIGURES

TABLES

CHAPTER 4
ABO, Lewis, Ii and P Groups

FIGURES

TABLES

CHAPTER 5
The Rh Blood Group System (and LW)

FIGURES

TABLES

CHAPTER 6
Other Red Cell Antigens

FIGURE

CHAPTER 7

Red Cell Antibodies Against Self Antigens, Bound Antigens and Induced Antigens

CHAPTER 8

Detection of the Reaction Between Red Cell Antigens and Antibodies

TABLES

CHAPTER 9
The Transfusion of Red Cells

FIGURES

TABLES

CHAPTER 10

Red Cell Incompatibility *in vivo*

FIGURES

CHAPTER 11

Haemolytic Transfusion Reactions

CHAPTER 12

Haemolytic Disease of the Fetus and the Newborn

FIGURES

TABLES

CHAPTER 13
Immunology of Leucocytes, Platelets and Plasma Components

FIGURES

TABLES

CHAPTER 14
The Transfusion of Platelets, Leucocytes and Plasma Components

CHAPTER 15
Some Unfavourable Effects of Transfusion

CHAPTER 16
Infectious Agents Transmitted by Transfusion

FIGURES

Appendices

TABLE

PREFACE TO NINTH EDITION

In the first edition of this book, published more than 40 years ago, the emphasis was very heavily on the transfusion of red cells; a good deal was known about their survival *in vivo*, their behaviour during storage and their immunology. In contrast, at that time, no attempts were being made to transfuse leucocytes or platelets, no leucocyte or platelet antigens had been described and no plasma fractions were available. The only diseases known to be transmitted by transfusion were hepatitis, for the infectious agents of which no tests were available, and syphilis and malaria; only four pages were devoted to the subject in a general chapter on the ill effects of transfusion.

The developments since then are reflected in the changed contents of the present edition. The immunology of leucocytes and platelets is considered in detail, as are therapeutic aspects of transfusions of leucocytes, platelets and plasma fractions. The longest chapter in the book is now that devoted to infectious agents transmitted by transfusion. At the same time, since the book has always tried to give a thorough account of the transfusion and immunology of red cells these topics are still given a good deal of space.

We have, in general, used SI units, although in referring to published work we have sometimes kept to the units used in the original publication; when the relation between old and new units is not obvious we have given the SI equivalent in parentheses. The meaning of abbreviations is explained on the first occasion on which they are used and can be discovered by consulting the index. The order of the chapters has been slightly changed so as to bring together those chapters dealing predominantly with red cells and those dealing mainly with leucocytes, platelets and plasma.

We should like to thank the many colleagues who have given us advice, particularly J.A. Barbara, N.C. Hughes-Jones and A. Lubenko; those who have typed the text and helped to find references, particularly Miss Joan Foley, Mrs Cynthia Freedman, Miss M. Mobed, Miss M.A.H. Mol and Mrs L.E.C. Snethlage; and John Robson of Blackwell Scientific Publications from whose expertise and enthusiasm we have once again benefited.

PREFACE TO FIRST EDITION

Blood was once regarded as a fluid of infinite complexity, the very essence of life. The blood of each person seemed to carry in it the secrets of individuality. As recently as 1666 it was natural for Mr Boyle, in writing to Dr Lower, to speculate in the following terms about the possible effect of cross-transfusion: '. . . as whether the blood of a mastiff, being frequently transfused into a bloodhound, or a spaniel, will not prejudice them in point of scent'.

If each person's blood were as individual as this, transfusion would indeed be complex and would deserve to rank as the most refined branch of medicine. However, this early view of the subtlety of transfusion was eclipsed at the beginning of the century by the discovery that the blood of all human beings could be divided into four groups. It seemed that, provided blood of the same group was transfused, one person's blood was indistinguishable from another's. Indeed, it came to be believed that people who belonged to the common group O could give their blood to anyone whatsoever. This point of view reached its widest acceptance in the early 1940s, when hundreds of thousands of bottles of group O blood were given as a general panacea for the injuries of war, with remarkably satisfactory effects. As a result of this experience, a generation of medical men has grown up believing that blood transfusion is one of the simplest forms of therapy.

And yet, this view of the interchangeability of blood has to be reconciled with the growing knowledge of its immense complexity. There are so many possible combinations of blood group antigens that the commonest of them all occurs in only 2% of the English population. Indeed, such is the individuality of the blood that, in Race's striking phase, certain combinations 'may never have formed the blood of an Englishman'.

The explanation of this apparent paradox—the potential complexity of transfusion and its actual simplicity—lies in the fact that many blood group factors are so weakly antigenic in man that they are not recognized as foreign by the recipient. However, it can no longer be maintained that a knowledge of the ABO system constitutes an adequate equipment for the transfusionist, for the role of some of the other systems is by no means negligible. Thus, a book on blood transfusion requires a special account of blood groups, in which the emphasis laid on any one of the antigens depends upon the part that it plays in incompatibility.

A good understanding of the effects of transfusion requires two further accounts: one of the regulation of blood volume and of the effects of transfusion on the circulation, and one of the survival of the various elements of blood after transfusion. The survival of transfused red cells has become a matter of special interest. Red cells survive for a longer period than any of the other components of blood, and their survival can be estimated with comparative precision by the method of differential agglutination. A study of the survival of transfused red cells has proved of great value in investigating haemolytic transfusion reactions. In addition, it has contributed strikingly to fundamental knowledge in haematology by demonstrating the diminished survival of pathological red cells and the existence of extrinsic haemolytic mechanisms in disease. Transfusions are now not uncommonly given for the purpose of investigation as well as of therapy.

This book is thus composed mainly of an account of blood groups from a clinical point of view and of descriptions of the effects of transfusion on the circulation and of the survival of transfused red cells; it also contains chapters designed to fill in the remaining background of knowledge about the results of transfusion in man. Finally it contains a rather detailed account of haemolytic disease of the newborn. It is addressed to all those who possess an elementary knowledge of blood transfusion and are interested in acquiring a fuller understanding of its effects.

In preparing this book I have had the help and advice of many friends. Dr J.V. Dacie read through almost all the typescript and made innumerable suggestions for improvements. Dr A.C. Dornhorst gave me the most extensive help in writing about the interpretation of red cell survival cures, and he is responsible for the simple rules for estimating mean cell life, which I hope that many besides myself will find useful; he has also read through the book during its preparation and given me the benefit of his very wide general knowledge. Dr J.F. Loutit, Dr I.D.P. Wootton and Dr L.E. Young are amongst those who have read certain sections and helped me with their expert advice.

I am even more indebted to Miss Marie Cutbush, who has given an immense amount of time to helping to prepare this book for the press and has, on every page, suggested changes to clarify the meaning of some sentence. In addition she has most generously encouraged me to quote many joint observations which are not yet published.

Miss Sylvia Mossom was responsible for typing the whole book, often from almost illegible manuscript. I am indebted to her for her skill and patience.

The *British Medical Journal, Clinical Science* and *The Lancet* have been so good as to allow the reproduction of certain figures originally published by them.

CHAPTER 1

THE WITHDRAWAL OF BLOOD

FIGURES

Safety of blood letting

The harmlessness of blood letting is attested by very long experience. As a form of medical treatment it found, perhaps, its most enthusiastic advocate in Benjamin Rush, physician, politician and most justly celebrated venesector. Rush not only believed in blood letting as a remedy for many common medical conditions including fever, but he also believed that it was valuable in the treatment of insanity, the primary site of which he believed resided in the blood vessels of the brain. One of his patients lost over 30 litres in the course of 47 venesections (Goodman, 1934).

In the last decade blood letting, as a form of therapy, has come back into fashion although in the more sophisticated form of plasma or red cell exchange. This chapter includes a discussion of this subject but is mainly concerned with the withdrawal of blood or its constituent parts from healthy donors for transfusion to patients.

BLOOD DONATION

The blood donor

Although in many countries, e.g. the UK, some 60% of the population are healthy adults aged 18–65 years and thus qualified to be blood donors (see below), the maximum frequency of donation in the world corresponds to about 10%, as in Switzerland (Hässig, 1990) and the frequency in most underdeveloped countries is less than 1% (Leikola, 1987). As a general rule, most adults between the ages of 18 and 65 who are in good health, have no history of serious illness, and do not recognize themselves as being at risk of transmitting any dangerous infectious agents particularly human immunodeficiency virus (HIV) are suitable as blood donors. Blood donors should be voluntary and unpaid; unpaid donors are safer than paid ones (Beal and van Aken, 1992). Most transfusion services have regulations for the selection of donors, designed for the protection of either donor or recipient (e.g. Department of Health, 1989; AABB, 1990). For example, some countries like the USA and Scotland accept blood donors from the age of 17, and others like Denmark and England extend the age of donation up to 70 years. Some accept donors from the age of 16 without parental consent. A medicolegal aspect of venesection may be briefly mentioned. A donor who becomes seriously ill shortly after giving blood may believe, or relatives may believe, that the illness is due to the donation. For this reason, among others, it is important to ensure that potential donors are in good health and that they have no history of conditions that would normally lead to their rejection as donors, such as anaemia, tuberculosis, cancer (except for cured carcinoma of the cervix), stroke, epilepsy, diabetes, liver cirrhosis, and cardiac, respiratory or renal disease. Individuals with significant hypertension should not be accepted as donors in view of the possibility of precipitating vascular accidents due to a sudden lowering of blood pressure; venesection as a therapeutic measure should not be carried out in a donor session.

Donors should sign a consent form before giving blood and should satisfy themselves and the blood transfusion service that they are not placing themselves or others at risk through their donations. The blood transfusion service should provide literature for the information of prospective blood donors.

Voluntary blood donors are highly suitable to become unrelated bone marrow donors and many transfusion services now recruit them for this purpose. It is estimated that over 400 000 HLA-typed bone marrow donors are now available in the different registeries of the World Marrow Donors Association (Buskard, 1991).

It should be possible to trace the origin of every blood donation. For this reason, records of donors should be kept safely for a period of years. Information on previous donations such as blood group, evidence of alloimmunization, presence of microbial antibodies, previous fainting, etc. will be of use for subsequent attendances. Information on current and previous blood donations by large panels of donors can be safely stored in computers, permitting prompt retrieval. Entry of data has been facilitated greatly by the use of bar-codes; verification of data through an in-built system to verify that labels have been read correctly, i.e. 'check digits', operator checks of eye-readable labels or laser readers, should be included to avoid the introduction of errors into the database (Roberts, 1989; Smit Sibinga, 1990).

Volume of donation
The volume of anticoagulants and preservative solutions in collection bags is calculated to allow for collection of a pre-set volume of blood which in the UK is 450 ± 45 ml. Additional volumes of 20–30 ml are taken into pilot tubes at the time of donation. From donors weighing 41–50 kg it is possible to collect a reduced volume of 250 ml of blood in packs in which the volume of anticoagulant has been appropriately adjusted; these packs may be obtained with attached satellite packs so that the donation may be subdivided for transfusions to infants.

In some countries, the volume collected routinely is less than 450 ml, e.g. 350–400 ml in Turkey, Greece and Italy, and is lower still (250 ml) in some Asian countries, where people are smaller than elsewhere.

Conditions that may disqualify a donor

Carriage of transmissible diseases
The most important diseases transmissible by transfusion are viral hepatitis in its several forms, acquired immune deficiency syndrome (AIDS) and other syndromes caused by HIV, human T-lymphotropic virus (HTLV), malaria, Chagas' disease, brucellosis, syphilis, kala-azar and Creutzfeld–Jakob disease. Steps that should be taken to minimize the risk of infecting recipients with the agents of these and other diseases are discussed in Chapter 16. If donors have been in contact with an infectious disease and are at risk of developing it, donation should be deferred for the length of the incubation period. The deferral periods appropriate for various infectious diseases are discussed in Chapter 16.

Units of blood collected 4 weeks to 3 months after recovery from one of the childhood infections (e.g. mumps) may be useful for the manufacture of specific immunoglobulin preparations.

Recent inoculations, vaccinations, etc.
To avoid the possibility of transmitting living viruses (e.g. those of measles, mumps, BCG, Sabin oral polio vaccine, yellow fever, vaccinia), donors should not give blood during the 2 weeks following vaccination. In the case of rubella, the interval should be 4 weeks. In subjects immunized with killed vaccines (cholera, influenza, typhoid, hepatitis B, Salk polio, rabies, anthrax, tick-borne and Japanese encephalitis) or toxoids (tetanus, diphtheria) the interval is normally only 48 h although some centres prolong it for 1 week for no apparent reason. As stated above, plasma from recently immunized donors may be useful for the manufacture of specific immunoglobulin preparations. Donors who have received immunoglobulins after exposure to infectious agents should not give blood for a period slightly longer than the incubation period of the disease in question. If hepatitis B immunoglobulin has been given after exposure to the virus, donation should be deferred for 9 months to 1 year; similarly, if anti-tetanus Ig has been given, donation should be deferred for 4 weeks. The administration of normal human immunoglobulin before travelling to countries where hepatitis A is endemic is not a cause for deferral. If rabies vaccination follows a bite by a rabid animal, blood donations should be suspended for 1 year. Donors who have received an injection of horse serum within the previous 3 weeks should not donate blood because of the risk

that their blood may still contain traces of horse serum which might accidentally immunize a recipient. (Although it is now the rule in developed countries to use anti-tetanus and anti-diphtheria immunoglobulin produced in humans rather than in horses, horse serum is still used in some parts of the world.)

Group O subjects may develop very potent haemolytic anti-A following an injection of materials which contain traces of hog pepsin; such materials include tetanus toxoid, TAB vaccine and pepsin-digested horse serum (see Chapter 4). In the past, the use of such subjects as 'universal donors' sometimes led to severe haemolytic transfusion reactions in subjects of other ABO groups.

Ear-piercing, electrolysis, tattooing, acupuncture
All these procedures carry a risk of transmission of hepatitis or HIV infection and, following them, blood donation should be deferred for at least 12 months.

'Allergic' subjects
Subjects who suffer from very severe allergy are unacceptable as donors because their hypersensitivity may be passively transferred to the recipient for a short period (see Chapter 15). On the other hand, subjects with seasonal allergy (e.g. hay fever) may donate when not in an active phase of their hypersensitivity.

Blood transfusions and tissue grafts
Donations should not be accepted for at least 12 months after the subject has received blood, blood components or grafts.

Surgery and dental treatment
Where surgery has been carried out without blood transfusion, donation may be considered when the subject has fully recovered. Uncomplicated dental treatments and extractions should not be a cause for prolonged deferral since the risk of bacteraemia persisting for more than 1 h is negligible (Nouri *et al.* 1989).

Drugs
Many subjects taking medication are not suitable as donors because of their clinical condition, e.g. subjects with heart disease. Others are unsuitable as donors because the drugs they are taking, e.g. anticoagulants or antibiotics, are potentially harmful to recipients (Mahnovski *et al.* 1987). Subjects who have taken aspirin within the previous week are unsuitable as sole platelet donors to a recipient (see p. 28). The taking of contraceptive pills or replacement hormones such as thyroxine is not a disqualification for blood donation. On the other hand, recipients of human growth hormone (non-recombinant) should be permanently debarred from blood donation (Contreras and Barbara, 1991). Subjects addicted to drugs injected by the parenteral route should not be accepted as donors.

Coagulation factor deficiencies or abnormal bleeding
Subjects with an abnormal bleeding tendency should be disqualified as blood donors.

Donors with relatively minor red cell abnormalities
In some populations a considerable number of donors have an inherited red cell abnormality. The three conditions most likely to be encountered are:

Glucose-6-phosphate dehydrogenase (G-6-PD) deficiency. The survival of G-6-PD-deficient red cells is, as a rule, only slightly subnormal (Brewer *et al.* 1961; Bernini *et al.* 1964) and, on storage, viability is only slightly less well maintained than in normal cells (Orlina *et al.* 1970). However, if the recipient ingests fava beans or one of a series of drugs (phenacetin, sulphonamides, vitamin K, primaquine, etc.) there may be rapid destruction of the donor's G-6-PD-deficient cells. In Blacks with the deficiency, the haemolytic process affects only the older red cells with the lowest enzyme content, thus limiting the haemolytic episode, but in Whites it seems that almost the whole red cell population is susceptible to destruction (Pannacciulli *et al.* 1965).

Sickle cell trait. In this condition red cells survive normally, even after storage, in normal subjects (Singer *et al.* 1948; Callender *et al.* 1949; Ray *et al.* 1959), although in patients with various types of anoxia they survive poorly, being trapped in the spleen (Krevans, 1959). Blood from donors with sickle cell trait should not be used for infants or for exchange transfusion in patients with sickle cell disease. Patients, other than those with sickle haemoglobin, requiring surgery under general anaesthesia should have no problems if transfused with Hb AS red cells provided that adequate oxygenation is maintained. Blood from donors with sickle cell trait should not be frozen due to problems during deglycerolization (see Chapter 9).

Thalassaemia trait is associated with little or no reduction in red cell life span in most subjects with a normal Hb concentration (Hamilton *et al.* 1950; Kaplan and Zuelzer, 1950; Bernini *et al.* 1964). There is no reason to disqualify subjects with thalassaemia trait from donation provided they have a normal Hb concentration.

Individuals with polycythaemia vera are sometimes treated by regular venesection and it is not uncommon for the blood to be offered to a transfusion service. It is known that red cells from such patients survive normally in the circulation of normal recipients (Merskey, 1949) and in the subject's own circulation (London *et al.* 1949), but in view of the fact that these patients sometimes develop leukaemia the blood is not as a rule used for transfusion. However, the risk of acquiring a graft of malignant cells from the donor seems to be negligible, except in recipients whose immune mechanisms are suppressed by disease or drugs (see Chapter 14).

Special conditions in which normally disqualified donors may donate
There are some circumstances in which a donor may give blood to be used for a special purpose, even though he or she does not meet the requirements for normal donation. For example, a donor who is mildly anaemic or who has recently given birth may give plasma or platelets by apheresis; the plasma may be needed for many special purposes, e.g. it may be the source of an antibody with a rare HLA specificity or the platelets may have a rare phenotype such as HPA-1(a –). Donors at risk from carrying malaria

may give blood provided that only plasma is harvested and is then used only for fractionation.

DONATION OF WHOLE BLOOD

Frequency of donation
Many transfusion services (e.g. the National Blood Tranfusion Service in the UK; see Department of Health, 1989) bleed donors not more than two or three times a year and do not bleed women who are pregnant or who have been pregnant within the previous year. The major object of this policy is to protect the donor from iron deficiency.

There is a wide variation in the recommended minimum interval between donations. For example in the USA, in line with WHO recommendations, the interval can be as short as 8 weeks with a maximum annual volume of 2 litres of blood collected (AABB, 1990). It is recommended that pre-menopausal women should not donate as frequently as men (WHO, 1989). In the Netherlands male donors are bled every 3 months and females every 6 months (cf. following paragraph).

Effect of blood donation on iron balance
Moore (1948) pointed out that the donor who gives blood twice a year loses more blood than the average menstruating woman whose annual loss does not normally exceed 650 ml. Finch (1972) stated that, in males, iron lost from a 400-ml donation is made up by enhanced absorption of dietary iron in 3 months, although in females in a longer time. He suggested that the interval between donations should be 3 months for males and 6 months for females. Nevertheless, even when these intervals are observed, blood donation does seem to be a cause of iron deficiency. For example, iron stores are exhausted in virtually all female donors regardless of the frequency of blood donations (Kaltwasser, 1981). In a group of healthy young males who gave blood every 2 months and received no iron therapy, after four donations one-third had no stainable iron in the marrow (Liedén, 1975).

In a study of donors who had given blood either 15 times or 50 times at the rate of five donations a year and had received a supplement of 600 mg Fe^{2+} after each donation, although the subjects were not anaemic and had normal serum iron levels, about 75% had no stainable iron in the marrow (Liedén, 1973). In a further study in which blood was donated every 2 months, resulting in an average daily loss of 3.5 mg iron, even when the subjects received 100 mg iron a day iron stores were not maintained at the initial level (Liedén et al. 1975).

Similarly, even in male donors who gave blood only twice a year, those who had given more than ten donations had a significant fall in mean ferritin levels accompanied by a lower Hb, red cell count and MCHC (Green et al. 1988). On the other hand, in 12 regular blood donors with subnormal serum ferritin levels who gave blood every 8 weeks, the ingestion of 5600 mg iron between phlebotomies was sufficient to restore serum ferritin levels to normal and to provide a small store of iron in the bone marrow (Birgegård et al. 1980). Despite this finding, some experts believe that frequent bleeding even with iron supplementation is not justified and that the maximum annual rate of donation should be twice for men and once for women (Jacobs, 1981).

In normal, well nourished subjects, serum ferritin concentration is in practice a good indicator of iron stores (Worwood, 1980; 1989), although some have shown that red cell ferritin is a better reflection of body iron status (Cazzola and Ascari, 1986). Red cell ferritin is affected only slightly by factors other than tissue iron stores (e.g. inflammation, increased red cell turnover) whereas these factors may cause a rise in serum ferritin. There are now several studies of ferritin estimations in large series which confirm that iron stores may be seriously depleted in blood donors (Finch *et al.* 1977; Bodemann *et al.* 1984; and see Skikne *et al.* 1984).

There is no doubt that, when the interval between donations is 3 months or less, iron supplementation in the form of ferrous iron should be given to try to prevent iron deficiency in blood donors. However, supplementation programmes are difficult to implement and maintain (see Skikne *et al.* 1984), and, even when they are implemented, the role of supplemental iron in donors who give blood frequently and have a normal diet seems to be minimal (Monsen *et al.* 1983). There is certainly a need for systematic, controlled studies of absorption of supplemental iron in donors who give blood frequently (Finch and Huebers, 1987).

Screening test to detect anaemia

Subjects should be tested before donation to make sure that they are not anaemic. A convenient test is to take a drop of blood and allow it to fall from a height of 1 cm into a selected solution of copper sulphate and thus to determine its Hb concentration from the specific gravity. In some countries, such as France, the Hb level is no longer determined before donation; instead, the Hb level and haematocrit of blood donations are estimated, and donors found to be anaemic are contacted.

The lowest acceptable Hb levels for male and female blood donors, defined by the specific gravity of whole blood, correspond reasonably well with limits defined by conventional haemoglobinometry on venous samples. In a series of 200 healthy subjects, the range (mean ± 2 SD) was 121–165 g/l for males and 120–147 g/l for females (Bain and England, 1975). Fairly similar values were reported by Garby (1970) in reviewing normal Hb concentrations, based on published data.

In the UK, the National Blood Transfusion Service accepts male donors whose blood contains at least 135 g Hb/l as judged by the fact that a drop sinks in a copper sulphate solution of specific gravity 1.055, and female donors whose Hb concentration is not less than 125 g/l as judged by the fact that a drop of their blood sinks in a copper sulphate solution of specific gravity 1.053. If a donor fails the copper sulphate test, rapid microhaematocrit or haemoglobin determinations can be done at the donor clinic from skin-prick blood, using portable machines. These supplementary determinations often reveal that a donation can be taken, thus saving the donor from unnecessary anxiety. When donors are found to be anaemic, venous samples should be taken and retested by conventional haemoglobinometry. Donors who are confirmed as anaemic should be referred to their general practitioner.

In the USA, the minimum acceptable levels of Hb for donors have recently been changed to 125 g Hb/l for males and 120 g/l for females (AABB, 1990).

Errors in technique in using the copper sulphate method, e.g. incorporation of air bubbles or the use of an inadequate height for dropping the blood, tend to result in underestimating the Hb concentration so that donors may be rejected unnecessarily (Pirofsky and Nelson, 1964). On the other hand, in rare cases in which the plasma protein concentration is greatly raised, anaemic donors may be accepted as normal, each extra g/dl of plasma protein being equivalent to 0.7 g/dl Hb (Mannarino and McPherson, 1963). Falsely high positive results in the copper sulphate method may also be due to a high white cell count associated with leukaemia.

The source of the blood sample may determine acceptance or rejection of a donor in borderline cases. Based on microhaematocrit methods, blood obtained by ear lobe puncture was found to give values about 6% higher than those obtained simultaneously by fingerprick puncture (Avoy *et al.* 1977), and blood from fingerprick was found to have an Hb value 2% lower than that of venous blood obtained simultaneously (Moe, 1970).

Haemoglobin regeneration after normal blood donation
In 14 normal healthy subjects bled of about 400 ml blood (8% of their blood volume) there was a small but significant increase in the reticulocyte count, with a peak on the ninth day after bleeding. The Hb level was lowest 1 or 2 weeks after bleeding; thereafter there was a rapid increase and pre-donation levels were reached at 3–4 weeks (Fig. 1.1).

Untoward effects during or shortly after venesection

Fainting or the vaso-vagal attack
The 'vaso-vagal attack' may be induced in certain subjects by the mere sight of blood being taken from another person and can be provoked in all subjects by

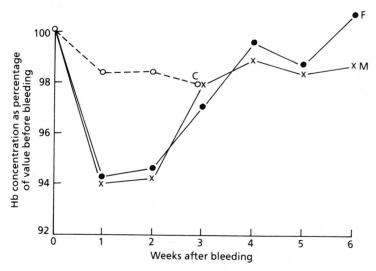

Figure 1.1 Mean Hb concentration in seven women (F) and seven men (M) at weekly intervals after being bled of about 8% of their blood volume. The dotted line indicates the change in mean Hb concentration for four men and four women who were not bled (C) (from Wadsworth, 1955).

withdrawing a sufficient quantity of blood. Even after the loss of as little as 400 ml blood, some subjects remain liable, for a few hours, to faint if they get up suddenly from a sitting or lying position. In view of this, all donors should be observed for at least 15 min after donation and they should be questioned about their occupation; those donors in whom fainting would be specially hazardous to themselves or to others (e.g. aircrew, bus drivers, machine operators) should probably not return to work or potentially dangerous hobbies for at least 12 h after giving blood. Donors who experience a delayed faint should be permanently debarred from blood donation regardless of their occupation.

The faint, or vaso-vagal attack appears to be a hypothalamic response. Its features are as follows: the subject starts to sweat and turns pale; the skin feels cold, the pulse slows strikingly and the heart rate may fall to 30 per min; the blood pressure may become unrecordable; there may be vomiting and involuntary defaecation. When taking blood, warning of oncoming fainting is often given by a fall in flow, as Harvey (1628) noted. As fainting develops the subject feels weak and objects start to appear dim. Loss of consciousness may follow and convulsions are occasionally seen.

It appears that these effects are produced mainly by the action of the autonomic system, causing slowing of the heart, vomiting and sweating and, perhaps most important, dilatation of the arterioles, leading to a sudden fall in blood pressure (Barcroft et al. 1944).

Fainting commonly occurs in subjects who have lost blood; moreover some of the signs produced by severe haemorrhage, such as a fall in blood pressure, also occur in the vaso-vagal attack. It is, therefore, important to be familiar with the vaso-vagal attack and to appreciate that an apparently grave clinical picture can be produced by emotion alone. In patients who display these signs but who have not lost blood, rapid recovery occurs when the patient is placed in the supine position and tilted so that the head is lower than the rest of the body. The slow pulse rate (30–60 per min) in the vaso-vagal attack is the most useful single sign in differential diagnosis.

Estimates of the frequency with which fainting occurs in blood donors vary according to the definition of the term 'faint': in the Medical Research Council's inquiry (1944), 'fainting' was defined as the manifestation of any of a series of signs or symptoms such as pallor, sweating, dizziness or nausea. In this sense of the word some 5–6% of donors fainted. Pole and Boycott (1942) found that in their first 10 000 cases only 2.8% of donors fainted, but they applied the term only to those who lost consciousness or could not stand or sit without doing so.

Vaso-vagal reactions are commoner on the first occasion of giving blood: Beal (1972) found that amongst 1000 donors studied over a period of several years more than one-half experienced their only symptoms at the time of their first donation; the incidence of reactions fell progressively over a period of 6 years. In 40 437 donations studied, fainting was found to be more common in female donors; 4.9% of first-time female donors had vaso-vagal reactions compared with 3.8% of first-time male donors. The figures were less than half of these in regular donors of both sexes, i.e. 1.9% and 1.1% respectively (Tomasulo et al. 1980).

Poles and Boycott (1942) found a definite relation between the incidence of fainting and the amount of blood donated. While only 3.8% of a series of 341 donors who gave 440 ml fainted, the incidence rose to 8.5% in 410 donors who gave 540 ml blood.

Barcroft *et al.* (1944) reported that fainting occurred in 11 of 28 normal males who lost 800–1000 ml blood and in 15 of 29 who lost 1000–1200 ml. Ebert *et al.* (1941) observed loss of consciousness in five of six volunteers from whom 780–1200 ml blood were withdrawn in 6–13 min. Howarth and Sharpey-Schafer (1947), who withdrew up to 1500 ml blood from normal volunteers, noted that fainting could be produced in all subjects provided that enough blood was withdrawn within a limited time.

Some other untoward effects

Bruising is one of the commonest complications of blood donation. In the majority of cases the haematoma is restricted to a small area in the antecubital fossa; however, very large, incapacitating and painful haematomas are seen occasionally following blood donation.

Tetany is occasionally observed in blood donors (incidence 1 in 1000) and is thought to be due to hyperventilation; it is characteristically observed in nervous subjects. Its manifestations may include carpopedal spasm, laryngismus stridulus and a positive Chvostek's sign. Rapid relief can be obtained by rebreathing from a paper bag, or inhaling 5% carbon dioxide from a cylinder (Frazer and Fowweather, 1942).

Convulsions are rare. If they occur, the donor should be held on the bed or on the floor, ensuring the airway is clear.

Puncture of an artery leads to an unusually rapid flow of bright red blood; when the needle is withdrawn there may be severe leakage of blood, followed by extensive bruising. If an arterial puncture is suspected, the needle should be withdrawn immediately and firm pressure applied for 5–10 min followed by a pressure dressing. If the radial pulse is not palpable, the donor should be referred to a vascular specialist.

Three months after an unusually rapid but uneventful donation, a donor presented with an arteriovenous fistula causing an aneurysm in the antecubital fossa which rapidly grew to the size of a tennis ball and needed operative repair (unpublished observations, MC; see also Lung and Wilson, 1971).

Air embolism during blood donation. When blood is taken into plastic bags which contain no air, there is no possibility of air embolism. On the other hand when blood is taken into glass bottles (as is still the practice in some countries), air embolism is occasionally encountered, the prime cause being obstruction to the air vent of the bottle. For details and further references see Mollison (1983, p. 6).

Fatalities attributed to blood donation. In 1975 the Food and Drug Administration (FDA) of the USA published regulations requiring the report of deaths associated with blood collection, plasmapheresis and transfusion. In the 10 years from 1976 to 1985 three deaths attributed to blood donation were reported out of 100 million units of donated blood. Two deaths were due to myocardial infarction and one was in a patient with phaeochromocytoma (Sazama, 1990).

Fatalities due to withdrawing too much blood. Many versions exist of the story of the three boys who were venesected to provide youthful blood for the ailing Pope Innocent VIII in 1492. Although it is often stated that the blood was infused into the veins of the Pope, the most plausible account states that the blood was offered as a draught and refused with horror, and that meanwhile all three boys had died. (For references see Ogle, 1881 and Matthew, 1912. For a scholarly account of the origins of this probably mythical story, see Gottlieb, 1991.)

Autologous transfusion

With the recognition that HIV, as well as other infectious agents such as those of hepatitis, can be transmitted by blood transfusion (see Chapter 16), the practice of autologous transfusion in its various forms has grown considerably in recent years, especially in the USA (Sandler, 1983; AuBuchon, 1989). For example, members of the American Association of Blood Banks collected 18 737 units of autologous blood in 1982 and almost 290 000 in 1987 (Maffei and Thurer, 1988). In fact, by 1990, approximately 5% of blood collected in the USA was for autologous transfusion (Silvergleid, 1991).

The advantages of autologous transfusion seem very substantial: all risks of incompatibility, of alloimmunization, of immunosuppression and of the transmission of infections such as viral hepatitis and HIV are avoided and donor blood is saved for other patients. The mere discussion of the possible use of autologous transfusion may serve to increase awareness of the advantages of a conservative approach to trans-fusion. On the other hand, clinicians may overuse autologous donation and transfusion without thinking of alternatives to reduce blood loss (Axelrod *et al.* 1988; AuBuchon, 1989). Some of the risks of blood transfusion, for example the risks of mistakes in identification, of bacterial contamination, of overloading the circulation or of improper handling of frozen units do not disappear with the use of autologous blood (Cregan *et al.* 1991; Silvergleid, 1991).

Although in some countries the use of autologous transfusion has increased greatly in the last few years at the expense of allogeneic blood transfusions (Surgenor *et al.* 1990), in others, such as the UK, it has remained low. Perhaps, one of the main reasons for this low usage is the additional cost associated with the collection and handling of autologous blood. Some other reasons may be that prospective recipients are often not well enough to act as donors; that special arrangements, which are more cumbersome than those needed for bleeding large numbers of healthy donors, have to be made for bleeding patients; that more thorough clinical examinations are needed; and, finally, that it is difficult to predict the amount of blood a particular patient will need so that either too much will be taken or too little and, in the latter case, the main advantage of autologous transfusion will be lost. In addition, the risks of contracting serious infectious disease through allogeneic transfusion have decreased considerably in the western world: HIV is now very seldom transmitted in this way and the risk of transmitting non-A, non-B post-transfusion hepatitis has fallen, e.g. in the USA from 7–10% in the late 1970s to approximately 1% by the late 1980s (Alter, 1989).

Pre-operative ('pre-deposit') autologous blood collections

The transfusion requirements of a significant number of surgical patients can be met completely with autologous blood (for references see Anderson and Tomasulo, 1988; Maffei and Thurer, 1988). The criteria for accepting donors for autologous transfusion need not be as strict as those for allogeneic transfusion. For example, there is a vast experience of including patients over the age of 70 and under the age of 17 years in autologous donation programmes (Mann *et al.* 1983; Ness *et al.* 1987; Silvergleid, 1987; Baker *et al.* 1988; Daneshvar, 1988); patients on medication as well as pregnant women with a high risk of bleeding during delivery and patients with a history of cardiac disease or recent surgery are acceptable in specialized centres for the collection or autologous blood (Britton *et al.* 1989; McVay *et al.* 1989; Owings *et al.* 1989). A study conducted by the American Red Cross showed that in 5660 pre-operative autologous donations given in donor clinics outside hospitals, serious untoward effects occurred in less than 1%. Patients not meeting the usual criteria for donors had an overall rate of reaction (mostly fainting) of 4.2% compared with 2.7% of those who met the criteria. Patients not meeting criteria for donors, e.g. those who were less than 17 years old, weighed less than 100 pounds (45.4 kg) or had suffered previous reactions, were more likely to have a reaction. On the other hand, donors over 75 years of age, with a history of cardiac disease, medication or surgery did not have an increased risk of reacting adversely to donation (AuBuchon and Popovsky, 1988).

When planning an autologous donation programme, it is important to select patients who are very likely to need blood. There are now several reports showing that a significant number of units of blood collected pre-operatively have not been transfused to the patient-donor; in fact the number can be as high as 50% (Axelrod *et al.* 1988; Eisenstaedt *et al.* 1988; McVay *et al.* 1989). Hospitals without surgical blood ordering schemes should not consider a programme of autologous transfusion until they know for which surgical procedures blood is needed routinely and the mean volume of blood used locally for each type of procedure.

When several units of blood need to be collected within a short period of time, oral iron therapy, e.g. 320 mg ferrous sulphate three times a day, should be given (AuBuchon, 1989). When the patient's Hb level does not rise as quickly as expected before the next autologous donation, recombinant erythropoietin, in addition to oral iron, has been tried by some with success; in clinical trials, erythropoiesis has increased after a lag of approximately 1 week, allowing a larger number of units of blood to be collected pre-operatively (Goodnough *et al.* 1989; Graf *et al.* 1990). However, it is questionable whether patients should be exposed to the risks and expense of erythropoietin for the sake of collecting one or two additional units of blood (Bell and Gillon, 1990).

Not all patients are eligible for autologous donation. Although the restrictions vary in different countries, with the USA taking a more liberal approach than the UK, there are absolute contraindications for pre-deposit autologous transfusion: (1) bacteraemia; (2) significant cardiovascular problems (e.g. unstable angina, cardiac failure, severe aortic stenosis, hypertension with a systolic BP of over 180 mm Hg), or respiratory or cerebrovascular diseases; (3) pregnancy with anaemia, hypovolaemia, pre-eclampsia or retardation of fetal growth. Patients who would not qualify as blood donors must be bled in a hospital under the supervision of a clinician. In some parts of the USA, when patients with moderate to severe cardiovascular disease are bled, saline is infused as the blood is drawn. Pregnant women likely to need blood transfusion for conditions such as placenta praevia and bleeding in the third trimester are bled in the left lateral position by some but with no special precautions by others (McVay *et al.* 1989). Although it has been shown that pregnant women can give blood with no significant adverse effects on themselves, very few data are available on the effect of blood collection in the third trimester on fetal circulation and iron status.

Only 2% of children between the ages of 8 and 18 years had adverse reactions to autologous donation, provided they had no cardiac or respiratory problems (DePalma and Luban, 1990). However, the collection of blood from children is difficult with current equipment; there is a need for suitable packs with smaller needles. Children weighing between 28 and 50 kg can be bled of 250 ml into Pedi-Paks, which contain 35 ml CPD-A1. If these packs are not available, a standard-sized pack can be used with a satellite pack attached so that excess anticoagulant can be removed whilst retaining a closed system.

The amount of blood to be taken is calculated as weight (kg)/50 × 450 ml, and the volume of anticoagulant to be used as volume of donation (ml)/450 × 63 ml.

It is advisable to perform the same tests on autologous blood as on blood given by routine blood donors. The main reasons for this recommendation are: (1) to cover the possibility that a mistake in identification may be made, leading to the transfusion of blood of the wrong ABO group or of blood contaminated with the viruses HBV, HCV or HIV; and (2) to discover whether the patient is already infected with a virus which he or she fears might be acquired if transfused with allogeneic blood. Several hospitals and transfusion centres will not store autologous units found positive for HBsAg or for anti-HIV, -HCV or -HTLV. In any case, autologous donations should be stored separately from routine blood donations.

Subjects for whom autologous transfusions are indicated are: (1) patients undergoing elective surgical procedures with a high probability of needing blood, provided they are fit enough to donate several units pre-operatively; and (2) some bone marrow donors, especially children likely to become anaemic after donating marrow for a sibling. In most cases autologous blood will be kept in the liquid state for up to 5 weeks; however, when more than 4–6 units are needed or when there is a cancellation or postponement of surgery, the red cells can be frozen for longer periods. With either method of storage, it is preferable to collect the blood into double packs in order to freeze the fresh plasma until required. The prolonged shelf-life of blood with modern preservative solutions has made the 'leap-frog' technique obsolete (see Mollison, 1983, p. 8, for a description and references), except when surgery is postponed and there are no facilities for freezing red cells already collected. Although the use of platelets is rarely indicated in elective surgery, except perhaps in complicated cardiac or vascular surgery, the collection of platelets with cell separators taken either 1–2 days or immediately before surgery has been reported (Giordano *et al.* 1988; Pineda and Valbonesi, 1990).

There has been some interest in the expensive practice of taking blood from healthy subjects for long-term storage in case they should require transfusion in the future. It is unlikely that such blood will ever be needed, or, if really needed in emergency, will then be readily available. On the other hand, long-term storage of autologous blood is indicated for: (1) subjects with rare blood groups or with multiple red cell antibodies, for whom it is difficult to find compatible blood; and (2) those rare patients who have had more than one unexplained haemolytic transfusion reaction.

In the UK, it is not recommended that blood taken for autologous transfusion should, if unused, be put into the general stocks of allogeneic blood ('crossover'). The main reasons for this recommendation are: (1) that since, at the time of withdrawal, the donation was not intended for allogeneic transfusion, the criteria for donor acceptance could have been less stringent (e.g. the patient might have been taking drugs, or might have been transfused within the last year); (2) that the labelling will be inappropriate; (3) that most autologous blood is collected in hospitals, using different documentation from that used at transfusion centres; (4) that the risks of making mistakes are increased by the mere fact of transferring donor details from one database to another; (5) that the donor may have an increased chance of being positive for markers of infectious disease (Grossman *et al.* 1988; Starkey *et al.* 1989); and (6) that a considerable proportion of the autologous units will be near expiry date when it is finally decided that they will not be needed for the patient-donor. In any case, if programmes of autologous transfusion are properly planned, the volume of blood left unused after surgery should be small. In fact, in well conducted programmes, not less than 3% and at the most 9% of autologous units would be available for allogeneic blood transfusion, and many of these would be nearing expiry. The complexities of record keeping to enable the transfer of such small numbers of units to the voluntary donor pool argue against the practice of 'crossover' (Silvergleid, 1991).

Intra-operative haemodilution
The practice of producing haemodilution by withdrawing relatively large amounts of blood from the patient immediately before surgery and replacing it by a colloid or crystalloid solution, and later returning the blood to the patient to replace operative losses, is described in Chapter 2.

Red cell salvage

Intra-operative red cell salvage. It was once a fairly common practice to collect blood shed into the peritoneal cavity, particularly when operating on patients with a ruptured ectopic gestation or ruptured spleen, and to reinject the blood immediately, or after filtration and citration, into the patient's circulation (for details see Mollison *et al.* 1987). Nowadays, when blood is salvaged at operation, special devices are used for the purpose. At least two types are available: (1) the simpler type (e.g. Solcotrans) only anticoagulates and filters the shed blood before returning it to the patient; and (2) the more automated type, based on semi-continuous flow technology requiring technical expertise, anticoagulates, washes and concentrates the red cells before reinfusion. Since the simpler system has the potential for the transfusion of activated clotting factors, complement components, haemolysed blood, excess anticoagulant, particulate matter and tissue fluids as well as for producing air embolism, large volumes of blood salvaged in this way cannot be used (Glover and Broadie, 1987; Dzik, 1988; Pineda and Valbonesi, 1990). However, although salvaged, unwashed blood contains increased levels of C3a, C5a and terminal complement components, there is no risk of systemic complement activation if fewer than 500 ml of unwashed salvaged blood are reinfused (Bengtson *et al.* 1990). In some places, red cells collected in this way are routinely washed in the blood bank. Cell salvage machines of all types induce mechanical injury to the red cells collected, reducing the Hb level and haematocrit, although 2, 3-DPG levels and survival of ^{51}Cr-labelled cells are satisfactory (see Pineda and Valbonesi, 1990).

Salvaged red cells should not be used if the blood is contaminated by micro-organisms or tumour cells or if topical disinfectants are being applied during suction (for references see AuBuchon, 1989). Favourable results, with significant volumes of salvaged washed red cells transfused during operation, have been reported in patients with trauma or ruptured ectopic pregnancy and in patients receiving liver transplants or undergoing cardiovascular or orthopaedic surgery (Mattox *et al.* 1975; Merril *et al.* 1980; Kruger and Colbert, 1985; Dale *et al.* 1986; Popovsky, 1987). When very large volumes of salvaged red cells are transfused, supplementary transfusions of platelets and fresh frozen plasma (FFP) are likely to be needed, although new devices for the salvage of platelets and plasma proteins are being developed. Alternatively, the intermittent-flow cell separator devices used for intra-operative blood salvage can be adapted to collect plasma and platelets (as well as red cells) in the immediate pre-operative period; at the end of collection, the tubing is connected to the suction cannula for intra-operative salvage. The devices can also be used to concentrate the red cells that remain in the oxygenator after cardiac surgery.

Recently, systems have been developed which salvage and wash red cells within 3 min, e.g. the Haemonetics Cell Saver 4. Blood salvage has been used successfully in vascular, cardiac, obstetric and orthopaedic surgery as well as in surgery for trauma and for liver transplantation. More than 8000 cases of red cell salvage with no major untoward effects have been reported from the Mayo Clinic (Williamson and Taswell, 1988). Machines which can handle with the necessary speed the large amounts of blood used only rarely now in liver transplantation (up to 250 units in adults) have yet to be developed (Williamson *et al.* 1989).

Post-operative red cell salvage. It has yet to be decided whether it is safe and cost-effective to reinfuse filtered or washed defibrinated blood which has been shed into the mediastinum or pleural cavities after cardiothoracic surgery. In most cases, the volume of blood saved is small and is reduced even further after processing (AuBuchon, 1989).

Directed donations
Directed donations are those given exclusively for named patients, usually by relatives or friends. This practice contravenes the normal principles of voluntary blood dona-tion, does not increase safety (Cordell *et al.* 1986; Strauss, 1989) and is justified only in a few circumstances; for example: (1) for patients with rare blood groups when the only available compatible donors may be close relatives; (2) in occasional patients awaiting renal transplants, in whom there may still be a place for donor-specific transfusions (Salvatierra *et al.* 1981a; Anderson *et al.* 1985a; see also Chapter 14); (3) in infants with neonatal alloimmune thrombocytopenia or haemolytic disease of the newborn, for whom maternal blood may occasionally be invaluable; (4) in children with haemophilia A or B, or with von Willebrand's disease, in whom plasma from

single designated donors collected by apheresis may satisfy the total replacement needs for coagulation factors (McLeod *et al.* 1988; Strauss, 1989); (5) in children requiring open-heart or extensive orthopaedic surgery, for whom the total requirements for blood and components can be collected pre-operatively, as for autologous transfusion but from designated relatives or parents, thus minimizing the number of donor units to which the children are exposed (Brecher *et al.* 1988); and (6) in patients with acute leukaemia who are relapsing after bone marrow transplantation, for whom donor granulocytes collected by apheresis are used as adoptive immunotherapy, to induce graft versus host disease (GvHD) (Sullivan *et al.* 1989); or in patients with chronic myeloid leukaemia, for whom donor granulocytes are used, together with α-interferon, to induce a graft-*versus*-host reaction against minor histocompatibility antigens of the host (Kolb *et al.* 1980).

The practice of transfusing parental blood to premature newborn infants is not without risks. Mothers may have antibodies against antigens (inherited from the father) on the infant's red cells, platelets or white cells. For this reason, ideally, maternal plasma should not be used. Fathers should not serve as cell donors because they may have antigens present on their red cells, leucocytes or platelets which are incompatible with maternally derived antibodies present in the fetus. Moreover, in view of partial histocompatibility, transfusion of cells from parents and close relatives may result in GvHD in the infants, especially if the infants are immunodeficient (Bastian *et al.* 1984; Strauss, 1989). Circumstances such as these, in which blood or platelet suspensions should be irradiated or depleted of white cells before transfusion, are described in Chapter 15.

The practice of transfusing parents with blood from their offspring could also be dangerous. Fatal GvHD occurred in two immunocompetent adult patients who were transfused with fresh whole non-irradiated blood from their children during cardiac surgery. In both cases, one of the donors was homozygous for one of the recipient's HLA haplotypes (Thaler *et al.* 1989).

Use of cadaver blood
The collection of blood from cadavers (for further details see Mollison 1983, p. 9), is practised in only a few centres in Russia nowadays (Agranenko and Maltseva, 1990).

EXCHANGE TRANSFUSION

A very impressive exchange transfusion was carried out in dogs by Dr Richard Lower of Oxford in February 1666.

The donors were two very large mastiffs and the recipient was a smaller dog. After drawing a large quantity of blood from the jugular vein of the smaller dog, blood from one of the donors was taken from its cervical artery and allowed to flow through a silver tube into the vein of the smaller dog. Blood was drawn from the recipient at intervals. After the first donor had been exsanguinated, the second was used in like fashion. Lower calculated that by the end of the experiment the recipient had received (and lost) an amount of blood equal to the weight of the whole body. 'Yet, once its jugular vein was sewn up and its binding shackles tossed off it promptly jumped down the table and apparently oblivious of its hurts soon began to fondle its master and to roll on the grass to clean himself of the blood, exactly as it would have done if it had merely been thrown into a stream and with no more sign of discomfort or displeasure' (Lower, 1669, translated from the Latin by Keynes, 1949).

Another account of Lower's experiments was communicated through the Royal Society by Robert Boyle (*Phil. Trans.* 1666, **20**, p. 353). Some practical notes of the method are followed by some reflections, the final one of which reads: 'The most probable use of this Experiment may be conjectured to be that one Animal may live with the bloud of another: and consequently that those Animals, that want bloud, or have corrupt bloud, may be supplyed from other with a sufficient quantity, and of such as is good, provided the Transfusion be often repeated, by reason of the quick expence that is made of the bloud.' Following the account of the operation it was mentioned that it was planned to exchange the blood of old and young, sick and healthy, hot and cold, fierce and fearful, tame and wild animals, etc., although it was predicted 'that the exchange of bloud will not alter the nature or disposition of the animals on which it shall be practised'.

In a later volume of the *Philosophical Transactions* (1666, **22**, p. 385) Boyle proposed various questions to Dr Lower which might be answered by transfusion experiments, for example: 'Whether a Dog that is sick of some disease chiefly imputable to the mass of bloud, may be cured by exchanging it with that of a sound Dog? And whether a sound Dog may receive such diseases from the bloud of a sick one, as are not otherwise of an infectious nature?'

As described later, blood transfusion fell into disrepute round about the year 1668 and did not become a relatively common procedure until about the time of the First World War (1914–18). Robertson (1924) had the idea of using exsanguino-transfusion for the treatment of severe toxaemias. He first experimented in rabbits, removing as much blood as the animal could stand before transfusing with blood from another animal, but since with this approach the amount of blood exchanged was limited by the amount of blood that could be withdrawn at any one time, he developed the technique of drawing blood from one vein and simultaneously transfusing blood into another. He applied this method to humans and reported that he had carried out 501 procedures including some in patients with various toxaemias (one with resorcin poisoning), and considered that the procedure substantially reduced the mortality rate.

Although exchange transfusion continued to be used up to about 1975 for removing toxic substances from plasma, for this purpose the procedure has now been replaced by plasma exchange (see below). On the other hand, there are a few conditions in which there is a need to remove the subject's red cells, e.g. haemolytic disease of the newborn (see Chapter 12) and sickle cell anaemia (see Chapter 9), and in these conditions exchange transfusion using blood is indicated.

Exchange transfusion of whole blood is more practicable than plasma exchange for removing toxic substances from the plasma of infants, since at the present time cell separators suitable for use in small children have not been developed.

Calculation of volume replaced

Formulae that predict the percentage of blood exchanged in replacement transfusion were given by Wallerstein and Brodie (1948). When replacement is being carried out continuously and one homogeneous fluid is being replaced by another, e.g. plasma by 5% albumin, the percentage of original plasma remaining at time $t = 100e^{(-v/V)t}$. The exchange of a volume equivalent to the subject's blood volume leaves 37% of the original fluid and an exchange equivalent to twice the blood volume leaves 13.5%.

When exchange is carried out by an intermittent method, as for example in exchange transfusion in newborn infants, and again assuming that one homogeneous fluid is being replaced by another, the percentage of the original blood remaining after n operations, where V = the original blood volume and v the volume of blood removed at each operation = $[(V - v)/V]^n$. Even when the packed cell volume (PCV) of the transfused blood and of the patient's blood happen to be the same, the formula is not applicable because the red cells are not uniformly distributed throughout the vascular system; a more elaborate formula is needed to predict the rate of red cell exchange. If the blood volume of the infant (assumed to be constant during exchange transfusion) is V ml, v ml is removed and replaced at each operation, H_0 is the initial venous haematocrit of the infant's blood, H_d is the haematocrit of the donor's blood and k is the ratio of the whole body haematocrit to the venous haematocrit (see Appendix 4), it can be shown that after n operations the fraction of the infant's original cells remaining is given by the formula:

$$\frac{H_n}{H_0} = \left(1 - \frac{v}{kV}\right)^n$$

where H_n is the venous haematocrit of the recipient's own red cells after n operations. The total PCV after n operations is given by:

$$H_n = H_0\left(1 - \frac{v}{kV}\right)^n + H_d\left(1 - \left(1 - \frac{v}{kV}\right)^n\right)$$

The first term represents the patient's residual red cells and the second term the donor's red cells (Veall and Mollison, 1950).

When the method of intermittent substitution is used for plasma exchange, a similar formula can be derived for calculating the rate of exchange (see Veall and Mollison, 1950).

Indications for red cell exchange

Exchange transfusion in sickle cell disease is considered in Chapter 9.

Exchange transfusion in haemolytic disease of the newborn is described in Chapter 12; see also Appendix 10.

Exchange transfusion in other conditions

Red cell exchange with or without plasma exchange has been used as an emergency measure in life-threatening, refractory syndromes. Automated red cell exchange has been used successfully in, for example, refractory warm autoimmune haemolytic anaemia, in the acute severe stages of malaria and babesiosis, in porphyria and, pre-operatively, in patients with paroxysmal nocturnal haemoglobinuria undergoing cardiac surgery (for references see Urbaniak, 1984). Red cell exchange is occasionally indicated when a patient is found to have been recently transfused with incompatible red cells or when a D-negative woman of child-bearing age who is not already immunized to D has been inadvertently transfused with a large volume of D-positive cells (see Chapter 5). Apheresis of red cells with return of the patient's plasma has been used successfully in polycythaemia secondary to hypoxic lung disease (Wedzicha *et al.* 1983) and in idiopathic haemochromatosis (Conte *et al.* 1983).

Technique of exchange transfusion
When the target is an exchange of 75–90% of red cells, continuous or intermittent-flow cell separators should be used (Klein, 1982). Automated procedures provide a rapid, effective and probably safer means for partial exchange transfusion. A further advantage is that the extracorporeal volume can be easily controlled. Whenever possible it is advisable to reinfuse the patient's own platelets and plasma along with donor concentrated red cells.

PLASMAPHERESIS

The term 'plasmapheresis', which simply means 'taking away plasma', was first used by Abel *et al.* (1914) to describe the removal of plasma with the return of the red cells to the donor, but these authors were not the first to carry out this manoeuvre.

As described on p. 431, transfusions of washed red cells were used in animal experiments as early as 1902 by Hédon, although this was because the transfusion of whole defibrinated blood was at that time regarded as highly dangerous and not because there was any intention of washing out some substance from the recipient's blood stream. On the other hand, Fleig (1910) experimented with plasmapheresis as a method of removing toxic substances from the blood. He demonstrated that in rabbits large amounts of blood could be withdrawn and replaced by the animal's own red cells suspended in isotonic spa water. His paper makes delightful reading since he compared the value of water from various romantic-sounding spas, such as Kreuznasch Elizabethquelle and Kissingen-Schönbornsprudel. Fleig went on to try his method in humans and showed that in a uraemic subject who, on three occasions, was bled of about 600 ml and then given back his own washed red cells suspended in isotonic spa water, there was substantial clinical improvement.

Plasmapheresis vs. plasma exchange
When relatively small amounts of plasma, e.g. 500–650 ml, are removed, saline may be infused as a replacement and plasmapheresis is then the appropriate term for the whole operation. Evidently, when more than a certain amount of plasma is removed it will become advisable to infuse plasma or albumin to replace part or all of the lost plasma protein. This operation constitutes plasma exchange.

Since the need for plasma is greater than the need for red cells, plasmapheresis is used as a method of collecting fresh plasma from normal donors for fractionation into plasma derivatives. Plasma from particular donors, for example donors hyperimmunized to Rh D, tetanus or HBsAg, needed to obtain specific immunoglobulins, is also collected by plasmapheresis. As described in a later section, plasma exchange is carried out with the object of removing some particular constituent from a patient's plasma.

Plasmapheresis using multi-unit bag manual procedures
Plasmapheresis became an easy procedure only after the introduction of plastic transfusion equipment (Walter and Murphy, 1952).

Normal practice is to take an ordinary donation (e.g. 450 ml blood) into a multi-unit plastic bag containing acid-citrate dextrose (ACD) or citrate-phosphate-dextrose (CPD) and then to centrifuge the blood whilst keeping open the line into the patient's vein with a saline drip. When the blood has been centrifuged, the plasma or platelet-rich plasma (PRP) is extracted and retained, and the red cells are then returned to the donor. The whole procedure may then be repeated ('double plasmapheresis') yielding a total of approximately 500 ml citrated plasma. With modern blood bank refrigerated centrifuges, double plasmapheresis can be completed in less than 1 h.

Plasmapheresis normally causes no more disturbance than an ordinary donation, except for the time expended. However, since the manual procedure carries some additional hazards, automated equipment is normally used (see below). The most serious hazard is that red cell units may be interchanged so that a donor suffers a haemolytic transfusion reaction. A case in which a plasmapheresis donor was accidentally transfused with the wrong red cells is described in Chapter 11; another case, with a fatal outcome, was described by Cumberland *et al.* (1991). Other possible, though remote, hazards are those of infection of the anticoagulant in the plastic bag into which the blood is originally drawn and from which the red cells are retransfused, and of contamination of the saline or administration sets used for i.v. infusion.

Plasmapheresis using automated equipment

There are several machines designed exclusively for plasma removal based either on the principle of separation of blood components by centrifugal force or by filtration. These machines require special sterile disposable tubing and containers. The anticoagulant is added in a controlled way. One of the first machines used for plasma collection was the modified Haemonetics machine (Model 50) assessed by Rock *et al.* (1981). Five hundred millilitres of plasma can be obtained within an average of 32 min. The advantages of automated plasmapheresis are that donors are never disconnected from their own red cells, thus eliminating the risk of transfusion of the red cells of another donor, that the speed of collection is considerably faster than in manual plasmapheresis, that the procedure appears to be preferred by donors to manual plasmapheresis, and that the total extracorporeal volume at any one time, particularly with filtration plasmapheresis, is less than in double (manual) plasmapheresis. The main disadvantage (apart from expense) of the Model 50 method appears to be that the plasma contains platelets which are smaller than average and which, if they are not removed, detract from the quality of the plasma intended for fractionation. At the same time, these small platelets give a poor response to aggregation and are therefore not suitable for the preparation of platelet concentrates. If the centrifugation force is decreased, the Haemonetics 50 can be adapted for the collection of PRP (Rock *et al.* 1983a; Penny *et al.* 1984).

For plasma collection, the Model 50 has been replaced by the Plasma Collection System, or PCS, and its mobile version, the Ultralite, produced by Haemonetics. These semi-automated machines need a single venous access, use a disposable bowl and can collect, by intermittent flow, 600 ml platelet-poor plasma (PPP) or PRP in 30 min. From the PRP, 450 ml plasma for fractionation and 150 ml platelet concentrate, containing $1-2 \times 10^{11}$ platelets can be obtained (Ciavarella, 1989).

PPP or PRP can also be obtained by filtration through a spinning cylindrical membrane with the Fenwal Autopheresis C (APC) machine which also needs a single venous access and operates on a semi-automated intermittent-flow system. The APC can collect 500–600 ml plasma within 30 min (Ciavarella, 1989). Both the PCS and the APC are simple to operate and suitable for the collection of large volumes of plasma for fractionation. The portable versions facilitate the collection of PPP and PRP at mobile donor clinics. The cost of plasma collected with these machines has decreased considerably but is still greater than that of plasma recovered from routine donations. Both plasmapheresis devices, i.e. the PCS and APC, provide plasma which gives satisfactory yields of Factor VIII and Factor IX (Collins et al. 1989).

Care of plasmapheresis donors
The criteria for the acceptability of plasmapheresis donors are slightly stricter than those for routine donors. In the UK, plasma donors are accepted for the first time only if they have given blood previously on at least two occasions, if they are under 50 years of age and if their full blood count and total serum protein are within the normal range. Laboratory tests should be carried out periodically and should include a full blood count, estimation of total serum proteins, of serum albumin, and of immunoglobulins as well as of urinary protein and glucose.

No donor should be subjected to plasmapheresis until he or she has been informed, in detail, about the possible hazards and has given written consent (WHO, 1989). If donors are to undergo immunization with vaccines, red cells or blood group substances for the provision of specific immunoglobulins, guidelines to safeguard the donor should be followed (WHO, 1975; 1989).

Plasmapheresis of donors may be performed at three levels (WHO, 1989):
1   The donor gives plasma at the same frequency as that allowed for whole blood.
2   The volume of plasma taken and the frequency of donations are two or three times that allowed for routine donations.
3   1000–1200 ml plasma are collected weekly, reaching an annual volume of 50–60 litres of plasma per donor, depending on whether the weight of the donor is below or above 80 kg. With this programme, protein levels do not return to initial values although, in most healthy well nourished donors, they remain within the normal range.

If a plasma donor gives whole blood or does not have their red cells returned during apheresis, a period of 8 weeks should elapse before the next plasma donation, unless the physician in charge decides otherwise (WHO, 1989).

Effects of intensive or long-continued plasmapheresis
Intensive plasmapheresis equivalent to levels 2 and 3 above, and long-term plasmapheresis, are well tolerated in healthy subjects (Cohen and Oberman, 1970; Friedman et al. 1975).

When 1000 ml plasma are removed weekly for long periods, if equilibrium is to be maintained an extra 6 g albumin and 2 g immunoglobulin G (IgG) must be produced daily. These amounts are considerable in relation to the normal production of these proteins, estimated at approximately 12 g albumin and 2 g IgG per day (Schultze and Heremans, 1966).

The maximum amount of plasma which should be donated was discussed by Lundsgaard-Hansen (1977a) who pointed out that regulations in the USA allow up to

50–60 litres a year but European regulations allow only 15 litres a year. When 1 litre of plasma is taken each week, as discussed above, albumin synthesis must increase by 50% if equilibrium is to be maintained; this figure seems uncomfortably close to the maximum possible increase in albumin synthesis which both in humans and experimental animals seldom exceeds 100%. Lundsgaard-Hansen pointed out that donors who give 1 litre of plasma a week lose as much albumin in this way as does a patient with nephrosis and severe proteinuria. Other possible risks of intensive plasmapheresis are atherosclerosis due to increased synthesis of low density and very low density lipoproteins stimulated by enhanced protein synthesis and platelet aggregation (Lundsgaard-Hansen, 1977b; 1981). Moreover, the levels of immunoglobulins, especially IgM, are reduced in such donors although the capacity to mount a normal immune response is maintained (Friedman et al. 1975). In donors undergoing long-term third level plasmapheresis, the plasma concentrations of antithrombin III, plasminogen and Factor VIII are not significantly affected (Cohen and Oberman, 1970; Jaffe and Mosher, 1981). In view of the fact that there is relatively little scientific information about the long-term effects of the considerable extra load on protein synthesis and of a depleted total albumin pool, it may be wise to accept the limit of 15 litres plasma a year and 600 ml per session with an interval not shorter than 2 weeks between donations. Several hundreds of donors in London have been undergoing level 2 plasmapheresis for more than 10 years with no adverse effects; reduced total protein and albumin concentrations have been found only in donors on 'slimming' diets (Brozovic, 1984). The socioeconomic background and protein intake of donors are important factors in any programme of intensive plasmapheresis (Oberman, 1984). In any case, it is better to increase the total number of plasma donors than to subject a smaller number to larger or more frequent donations.

In plasmapheresis it is possible to return most of the platelets to the donor. When PRP is harvested, the donor's platelet count is well maintained until about 5 litres plasma are collected per week; even then, platelet counts return to normal within 3 d of the last donation (Kliman et al. 1964).

HARVESTING OF PLATELETS, LEUCOCYTES AND STEM CELLS

Collection of platelets
Plastic containers are used exclusively for the collection of platelets, firstly because their use is almost essential in preparing platelet concentrates, and secondly because their use is absolutely essential if the concentrates are to be stored. In the latter case, the platelets are separated in a closed system and gas exchange through an appropriate plastic is vital to avoid hypoxic conditions leading to an accelerated production of lactic acid. The availability of more permeable or thinner plastics has prolonged the shelf-life of platelet concentrates by facilitating gas exchange even further (see Chapter 14).

Preparation of platelet concentrates from single units of whole blood
In deciding on the optimum method for producing platelet concentrates, all of the following considerations should be taken into account (Slichter and Harker, 1976a):

(1) centrifugation time and force; (2) yield; (3) platelet viability; (4) platelet function; (5) resuspension time; (6) storage capability; and (7) recovery of Factor VIII from the residual PPP. In addition, the temperature at which the blood is kept before and during processing, the time between collection and preparation of the platelet concentrate, the volume of plasma left to resuspend the platelets, the white cell and red cell contamination, and the temperature and mode of agitation during storage should be considered (Slichter, 1985). Two methods for preparing platelet concentrates are described briefly in Appendix 1; one method involves an initial gentle centrifugation to obtain PRP and concentration of platelets by further centrifugation; the second method involves an initial hard centrifugation to obtain buffy coats from whole blood and the subsequent recovery of the platelets by gentle centrifugation. Two types of machine, (1) the Optipress or Biopack, using two outlets in the primary collection pack ('bottom and top'), and (2) the Compomat or Ex 30, using traditional multiple packs, have been developed to automate platelet collection from buffy coats as well as plasma separation (see Chapter 14). Each platelet concentrate should have at least 5.5×10^{10} platelets in 50 ml plasma or an appropriate platelet suspension medium and the pH should not be allowed to fall below 6.4 or rise above 7.4. Platelet concentrates prepared under these conditions have 0.09 ± 0.04 leucocytes $\times 10^8$/unit. A proportion of the platelet concentrates produced each month should be selected at random at the end of the allowable storage period, for platelet count, platelet function tests, red cell content, Hb estimation, white cell content and measurement of pH. Recently, special filters have become available that remove more than 90% of leucocytes from pooled platelets or from platelet concentrates collected by cell separators with a loss of less than 15% of platelets (see Chapter 13).

Use of cell separators

Intermittent-flow cell separators

The donor's or patient's anticoagulated blood is drawn in successive batches and separated into its components in a disposable bowl (Fig. 1.2). The cycles are repeated as often as necessary to obtain the required volume of PPP or PRP. Advantages of these methods are the simplicity of operation, the portability of the machines, and the possibility of a single venous access, although a double access is preferred for speed and security. The disadvantages are the slowness of operation, the relatively large amount of blood (600 ml or more) which is outside the donor in the final stages of the procedure, and the contamination of the platelet concentrates with lymphocytes (see Huestis *et al.* 1981; Huestis, 1983a). Most users of the intermittent-flow Haemonetics H-30 cell separator reprocess the platelet concentrates by centrifugation in order to reduce the volume and remove white cells and red cells.

By using a centrifugal force of 650 *g* and a ratio of ACD to blood of 1:12 with the Haemonetics V-50, Rock *et al.* (1983a) were able to collect in less than 50 min, 600 ml PRP which was later separated by centrifugation into 500 ml PPP and 100 ml platelet concentrate with an average yield of 2.21×10^{11} platelets. A similar system, but with an integral platelet collection pack, was used by Penny *et al.* (1984), resulting in the final collection of approximately 360 ml PPP and 140 ml platelet concentrate with an average yield of 1.06×10^{11} platelets and minimal white cell contamination. In the

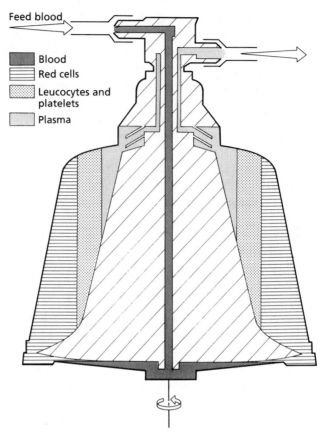

Figure 1.2 Cross-section of an intermittent-flow cell separator bowl (Haemonetics Model A-30 Latham bowl) redrawn from a diagram supplied by the Haemonetics Corporation. Blood is fed into the bottom of a disposable, polycarbonate, rotating bowl and, after separation of the components of blood into layers, different fractions may be harvested sequentially into separate plastic bags. The required fraction, e.g. that containing the platelets, is retained for transfusion to a patient and the remaining components are returned to the donor. The whole operation may then be repeated.

more advanced and faster V-50 model, the 'surge' procedure, by combining centrifugation with elutriation, has improved cell separation with higher yields of platelets ($3–5 \times 10^{11}$ platelets per procedure) which are minimally contaminated with leucocytes. The V-50 model has variable centrifuge speeds, automated collection assisted by optical density sensors, and automated on-line monitoring capabilities. It also offers the possibility of extended storage of platelet concentrates by guaranteeing sterility; the introduction of a pressure sensor ensures the integrity of the rotating seal and the disposables used are pre-connected by the manufacturer (Ciavarella, 1989).

Continuous-flow cell separators were developed primarily for the collection of granulocytes (Freireich *et al.* 1965). Anticoagulated blood is fed continuously into a rapidly rotating bowl or channel in which red cells, leucocytes, platelets and plasma separate into layers (Figs 1.3 and 1.4). Any layer or layers can be removed, and the remainder, together with a replacement fluid, returned to the patient. Models in use at the present time include the Fenwal CS-3000, the COBE 2997 and the Spectra COBE.

The CS-3000 has two chambers within one centrifugation bowl; citrated blood enters into the first (separation) chamber followed by separation, in the second (collection) chamber, of the platelets or white cells from plasma depending on the computerized programme and the collection chamber selected. The red cells are returned to the donor and most of the processing is carried out through computer-assisted devices. The donor's extracorporeal volume is much lower, i.e. about 300 ml, than with intermittent-flow machines. The absence of a seal in the CS-3000 permits collection of platelets in a closed system, making it safe to store them for more than 24 h. High platelet yields ($3–5 \times 10^{11}$ per 90–110 min procedure) are obtained with the standard platelet separation chamber. Higher platelet yields of more than 6×10^{11} in 70–90 min seem possible with a high-efficiency separation chamber insert, although with considerably greater white cell contamination. For this reason, the manufacturer has developed the Fenwal CS Plus TNX-6 machine which supersedes the CS-3000 in all aspects of platelet collection, i.e. better yields, sufficient for two therapeutic doses, with less white cell contamination and possibility of storage for a period longer than 24 h.

The operator-dependent Spectra 2997 and the more automated Spectra COBE also use a rotating seal to connect the tubing with the centrifuge. These machines separate the different components of blood on the basis of their individual densities; they have a hollow, loop-like, rotating channel in which the blood travels circumferentially and in which centrifugal forces act radially. The centrifugal force and flow rate can be varied by the operator to adjust the composition of the buffy coat which is then extracted via a tubing manifold into a collection chamber. The outlet port of each component is controlled by a separate pump. There are two types of channel with different positionings and sizes of the exit ports, which are used to collect white cells or platelets by one type of channel or to perform plasma or lympho-plasma exchange by the other. A two-stage channel is available to collect a purer preparation of platelets; in the first stage PRP is separated from the red cells, and in the second stage the PRP enters a spiral and narrow channel in which the concentrated platelets and PPP are separated. After separation, the concentrated red cells flow clockwise against the flow of whole blood and are returned with or without the plasma to the donor (Hester, 1979; Ciavarella, 1989; see Fig. 1.4). The Spectra COBE AS-104 cell separator is the most advanced, computerized, automated and transportable of the COBE models and can use any of the three channel designs; the platelets collected with the dual-stage separation channel have a very low white cell contamination (less than 0.5×10^7 per concentrate) with a yield, after 90 min collection (often above 6×10^{11}) that provides enough platelets to enable division of the concentrate into two full therapeutic doses. The use of submicron filters for the anticoagulant and saline make extended platelet storage safe. The COBE machine has the lowest extracorporeal volume of all continuous-flow cell separators but it cannot be used for red cell exchanges or for single venous access procedures. Both the 2997 model and the Spectra COBE use more citrate per procedure and this use is associated with a greater incidence of hypocalcaemic symptoms.

Continuous-flow cell separators (COBE 2997, Fenwal CS-3000, Celltrifuge II, Dideco 'Viva') have the advantage of speed and also, because of the small extracorporeal volume involved, of causing minimum blood volume fluctuations. The disadvantages of these separators are that, except for the lighter Spectra COBE AS104, they are relatively immobile, require two sites of vascular access and have rates of extraction of platelets or granulocytes which are lower than those of intermittent-flow systems. Detailed descriptions of both centrifugal systems of cell separation can be found in Huestis (1983b) and Ciavarella (1989).

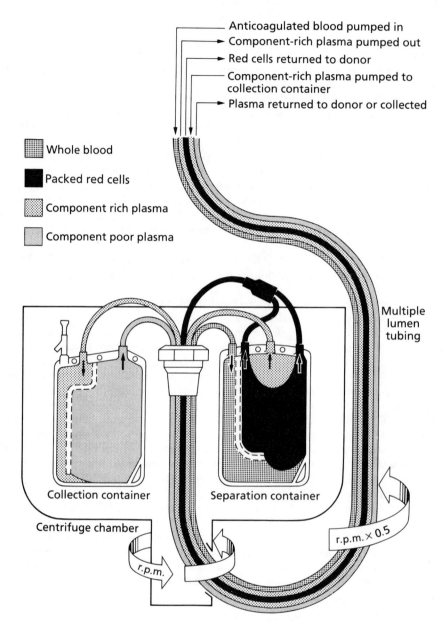

Figure 1.3 Diagram of continuous-flow blood cell separator (Fenwal CS-3000). Blood is pumped through one of the five channels of the multiple lumen tube into the separation container.

As the centrifuge chamber revolves, the multiple lumen tube revolves round the outside of the chamber at half the speed so that twisting of the tube is avoided and there is no need for a rotating seal.

Component-rich, e.g. platelet-rich, plasma is pumped out of the separation container and back into the collection chamber, which can be used directly for transfusion. For further details, see text (diagram supplied by Fenwal Laboratories).

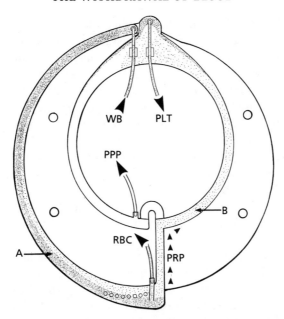

Figure 1.4 Diagram of the Spectra COBE AS-104 dual-stage blood separation channel: citrated whole blood (WB) flows counter-clockwise in a circular half-channel (A) and is separated into concentrated red cells (RBC) and platelet-rich plasma (PRP) when it reaches a channel offset. The PRP continues to flow in an annular half-channel (B) in the same direction, where platelets are separated and collected through an outer port (PLT), plasma (PPP) being collected at a medial port. The concentrated red cells flow clockwise towards the inlet tube for whole blood and are returned to the donor with saline or plasma (diagram supplied by Fresenius).

Collection of platelets by cell separators

Large quantities — at least a full dose of 3×10^{11} platelets — can be collected from single donors using intermittent-flow centrifugation or continuous-flow centrifugation (Huestis *et al.* 1975; Mishler *et al.* 1976; Buchholz *et al.* 1983; Ciavarella, 1989). In both cases the procedure normally requires 1–2 h and a relatively large volume of citrate anticoagulant is returned to the donor. Obviously, regardless of the system used, the platelet count will depend mainly on the donor's platelet count before thrombapheresis and on the volume of blood processed. On the other hand, the volume of the platelet concentrate and the degree of white cell contamination will depend on the machine used. For platelet collection by apheresis, as for plasmapheresis and leucapheresis, anticoagulant must be added in the correct proportion to donor blood before it enters the cell separator.

As described above, the more modern versions of cell separator allow the possibility of extended storage of large numbers of platelets in appropriate large platelet containers. However, the disposables for these systems are expensive and in most countries, platelet concentrates collected with cell separators are used mainly for special purposes, e.g. collection of HLA-compatible platelets for patients who have become refractory to the transfusion of platelet concentrates from random donors. The systems are too expensive and laborious for general use, although some centres, due to increasing demands, have to collect platelets by apheresis to supplement supplies of platelets obtained from whole blood donations. Two machines, the Autopheresis C from Baxter and PCS from Haemonetics, are suitable for this purpose because they have programmes for collecting plasma for fractionation and platelets simultaneously, as required. Hence, donors can be switched from plasmapheresis only to plasmapheresis and thrombapheresis according to platelet demands. Some centres, such as the Mayo Clinic, advocate the routine use of platelet concentrates collected by apheresis because the patient is then exposed to fewer donors, an important advantage, especially when the patient is immunosuppressed (A. Pineda, personal communication).

When platelets from only one or two donors are needed, as when transfusing infants or using HLA-matched platelets collected by apheresis, it is important that the donors should not have taken aspirin within the previous week since aspirin impairs platelet function. On the other hand, when transfusing pooled concentrates obtained from many different donors, it seems unnecessary to reject platelets from donors taking aspirin since it is unlikely that all donors contributing to a pool will be taking the drug (Slichter, 1985).

On the whole, different modern cell separators all give similar yields of platelets. The lowest white cell contamination is achieved with the Spectra COBE: fewer than 10^6 white cells per platelet concentrate have been reported (see Ciavarella, 1989). Special filters such as the PALL PL100 can be used to decrease the number of leucocytes in platelet concentrates collected by systems other than the Spectra COBE (Anderson et al. 1991b).

Autologous platelets collected by thrombapheresis have normal recovery and survival (Slichter, 1978). Several studies have shown that platelets collected by apheresis have in vitro and in vivo functions similar to platelets obtained from units of whole blood. Platelets intended for extended storage should be placed into the appropriate large plastic containers at a concentration suitable to maintain their pH between 6.4 and 7.4. In the case of high platelet yields, this will require separation of the concentrate into two storage containers (Ciavarella, 1989).

In this edition, the subject of bone marrow transplantation is not covered in detail but, as stated earlier, blood donors and especially donors who give platelets by apheresis often volunteer to be included in national or international panels of bone marrow donors for transplantation. Volunteers in such panels need to meet stricter selection criteria than routine blood donors, i.e. they are required to be under 50 years of age and are made aware of the requirement for a general anaesthetic if asked to give their marrow. Their HLA type is kept in a central computer with a programme adapted to search for donors compatible with prospective recipients of allogeneic bone marrow grafts. These donors are often asked to give HLA-compatible platelets for patients who have become refractory to transfusions of random platelets (see Chapter 14).

Collection of granulocytes by leucapheresis

The harvesting of granulocytes with the return of the rest of the blood to the donor is described as leucapheresis. Since the indications for supportive therapy with granulo- cytes for patients with malignant disease or leukaemia are very limited and still controversial, the collection of granulocytes by leucapheresis is restricted to specialized centres.

Methods of collecting granulocytes from individual routine blood donations have been described but, for adult recipients, they do not provide a reasonable alternative to leucapheresis because the leucocyte yields are very poor (Waldman and Shander, 1980) or because the addition of sedimenting agents such as hydroxyethyl starch (HES) to whole blood makes the remaining red cells and plasma unsuitable for transfusion (Poon and Wilson, 1980). On the other hand, for newborn infants, granulocytes separated within 24 h of collection from single routine blood donations after the addition of HES or gelatin can be useful in the treatment of septicaemia (Rock et al. 1984c).

The preferred spellings for the collection of granulocytes and platelets by apheresis are leucapheresis and thrombocytapheresis (abbreviated to thrombapheresis), respectively. (For discussion, see Mollison et al. 1987.)

Collection of granulocytes by cell separators

Two methods have been widely used, separately or in combination, to increase the yield of granulocytes: the administration of steroids to the donor to increase the peripheral granulocyte count, and introduction into the donor or cell separator of a red cell sedimenting agent, i.e. HES, dextran or modified fluid gelatin, to improve the separation between red cells and leucocytes. The need for agents which cause rouleaux formation and thus help to separate red cells from granulocytes arises from the fact that the specific gravity of red cells and granulocytes is very similar (1093–1096 for red cells; 1087–1092 for granulocytes), so that centrifugation alone is a very inefficient means of separation (Mishler et al. 1975; Huestis et al. 1981).

Use of steroids and rouleaux-forming agents

The administration of corticosteroids increases the granulocyte count by stimulating the release of neutrophils from the bone marrow reserve, by causing a shift of cells from the marginated to the circulating granulocyte pool and by inhibiting the escape of granulocytes from the circulation (see review by Mishler, 1977).

If 40 mg prednisolone are given orally to normal subjects, the increase in granulocyte count reaches a peak at 5 h; the increase varies widely in different donors but is at least 2×10^9 neutrophils per litre with a mean increase of about $5.8 \times 10^9/l$ in subjects under the age of 60 years (Cream, 1968). Suitable doses of steroids are: dexamethasone 6–12 mg, or prednisone 40–60 mg orally, given 10–12 h before collection of granulocytes. These doses may very rarely give rise to transient side-effects such as headache, palpitations, flushing, insomnia and euphoria.

As discussed above, the yield of granulocytes can also be increased by adding a rouleaux-forming agent with the citrate anticoagulant to the input line of the cell separator. HES has been used extensively. The increased granulocyte yield caused by HES is not solely due to its sedimenting properties; it appears to have a specific effect in some cell separator devices which is independent of an increase in erythrocyte sedimentation rate (ESR) (Mishler, 1982).

From a review of nearly 2000 leucaphereses on more than 500 donors it was concluded that HES was devoid of serious side-effects, causing only an occasional pyrogenic reaction or mild urticaria (Mishler, 1975). Due to its high water-binding capacity HES has the disadvantage of causing transient plasma expansion which can lead to headache and oedema if used in large volumes or on consecutive days (Mishler, 1982). When 160–500 ml (15–60 g) HES are added to the input line of the cell separator and 4–10 litres blood are processed, a total of $7–10 \times 10^9$ granulocytes can be collected in 2–4 h. The yield of granulocytes can be increased two- to four-fold if HES is used in combination with corticosteroids (Mishler, 1977). Best results are obtained if HES is given continuously during the collection procedure and if the dose is not decreased on sequential days of collection (Rock and McCombie, 1985). Plasmagel (a modified fluid gelatin) has been used widely in France (see, for example, Bussel *et al.* 1976) and seems also to be a good red cell sedimenting agent. It has the advantage over HES that it is eliminated more rapidly from the body, although allergic reactions are more frequent (Huestis *et al.* 1985; see also Chapter 2), granulocyte yields are lower with some models of cell separators (Mishler *et al.* 1983) and plasma volume is expanded (Rock *et al.* 1984b). For further data on the frequency of reactions after the infusion of plasma substitutes see Chapter 2.

Large numbers of granulocytes can be collected from donors with chronic granulocytic leukaemia with or without the use of sedimenting agents (Huestis *et al.* 1976; Lowenthal, 1977).

Although few comparative studies are available, all cell separators can produce adequate yields, viz. $10–20 \times 10^9$ granulocytes per $1–2$ h procedure in steroid-stimulated donors with the addition of sedimenting agents. The concentrates have a high content of platelets ($2–4.5 \times 10^{11}$) and red cells ($15–28$ ml). Continuous-flow cell separators such as the CS-3000 and Spectra COBE have been shown to give higher yields of granulocytes than intermittent-flow machines such as the H-30 and V-50.

When compared with granulocytes collected from whole blood donations, granulocytes collected by apheresis have shown little or no impairment in function (Ciavarella, 1989).

Effects of repeated cytapheresis
In subjects undergoing repeated apheresis, levels of red cells, platelets and lymphocytes should be carefully monitored and not allowed to fall below normal limits. Neutrophils are so rapidly produced and released that their level is unchanged.

Platelets
When platelets or granulocytes are collected with cell separators the donor's platelet count will not return to its pre-donation level for 6–7 days. This fact limits the frequency of platelet donations by relatives of patients requiring HLA-compatible platelets. Sometimes the platelet count can fall below 100×10^9/l and, although this is not dangerous for the donor, it may make it unprofitable to collect further platelets (Huestis, 1983a). Platelet donation should not be allowed if the pre-apheresis platelet count is $< 150 \times 10^9$/l (Strauss *et al.* 1983b).

Lymphocytes
High losses of lymphocytes are possible during intensive thrombapheresis owing to the similar density of lymphocytes and platelets.

Donors from whom platelets, or granulocytes, were harvested by intermittent-flow cytapheresis (IFC), using a six-cycle procedure, were found to lose an average of 3.5×10^9 lymphocytes (Koepke *et al.* 1981). Broadly similar estimates of the loss of lymphocytes were obtained by Fratantoni and French (1980), who estimated that when sedimenting agents were used, 6×10^9 lymphocytes were lost per platelet donation, and by Dwyer *et al.* (1981), who estimated that when the donor was given prednisone and a sedimenting agent the mean loss of T lymphocytes per donation was

3×10^9. The long-term effects of this loss of lymphocytes are potentially serious. After 10-weekly donations a fall in the lymphocyte count of 20%, with a decrease in B cells in half of the donors, was found by Koepke *et al.* (1981).

In a study of 21 healthy blood donors subjected to 9–17 cytaphereses over a period of 12 months there was a 23% decrease in absolute lymphocyte count, a 25% decrease in T cells, and a 46% decrease in B cells, with a reduction of 14% in serum IgG concentration; the donors had not been given steroids in connection with their donations. The authors concluded that frequent cytapheresis may pose long-term hazards to the immune status of donors (Senhauser *et al.* 1982).

Similar results were obtained by Robbins *et al.* (1985), who reported lymphocytopenia in 21 of 113 donors who gave platelets regularly by apheresis with the Haemonetics H-30 model with a mean number of 13.1 procedures per annum over a mean period of 162.7 weeks. The lymphocyte count was inversely related to the total number of thrombaphereses and the T4 + and T8 + lymphocyte subsets were reduced in all 13 lymphocytopenic donors tested. However, T4 : T8 ratios were found to be normal and no adverse effects were noted in any of the donors. Lymphocytes are also lost in large numbers when the CS-3000 is used to collect platelets, particularly with the isoradial chamber. It is recommended that any donor who develops lymphocytopenia (lymphocyte count $< 1 \times 10^9/l$) should be excluded from donation until the lymphocyte count is $> 1.5 \times 10^9/l$. Donors who fail to revert to normal within 8 weeks should be referred to their doctor for further investigations (Strauss *et al.* 1983). On the other hand, short-term removal of lymphocytes may not have adverse effects. Following a total of six lymphapheresis procedures over a 12-d period in 12 blood donors with a mean removal of 41.6×10^9 lymphocytes, there were no significant changes in absolute lymphocyte counts, immunoglobulin levels or *in vitro* tests of the immune response (Blanchette *et al.* 1985b).

Symptoms and signs in donors giving blood via cell separators

Many of the symptoms and signs such as vaso-vagal reactions are similar to those experienced by donors giving a routine blood donation or by patients during plasma exchange. Factors that may cause symptoms or signs are changes in the donor's blood volume, chilling of blood and the introduction of foreign substances such as citrate or HES. Of a total 195 372 donor apheresis procedures, complications were reported in 9.6% of cases, including 5.2% donor-related problems (e.g. fainting, citrate toxicity), 4% machine and harness problems, and 0.4% operator errors (Robinson, 1990a). Most of the immediate complications can be handled by the operator and apheresis need not be halted; the reactions can usually be controlled by increasing the return flow of blood or the rate of saline infusion into the receiving arm.

A decrease in certain complement components has been observed in donors undergoing leucapheresis on intermittent-flow cell separators, possibly due to absorption on to the surface of the disposable plastics used in the procedure (Strauss *et al.* 1980).

Syncope occurs more frequently when using IFC machines as the extracorporeal blood volume is larger than with continuous-flow cytapheresis (CFC) cell separators. It has been recommended that the extracorporeal volume should not exceed 15% of the donor's own volume at any time (Huestis, 1989). Severe vaso-vagal attacks were reported in 32 donors undergoing leucapheresis; ten donors lost consciousness and had seizures (Sandler and Nusbacher, 1982). However, if, as in the UK, experienced blood donors are used for plasmapheresis and thrombapheresis, syncope occurs in only 0.2% of procedures although fainting and nausea are ten times more likely when cells are collected rather than PPP or PRP. From the UK apheresis registry, the chance of severe syncope requiring resuscitation has been estimated at 1 in 100 000 procedures (Robinson, 1990a; supplemented by personal communication).

Chills are relatively common and may be due partly to extracorporeal chilling of blood and partly to undetermined factors. In most cases, a blanket or a blood warmer will prevent the chills.

Citrate toxicity is related to the concentration of citrate used, the rate of reinfusion, the duration of the procedure, and to whether a continuous or discontinuous procedure is used. In the collection of PRP or PPP, the return of citrated plasma is small and the incidence of toxicity is ten times lower than when leucocytes or platelets are collected (Robinson, 1990a) Common manifestations are as follows: circumoral paraesthesia, vibratory feeling in the chest, nausea, vomiting and, rarely, overt tetany which may be made worse by hyperventilation. Signs of citrate toxicity closely parallel the fall in ionized calcium when standard concentrations of ACD-A (Olson *et al.* 1977) or sodium citrate (Mishler *et al.* 1976) are used. Signs of toxicity may be avoided by slowing the rate of infusion or by using a lower concentration of citrate, combined if necessary with a small amount of heparin (Huestis, 1986b). 'Half-strength' ACD-A contains half the amount of trisodium citrate but the same amount of citric acid as ACD-A so that the total citrate in a unit is 5.1 mmol compared with 7.7 mmol in a unit of ACD-A blood. The use of this modified ACD-A does not lead to clotting and does not impair platelet function (Mishler *et al.* 1977).

In the treatment of citrate toxicity, the administration of calcium is not recommended as it can cause clotting in the extracorporeal system or severe arrhythmia in the donor (Westphal, 1984). However, in the USA, where it is recommended that the citrate load (ACD-A) should not exceed 1 ml/l of the total blood volume, i.v. calcium gluconate is offered to all donors who develop symptoms of citrate toxicity. In the UK, there are guidelines for maximum flow rates for the different anticoagulant ratios in IFC and CFC machines which avoid the need to use calcium gluconate (Robinson, 1990b).

Haematoma formation occurs more frequently in apheresis donors owing to the pumped red cell return (Robinson, 1990a).

Adverse effects of hydroxyethyl starch. Febrile and allergic reactions due to HES are discussed in Chapter 2. The potential hazard of receiving frequent infusions of HES over a short period is illustrated by the experiments of Rock and Wise (1979). Four healthy donors were given infusions of 500 ml HES (mol. wt. 450 000) daily for 4 d. After the fourth infusion, the average increase in plasma volume was 0.85 litres; 24 h later, in all but one of the donors, plasma volume was still 0.5 litres above the donor's initial value.

In donors who give blood regularly by cell separator and receive repeated injections of HES, serum HES levels are still raised 3 months after the last infusion (Ring *et al.* 1980). In such donors, headache, mild hypertension, swollen fingers, and peripheral or peri-orbital oedema may be present (Westphal, 1984). Some countries do not allow the use of HES (and, or steroids) in voluntary donors but allow the use of dextran or gelatin as alternative sedimenting agents (Robinson, 1990b).

Transitory side-effects due to *steroid administration* such as headache, insomnia, flushing, palpitations and euphoria occur in some donors and are dose-related. Subjects who cannot tolerate steroids or in whom steroids are contraindicated (e.g. those with diabetes or peptic ulcer) should not be used for leucapheresis (Huestis, 1989).

Allergic reactions consisiting of sneezing, urticaria or even angioedema are seen in occasional donors (Huestis, 1983a) and are five times more likely to occur in donors giving cells than in donors giving PPP or PRP (Robinson, 1990a). Severe reactions due to sensitization to ethylene oxide are mentioned in Chapter 15.

Mild haemolysis is occasionally seen and is caused by kinks in the plastic tubing (see p. 37).

Infections at the site of venesection are more likely to occur in cytapheresis donors who have two needles in their veins for a period of 1–3 h. There is also the more remote, although more serious, danger of infection from contaminated bottles of solutions used in cytapheresis or from leaking harnesses (Kosmin, 1980; Robinson, 1990a).

Mortality
Fatalities attributed to the donation of plasma or cells by apheresis are rare. Nine deaths were reported to the FDA for the 10 years between 1976 and 1985; eight of these were attributed to plasma donations and one to leucapheresis (Sazama, 1990). No deaths attributed to apheresis have occurred in 289 385 procedures analysed in the UK registry from mid-1985 to April 1989 (A. Robinson, personal communication, 1991).

Medical supervision of donors who give blood via cell separators
Compared with simple blood donation, giving blood components routinely via cell separators involves extra hazards and the donors should receive extra surveillance. Potential long-term side-effects of plasmapheresis have been postulated, such as chronic protein depletion with increased protein synthesis and overproduction of α_2-globulins, β-lipoproteins, fibrinogen and other coagulation factors which could lead to accelerated atherosclerosis or to a hypercoagulable state (see Robinson, 1990a). The clinical and laboratory examinations considered to be necessary vary in different countries but a minimum, at the time of recruitment, might include the following: a medical examination, including chest radiography and, for those over 40 years, electrocardiography; a full blood count, a prothrombin time and partial thrombo-plastin time; estimation of total serum proteins together with estimates of albumin and immunoglobulin concentrations. At the time of each donation a full blood count with a

platelet count greater than $150 \times 10^9/l$ and a white cell count greater than $4.0 \times 10^9/l$ is essential and, for level 2 and 3 plasma donors (see p. 21), an estimation of total serum protein and albumin concentrations. The fitness of donors should be assessed at least once a year, especially in those over 45 years of age.

Some countries have recommendations regarding the maximum number of cytapheresis procedures permitted in normal donors; in the UK the number per year is 12 leucapheresis donations and 24 thromapheresis donations when collected with the PCS or APC.

There are many (e.g. the UK Blood Transfusion Service), who consider that cell separators such as the CS-3000 and Spectra COBE, should be used only in places where a cardiac arrest team is immediately available in case the donor collapses during donation. On the other hand, plasmapheresis machines such as the PCS and APC, as well as their portable versions, are suitable for use in plasma clinics remote from hospitals and in mobile clinics.

PLASMA EXCHANGE

The exchange of large volumes of plasma became possible with the introduction of cell separators. The advantage of most systems available today is the use of totally disposable software.

Use of membrane filters for plasma exchange
Plasma can be separated from the cellular components of blood by filtration at a high flow rate through continuous-flow systems using either flat-bed filters or hollow fibres (Castino *et al.* 1981; Smith *et al.* 1981; Buffaloe *et al.* 1983). The blood passes by membranes of varying composition and design, allowing the plasma to filter through and leaving the cells resuspended in a replacement fluid to be returned to the patient. Compared with cell separators, membrane filters have the advantages of simplicity and of being usable with only small volumes of blood, so that less of the subject's blood has to be outside the body at any one time. On the other hand, membrane filters have potential problems such as their liability to leak, to damage cells and to activate complement. Cellulose diacetate membranes, especially of the double filtration type, seem to cause much more activation of the alternative pathway of complement than the newer polycarbonate membranes, resulting in a significant return of C3a and C5a to the patient. The release of these anaphylatoxins may be responsible for the initial leucopenia and lymphocytopenia in donors undergoing filtration plasmapheresis (Jørstad *et al.* 1985). However, the clinical significance of complement activation by membranes has yet to be determined. In order to obtain a high flow rate with an adequate filtration coefficient, some of the filtration machines require an arteriovenous shunt but there are now systems available which require only a two-vein access in order to obtain yields of filtered plasma of 30 ml/min (Bussel *et al.* 1982). Some of these newer machines need large-scale trials and the operational procedures need to be simplified. Attractive innovations in the membrane systems, which allow the return of the patient's own plasma, include the selective removal of large molecules by cascades of filters of different pore size (Sieberth, 1981) and the addition of cryoprecipitation chambers to remove cryoglobulins or immune complexes (Malchesky *et al.* 1980).

Volumes of fluid exchanged

In therapeutic plasma exchange, the amount of a specific pathogenic substance removed depends on the volume of plasma exchanged and on the frequency of the procedure. The concentration X_t of a pathogenic substance X after a time t (in h) of plasma exchange is given by the equation:

$$X_t = X_0 e^{-rt}$$

where X_0 represents the initial concentration of the pathogenic component and r the fractional rate of exchange or volume of plasma exchanged per hour divided by the plasma volume (Calabrese *et al.* 1980). The equation is valid only if the following conditions are met: complete mixing, no change in the patient's blood volume and no influx of the component from the extravascular space. If these conditions are met, each plasma exchange equivalent to one plasma volume will remove approximately 60% of a (pathogenic) intravascular component. The removal of 40 ml plasma per kg of body-weight gives roughly the same results as predicted by the equation (Huestis, 1986a). However, in practice, the conditions outlined above are rarely met. For molecules that are mainly intravascular, such as immune complexes or IgM, the final concentration is nearer the calculated value than for smaller molecules such as IgG which diffuse freely to the extravascular space. Other factors that need to be taken into consideration are the catabolism, half-life and rate of renewal of the substance being removed. If resynthesis is very rapid, greater numbers of procedures will be required. Rebound phenomena tend to occur after plasma exchange when antibodies or immune complexes need to be removed. In these cases the concurrent use of immunosuppressive therapy has proved the treatment of choice since plasma exchange reduces the required dose of immuno-suppression with a consequent reduction in hazards (Huestis, 1986a). The volume of plasma exchanged in most therapeutic procedures is equivalent to the patient's plasma volume. The usual practice consists of a course of four or five procedures carried out within 7–10 days, although the volume and frequency of plasma exchanges vary depending on the individual patient, the clinical condition and the protocols of each centre. As plasma exchange has short-lived benefits and because it is a complex and expensive form of therapy, its use should be limited to conditions in which there is good evidence of its efficacy.

Rationale of plasma exchange

The main criteria for the rational application of therapeutic plasma exchange are: (1) the existence of a known pathogenic substance in the plasma; and (2) the possibility of removing this substance more rapidly than it can be renewed in the body. However, clinical improvement does not necessarily follow the removal of a pathogenic sub-stance. On the other hand, some conditions improve after plasma exchange even when the concentration of the substance in the plasma does not fall (Huestis, 1986a). Moreover, in rare conditions such as thrombotic thrombocytopenic purpura (TTP), there appears to be a missing plasma factor which is supplied in sufficient quantities by plasma exchange (see pp. 40 and 660). In general, plasma exchange is used to treat severely ill patients not responding to conventional therapy (Huestis, 1989).

Vascular access
An antecubital vein is used whenever possible; if a larger blood flow is needed, a catheter can be passed into a femoral or subclavian vein, or arteriovenous shunts, arteriovenous fistulae or prosthetic grafts can be established (Pusey, 1983). The morbidity associated with these procedures is not negligible and includes thrombosis, infection, gangrene, formation of an aneurysm, cardiac arrhythmia, pneumothorax, perforation of great vessels and even of the heart (see Bell *et al.* 1983; Huestis, 1986b).

Some effects of plasma exchange
The effects of intensive plasmapheresis in which small amounts of plasma are removed on numerous occasions have been considered above. In plasma exchange, large amounts of plasma are removed on any one occasion.

Effects on the circulation
Pronounced tiredness and malaise, presumably due to the shifts in fluid balance and extracorporeal circulation, are seen not infrequently in patients undergoing plasma exchange. Hypotension, hypovolaemia and vaso-vagal attacks seem to be commoner after plasma exchange than after routine blood donations. Most of these reactions can be controlled by temporary interruption of the procedure and by the reinfusion of some extra fluid (Huestis, 1986b).

Plasma protein levels
The extent of protein depletion will depend on the volume exchange, the number of procedures and the replacement fluid. Several studies have shown that plasma levels of immunoglobulins, C3, cholesterol, alkaline phosphatase and serum glutamic oxalo-acetic transaminase (SGOT) are considerably reduced after plasma exchange and that it may take weeks for them to return to normal levels (see Keller and Urbaniak, 1978; Orlin and Berkman, 1980; Stellon and Moorhead, 1981; Nilsson *et al.* 1983). Immuno-globulin depletion combined with immunosuppression increases the possibility of infection.

Coagulation factors
Intensive or prolonged plasma exchange results in a decrease of coagulation factors with a low turnover rate. In a series of patients in whom repeated plasma exchanges of 4–5 litres were carried out, fibrinogen levels fell to 25% after one exchange, to about 11% after five exchanges, and to about 1% after ten exchanges; haemorrhagic phenomena were seen very rarely although prophylactic platelet transfusion was sometimes given when the platelet count was low (Keller *et al.* 1979). After large-volume plasma exchange (1–1.5 plasma volumes), fibrinogen and platelets return to normal levels in 2–4 d (Urbaniak, 1984).

    Repeated plasma exchanges may carry some risk of induction of a hypercoagulable state. Antithrombin III (AT III) levels fell by about 84% in myasthenic patients undergoing 5-litre plasma exchanges. Prothrombin and thrombin times shortened progressively and two patients showed hypercoagulability. Since AT III is depleted and, due to stress, Factor VIII is elevated, there is a danger of thromboembolic episodes (Sultan *et al.* 1979). However, a study of seven alloimmunized pregnant women, undergoing plasma exchanges equivalent to 60% of their plasma volume five times per week during pregnancy, showed that coagulation factors remained within normal limits: AT III was considerably decreased in only one patient who had a low level of AT III before plasma exchange was started (Nilsson *et al.* 1983).

Despite gross disturbances in fibrinogen, platelets and AT III levels after repeated plasma exchange, very few thrombotic or haemorrhagic complications have been reported (Huestis, 1986b). It is impossible to discern whether these complications can be attributed to the plasma exchange or to the underlying disease. An analysis of coagulation studies on patients undergoing repeated plasma exchanges of 1–1.5 plasma volumes with plasma-free solutions showed that 10% of patients have levels of fibrinogen below the pre-exchange level and that in 23% of patients platelet counts fell below 30×10^9/l. AT III levels were reduced to 40–50%. Only five bleeding episodes, attributed to thrombocytopenia, were observed in 815 procedures (0.6%). It was concluded that adequte platelet levels are more important in maintaining haemostasis than the levels of procoagulant factors; the fact that thrombotic complications are rare in the presence of low levels of AT III may be due to the concomitant reduction of fibrinogen and other procoagulant factors (Urbaniak, 1984).

Haemolysis
In intermittent-flow cell separators especially, kinking of the plastic tubing may force the blood at high pressure through very narrow orifices, leading to haemolysis. The procedure should be stopped as soon as any signs of haemolysis are seen (Huestis, 1986b; 1989).

Citrate toxicity
The manifestations of citrate toxicity have been considered in the section on cell separators (see p. 32). The effects are exacerbated if the plasma is infused without first being warmed and if it is delivered through catheters close to the heart (Sutton *et al.* 1981).

Infection
As stated above, depletion of immunoglobulins, concomitant immunosuppressive therapy and complications of vascular access are all contributory factors to bacterial infection. In intensive plasma exchange, the progressive decrease of plasma fibronectin may also contribute to the increased susceptibility to infection (Norfolk *et al.* 1985).

There is a risk of transmission of hepatitis viruses, cytomegalovirus (CMV) and HIV when plasma is used as a replacement fluid.

Mortality
Plasma exchange is used to treat severely ill patients and it is difficult to decide from most of the published reports whether to attribute a particular death directly or indirectly to the exchange procedure or to the patient's underlying condition. Since 1982, Huestis has been compiling worldwide information on mortality of plasma exchange and has estimated the fatality rate to be 3 per 10 000 procedures. Up to March 1984, the number of deaths reported to be associated with plasma exchange was 59. Thirty of the reported deaths were attributed to cardiac arrhythmia leading to

cardiac arrest or to severe respiratory complications such as the adult respiratory distress syndrome; plasma was used as a replacement fluid in the majority of these cases (see Huestis, 1989). In the UK, where albumin is the main replacement fluid and plasma is seldom used, no deaths attributed to plasma exchange have been reported. In France, five deaths attributed to plasma exchange were reported in 9437 procedures carried out in 1130 patients, and in Canada one death was reported in 3840 procedures in 640 patients (Robinson, 1990a).

From the above, it is evident that plasma exchange is associated with some immediate and delayed morbidity and a not negligible mortality rate. However, it is thought that the mortality rate is now less than the 3 per 10 000 procedures mentioned above (Huestis, 1989).

Replacement fluid
Except for thrombotic thrombocytopenic purpura (TTP), for which plasma is the treatment of choice, there is no condition for which the optimal replacement fluid has been chosen on the basis of scientific data. In most cases the choice is based on cost, convenience, availability and volume of plasma removed (Urbaniak, 1983). Albumin, FFP, stored or cryoprecipitate-poor plasma singly or in combination are used in different centres. Plasma volume expanders, especially modified fluid gelatin, are also used (Stellon and Moorhead, 1981; Urbaniak, 1983). If the patient's albumin and protein levels are normal, crystalloids may be used at the beginning of the procedure to replace part, say 1 litre, of the plasma; the replacement fluid given first will be partially removed at the end of the exchange (Urbaniak, 1983).

Most centres use albumin or plasma protein fraction (PPF) as the major replacement fluid to maintain normal colloid osmotic pressure during intensive plasma exchange. Febrile, urticarial or hypotensive reactions are seen very occasionally with these products. Hypotension, presumably due to pre-kallikrein activator, is more common with certain batches of PPF. The main disadvantages of replacement with albumin preparations are that the preparations may not include the constituent that the patient lacks as, for example, in TTP, or that they may dangerously lower the plasma levels of certain constituents such as coagulation factors (see above) or of cholinesterase, leading to apnoea in patients injected with suxamethonium (Evans et al. 1980).

Patients treated with plasma as a replacement fluid are at greater risk (see section on mortality). The disadvantages of the use of plasma include: increased incidence of citrate toxicity and of urticarial and anaphylactic reactions, transmission of viral infections and passive transfer of antibodies such as leucoagglutinins, which are thought to be responsible for the severe and even fatal pulmonary complications of plasma exchange. If plasma is to be used, it is preferable to obtain it from untransfused men. However, in most conditions, the ideal replacement fluid is the patient's own plasma from which the pathogenic component has been removed.

Indications for plasma exchange
Plasma exchange can be considered to be of confirmed value only if: (1) there is evidence that, in the condition concerned, there is a plasma component that can be removed or replaced by plasma exchange; and (2) well controlled clinical trials

demonstrate benefit. Although therapeutic plasma exchange has been claimed to be beneficial in more than 100 disorders (see Hamblin, 1983; Shumak and Rock, 1984; Urbaniak, 1984), scientific studies and well controlled clinical trials are sparse. There are only a few conditions in which plasma exchange has been shown to be of definite benefit, namely the hyperviscosity syndrome, cryoglobulinaemia, myasthenia gravis, hypercholesterolaemia, Goodpasture's syndrome, post-transfusion purpura, Refsum's disease, haemophilia with high-titre Factor VIII antibody unresponsive to Factor VIII therapy, cold antibody autoimmune haemolytic anaemia with acute haemolysis and TTP. There are also many conditions in which suggestive evidence of the value of plasma exchange has been obtained but in which it is impossible to reach definite conclusions owing to the absence of controlled trials; plasma exchange in D-immunized pregnant women is a good example. For reviews of the effects of plasma exchange in various other conditions see Hamblin (1983), Urbaniak (1984), Shumak and Rock (1984) and Huestis (1986b). In general, therapeutic plasma exchange is used to treat symptomatically those acute conditions for which conventional therapy has failed; only in occasional circumstances is it used as chronic maintenance therapy.

Possible indications for plasma exchange may be considered under the following headings (modified from Shumak and Rock, 1984; Huestis, 1986a):

1 *Removal of antibodies.* (a) Alloantibodies, e.g. anti-HPA-1a in post-transfusion purpura (see Chapter 15); anti-D in pregnant women (see Chapter 12) and HLA antibodies in immunized uraemic patients before renal transplantation (Wikström *et al.* 1990). The removal of anti-A and anti-B in ABO-incompatible bone marrow transplants is now seldom necessary since the donor's red cells can be efficiently removed from the marrow before grafting (see Chapter 14). (b) Autoantibodies, e.g. anti-acetylcholine receptor (AChR) in myasthenia gravis; anti-basement membrane in Goodpasture's syndrome; Factor VIII inhibitor in unresponsive haemophiliacs with severe haemorrhage (Slocombe *et al.* 1981); red cell autoantibodies in cold antibody autoimmune haemolytic anaemia with acute haemolysis (Rosenfield and Jagathambal, 1976) and in the rare antibody-mediated, pure red cell aplasia; autoantibodies to epidermal cell-membrane glycoproteins in pemphigus; platelet autoantibodies in refractory autoimmune thrombocytopenia; and peripheral-nerve myelin autoantibodies in Guillain–Barré syndrome.

In myasthenia gravis, removal of AChR antibody by plasma exchange is associated with short-term clinical improvement, which may be dramatic (Newsom-Davis *et al.* 1978). However, in a controlled trial, no cumulative long-term benefit was conferred by plasma exchange (Hawkey *et al.* 1981).

In Goodpasture's syndrome, autoantibodies to the glomerular and alveolar basement membranes should be rapidly removed by plasma exchange in the early stages of the disease; suppression of further antibody synthesis can be achieved with cyclophosphamide and corticosteroids. Early treatment is essential since renal impairment is irreversible once the patient becomes dependent on dialysis (Savage *et al.* 1986). On the other hand, the same combination of plasma exchange plus immunosuppression proved successful in a controlled study of rapidly progressive glomerulonephritis excluding Goodpasture's syndrome even when patients had become dependent on dialysis. In severe systemic vasculitis with pulmonary haemorrhage even in the absence of renal involvement, plasma exchange combined with immunosuppression proved to be successful in inducing remission in most cases. Plasma exchange would remove anti-neutrophil cytoplasm autoantibodies (ANCA) or immune complexes as well as inflammatory mediators such as cytokines, complement factors and coagulation components (for references see Jayne, 1990).

2 *Removal of immune complexes*, e.g. rapidly progressive nephritis, systemic lupus erythematosus, cryoglobulinaemia and hypothetically in Guillain–Barré syndrome.

Symptomatic treatment of cryoglobulinaemia with plasmapheresis or plasma exchange has proved successful on a short-term basis (Berkman and Orlin, 1980; Haworth and Pusey, 1983). The cold-precipitating properties of cryoglobulins open the possibility of their selective depletion although the efficiency of presently available methods has been questioned (Rock *et al.* 1982).

3 *Removal of inflammatory mediators*, e.g., possibly, factors contributing to the pruritus of cholestasis.

4 *Removal of exogenous toxins which are protein-bound*, e.g. paraquat poisoning, aluminium toxicity (encephalopathy), metabolites in patients on dialysis, other drug poisonings (sodium chlorate, digoxin). Plasma exchange was used successfully as an adjunct to conventional therapy in 11 of 15 patients with severe progressive disseminated intravascular coagulation (DIC) and renal failure due to septic shock (Stegmayr *et al.* 1990).

5 *Removal of monoclonal proteins*, e.g. hyperviscosity syndrome. The hyperviscosity syndrome is most commonly due to an increase of serum IgM (Waldenström's macroglobulinaemia), although it is occasionally due to high mol. wt. polymers of IgG or IgA (in patients with multiple myeloma). In normal subjects the serum viscosity relative to water is 1.4–1.8 (MacKenzie *et al.* 1970a,b) but in patients with hyperviscosity syndrome may be as high as 8–33, in association with a greatly increased plasma volume. One of the most effective applications of plasma exchange is the treatment of the acute cardiovascular, neurological and haemorrhagic complications of this disease before there has been time for chemotherapy to become effective. In most cases only two or three plasma exchanges are needed; the replacement fluid should be plasma free and if the volume replaced is moderate it is usually not necessary to include albumin. Patients who are refractory or intolerant to chemotherapy can be maintained on plasma exchange at regular (4–6-weekly) intervals.

6 *Removal of excess plasma constituent*, e.g. phytanic acid as an adjunct to restrictive diet in Refsum's disease (Gibberd *et al.* 1979), ceramide trihexoside in Fabry's disease, cholesterol and low density lipoproteins (LDL) in familial hypercholesterolaemia.

Familial hypercholesterolaemia is characterized by a high level of LDL which is virtually confined to the plasma. Treatment with plasma exchange has been shown to be very effective in reducing the levels of cholesterol and LDL (King *et al.* 1980; Thompson, 1981) but there are no controlled trials showing the benefits of plasma exchange in this condition.

7 *Replacement of a specific plasma component*, e.g. in TTP, a disorder possibly resulting from lack of some normal plasma constituent (Byrnes and Khurana, 1977) which is probably prostacyclin-related (Machin *et al.* 1980; Remuzzi *et al.* 1980). Others claim that TTP is due to a platelet-aggregating factor which is inhibited by normal plasma (Lian *et al.* 1979). These two pathogenetic theories provide a rational basis for the use of plasma as a form of therapy in this condition and there are several reports of the successful treatment with either plasma infusion alone, exchange transfusion or with plasma exchange. A recent prospective, controlled trial in 102 patients seems to have shown that plasma exchange is the treatment of choice. On 7 of the first 9 d of entry into the trial, patients received either a plasma exchange (with FFP) or a simple infusion of FFP. All patients received aspirin and dipyridamole. At the end of 9 d, platelet counts had risen in 24 of 51 patients in the plasma exchange group but in only 13 of 51 in the infusion group; after 6 months, 11 patients in the plasma exchange group and 19 patients in the infusion group had died. The authors concluded that plasma exchange with FFP should be used in the treatment of TTP but mentioned that the results did not exclude the possibility that exchange had given better results than simple infusion because it resulted in the administration of larger amounts of plasma (Rock *et al.* 1991b).

The use of cryo-depleted plasma rather than FFP for plasma exchange may be more beneficial in life-threatening TTP; see p. 660.

8 *Placebo effect*, e.g. rheumatoid arthritis (RA). Controlled clinical trials are needed in RA as the disease is widespread and plasma exchange is expensive. Moreover, sham plasma exchange has shown a strong placebo effect in this disorder (Shumak and Rock, 1984).

Methods for the selective removal of plasma components

It is desirable to develop methods for the selective removal of unwanted substances from the patient's plasma to be followed by the return of the remaining plasma to the patient, thus completely avoiding the need for transfusing large volumes of normal donor plasma. Several methods for the selective removal of plasma components have already been described, based either on separation according to the physical characteristics of the component or on affinity binding. The combination of apheresis with column technology (see below) has several advantages: (1) because only separated plasma is passed through the column, there is no danger of platelet depletion; (2) there is no danger of depletion of coagulation factors either, allowing more intensive plasma exchange; (3) there is a wider choice of type and concentration of anticoagulants; and (4) the possibility of using smaller bead packings allows faster and more efficient adsorption (Pepper, 1983). There is one main condition, as described above, in which the selective removal of an unwanted pathogenic substance is easily achieved; in cryoglobulinaemia the abnormal protein precipitates in the cold and can be easily removed (McLeod and Sassetti, 1980).

Selective removal of antibodies

Removal of anti-A and anti-B by passage through immunoadsorbent columns. A method of selectively removing anti-A and anti-B from the recipient's plasma was described by Bensinger *et al.* (1981). This method is no longer needed since it is possible to deplete bone marrow of 95–98% of its red cells; see Chapter 14.

Adsorption of alloantibodies on to red cells. In a pregnant woman with relatively potent anti-M and a history of previous stillbirths, 51 litres plasma were withdrawn, absorbed with M-positive red cells and reinfused. Although this treatment resulted in only a small fall in antibody titre, the woman was delivered of a normal infant (Yoshida *et al.* 1981a). A group P^k pregnant woman with potent IgG anti-P and a history of repeated abortions was treated similarly. A total of 215 litres plasma were treated, as a result of which the antibody was maintained at a low level. A healthy infant was delivered at 35 weeks (Yoshida *et al.* 1984). On the other hand, in a case in which plasma from an Rh D-immunized woman was treated *in vitro* with D-positive red cells before being centrifuged and reinfused there was a dramatic increase in anti-D concentration which may well have been due to the presence of D-positive material in the reinfused plasma (Robinson, 1981). The potential hazard of introducing foreign red cells can be overcome by passing the plasma through a micropore filter (Yoshida *et al.* 1984).

A method of general application

A method that may be applicable to the elimination of any plasma component with antigenic properties was described by Stoffel and Demant (1981). To determine the effectiveness of the method, antibodies were prepared in swine against LDL and covalently linked to sepharose. By passing plasma through the anti-LDL–sepharose column large amounts of LDL could be removed from the plasma. The advantages of this method are that the high density lipoproteins are not removed from the plasma.

However, there is a danger of leakage of affinity ligands and the patient may become immunized to antibodies raised in animals. Human monoclonal antibodies should provide the solution to this problem (Pepper, 1983).

Selective removal of other unwanted substances

Other examples of unwanted substances which can be selectively removed are as follows: bilirubin, by adsorption on to ion-exchange resins (Sideman *et al.* 1981); bile acids, by the circulation of plasma over charcoal-coated glass beads (Lauterburg *et al.* 1978); lipoproteins, by the passage of plasma through a heparin–agarose column (Burgstaler *et al.* 1980); toxic substances (drugs), from plasma by the circulation of blood over amberlite resin columns (Lynn *et al.* 1979); anti-DNA (from a patient with lupus erythematosus), by circulation over a column containing immobilized DNA (Terman *et al.* 1977); IgG (only subclasses 1, 2 and 4) and immune complexes by specific binding of the Fc region to staphylococcal protein A (or SpA) (Sandor and Langone, 1982; Gjörstrup and Watt, 1990; Verrier Jones, 1990); fibronectin and Factor VIII, by binding to gelatin or collagen (Pepper, 1983); myeloma proteins, by binding to concanavalin A (Ray and Raychaudhuri, 1982); and rheumatoid factor by the passage of plasma through plates with chemically attached aggregated IgG (Lazarus *et al.* 1991). Enzymes are a further attractive source of ligands although few have found a clinical application so far. Immobilized bacterial heparinase has been used to de-heparinize blood after passing through extracorporeal circuits and before it is returned to the patient (Langer *et al.* 1982). Another possible approach to the removal of particular proteins, e.g. euglobulins, is the use of electrodialysis (Gurland *et al.* 1981). All methods of selective removal are promising and attractive but at present they are more expensive than conventional plasma exchange (Hamblin, 1983). For example, although SpA used as an immunosorbent on-line has been shown to be successful in the treatment of some patients with resistant autoimmune thrombocytopenic purpura (AITP) and with haemolytic uraemic syndrome, the absorptive capacity of the columns appears to be only 2% of the body's total IgG pool. Efficiency of removal is greater for immune complexes. Up to 30% of patients treated have adverse effects consisting of nausea, vomiting, fever, rash and hypotension (Verrier Jones, 1990).

Removal of leucocytes or platelets as a therapeutic procedure

In chronic granulocytic leukaemia, leucapheresis, performed two or three times weekly using a suitable sedimenting agent, can abolish symptoms of leucostasis and occlusion of the microcirculation especially in the nervous and respiratory systems, reduce the size of the liver and spleen, and restore the peripheral blood leucocyte count to normal. The reduction in leucocytes will decrease the risk of hyperuricaemia due to chemo-therapy. It is not always necessary to use sedimenting agents for these patients. Although patients can be treated by leucapheresis alone on a long-term basis, there is no evidence that the avoidance of radiotherapy or of cytotoxic drugs prolongs the duration of the chronic phase of the disease.

Long-term leucapheresis does not delay the onset of the blast crisis (Hester *et al.* 1982). It may, however, be useful in the short term for rapid reduction of initial very high leucocyte counts or for managing patients who are pregnant at the time of diagnosis (Goldman *et al.* 1975; Lowenthal, 1977a), who are allergic to chemotherapy or who have drug-resistant leukaemia (Radovic *et al.* 1991).

In promyelocytic leukaemia, leucapheresis will help to avoid DIC before chemotherapy is effective.

In acute myelocytic leukaemia, it has been claimed that cytapheresis, by reducing the initial leukaemic mass before chemotherapy, will improve the chance of remission and survival (Cuttner *et al.* 1983).

In chronic lymphocytic leukaemia (CLL), continuous-flow leucapheresis may be very effective in reducing the size of the spleen and lymph nodes. Its principal use in this condition may be in patients with high lymphocyte counts whose disease appears to be refractory to corticosteroids, alkylating agents and radiotherapy. For example, patients with prolymphocytic leukaemia initially respond favourably to leucapheresis. In Sézary syndrome, repeated leucapheresis may effectively remove the abnormal lymphocytes from the skin, relieving the intensively pruritic erythroderma (Marcus and Adams, 1983). Thirty-one patients with CLL and marked lymphocytosis were treated with intensive leucapheresis as an emergency procedure. There was an average fall in white cell count of 78.5%, followed by regression of splenomegaly and lymphadenopathy and relief of symptoms and signs induced by lymphocytosis (Radovic *et al.* 1991).

In hairy cell leukaemia transient improvement of the skin lesions and reduction of lymphadenopathy and splenomegaly have been obtained in refractory patients (Worsley *et al.* 1982).

In active severe rheumatoid arthritis, lymphapheresis carried out two to three times a week for 6 weeks produced substantial rapid improvement in four subjects. During each procedure the number of lymphocytes removed was equivalent to the number in 8–14 litres blood. In all, more than 10^{11} lymphocytes were removed. Lymphocytopenia gradually developed and persisted for at least 1 month after the last lymphapheresis (Karsh *et al.* 1979). In patients with rheumatoid arthritis subjected to three lymphaphereses a week for 5–6 weeks, there was a profound lymphocytopenia which in some cases lasted for 1 year (Fratantoni and French, 1980). Similar results were obtained by Wright *et al.* (1981) who found persistent lymphocytopenia lasting for more than 1 year in five of eight patients treated with 2–3-weekly CFC lymphaphereses for 5–7 weeks. The authors also reported a fall in serum IgM which was consistent with the lymphocytopenia. The number of lymphocytes removed during lymphocytapheresis is markedly influenced by the model of cell separator used. In one study, the IBM 2997 gave significantly higher lymphocyte yields than the Fenwal CS-3000 or the Haemonetics 30 cell separators (Blanchette *et al.* 1985a).

Severe thrombocytosis. In a patient with polycythaemia vera whose platelet count varied between 3410 and 4500 × 10^9/l following splenectomy and who was suffering from gastrointestinal bleeding, thrombapheresis using the Haemonetics machine reduced the platelet count by about one-third. After three thrombaphereses in 6 d the count fell to 1800 × 10^9/l and the rate of bleeding decreased notably (Greenberg and Watson-Williams, 1975).

Severe thrombocytosis can also be present in chronic granulocytic leukaemia and in essential thrombocythaemia. Before conventional therapy is effective in reducing the platelet count, thrombapheresis daily or on alternate days may prove useful in helping to control haemorrhagic or thrombotic complications or in preventing bleeding in patients needing surgery (Pineda *et al*. 1977; Taft, 1981).

Plasmapheresis and leucapheresis in cancer immunotherapy
The removal of large volumes of autologous plasma followed by its treatment *in vitro* to remove suppressor factors and, or, to generate activators of the immune system, with subsequent return of the plasma to the donor has been used in the treatment of cancer in experimental animals and in humans (Ray, 1982).

Autologous lymphokine (IL-2)-activated killer cells (LAK) cells and activated mono-cytes have been used in cancer therapy (Osband *et al*. 1990; Hamblin; 1991).

Collection of stem cells
Pluripotent colony forming units (CFU-MIX) can be harvested from peripheral blood using cell separators and have been used to reconstitute bone marrow. Autologous stem cells are collected, as part of the mononuclear cell fraction from peripheral blood, during either (1) the period of marrow recovery from chemotherapy, or (2) a hae-matopoietic steady state, and frozen. In subsequent episodes of pancytopenia following further chemotherapy, the stored stem cells, obtained from several collections, are transfused (for references see McCarthy and Goldman, 1984; Lasky, 1986). More recently, three groups have reported the successful restoration of haematopoietic function after the transfusion of cryopreserved stem cells collected from peripheral blood by CFC using the Fenwal CS-3000 or Spectra COBE. The procedure is particu-larly useful in patients with metastatic tumours involving the bone marrow or with a hypocellular bone marrow after high dose chemotherapy resulting in bone marrow ablation (Kessinger *et al*. 1988; Williams *et al*. 1990; Sniecinski, 1991). In view of the requirement to process large volumes of blood (8–10 litres) per collection during several (6–20) procedures, long-term venous access through a catheter is required. Mononuclear cell yields of 5^{10}–10^{10} can be obtained depending on the donor's initial lymphocyte count and the total volume of blood processed. A mononuclear cell dose of 7×10^8/kg seems to ensure complete haematopoietic reconstitution. An increase in the number of stem cells in the circulation, or 'mobilization', 100-fold above baseline levels is achieved after the administration of marrow toxic drugs and, or by infusing growth factors such as recombinant human granulocyte macrophage colony stimulating factor (rhGM-CSF) and appropriate timing of collection by apheresis. In addition, the possibility of immunophenotyping immature haemopoietic cells bearing the CD34 and CD33 differentiation antigens offers a rapid method of identifying and quantitating pluripotent stem cells, in view of the good correlation between total CD34- and CD33-positive cells and committed progenitor CFU-GM (see Kessinger and Armitage, 1991; Siena *et al*. 1991; Sniecinski, 1991). Immediately after collection, the mononuclear cells, with or without Percoll or Ficoll-hypaque sedimentation, are suspended in autologous plasma, mixed with dimethyl sulphoxide (DMSO) and stored frozen in liquid nitrogen. When required, i.e. 48–72 h after high dose chemotherapy, the mononuclear cells are thawed rapidly and transfused to the patient. Granulocyte recovery seems to occur more rapidly and regularly than platelet recovery (Williams *et al*. 1990) although the period of thrombocytopenia was shortened significantly when stem cells collected after mobilization with growth factors were used (Sniecinski, 1991).

Gene therapy
Treatment of severe combined immunodeficiency caused by adenosine deaminase deficiency (ADA) by the insertion of a normal *ADA* gene into autologous cultured T cells has been successful, with complete immunologic reconstitution after therapy (Blaese and Culver, 1991). Stem cells, when collected in sufficient quantity, will be the ideal targets for gene insertion.

ANTICOAGULANTS

Transfusions carried out in the nineteenth century were hampered by the occurrence of clotting in the transfusion apparatus (which was usually some kind of syringe). It was therefore a great advance when Carrel (1902) developed a technique, in animals, for joining arteries to veins; a few years later, he demonstrated in a dramatic case that this method could be used for saving lives in humans.

The patient was a newborn infant who had developed signs of haemorrhagic disease of the newborn within hours of birth. By the fifth day of life the infant was bleeding from the nose and the gut, and was near to death. Transfusion of so small a recipient had not been attempted before, but it occurred to the father, who was a Professor of Surgery at Columbia University, that Dr Alexis Carrel, a Research Fellow at the Rockefeller Institute, who was carrying out experiments involving the anastomosis of blood vessels in dogs and cats, might have the necessary skill. Carrel anastomosed the father's left radial artery to the infant's right popliteal vein and within a very short time the baby's colour changed from 'white to pink and finally to red all over'. The infant stopped bleeding immediately and had no further trouble (Lambert, 1908; Clarke, 1949; Walker, 1973).

Carrel's technique was too difficult for most surgeons to apply but Crile made it much easier by using a ring over which the intima could be cuffed, and in 1907 he reported briefly that he had used the method in 32 clinical cases. In a book published shortly afterwards he reported many more successes (Crile, 1909). Direct artery to vein transfusions were still in use during the First World War (Keynes, 1949), although the introduction of citrate made them increasingly rare thereafter.

Citrate is by far the most widely used anticoagulant in transfusion. Among its many advantages are the facts that it prevents coagulation over a long period in stored blood and that it is toxic only when given in very large amounts over short periods (see Chapter 15). By contrast, heparin, the least toxic anticoagulant, is progressively inactivated during storage after addition to blood.

Heparin
Heparin prevents coagulation by inactivating the proteolytic activity of thrombin after complexing with AT III and thrombin (Barrowcliffe *et al.* 1978). By increasing the activity of AT III, which is a serine-protease inhibitor, heparin also inactivates Factors Xa, IXa, XIa XIIa and plasmin (Wessler and Gitel 1979).

Although 1000 iu is approximately equal to 10 mg, iu and mg are not strictly interchangeable because commercial preparations of heparin vary in composition.

The dose of heparin required for anticoagulation is 0.5–2.0 iu/ml, e.g. approximately 500 units for 500 ml blood. However heparinized blood is rarely used at present and heparin is not recommended for routine blood collection because it has no preservative properties and its anticoagulant properties are neutralized by normal plasma. Heparinized blood should be transfused within 24 h of collection. Heparin is used in some apheresis systems.

The low toxicity of heparin is indicated by the fact that a subject may be 'heparinized', i.e. given a sufficient dose of heparin to render his or her blood temporarily incoagulable, with very little risk. Heparinization is a routine practice in many open-heart surgery units but heparin is now infrequently added to the blood, as extracorporeal pumps are usually primed with crystalloids and not with blood. It is not uncommon to attribute bleeding of patients on bypass to DIC when, in fact, it is often due to over-heparinization of the patient (Umlas, 1979).

Circulating heparin can be neutralized by injecting protamine sulphate; the usual dose is 1 mg to neutralize 1 mg heparin; e.g. to neutralize 5000 units heparin (50 mg), 5 ml of a 1% solution of protamine sulphate would be needed. The rapid injection of protamine produces transient hypotension but this may be avoided by taking not less than 5 min over the injection.

Heparin is not a suitable anticoagulant for plasma fractionation since it reduces the yield of Factor VIII by allowing the formation of fibrinogen in stored plasma (J. K. Smith, personal communication). However, small-pool, high-yield cryoprecipitate which can be freeze-dried and heat-treated in blood transfusion centres has been successfully produced after double cold precipitation of heparinized plasma (Smit Sibinga, 1989).

Citrate

Sodium citrate was used as an anticoagulant for blood transfusion in animals (e.g. Todd and White, 1911) before it was used in humans. The safety of citrate in humans was described by Hustin (1914), who probably gave the first transfusion of citrated blood to a human. Very soon afterwards papers describing the use of citrate were published by Agote (1915), Lewisohn (1915) and Weil (1915). According to Rosenfield (1974), Agote was responsible for a newspaper release in the *New York Herald* in November 1914 which stimulated both Lewisohn and Weil to publish their experiences. Lewisohn had been working on citrate toxicity since about 1911 and had concluded that a final concentration of 0.2% was sufficient to prevent clotting and that in this concentration as much as 2.5 litres could be given with safety in a brief period. Weil (1915) had not made a special study of dosage but he had made the important observation that animals which had been practically exsanguinated could be rapidly restored by the transfusion of citrated blood which had been kept in an icebox for several days.

In commenting on this early work, Ottenberg (1937) pointed out that the technique of Hustin was inappropriate, that the dose chosen by Weil was so large that for an ordinary-sized transfusion it might have been fatal, and that it was Lewisohn who worked out the upper and lower limits of the dosage so carefully and devised so simple a technique that it hardly needed to be changed during the following 20 years and that, as a result, he has generally been given most of the credit.

Citrate acts as an anticoagulant by chelating calcium but the amount required is very much more than would be needed if one mole of citrate firmly chelated one atom of ionized calcium. For example, if 2 g disodium citrate in 120 ml water are added to 420 ml blood, the concentration of citrate in the final citrate–plasma mixture will be approximately 0.57% or 0.022 mol/l, and the final calcium concentration will be 0.0025 mol/l. Although the molar ratio of citrate to calcium is thus approximately 10 : 1, with glass containers it is necessary to mix the blood and citrate thoroughly if clot formation is to be completely avoided. With plastic containers lower concentrations of citrate are satisfactory.

Subjects with unimpaired liver function will tolerate the transfusion of one unit of CPD or CPDA-1 blood in 5 min and it is therefore unnecessary to add calcium (and heparin) to CPD blood routinely for patients having massive transfusions. In special circumstances, 1500 units heparin may be added to each unit, followed by 500 mg calcium chloride.

At present, citrate anticoagulants, namely CPD and CPDA-1, are the anticoagulants of choice for whole blood collection (see Chapter 9). In donor apheresis procedures, various anticoagulants are used at different ratios of citrate solution to blood. For the collection of PPP and PRP with the PCS or Auto-C machines, the anticoagulants of choice in the UK are CPD-50 at a ratio of 1:16 or ACD-A at 1:12–1:16. For the simultaneous collection of platelet concentrates and PPP, the following are used in the UK: ACD-A at 1:8–1:12, ACD-B at 1:8, and acid CPD at 1:12 (A. Robinson, personal communication, 1991). The composition of acid CPD-50 is: sodium citrate, 22.0 g; citric acid monohydrate, 12.0 g; dextrose monohydrate, 50.0 g; sodium acid phosphate, 33.76 g; water for injection to 1000 ml. The composition of CPD-50 is as follows: trisodium citrate dihydrate, 39.5 g; citric acid monohydrate, 4.9 g; sodium acid phosphate, 3.76 g; dextrose monohydrate, 50.0 g; water for injection to 1000 ml. The composition of ACD-A, ACD-B, CPD and CPDA-1 are given in Appendix 8.

In selecting the optimum concentration of citrate to use when PRP is collected by apheresis, two requirements must be balanced. A lower than usual citrate concentration minimizes irreversible platelet aggregation, enhancing the efficacy of the platelets in the concentrate. On the other hand, when the PPP is to be used for the production of clotting factor concentrates, too low a citrate concentration (as when ACD-B is used) leads to incipient clotting and generation of thrombin with the consequent activation of Factor IX and potential thrombogenicity *in vivo*, as well as to decreased yields of Factor VIII. Consequently ACD-A, CPD-50 and 'acid CPD' are the anticoagulants of choice for the collection of PRP by apheresis (Duguid *et al.* 1989). For plasma exchange many people still use ACD and some heparinize the donor and add ACD to the blood in the extracorporeal circuit. This latter combination seems to reduce the side-effects of both heparin and citrate.

EDTA (edetic acid)

The sodium salts of ethylene diamine tetra-acetic acid (EDTA) are powerful chelating agents and prevent coagulation by binding calcium. The binding of EDTA with calcium is more powerful than that of citrate with calcium. In fact, the amount of EDTA required to prevent clotting is only slightly greater than the amount required if one assumes that 1 mol EDTA binds 1 mol calcium. EDTA is no longer used in blood transfusion as it has no advantage over citrate and damages platelets.

CHAPTER 2

TRANSFUSION IN OLIGAEMIA

TABLES

History

It was realized in the nineteenth century that the most dramatic effects that could be achieved with blood transfusion would be in the treatment of acute blood loss. Dr J. Blundell, who was an obstetrician on the staff of the United Hospitals of St Thomas and Guy, is generally given credit for having been the first to perform a human to human blood transfusion. Before he gave his first transfusion to a human he had established two very important points: the first was that a dog which had been bled could be revived by a transfusion of dog's blood, and the second was that a transfusion to a dog of even a small amount (114 ml) of the blood of another species (human) could be fatal (Blundell, 1824).

Convinced that only human blood was suitable for transfusion to humans, Blundell began very cautiously experimenting in humans not daring to attempt transfusion until the patient was beyond hope (Blundell, 1818; 1824). Finally, he recorded a successful case in which a patient who had had a postpartum haemorrhage was transfused by means of a special syringe with some 8 oz (227 ml) of blood. The patient reported that 'she felt as if *life* were infused into her body' (Blundell, 1829).

It seems that Dr Blundell may not, in fact, have been the first physician to carry out a transfusion from one human to another. Schmidt (1968) recounts that Dr Philip Syng Physic almost certainly carried out such a transfusion in Philadelphia in 1795. Few details are known about the operation and no formal publication was made—there was simply a reference in a footnote. Dr Blundell seems to deserve the main credit for initiating human to human transfusions since he carried out careful preliminary experimental studies and published full details of his work.

Blood transfusions—though not from human donors—were first carried out in the seventeenth century. The bold concepts which lay behind this early work and the great skill with which it was carried out still seem astonishing.

Notes on the early history of transfusion

Intravenous injection. It is generally accepted that it was the work of William Harvey on the circulation of the blood which provided the essential climate for the trial of blood transfusion. Christopher Wren, who, at the age of 16, assisted in dissections by Charles Scarburgh, a pupil of Harvey's, studied at Oxford University for the following 7 years. In his last year there, in 1656, he had as friends Wilkins, who was the head of his college (Wadham), and Robert Boyle, later to become famous for his work in physics. These three discussed the possibility of administering poisons directly into the blood stream. After Boyle had procured a dog, Wren injected morphia suspended in sack (sherry) i.v. and the dog very rapidly became lethargic. Although Wren subsequently tried the effect of several other drugs i.v., his work in this field was interrupted by his move to Gresham College, London, as Professor of Astronomy in 1657. Wren was one of the small group of men who founded the Royal Society in 1660.

When Sprat (1667) wrote the early history of the Royal Society he decided that it would be invidious to describe the part played by each one of the founder members, but when he came to Wren he made an exception. After many references to the tremendous part which Wren had played in many other discoveries of the time, he went on to say of him:

> He was the first author of the Noble Anatomical experiment of injecting liquors into the veins of animals, an experiment now vulgarly known but long since exhibited by the meetings at Oxford. By this operation divers creatures were immediately purged, vomited, intoxicated, killed or revived. Hence arose many new experiments and chiefly that of transfusing blood which the Society has prosecuted in sundry instances that will probably end in extraordinary success.

The first transfusion was carried out between dogs and is described in Chapter 1.

The first transfusion to a human. The first transfusion from an animal to a human was performed by Professor J. Denis with the help of a surgeon, Mr C. Emmerez, in France in June 1667 (see Chapter 10), and the first transfusion of this kind was performed in England in November of the same year by Lower and King, the recipient being an impoverished Bachelor of Divinity by the name of Arthur Coga (*Phil. Trans.*, 1667, p. 557).

THE RESPONSE TO BLOOD LOSS

Normally, the picture of acute haemorrhage in humans is confused by other signs connected with the cause of the haemorrhage; for example, by pain. Moreover, it is seldom possible to form any precise estimate of the amount of blood that has been lost. However, studies of the effect of sudden loss of blood, produced by the venesection of volunteers, have provided valuable information about the effects produced by haemorrhage alone.

Circulatory effects of blood loss

In adults, the loss of 430 ml blood in 4 min usually produces only trivial effects on the circulation. As a rule there is no change in blood pressure or pulse rate, although the venous pressure may fall slightly and take more than 30 min to regain its initial level (Loutit *et al.* 1942).

In normal subjects the rapid withdrawal of about 1 litre blood often produces no fall in blood pressure as long as the subject remains supine, but if the subject sits up blood pressure may fall and consciousness may be lost (Ebert *et al.* 1941; Wallace and Sharpey-Schafer, 1941). The loss of 1500–2000 ml leads to a fall in right atrial pressure and a diminished cardiac output; the subject becomes cold and clammy and may display air hunger (Howarth and Sharpey-Schafer, 1947).

Changes in central venous pressure (i.e. right atrial pressure) reflect changes in blood volume; a fall in central venous pressure leads to a fall in cardiac output which in turn leads to a fall in arterial pressure. This produces adrenergic stimulation, an increase in the force and rate of the heart, constriction of the veins and venules, and regional increases in peripheral resistance, chiefly in the skin, muscles, kidney and gut. The increase in resistance is mainly pre-capillary so that capillary pressure is reduced and plasma volume is restored at the expense of tissue fluid. If the inadequate peripheral flow continues, pre-capillary resistance ceases to respond to adrenergic stimulation while the veins still respond so that there is still further loss of fluid from the circulation (Mellander and Lewis, 1963).

Spontaneous restoration of blood volume

In healthy normal males, after the sudden loss of about 1 litre blood, restoration of blood volume may take more than 3 d (Adamson and Hillman, 1968). The rate at which packed cell volume (PCV) falls seems to depend to some extent on the activity of the subject. In the experiments just referred to, subjects were encouraged to walk immediately after venesection and PCV had not fallen significantly at 10 h in four of six subjects; the average plasma volume replacement at about 3 d was only 76%. On the other hand, in a series in which subjects rested in bed for 24 h after venesection, blood volume was usually restored at 36 h (Ebert *et al.* 1941). Even after the loss of as little as 0.5 litre only about half of the decrease in blood volume has been replaced at the end of 24 h (Pruitt *et al.* 1965). In summary, for at least 48 h after haemorrhage, the PCV alone is misleading as an index of the extent of acute blood loss in normal people.

Following acute haemorrhage, plasma protein concentration falls only to a trivial extent due to the fact that protein is transferred to the plasma from the extravascular space (Adamson and Hillman, 1968).

Oligaemic shock

When the amount of blood lost rapidly is equivalent to 30% of the blood volume, a subject may pass into oligaemic shock. The term 'shock' may be defined as 'loss of effective circulating blood volume which produces abnormal micro-circulatory perfusion and attendant cellular metabolic derangements' (Schumer and Nyhus, 1974) or more simply as 'inadequate capillary perfusion' (Hardaway, 1974). Shock may be classified as hypovolaemic, cardiogenic, septic or anaphylactic.

Investigations carried out during the First World War showed that in 'wound shock' blood volume was reduced and that the severity of the clinical picture was roughly paralleled by the degree of reduction in blood volume (Keith, 1919; Robertson and Bock, 1919).

Assessment of the degree of haemorrhage

It is only rarely that the amount of blood lost is immediately obvious to the observer. Usually, the extent of bleeding has to be deduced from the nature of the injury which caused the haemorrhage, from the physical signs in the patient's cardiovascular system, from any evidence of impaired organ perfusion and from the patient's response to treatment of the oligaemia.

Estimates of blood loss

Assessment of haemorrhage around the site of injury. Swelling surrounding the area of the wound is due to loss of blood into the tissues and thus often indicates a gross reduction in circulating blood volume. In severe injuries without external blood loss there is a tendency to underestimate the amount of blood that has been lost into the tissues (Noble and Gregersen, 1946).

Patients with wounds of the extremities involving large muscles may require very large transfusions. Prentice *et al.* (1954) found that such patients frequently needed the transfusion of an amount of blood equal to their initial blood volume; they considered that the continued loss of blood into the tissues was important in bringing about the extensive loss of blood from the circulation. Clarke *et al.* (1955) found that a single injury to the thigh might be associated with a blood loss of 2.5 litres or even more.

Perforating wounds of the chest or abdomen are usually associated with considerable haemorrhage into the pleural or peritoneal cavities, and pelvic fractures often cause massive haemorrhage into retroperitoneal tissues.

In battle casualties where there is gross disruption of tissue, the size of the wound itself is fairly well correlated with the degree of blood loss. Thus, Grant and Reeve (1951) found that for each area of tissue damaged corresponding to the size of the patient's hand, a loss of 10% of the patient's blood volume should be assumed. Patients with extensive soft tissue injuries have a high death rate, often from pulmonary insufficiency; there is a good correlation between the general severity of the clinical picture and signs of disseminated intravascular coagulation (DIC) (String *et al.* 1971).

Oligaemia in 'accidental' haemorrhage. Tovey and Lennon (1962) estimated plasma volume in 29 cases of 'accidental' (placental) haemorrhage and concluded that when the blood pressure had fallen by 20 mm Hg or more and the pulse rate had risen to 100 or above, the chance was at least six to one that the patient had suffered a loss of 30% or more of blood volume.

Blood loss at operation. There is some evidence that even operations associated with very little apparent blood loss are accompanied by a decrease in circulating red cell volume. Davies and Fisher (1958) in a series of nine patients undergoing meniscectomy found that on average red cell volume decreased by 7% in the period between the day before operation and 3 d after operation. In the following week there was a further fall of 2%.

Measurement of blood volume changes after other operations have confirmed that the decrease is greater than expected from the amount of blood lost externally. For example, Wiklander (1956) found that the average total blood loss associated with partial gastrectomy was about 1400 ml; of this about 650 ml was lost at operation, a further 300 ml was lost from the circulation in the next 24 h, and a further 450 ml in the week after that. The loss determined by weighing swabs at operation was usually only about 70% of that determined from estimates of blood volume. This agrees well with the conclusion of Cáceres and Whittembury (1959) who found that the weighing of the sponges at operation underestimated blood loss by 25%, due partly to evaporation of fluid from the sponges before weighing and partly to bleeding into tissues which was not allowed for. The authors concluded that the relation between the true reduction in blood volume and the apparent reduction, as estimated from weighing swabs, was constant enough to enable satisfactory estimates to be made, i.e. apparent loss plus 25%.

Circulatory signs
The cardinal signs of oligaemia are tachycardia, peripheral vasoconstriction, hypotension and a reduced jugular venous pressure.

Peripheral vasoconstriction. In subjects who have lost large amounts of blood, the skin remains cold even after the subject has been lying for some time in reasonably warm surroundings. In subjects suffering from shock of diverse aetiology there is a close correlation between toe temperature and cardiac index. For example, if within 3 h of admission to the resuscitation ward the temperature of the big toe remains less than 2°C higher than that of the ambient temperature, prognosis is bad (Joly and Weil, 1969).

Hypotension does not occur in mild oligaemia, which is adequately compensated for by tachycardia and vasoconstriction. It is a reliable guide to the degree of hypovolaemia only if the patient's blood pressure before haemorrhage is known. A young man with a systolic pressure of 100 mm Hg may be perfectly well; in an elderly patient with arterial disease such a figure represents severe decompensation.

Central venous pressure. Empty peripheral veins and low jugular venous pressure are features of poor circulatory filling. The right atrial pressure (central venous pressure, CVP) may be measured directly by cannulating the vena cava through a peripheral vein. The normal range of values is wide and the zero level (that of the right atrium) difficult to estimate consistently. It is usually taken as the angle of Louis in a patient propped up at an angle of 45°, and as the mid-axillary line in one lying flat, so that the level has to be moved as the patient's position changes. A single measurement of the CVP is, therefore, almost useless in assessing the degree of haemorrhage. Changes in CVP in response to circulatory refilling are, however, a useful guide to the adequacy of therapy (Sykes, 1963).

The need to check the position of CVP lines radiologically was stressed by Johnston and Clark (1972); without such a check they found that only 64% were correctly positioned.

Left atrial pressure. The use of CVP measurements as a guide to cardiac performance or to circulatory filling rests on the assumption that the right and left ventricles function similarly. The right and left atrial pressures would thus be similar; at the very least, they could be expected to move in the same direction at the same time. In a number of circumstances, this underlying assumption may be false; there are many cardiac disorders which affect predominantly one side of the heart. In oligaemia, especially in the elderly, hypotension and tachycardia impair coronary perfusion, affecting mainly the performance of the left ventricle. Continued filling of the normally functioning right ventricle will thus overfill the left atrium and pulmonary oedema will result. There is a place, therefore, for measuring left atrial pressure itself. The least invasive method of doing so is to float a catheter through the superior vena cava, right atrium and right ventricle into the pulmonary artery for as great a distance as possible. The inflation of a balloon at the end of the catheter wedges it into a pulmonary capillary and the pressure is then recorded. Pulmonary capillary wedge pressure, or PCWP, is a good indication of left atrial pressure (Swan *et al.* 1970). It is certainly not necessary to measure the PCWP in every bleeding patient and its value is, in any case, questionable in patients who are being artificially ventilated with positive end-expiratory pressure (PEEP) (Lozman *et al.* 1974; see also Leading Article, 1980).

Further uses of pulmonary artery catheters. Catheterization of the pulmonary artery is an essential step towards measuring cardiac output; if the catheter is fitted with a thermistor, the method of thermodilution may be employed. Cardiac output computers, if primed with appropriate data, will derive other variables; for example, the systemic vascular resistance can be calculated if the cardiac output and blood pressure are known, and oxygen delivery if the arterial oxygen content is measured as well as cardiac output. Fibreoptic oximeters have been incorporated into pulmonary artery catheters and can provide a continuous estimate of mixed venous oxygen saturation, a useful guide to the adequacy of tissue oxygenation (Armstrong *et al.* 1978).

Organ damage secondary to oligaemia
The combination of hypotension and arterial vasoconstriction causes a reduction of blood flow in most organs. The blood supply to some vital organs, notably the brain and kidneys, is protected to some extent by local vasodilatation ('autoregulation'), but severe oligaemia invariably leads to underperfusion.

Impaired renal perfusion is associated with a low output of concentrated urine. Renal failure may ensue if oligaemia is not corrected. One of the aims of resuscitation is to restore the urine output to at least 0.5 ml/kg body-weight per min.

Cerebral and myocardial damage may also follow oligaemia, especially in elderly patients whose arteries are atheromatous (Weisel *et al.* 1978). Hepatic hypoperfusion associated with severe hypovolaemia may determine the onset of jaundice in patients transfused with non-viable red cells in stored blood (see p. 524). Splanchnic vasoconstriction may, if prolonged, cause ischaemic damage to the bowel mucosa, and toxic substances may be absorbed from the lumen. Hypovolaemia may then be complicated by bacteraemia and, or, endotoxaemia.

The adult respiratory distress syndrome (ARDS) (Petty and Ashbaugh, 1971). ARDS is a diffuse pulmonary parenchymal injury which may be acute or chronic, moderate or severe. Microvascular endothelial damage with increased capillary permeability and oedema are constantly found, and the clinical features are of progressive hypoxaemia, with widespread radiological shadowing and reduced compliance (Murray *et al.* 1988). (Some would also insist that the left atrial pressure must be established as being within normal limits, to exclude pulmonary oedema due to left ventricular failure.)

It has been proposed that the diagnosis of ARDS in any patient should be accompanied by some reference to its underlying cause and that the possible underlying causes fall into two categories. In the first are specific agents such as toxic gases, fat emboli, gastric contents and infectious micro-organisms which damage the lungs directly, the resultant injury being confined to the lungs. The second category comprises generalized disorders, involving many organs as well as the lungs, with a high mortality rate due to multiple organ failure. For example, systemic sepsis, acute pancreatitis and multiple injuries are frequent precursors of ARDS, DIC and hepatic and renal dysfunction (Murray *et al.* 1988).

The mechanism by which these diverse causes produce the lesions of ARDS remains obscure, and may not always be the same. Indeed, since the definition of ARDS now proposed (Murray *et al.* 1988) embraces almost every inflammatory disorder which may affect the lungs, it would be amazing if the pathophysiology were identical in every case. Complement activation, with raised levels of C5a in the plasma causes the aggregation of granulocytes in pulmonary capillaries in patients who develop ARDS (Hammerschmidt *et al.* 1980). It has been argued that, after aggregating, the activated neutrophils generate and release free radicals of oxygen which damage the lung capillaries and cause the leakage of fluid into the lung (Flick *et al.* 1981). However, there have been several studies which demonstrate that ARDS may develop in patients with neutropenia (see Rinaldo and Rogers, 1986). More recently, it has been shown that bacterial endotoxin may damage the pulmonary endothelium (Meyrick *et al.* 1986); endotoxin has been found in the plasma of patients at risk of ARDS who developed the syndrome (Parsons *et al.* 1989). It is postulated that endotoxin stimulates macrophages to release peptide cytokines which are responsible for the capillary leak in ARDS, and for the multiple organ failure associated with systemic sepsis (see Rinaldo and Christman, 1990).

Repeated large transfusions have been associated with the development of ARDS, suggesting the possibility that blood loss is an important factor, but in experimental animals oligaemia alone does not seem to produce the syndrome (Tobey *et al.* 1974). It may be that it is the translocation of bacteria and endotoxin from the bowel into the circulation, during an episode of hypovolaemia needing transfusion, which is responsible for the relationship between transfusion and ARDS (Parsons *et al.* 1989).

A very severe type of reaction, known as transfusion-related acute lung injury (TRALI), due to granulocyte antibodies and characterized by fever, dyspnoea, hypotension and radiographic changes in the lungs, is described in Chapter 15.

Evidence that micro-aggregates infused with stored blood cause pulmonary damage is inconclusive (see Chapter 15).

ARDS carries a high mortality rate and treatment consists only of supportive measures, namely, fluid restriction to prevent exacerbation of the oedema, oxygen therapy with artificial ventilation if necessary and antibiotics to control infection. As protein leaks through the damaged pulmonary capillaries in ARDS (Anderson *et al.* 1979; Fein *et al.* 1979), the use of albumin infusions in its management seems contraindicated. The early administration of corticosteroids has been shown to prevent the increase in pulmonary capillary permeability in experimental animals (Pingleton *et al.* 1982; Brigham *et al.* 1981). In patients with sepsis, however, the use of corticosteroids has been shown to be of no value in the prevention of ARDS (Weigelt *et al.* 1985; Luce *et al.* 1988; see also Editorial, 1986).

A human monoclonal IgM antibody against endotoxin has been tested, in a randomized double-blind placebo-controlled trial, in patients with sepsis suspected of having Gram-negative infection (Ziegler *et al.* 1991). A significant reduction in the mortality rate was found in patients with positive blood cultures who were treated with the antibody.

RESTORATION OF BLOOD VOLUME BY
TRANSFUSIONS OR INFUSIONS

Physiological considerations in fluid replacement

The aim of i.v. fluid replacement in the oligaemic patient is to provide an adequate supply of oxygen to the tissues. Oxygen delivery is given by the equations (Nunn and Freeman, 1964a):

$$\text{oxygen delivery (ml/min)} = \text{cardiac output (ml/min)} \times \text{arterial } O_2 \text{ content}$$

and

$$\text{arterial } O_2 \text{ content (ml/dl)} = \text{Hb concentration (g/dl)} \times \text{ml } O_2 \text{ carried/g Hb}$$

If normal values are substituted in the equations above, a healthy adult male of 70 kg body-weight will have an oxygen delivery of about 1000 ml/min; his basal oxygen consumption at rest, which is given by the equation:

$$\text{oxygen consumption} = \text{cardiac output} \times \text{arteriovenous oxygen content difference}$$

will be about 250 ml/min. It seems reasonable to conclude that, provided the cardiac output and arterial oxygen saturation are maintained within the normal range, a degree of anaemia should be tolerated.

There is, furthermore, evidence that oxygen delivery is enhanced by a moderate degree of acute normovolaemic anaemia. In dogs rendered acutely anaemic by the withdrawal of blood, and kept normovolaemic by the simultaneous infusion of dextran, oxygen delivery was at its peak at an Hb level of 100 g/l, and fell below the pre-phlebotomy level at an Hb level of about 85 g/l. The improvement in oxygen delivery was attributed to a fall in blood viscosity and a doubling of the cardiac output (Messmer et al. 1972). Subsequent human studies have confirmed these findings (see Messmer, 1987). At lower Hb levels, when oxygen is reduced, demand for oxygen is met by increased extraction of oxygen from the blood perfusing them. The mixed venous oxygen content then falls (see Wilkerson et al. 1987). In chronic normovolaemic anaemia, the low arterial oxygen content is further compensated by a shift of the oxygen dissociation curve to the right (see Chapter 9).

Some organs normally extract more oxygen from the blood which perfuses them than others. Thus, although the whole body arteriovenous oxygen content difference is normally 5 ml/dl at rest, corresponding to an extraction ration of 25%, the heart normally extracts 55% of the oxygen from the blood it receives and the brain 35–40%. Substantial increases in coronary and cerebral blood flow will therefore be required to maintain oxygen delivery to the heart and brain in the presence of normovolaemic anaemia. In normovolaemic humans, cerebral blood flow rises when the PCV is reduced to 0.28 (Paulson et al. 1973). The reduction in blood viscosity which results from haemodilution of this order appears to be beneficial in patients with focal cerebral ischaemia (Kee and Wood, 1984). Animal studies suggest that coronary blood flow increases out of proportion to the rise in cardiac output in normovolaemic anaemia (von Restorff et al. 1975; Biro, 1982), but that the combination of severe acute anaemia with coronary stenosis results in myocardial ischaemia (Most et al. 1986; Biro et al. 1987).

The implications for the restoration of blood volume in oligaemic patients are, first, that it is crucial to maintain the cardiac output by prompt restoration of the circulating blood volume; second, that a moderate degree of anaemia should be well tolerated at least in previously healthy subjects; and third, that in patients whose coronary or cerebral arteries are diseased, or whose cardiac reserves are already depleted, any diminution in the oxygen delivery may be damaging.

Choice of intravenous fluid in oligaemia; use of whole blood

On first thoughts, it might seem obvious that no other fluid could be better than whole blood in the treatment of haemorrhage, even when it is remembered that blood which has been stored in the cold is devoid of functioning platelets and may, after 2 weeks' storage, have 2,3 DPG-depleted red cells which are temporarily less effective than fresher red cells in giving up oxygen to the tissues.

In fact, several additional factors militate against the routine use of whole blood. Blood is a scarce resource and should not be used when an adequate substitute is available. Blood transfusion involves many hazards, of which the transmission of human immunodeficiency virus (HIV) is but the latest. Because, as argued above, a degree of anaemia can be tolerated by most patients, moderate haemorrhage can frequently be dealt with adequately by the infusion of a plasma substitute or of Ringer's lactate solution. Plasma substitutes are considered later in this chapter. If a haemorrhage is large enough to require the transfusion of red cells, the use of red cell concentrates with crystalloid or artificial colloid solutions may be more appropriate than the transfusion of whole blood; the infusion of albumin with red cells is clearly extravagant.

The argument for using only that fraction of whole blood which is needed by the patient is clearly that other fractions of the blood can be used for other patients. When red cell concentrates are used by clinicians instead of whole blood, platelets and plasma become available to the transfusion services for the preparation of platelet concentrates and plasma derivatives, notably albumin and Factor VIII. The need for plasma fractionation is discussed below.

Whole blood may still be appropriate in the treatment of massive haemorrhage. Many clinicians treating heavily bleeding patients would agree with Schmidt (1978) that, in hospital practice, there is a real need for whole blood. On the other hand, Lundsgaard-Hansen et al. (1978), found it possible to issue 80% of units as packed cells by giving modified fluid gelatin at the same time when treating large haemorrhages.

Transfusion in Jehovah's witnesses. Jehovah's witnesses will not accept blood or blood products for themselves or their children. This refusal obviously poses medicolegal problems. In an unconscious adult in urgent need of a transfusion, most clinicians would feel bound to give the transfusion even though relatives opposed it. On the other hand, the clearly expressed wishes of a conscious patient must be respected. For children below the age of consent, the general opinion (at least in the UK) is that clinicians should seek a court order for doing what is needed for the child's welfare, irrespective of the wishes of the parents. A full discussion of the problems raised when transfusion is clinically indicated for Jehovah's witnesses, and evidence that the decisions of courts in different countries may well differ, can be found in a series of articles in *Transfusion Medicine Reviews* (1991) vol. 5, no. 4).

The need for plasma fractionation; the use of albumin

At present, there is a massive demand for three plasma fractions: albumin, Factor VIII and immunoglobulin. Of the need for the last two there is no doubt but the need for albumin is a more controversial matter. Albumin is an effective plasma substitute but it is easily the most expensive available and there are plenty of alternatives to choose from. In a prospective, randomized study of 475 patients admitted to an intensive care unit, albumin was found to offer no advantage over gelatin in terms of mortality within the unit, length of stay there, or incidence of pulmonary oedema or renal failure, although serum albumin levels were lower in the patients who received gelatin (Stockwell *et al.* 1992a,b).

Infusions of albumin are widely used in the treatment of burns, and albumin is in great demand for plasma exchange. Confusion about the amount of albumin that is needed is emphasized by the fact that its use varies widely in countries with highly developed health care systems. For example, the consumption of albumin (per million inhabitants) in Denmark and the USA is twice that in Canada and four times that in England and Wales (Myllylä, 1991).

Infusions of saline; the crystalloid vs. colloid controversy

Argument has raged as to whether saline or a colloid solution should be used in the initial management of haemorrhagic shock. The proponents of both views base their case on the Starling equation, which states that the flow of fluid outwards through the walls of the capillaries (J_v) is proportional to the hydrostatic pressure (*P*) gradient between the capillaries and the interstitial space and inversely proportional to the protein oncotic pressure (*π*) gradient, namely:

$$J_v = Kf(P_c - P_t) - \sigma(\pi_c - \pi_t)$$

where P_c is capillary hydrostatic pressure; P_t is interstitial fluid hydrostatic pressure; π_c is plasma protein oncotic pressure; π_t is interstitial fluid oncotic pressure; Kf is the filtration coefficient representing the permeability of the capillary membrane to fluids; and σ is the reflection coefficient representing the permeability of the capillary membrane to proteins.

The protein concentration of plasma is normally considerably higher than that of interstitial fluid, so it seems logical to suppose that infusions of albumin, or of other substances of equal or greater mol. wt., would, given normal capillary permeability, remain in the intravascular space for longer than would saline, which diffuses throughout the extracellular compartment. Smaller volumes of colloid than of crystalloid should be required to restore the circulating volume of the oligaemic patient, and oedema should be less likely to develop if colloids are employed.

Measurements in rabbits (see Table 2.2 on p. 69) have suggested that colloid solutions are more effective and persistent expanders of the plasma volume than isotonic saline. In a group of sheep, which had had about half their own blood volume removed, restoration of the left atrial pressure and cardiac output to baseline values with Ringer's lactate required the infusion of two and a half times the volume of the blood withdrawn, whereas a second similarly bled group needed only to have the shed blood returned to achieve the same result. The authors could find no evidence of pulmonary capillary damage after this degree of haemorrhage

(Demling *et al.* 1980). In a study of shocked elderly patients resuscitated with either hydroxyethyl starch or Ringer's lactate, together with packed cells, much smaller volumes were required and there was a lower incidence of pulmonary oedema in the group receiving colloid (Rackow *et al.* 1983). The case for colloids has been put forcefully by Twigley and Hillman (1985).

However, an opposing case has also been presented. In the first place, several estimates of the protein concentration of pulmonary interstitial fluid (see Staub, 1974) have suggested that it is higher than in interstitial fluid elsewhere in the body. In baboons subjected to haemorrhage, and treated with either albumin or Ringer's lactate plus their own shed blood, pulmonary oedema was more frequent when albumin was used, and albumin appeared to be extravasated into the pulmonary tissue (Holcroft and Trunkey, 1974).

Numerous clinical studies support these animal findings. For example, Virgilio *et al.* (1979) compared the results of infusing albumin and Ringer's lactate, both with packed red cells, in two groups of patients undergoing major vascular surgery. To achieve a pre-determined circulatory state and urine output, the patients who were given albumin required the infusion of smaller volumes than did those who were given crystalloid, but showed a higher incidence of pulmonary oedema. Moss *et al.* (1981) studied a series of young injured patients who were given washed red cells and Ringer's lactate, supplemented in half the cases with albumin. No patient developed pulmonary oedema and the total volume of Ringer's lactate required to correct hypovolaemia was not reduced by the addition of protein (see also Pearl *et al.* 1988).

In the face of such conflicting evidence, conclusions are difficult to draw. The human studies were conducted on widely differing groups of patients, often involved different measurements, and all had different end-points. In a few instances, they seem designed to reinforce the pre-conceived ideas of the workers concerned. The results of animal studies are also at variance, and, illuminating though such studies may be, they are not necessarily applicable to humans. It seems reasonable to conclude that, in previously fit young patients, it does not matter how restoration of the blood volume is accomplished, and therefore cost and convenience should dictate the choice of solution infused. In the elderly, or in patients with poor renal function, it may be wise to avoid massive infusions of saline.

Infusions of hypertonic saline
Infusions of small volumes (about 4 ml/kg body-weight) of hypertonic solutions (7.2–7.5% sodium chloride) over a short period (2 min) have been used in the initial resuscitation of both patients and experimental animals with hypovolaemic shock. Dramatic instantaneous improvements in cardiac output, arterial pressure, acid–base balance and urine flow, persisting for a few hours, have been observed. Hypertonic solutions produce their beneficial effects by expanding the circulating volume at the expense of the intracellular volume. Several studies have shown that the efficiency of hypertonic saline may be enhanced by the addition of dextran. Hypertonic saline solutions, with or without supplementary colloid, appear to have a place in the immediate management of an injured patient; an infusion may be started at the site of the accident before the patient is removed to hospital (see Messmer, 1988).

The rate of transfusion

It has already been emphasized that, in treating oligaemia of any kind, the primary aim is to maintain an adequate supply of oxygen to vital organs, and that, provided the cardiac output is maintained, some degree of anaemia can be tolerated. If haemorrhage is moderate or severe, it is much better to restore the circulating volume immediately with a rapid infusion of crystalloid or colloid than to delay resuscitation until blood has been crossmatched.

It may well be necessary to transfuse a unit of blood in a few minutes or less and rapid transfusion is safe if the patient is carefully monitored. Very fast rates of transfusion cannot be attained by simply allowing the blood to run in under gravity through a small cannula lying in a peripheral vein. Ways of increasing the rate of flow are discussed below.

Technique of rapid transfusion

The bore of the cannula is a very important factor in limiting the rate of flow. Krestin (1987) measured the flow rates generated through all the intravenous cannulae available in the UK using a test prescribed by the British Standards Institution (BSI, 1972). Distilled or deionized water was run under a pressure of 10 kPa (76 mm Hg) from a constant level tank at 22°C via 110 cm tubing with an internal bore of 4 mm. The mean flow obtained through 14 SWG cannulae of all brands was 286 ± 35 ml/min, whereas through 16, 18 and 20 SWG cannulae it was 162 ± 35, 91 ± 17 and 54 ± 14 ml/min, respectively.

The viscosity of the blood. Blood is more viscous than water, and under test conditions and at room temperature, the flow of blood with a PCV of 0.45 through cannulae is only 50–60% of the flow of water (Farman and Powell, 1969). The viscosity of blood varies with PCV and with temperature. Raising the Hb concentration of blood infused at constant pressure through needles of various bore sizes from 12.6 g/dl to 14.3 g/dl slowed the flow rate by about 10% (Chaplin and Chang, 1955). Warming blood with a PCV of 0.42 from 10°C to 36°C doubles the rate of flow (Knight, 1968).

Venous spasm. The giving of very cold blood may cause local discomfort and venespasm, which will slow transfusion. The transfusion of warm blood or plasma may also induce venous spasm due to vasoconstrictor substances in plasma (see Mollison, 1983, pp. 746–747). In patients with peripheral circulatory failure due to oligaemia, the veins are constricted, so that the rate of flow of transfusion may be slower than is required. Local warming of the arm helps to relieve venous spasm, as does transdermal nitroglycerine applied as a patch distal to the infusion site (Wright *et al.* 1985a).

Despite its potential disadvantages, the transfusion of 1–2 units of blood taken straight from the refrigerator seems to be quite safe; the transfusion of large amounts of very cold blood is undesirable (see Chapter 15).

Positive pressure. Quadrupling the pressure gradient from a litre bag of 0.9% saline down a giving set and cannula by enclosing the bag in a pressure infusor at 300 mm Hg only doubles the flow rate through the cannula. The rather small increment in flow rate may be due to the development of turbulence (Krestin, 1987). When rapid transfusion is required, it is more efficacious to insert a large cannula than to rely on pressurizing the infusate through a smaller one. Central venous cannulation with catheters of wide bore (for example, a pulmonary artery catheter introducer is of 8.5 French gauge) is generally performed in the management of severe haemorrhage. Pumps may be employed to transfuse or reinfuse blood at operations where blood loss is massive, e.g. liver transplantation.

How long to continue transfusion in oligaemia
Transfusion with appropriate fluids should be continued until haemorrhage has stopped and there is clinical evidence of relief of hypovolaemia; i.e. until the signs described on p. 52 have disappeared.

A rise in systolic BP to 100 mm Hg is not an indication for stopping the transfusion. A relatively small transfusion given to an injured person may produce considerable clinical improvement without fully restoring blood volume. Evans *et al.* (1944) made serial estimations of plasma volume in injured subjects with signs of peripheral failure. They noted that after a small transfusion, say 500 ml blood, BP might rise and, superficially, the patient appear much improved. Nevertheless, blood volume remained low for as long as 4 d. During the intervening period the patient might easily pass into shock again. It was estimated that the subjects should have received 1000–1500 ml blood initially. Grant and Reeve (1951) suggested that the patient's blood volume should be raised to at least 80% of normal before the operation is begun.

Failure to respond to transfusion
If an injured person whose BP is low fails to respond to transfusion, it is usually for one of two reasons. First, the patient may still be losing blood, so that transfusion is not succeeding in restoring blood volume to an adequate level. Second, there may be infection, so that the patient is septic as well as hypovolaemic. Operation should not be further delayed if the patient's condition does not improve after a transfusion of reasonable volume, since surgery may help to deal with both underlying causes.

Overloading of the circulation
Although, probably, the usual tendency is to underestimate blood loss and although there is evidence that it is difficult to overload the circulation of a patient who has lost blood through an injury, overloading, characterized by engorgement of the neck veins and moist sounds on auscultation, is occasionally observed.

Overloading is best prevented by close attention to the state of the patient's circulation. Frequent or continuous monitoring of the heart rate, the arterial and venous pressures, and core and peripheral temperatures usually give a reliable guide to the degree of filling.

Intra-arterial transfusion
It was once believed that, when blood is introduced into the arterial side of the circulation, there

may be a small but decisive advantage because the coronary circulation is filled directly. However, in dogs which had been made hypotensive by bleeding, the coronary flow and arterial pressure responded just as rapidly, and to the same extent, whether the blood was returned by the intravenous or intra-arterial route (Case *et al.* 1953).

Transfusion in burns

After thermal injury, there is a considerable and continual leakage of salt- and protein-containing fluid from the damaged tissue, with consequent falls in circulating volume and cardiac output. The volume of fluid lost depends on the size and thickness of the burn.

Arturson (1961) showed that, in dogs, extensive third degree (full thickness) burns were associated with an increase in capillary permeability in unburned areas. He emphasized, however, that the capillary membrane in such areas remained impermeable to protein molecules, although there was a leakage of dextran of mol. wt. 40 000.

It is generally agreed that the patient's circulating volume should be restored with i.v. fluids containing salt and water. Many schemes have been suggested for the way in which this restoration should be carried out, some of which are summarized in Table 2.1. All these schemes agree that the volume of fluid infused should be related to the surface area of the burn, and that most of this large volume must be given in the first 24 h after injury. It is usually recommended that half the total requirement of the first 24 h should be administered during the initial 8 h and the rest over the next 16 h. The patient's circulatory state, PCV and urine output must be carefully monitored.

In calculating the area of the burn, the following figures for the relative areas of the different parts of the body are helpful (Berkow, 1931):

Head	6%	6
Trunk and neck (back and front together)	38%	38
Upper limb: hand alone, 2.5%	9% × 2	18
Lower limb: thigh alone, 9.5%		
leg alone, 6.5%		
foot alone, 3.0%	19% × 2	38
		100

There is disagreement about the desirability of giving colloidal solutions such as albumin to burned patients. The formulations of Bull (1954) and Evans *et al.* (1952) recommended that half of the fluid infused should contain protein, or be given in the form of a plasma substitute. This plan is still followed in the UK (Settle, 1982). A mixture of a gelatin solution and Ringer's lactate was used successfully in the Falkland Islands campaign (Williams *et al.* 1983). In the USA, following the finding that the infusion of plasma into burned patients is not followed by a significant and persistent rise in blood volume until 24 h after injury (Baxter, 1974), there has been widespread acceptance of the case for giving no colloid until the protein leak has ceased (Pruitt, 1978); only saline solutions are used for fluid replacement during the first 24 h. A number of centres in the USA now follow this practice, accepting that larger volumes must be infused in resuscitation than if albumin is used as well as electrolytes (Goodwin *et al.* 1983).

Table 2.1 Some classical regimens* for intravenous fluid therapy in the first 24 h after thermal injury in adults

Regimen	Colloid	Crystalloid
Evans *et al.* (1952)	Plasma or plasma substitute initially; then whole blood to total 1 ml/1% area burned/kg	Normal saline 1 ml/1% area burned/kg Dextrose 5% 2 litres
Bull (1954)	Plasma or dextran 1 ml/1% area burned/kg	Half normal saline 3–4 litres
'Parkland' (Baxter and Shires, 1968)	None	Ringer's lactate 4 ml/1% area burned/kg
Monafo *et al.* (1973)	None	Hypertonic saline solutions (250–300 mmol sodium/litre) infused to produce urine output of 30–40 ml/h

* Present-day regimens are essentially minor variants of these original ones. For a recent review, see Demling (1990), who emphasized that no single regimen is suitable for all patients, or at all stages.

In order to keep the volume of fluid infused to a minimum, Monafo *et al.* (1973) suggested that hypertonic saline solutions might be infused. The extracellular fluid volume would then be maintained at the expense of some intracellular dehydration.

Red cells are destroyed in burned tissue (Shen *et al.* 1943). In patients with large burns, transfusions of red cells may be needed (Topley *et al.* 1962).

Massive transfusion
A transfusion is conventionally regarded as massive when a volume equivalent to the patient's normal blood volume is given within 24 h.

The clinical problems which arise in patients receiving massive transfusions are due first to the condition which caused the haemorrhage, and second to the effect of replacing normal whole blood with stored citrated blood, possibly supplemented by plasma substitutes. Although a detailed consideration of clinical conditions associated with haemorrhage is outside the scope of this book, it is relevant that some of these conditions produce effects which may be attributed to massive transfusion, e.g. DIC and pulmonary microembolism.

Some of the effects of replacing large volumes of the patient's blood with similar volumes of stored citrated blood are as follows:
1 There is a shift to the left in the oxygen dissociation curve due to the fact that stored red cells have a diminished 2,3-DPG content; see Chapter 9.
2 There may be toxic effects from citrate; there may also be changes in electrolytes and in plasma pH.
3 There may be a fall in the recipient's temperature which may reach dangerous levels if blood is transfused straight from the refrigerator.
4 Microaggregates may be transfused from stored blood into the recipient.
    (Points 2, 3 and 4 are discussed in Chapter 15.)
5 Dilutional thrombocytopenia occurs since platelets do not survive in stored blood. Moreover, the residual population of the patient's own platelets may be damaged.

There may be a diminution in clotting factors, particularly those that deteriorate rapidly in blood during storage, such as Factor V.

A haemorrhagic state following massive transfusion

In adults transfused with large amounts of stored blood, excessive bleeding is commonly observed. Abnormal bleeding associated with thrombocytopenia has been observed after transfusions of volumes of stored blood as small as 5 litres (Stefanini et al. 1954; Krevans and Jackson, 1955). In a later series of 27 patients with major trauma, massive gastrointestinal haemorrhage or ruptured aortic aneurysm, who received an average of 33 units blood, eight had a haemostatic abnormality within 48 h of admission, i.e. uncontrolled oozing at multiple sites. In three subjects there was evidence of DIC and in these and four further subjects platelet counts were $90 \times 10^9/l$ or less. In six of the seven subjects who were treated with platelet concentrates, bleeding was rapidly controlled (Counts et al. 1979). It was concluded that thrombocytopenia, most frequently due to the loss of large numbers of the patient's own platelets from the circulation with replacement by non-viable platelets in stored blood, was the most important factor in causing the haemostatic abnormality seen in massively transfused patients.

The view that the thrombocytopenia is simply dilutional has since been modified. In a prospective study, two groups of massively transfused patients were compared. The first group (17 patients) was prophylactically given 6 units platelets for every 12 units blood, while the second group received 2 units fresh frozen plasma (FFP) for every 12 units blood. There was no significant difference between the two groups, either in platelet counts or in the incidence of clinically abnormal bleeding (three cases in each group). The authors calculated that dilution could not account for the degree of thrombocytopenia they observed in all but one of the patients who developed a haemorrhagic tendency. They argued that, in such cases, platelet consumption due to the injuries necessitating transfusion is most likely to be responsible (Reed et al. 1986). In another study of 22 massively transfused injured patients, not one showed any clinical evidence of abnormal bleeding, although all showed thrombocytopenia, which was most marked (mean level $76 \times 10^9/l$) 24–48 h after the transfusion, and all had a prolonged bleeding time (Harrigan et. al. 1985). A Consensus Development Conference (NIH, 1987) concluded that, at platelet counts of $50 \times 10^9/l$ and above, any bleeding was unlikely to be due to thrombocytopenia. Massive transfusion is sometimes followed by platelet counts of this order, and such thrombocytopenia is more often due to DIC than to simple dilution. There is no place for the prophylactic administration of platelets, whose use should be restricted to patients with abnormal bleeding and a platelet count of less than $50 \times 10^9/l$.

Collins (1987) has argued for some years that prompt treatment of haemorrhage with adequate and appropriate transfusions will prevent the development of a haemorrhagic diathesis following massive transfusion. This conclusion is supported by a study of 36 patients which revealed no correlation between the degree of coagulopathy and the volume of blood transfused, but demonstrated that the longer that patients are allowed to remain hypotensive after severe haemorrhage, the more severe the ensuing coagulopathy will be (Harke and Rahman, 1980).

Finally, there is some evidence that hypothermia, a frequent concomitant of massive transfusion, may cause platelet dysfunction and contribute to a tendency to bleed abnormally. It has been demonstrated that such platelet dysfunction is reversible in baboons (Valeri *et al.* 1987). In a retrospective study of 45 injured patients who required massive transfusion, those who were hypothermic and acidotic developed abnormal bleeding despite adequate blood, plasma and platelet replacement (Ferrara *et al.* 1990).

Indications for fresh frozen plasma (FFP)

A definition of FFP and a discussion of the indications for giving FFP to normovolaemic patients can be found in Chapter 14. In the present chapter only the indications for giving FFP to oligaemic patients are discussed. A conference of the National Institutes of Health (NIH, 1985) concluded that there was no justification for the use of FFP as a volume expander or nutrition source, although it had been reported that 50% of FFP was given solely for such reasons (Silbert *et al.* 1981). The NIH conference also confirmed that, in treating abnormal bleeding after massive transfusion (see above), FFP should be used only after demonstrating an abnormality of blood coagulation.

It seems to be difficult to predict whether a deficiency of clotting factors will occur during a massive transfusion. Counts *et al.* (1979) in a prospective study of 27 massively transfused patients were unable to find any correlation between the levels of labile clotting factors and the number of units of whole blood transfused. Oberman (1985) thought that this lack of correlation might be due to the fact that the plasma of some units of whole blood contains small, but perhaps effective, amounts of labile clotting factors, as does the plasma infused with platelet concentrates, which many massively transfused patients receive.

It is, furthermore, uncertain whether the correction, with FFP, of a deficiency of clotting factors in patients who have been massively transfused will reverse a tendency to abnormal bleeding. For example, Bove (1978) concluded that, in the haemorrhagic complications of trauma, shock and massive blood replacement, multiple factors, particularly DIC, are operative and that simple dilution of plasma clotting factors is rarely sufficient to explain the bleeding. He pointed out that the transfusion of 15 or more units of blood is almost always associated with abnormal prolongation of both prothrombin time (PT) and the partial thromboplastin time (PTT), and that the transfusion of FFP returns the PT and the PTT to normal but does not alter the bleeding tendency (see also Miller *et al.* 1971). Mannucci *et al.* (1982), in a comparative study, found that the administration of 1 unit FFP for every 3 units whole blood or packed red cells was not associated with any reduction in the amount of blood transfused, nor with any improvement in the coagulation test results. In a controlled experiment in which dogs were resuscitated by massive transfusion after severe haemorrhage, it was demonstrated that the prophylactic administration of FFP made no difference to the results of coagulation tests (Martin *et al.* 1985). Exchange transfusion in infants with red cells suspended in albumin does not give rise to any bleeding problems (Kreuger and Blombäck, 1974).

TRANSFUSION IN ELECTIVE SURGERY

Pre-operative haemoglobin levels in the surgical patient

It was for long considered that a pre-operative Hb concentration of 100 g/l was the lowest value acceptable for safe elective surgery. If the three determinants of oxygen availability — cardiac output, arterial oxygen saturation and Hb concentration — are all reduced by one-third, oxygen availability will be only 300 ml/min (Nunn and Freeman, 1964a). The work of Messmer, which has already been referred to, lent a value of 100 g/l some theoretical support (see p. 55). There was no agreement as to what should be done when a patient presented for surgery with a Hb concentration below 100 g/l. Some clinicians, mindful that anaesthesia may be associated with a fall in cardiac output and arterial desaturation, and that surgery often causes haemorrhage, might insist on pre-operative transfusion to attain 100 g Hb/l. Others might be more flexible, accepting some patients with lower Hb concentrations, and referring others for investigation. Nunn and Freeman (1964b) pointed out that a great deal of surgery throughout the world is performed on patients with Hb concentrations of less than 80 g/l, and most of them survive.

In recent years, there has been increasing difficulty, in some areas, in collecting sufficient blood for transfusion and an increased awareness on the part of the medical profession and its patients that transfusion is hazardous. Opinion has swung away from pre-operative transfusion and towards a more conservative approach (Stehling, 1990). A Consensus Conference (1988) suggested acceptance, in certain circumstances at least, of Hb levels as low as 70 g/l. It was not proposed that a figure of 70 g/l should be universally applied; there is even less theoretical support for 70 g/l than there is for 100 g/l.

In practice, each case must be considered on its merits, and clinicians must satisfy themselves that they are bringing patients to surgery in the best possible condition that the circumstances permit, and are not accepting unnecessary risks because they will probably 'get away with it'. For example, an Hb concentration of 70 g/l would be perfectly acceptable as part of a normocytic normochromic picture in a patient with chronic renal failure. If a patient booked to have minor elective surgery unexpectedly turns out to have a pre-operative Hb level of 70 g/l, it is more important to discover the cause of his anaemia and treat it than it is to ligate his varicocoele. If an Hb concentration of 70 g/l is due to recent bleeding which surgery is expected to stop and the patient is known to have coronary artery disease, transfusion is indicated.

Haemodilution

The term normovolaemic haemodilution has been used to describe the deliberate production of a low Hb level immediately before surgery, by taking blood from the patient, with the objects of (1) improving the micro-circulatory flow due to a reduction in the viscosity of the blood, and (2) obtaining autologous blood and so reducing the amount of allogeneic blood required for transfusion, since the blood is returned to the patient as needed. The theoretical basis for the practice is discussed on p. 55. Although, in this form of autologous transfusion, blood is taken before surgery, because bleeding is carried out in the operating suite, it is widely (though slightly confusingly) referred to as 'intra-operative haemodilution'.

Messmer (1975) described the way in which haemodilution could be used in patients immediately before surgery: 1800–2000 ml blood are withdrawn with simultaneous infusion of a colloid solution, producing a fall in the PCV to about 0.25. Cardiac output increases, but heart rate, CVP and mean arterial pressure remain essentially unchanged. When the intra-operative blood loss exceeds about 300 ml, retransfusion of autologous blood is started. It is claimed that this method is adequate for dealing with intra-operative blood losses up to about 2000 ml, and that additional blood (i.e. allogeneic) is seldom needed. Messmer et al. (1972) emphasized that: (1) an increase in cardiac output must be regarded as an indispensable compensatory mechanism; (2) the tolerance and safe limits of clinical haemodilution are dependent on the contractile state of the myocardium; and (3) the following are to be regarded as contraindications: myocardial failure, coronary artery disease, obstructive lung disease and pre-existing anaemia.

Renewed interest has been given to all forms of autologous transfusion since allogeneic transfusion was shown to be a possible vehicle for HIV transmission. Although intra-operative haemodilution does not make very large amounts of autologous blood available, it is much more convenient for the patient than pre-operative deposit, and the blood itself is fresh, with viable platelets, if kept at room temperature. Intra-operative haemodilution to PCV levels of 0.27–0.30 has been used successfully in a wide range of patients and operations (see Messmer, 1987).

Cardiopulmonary bypass

Since the introduction of coronary artery bypass grafting with veins taken from the leg or arm (CAVG or CABG), there has been a great increase in the number of operations involving cardiopulmonary bypass. The annual requirement for CABG in the UK has been estimated as 400–450 per million of the population (Joint Cardiology Committee, 1985). The number of such operations performed in the USA far exceeds this figure. As the number of operations has risen, the number of units of blood used at each operation has fallen. In 1971, a survey of 88% of hospitals performing cardiopulmonary bypass in the USA revealed an average use of almost 8 units per operation (Roche and Stengle, 1973). In 1974, however, Sandiford et al. referred to a previously published series of 100 consecutive patients who underwent open-heart surgery at the Texas Heart Institute with an average transfusion requirement of 1.4 units blood per patient; 35 of the 100 patients required no blood whatever and a further 31 received only a single unit. They also stated that among more than 2500 patients who underwent coronary bypass surgery about 30% did not require blood transfusion at all. Finally, they reported a series of aortocoronary bypass operations on 36 Jehovah's witnesses in whom no blood was used. The estimated blood loss during operation was 530 ml range (range 200–1200 ml) and the mean blood loss from chest tubes during the first two post-operative days was 250 ml in all but one patient. Only two patients died and in neither case was the death related to the lack of transfusion. The average Hb concentration fell from 149 g/l before operation to 112 g/l in the immediate post-operative period, and was at its lowest about 6 d after operation with an average of 92 g/l.

Numerous later reports have confirmed an average use of 3 units or fewer per patient, and state that a significant proportion of patients require no allogeneic blood at all (Cosgrove *et al*. 1981; McCarthy *et al*. 1988). Several factors have helped to reduce the need for blood.

Priming of pump-oxygenators with electrolyte solution

Pump-oxygenators are normally primed with electrolyte solution but in exceptional circumstances, e.g. in children or patients with severe renal failure, it may be necessary to use blood.

Use of autologous transfusion

A number of centres now permit patients booked for elective cardiac surgery to pre-deposit blood (Owings *et al*. 1989). Haemodilution is widely practised and, together with the use of electrolyte priming solution, can produce PCVs as low as 0.20 during bypass (Cosgrove *et al*. 1981). The safety of such low PCV levels is disputed (Messmer, 1987).

Post-operatively, it is possible to collect defibrinated blood shed through mediastinal drains and retransfuse it without washing the red cells (Thurer *et al*. 1979). Because the blood loss after cardiac surgery is usually small, the adoption of this manoeuvre is unlikely to bring about a great saving in transfusion requirements. The return of unwashed red cells is also liable to criticism (Griffith *et al*. 1989; see also Chapter 1).

Haemostasis after cardiopulmonary bypass

Haemorrhage does not occur through the walls of intact blood vessels, and it is reasonable to suppose that improved surgical technique has contributed to the diminished need for allogeneic blood transfusion that has been observed in cardiac surgical patients over the past 20 years. In 1964, the commonest cause of serious bleeding after cardiopulmonary bypass was found to be failure to ligate blood vessels (Bentall *et al*. 1964). The use, now routine, of vasodilators to prevent hypertension after cardiac surgery may also help to reduce blood loss. There has been a suggestion, not entirely convincing, that application of positive end-expiratory pressure (PEEP) may reduce severe bleeding in cardiac surgical patients (Ilabaca *et al*. 1980).

Defective haemostasis may be due to a reducton in the number of platelets and to an impairment of platelet function (Moriau *et al*. 1977; Mammen *et al*. 1985; Musial *et al*. 1985). Platelets may be damaged in the oxygenator, and pre-operative factors such as the administration of aspirin or calcium channel blockers may contribute to a prolonged bleeding time. Bleeding after cardiopulmonary bypass may also be due to inadequate neutralization of heparin or overneutralization with protamine. Dilution of clotting factors occurs in oxygenators primed only with electrolytes, but seldom affects tests of coagulation.

Desmopressin acetate (DDAVP), which increases the plasma concentration of von Willebrand factor, has been shown to reduce bleeding in patients who have undergone cardiac surgery (Czer *et al*. 1985; Salzman *et al*. 1986). However, a double-blind, randomized trial involving 150 patients undergoing cardiac surgery failed to demonstrate any favourable effect when DDAVP was administered after bypass in place of a placebo (Hackmann *et al.* 1989).

Aprotinin, a serine proteinase inhibitor, when administered in very large doses, has brought about striking reductions in blood loss and transfusion requirements in both complicated cardiac surgery (Royston *et al.* 1987; Bidstrup *et al.* 1988) and in routine CABG (Dietrich *et al.* 1990). Aprotinin is believed to inactivate kallikrein (Emerson, 1989) and to preserve platelet function (Aoki *et al.* 1978). Because aprotinin is a bovine protein, its administration may possibly cause antibody formation.

Fibrinolysis is commonly associated with cardiopulmonary bypass, and fibrinolytic agents might, therefore, be expected to reduce blood loss. Small but significant, reductions have been demonstrated in randomized, double-blind studies using ε-aminocaproic acid (van der Salm *et al.* 1988) and tranexamic acid (Horrow *et al.* 1990).

Complement activation during cardiopulmonary bypass
During cardiopulmonary bypass, plasma levels of C3a increase steadily; although plasma levels of C5a do not increase, granulocytopenia follows the re-establishment of cardiopulmonary circulation, suggesting that C5-activated granulocytes are trapped in pulmonary vessels. Complement activation is promoted by contact of blood with plastic surfaces (e.g. nylon-mesh liner and bubble oxygenator) as well as by vigorous oxygenation of the whole blood. The production of C3a and C5a during extracorporeal circulation may contribute to the pathogenesis of the so-called post-pump syndrome (Chenoweth *et al.* 1981). The interaction of heparin and protamine is another potential source of complement activation (Rent *et al.* 1975; Chenoweth 1981; White, 1981).

BLOOD SUBSTITUTES

Plasma substitutes
The good effect of blood transfusion in haemorrhage is due mainly to the sustained increase in blood volume which it produces. Bayliss (1919) showed that a fluid which contained colloids with an osmotic pressure similar to that of plasma proteins could be used as a substitute for blood.

Many substances have been tried as plasma substitutes but not one of these has entirely fulfilled the theoretical requirements. For example, gum arabic, introduced by Bayliss (1919), later fell into disrepute because it was found to be stored in the tissues.

The main qualities required of a plasma substitute are: (1) retention in the circulation for relatively long periods after infusion; (2) freedom from causing allergic reactions; (3) freedom from causing unwanted side-effects; (4) complete metabolism after clearance from the circulation; and (5) low cost.

A problem that arises with all artificial colloids is that they are polydisperse, that is to say, they are composed of mixtures of molecules of widely varying size. Ideally, a preparation should contain no molecules of mol. wt. below 70 000, since these will be rapidly excreted by the kidney. On the other hand, to ensure that only a small proportion of such molecules are present, it may be necessary to accept some molecules with a mol. wt. greater than 250 000.

In describing the average mol. wt. of preparations which contain molecules of widely varying size it makes a substantial difference whether one gives the number average ($\overline{M}_n$) or weight average ($\overline{M}_w$).

$\overline{M}_n$ is obtained by dividing the total weight of all molecules present by the total number of molecules. $\overline{M}_w$ is obtained by summing the products of the weights of all molecules of a particular size multiplied by their mol. wt. and dividing the sum by the total weight of all the molecules. For mixtures of different molecular weight, $\overline{M}_w$ is always greater than $\overline{M}_n$ and the ratio $\overline{M}_w/\overline{M}_n$ gives a good measure of the degree of scatter of mol. wts in the mixture. Values of $\overline{M}_w$ and $\overline{M}_n$ for dextran and gelatin preparations given in this chapter are either taken from the monograph by Gruber (1969) or have been obtained from manufacturers.

Clinical dextran

Only two preparations of clinical dextran are now available, namely dextran 70 ($\overline{M}_w$ 70 000, $\overline{M}_n$ 39 000) and dextran 40 ($\overline{M}_w$ 40 000, $\overline{M}_n$ 25 000). The effects on the plasma volume of rabbits of these two dextrans, and also of dextran 110, modified fluid gelatin, 'plasma protein preparation', i.e. albumin, were compared by Farrow (1967; 1977); see Table 2.2. The main conclusions were as follows. The expansion of plasma volume depends mainly upon the weight of dextran in the circulation and is not directly related to the mol. wt. of the preparation. However, in terms of maintenance of expanded plasma volume the average mol. wt. of the infused dextran is very important because of the rapid excretion of small molecules. Dextran 40 is supplied as a 10% solution whereas other dextran preparations are supplied as 6% solutions so that for equivalent volumes the immediate effect of Dextran 40 is considerably greater; the infusion of a volume equivalent to 22% of the rabbit's plasma volume produces an immediate increase of about 35%. Nevertheless, the effect is maintained for only a few hours. Compared with Dextran 110, Dextran 70 has the advantage of producing

Table 2.2 Plasma volume expanding capacity of several products (from Farrow, 1967)*

	Isotonic saline	Physiogel[†] 4.2 g/dl	Dextran 40[‡] 10 g/dl	Dextran 40[‡] 6 g/dl	Dextran 70 6 g/dl	Dextran 110 6 g/dl	Plasma protein fraction 4.3 g/dl
Maximum expansion as percentage of infused volume	30	65	175	118	146	110	59
Maximum expansion as ml per g of material infused	—	15.1	17.7	20.0	24.4	18.6	11.6
Time for which expansion maintained at 50% or more of maximum (h)	Few minutes	1.5	1	1.5	4.5	14	15

* Further details of these experiments were published by Farrow (1977).
† A commercially available preparation of modified fluid gelatin (see below).
‡ Normally supplied as a 10 g/dl solution.

negligible rouleaux formation, but on the other hand the duration of plasma volume expansion is sacrificed and the material remains effective for only about 24 h whereas at the end of this period Dextran 110 continues to produce some increase in plasma volume. Plasma protein fraction produces a much smaller increase in plasma volume than an equivalent volume of 6% dextran but the effect is well maintained. Physiogel has a very short survival in the circulation, similar to that of Dextran 40 and is, therefore, not particularly effective as a plasma volume expander.

In the treatment of shock, Dextran 40 as a plasma volume expander is absolutely contraindicated because it may obstruct the renal tubules (Rush, 1974). Similarly, the infusion of large amounts of Dextran 40 in patients who already have slight impairment of renal function may precipitate acute renal failure; six cases were reported by Feest (1976) who advised that not more than 1 litre a day should be given and that, if urinary output falls, the infusions should be stopped and the patient given diuretics and a high fluid intake.

Allergic reactions to dextran

Many types of clinical dextran are capable of acting as antigens in humans; moreover anti-dextrans may be found in the serum of individuals who have never received dextran infusions (Kabat and Berg, 1953). Palosuo and Milgrom (1980) found dextran to be a widely distributed antigen in human serum. The sera of elderly people and of patients with inflammatory disease of the digestive tract sometimes contain large quantities of dextran and reactive antibodies of the IgG class. The authors inferred that dextran might be ingested in food or produced by micro-organisms in the gut.

Severe reactions to dextran infusions are confined to individuals who have high titres of IgG anti-dextran before they receive any dextran (Hedin and Richter, 1982). Hedin et al. (1979) postulated that the clinical manifestations are due to the formation of immune complexes between the dextran infused and the antibodies already present (type III anaphylaxis). The inhibition of immune complex formation by a hapten (Dextran 1) prevents severe dextran-induced anaphylactic reactions (Messmer et al. 1980). The routine use of Dextran 1 immediately before the infusion of Dextran 70 or Dextran 40 has been associated with a reduction in the reported incidence of severe reactions in Sweden (from 22 per 100 000 units between 1975 and 1979 to 1.2 per 100 000 units between 1983 and 1985) (Ljungstrom et al. 1988), although cases continue to be reported (Berg et al. 1991).

Unwanted side-effects of dextrans

Abnormal bleeding. Dextran may interfere with haemostasis, apparently by affecting platelet function. In experiments in which subjects were given infusions of 1000 ml dextran (mol. wt. 50 000–55 000) at a rate of 20 ml/min, the bleeding time was prolonged (more than 10 min) in 30–50% of subjects. The maximum effect was seen 3–9 h after infusion. With dextran of mol. wt. 180 000 (no longer used) bleeding time was prolonged in 50% of subjects. In a control series of subjects receiving 5% albumin, bleeding time was prolonged in nearly 2.5% of cases. Of 77 subjects in the series with a prolonged bleeding time, only two developed spontaneous bleeding or bruising (Langdell *et al.* 1958).

In a comparison in dogs between 6% Dextran 75, 10% Dextran 40 and 6% hydroxyethyl starch (HES, see below), the animals were given infusions of a total volume of 30 ml/kg, containing either 10, 20 or 30 ml/kg of expander with the volume made up with saline. The animals were first bled of an amount of blood considered to be osmotically equal to the amount of plasma expander to be infused. The bleeding time was measured before and after infusion by making incisions in the animal's flank and the volume of blood lost from these skin wounds was measured. After 10 ml/kg of expander the bleeding time increased by about 50%, and the blood loss from the incisions doubled. After 20 ml/kg of expander the bleeding time increased 5-fold and blood loss increased 5–14-fold (most with Dextran 75). After 30 ml/kg bleeding time increased 3–7-fold and blood loss 5–27-fold. The lowest figures were with HES, and with this expander blood loss was significantly less than with either dextran preparation (Karlson *et al.* 1967).

Interference with crossmatching. The tendency of dextran to cause rouleaux formation increases with mol. wt.; with a mol. wt. of 60 000, a concentration of 2% is needed, but with a mol. wt. of 270 000 only 0.4% (Thorsen and Hint, 1950). Despite the wide range of mol. wts in dextran preparations, in practice the infusion of presently available preparations does not lead to rouleaux formation in tests with untreated red cells. On the other hand, if enzyme-treated cells are used, even infusions of Dextran 40 can lead to intense aggregation (see Chapter 8). When there is a possibility that large amounts of dextran may be given, blood should be taken for crossmatching before the infusion is begun.

The safety of dextran as a plasma substitute is attested by an early experience. Using a relatively high mol. wt. preparation (Dextran 150) in patients with burns, provided that the amount given did not exceed the patient's own plasma volume, supplementary plasma or blood being given as necessary, the mortality rate was no higher than in patients treated entirely with plasma or blood (Bull and Jackson, 1955). It is often stated that not more than 1 litre dextran should be given but the scientific basis for this assertion is unknown.

Gelatin

Preparations of a molecular size large enough to be well retained in the circulation do not remain fluid at low temperatures and this is a serious disadvantage in a preparation that is essentially needed for emergency conditions.

Three preparations that remain fluid under normal ambient temperatures are available. In these the range of mol. wts is wide; about 70% of molecules are below the renal threshold (see review by Rudowski and Kostrzewska, 1976).

The $t_{\frac{1}{2}}$ of injected modified fluid gelatin, like that of Dextran 40, was found to be 2–3 h compared with 6 h for Dextran 60 and HES (Ring *et al.* 1980).

The following details are taken from the monograph by Gruber (1969):

Modified fluid gelatin, e.g. (a) Physiogel (4.2% in electrolyte solution), $\overline{M}_w$ 35 000, $\overline{M}_n$

16 000. Some results obtained with this solution are shown in Table 2.2. (b) Plasmagel (3% in electrolyte solution), mol. wt. distribution: 60% between 20 000 and 60 000.

Gelatin crosslinked by means of urea bridges, supplied as Haemaccel (3.5% in electrolyte solution), $\overline{M}_w$ 35 000, $\overline{M}_n$ 20 000.

As mentioned below, allergic reactions seem to be somewhat commoner after gelatin than after other plasma substitutes.

Perhaps the greatest advantage of modified fluid gelatin over other plasma substitutes is its lower tendency to produce haemorrhagic manifestations. Compared with dextran and HES it has only a slight effect on platelets; moreover, whereas both dextran and HES depress the partial thromboplastin time, gelatin has no effect (Harke *et al.* 1976). In experiments on irradiated thrombocytopenic dogs which were submitted to rapid haemorrhage of 25 ml blood per kg, replaced either by oncotically equivalent volumes of 15 ml/kg 6% dextran or 4% modified fluid gelatin, the output of red cells into the thoracic duct lymph was three times greater in three of six dogs treated with dextran, but was no greater than before bleeding in the dogs treated with gelatin (Lundsgaard-Hansen and Tschirren, 1978). Furthermore, in a controlled prospective study of patients undergoing elective surgery, in those patients receiving 1000 ml of 6% dextran 70, bleeding times post-operatively were 50 s greater than pre-operatively, whereas in patients receiving 1500 ml of 4% modified fluid gelatin the increase was insignificant (3.8 s). It was mentioned that three patients had survived after receiving more than 10 litres of modified fluid gelatin within 24 h (Tschirren *et al.* 1973/74).

Hydroxyethyl starch
HES is supplied as a 6% solution in 0.9% saline ($\overline{M}_w$ 450 000, $\overline{M}_n$ 65 000).

So far as initial retention in the circulation is concerned, HES appears to be similar to Dextran 70 (Gruber, 1969, p. 140), although small amounts of HES tend to persist in the circulation for long periods (see below).

HES has a relatively low tendency to cause allergic reactions. In one study, only eight untoward reactions were observed in just over 10 000 recipients; only one of the reactions was of a severe anaphylactic type (see below).

Like dextran, HES interferes with blood coagulation, although to a lesser extent (Karlson *et al.* 1967).

HES is commonly used to increase the yield of granulocytes from donors giving blood via cell separators (see Chapter 1).

Comparisons between plasma substitutes
Comparisons may be made on the grounds of retention in the circulation, incidence of allergic reactions, unwanted side-effects, such as interference with platelet function, catabolism and excretion from the body, and cost.
1   As mentioned above, Dextran 70 and HES appear to be retained about equally well but gelatin preparations, with smaller molecular weights, are excreted more rapidly.
2   All plasma substitutes have been associated with allergic reactions. In a prospective survey, reported in 1977, the incidence of reactions of all kinds, i.e. from skin

symptoms alone at one extreme to cardiac arrest at the other, was 0.69% for Dextran 60/75; 0.007% for Dextran 40; 0.085% for HES; 0.115% for gelatin; and 0.014% for plasma protein solutions (either whole serum or albumin). Only about one-quarter of the reactions were life-threatening; the highest incidence was found with gelatin solutions (0.039%), the next with Dextran 60/75 (0.017%), then HES (0.006%) followed by plasma protein solutions (0.004%), with Dextran 40 last with 0.002% (Ring and Messmer, 1977).

3   As described above, gelatin is less likely than the other two plasma substitutes to interfere with platelet function and it is thus less likely to provoke bleeding.

4   Gelatin is rapidly catabolized, and dextran is also completely broken down, but some doubts remain about HES which, in any case, tends to persist for long periods in the circulation. In volunteers infused with 7 ml/kg HES or Dextran 60, after 17 weeks the plasma HES concentration was still 1% of the post-infusion level whereas after 4 weeks, dextran was undetectable (Boon et al. 1977; see also Chapter 1).

5   HES is an expensive product. Its present cost in the UK is half that of albumin but five times that of gelatin. Dextran 70 is somewhat more expensive than gelatin.

Red cell substitutes

Unmodified and modified haemoglobin

Solutions of unmodified Hb can largely replace whole blood for short periods in cats (Amberson et al. 1934) and stroma-free Hb solutions have been claimed to be harmless to the kidney (Rabiner et al. 1970). However, serious ill effects have been reported: in eight volunteers infused with 250 ml stroma-free Hb there was gross haemoglobinuria, accompanied by bradycardia, a fall in creatinine clearance and urine output, and prolongation of the activated PTT (Savitsky et al. 1978).

In any case, unmodified Hb suffers from two serious disadvantages:

1   Hb in solution has a far higher oxygen affinity (P_{50} about 15 mm Hg) than that of red cells (P_{50} 28 mm Hg); as a consequence less oxygen is released to the tissues.

2   Unmodified Hb is rapidly cleared from the plasma. Both these disadvantages can be overcome, at least to some extent. Pyridoxylation of Hb lowers its oxygen affinity (Benesch et al. 1972), and subsequent polymerization with glutaraldehyde yields a product which is cleared from the plasma far more slowly than unmodified Hb (Greenburg et al. 1979; Sehgal et al. 1980; DeVenuto and Zegna, 1983), although its half-life in the circulation is still only 25 h.

Gould et al. (1990) reported that six baboons survived an exchange transfusion with a new preparation of polymerized pyridoxalated Hb. The preparation (Poly SFH-1) had a P_{50} of 16–20 mm Hg and a plasma $t_{1/2}$ of 40–46 h. The same group of workers infused Poly-SFH-1 into six well hydrated human volunteers, only one of whom developed an adverse reaction, described as a 'mild allergic response' (Moss et al. 1989). No further tests of this product have been published in scientific journals. The Center for Biologics Evaluation and Research has expressed concern about the intensity and severity of unexplained reactions in human recipients of haemoglobin solutions (FDA, 1991a).

Haemoglobin solutions with an appropriate P_{50} and adequate $t_{1/2}$ in the circulation are an enticing prospect at a time when the supply of allogeneic red cells is short and the public's fear of possible infection from their transfusion is considerable. Even if a safe product with the necessary characteristics were available, several steps would have to be taken before it could replace red cells in the treatment of haemorrhage. First, the haemoglobin solution would have to be shown to be effective as an oxygen carrier in oligaemic patients. Given that red cells are known to be effective in such patients, it would be difficult to design and carry out an ethical clinical study in which selected bleeding patients were transfused with a haemoglobin solution instead. Second, large-scale production of the Hb solution would have to be feasible. A large supply of Hb would be needed as starting material and it is difficult to see how the transfusion services could provide enough human Hb for the purpose (see Zuck, 1990). The perspective has recently been altered by the demonstration that human Hb can be synthesized, and correctly assembled into $\alpha_2\beta_2$ tetramers, in a yeast (Ogden *et al.* 1991). Bovine Hb, which has a P_{50} of less than 30 mm Hg when stroma free and polymerized, would be easier than human Hb to obtain in quantities great enough to support a commercial process. Sheep have been shown to survive a 95% exchange transfusion with bovine Hb and to be in good health with normal renal function a month later, whereas sheep exchange-transfused with HES died during the experiment (Vlahates *et al.* 1990).

Encapsulated haemoglobin

Haemoglobin can be enclosed in lipid vesicles (liposomes). Such encapsulated Hb has been shown to be as effective as red cells in transporting oxygen; the dissociation curve is similar to that of whole blood with a P_{50} of 26–28 mm Hg.

Rats can live for several hours after exchange transfusions with liposomes (Djordjevich and Miller, 1980), but they can also survive an exchange of up to 95% with crystalloid or colloid solution.

The half-life of liposomes in the circulation is short (Farmer and Gaber, 1984). However, if the composition of the liposomal membrane is altered, the clearance of liposomes may be reduced; for instance, the incorporation of glycoproteins into the membrane has been shown to reduce their hepatic uptake (Jonah *et al.* 1978). Encapsulated Hb has never been administered to humans and its future as a blood substitute appears to depend on the development of a membrane of superior composition to any known at present (see Kahn *et al.* 1985).

Perfluoro compounds

Oxygen (like carbon dioxide) is highly soluble in perfluoro compounds. For example, the compound known as FC-80, when equilibrated with 95% O_2 and 5% CO_2, contains about the same amount of oxygen as an equal volume of packed red cells under the same conditions (Colman *et al.* 1980).

The ability of perfluoro compounds to deliver oxygen in intact animals was first demonstrated by Sloviter *et al.* (1969). Total blood replacement with a compound FC-47 was carried out in rats by Geyer (1975). The rats were initially kept in 95% O_2 but the concentration was reduced progressively as red cells (and serum proteins) were regenerated and the animals were returned to air at 7 d. Some of the animals were alive 1 year later. An emulsion of two different perfluoro compounds described as Fluosol–DA, with an oxygen carrying capacity at 37°C about 40% as great as that of red cells, was given as an i.v. infusion, in a dose of about 20 ml/kg, to 186 patients without ill effects except in one patient who received repeated infusions (Mitsuno *et al.* 1982).

Perfluoro compounds have great limitations. They can carry substantial amounts of oxygen only when exposed to high oxygen tensions (Tremper *et al.* 1982) which may be toxic (Frank and Macaro, 1980). The infusion of Fluosol-DA in doses up to 40 ml/kg was found to be ineffective as an oxygen carrier in a small group of acutely anaemic surgical patients who had refused blood transfusion on religious grounds (Gould *et al.* 1986). The emulsified compounds must be stored in the frozen state; they have only a brief survival time in the circulation but are retained for long periods in the mononuclear phagocyte system (MPS) (Ohnishi and Kitazawa, 1980; Kitazawa and Ohnishi, 1982). There is evidence that macrophages which have accumulated perfluoro compounds show loss of phagocytic function (Bucala *et al.* 1983; Virmani *et al.* 1983). The emulsifying agent in Fluosol–DA (Pluronic 68) may activate the complement system and cause pulmonary damage (Vercelloti *et al.* 1982).

It is possible, however, that perfluorocarbons may find a place in more restricted circumstances. For example, oxygenated Fluosol-DA was shown to prevent myocardial ischaemia when infused into the distal coronary artery during ballon angioplasty (Jaffe *et al.* 1988), whereas infusions of oxygenated Ringer's lactate solutions and non-oxygenated Fluosol–DA conferred no such benefit.

CHAPTER 3

IMMUNOLOGY OF RED CELLS

In this chapter blood groups as a whole are discussed with special emphasis on immunological aspects; in subsequent chapters some of the blood group systems are considered in more detail.

Although all inherited differences in the blood may fall within the widest meaning of the term blood groups, in this book the term is usually used simply for red cell antigens. When the inheritance of one series of antigens is independent of another series the antigens are said to belong to different blood group systems.

Discovery of the blood group systems (Table 3.1)

The ABO system

Antigenic differences between different species were recognized before differences within a species. Landois (1875, p. 185) discovered that when the red cells of an animal, e.g. a lamb, were mixed with the serum of another animal (a dog) and incubated at 37°C they might be lysed within 2 min.

Table 3.1 Discovery of main blood group system*

Blood group system		First examples of antibody defining system		
			Detected by:	
Name (abbreviation)	Year of discovery	Found in serum of	Agglutination of red cells in saline	Antiglobulin test
ABO	1901	Normal subjects	Yes	—
Lewis (Le)	1946			
MN	1927	Rabbits injected with	Yes	—
P	1927	human red cells		
LW	1930s (see text)	Rabbits and guinea pigs injected with rhesus monkey red cells	Yes	—
Rhesus (Rh)	1939	(i) Mother of stillborn infant	Yes	—†
	1940	(ii) Transfused patients	Yes	—†
Lutheran (Lu)	1945	Transfused patient	Yes	—
Kell (K)	1946	Transfused patients or mothers of infants with haemolytic disease of the newborn	No‡	Yes
Duffy (Fy)	1950			
Kidd (Jk)	1951			
Diego (Di)	1955			
Cartwright (Yt)	1956			
Xg	1962			
Dombrock (Do)	1965			
Colton (Co)	1967			

* Systems omitted from the table include Sc, Chido/Rodgers, Hh, Kx, Gerbich and Cromer.
— not done.
† The antiglobulin test was introduced into clinical work in 1945; it was soon realized that many Rh antibodies which could be detected by this test would not agglutinate red cells suspended in saline.
‡ In most of the blood group systems, potent examples of antibodies will agglutinate red cells in saline.

Landsteiner (1900; 1901) was prompted by the work of Landois to see whether it was possible to demonstrate differences, although presumably slighter ones, between individuals of the same species. As he later explained (Landsteiner, 1931), he chose the simplest plan of investigation and simply allowed serum and red cells from different human individuals to interact. For his resulting discovery of the ABO blood group system, which proved to be of vast importance for blood transfusion, he received the Nobel prize, although it is said that he would much rather that it had been awarded to him for his work on the chemical basis of the specificity of serological reactions.

MN and P systems

After the discovery of the ABO system no new blood group systems were found for 25 years. Landsteiner and Witt (1926) examined human sera for antibodies other than anti-A and anti-B but could find only weak agglutinins active at low temperatures. It occurred to Landsteiner and Levine that they might be able to reveal other antigens by injecting different samples of human red cells into rabbits. Antibodies identifying three new human antigens were obtained (Landsteiner and Levine, 1927); to the first of these the letter M was given to indicate that the antigen had been identified with immune serum ('I' was avoided because of confusion with the numeral 1 (Levine, 1944)).

The Rh system

Antibodies demonstrating Rh polymorphism in humans were found in two different ways. Landsteiner and Wiener (1940; 1941) injected the red cells of rhesus monkeys into rabbits and guinea pigs and tested the resulting serum against human red cells. Meanwhile, Levine and Stetson (1939) found an antibody (which subsequently proved to be anti-Rh D) in the serum of a recently delivered woman whose fetus had died *in utero*. Although the dates quoted here seem to establish priorities clearly, it is in fact very difficult to give a short answer to the question 'who discovered the Rh blood group system?'

According to R.E. Rosenfield (1977, supplemented by personal communication), L. Buchbinder, a PhD student of Karl Landsteiner, had discovered Rh polymorphism at some time in the 1930s, but Landsteiner had refused to permit further studies or publication (Buchbinder's studies on the antigenic structure of erythrocytes of humans and *Macacus rhesus* were published in 1933).

A.S. Wiener, who worked with Landsteiner in the late 1930s, stated, in the preface to his book *Rh–Hr Blood Types* published in 1954, that he had known about Rh polymorphism in 1937. In 1940, he described the results of tests on three patients who had had severe transfusion reactions; with the rabbit anti-rhesus serum available in Landsteiner's laboratory, the patients typed as D negative and the donors as D positive; moreover, haemagglutinins of the same specificity as the rabbit anti-rhesus serum were present in the patients' plasma (Wiener and Peters, 1940). Landsteiner now agreed to publish the results of human blood typing with the animal anti-rhesus sera (Landsteiner and Wiener, 1940). Rosenfield (1977) pointed out that in this latter paper no data were published on adsorption and elution experiments; Rosenfield added, 'if Landsteiner remembered that this had been done by Buchbinder he forgot that it had not been published by Buchbinder [in 1933]'. Rosenfield concluded that if only Landsteiner and Wiener had published their findings in 1937 the question of priorities would not have arisen. As it was, Levine and Stetson's (1939) case (see Chapter 12) was the first published evidence of polymorphism related to Rh and thus could be claimed to take priority over the rabbit anti-rhesus data not published by Landsteiner and Wiener before 1940, even though Levine and Stetson failed to give a name to the specificity they had discovered. For further details of the Levine–Wiener argument, see Rosenfield (1989).

Other blood group systems

Between 1946 and 1967 the Kell (K), Duffy (Fy), Kidd (Jk), Diego (Di), Cartwright (Yt), Xg, Sc, Dombrock (Do) and Colton (Co) blood group systems were discovered, in every case by the use of the indirect antiglobulin test. During this period two new systems, Lewis and Lutheran, and one family of antigens (Ii) were discovered by the use of agglutination tests in saline. Discoveries since 1967 are mentioned in later parts of this book.

Terminology of blood groups

Blood group terminology is inconsistent. In some systems, e.g. ABO, antigens are given capital letters (e.g. B) or capital letters with subscripts (e.g. A_2); the corresponding alleles are denoted by italics, with superscripts when relevant (e.g. A^2). Although the alleles of the ABO system are all thought to be alternative forms at a single locus, this is not indicated by the nomenclature (e.g. one allele of A^2 is O). In other systems (e.g. Kell) the main alleles are denoted respectively by large and small letters, thus K and k; here the terminology indicates that the alleles are alternative forms. The MNSs system follows a blend of these two systems of nomenclature, the first antigens to be described being called M and N, and the next pair S and s. The Lewis, Lutheran, Duffy, Kidd, Diego, Cartwright, Dombrock and Colton systems follow a uniform pattern. The system is denoted by a capital letter followed by a small letter, thus: Le, Lu, Fy Jk, Di, Yt, Do and Co; alleles are denoted thus: Lu^a; phenotypes are written Lu(a + b –) and antibodies thus: anti-Lu^a. In the Xg, P_1, Hh and Kx systems only one antigen has been demonstrated so far and the alleles are therefore termed, for example, Xg^a and Xg. In the Scianna system the antigens are termed Sc1 and Sc2. In most cases the name of the system is that of the patient in whom the antibody which led to the recognition of the system was found.

For the Rh system there are two different nomenclatures in addition to a numerical notation (see Chapter 5). Numbers are also used for several of the other systems described above, e.g. Kell. A standard numerical nomenclature, consisting of six numbers and suitable for computerization has been devised by a working party of the International Society of Blood Transfusion (Lewis et al. 1985; 1990). The first three numbers represent the blood group system, e.g. 001, ABO; 002, MNSs; 003, P; 004, Rh, and the second three numbers represent a particular antigenic specificity within that system, e.g. 001001, A; 004001, D.

Twenty-one blood group systems have been given numbers so far. In numerical order, systems 001–021 are: ABO, MNSs, P_1, Rh, Lu, Kell, Lewis, Fy, Jk, Di, Yt, Xg, Sc, Do, Co, LW, Chido/Rodgers, Hh, Kx, Ge (Gerbich) and Cromer. The numbers of antigens within each system vary from only one (P_1, Xg^a, H, Kx) to 48 (Rh). The Ge system incorporates the low frequency antigens Wb and Ls^a, previously considered to be 'private' antigens, i.e. low frequency antigens unlinked to a known blood group system. The antigens of the Cromer system (Cr^a, Tc^{a,b,c}, Dr^a, Es^a, IFC, WES^{a,b} and UMC) reside on the red cell membrane protein DAF (decay accelerating factor) which

regulates membrane-bound C3b activity. Further series of numbers have been established to encompass related families of antigens ('the collections') as well as those high
incidence antigens ('publics'; the 900 series) and those low frequency antigens
('privates'; the 700 series) that are not currently known to be genetically linked to any
of the 21 established blood group systems. At present, the 'collections' comprise the
Indian (203), Cost (205, which includes York, Knops and McCoy antigens), Gregory
(206 series, including Gy and Hy), Ii (207 series), Er (208 series including Er^a and Er^b),
P (209 series which includes P, P^k and LKE), Lewis-like (210 series for Le^c and Le^d) and
Wright (211 series). The antigens of the collections are grouped together on the basis of
their genetic (e.g. In^a, In^b; Er^a, Er^b), phenotypic (Ii; P, LKE; Wr^a, Wr^b) or biochemical
(Gy, Hy) interrelationships (Lewis *et al.* 1991).

The relative clinical importance of different blood group systems
The clinical importance of any particular blood group system depends on (a) the
frequency with which alloantibodies of the system occur, and (b) the characteristics of
the alloantibody, namely, immunoglobulin (Ig) class and, if IgG, subclass and ability to
activate complement. These characteristics in turn determine the capacity of the
antibody to cause red cell destruction and to pass the placenta and cause haemolytic
disease of the newborn.

The ABO system is easily the most important because anti-A and anti-B are found
in virtually all subjects who lack the corresponding antigens and these antibodies often
cause intravascular haemolysis if incompatible red cells are transfused.

The Rh system comes next in importance because Rh D-negative subjects readily
form anti-D and the antibody is capable of causing severe haemolytic transfusion
reactions and haemolytic disease of the newborn.

There are some systems in addition to ABO in which antibodies are commonly
found in the serum of subjects who have not been transfused or been pregnant; by
convention such antibodies are described as naturally occurring. It may be objected
that the term 'naturally occurring', to describe an antibody found in the plasma of a
subject who has never been exposed to red cells containing the corresponding antigen,
is misleading since it may seem to imply that the antibody has appeared in the
subject's plasma without known cause. Many, if not all, naturally occurring antibodies
are believed to be formed in response to bacterial antigens (p. 101). The number of
chemical structures found on the cell membranes of bacteria and animals is limited,
and the same structures may be found in animals widely separated on the evolutionary scale. As a consequence, antibodies provoked by bacterial antigens commonly
react with the red cells of several animal species, e.g. humans. The term 'non-red cell
immune' has been coined to indicate the origin of such antibodies. This term is rather
cumbersome and since, in any case, exposure to bacteria can scarcely be regarded as
unnatural, the authors prefer to retain the term naturally occurring.

In general, naturally occurring antibodies other than anti-A and anti-B are of
negligible importance because they are usually inactive at body temperature and are
then incapable of causing clinically significant red cell destruction. A minor exception
is anti-Le^a, which is normally active at 37°C but, for reasons described below, very
seldom causes haemolytic transfusion reactions.

There are other systems that have some similarities with Rh in that naturally occurring antibodies are rare and immune antibodies relatively frequent, particularly in patients who have been transfused many times. The most important of these systems, Kell, is very much less important than Rh, and the importance of the many other blood group systems, also described in Chapter 6, becomes progressively less until one reaches a system such as Colton in which very few antibodies have ever been encountered.

RED CELL ANTIGENS

The red cell membrane

Like other cell membranes, the red cell membrane is an assembly of lipid and protein molecules. The lipids, which together make up almost half of the mass of the membrane, are phospholipids (60%), cholesterol (30%) and glycolipids (10%). The lipid molecules are arranged as a continuous double layer, 4–5 nm thick. This lipid bilayer forms the basic structure of the membrane and various proteins, such as band 3 glycoprotein, the anion transporter, sialoglycoproteins (SGP), and the protein carrying the Rh D antigen are inserted into it. About 60% of the inner aspect of the lipid bilayer is attached directly to the cytoskeleton, the structure of which has been compared to a hairnet; the 'knots' in the hairnet are the junction complexes, composed of an actin oligomer, proteins 4.1, 4.9 (dematin), adducin and tropomyosin. In addition, at this site, the spectrin lattice, consisting of α–β-heterodimers forming mainly hexagons with some pentagons and heptagons, is tied to a transmembrane protein, glycophorin C (β-SGP), and perhaps also to glycophorin A or α-SGP (Nagel, 1990). The transmembrane protein, band 3, is anchored to the cytoskeleton through bands 2.1 (ankyrin) or 4.1 (see Fig. 3.1).

The protein carrying the D antigen is believed to be attached to the cytoskeleton but to which protein is not yet known.

Band 3 protein, which constitutes about 25% of the total membrane protein, is a thread-like structure which makes many traverses of the lipid bilayer (Kopito and Lodish, 1985); it is present in about one million copies per red cell. The whole molecule is a dimer with a channel between its two halves which is the main route through which anions are transported (Jennings, 1984; Palek and Lambert, 1990). Band 3 is also an important binding site for glycolytic enzymes, Hb and haemicromes or Heinz bodies (Low, 1986).

Sialoglycoproteins or glycophorins have most of their mass on the external surface of the red cell membrane; most of the surface carbohydrate, including more than 75% of the sialic acid and therefore most of the negative charge of the cell surface, is carried by glycoprotein molecules (see Anstee, 1981), whereas Rh D is mostly in the membrane.

Chemical nature of red cell antigens

A, B and H antigens are determined by terminal sugars which are attached to at least four kinds of structure on the red cell surface: band 3 (mentioned above), SGPs, polyglycosyl ceramides and simple glycolipids; the greatest number of A B and H antigen sites are on band 3 glycoprotein. Further details of the chemistry of the ABH antigens, and also of Lewis, Ii and P antigens are given in Chapter 4.

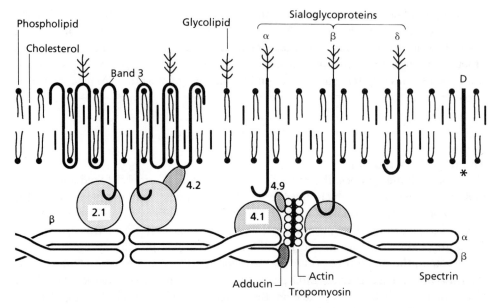

Figure 3.1 Diagram of the red cell membrane showing the lipid bilayer, some of the transmembrane proteins, namely band 3 (see text), α-, β- and δ-sialoglycoproteins (SGP) (glycophorins A, C and B respectively), the Rh D protein and the cytoskeleton. Carbohydrate molecules with their side-chains are shown as part of band 3, glycolipids and SGPs. Some of the transmembrane proteins are attached to the proteins of the cytoskeleton on the inside of the cell membrane, e.g. band 3 is attached to band 2.1 (ankyrin) and to protein 4.2, and β-SGP to band 4.1 (the term 'band' applies to identification on SDS-PAGE electrophoresis) and to actin. The heterodimer adducin binds to actin and spectrin, and promotes the binding of spectrin to actin. * indicates that the Rh D protein is attached to the cytoskeleton but that the site of attachment is not yet established.

The Rh D antigen is on a protein of approximate mol. wt. 30 000 containing no carbohydrate; LW is a glycoprotein distinct from Rh; for further details, see Chapter 5. Kell antigens are carried on a glycoprotein of mol. wt. 93 000 and Duffy antigens on a heavily glycosylated protein of mol. wt. about 30 000. MN and Ss antigens are carried on the α- and δ-SGPs (glycophorins A and B). For further details of the molecular biology of these and other blood group antigens, see Chapter 6.

The antigenic determinant
The antibody-binding portion of an antigenic determinant, the 'epitope', which is the region of the antigen that is complementary to the combining site of the antibody, has an area of between one and seven sugar residues (0.5–3.5 nm) for the carbohydrate moiety of glycoproteins or glycolipids, and of four or five amino acids for protein antigens. That part of the antigenic determinant which is bound most strongly is called the immunodominant group and is often the terminal non-reducing sugar residue or terminal amino acid. The relative binding contribution of the remaining residues decreases proportionately with the distance from the immunodominant group. Antigenic determinants may be sequential, as in linear polysaccharides or polypeptides, or may be conformational and involve structures brought into proximity by folding, as in proteins. Even to a single homogeneous polysaccharide such as dextran, the antibody

response is heterogeneous; antibody molecules with complementarity to different numbers of glucose residues are produced (Kabat, 1973).

Number of antigenic determinants on red cells

The number of available antigenic determinants per red cell varies widely between different systems: there appear to be between $1-2 \times 10^6$ sites for ABH; 1×10^6 for M and N (actually glycophorin A); $1-5 \times 10^5$ for I; 3×10^4 for Rh D, S, s, Fy^a, Jk^a and Di^a; and $2-5 \times 10^3$ for Le^a, K and Lu^b. References will be found in the relevant chapters.

Distribution of antigen sites on the red cell membrane

Clustering. When lymphocytes or granuloctyes (Ackermann and Terasaki, 1974) are incubated with serum containing an appropriate antibody certain antigen sites aggregate and move to one pole of the cell, the so-called capping phenomenon. In contrast, intact adult human red cells do not exhibit capping.

No evidence of clustering of Rh D antigen sites was found by Singer and Nicholson (1972) or by Romano *et al.* (1974). The latter authors used gold-labelled anti-IgG added to anti-D-sensitized red cells which were then lysed and prepared for electron microscopy.

Clustering has been demonstrated with enzyme-treated cells incubated first with anti-D and then with anti-IgG (Romano *et al.* 1975) and with enzyme-treated red cells incubated simply with ferritin-labelled IgG anti-D (Victoria *et al.* 1975). Clustering has also been found with untreated red cells of phenotype –D– following incubation first with anti-D, then with anti-IgG (Romano *et al.* 1975; Victoria *et al.* 1975). In all these cases red cell membranes from lysed red cells were examined; antigens on intact red cells are insufficiently mobile to form clusters (see Fig. 3.1).

In the intact red cell membrane the movement of glycoproteins is severely restricted by the cytoskeleton which has multiple attachments to the inner surface of the membrane. The maximum possible lateral movement is probably no more than $0.3 \ \mu m$ (Sheetz, 1983).

Relation between antigens of the same blood group system

As described in Chapter 4, different antigenic determinants of some blood group systems, i.e. those in which particular sugars are added to an oligosaccharide chain, may be present on the same molecule. In the Rh D system, in which the antigens are determined by structural genes, the antigens seem to be spatially separated on the red cell surface. In fact, D sites on the one hand and c and E sites, on the other, appear to be on separate proteins (see Chapter 5).

Effect of enzyme treatment on red cell antigens

Treatment of red cells with neuraminidase, which removes N-acetylneuraminic acid from the surface, diminishes the reactions of red cells with some anti-M and anti-N reagents but has no effect on the A, B, H, Le^a, Le^b, P_1, C, D, E, c, e, Lu^a, K, k, Fy^a and Jk^a antigens (Springer and Ansell, 1958). In confirming these observations, Bird and Wingham (1970b) also found that S, s and U were unaffected and that the reactions of red cells with the lectins from *Ulex europaeus*, *Vicia graminea* and *Bauhinia variegata* were enhanced.

Red cells treated with proteolytic enzymes (e.g. ficin) are more readily agglutinated by antibodies of certain specificities and advantage is taken of this effect in serological tests. Details of tests are given in Chapter 8, where there is also a list of red cell antigens that are destroyed by proteolytic enzymes.

Inheritance of red cell antigens

Two similar sets of chromosomes—one set inherited from each parent—are present in all cells of the body except the germ cells; each set is composed of 22 'autosomes' and one sex chromosome so that the total number of chromosomes per cell is 46. In the female the sex chromosomes are equal in size and are termed X chromosomes but in the male there is one X chromosome and one much smaller chromosome, termed Y.

The term gene is used for that part of chromosomal DNA which determines the inheritance of the characters of some identifiable system, such as ABO. The alternative forms of genes at a particular locus are termed alleles, e.g. *A* and *B*.

The genes controlling the structures of the antigens in any particular blood group system are assumed to occupy corresponding loci on a pair of homologous chromosomes. Thus, for all genes carried on autosomes, an individual may be homozygous (both alleles the same, e.g. *AA*) or heterozygous (alleles dissimilar, e.g. *AO*); *AA*, *AO*, etc. are referred to as genotypes; see Table 3.2. In almost all the systems carried on autosomes, the alleles are co-dominant. The only blood group gene not carried on an autosome is that of the Xg system, which is carried on the X chromosome. Females may be homozygous or heterozygous for Xg^a (*e.g.* Xg^aXg^a or Xg^aXg) but males can only be Xg^a or Xg and are said to be hemizygous.

In some systems, e.g. Rh (also HLA, see Chapter 13), the inheritance of antigens is determined by a series of alleles which are so closely linked that crossing over between them is very rare. The alleles which encode various combinations of the antigens D, C (or c) and E (or e) are inherited together. Thus, inheritance of DCe from one parent is determined by the haplotype (haploid genoytype) *DCe*.

Red cell antigens which are proteins (e.g. Rh and K) are, presumably, direct gene products, but those which are carbohydrate (e.g. A and Le^a) are determined indirectly by enzymes (transferases) which are the gene products; these enzymes transfer the appropriate sugar, determining specificity, on to a structure whose synthesis may be determined by one or more unrelated genes.

In most cases there appears to be a simple correspondence between genes and antigens, so that if a person inherits a given gene the antigen can be detected on his or

Table 3.2 Phenotypes and genotypes, illustrated by the ABO system (ignoring subgroups)

Phenotypes	Genotypes*
AB	*AB*
A	*AA* or *AO*
B	*BB* or *BO*
O	*OO*

* It is customary to denote genes and genotypes by italic letters.

her red cells. The main exceptions to this rule are provided by cases in which the expression of one gene is suppressed or modified by a gene carried on a different chromosome. Examples of both of these exceptions are described in Chapter 4 (*A* and *B* modifying the expression of *Le*) and in Chapter 6 (expression of *Lu* genes).

Some alleles do not produce any recognizable effects, and are termed amorphs. For example, ignoring the existence of subgroups, the inheritance of the ABO groups is thought to depend upon the alleles *A*, *B* and *O*, *A* and *B* code for transferases which determine A and B specificities but *O* gives rise to no enzymic activity. Accordingly, although there are six possible genotypes, only four phenotypes can be recognized in tests with anti-A and anti-B (see Table 3.2). (The term genotype is used for the sum of inherited alleles whereas phenotype refers only to recognizable characteristics.)

In some blood group systems the red cells of homozygotes and heterozygotes can be distinguished by the strength of their reactivity with antisera. For example, using antibodies of the Rh, K, Jk, Ss and Fy systems, flow cytometry could distinguish between homozygotes and heterozygotes without overlap with 11 of 14 sera. With manual titration methods, although homozygotes reacted more strongly than heterozygotes, there was overlap with 10 of 11 sera (Oien *et al.* 1985).

Gene (allele) frequencies

By gene frequency is meant simply the frequency of the allele in the population as a whole; the term allele frequency would be more precise but it is not generally used. From a knowledge of the frequencies of the gene (allele) frequencies in a blood group system, phenotype frequencies are readily derived. For example, based on testing almost 200 000 British subjects, the frequencies of the three main alleles in the ABO system were calculated to be: *A*, 0.2573; *B*, 0.0600; and *O*, 0.6827 (Dobson and Ikin, 1946). (Note that in calculating the frequency of the *O* allele one must count not only people of group O with a double dose of the allele but also those people whose genotype is *AO* or *BO*.) From the above gene frequencies, the frequency of group O is 0.6827 × 0.6827, or 0.47 (47%); that of group AB is (0.2573 × 0.0600) × 2, or 0.03 (3%). The '× 2' is accounted for by the fact that *A* can combine with *B*, as well as *B* with *A*. In this book, unless otherwise stated, frequencies of alleles and phenotypes refer to the UK. Frequencies for many other parts of the world are given by Mourant *et al.* (1976).

In different races the proportion of individuals belonging to a particular blood group varies widely; some examples of differences between Chinese, Europeans and West Africans are given in Table 3.3.

Independent inheritance of different blood group systems

Alleles of genes on different chromosomes are inherited independently of one another. Figure 3.2 illustrates the independent inheritance of alleles of the ABO and Kell systems. *Rh*, *Fy*, *Sc*, *Rd* and *Cr* are on chromosome 1; *Jk*, *Co* and *Ge* are on chromosome 2; *MNSs* is on chromosome 4; *HLA*, genes for several complement components including C2 and the C4A and C4B markers Ch and Rg are on chromosome 6; *Co* is on chromosome 7; *ABO* is on chromosome 9; *Jk* is on chromosome 18; *Le*, *Lu*, *H*, *Se* and *LW* are on chromosome 19; P_1 is on chromosome 22; and *Xg*, together with the X-linked suppressor of *Lu*, and *Xk*, the gene determining Kx, are on the X chromosome.

Table 3.3 Frequencies (as percentages) of some blood group antigens in Chinese, Europeans and West Africans

	Chinese	Europeans	W. Africans
B	35	14	20
P_1	31	80	95
Rh D	100	84	95
V(ce^s)	?0	0	40
K	0	9	<1
Js^a	0	0	20
Fy^a	99	65	20
Di^a	5	0	0

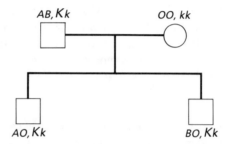

Figure 3.2 Independent inheritance of the ABO and Kell genes. In this example, the father passes on *A* to one son and *B* to the other, but passes on *K* to both.

The chromosomal locations of the genes determining the Di and Do systems remain to be determined (Lewis *et al.* 1991). Linkage between *K* and the locus for prolactin-induced protein indicates that *K* is on chromosome 7 (Zelinski *et al.* 1991a); since *Yt* is linked to *K*, *Yt* is also on chromosome 7 (Zelinski *et al.* 1991b).

Short lengths of DNA adjacent to blood group genes can be used as substitute markers for the gene. Such markers, 'restriction fragment length polymorphisms (RFLPs)', have already served to assign some blood group genes to particular chromosomes. They are certain to prove valuable in excluding or establishing linkage between genes for blood group antigens so far unassigned to a blood group system and genes of established systems; see review by Zelinski (1991) and Table 3.4.

Genetic markers on blood cells and predisposition to disease

The relation between a genetic marker and disease may be expressed as linkage, i.e. the marker and disease susceptibility are inherited together, or as association, i.e. the particular marker is more frequent in subjects with the disease than in normal subjects.

The majority of HLA-associated diseases display a higher frequency of a particular HLA-DR antigen, e.g. in IgA deficiency and in several autoimmune diseases, the frequency of HLA-DR3 is increased (see Svejgaard *et al.* 1983).

The associations between red cell groups and disease are not as strong as those between HLA groups and disease, and the risk, for individuals carrying the associated red cell group, of acquiring a particular disease is never very much larger than for

Table 3.4 DNA markers as substitutes for red cell antigens (data kindly supplied by T. Zelinski)

Blood group system	Locus of substitute marker		Chromosomal location of substitute marker
	Abbreviation	Full name	
Cloned blood group genes			
MNSs	GYPA	Glycophorin A	9q34.1–q34.2
Ge	GYPC	Glycophorin C	2q14–q21
Cr	DAF	Decay accelerating factor	1q32
Hh	FUT1	Fucosyl transferase 1	19q
*Closely linked DNA markers**			
Lu	APOC2	Apolipoprotein C-II	19q13.2
Co	D7S135	DNA segment, single copy, probes TM102L, HSC-TM102L	7pter–p14
K	PIP	Prolactin-inducible protein locus	7q32–qter
Yt	COL1A2	Collagen, type 1, alpha-2	7q21.3–q22.1
Yt	D7S13	DNA segment, single copy, probe pB79a locus	7q22.3–q31.2
LW	LDLR	Low density lipoprotein receptor locus	19p13.2–p13.1
Recombination established†			
Rh	FUCA1	Fucosidase, alpha-L-1, tissue	1p35–p34
Fy	SPTA1	Spectrin, alpha, erythrocytic 1	1q21
Jk	D18S6	DNA segment, single copy, probe L 2.7	18p11
Co	ASSP11	Argininosuccinate synthetase pseudogene 11	7p
Ch/Rg	HLA	Major histocompatibility complex	6p21.3
Sc	MYCL1	Avian myelocytomatosis viral (v-myc) oncogene homologue 1, lung carcinoma-derived	1p32

* Recombination between the blood group locus and the DNA markers has yet to be observed.
† Recombination fraction 1–10%.

those subjects negative for the red cell group (Mourant, 1977). The first of such associations to be established was that between group A and carcinoma of the stomach (Aird and Bentall, 1953), the risk of group A subjects being 1.2 times that of group O or B subjects (see review by Roberts, 1957). An association of interest to haematologists is that between the level of Factor VIII and ABO group, the level being slightly higher in A than in O subjects (Preston and Barr, 1964).

Red cell markers on functionally important membrane structures

Some red cell antigens are situated on important structures on the cell membrane so that absence or presence of the antigen is associated with some structural abnormality of the cell, associated with functional change. Examples of such associations are as follows: (a) between Rh_{null} or Rh_{mod} and haemolytic anaemia (see Chapter 5); (b) between the rare McLeod phenotype (see Kell blood group system, Chapter 6) and acanthocytosis; (c) between absence or depression of certain red cell antigens and elliptocytosis (see Chapter 6); (d) between Fy-related antigens and susceptibility to malaria (see Chapter 6); (e) between Cr-null (Inab phenotype) red cells and absence of decay accelerating factor (see Chapter 6); and (f) between expression of the normally hidden antigen Tn and deficiency of sialic acid (see Chapter 7).

A P-like structure acts as a receptor on uroepithelial cells for strains of *Escherichia coli* responsible for pyelonephritis, and p individuals may be protected against infections with such bacteria (Källenius *et al.*1981).

Effect of neoplastic change and dyserythropoiesis on blood group antigens

Cell surface antigens and neoplastic change
Neoplastic change in cells may be accompanied by changes in cell surface antigens. Some of these changes are due to incomplete synthesis of antigens normally present; others are due to abnormal synthesis, giving rise to neoantigens. As an example of the first kind of change, in some subjects with acute leukaemia, A, B and I antigens may be depressed (see Chapter 4); similarly, in some subjects with carcinoma, ABH determinants are lost due to incomplete synthesis, and precursor substances accumulate (Hakomori, 1984a).

The first recorded example of the production of a neoantigen by malignant tissue was that of Levine *et al.* (1951a). The patient was a woman with a gastric adenocarcinoma whose serum contained the rare antibody anti-Tj^a (later renamed anti-PP$_1$P^k). As expected, the patient's red cells were Tj(a −) but a dried extract of the tumour specifically inhibited the antibody in her serum, suggesting that Tj^a antigen had been formed by the malignant tissue and might have evoked production of the anti-Tj^a. Thirty years later, biochemical analysis on lyophilized tumour tissue showed that glycolipids with P and P$_1$ activity were present (Hakomori, 1984a). Similarly, some tumours derived from gastrointestinal tissue of group O or B individuals contain an A-like antigen, different from Forsmann antigen, and some tumours from Forsmann-negative tissue contain Forsmann antigen, which is similar to blood group A (Hakomori, 1984a). The overlapping functions of *A* and *B* transferases provide an explanation for the apparent expression of blood group antigens in certain tumours; changes in biochemical pathways in tumour tissue may provide appropriate substrates for the transfer of the 'wrong' sugars, giving rise to A or B antigens not expected from the ABO genotype of the individual (Yates *et al.* 1983).

Various types of human adenocarcinoma accumulate a large quantity of fucolipids and their sialylated derivatives as well as fucosylated glycoproteins with type II chains (see Chapter 4). Various monoclonal antibodies directed against these structures have been produced and may prove to be useful diagnostic and therapeutic tools.

Dyserythropoiesis
In acquired dyserythropoiesis associated with a variety of haematological disorders (e.g. megaloblastic anaemia, sideroblastic anaemia) there is an increase in i and, in tests with some antisera, of I. In inherited dyserythropoietic anaemia of type I and type II (HEMPAS), i is increased but I is probably not increased; see review by Worlledge (1977).

Myeloproliferative disease
Myeloproliferative disease is thought to be due to a mutation of haemopoietic stem

cells, giving rise to an abnormal clone of cells. In several cases, Rh mosaicism has been observed; e.g. in a patient whose probable genotype was originally *CDe/cde*, a proportion of the red cells typed as D negative (Mannoni *et al.* 1970). In a case described by Copper *et al.* (1979), a man who had originally been D positive was found to have become D negative (his red cells still reacted with anti-c and anti-e). An anomaly was found involving chromosome 1, on which the *Rh* gene is known to be located. The patient developed anti-D (and -C) following transfusion, demonstrating loss of immunological tolerance to self antigens following the loss of ability to express these antigens.

Tn polyagglutination (Chapter 7), which is a form of mosaicism affecting red cells (and other blood cells), has also been observed in myelofibrosis (Bird *et al.* 1985).

Development of red cell antigens

Red cell antigens in embryos and newborn infants
During ontogeny, ABH and Lewis activity is at its highest from the fifth week after fertilization. ABH antigens are found in large amounts on endothelial cells, on most epithelial primordia, and in practically all early organs, e.g. in the blood islands of the yolk sac, on digestive tube epithelia, etc. The central nervous system, liver, adrenal glands and secretory tubules show no activity at this stage. From the end of the 12th–14th week of gestation, there is regression of ABH expression from epithelial cell walls and from thyroid and other glands and organs (Szulman, 1980). Similarly, although P_1 is only weakly expressed on the red cells of newborn infants, on the red cells of embryos with a crown–rump length of less than 10 cm it is expressed almost as strongly as in the adult (Ikin *et al.* 1961). The reason for the regression of expression of these various antigens is unknown.

I, Le^a, Le^b and Sd^a are very weakly expressed on the red cells of newborn infants, and A, B, P_1, Lu^a, Lu^b, Yt^a, Xg and Vel are more weakly expressed on infants' red cells than on adults' red cells.

The antigens of the Rh, K, Fy, Jk, MNSs, Di, Do and Sc systems, as well as Co^a and Au^a, appear to be fully developed at birth (Race and Sanger, 1975).

Red cell antigens on red cell precursors
Reticulocytes appear to be as strongly agglutinated as mature red cells by anti-A and anti-B (Maizels and Patterson, 1940; Winkelstein and Mollison, 1965). Although A can be demonstrated even on early erythroblasts (Reyes *et al.* 1974; Gourdin *et al.* 1976), anti-A and anti-B do not inhibit the growth of colony forming units (CFU-c) or blood forming units (BFU-E) *in vitro* (Hershko *et al.* 1980), nor do they delay the engraftment of ABO-incompatible bone marrow *in vivo* (Dinsmore *et al.* 1983). The following red cell antigens have also been demonstrated on erythroblasts: A_1, B and H (Yunis and Yunis, 1963), I and those of the Rh, MNSs, P, Lu, K, Le Fy and Jk systems (Yunis and Yunis, 1964). The amount of D antigen on pronormoblasts is about one-quarter as great as that on mature red cells (Rearden and Masouredis, 1977).

It seems that the onset of Hb synthesis and expression of glycophorin at the cell surface occur at the same stage of differentiation (Gahmberg *et al.* 1978).

RED CELL ANTIBODIES

Antibodies are Igs, a family of proteins that are structurally related and all of which have two functions: (1) to combine with antigen; and (2) to mediate various biological effects. Thus, all antibody molecules have antigen-combining sites and various effector function sites.

The common structural feature of all Ig molecules is an arrangement of a pair of identical, relatively large, 'heavy' (H) polypeptide chains joined, by covalent (disulphide) and non-covalent bonds, to each other and to a pair of identical 'light' (L) chains (Fig. 3.3). The covalent bonds are mainly in the hinge region (see below). Five different classes of Ig are recognized, IgG, IgM, IgA, IgD and IgE, and these have different H chains, termed γ, μ, α, δ and ε. Igs of all five classes have the same L chains, although these may be either kappa (κ) or lambda (λ). In each IgG molecule the two L chains are the same, e.g. a molecule may be $\gamma\gamma\kappa\kappa$ or $\gamma\gamma\lambda\lambda$. IgG molecules occur as monomers, IgM molecules as pentamers, e.g. $(\mu_2\lambda_2)_5$ (see below), and IgA molecules as monomers or dimers. All Ig molecules have carbohydrate (CHO) attached to their H chains. For example, in IgG there is a short-branched CHO chain (approximately nine residues) attached to each H chain in the $C\gamma2$ domain (see Fig. 3.4). The CHO chains lie in

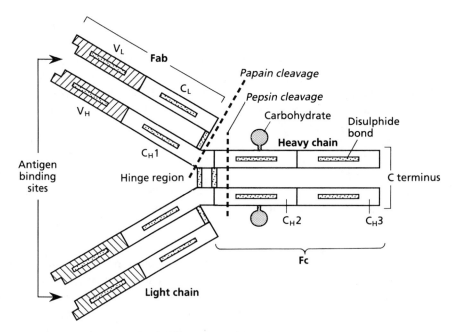

Figure 3.3 Diagram of IgG molecule. The constant (C) and variable (V) domains of the heavy (H) and light (L) chains are shown, together with the intra- and inter-chain disulphide bonds (⊏⊐) which hold them together. The antigen-binding site is situated in the groove between the terminal parts of the V_H and V_L regions. The sites of attachment of carbohydrate chains are shown (◯), although the diagram does not indicate that these chains are more than half as long as the domain to which they are attached. After treatment with papain, the IgG molecule is cleaved into two Fab fragments and one Fc fragment; after treatment with pepsin, the two Fab fragments remain joined by disulphide bonds as a (Fab)$_2$ fragment and the Fc fragment disintegrates. Slightly modified from Roitt *et al.* (1989).

the space between the two $C\gamma2$ domains and may help to keep them apart. IgM has short CHO chains attached to each of the constant domains. The function of these CHO chains is not definitely known although there is often loss of functional activity when the CHO is absent.

H and L chains are made up of regions ('domains'), each of about 110 amino acids with the same basic structure. Both H and L chains take part in combining with antigen. The first 110–120 amino acids at the amino-terminal end of each chain form the variable (V) domains, each of which contains hypervariable regions (four for H chains and three for L chains). The hypervariable regions on a pair of H and L chains, each consisting of fewer than ten amino acids, come together in the folded molecule to form the antigen-binding site. The peptide sequences joining the hypervariable regions do not take part in binding to antigen but form an essential framework. The rest of the H and L chains are constant regions (C_H and C_L) with characteristic amino acid sequences. IgG and IgA have three constant regions per H chain but IgM and IgE have four; L chains each have only one C region. The different biological activities of each class of Ig molecule are affected by the amino acid sequences of the C regions. Flexibility is conferred on Ig molecules by a hinge region which, in IgG, is situated between the $C\gamma1$ and $C\gamma2$ domains (see Figs 3.3 and 3.4) and in IgM in the $C\mu2$ domain (Fig 3.5). Flexibility is believed to be very important in enabling the molecule to fulfil its effector functions.

In IgG1 and IgG3, the site for binding C1q, and thus for activating the complement pathway (see later), is found on $C\gamma2$, as is the site for binding to Fc receptors on mononuclear phagocytic cells. Sites on both the $C\gamma2$ and $C\gamma3$ domains are involved in binding IgG to Fc receptors on placental tissue. The CHO of IgG molecules is also attached to the $C\gamma2$ domain. In IgM, the site for binding C1q is on the C_H3 domains.

By treatment with papain, the IgG molecule can be split, between the $C\gamma1$ and $C\gamma2$ domains (Fig. 3.3), into two Fab (fragment antigen-binding) fragments, each of which carries a single antigen-combining site, and one Fc (fragment crystallizable) fragment which carries sites for various effector functions (see above). As Fig. 3.3 implies, the Fab fragment consist of the whole of the L chain and part of the H chain; in both chains, regions (V_L and V_H) at the amino-terminal end of the fragment are joined to the single C region of the L chain and the $C\gamma1$ region of the H chain. IgG can also be split into fragments by pepsin but in this case the molecule is cleaved nearer the carboxy-terminal end (Fig. 3.3) and the two Fab fragments are left joined together to form an F(ab')$_2$ fragment, the rest of the molecule being broken up.

Some characteristics of different immunoglobulins

IgG

IgG is the most abundant Ig in plasma, having a mean concentration of about 12 g/l (range 8–16 g/l), so that the total plasma content, taking the plasma volume to be 40 ml/kg, is about 0.5 g/kg or, in a subject weighing 70 kg, 35 g; there is an approximately equal amount of IgG in the extravascular space, so that, in the example taken, total body IgG would be about 70 g, or 1 g/kg. The rate of transfer of IgG between the extra- and intravascular compartments is described briefly in Chapter 14 and the daily production in Chapter 1.

IgG is the only Ig to be transferred across the placenta from mother to fetus, a fact which explains the role of IgG antibodies in the aetiology of alloimmune cytopenias of the fetus and newborn.

Four subclasses of IgG are recognized and their mean concentrations in normal adult serum (in g/l) are as follows: IgG1, 6.63; IgG2, 3.22; IgG3, 0.58; IgG4, 0.46 (Morell *et al*. 1971). The subclasses differ in structure and function; thus, the number of inter-H-chain disulphide bonds varies in the different subclasses and, for example, IgG3 differs from the other subclasses in having a much larger hinge region (Fig. 3.4). Monomeric IgG1 and IgG3 bind to the Fc receptor, FcRI; polymeric IgG1 and IgG3 bind, in addition, to FcRII and FcRIII (see p. 132). IgG2 and IgG4 bind only weakly to FcRII. IgG1 and IgG3 activate complement strongly but IgG2 activates only weakly and IgG4 not at all. IgG1, IgG2 and IgG3 have catabolic rates which are similar to those of total IgG, i.e. they have a $t_{1/2}$ of about 21 d but the $t_{1/2}$ of IgG3 is about 7 d (Morell *et al*. 1970). These estimates are derived from studies with myeloma proteins and will not necessarily be confirmed by studies with monoclonal antibodies.

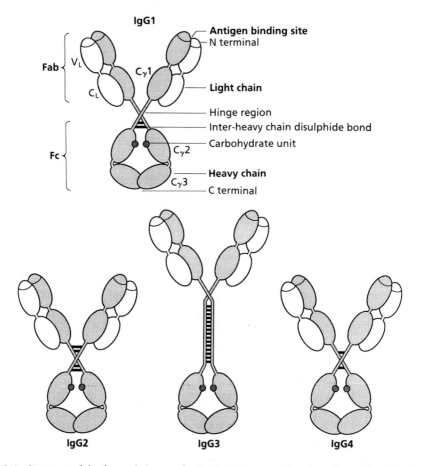

Figure 3.4 Structure of the four subclasses of IgG. The arrangement and number of the inter-heavy-chain disulphide bonds are different in each of the subclasses. In IgG3 the hinge region is much longer than in the other subclasses (from Roitt *et al*. 1989).

IgM

The plasma concentration of IgM is 0.5–2.0 g/l; about 74% of total body IgM is intravascular; the plasma $t_{1/2}$ is 5 d. IgM molecules are held together by a J (joining) chain (Fig. 3.5).

IgM is more effective than IgG in activating complement. The difference is due to the fact that C1 is activated only when it is attached by two of its C1q heads to the activating molecule. Thus, whereas a single bound IgM molecule can activate C1, two IgG molecules bound at closely adjacent sites are needed. Several of the antigen-binding sites on a single IgM molecule may bind to antigen sites on the cell surface, giving the molecule the appearance of a staple (Fig. 3.5b), in contrast to the normal star form shown in Fig. 3.5a.

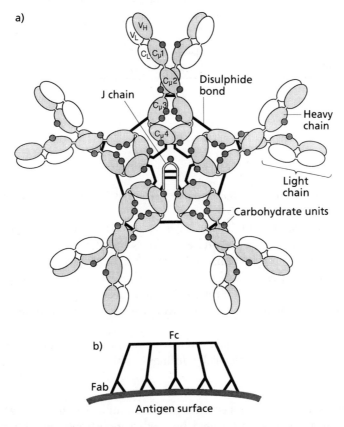

Figure 3.5 (a) Diagram of IgM molecule, to show the way in which the five subunits are held together by disulphide bonds and joined by joining, J chain. As in Fig. 3.3, the position of attachment of carbohydrate chains is shown but their size and structure are not indicated. Slightly modified from Roitt *et al.* (1989).

(b) Staple form (as opposed to star form shown in (a)) of IgM molecule. This configuration is observed when the molecule binds to a surface on which antigen sites are sufficiently close together to permit two or more antigen-combining sites of the same IgM molecule to bind (Feinstein *et al.* 1971).

Table 3.5 The main immunoglobulins in serum

	IgG	IgM	IgA
Heavy chains	γ	μ	α
Light chains	κ and λ	κ and λ	κ and λ
Molecular forms	$\gamma_2\kappa_2$	$(\mu_2\kappa_2)_5$J	$\alpha_2\kappa_2$
	$\gamma_2\lambda_2$	$(\mu_2\lambda_2)_5$J	$\alpha_2\lambda_2$
Mol. wt.	150 000	970 000	160 000
Sedimentation coefficient	7S	19S	7S
Concentration in plasma (g/l)			
Adult*	8–16	0.5–2.0	1.4–4.0
Newborn	Similar	Approx. 0.1	Undetectable
Catabolic rate, $t_{1/2}$ (d)[†]	21	5	6
Percentage of total which is intravascular[†]	52	74	40
Transferred across placenta?	Yes	No	No
Usual serological behaviour as red cell antibody	Incomplete antibody	Agglutinin	?
Serological activity after heating to 56°C for 3 h	Unaffected	Reduced	Unaffected
Effect of reducing agents on serological activity	May develop agglutinating activity	No longer agglutinates	Partially inactivated

* Roitt (1988).
[†] Wells (1980).
J = J chain.

IgA

The plasma concentration of IgA is 1.4–4.0 g/l; about 40% of total body IgA is intravascular; the plasma $t_{1/2}$ is 6 d.

IgA is the only Ig present in epithelial secretions. Whereas, in plasma, IgA is predominantly monomeric, in secretions it occurs mainly as dimers, which are held together by a J chain. In secretions, IgA has a 'secretory piece' which prevents the molecule from being digested. The presence of IgA in secretions is believed to be due almost entirely to local production rather than to transport from plasma. The function of IgA is evidently to neutralize antigens which might otherwise enter the body via mucosal routes.

There are two subclasses of IgA, a major component, IgA1, and a minor component, IgA2, which has two serologically distinguishable variants, A2m(1) and A2m(2).

IgD and IgE

Both of these Igs act mainly as cell receptors. No antibodies made of IgD have been described, although IgD is synthesized by, and demonstrable on, the surface of B lymphocytes and is probably involved in the activation of these cells by antigen.

IgE is synthesized by plasma cells and is present in the plasma in very low concentrations. It has a very high affinity for Fc receptors on basophils and mast cells. The binding of antigen to IgE antibody on the surface of these cells produces release of histamine and other substances, e.g. leukotrienes, known to have far greater vaso-active effects (Dahlen *et al.* 1981) and to be responsible for producing such atopic phenomena as asthma and hay fever. The role of IgE antibodies in reactions to atopens is discussed in Chapter 15.

Markers on immunoglobulin molecules

Idiotypic markers. Idiotypic determinants arise from the unique configuration of the antigen-combining site of an antibody molecule which gives the molecule its specificity.

The idio*type* of a particular antibody specificity is composed of several individual determinants called idio*topes*, in much the same way that the Rh antigens expressed by the R^1 haplotype encompasses several Rh determinants (e.g. C, D, G, e, Rh34, Hr_o, Rh17, Rh29, Rh44, Rh46, Rh47, etc.). Some of the individual idiotopes arise from the unique amino acid sequences in the hypervariable region that come into contact with the antigen in the antibody-binding site; others arise from framework amino acid sequences. Antisera can be raised to both sets of idiotopes.

Some idiotypes (public idiotypes) are common to all antibodies of a single specificity; each individual can make 10^6–10^7 different antibody specificities. Other idiotypes (private idiotypes) are restricted to only a few clones producing antibodies of similar specificity but each differing slightly (by one or two amino acids) in their hypervariable region; a typical polyclonal immune response can be composed of 10^4 different species of antibody molecules of similar specificity, each species being the product of a separate B cell clone. Sometimes, antibodies of quite distinct specificities, e.g. anti-albumin and anti-influenza virus, can exhibit common idiotypes; these are called the major crossreactive idiotypes (CRI) and represent common amino acid sequences in the framework regions of their binding sites.

Every antibody is capable of inducing the formation of auto- or allo- anti-idiotype antibodies. The formation of auto-anti-idiotypes is believed to be important in regulating the immune response.

Allotypic markers are antigens, found on γ, α and κ chains, the inheritance of some of which is controlled by alleles of the gene coding for a particular Ig chain. For example, H chains of IgG subclass 1 can carry either G1m(z) or G1m(f), the difference being determined by a single amino acid substitution. Further details are given in Chapter 13.

Isotypic markers are antigenic determinants on H chains and on certain L chains which define and characterize the class or subclass of Ig molecules and which are sequences on the C region of γ and μ chains or on the C region of κ and λ chains. Isoallotypic markers (formerly called non-markers) are those which are isotypic markers for one subclass but are allotypic markers in another subclass. For example, G4m(a) is an allotype in subclass IgG4 but is an isotype in IgG2.

Immunoglobulins in fluids other than plasma

Colostrum and saliva. In colostrum the IgA concentration is about 90% and in saliva is about 20% of that in normal serum (Chodirker and Tomasi, 1963). By contrast, concentrations of IgG and IgM in colostrum are respectively 1% and 5–10% of the amounts in normal serum, and in saliva only faint traces of IgG and IgM are present (Adinolfi *et al.* 1966).

The titre of IgA antibody tends to be higher in colostrum than in serum (Tomasi *et al.* 1965; Adinolfi *et al.* 1966). Colostrum frequently contains potent IgA anti-A and anti-B, but in saliva these antibodies are usually present only in low concentration (see Chapter 4).

Ascitic fluid. Several alloantibodies have been harvested from ascitic fluid; anti-Yt[a] (Eaton *et al.* 1956); anti-c and -Le[a] (M.M. Pickles, quoted by Race and Sanger, 1968, p. 255); anti-E (Zeitlin *et al.* 1958) and anti-K (Longster and Major, 1975). In the last mentioned case the titre of the antibody was about the same in serum as in ascitic fluid and the antibody was probably IgG; in contrast to those of anti-K, the titres of anti-A and anti-B were slightly lower in ascitic fluid than in serum.

Amniotic fluid. The IgG concentration at or near term is about 0.1–0.2 g/l, i.e. 1/50–1/100 of that in normal adult serum.

Production of immunoglobulin in the fetus and infant
Changes in Ig levels in the first year of life are summarized in Fig. 3.6.

IgG. Although most of the IgG in the serum of newborn infants is derived from the mother by placental transfer, a small amount is of fetal origin as shown by the fact that it has the father's Gm allotype (Mårtensson and Fudenberg, 1965).

The time at which the synthesis of substantial amounts of IgG begins after birth was studied by Zak and Good (1959) in two normal infants born to mothers with severe hypogammaglobulinaemia. The IgG level, which was negligible at birth, started to increase between 3 and 6 weeks; antibodies were first demonstrable at about 2 months, by which time the IgG level had reached 2 g/l. At 10–18 months, IgG levels are about 60% of adult values (Buckley *et al.* 1968).

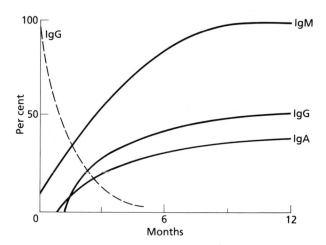

Figure 3.6 Concentration of IgG, IgM and IgA in the first year of life, as percentages of the normal adult levels (based on the data of West *et al.* 1962). The dotted line indicates IgG derived from the mother by placental transfer.

IgM. IgM is not transferred across the placenta. The concentration in cord serum is between 5% and 10% of that found in adult serum (Franklin and Kunkel, 1958; Polley *et al.* 1962).

IgM antibodies of various specificities can be found in cord serum: anti-I in most infants (see Chapter 7); anti-A and anti-B in occasional infants (see Chapter 4); anti-Gm in most infants (see Chapter 13) and anti-λ chain in about 10% of infants (Epstein, 1965).

Within 2 or 3 d of birth the concentration of IgM starts to rise and reaches 50% of the adult level at 2–3 months and 100% at about 9 months; between the ages of 9 months and 3 years values remain at the adult level, although between 5 and 9 years they are at the lower end of the adult range (West *et al.* 1962).

IgA. This protein cannot be detected in cord serum. By the age of 2 months the amount in the serum has reached about 20% of the adult level (West *et al.* 1962), and by the age of 5 years about 50% (Buckley *et al.* 1968).

Immunoglobulin class and subclass of red cell alloantibodies
Red cell alloantibodies may be naturally occurring or immune. When naturally occurring they are most often IgM but may be partly IgG or, occasionally, predominantly IgG (see also p. 102); when immune they are most often IgG but may be IgM or a mixture of IgM and IgG; they are sometimes partly IgA. The cells of a single clone can make IgM and IgG antibodies of the same specificity.

Determination of the subclass of antibodies is difficult. There is more than 95% sequence homology between most of the C regions of human IgG subclasses. There are therefore few subclass specific epitopes and it is difficult to raise antibodies against them (Michaelsen and Kornstad, 1987). If insufficiently absorbed sera are used, false-positive results are obtained. If well absorbed sera are used, some antibodies fail to react with any subclass sera.

Investigations of the subclass composition of different blood group antibodies are referred to in the three following chapters.

Immunoglobulins on B lymphocytes
The Ig on the surface of lymphocytes gives them the capacity to react with an antigen of corresponding specificity and to develop into active antibody-secreting cells. The two major classes of Ig demonstrable on the surface of immature B lymphocytes are IgM and IgD; the latter appears to have a role in triggering the cell's response to antigen.

In subjects immunized to Rh D, anti-D-bearing lymphocytes can be demonstrated by incubating D-positive red cells with the blood of the immunized subjects and observing 'rosettes', i.e. single lymphocytes surrounded by many adherent erythrocytes. Rosetting could be demonstrated in two of eight women immunized by pregnancy and in five of five hyperimmunized volunteers following a booster injection of red cells; in these latter subjects the number of rosettes increased to a maximum on about the tenth day after restimulation (Elson and Bradley, 1970).

Methods of separating and identifying immunoglobulins
Immunoglobulins may be separated according to their different charges, e.g. by

ion-exchange chromatography, or by their different sizes, e.g. by passage through a 'molecular sieve' as in gel filtration.

Some of these methods are employed in plasma fractionation, e.g. separation on diethylaminoethyl (DEAE)-cellulose is used in one method of preparing anti-D Ig (Hoppe *et al.* 1973). The method gives a high yield of a product suitable for i.v. use.

Some IgG antibodies can be separated from one another by fractionation on carboxymethyl (CM) cellulose or hydroxyapatite columns, and results with these methods will be briefly described since the methods do not seem to have been fully exploited so far.

Fractionation of IgG on carboxymethyl cellulose or hydroxyapatite columns. Anti-D is more positively charged than the bulk of the IgG in serum (Abelson and Rawson, 1959; Frame and Mollison, 1969), and can thus be partially separated from it by fractionation on an appropriate ion-exchange column. For example, if serum containing anti-D is fractionated on a CM-cellulose column by elution with phosphate buffers, pH 6.6, of increasing molarity, the bulk of the IgG is eluted with 60–80 mmol/l-phosphate whereas most of the anti-D is eluted with 150 mmol/l-phosphate (Fig. 3.7). Other antibodies eluted with 150 mmol/l-phosphate are anti-E, anti-Fy[a] and anti-Jk[a] (Frame and Mollison, 1969) and anti-C (Skov and Hughes-Jones, 1977). Examples of anti-c were eluted with 60–100 mmol/l-buffer (Frame and Mollison, 1969). Similarly, anti-f (ce) was found to have a charge intermediate between anti-D and the bulk of the IgG; isoelectric points were as follows: IgG, 8.6–8.9; anti-f, 8.8–9.1; and anti-D, 8.8–9.6 (R. Perrault, personal communication). Anti-A, -B and -K are eluted with the bulk of the IgG (Frame and Mollison, 1969).

Concordant results have been reported using hydroxyapatite columns, with phosphate buffers pH 6.8 (Jungfer, 1970). With 80 mmol/l-buffer, anti-A, anti-B and anti-K were eluted and with 250 mmol/l-buffer, anti-D, anti-E, anti-C and anti-c. One

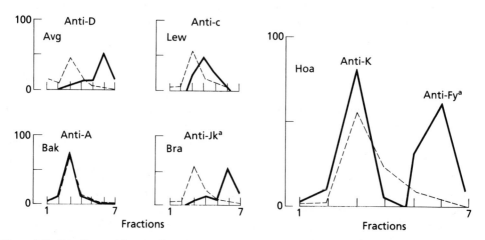

Figure 3.7 Distribution of total IgG (– – – –) and of particular antibodies (——) in fractions eluted from carboxymethyl-cellulose (using buffers of increasing molarity), expressed as percentages of the total amount recovered from the columns. The letters on each small figure (e.g. Avg) identify the donor of the serum. The four small figures show the distribution of single antibodies in four sera; the larger right-hand figure shows the elution of two antibodies from one serum (from Frame and Mollison, 1969).

example of anti-M was eluted mainly with 125 mmol/l-buffer and one example of anti-e was found in all three fractions.

Sela and Moses (1966) presented evidence of a relation between the net electric charge on antigens and the electric charge on the antibodies which they elicited in rabbits. This observation suggests that the differences in the charge on the antibody are determined by differences in the antigen-combining site. It is not known whether this interpretation applies to the differences observed with human alloantibodies or whether the charge differences are due to differences in other regions of the antibody molecule, e.g. differences in IgG subclass.

Identification of immunoglobulins using the antiglobulin test
Determination of the Ig class of red cell antibodies is most conveniently performed using Ig class-specific antiglobulin reagents (Polley *et al.* 1962; Adinolfi *et al.* 1966; see also Chapter 8).

Selective inactivation of IgM antibodies by treatment with sulphydryl compounds
Treatment of serum with sulphydryl compounds is a convenient method of inactivating IgM antibodies (see below).

Effect on IgM. Mild reduction of human IgM with sulphydryl compounds cleaves intersubunit (IgMs–IgMs), intersubunit-J chain, and intrasubunit (H-H, H-L) disulphide bonds. Intersubunit bonds are more sensitive than intrasubunit bonds to reduction. Mild reduction releases J chain from the IgM molecule.

IgM subunits (e.g. $\mu_2\lambda_2$) produced by mild reduction of IgM have a greatly reduced agglutinating activity (see review of Metzger, 1970); in fact, treatment of serum with a reducing agent abolishes the agglutinating activity of most IgM antibodies (Grubb and Swahn, 1958).

IgM subunits of anti-D, anti-A and anti-B retain their ability to combine with red cell antigens (Chan and Deutsch, 1960; Jacot-Guillarmod and Isliker, 1964; Economidou *et al.* 1967c; Holburn *et al.* 1971b) but subunits of IgM anti-Le[a] have no serological activity, indicating that their binding affinity is very low (Holburn, 1973).

If a monoclonal IgM is mildly reduced and then dialysed against saline to remove the reducing agent, the subunits may slowly reassemble, if the suspending medium does not contain non-specific IgM. It would therefore be expected that if a purified IgM antibody, e.g. an eluate, were treated in the same way, the serological activity of the antibody would be partially restored. On the other hand, when an IgM antibody in whole serum is mildly reduced and the serum is then dialysed, restoration of serological activity is not expected, because the subunits of IgM reassemble at random and most of the IgM molecules in the serum are of different antibody specificities.

The reassembly of IgM subunits to form 19S IgM can be prevented by treatment with alkylating agents, such as iodoacetamide (IAA). Such agents irreversibly block the SH groups which have been liberated by reduction of the protein, as well as any free SH groups originally present.

Effect on IgG. After mild reduction, some IgG incomplete antibodies such as anti-D become weakly agglutinating (Chan and Deutsch, 1960; Pirofsky and Cordova, 1963; Romans *et al.* 1977). The changes in the properties of the IgG molecule are brought about by the breaking of the disulphide bonds in the hinge region of the molecule, permitting the two antigen-binding sites to move further apart and thus bridge the distance between red cells. The two halves of the molecule remain held together by strong non-covalent bonds between the C_H3 domains (see Fig. 3.3). Reduced IgG3 anti-D monoclonals are more potent direct agglutinators than reduced IgG1 anti-D monoclonals (Scott et al. 1989).

The modification of the properties of the IgG molecule produced by mild reduction are stabilized by treatment with alkylating reagents (e.g. IAA).

Treatment of IgG antibodies with reducing agents diminishes the ability of the antibody to bind complement but the effect seems to vary with different antibodies (Schur and Christian, 1964; Nagashima et al. 1965). Dithiothreitol (DTT) treatment also reduces reactivity with some monoclonal subclassing reagents (S. Garner, personal communication).

Practical applications. Treatment of serum with the reducing agents 2-mercaptoethanol (2-ME), DTT or its isomer dithioerythritol (DTE), is commonly used in blood-group serology to distinguish between IgG and IgM antibodies since if the agglutinating activity is abolished it is virtually certain that the antibody in question is IgM.

DTT is preferred to 2-ME for the following reasons: first, it is more efficient in maintaining reduction; second, it is more resistant to oxidation in air; and third, it lacks an offensive odour. Nevertheless, treatment of serum with an equal volume of 0.2 mol/l 2-ME was found to be slightly better than treatment with an equal volume of 0.01 mol/l DTT in reducing IgM antibodies by Freedman et al. (1976). These authors noted that higher concentrations of these reducing agents could not be used because they caused gelling of the serum. They also emphasized the advantage of treating serum at 37°C rather than at room temperature.

Serum that has been treated with 2-ME may be tested for agglutination without preliminary dialysis (Reesink et al. 1972), although if the mixture of undiluted serum and 2-ME is tested by the indirect antiglobulin test, false-positive reactions occur (Freedman et al. 1976). False-positive reactions also occur occasionally if DTT-treated undiluted serum is left with red cells for more than 2 h. False-positive reactions are not observed when dilutions of 2-ME-treated or DTT-treated serum are tested. Details of methods of treating serum with DTT are given on p. 371. The use of reduced IgG anti-D in agglutination tests is discussed on p. 329.

Heat lability of different immunoglobulins

Heating at 56°C for 3 h has little effect on anti-D (IgG) but produces a just detectable fall in anti-P_1 titre (IgM). Heating at 63°C for 3 h decreases the IgG anti-D titre by about one-third whereas heating at 63°C for only 1 h almost completely inactivates anti-P_1 (Adinolfi, 1965a). IgA antibodies, like IgG antibodies, are unaffected by heating at 56°C for 3 h (Adinolfi et al. 1966).

Naturally occurring antibodies

An antibody is said to be naturally occurring if it is found in the serum of an individual who has never been transfused or injected with red cells containing the relevant antigen or been pregnant with a fetus carrying the relevant antigen.

Specificities of naturally occurring antibodies

ABO, Lewis and P systems. Apart from anti-A, -B, -H, $-PP_1P^k$ and $-P^k$, found in virtually all subjects who lack the corresponding antigens, antibodies of several specificities, e.g. anti-A_1, -Le^a and -P_1 occur relatively frequently and others, e.g. anti-HI, rarely. For further details see Chapter 4.

Rh system. Antibodies of several specificities are found, the commonest being anti-E. For further details see Chapter 5.

Other blood group systems. The commonest are anti-Sd^a, found in 1–2% of normal people, and anti-V^w and anti-Wr^a, each found in about 1%. Others found much more rarely include, in approximate descending order of frequency, anti-M, -S, -N, -Ge, -K, -Lu^a, -Di^a and -Xg^a. For further details see Chapter 6.

What is the stimulus for production of naturally occurring antibodies?
Two explanations may be offered for the presence in serum of naturally occurring alloantibodies reacting with red cells: (1) they may be heteroagglutinins produced as an immune response to substances in the environment which are antigenically identical with, or similar to, red cell alloantigens; this explanation was offered by Wiener (1951b) to explain the presence of anti-A and -B in human serum. Evidence that some naturally occurring antibodies are of this kind is supplied by the observation that their formation is prevented by rearing animals in a germ-free environment.

In 'germ-free' chicks, no heteroagglutinins against group B human red cells developed in the first 60 d of life whereas in ordinary chicks such agglutinins usually develop within the first 30 d. In germ-free chicks anti-B developed promptly after the administration by mouth of *Escherichia coli* O_{86}, the antibodies had serological characteristics similar to the 'naturally occurring' agglutinins; that is, they reacted slightly more strongly at 0°C than at 37°C. In germ-free chicks, very weak agglutinins developed 2–3 months after hatching but this was attributed to traces of non-living antigenic contaminants.

Although the stimulus to the formation of these naturally occurring agglutinins was traced to the environment, the authors pointed out that there was evidence that the time of onset and extent of the response depended upon genetic factors (Springer *et al.* 1959).

A direct demonstration that anti-B titres can be increased in humans by the ingestion or inhalation of suitable bacteria was provided by Springer and Horton (1969). In one series of experiments, killed *E. coli* O_{86}, with blood group B specificity, were fed to infants in the first few months of life. An eight-fold increase in anti-B titre was observed in 11 of 16 infants with diarrhoea but in only one of seven healthy infants. When the same bacteria were fed to adults, increases in anti-B titre were observed in several healthy subjects and in four of four subjects with intestinal disease. Four of 12 adults showed an increase in anti-B titre after receiving a nasal spray of *E. coli* O_{86}. Similar observations have been reported for anti-T and anti-Tn (Springer and Tegtmeyer, 1981).

The formation of naturally occurring anti-K may be due to infection with an organism producing K-like substance (see Chapter 6).

Although substances other than red cells capable of stimulating the formation of Rh antibodies in humans have not been described, it seems possible that they exist; see, for example, the finding of anti-E in only one of identical twins (Hopkins, 1971).

(2) The possibility that some naturally occurring antibodies are made without an environmental stimulus seems to be raised by the finding that antibodies against a great variety of antigens (many of them self antigens) are present in normal serum (Guilbert et al. 1982). Moreover, many alloantibodies against antigens which seem unlikely to be present in the environment are now known to be relatively commonly present in human serum, e.g. anti-E in about 0.1% of D-positive donors (see Chapter 5) and anti-HLA in about 1% of normal donors (see Chapter 13).

An example of the production of specific red cell alloantibodies without a corresponding specific stimulus is provided by the formation of antibodies to low-incidence antigens in autoimmune haemolytic anaemia; in such patients antibodies to Wr^a, Sw^a, C^x, Mi^a and Vw are commonly present (Cleghorn, 1960).

Naturally occurring antibodies and class of immunoglobulin
Most, but by no means all, naturally occurring antibodies are cold agglutinins even though immune antibodies of the same specificity are either warm agglutinins or warm incomplete antibodies. As expected from this observation the majority of naturally occurring antibodies are IgM.

Anti-A and anti-B are always partly IgM and may be wholly IgM; in group O subjects anti-A and -B are always partly IgG and may be partly IgA. Anti-A_1 in A_2 and A_2B subjects seems always to be wholly IgM, but anti-A_1 separated from group O serum may be only IgG (see Chapter 5). Examples of anti-HI and -H have been solely IgM (Adinolfi et al. 1962; Chattoraj et al. 1968a).

Although most examples of anti-Le^a behave on ordinary serological testing as if they were solely IgM, an IgG component can often be demonstrated by appropriate methods. Rare examples of anti-Le^a and -Le^b are solely IgG.

Naturally occurring antibodies of the MNSs system are usually IgM but some examples of naturally occurring anti-M have been at least partly IgG.

In the past, many examples of naturally occurring anti-E were considered to be solely IgM because they gave a negative indirect antiglobulin test but, with the introduction of more sensitive methods, an IgG component is usually detectable and some examples may be solely IgG. Rather surprisingly, cold-reacting anti-D, demonstrable in the AutoAnalyzer, has been found to be IgG. References supporting the foregoing statements and further details will be found in Chapters 4–6.

Naturally occurring antibodies to low-frequency antigens (e.g. anti-Wr^a) are mainly IgM but a large proportion of them have an IgG component and some are solely IgG (Lubenko and Contreras, 1989).

IMMUNE RESPONSES TO RED CELL ANTIGENS

Primary and secondary responses
Primary responses to any particular antigen can, by definition, be studied only in subjects who have not previously encountered the antigen and who have no trace of

the antibody in their plasma. These restrictions imply that primary responses to antigens such as A, B and, often, Le^a, Le^b and P$_1$ cannot be studied, whereas those to antigens of many other systems (Rh, K, Fy, Jk, etc.) can. Since Rh D is the most immunogenic of the latter antigens, it has been used in most of the systematic work that has been done. As described in Chapter 5, after a first injection of 1 ml D-positive red cells to D-negative subjects who have not previously been exposed to the antigen and who have no trace of anti-D in their serum, antibody can first be detected in some subjects after about 4 weeks; in these subjects, the concentration of antibody increases slowly and after 6–10 weeks reaches peak values not exceeding about 4 μg/ml (Samson and Mollison, 1975; Contreras and Mollison, 1981). In other subjects, antibody can first be detected only after two injections, given at an interval of 3 months or more; less commonly, antibody is first detected only after three or more injections. There is evidence that in all subjects in whom antibody is ultimately detected, primary immunization is induced by the first injection of red cells because in such subjects red cells injected on the second occasion invariably have a shortened survival (see Chapter 10). There are some subjects in whom no antibody is formed even after many injections given over a period of 2–3 years, and these subjects are classified as non-responders. In these subjects, D-positive red cells have a strictly normal survival even after many injections of D-positive red cells have been given.

The production of anti-D after a first injection of D-positive red cells cannot be hastened by injecting a much larger amount of red cells, although the number of responders increases, as does the amount of antibody produced in the primary response (see Chapter 5).

It is known that in animals, after a first injection of antigen has been given, there is a certain period during which the animal will not respond well to a second injection. For example, in horses injected with tetanus toxoid, the period was at least 3 months, although less than a year (Barr and Glenny, 1945). In humans the number of D-negative subjects forming anti-D within 6 months did not appear to be greater when injections were given every 6 weeks than when only a single injection was given (Archer et al. 1969).

In subjects already immunized to Rh D, following a (further) transfusion of D-positive red cells, the concentration of anti-D in the serum starts to increase about 3 d after transfusion and then rises logarithmically to reach a peak value, which may be as high as about 1000 μg/ml (i.e. 10% of the total IgG), some 10–20 d later (see Chapters 5 and 11). The response to a first injection of group A or B red cells in a group O subject is similar in that antibody concentration rises rapidly and reaches a peak within about 12 days (see Figs 4.2 and 4.3), indicating that these responses should be regarded as secondary.

The differences between primary and secondary responses to the D red cell antigen in humans are very similar to those between primary and secondary responses to bacterial toxins in animals (Burnett and Fenner, 1949).

There have been few systematic studies of immune responses to alloantigens other than D; the production of serologically detectable anti-K, -E and -C within 4 weeks of a first transfusion has been reported in children with burns (Bacon et al. 1991).

Class of immunoglobulin produced
'In the primary response it is usual for IgM antibody to be formed initially and for production then to be switched to IgG antibody' (Bauer and Stavitsky, 1961).

It has proved difficult to confirm that this generalization applies to the production of red cell alloantibodies in humans. For example, in investigating responses to the Rh D antigen, using manual tests, anti-D can often first be detected by the agglutination of enzyme-treated red cells at a time when the indirect antiglobulin test is negative. Since it is known that both IgM and IgG anti-D in low concentrations will agglutinate enzyme-treated cells, and since all serological reactivity is usually lost if attempts are made to fractionate serum containing such antibodies, it is usually impossible to decide the Ig class of the antibody present.

Although it is not known with certainty whether IgM antibody is the first to be made in subjects responding to the Rh D antigen, it is quite clear that in the majority of subjects IgG antibody soon predominates and is often the only type that can be identified at any time. In a minority of subjects IgM is also produced in substantial amounts. In hyperimmunized donors anti-D is also quite often partly IgA (see Chapter 5).

Responses to several other red cell antigens, e.g. K, Fy^a and Jk^a, appear to be similar to responses to D; that is to say, most antibodies are predominantly IgG, although in some subjects a mixture of IgM and IgG antibodies is found (Abelson and Rawson, 1961; Adinolfi et al. 1962; Polley et al. 1962). Lutheran antibodies may sometimes be partly IgA (see Chapter 6).

Blood group systems in which naturally occurring antibodies are found demand separate consideration. In the ABO system perhaps all subjects should be regarded as immunized. Moreover, ABO-incompatible pregnancies and injections of various animal products cause both quantitative and qualitative changes in anti-A and anti-B (see Chapter 4). Perhaps the most interesting fact about the production of ABO antibodies is that immune anti-A and anti-B are predominantly IgM in A or B subjects but may be largely IgG (and partly IgA) in group O subjects.

Alterations in binding constant. IgG antibody formed late in the immune response tends to have a higher binding constant than antibody formed early in the response (Eisen and Siskind, 1964). An increase in the binding constant of anti-D during the response to secondary Rh D immunization was demonstrated by Holburn et al. (1970).

Increased heterogeneity of antibody in hyperimmunized subjects
There is evidence that as immunization progresses the antibody tends to be more diverse with regard to Ig class and subclass. Data with regard to anti-D are given in Chapter 5.

Persistence of IgM and IgG antibodies
IgM antibodies tend to decline rapidly in concentration after the last stimulus and usually become undetectable after 1–2 years (cf. p. 234). Some IgG antibodies (e.g. anti-Rh D) decline far more slowly and may be readily detectable 30 years after the last stimulus (see Chapter 5); others (e.g. anti-Jk^a) may become undetectable a few months after the last stimulus. In a follow-up with a median period of 10 months, of 160 patients in whom 209 antibodies had been detected, some of the findings were as

follows: of 39 antibodies belonging to the Lewis, MN or P_1 systems (presumably IgM), 28 became undetectable, whereas of 170 belonging mainly to the Rh, K, Fy and Jk systems, which were presumably IgG, only 49 became undetectable. Antibodies of the Kidd system became undetectable more frequently than those of the Rh system, in 11 of 21 compared with 27 of 98, although this difference may have been partly due to the relative potency of the antibodies concerned; of antibodies (of all specificities) with initially weak reactions, 41 of 84 became undetectable whereas of those with initially very strong reactions, only 1 of 18 became undetectable (Ramsey and Larson, 1988).

Relation between immunoglobulin class of antibody and serological behaviour

IgM antibodies. Most IgM antibodies will agglutinate red cells suspended in saline. Agglutination by some IgM antibodies, e.g. anti-A (Polley *et al.* 1963) is not enhanced in a medium of serum whereas that of some other antibodies is. Using purified IgM anti-D, it was found that the agglutinin titre was greater by four or five doubling dilutions when using serum rather than saline as a diluent; the effect was observed with serum diluted up to 1 in 32 (Holburn *et al.* 1971a). The enhancing effect of serum is, therefore, important only when comparing sera with titres of more than 32 or when determining the titre of purified antibodies.

The titre of IgM antibodies is about four times higher with enzyme-treated red cells than with untreated cells (Aho and Christian, 1966; Holburn *et al.* 1971a). Evidently, very weak IgM antibodies may be detectable only with enzyme-treated red cells.

Naturally occurring IgM antibodies of the ABO, Lewis and P systems agglutinate red cells more strongly at 0°C than at higher temperatures. For example, the titre of anti-A and anti-B is about eight times higher at 0°C than at 37°C (Kettel, cited by Wiener, 1943, p. 19). Although anti-A and -B almost invariably agglutinate appropriate red cells at 37°C, other antibodies of the aforenamed systems, e.g. anti-A_1, -HI, -Le^a -Le^b and -P_1, do not usually agglutinate red cells above 20–25°C; occasional examples of these antibodies will agglutinate up to about 30°C and even give trace reactions at 37°C; examples with such a wide thermal range as this will invariably bind complement. The behaviour of anti-Le^a is slightly different in that although it will usually not agglutinate cells above a temperature of about 20–25°C, it will usually fix complement at 37°C and thus give a strongly positive indirect antiglobulin test.

Anti-D agglutinins produced in an immune response are 'warm', i.e. they are as active at 37°C as at lower temperatures (Levine *et al.* 1940). A few IgM antibodies are 'incomplete', e.g. occasional examples of anti-Jk^a (Adinolfi *et al.* 1962; Polley, 1964).

IgG antibodies. In most blood group systems IgG antibodies will not agglutinate untreated red cells suspended in saline; such non-agglutinating antibodies are sometimes described as 'incomplete'.

The term 'incomplete' was introduced by Pappenheimer (1940) for horse antibodies against ovalbumin that produced no visible precipitation but inhibited the reaction of precipitating antisera. The term was subsequently introduced into blood group serology by Race (1944) to describe the behaviour of Rh D antibodies which failed to agglutinate D-positive red cells suspended in saline but blocked the subsequent agglutination of the red cells by an agglutinating anti-D serum; such antibodies were described as 'blocking' by Wiener (1944).

Potent examples of IgG anti-D either in undiluted serum, or in some case in serum diluted 1 in 2 in saline, will agglutinate saline-suspended red cells (Hopkins, 1969b; 1970a). In fact, it has subsequently become clear that really potent IgG anti-D even at a dilution of 1 in 10 or more will agglutinate saline-suspended cells (unpublished observations, MC).

The titre of those IgG antibodies, such as anti-A, which, when diluted more than 1 in 2 in saline, and when sufficiently potent, agglutinate saline-suspended red cells is about 16 times higher with enzyme-treated cells than with untreated cells (Aho and Christian, 1966); with untreated cells the titre is increased about 30-fold when the indirect antiglobulin test is used rather than simple agglutination (see Chapter 8). IgG anti-M also agglutinates red cells suspended in saline; the reactions are enhanced in a medium of albumin or serum.

IgA antibodies. IgA fractions containing anti-A and anti-B will agglutinate red cells suspended in saline; the titre is increased about four-fold by using the indirect antiglobulin tests with an anti-IgA serum (Adinolfi *et al.* 1966). Sera containing IgA anti-D as well as IgG anti-D do not as a rule agglutinate red cells suspended in saline although they sensitize red cells to agglutination by anti-IgA. A serum containing potent IgA anti-D which, like a purified IgA fraction from the same serum, did agglutinate saline-suspended red cells is mentioned in Chapter 5. In tests on five murine IgA monoclonals, three anti-A and two anti-A,B, agglutinating activity was associated only with tetramers or higher polymers (Guest *et al.* 1992).

Individual differences in response

Individuals vary widely in their response to different antigens. The recognition of many antigens depends on the simultaneous presence of class II HLA antigen and of foreign antigen on antigen-presenting cells, i.e. dendritic cells. Evidently then, specific immune responsiveness is influenced by the products of the HLA-DR alleles (see review by Benacerraf, 1981; see also Chapter 13). Genetic control of antibody responses is also influenced by genes outside the HLA system and segregating independently from it, which control the quantitative production of antibody (Gill *et al.* 1970).

Alterations in antibody response in disease

Subjects with autoimmune disease appear to have an increased risk of forming red cell alloantibodies. One early example was a patient with systemic lupus erythematosus who formed five different immune alloantibodies (Callender and Race, 1946; Race and Sanger, 1950, p. 240). Patients with autoimmune haemolytic anaemia (AIHA) also seem to have an increased risk (Laine and Beattie, 1985). In one series, among 26 patients with AIHA who had been pregnant or had received between one and five transfusions, as many as eight (31%) had clinically significant antibodies (James *et al.* 1988).

Subjects with hypogammaglobulinaemia have a greatly diminished capacity to form all antibodies. As described in Chapter 4 their serum may lack anti-A and anti-B. In one case a patient of group A whose serum lacked anti-B was given a series of injections of B substance of animal origin but failed to form anti-B (Barandun *et al.* 1956).

Among patients with various diseases, receiving regular transfusion over a period of a year or so, only those with chronic lymphocytic leukaemia failed to produce any new red cell alloantibodies; in contrast, patients with acute myeloid leukaemia on intensive chemotherapy produced alloantibodies as frequently as those with aplastic anaemia or gastrointestinal bleeding (Blumberg *et al.* 1983).

In another study of patients receiving regular transfusions, the frequency of formation of red cell alloantibodies was significantly lower in patients with chronic lymphocytic leukaemia than in those with other diagnoses (Blumberg *et al.* 1984b). Patients on haemodialysis may have a reduced tendency to form red cell alloantibodies; of 405 patients who had received a total of almost 7000 red cell transfusions, only seven developed alloantibodies attributable to the transfusion (Habibi and Lecolier, 1983).

Formation of immune red cell alloantibodies in infants
It is uncommon for red cell alloantibodies other than anti-A and anti-B to be produced in the first few months of life. Three cases have been recorded: (1) anti-c in a 7-week-old child of phenotype CCDee, who had been transfused during surgery 6 weeks previously (S. Kevy, unpublished observations, reported by Konugres, 1978); (2) anti-Lu^b in a 2-month-old infant who had been transfused 1 month previously (unpublished observations, MC); and (3) IgG anti-E in an infant aged 11 weeks who had received 31 transfusions in the previous 6 weeks, all from donors whose plasma had been screened for alloantibodies (DePalma *et al.* 1991).

In two series of newborn infants transfused with blood from an average of nine donors during the first few months of life no unexpected red cell antibodies were detected. The first series consisted of 53 premature infants, about half of whom were tested at least 5 months after birth (Floss *et al.* 1986) and the second of 90 full-term infants tested not less than 3 weeks after their last transfusion (Ludvigsen *et al.* 1987). The interpretation of these observations is not obvious since there is very little information about the frequency with which red cell alloantibodies are formed in adults within the few months following a first series of transfusions.

Role of the spleen
In splenectomized subjects the response to sheep red blood cells (SRBC) is much lower than in control subjects (Rowley, 1950; McFadzean and Tsang, 1956). However, the spleen is not essential in the formation of antibodies against red cell antigens. For example, the patient described by Collins *et al.* (1950), who formed so many blood group antibodies, had had her spleen removed before receiving the series of blood transfusions which immunized her. Moreover, in subjects with sickle cell disease, whose spleens are usually infarcted and functionless, alloimmunization is no less frequent than in other patients (see later).

Association between weakening of red cell antigens
and the appearance of allo- or autoantibodies in the serum
Six examples can be given. (1) In pregnant women the agglutinability of red cells with

Lewis antibodies tends to diminish (see Chapter 4), a change that appears to be correlated with an increase in the frequency with which Lewis antibodies are detected. (2) Transient weakening of Rh D antigens has been observed in an infant with AIHA; when the infant recovered and the direct antiglobulin test (DAT) became negative, the antigens became normally reactive (Issitt *et al.* 1983). (3) Temporary weakening of LW may be associated with the appearance of anti-LW in the serum (see Chapter 5). (4) The appearance of Kell antibodies in the serum may be associated with weakening of Kell antigens (see Chapters 6 and 7). (5) In a patient whose red cell phenotype changed from Jk(a + b –) to Jk(a – b –), loss of Jk^a was associated with the appearance in the serum of anti-Jk3 (see Chapter 6). (6) In a patient in whose serum anti-β-SGP appeared, β-SGP was temporarily absent from the red cell membrane; when β-SGP reappeared, the antibody disappeared; the cells now reacted with serum taken earlier (Daniels *et al.* 1988).

Monoclonal antibodies

When an animal is injected with an antigen it responds by producing antibodies which react with many different determinants (epitopes) on the antigen. Moreover, of the antibodies that react with any one of the determinants, some have a much higher affinity than others, i.e. the fit of the individual antibody molecules to the antigenic determinant varies widely. When the same antigen is injected into two different animals it is not surprising that the resulting population of antibodies varies from one animal to another. Each kind of antibody molecule is made by a line of plasma cells derived from a single lymphocyte. The progeny of a single cell is called a clone and the identical molecules produced by such a clone constitute a monoclonal antibody. In 1975 Köhler and Milstein described a method of obtaining monoclonal antibodies which depended on fusing mouse lymphocytes with mouse myeloma cells. The lymphocytes were obtained from the spleen of mice immunized with a particular antigen. The fused 'hybridoma' cells secreted specific antibody and grew indefinitely in culture. Hybrid cells were plated out and grown, and numerous clones were tested to find those containing the wanted antibodies. Subsequent work has shown that the culture fluid may have antibody concentrations of about 0.05 mg/ml. Much higher concentrations of antibody can be obtained by injecting the hybrid cells intraperitoneally into a mouse, in which they form a tumour, with the neoplastic cells producing virtually pure antibody. Ascitic fluid from such a mouse may have a protein concentration as high as 5 mg/ml, of which 90% is antibody. (See reviews by Milstein (1980; 1981) and Diamond *et al.* (1981).)

Mouse monoclonal antibodies

Numerous murine monoclonal antibodies reacting with previously recognized and unrecognized specificities have been described: anti-A, -B, -A,B, -H type 1, -H type 2, -P, -P$_1$, -P^k, -I, -Y (as in Le^y), -Le^a, -Le^b, -M, -N, -S-like, -T, -Tn, -k, -Lu^b, -Rh e-like, -glycophorin A (GPA), -GPB, -GPC, Ge-like, -Band 3, and -En^a TS (First International Workshop on Red Cell Monoclonal Antibodies, 1987; Second International Workshop on Red Cell Monoclonal Antibodies, 1990).

Murine monoclonal antibodies specific for various human complement components, e.g. anti-C3c, -C3dg, -C4b as well as anti-IgG and anti-IgG1–IgG4 have proved to be very satisfactory as laboratory reagents and, as with murine monoclonal anti-A and -B, have largely replaced polyclonal reagents; see Chapter 8.

Human monoclonal antibodies

The first human monoclonal antibodies with blood group specificity were produced by transformation of human B lymphocytes with Epstein–Barr virus (EBV). The lymphoblastoid cells which result have the property of growing in tissue culture and of secreting antibody. By taking lymphocytes from Rh D-immunized donors, both IgG (Koskimies, 1980; Crawford et al. 1983; Rouger et al. 1985) and IgM (Boylston et al. 1980) anti-D have been obtained. EBV-transformed cell lines are unstable, often ceasing to produce antibody after a few months (Melamed et al. 1985), although many stable EBV-transformed cell lines have been described (Goosens et al. 1987; Kumpel et al. 1989a). Another way of obtaining stable cell lines is to fuse human lymphocytes with murine myelomas or with heteromyelomas (see review by Thompson and Hughes-Jones, 1990).

Examples of monoclonal anti-D have been used in analysing the different D epitopes (see Chapter 5) and in the experimental clearance of D-positive red cells from the circulation of volunteers (see Chapter 10); they are used routinely in blood grouping (see Chapter 8).

Human anti-E, -c, -Jk^a and -Jk^b are also now available (Second International Workshop on Red Cell Monoclonal Antibodies, 1990).

Some disadvantages of monoclonal antibodies

As mentioned elsewhere in this chapter changes in pH alter the binding affinity of antibodies. Mosmann et al. (1980) found that the effect was particularly striking with monoclonal antibodies and they pointed out that this might have a profound effect on apparent specificity in tests in a system such as HLA, which involves many similar but non-identical antigens. Two monoclonal antibodies which gave non-specific reactions at normal pH could be made monospecific by lowering pH to 6.0.

A problem associated with some high-affinity monoclonal antibodies is crossreactivity. It may seem paradoxical that an antibody apparently specific for a single antigenic determinant should crossreact at all. Nevertheless, single antibody molecules are not specific for one particular epitope. The combining site on the end of the Fab arm is capable of binding closely with a number of different epitopic configurations (Talmage, 1959; Richards et al. 1975). The higher the affinity of an antibody, the more it tends to crossreact (Steiner and Eisen, 1967). Presumably, the more strongly an antibody combines with any particular determinant, the more certain it is to bind to some extent to related antigenic determinants. By no means all monoclonal antibodies have a high affinity. Indeed, the affinities of monoclonal antibodies are similar to those of polyclonal antibodies, although all antibodies of a single clone have the same affinity whereas the antibodies in a polyclonal population have a range of affinities.

Crossreactivity explains the demonstration that certain examples of monoclonal anti-D react with the cytoplasmic component vimentin (Thorpe 1989; 1990), giving rise to the false conclusion that D is present on tissue cells. On the other hand, the reaction of certain monoclonal anti-As with B cells and of certain monoclonal anti-Bs with A cells is due to the potency of the antibodies concerned which enables them to detect the small amounts of B and A, respectively produced by A and B subjects (see Chapter 4).

A different problem is provided by monoclonal antibodies with 'pseudo-specificity'; for example: (1) an anti-glycophorin B which in agglutination tests behaved as anti-S but in other tests reacted both with s + and with S + red cells (Green *et al.* 1990a); and (2) an anti-J chain which reacted more strongly with Gm(a +) than Gm(a –) molecules but could be shown to be reacting with the same determinant on the chain in both cases (De Lange, 1988).

Copying variable regions and constructing new antibodies
A way of insuring against the loss of particular monoclonals and of selecting V regions for the construction of new antibodies has been described. V regions are amplified using the polymerase chain reaction and are then cloned into expression vectors (e.g. bacteriophage). Complete antibody V domains with specificity identical to the parent antibody can then be displayed on the surface of the bacteriophage. Completely new antibodies can be constructed (McCafferty *et al.* 1990).

Other methods of constructing new antibodies, e.g. monomeric IgM, molecules composed of murine variable regions and human constant regions, drug–antibody conjugates, etc. have been described; see Yap and Williams (1990).

Frequency of immune red cell alloantibodies

By definition, an immune red cell alloantibody is one that develops in a subject who has been exposed to a red cell alloantigen. Evidently then, the frequency of immune red cell antibodies will be zero in subjects who have never been transfused or been pregnant and will be greatest in subjects who have received many transfusions. For two reasons, pregnancies constitute a smaller stimulus than transfusions: first, the number of foreign antigens is limited to those possessed by the father of the fetus (although, of course, some women have infants by more than one man), and, second, in many pregnancies the amount of red cells transferred from fetus to mother is too small to stimulate a primary response.

The frequency of alloantibodies is expected to be relatively low in blood donors compared with patients in hospital requiring blood transfusion; blood donors have a lower average age and are far less likely to have received blood transfusions in the past. Patients who have been transfused on only a single occasion, some years previously, may either not have formed any red cell antibodies or, if they have, may have made only a weak antibody which can no longer be detected. On the other hand, patients who have, over the previous few months, been transfused repeatedly are likely to have detectable antibodies. The frequency with which particular antibodies are found is much affected by the ethnic origin of the population being tested. For example, the frequency of anti-D is very low in Chinese people in whom the D-negative phenotype is rare.

D is the most immunogenic red cell antigen but the frequency with which D-negative subjects make anti-D has diminished progressively since the 1940s. The practice of determining the Rh D group of donors and recipients spread rapidly after the end of the Second World War (i.e. in 1945) and now D-positive red cells are transfused to D-negative recipients only accidentally or occasionally, for example in elderly male recipients, when D-negative blood is not readily available. Immunization to D by blood transfusion has become rare and most subjects in whom anti-D is found are women who have been immunized by pregnancy. Before the introduction of immunoprophylaxis with anti-D Ig in the late 1960s, about one in six D-negative women who had two D-positive infants (the first ABO-compatible) formed anti-D, and the overall frequency of anti-D in women (i.e. of unknown D group) who had had two pregnancies was more than 0.5%. The postnatal administration of anti-D Ig reduced the frequency of D immunization to about one-tenth of the previous rate. Antenatal administration seems capable of reducing this figure by a further factor of ten (see Chapter 12) but, although used widely in some countries, e.g. Canada, it is still used only to a small extent in others, e.g. the UK.

In contrast to the diminishing frequency of anti-D, that of anti-K, -Fy^a, etc. has increased, evidently due to the increased number of multi-transfused patients and the absence of measures for preventing immunization to antigens other than D.

Frequency of immune anti-D (including anit-CD and anit-DE)

In healthy blood donors. In more than 200 000 donors screened between 1971 and 1975 in Seattle, the frequency was 0.22% (Giblett, 1977). In 36 000 donors screened in London in 1988, the frequency (0.25%) was almost identical although in 35 000 screened in 1990 the frequency was 0.16% (R. Knight, personal communication).

In pregnant women. Before the introduction of immunoprophylaxis, anti-D was found in approximately 1 in 170 pregnant white women, both in England (Walker, 1958) and in North America (Walker, 1984). Following the introduction of immunoprophylaxis with anti-D in the late 1960s, the frequency with which anti-D is found has fallen progressively and was, for example, 1 in 963 in 1988 in one North American survey (R.H. Walker, personal communication, 1991). The frequency in one English region for 1988 was substantially higher than this, namely 1 in 497 (G.J. Dovey, personal communication).

In transfusion recipients. Although there appears to have been a fall between the mid-1950s and mid-1970s in the frequency with which anti-D has been found in transfusion recipients, there has been no obvious fall since then. Some figures are as follows: in 1956–7, 0.77%; in 1974–5, 0.52%, based on testing 60 000 patients in Seattle (Giblett, 1977); in 1976–81, 0.29% and in 1982–7, 0.27%, based on screening about 100 000 patients in each 5-year period in Michigan (Walker *et al.* 1989). In a smaller series (more than 12 000 patients) tested in England in 1990, 0.56% (J. Sangster, personal communication).

Frequency of immune red cell antibodies other than anti-D

In healthy blood donors. In the two series referred to above, the frequencies were 0.10% in Seattle in 1975 (Giblett, 1977) and in London 0.19% in 1988 and 0.18% in 1990 (unpublished observations, MC). In the London series, about 30% of the antibodies were anti-E and 20% were anti-K.

In pregnant women. In approximately 175 000 women (about 85% of whom were D positive) antibodies other than anti-D were found in 0.14%; rather more than half of these were within the Rh system and, of these, one half were anti-E; the next commonest antibody, found in 0.025% of the women, was anti-K (Kornstad, 1983).

In transfusion recipients. Frequencies were: in 1956–7, 0.33%; in 1974–5, 1.12% (Giblett, 1977); in 1970–5, 0.39%; in 1976–81, 0.45% and in 1982–7, 0.6% (Walker *et al.* 1989).

Relative frequencies of antibodies other than anti-D. Combined figures from 20 different blood grouping laboratories were reported by Grove-Rasmussen (1964); these figures and those from a much smaller series reported by Tovey (1974) are shown in Table 3.6. No information was given as to the relative numbers of parous women and transfusion recipients in the two series. As will be seen, Rh antibodies (other than anti-D) constituted about 54% of the total and anti-K and -Fy^a about 40%, leaving only 5% for all other specificities. In the series of Walker *et al.* (1989), if the figures for the three 5-year periods (in each of which approximately 100 000 patients were screened) are pooled, the absolute frequencies for antibodies of various specificities were as follows: Rh antibodies other than anti-D, 0.17%; anti-K, 0.15%; anti-Fy^a, 0.06%; anti-Jk^a, 0.03%.

Patients with thalassaemia are usually transfused about once a month, starting in the first few years of life. In some series in which patients have been transfused with blood selected only for ABO and D compatibility, antibodies, mainly of Rh or K specificities, have been found in more than 20% of patients. For example, of 973 thalassaemics transfused with an average of 18 units a year from about the age of 3 years, 21.1% had formed clinically significant antibodies after about 6 years; 84% of the antibodies were within the Rh or K systems; about half the immunized patients made antibodies of more than one specificity. Of 162 patients transfused from the outset with red cells matched for Rh and K antigens, only 3.7% formed alloantibodies compared with 15.7% of 83 patients of similar age, transfused with blood matched only for D (Spanos *et al.* 1990).

Table 3.6 Relative frequency of immune red cell antibodies* (excluding anti-D, -CD and -DE): (a) and (b) in transfusion recipients (and some pregnant women); (c) associated with immediate haemolytic transfusion reactions; and (d) associated with delayed haemolytic transfusion reactions

	No. of cases	Blood group systems within which the various alloantibodies occurred (%)				
		Rh (excluding -D)[†]	K	Fy	Jk	Others
(a)	4523	51.8	28.6	10.2	4.2	5.2
(b)	705	61.4	24.7	10.2	2.4	1.3
(c)	142	42.2	30.3	18.3	8.5	0.7
(d)	82	34.2	14.6	15.9	32.9	2.4

(a) Grove-Rasmussen, 1964; (b) Tovey, 1974; (c) Grove-Rasmussen and Huggins, 1973; (d) data from the Mayo Clinic and Toronto General Hospital; for further details see Chapter 11.
* That is, excluding antibodies of the ABO, Lewis and P systems and anti-M and anti-N.
[†] Almost all anti-E or -c.

The incidence of antibody formation is less when transfusion is started in the first year of life (Economidou *et al*. 1971). The induction of immunological tolerance by starting repeated transfusions in the first year of life was believed to account for the low rate of alloimmunization, namely 5.2%, observed in a series of 1435 patients (Sirchia *et al*. 1985).

Alloimmunization in sickle cell disease
In a survey of 1814 patients from many centres, the overall rate of alloimmunization was 18.6%. The rate increased with the number of transfusions and, although alloimmunization usually occurred with less than 15 transfusions, the rate continued to increase as more transfusions were given. The commonest specificities were anti-C, -E and -K; 55% of immunized subjects made antibodies with more than one specificity (Rosse *et al*. 1990). In another series the incidence of alloimmunization was somewhat higher. Of 107 patients who received a total of 2100 units, 32 (30%) became immunized and 17 of these formed multiple antibodies; 82% of the specificities were anti-K, -E, -C or -Jk^b. Those patients who formed antibodies had had an average of 23 transfusions; those who did not had had an average of 13; 75% of antibodies had developed by the time of the 21st transfusion (Vichinsky *et al*. 1990).

The finding that the percentage of patients forming antibodies increases with the number of transfusions has been documented in previous series (Orlina *et al*. 1978; Reisner *et al*. 1987). In the latter series, 50% of patients who had received 100 or more transfusions had formed antibodies.

It has been suggested that in sickle cell disease the rate of alloimmunization is due partly to racial differences between donors (predominantly Whites) and patients (Blacks). The antibodies formed most commonly are anti-K, -C, -E and -Jk^b, and the frequencies of each of the corresponding antigens are significantly higher in Whites than in Blacks (Vichinsky *et al*. 1990). It has been pointed out that when one considers the probability of giving at least one incompatible unit when ten units are transfused, the differences for C, E, and Jk^b between White and Black donors become very small, only that for K remaining substantial, namely 0.178 with Black donors, and 0.597 with White (Pereira *et al*. 1990), so that the use of White donors for Blacks may not play a large role in inducing the formation of red cell alloantibodies. In any case, the conclusion is that for patients with sickle cell disease, as for those with thalassaemia, it is worth giving blood matched for Rh D antigens and for K. This conclusion is implied by the findings of Rosse *et al*. (1990) and was reached earlier by Davies *et al*. (1986). These latter authors found that two of their patients, both of the phenotype ccDee, which is much commoner in Blacks than in Whites, had developed anti-C and anti-E, and they recommended that ccDee patients with sickle cell disease should be given either ccDee or ccddee blood.

Relative importance of different alloantibodies in transfusion
As discussed in Chapter 11, anti-A and anti-B must be regarded as overwhelmingly the most important red cell alloantibodies in blood transfusion because they are most commonly implicated in fatal haemolytic transfusion reactions. Rh antibodies are the next most important mainly because they are commoner than other immune red cell alloantibodies. For example, in the series of Grove-Rasmussen and Huggins (1973), of

177 antibodies associated with haemolytic transfusion reactions (omitting 30 cases in which anti-A and anti-B were responsible and also omitting cases in which only cold agglutinins were found which were unlikely to have been responsible for red cell destruction), 95, including 35 examples of anti-D, were within the Rh system. Estimates of frequencies with which other red cell alloantibodies were involved in immediate and delayed haemolytic transfusion reactions are shown in Table 3.6.

The figures given in Table 3.6 show that the frequencies with which the different red cell alloantibodies were involved in immediate haemolytic transfusion reactions were similar to the frequencies with which the same red cell alloantibodies were found in transfusion recipients. On the other hand, the figures for delayed haemolytic transfusion reactions show one very striking difference in that antibodies of the Jk system were very much more commonly involved than expected from a frequency of these antibodies in random transfusion recipients. Possibly this discrepancy is due to the fact that red cell destruction by Kidd antibodies tends to be severe so that perhaps delayed haemolytic reactions are more readily diagnosed when these antibodies are involved, or, to put it in another way, delayed haemolytic transfusion reactions associated with other red cell alloantibodies may tend to be missed.

Perhaps a more important reason why Kidd antibodies tend to be relatively frequently involved in delayed haemolytic transfusion reactions may be that they are difficult to detect, particularly when present in low concentration. Moreover, unlike some antibodies, e.g. anti-D, which after having become detectable remain detectable for long periods of time, Kidd antibodies tend to disappear.

Although virtually all examples of anti-Le^a and some examples of anti-Le^b are active at 37°C *in vitro* they have very seldom been the cause of haemolytic transfusion reactions, mainly because Lewis antibodies are readily neutralized by Lewis substances which are present in the plasma of the transfused blood.

Although most antibodies which are active at 37°C *in vitro* are capable of causing red cell destruction, there are exceptions (see Chapter 11). In some cases the explanation may lie in the IgG subclass of the antibody and in others, perhaps, in the paucity of antigen sites.

Cold alloantibodies such as anti-A$_1$, anti-HI, anti-P$_1$, anti-M and anti-N are usually inactive *in vitro* at 37°C and are then incapable of bringing about red cell destruction. Occasional examples which are dubiously active at 37°C but active at 30°C or higher may bring about the destruction of small volumes of incompatible red cells given for the purpose of investigation. References to very rare examples of anti-A$_1$ and anti-P$_1$, anti-M and anti-N which have caused haemolytic transfusion reactions will be found in later chapters.

Relative potency (immunogenicity) of different antigens

An estimate of the relative potency of different red cell alloantigens can be obtained by comparing the actual frequency with which particular alloantibodies are encountered with the calculated frequency of the opportunity for immunization (Giblett, 1961). For example, suppose that in transfusion recipients anti-K is found about 2.5 times more commonly than anti-Fy^a (see Table 3.6, (a) and (b)). The relative opportunities for immunization to K and Fy^a can be estimated simply by comparing the frequency of the combination K-positive donor, K-negative recipient; i.e. $0.09 \times 0.91 = 0.08$, with the frequency of the combination Fy(a +) donor, Fy(a −) recipient; i.e. $0.66 \times 0.34 = 0.22$. Thus the opportunity for immunization to K is about 3.5 times less than that for Fy^a (0.08 vs. 0.22). In summary, although opportunities for immunization to K are 3.5 times less frequent than those to Fy^a, anti-K is in fact found 2.5 times more commonly than anti-Fy^a so that, overall, K is about nine times more potent than Fy^a. If a single transfusion of K-positive blood to a K-negative subject induces the formation of serologically detectable anti-K in 10% of cases (see pp. 250) it is, therefore, predicted that the transfusion of a single unit of Fy(a +) blood to an Fy(a −) subject would induce the formation of serologically detectable anti-Fy^a in about 1% of cases.

Using earlier data, Giblett (1961) calculated that c and E were about three times less potent than K, that Fy^a was about 25 times less potent, and Jk^a 50–100 times less potent.

Transfusion vs. pregnancy as a stimulus
In considering the risks of immunization by particular red cell alloantigens, the effect of transfusing multiple units of blood and the relative risks of immunization by transfusion and pregnancy must be discussed.

When an antigen has a low frequency, e.g. K, with a frequency of 0.09, the chance of receiving a unit containing the antigen increases directly with the number of the units transfused, up to a certain number (11 in this instance). On the other hand, when an antigen has a high frequency, e.g. c, frequency 0.8, the chance of exposure is high with only a single unit and increases only slightly as the number of units transfused increases. The point can be illustrated by calculating an example. For the transfusion of a single unit, the chance that the donor will be K positive and the recipient K negative is $0.09 \times 0.91 = 0.08$; the corresponding risk of incompatibility from c is $0.8 \times 0.2 = 0.16$; the relative risk from the two antigens (K/c) is thus $0.5 : 1.0$. When 4 units are transfused, the chance of K-incompatibility (at least one donor K positive and the recipient K negative) is $0.31 \times 0.91 = 0.28$ and of c-incompatibility $0.997 \times 0.2 =$ approximately 0.2, so that the relative risk (K/c) is now $0.28 : 0.2$ or $1.4 : 1$ (Allen and Warshaw, 1962). To summarize, the relative risk of exposure to K compared with c is about three times as great with a 4-unit blood transfusion as with a 1-unit transfusion.

When the antigen has a low frequency, opportunities for making the corresponding antibody are much lower from pregnancy than from blood transfusion if it is assumed that a woman has only one partner and that in transfusion many different donors are often involved. For example, in women who have three pregnancies the chance that in two of them the fetus will be c-incompatible with its mother is about three times greater than that two of them will be K-incompatible (Allen and Warshaw, 1962).

These theoretical considerations are supported by actual findings: among women sensitized by blood transfusion alone, anti-K was almost three times more common than anti-c (32 : 12) whereas among women sensitized by pregnancy alone the incidence of the two antibodies was similar (9 : 7) (Allen and Warshaw, 1962).

When a woman carries a fetus with an incompatible antigen she is far less likely to form alloantibodies than when she is transfused with blood carrying the same antigen. Presumably the main reason for the difference is simply that in many pregnancies the size of transplacental haemorrhage does not constitute an adequate stimulus for primary immunization.

In two different series in which anti-c was detected in pregnant women there was a history of a previous blood transfusion in over one-third of the women (Fraser and Tovey, 1976; Astrup and Kornstad, 1977).

The effect of Rh D immunization on the formation of other red cell alloantibodies
Among Rh D-negative volunteers deliberately injected with D-positive red cells, those who form anti-D tend also to form alloantibodies outside the Rh system, whereas those who do not form anti-D seldom form any alloantibodies at all. In one series, of 73 subjects who formed anti-D, six formed anti-Fy^a, four formed anti-Jk^a and four formed other antibodies; by contrast, amongst 48 subjects who failed to form anti-D, not one made any detectable alloantibodies (Archer *et al.* 1969).

An association between the formation of anti-D and that of antibodies outside the Rh system was previously noted by Issitt (1965) in women who had borne children.

Several series in which D-negative subjects have been deliberately immunized with D-positive red cells are available for analysis. In some series, donors and recipients were tested for other red cell antigens so that the numbers at risk from these other antigens are known. In other series, donors and recipients were not tested, or only donors were tested, for antigens other than D, so that it is only possible to estimate the numbers at risk from the known incidence of the relevant antigens in a random population. In Table 3.7 estimates of the immunogenicity of K, Fy^a, Jk^a and s in three circumstances are listed: (1) in subjects receiving D-compatible red cells; (2) in D-negative recipients receiving D-positive red cells but not making anti-D, and (3) in D-negative recipients receiving D-positive red cells and making anti-D.

The data summarized in Table 3.7 emphasize the tremendously increased response to antigens outside the Rh system in subjects responding to D. In subjects who formed anti-D and had the opportunity of making other antibodies, 50% formed anti-K. The

Table 3.7 Response to K, Fy^a, Jk^a and s in relation to Rh D-compatibility of injected red cells

	Proportion of subjects making antibodies outside the Rh system		
		Donor cells D-incompatible	
Recipients making	Donor cells D-compatible	Recipients not making anti-D	Recipients making anti-D
Anti-K	1/12*	0/20[‡]	6/12[‡]
Anti-Fy^a	1/19[†]	0/15[§]	9/49[§]
Anti-Jk^a	0/16[†]	0.19[§‖¶]	16/87[§‖¶]
Anti-s	0/21[†]	—	3/14[¶]

* Adner *et al.* (1963).
[†] Race (1952).
[‡] Freda Roberts (personal communication).
[§] Archer *et al.* (1969).
[‖] L.A.D. Tovey (personal communication).
[¶] R.S. Lane (personal communication).
For assumptions made in deriving these figures, see Mollison (1983, p. 238).

incidence of anti-Fy^a, anti-Jk^a and anti-s in those who could respond was about 20% in each instance. In deliberately immunizing Rh D negative subjects to obtain anti-D it is clearly very important to choose donors who cannot stimulate the formation of antibodies such as anti-K, -Fy^a or -Jk^a.

The question arises whether non-responders to D are also non-responders to other red cell antigens. The data shown in Table 3.7 do not answer the question, since although no alloantibodies were formed by non-responders to D only two such antibodies were made by recipients of D-compatible red cells, and much larger numbers are needed to discover whether there is any difference between the two categories.

The enhancing effect of antibodies other than anti-D on the formation of other red cell alloantibodies

Issitt et al. (1973) described three Rh D positive subjects, all of whom had previously been transfused and two of whom had been pregnant, who formed multiple red cell antibodies following a further transfusion. The first subject made anti-Fy^a after receiving 12 units blood and 1 year later, 3 d after receiving a further unit, was found to have made anti-CE and anti-Jk^b. The second subject who had had many previous transfusions but was not known to have formed any immune alloantibody at the time of her last transfusion, was found some months later to have made anti-E, anti-K and anti-Fy^a. A third subject, who had last been transfused 16 years previously, after a further transfusion developed anti-E, -Fy^a and -Jk^b within the following 2 weeks. It was suggested that the production of one antibody may augment the response to other alloantigens or alternatively that some subjects are simply good responders. The observations described above, relating to antibodies associated with the formation of anti-D, favour the first of these hypotheses.

Enhancing effect of 'strong' antigens: experiments in chickens

The great enhancing effect, on the immunogenicity of weak alloantigens, of a response to a strong alloantigen finds an exact parallel in experiments reported in chickens. In these animals B is a strong antigen and A is a weak one, so that when cells carrying only one of these antigens are given, responses to B are the rule, but to A are very infrequent. However, when red cells carrying both these antigens are given, recipients make both antibodies. The effect is not found when mixed A and B red cells are given and thus depends on both antigens being carried on the same red cells (Schierman and McBride, 1967).

Competition of antigens

If an animal is immunized to one antigen, X, and is subsequently reinjected with X, together with an unrelated antigen, Y, it may show a significantly lowered response to Y (see, for example, Barr and Llewellyn-Jones, 1953), a phenomenon known as antigenic competition. It has been suggested that control mechanisms, designed to prevent the unlimited progression of the immune response, may be responsible and that the phrase non-specific antigen-induced suppression may be a better description of the phenomenon. It is probable that the suppression observed is due to several different mechanisms varying with the antigens used, the time sequence of immunization and other factors (Pross and Eidinger, 1974).

In considering the possible interference of immunization to one red cell antigen on the response to another, the fact that both antigens may be carried on the same red cells must be taken into account. As soon as antibody has been formed to one antigen it will tend to bring about rapid destruction of the red cells and this process may interfere with the immune response to a second antigen.

There is quite extensive evidence that red cells carrying two antigens, for the first of which there is a corresponding antibody in the subject's serum, may fail to immunize against the second antigen. The best known example is the protective effect against Rh D immunization exercised by ABO incompatibility (see Chapter 5). ABO incompatibility has also been shown to protect against immunization to c (Levine, 1958), K (Levine, quoted by Race and Sanger, 1968, p. 283), and a number of other antigens including Fy^a, Jk^a and Di^a (Stern, 1975).

The following case illustrates the circumstances in which protection may be observed: a D-negative, S-positive woman was transfused with D-negative, S-negative blood. After two D-positive pregnancies she was found to have formed potent anti-s but only low-titred anti-D (Drachmann and Hansen, 1969; Stern, 1975). A similar phenomenon was reported by Stern et al. (1958). An R_1R_1 subject was injected with Be (a +), D-negative cells, and formed anti-Be^a. Two weeks after the appearance of anti-Be^a, anti-c was detected. After further immunization, anti-Be^a reached a high titre whereas the anti-c became weaker and was finally only just detectable. (Be^a is associated with weak c and e antigens; see Race and Sanger, 1975, p. 204.)

It has been suggested that the antibody which is made first diverts antigen to sites where the corresponding antibody is being made and that these sites are unfavourable for the formation of other antibodies carried on the same red cells (Stern et al. 1961; Stern, 1975). Thus, the mechanism is probably exactly the same as that of immuno-suppression by passive antibody (see p. 121).

It is possible that the mechanism of protection by ABO incompatibility is different in so far as it leads to intravascular lysis of red cells and in so far as lysed red cells seem to be less antigenic than intact ones (see below).

In any case, there is a paradox to be resolved: the enhancing effect, on immuniza-tion to a weak antigen such as Jk^a, of a response to a strong antigen such as D and the suppressive effect, on immunization to a relatively strong antigen such as D, of ABO incompatibility. Perhaps the important difference lies in the presence or absence of alloantibody in the serum at the time when induction of immunization to a second antigen is in question. During primary immunization the induction of a response to a weak antigen may be facilitated by a response to a strong antigen but once potent antibody is present in the serum it may be difficult to induce primary immunization to another red cell antigen. This would apply with special force when the antibody concerned is haemolytic.

Immunogenicity of red cell stroma. When whole lysed blood is injected, or stroma prepared from lysed blood, antibody production tends to be less than when whole intact red cells are injected. Schneider and Preisler (1966) gave two i.v. injections, each of 0.5 ml D-positive cord blood, at an interval of 1–7 weeks to D-negative subjects; the number of subjects forming anti-D was 4 of 15 in a series in which intact red cells were given but only 1 of 17 in a series in which lysed red cells were given. Similarly, sonicated human red cells are less immunogenic than intact cells (Pollack et al. 1968a);

and in rabbits less potent alloantibodies against the antigen Hg^A result from injecting lysed red cells than from injecting intact red cells (Mollison, 1967, p. 203).

Autoantibodies associated with alloimmunization

The development of cold red cell autoagglutinins has been observed in animals following repeated injections of red cells (see Chapter 7) and has occasionally been observed in humans in association with delayed haemolytic transfusion reactions (see Chapter 11).

A positive direct antiglobulin test is sometimes observed during secondary immunization to D (see Chapter 5) and has been noted in about 1 in 60 subjects who are developing secondary responses to other alloantigens, such as K (P.D. Issitt, personal communication). The development of a positive direct antiglobulin test affecting the recipient's red cells following a delayed haemolytic transfusion reaction is discussed in Chapter 11.

The development of autoantibodies has also been observed following an episode of red cell destruction induced by passively administered antibodies and following intensive plasma exchange (p. 238).

Immunological tolerance

Long-lasting immunological tolerance can be induced either by introducing into an embryo a graft which survives throughout life or by giving repeated injections of cells.

Examples of graft survival are provided by 'chimeras', i.e. individuals whose cells are derived from two distinct zygotes. Many examples of such permanent chimerism have been described in human dizygotic twins (see review in Watkins *et al.* 1980). Temporary chimerism may be observed in subjects who have received immunosuppressive therapy and have then been transfused or have received a bone marrow transplant. Occasionally, cells of two different phenotypes derived from a single zygote lineage are found, a phenomenon known as mosaicism. The commonest form of mosaicism encountered in blood grouping is due to somatic mutation, i.e. Tn polyagglutinability (see Chapter 7).

Examples of possible tolerance to blood cells in humans

In experiments in which weekly i.v. injections of whole heparinized blood not more than 24 h old were given from the same donors to the same recipients, in about 10% of cases there was a progressive decrease in the intensity of the antibody reponse to HLA antigens until humoral cytotoxic activity could no longer be demonstrated (Ferrara *et al.* 1974).

The induction of partial tolerance to skin grafts in newborn infants transfused with fresh whole blood but not stored blood was described by Fowler *et al.* (1960).

The development of fatal graft versus host disease (GvHD) following transfusion in newborn infants in whom a previous intra-uterine transfusion had apparently induced tolerance is described in Chapter 15.

Subjects with thalassaemia to whom transfusions are given from the first year of life onwards appear to be rendered partially tolerant to red cell antigens (see p. 112).

For tolerance to grafts and neoplasia induced by transfusion, see Chapter 13.

Suppression of the immune response by passive antibody

Practical aspects of the suppression of Rh D immunization by passively administered antibody are discussed in Chapter 5. Here, some theoretical aspects of the subject are considered briefly.

Von Dungern (1900) observed that if cattle red cells saturated with antibodies are injected into a rabbit, the immune response which would otherwise occur is prevented, and others found that the response to soluble antigens can be suppressed by giving 'excess' antibody (Smith, 1909; Glenny and Südmersen, 1921). 'Excess' in this context is usually thought of as literally an outnumbering of antigen sites by antibody molecules. The response to antigens carried on red cells can be suppressed by very much smaller amounts of antibody. For example, suppose that 25 μg anti-D is effective in suppressing immunization when 1 ml D positive red cells is injected (see Chapter 5). Assuming that the antibody is distributed within a space about twice as great as the plasma volume it can be calculated that, at equilibrium, only about 5% of antigen and about 1% of antibody will be bound. Similarly, the amount of passive antibody required to suppress the immune response in mice to SRBC was calculated to be 100 times less than the amount required to saturate the antigen site (Haughton and Nash, 1969). Evidently, in these circumstances, suppression of the immune response is not due to covering of antigen by antibody but is due to destruction of antigen in circumstances in which it cannot induce immunization; a possible mechanism of suppression is discussed below.

The suppressive effect of passive antibody against soluble antigen is antigen-specific. In an experiment in which a molecule carrying two antigenic determinants was injected, the response to one could be suppressed without affecting the response to the other (Brody *et al.* 1967). On the other hand, discrepant results have been observed with antigens carried on red cells. In rabbits and chickens it has proved possible to suppress the response to one antigen carried on the cells without suppressing the response to another (Pollack *et al.* 1968a; Schierman *et al.* 1969). However, in the only experiment reported in humans, when red cells carrying both D and K were injected together with anti-K, the response both to K and D was suppressed (Woodrow *et al.* 1975). Volunteers, all of whom were D negative, were given an injection of 1 ml D positive, K-positive red cells. In addition, half the subjects ('treated') were given an injection of 14 μg IgG anti-K, which was sufficient to clear the K-positive, D positive red cells from the circulation into the spleen within 24 h. At 6 months, 7 of 31 control subjects but only 1 of 31 treated subjects had formed anti-D. After a further stimulus 4 more control subjects but no more treated subjects developed anti-D.

The fact that ABO-incompatible D positive red cells induced D immunization far less frequently than ABO-compatible D positive cells has been mentioned above. It should be noted that the mechanism of destruction of red cells by anti-K and anti-A are quite different. Anti-K is a non-haemolytic antibody which, when also non-complement-binding, as in the example used in the experiment described above, brings about red cell destruction predominantly in the spleen. On the other hand, anti-A and anti-B bring about destruction predominantly in the plasma by direct lysis of red cells, with sequestration of unlysed cells predominantly in the liver.

It seems unlikely that the rate of clearance of D positive red cells is causally related to the probability of suppression of immunization. On the other hand, since the ratio of antibody to red cells determines both the rate of red cell clearance and the probability of suppression, clearance and suppression are expected to be correlated. From a review of published work it was concluded that clearance of a small dose of red cells within 5 d and of a large dose within 8 d was usually associated with suppression, slower rates of clearance being associated with failure of suppression (Mollison, 1984b).

There is one observation which, if confirmed, would demonstrate a relationship between splenic destruction — and perhaps between rapid destruction — and suppression: in a splenectomized, D negative subject injected with 4 ml D positive red cells together with 300 μg anti-D i.v., the red cells were cleared with a $T_{1/2}$ of 14.5 d and the subject developed anti-D within 4 months (Weitzel *et al.* 1974). Thus, slow clearance was associated with failure of suppression by a normally suppressive dose of anti-D.

Although the rate of clearance itself seems unlikely to be related to the probability of suppression of immunization, the interaction between antibody-coated red cells and macrophages may explain the relationship. For a start, it is known that the Fc part of IgG is essential for bringing about attachment to macrophages and that F(ab)$_2$ preparations made from IgG anti-D, when injected with small amounts of D positive red cells, fail to bring about red cell destruction (von dem Borne *et al.* 1977a). Fc is also essential for the suppression of primary responses by IgG antibodies (Heyman, 1990). Macrophages which engulf antibody-coated red cells are known to be poor presenters of antigen to the immune system, having very poor expression of class II HLA antigens on their surface. In contrast, dendritic cells have no Fc receptors and therefore do not engulf antibody-coated cells. Dendritic cells may be responsible for the destruction of red cells not coated with antibody; they have very good expression of class II antigens and are essential for antigen presentation and thus for the initiation of immune responses (Crowley *et al.* 1990). Because red cells sensitized with IgG antibodies adhere to and are engulfed by macrophages, they are kept away from dendritic cells which therefore cannot present red cell antigens to T helper cells.

A point of practical importance is whether immunization can be suppressed when antibody is administered at some time interval after antigen, and furthermore whether the immune reponse, once initiated, can be suppressed either partially or totally by passive administration of antibody.

So far as D immunization is concerned there is evidence that in a proportion of subjects the response to D can be suppressed by giving antibody as late as 2 weeks after the D positive cells have been injected (Samson and Mollison, 1975); see also Chapter 5. Passively administered anti-D is ineffective once primary D immunization has been initiated and also fails to suppress secondary reponses (see Chapter 5).

Augmentation of the immune reponse by passive antibody

The term augmentation, applied to immune responses, has been used to describe at least three apparently different effects observed when relatively small amounts of antibody are injected together with antigen:

1   When SRBC are injected into mice the number of plaque-forming cells (PFC) can be increased by injecting purified IgM anti-SRBC with the SRBC (Henry and Jerne, 1968). In confirming this observation, using monoclonal IgM antibody, it was found that the

effect was observed only when the dose was one, i.e. 1×10^5 red cells, which ordinarily elicited a negligible immune response (Lehner *et al.* 1983). The effect of passive IgM antibody is thus to turn an otherwise ineffective stimulus into an effective one. Note that in this system the antigen is heterologous and that the antibody response reaches a peak at about 5 d; the response is thus more like secondary than primary immunization.

In a different context, i.e. in newborn mice which have passively acquired IgG anti-malarial antibodies, passive monoclonal IgM antibody can overcome the suppressive effect of IgG antibody and induce responsiveness to malarial vaccine (Harte *et al.* 1983).

2   In mice injected with human serum albumin together with antibody, with antigen in slight excess, the effect of passive antibody is to accelerate primary immunization and to increase the amount of antibody formed (Terres and Wolins, 1959; 1961). Similar effects have been observed in newborn piglets (Hoerlein, 1957; Segre and Kaeberle, 1962).

3   The stimulus for memory (B_m) cell development appears to be the localization of antigen–antibody complexes on follicular dendritic cells, a process which, at least in mice, is C3-dependent (Klaus *et al.* 1980). Antigen–antibody complexes are 100-fold more effective than soluble antigen in priming virgin B cells to differentiate into B_m cells (Klaus, 1978).

The relevance of the foregoing observations to possible augmentation of immune response to human red cell alloantigens is uncertain. So far as responses to D are concerned, it is unlikely that passive IgM plays any part since the biological effects of IgM antibodies are believed to depend on complement activation and anti-D does not activate complement. Similarly, IgG D antibodies, if they can increase the formation of memory cells, must do it by a method other than that which has been shown to operate in mice. It might seem then, by exclusion, that the effect of small amounts of passively administered IgG anti-D would be to increase antibody formation in primary immunization but, in fact, this effect has not been observed. As described in Chapter 5 the only effect for which there is some evidence is the conversion of an ineffective stimulus into an effective one.

Different effects produced by different IgG subclasses. Experiments in mice indicate that one subclass of IgG (γ G1) when injected with antigen depresses the immune response, whereas another subclass (γ G2), over a certain range of dosage, actually augments the immune response (Gordon and Murgita, 1975). No information is available about possibly analogous differences between human IgG subclasses.

Tolerizing effect of oral antigen
As described above, it is believed that most, if not all, naturally occurring antibodies are formed in response to bacterial antigens carrying determinants which crossreact with red cell antigens. It is likely that bacterial antigens are absorbed mainly through the gut; mechanisms for limiting the immune response to antigens absorbed in this way may therefore be relevant. It seems that at least two mechanisms are involved: (1) the production of IgA antibodies in the gut may limit the uptake of subsequently-ingested antigen (André *et al.* 1974); and (2) oral administration of antigen induces the

formation of suppressor cells (Mattingley and Waksman, 1978). There is evidence that the complex of IgA antibody with antigen is tolerogenic (André *et al.* 1975). Under some circumstances the administration of an antigen by mouth to mice may completely abolish the ability to respond to a subsequent parenteral dose of antigen (Hanson *et al.* 1979). For further references, see Tomasi (1980). In an experiment in human volunteers the oral administration of Rh D antigen to previously unimmunized males failed to influence the subsequent primary response to D positive red cells given i.v. (see Chapter 5).

LECTINS

Although lectins are not antibodies they share two important properties with antibodies, namely, that of binding to specific structures and of causing red cells to agglutinate, and it is convenient to consider them here.

The red cell agglutinating activity of ricin, obtained from the castor bean, was described in 1888 (see reviews by Bird, 1959; Boyd, 1963) but the fact that plant extracts might have blood group specificity was first described 60 years later. Renkonen (1948) showed that some samples of seeds from *Vicia cracca* contain powerful agglutinins acting much more strongly on A than on B or O cells; and Boyd and Reguera (1949) found that many varieties of Lima beans contain agglutinins which are highly specific for group A red cells.

Lectins are sugar-binding proteins or glycoproteins of non-immune origin which agglutinate cells and, or, precipitate glycoconjugates (Goldstein *et al.* 1980). Although first discovered in plants, lectins have also been found in many organisms from bacteria to mammals, e.g. lectins for human red cell antigens are found in the albumin glands of snails and in certain fungi. Further criteria for the definition of lectins were discussed by Goldstein *et al.* (1980).

The simple sugars found on the red cell membrane are D-galactose, mannose, L-fucose, glucose, N-acetylglucosamine, N-acetylgalactosamine and N-acetylneuraminic acid. Although lectins can be classified according to their specificity for these simple sugars 'it must be realized that lectin specificity is not only dependent on the presence of the reactive sugar in terminal position but also on its anomeric configuration, the nature of the sub-terminal sugar, the site of its attachment to this sugar and, in cellular glycoproteins or glycolipids, on the number and distribution of receptor sites and the amount of steric hindrance caused by vicinal (neighbouring) structures. The most important factor is the outward display of the carbohydrate chain which may depend on its "native" configuration or on the configuration imparted to it by the structure of the protein or lipid to which it is attached' (Bird, 1981). Accordingly, each simple sugar may be associated with several different specificities. Since there is some similarity between the various combinations of simple sugars, crossreaction is not unusual amongst lectins.

Some plant seeds contain more than one lectin; e.g. *Griffonia simplicifolia* seeds contain three lectins GS I, GS II and GS III. GS I is a family of five tetrameric isolectins, of which one, A_4, is specific for N-acetyl-D-galactosamine and another, B_4, is specific for D-galactose (Goldstein *et al.* 1981). GS II is specific for N-acetyl-D-glucosamine.

Examples of simple sugars found on the red cell surface which react with lectins, are as follows:

D-*galactose.* D-galactose in α-linked position is the chief structural determinant of B, P_1 and P^k specificity. Lectins with this specificity include those from *Fomes fomentarius* and the B-specific isolectin of GS I. Most D-galactose-specific lectins, however, also react with this sugar in β-linked position and therefore agglutinate human cells regardless of blood group (e.g. the lectin from *Ricinus communis*). The lectins from *Arachis hypogaea*, *Vicia cretica* and *V. graminea* are exceptions and react specifically with certain β-galactose residues.

L-*fucose.* The specific lectins for this sugar include those of *Lotus tetragonolobus*, *Ulex europaeus*, and the lectin from the plasma of the eel *Anguilla anguilla*. All these three lectins are very useful anti-H reagents.

N-*acetylgalactosamine.* Lectins with a specificity for this sugar include those of *Dolichos biflorus*, which reacts with A_1, Tn and Cad determinants, *Phaseolus lunatus* (anti-A) and *Helix pomatia* (anti-A).

Further details about the reactions of lectins will be found in later chapters.

REACTION BETWEEN ANTIGEN AND ANTIBODY

In blood group serology the interaction between antigen on cells and the corresponding antibody is normally detected by observing specific agglutination of the cells concerned. Nevertheless, the fundamental reaction is simply a combination of antigen with antibody, which may or may not be followed by agglutination, and this combination must first be studied.

Combination of antigen and antibody

Antigen and antibody do not form covalent bonds. Rather, the complementary nature of the corresponding structures on antigen and antibody enable the antigenic determinants to come into very close apposition with the binding site on the antibody molecule, and antigen and antibody can then be held together by relatively weak intermolecular bonds. These bonds are believed to include: opposing charges on ionic groups, hydrogen bonds, hydrophobic (non-polar) bonds, and van der Waals forces. Probably, more than one type of bond is usually involved. In one example investigated by Nisonoff and Pressman (1957) an ionic bond at one end of the molecule contributed most to the strength of the bond but a substantial contribution was made by non-polar groups. The strength of the bond between antigen and antibody, measured as the free energy change, was calculated for examples of IgG anti-D, -c, -E and -e to lie within the range $-10\,200$ to $-12\,800$ cal/mol; that for IgG anti-K ($-14\,300$ cal/mol) was rather higher (Hughes-Jones, 1972) (1 cal $\equiv$ 4.2 J). Note that these figures are all for intrinsic affinities (see below). These figures indicate that the strength of the bond between antigen and antibody-combining site, for these particular antibodies, is about one-tenth as great as that of a covalent bond.

The reaction between antibody (Ab) and antigen (Ag) is reversible in accordance with the law of mass action (for review, see Hughes-Jones, 1963) and may be written thus:

$$Ab + Ag \overset{k_1}{\underset{k_2}{\rightleftharpoons}} AbAg$$

where k_1 and k_2 are the rate constants for the forward and reverse reactions respectively.

According to the law of mass action, at equilibrium:

$$\frac{[AbAg]}{[Ab] \times [Ag]} = \frac{k_1}{k_2} = K$$

where [Ab], [Ag] and [AbAg] respectively are the concentrations of Ab, Ag and the combined product AbAg, and K is the equilibrium or association constant. Similarly, at equilibrium:

$$\frac{[AgAb]}{[Ab]} = K[Ag]$$

That is to say, the higher the equilibrium constant the greater will be the amount of antibody combining with antigen at equilibrium.

The equilibrium constant of an antibody may be looked on as a measure of the goodness of the fit of the antibody to the corresponding antigen, and of the type of bonding; for example, hydrophobic bonds generally give rise to higher affinities than do hydrogen bonds. When the equilibrium constant is high, the bond between antigen and antibody will, as a rule, be less readily broken.

IgG antibodies have two antigen-binding sites (Eisen and Karush, 1949). When antigens are close together on cells, both the antigen-combining sites on an antibody may bind to the same cell, a process known as monogamous bivalency (Klinman and Karush, 1967). IgG anti-A and anti-B appear to bind to red cells by both their binding sites (Greenbury *et al.* 1965, but see p. 166) and there is evidence that IgG anti-M also binds bivalently (Romans *et al.* 1979; 1980). IgG anti-D binds to red cells monovalently (Hughes-Jones, 1970). Any anti-A, -B or -M which, at equilibrium, is bound to red cells by just one combining site rapidly dissociates on washing (Romans *et al.* 1979; 1980).

The strength of the bond between antigen and antibody is enormously increased when both combining sites on the antibody can bind to the red cell simultaneously. The bond between antigen and antibody is constantly being broken and, when only one site on the antibody is bound initially, the antibody molecule can drift away from the antigen. When two combining sites are bound, the breaking of one bond leaves the antibody joined to the antigen by the other combining site and there will be an increased opportunity for the first combining site to recombine with antigen before the antibody molecule drifts away. The equilibrium constant is increased approximately 1000-fold when both of the combining sites on an IgG antibody can bind to antigen (Hornick and Karush, 1972).

IgM molecules have ten binding sites, but with antigens of molecular weight greater than about 3000 they have an apparent valency of only five, due to steric hindrance and restricted mobility between the Fab regions of each of the five main subunits (van Oss *et al.* 1973). IgM anti-D appears to bind to individual red cells by only one site, presumably because the distance between two D antigens is too great to be bridged by the combining sites on a single antibody molecule (Holburn et al. 1971b).

With some antigens it has been found that fewer IgM than IgG molecules will combine with a red cell. One explanation for such a finding could be that the antigen sites are so closely packed that, at saturation, IgG molecules cover virtually the whole surface; since IgM molecules are much larger, the maximum number which could bind would clearly then be less. This explanation would apply to the observations of Humphrey and Dourmashkin (1965) that with SRBC the maximum of Forssman antibody molecules which will combine is about 600 000 for IgG and 120 000 for IgM.

Apart from differences between the average equilibrium constants of antibodies from different donors, considerable heterogeneity is always found amongst the antibody molecules of a particular specificity from any one donor (Hughes-Jones, 1967).

The difference between intrinsic and functional binding constants
The term intrinsic binding constant is used to refer to the affinity of a single antibody-combining site for a single antigenic determinant, i.e. monovalent binding, whereas the term functional affinity constant refers to binding of one or more combining sites on an antibody molecule to more than one antigenic determinant on a single carrier, i.e. ignoring valency. As already mentioned, when both combining sites on an IgG antibody are bound, the functional affinity constant may be 1000 times greater than the intrinsic binding constant. For one example of IgM, the enhancement value due to multivalency was of the order of 10×10^6 indicating that multivalent binding involved three or more combining sites (Hornick and Karush, 1972).

Factors affecting the equilibrium constant
The equilibrium constant (a term that includes both intrinsic and functional affinity constants) is affected by pH, ionic strength and temperature, and knowledge of the effect of these variables is helpful in predicting the optimal conditions for eluting antibodies from red cells on the one hand and for the detection of antibodies on the other.

Effect of pH. Hughes-Jones et al. (1964a) found that the equilibrium constant for anti-D was highest between pH 6.5 and 7, although there was relatively little change over the range 5.5–8.5.

A few red cell alloantibodies have been described which are detectable only when pH is reduced, e.g. examples of anti-I and anti-M (see relevant chapters).

Effect of ionic strength. The rate of association of antibody with antigen may be enormously increased by lowering ionic strength. For example, the initial rate of association of anti-D with D-positive red cells is increased 1000-fold by a reduction of ionic strength from 0.17 to 0.03 (see Hughes-Jones et al. 1964a). These authors pointed out that the use of a low-ionic-strength medium should be valuable in detecting antibodies with relatively low equilibrium constants. They found that, in practice, the titre of most blood group antibodies was enhanced by diluting the serum in a low-ionic-strength medium (0.2% NaCl in 7% glucose) rather than in normal saline.

Elliott *et al.* (1964) independently came to a similar conclusion. Using as a diluent a glycine–phosphate buffer to produce a final ionic strength of 0.07 they found that the titre of a number of antibodies was enhanced, although that of examples of anti-A, anti-B, anti-Le^a and anti-Le^b was not.

In studying the effect of low ionic strength on the reaction between anti-D and D-positive red cells, Atchley *et al.* (1964) noted that the enhancement observed was not additive to that observed with enzyme-treated red cells, and they suggested that in both cases the effect was due to a reduction in the electrostatic 'barrier' surrounding the red cells.

The practical value of using a low-ionic-strength medium in the detection of blood group antibodies is discussed in Chapter 8.

Effect of temperature. A distinction must be made between the effects of temperature on (1) the equilibrium constant, and (2) the rate of the reaction. For example, with anti-D, lowering the temperature from 37°C to 4°C slightly increases the equilibrium constant but, since it also slows the rate of reaction 20-fold, is not in practice advantageous (Hughes-Jones *et al.* 1964c).

Different considerations apply to the detection of cold agglutinins which by definition react much more strongly at low temperatures and may produce no detectable reaction at all above a temperature in the approximate range 15–30°C.

The reactions of all antibodies should, in theory, be exothermic, i.e. they should give out heat when combining with antigen. In fact, those of anti-A (Economidou *et al.* 1967b) and -I (Olesen, 1966) have been shown to be mainly exothermic. On the other hand, warm antibodies do not give out heat when combining with antigen and the interaction is instead accompanied by an increase in entropy (Hughes-Jones *et al.* 1963a). The nature of the bond at the combining site determines whether an antibody is warm or cold so that the chemical nature of the antigen is the determining factor; for example, hydrogen bonding is mainly exothermic and stabilized by lower temperatures whereas hydrophobic bonding is mainly associated with a change in entropy, which is increased by higher temperatures (Hughes-Jones, 1975).

In conformity with the view that antigen is the determining factor in deciding whether an antigen–antibody reaction is of a warm or cold type, Lalezari *et al.* (1973) found that seven examples of anti-s and one each of anti-S and -U, although IgG, were all cold-reacting. By contrast, examples of anti-D, -Fy^a and -k reacted more strongly at 37°C; see also pp. 344–345. Note, however, that one kind of naturally occurring IgG anti-D is cold-reacting.

Anti-I (like -i and -Pr), whether IgM or IgG, always reacts more strongly with human red cells at low temperatures. It has been suggested that the greater complementarity of I with its antibody at low temperature, justifying the description 'cold antigen' (Moore, 1976), may depend on the loss of fluidity of the red cell membrane at low temperature (Cooper, 1977). Although human red cells react strongly at 4°C with anti-I and, as a rule, do not react at all at 37°C, rabbit red cells are agglutinated at 37°C.

Non-specific attachment of IgG

If red cells are incubated with labelled serum proteins at a concentration of 20 g/l, about 5–15 μg protein is taken up per millilitre of packed cells. IgG is taken up to the greatest extent (Hughes-Jones and Gardner, 1962; Müller and Gramlich, 1965), which is not surprising since IgG is the most positively charged serum protein and red cells are negatively charged.

There is evidence that the IgG present on normal red cells interacts with anti-IgG serum. For example, in absorbing antiglobulin serum to remove heteroagglutinins, the use of untreated red cells leads to a definite fall in antiglobulin titre whereas the use of trypsin-treated cells does not (Stratton and Jones, 1955) because trypsin removes IgG from the red cells (Merry *et al.* 1982). When washed, but otherwise untreated, red cells are added to ^{125}I-labelled anti-IgG, a small amount of antiglobulin regularly binds to the cells (Rochna and Hughes-Jones, 1965).

Although anti-IgG fails to agglutinate normal red cells in manual testing, positive results are obtained in an AutoAnalyzer; the specificity of the reactions is demonstrated by their inhibition by IgG but not by other proteins (Burkart *et al.* 1974).

Factors involved in red cell agglutination

Red cells normally repel one another, the electric potential (zeta-potential) at the surface of red cells depends not only on the electronegative surface charge but on the ionic cloud which normally surrounds them. The electrostatic repulsion is such that red cells can only approach within about 8 nm of their sialoglycoprotein surfaces, leaving a distance between their actual red cell membranes of about 18 nm. IgM molecules (diameter 30 nm) can bridge the gap and thus bring about agglutination but IgG molecules, with a maximum distance between binding sites of 12 nm, cannot normally do so (van Oss and Absolom, 1983). Another factor besides net negative charge which may be important in keeping cells apart is vicinal water, i.e. water that is tightly bound to the cell surface (for a review, see Steane and Greenwalt, 1980). Although IgG antibodies often fail to agglutinate red cells, agglutination occurs under the influence of various potentiating mechanisms.

Influence of number of antigen sites

Although it is true that many human IgG antibodies fail to agglutinate red cells suspended in saline there are certain exceptions, notably IgG anti-A, anti-B and anti-M. The reasons why IgG anti-A will agglutinate saline-suspended cells whereas, e.g., IgG anti-D will not, may simply be that the number of A sites is about 100 times greater than the number of D sites. The agglutination of –D–/–D– cells by incomplete anti-D also suggests that site number is important.

Additional evidence was provided by experiments in which a hapten was covalently coupled to red cells in different amounts; it was found that a higher hapten density was required for agglutination by IgG antibodies than for IgM antibodies. When the hapten density fell below a certain level, the IgG antibodies behaved as incomplete antibodies and did not agglutinate untreated red cells (Leikola and Pasanen, 1970). Similar findings were reported by Hoyer and Trabold (1971).

It has also been shown that the density of receptors on the red cell surface can influence the thermal amplitude of cold agglutinins; red cells were treated with neuraminidase to remove sialic acid receptors and allowed to adsorb haematoside (sialyllactosylceramide). When fewer than 10^6 molecules of haematoside per cell had been adsorbed, the cells were agglutinated at 0°C but not at 37°C, but when more than 10^6 molecules of haematoside were adsorbed, the cells were agglutinated both at 37°C and at 0°C (Tsai *et al.* 1978).

Other factors besides site number may be: (1) the degree to which the antigen site projects beyond the cell membrane, e.g. A and B project substantially from the lipid bilayer of the red cell membrane (Fukuda *et al.* 1979) whereas Rh D may well not project, and (2) the proximity of the antigen sites to one another. This latter variable will depend, first, on the number of antigen sites per red cell, second on the extent to which the sites occur normally in clusters, and finally the extent to which they are capable of forming clusters after combining with antibody. However, clustering cannot be an absolute requirement since D-positive red cells are agglutinated by incomplete antibody in a medium of albumin (Diamond and Denton, 1945) in circumstances in which clustering does not occur (Victoria *et al.* 1975). Proximity of antigen sites does not necessarily favour agglutination since it makes it possible for antibody molecules to bind bivalently to sites on a single cell.

Minimum number of antibody molecules for agglutination in saline

Some estimates of the minimum number of antibody molecules per red cell required for agglutination by IgM antibodies are as follows: anti-A, about 50 (Economidiou *et al.* 1967b); anti-D, about 120 (Holburn *et al.* 1971b); anti-I (at 5°C), between 65 and 440 (Olesen, 1966). The number of molecules required for agglutination by IgG anti-A (in saline) was found to be much higher: about 7000 (Economidou *et al.* 1967b). Slightly different figures for anti-A were found by Greenbury *et al.* (1963), namely 25 for IgM and 20 000 for IgG.

Similarly, the minimum serum concentration required for agglutination was found to be approximately 0.001 μg/ml for IgM anti-A but 0.2 μg/ml for IgG anti-A (Economidou *et al.* 1967b); on a molar basis IgM anti-A is thus 100 times more effective than IgG anti-A. A similar difference was reported by Ishizaka *et al.* (1965), although the figures for the minimal concentrations of IgM and IgG anti-A for agglutination were about four times lower, presumably due to greater sensitivity of the tests employed. Incidentally, the same authors found that on a weight (and molar) basis IgG anti-A was about ten times less effective than IgM anti-A in producing agglutination.

The minimum concentrations of IgG and IgM anti-A required for agglutination were also determined by Moreno and Kabat (1969). Although on a weight basis IgM was 100 or more times as effective as IgG in two out of three cases, in the third case the IgG antibody was actually a better agglutinator.

Effect of centrifugation

The agglutination of red cells is enhanced by centrifugation (see Chapter 8). Furthermore, some IgG antibodies which will not agglutinate saline-suspended red cells under ordinary conditions may do so if the mixtures are centrifuged. Hirszfeld and Dubiski (1954) found that incomplete (IgG) anti-D would agglutinate D-positive cells after centrifugation at 12 000 rev/min but not at 6000 rev/min; Munk-Andersen (1956) found that agglutination by anti-A (IgG) from cord serum was greatly enhanced by centrifugation for 3 min at 3000 rev/min; the enhancement was striking only when the cells were suspended in saline.

Solomon (1964) confirmed that incomplete anti-D would agglutinate D-positive cells in saline at a sufficiently high centrifugal force. Agglutination began at 4430 g and there was no further enhancement above 17 750 g.

Effect of enzyme treatment of red cells

The action of enzymes on red cells may potentiate agglutination in at least two different ways: first by reducing surface charge, thus allowing cells to come closer to one another (Steane, 1982); for instance, almost all the sialic acid can be removed by treatment with neuraminidase (see review by Whittam, 1964). Although neuramini- dase is the most efficient of all enzymes in reducing the surface charge of red cells (Eylar et al. 1962; Pollack et al. 1965) it is not as effective as proteases (which also remove sialic acid) in increasing red cell agglutinability with certain antibodies. For example, with papain-treated red cells the titre of incomplete anti-D is far higher than with neuraminidase-treated cells (Stratton et al. 1973; Luner et al. 1975). A second way in which enzymes may potentiate agglutination is by removing structures which sterically interfere with the access of antibody molecules (Hughes-Jones et al. 1964b; van Oss et al. 1978).

The increased agglutinability of enzyme-treated red cells is much more pronounced with IgG antibodies than with IgM antibodies. Aho and Christian (1966) tested various agglutinating IgG antibodies and found that their titre was about 16 times higher with enzyme-treated cells than with untreated cells; by contrast, with IgM antibodies the increase was only about four-fold.

Effect of polymers

Red cells suspended in various water-soluble polymers, e.g. serum albumin, gelatin, dextran, polyvinylpyrrolidone (PVP), are agglutinated by IgG antibodies, but the way in which this effect is produced is uncertain. Pollack (1965) proposed that these polymers act by decreasing zeta potential but some of the polymers, e.g. dextran, actually increase zeta potential (Brooks and Seaman, 1973). Although albumin does increase the dielectric constant of water (thus diminishing zeta potential) its effect seems to be too small to account for the enhancement of agglutination observed (van Oss et al. 1978, citing Oncley, 1942). There is evidence that dextran and PVP potentiate agglutination by polymer bridging (Hummel, 1962; Brooks, 1973). Positively charged molecules such as polybrene potentiate agglutination by forming bridges, by virtue of their interaction with the negatively charged red cell surface.

Osmotic effects. Macromolecules, by increasing extracellular colloid osmotic pressure, even though to a much lower level than that prevailing within the red cells, may exert an influence on the shape of red cells and thus facilitate a closer approach between the surface of different cells (van Oss et al. 1978).

Effect of serum and plasma

A mixture of human plasma (or serum) and concentrated bovine albumin is superior to albumin alone as a medium for the agglutination of Rh D-positive red cells by 'incomplete' anti-D (Wiener *et al.* 1947; Pickles, 1949; Stratton and Dimond, 1955). Although these observations indicate clearly that plasma contains an agglutination-enhancing factor which is different from albumin, it is not possible to say exactly what the extra factor or factors may be.

The rouleaux-forming tendency of proteins depends on their shape, molecular weight and concentration; in plasma, fibrinogen is the most important protein and, in serum, Ig. Plasma greatly enhances the agglutination of A (and B) red cells by IgG anti-A (and -B). The enhancing effect of serum is negligible, suggesting that fibrinogen is responsible for the enhancing effect of plasma (Romano and Mollison, 1975).

Red cell spiculation
Another factor that may be important in bringing about agglutination is the formation of red cell spicules, i.e. protrusions of a small radius or curvature (van Oss *et al.* 1978). Spicules are induced by anti-A although not by anti-D (Salsbury and Clarke, 1967), which may account for the fact that IgG anti-A though not IgG anti-D will agglutinate red cells suspended in saline. Furthermore, red cells exposed to 10% dextran (mol. wt. 40 000) and red cells treated with a proteolytic enzyme, exhibit spiculation (van Oss *et al.* 1978).

Elution of blood group antibodies from red cells

Bonds due to ionic (electrostatic) forces are expected to be dissociated either at low or high pH (Hughes-Jones *et al.* 1963b). The van der Waals attraction between antigen and antibody can be turned into a repulsion by lowering the surface tension of the liquid medium to a value intermediate between the surface tension of the antibody-combining site and of the antigenic determinant (van Oss *et al.* 1979). Some red cell antibodies can be completely eluted from red cells by using a suitable medium in which surface tension is lowered and pH raised (van Oss *et al.* 1981).

Antibodies can also be eluted from red cells by heat (Landsteiner and Miller, 1925) partly because the reaction between antigen and antibody is in general exothermic (and heat elution is therefore most successful with cold antibodies) and partly because heating denatures some antigens, e.g. D (N.C. Hughes-Jones, personal communication). However, the methods which are most widely used involve the use of organic solvents. It has been suggested that these compounds produce their effects by lowering surface tension (van Oss *et al.* 1981). Results obtained with various methods of elution are discussed in Chapter 8.

Effects of antibodies on red cells

There is a good deal of evidence to suggest that red cell antibodies do not cause any direct damage to red cells. In theory the attachment of antibody molecules to the red cell surface might possibly interfere with the passage of substances across the red cell membrane or might alter red cell metabolism by stimulating or inhibiting enzymes situated at or near the cell surface. However, so far as human red cells are concerned, there is little evidence in favour of any of these possibilities.

Several authors have found that anti-A and anti-B do not affect the dextrose consumption of A and B red cells (Jandl, 1965; Palek *et al.* 1968) although with packed, incubated cells a decrease has been noted (Benbassat *et al.* 1966). On the other hand, red cells exposed to anti-A show a fall in ATP (Jandl, 1965; Palek *et al.* 1968).

No effect of anti-Rh on red cell glycolysis was found by Jandl (1965), who also observed that amounts of antibody that were more than adequate to cause red cell destruction *in vivo* had no appreciable effect on cation flux *in vitro*; this latter observation has been confirmed: Rh D-positive red cells coated with approximately 30 μg anti-D per ml were found to have a normal uptake of ^{42}K (A.M. Patel, personal communication). On the other hand Schrier *et al.* (1968) found that anti-D inhibited both glycolysis and ATP synthesis.

In sheep an antigen L acts as an inhibitor of active potassium transport (Tucker and Ellory, 1970). In the presence of anti-L the effect of L is neutralized and potassium transport is stimulated (Ellory and Tucker, 1969).

Interactions of antibody-coated red cells with monocytes, other phagocytic cells and lymphocytes

IgG red cell antibodies which are incapable of lysing red cells directly by activating complement to the C8/9 stage bring about red cell destruction by mediating inter-actions with macrophages and other phagocytic cells and, *in vitro* at least, with K lymphocytes. Antibody-coated red cells become attached to these various cells either by an interaction between a site on the Fc fragment of IgG1 or IgG3 molecules and an Fc receptor on the phagocytic or cytotoxic cell, or, if the antibody activates comple-ment but only to the C3 stage, by an additional interaction between C3b or iC3b and complement receptors on effector cells. The Fc-receptor binding site on IgG1 and IgG3 is on the Cγ2 domain, near the hinge region (Woof *et al.* 1986; Fig. 3.8).

Three Fc receptors have been identified: FcR I, found on monocytes and macro-phages, which has the highest affinity, and is the only Fc receptor with high affinity for monomeric IgG; FcR II, found on monocytes, macrophages, neutrophils, B lympho-cytes and platelets; and FcR III, which has the lowest affinity and is found on macrophages, neutrophils and K lymphocytes, although not on resting monocytes (Anderson, 1989).

In vitro, red cells sensitized with IgG anti-D (EA-IgG anti-D) adhere to all three Fc receptors (Klaassen *et al.* 1990). Only adherence to FcR I leads to lysis of EA-IgG anti-D, and adherence to this receptor is therefore probably also essential for cytotoxic lysis of IgG-sensitized cells *in vivo* (Klassen *et al.* 1990; Levy *et al.* 1990). However, it is not certain to which receptor or receptors EA-IgG adhere initially *in vivo*. FcR I, because of its high affinity for monomeric IgG, is probably blocked *in vivo*, whereas FcR II and FcR III are not. Possibly, therefore, EA-IgG adhere initially to FcR II and FcR III and subsequently to FcR I. For *in vitro* assays, e.g. the ADCC(M) assay (see below), it might therefore be preferable to use cultured monocytes on which all three Fc receptors are expressed as effector cells, rather than uncultured monocytes on which FcR III is lacking.

Many IgG-coated red cells may become attached to the same effector cell, giving rise to the appearance of rosetting. After attachment to monocytes, the red cells may be engulfed or may be lysed external to the monocyte membrane by lysosomal enzymes excreted by the monocyte (Fleer *et al.* 1978). The factors that determine whether the cell is engulfed or lysed are uncertain, although there is evidence that lysis

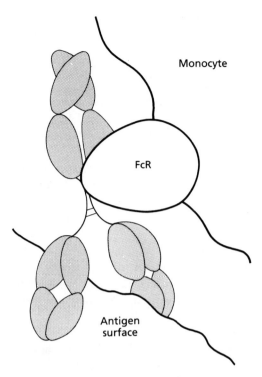

Monocyte

FcR

Antigen
surface

Figure 3.8   Model of the interaction between the monocyte Fc receptor (FcR) and an IgG1 molecule bound to an antigen surface. The two Fab arms are bound to the antigen and the monocyte Fc receptor binds to the inter-heavy-chain disulphide bridges as well as to part of the Cγ2 domain (slightly modified from Woof *et al.* 1986).

is associated with relatively high concentrations of antibody (Engelfriet *et al.* 1981). Presumably, the ratio of effector cells to red cells must be another important factor. IgG subclass and the ability to bind complement are also involved (see below). In animals, intense erythrophagocytosis is found in splenic macrophages after giving hetero-immune sera (Levaditi, 1902; Dudgeon *et al.* 1909) or after transfusing incompatible red cells to an animal which has developed a corresponding alloantibody (Swisher and Young, 1954). In these particular cases the antibodies were complement activating. Although red cells coated with IgG alone are also engulfed mainly by macrophages they may be engulfed by phagocytic cells other than monocytes and macrophages, e.g. granulocytes. Furthermore, following attachment to K lymphocytes, the red cell may be lysed by perforins excreted by the lymphocyte, although this interaction has been studied only *in vitro*. Most of the foregoing interactions have been used as the basis for cellular bioassays to assess the clinical significance of red cell alloantibodies.

In vivo, the main effector cells in the destruction of antibody-coated red cells are splenic and hepatic macrophages, but since these cells are not available for use in assays, alternatives must be found. The cells used include monocytes from peripheral blood, a cultured malignant cell line, e.g. 'U937' (Kumpel *et al.* 1989b), macrophages derived by culturing monocytes (Armstrong *et al.* 1987) or these cultured macrophages stimulated with γ-interferon to increase the number of IgG Fc receptors expressed on the phagocyte membrane (Wiener and Garner, 1987; Wiener *et al.* 1987). There are substantial differences in activity between the monocytes of different subjects (Munn and Chaplin, 1977; Douglas *et al.* 1985) and tremendous increases in phagocytic activity are noted in acute viral infections (Munn and Chaplin, 1977). In practice, standardization can be achieved by using a pool of monocytes, e.g. derived by elutriation from buffy coats of 50–100 donations from healthy subjects; the monocytes can be mixed with dimethyl sulphoxide and stored in ampoules in the frozen state (Engelfriet and Ouwehand, 1990). In two circumstances, the use of a pool is inappropriate: first, when using a bioassay to predict whether serologically incompatible red cells will be destroyed if transfused to a recipient whose serum contains an antibody of doubtful significance: in such a case, the recipient's own monocytes should be used in the assay; and second, when testing for the presence of Fc-receptor-blocking antibodies in a mother's serum, when monocytes from the father should be used.

Erythrophagocytosis in peripheral blood. Although tissue macrophages are the chief sites of engulfment of incompatible red cells, erythrophagocytosis by neutrophils may be observed in samples of peripheral blood (see Chapter 10). Erythrophagocytosis in blood films is also found in severe autoimmune haemolytic anaemia (see Dacie, 1962, p. 359).

Role of complement. Complement-coated red cells become attached to a variety of cells through various receptors. CR1 receptors are abundant on red cells and are also present on many other cells, including neutrophils and monocytes. CR1 binds C3b and C4b and binds weakly to iC3b. Other functions of CR1 are discussed in a later section. It is postulated that CR1 sites, with C3b molecules attached, undergo proteolytic digestion during contact with macrophages in the liver and spleen. In cold haemagglutinin disease there are only 50–200 CR1 receptors per red cell compared with the normal of 400–1200 per cell (Ross *et al.* 1985).

CR3 receptors are found on neutrophils, monocytes and large granular lymphocytes and bind primarily to iC3b. A closely related receptor, CR4, binds both iC3b and, with a much lower affinity, C3dg, and is the predominant type of C3 receptor expressed on tissue macrophages (see review by Ross, 1989). CR2 binds mainly to C3dg and presumably plays no significant role in red cell destruction.

C3b and iC3b play the most active role (in collaboration with Ig) in bringing about erythrophagocytosis. C3dg is a poor opsonizer, acting only through CR4. In cold haemagglutinin disease, red cells coated with as many as 20 000 C3dg molecules per cell are present in the circulation without being cleared by the mononuclear phagocyte system (MPS) (Ross, 1986).

The role of complement in erythrophagocytosis seems to be primarily to bring about attachment of red cells to macrophages. Red cells coated with C3b alone normally undergo little or no phagocytosis although they may be ingested by activated macrophages (see discussion on pp. 453–455).

Red cells incubated with IgM alone bind to monocytes only if complement is present (Huber *et al.* 1968). Red cells coated with approximately 80 000 molecules C3 per cell without Ig form abundant rosettes with monocytes but are not lysed (Kurlander *et al.* 1978).

There is a synergistic action between IgG and C3b (iC3b), and phagocytosis is enormously enhanced when both are attached to red cells (Ehlenberger and Nussenz-weig, 1977). Each pair of bound IgG molecules may bring about the binding of many C3b molecules. *In vivo*, the amount of bound IgG needed to produce a given rate of clearance is very much less if C3b is also bound (see Chapter 10).

Bioassays

Rosetting and phagocytosis

Rosetting. Fewer IgG3 than IgG1 molecules per red cell are required to bring about attachment to effector cells. Using monoclonal anti-D, estimates for the minimum number for attachment to monocytes have ranged from 100 to 600 for IgG3 and from 2000 to 10 000 for IgG1 (Wiener *et al.* 1987; Merry *et al.* 1988; 1989). Similar results have been observed with polyclonal anti-D (Zupanska *et al.* 1986). The rather wide range of results is due presumably to many factors such as heterogeneity in monocyte activity; heterogeneity of antibodies, since both IgG1 and IgG3 antibodies produced by different clones or different individuals differ in their capacity to adhere to Fc receptors (Armstrong *et al.* 1987; Engelfriet and Ouwehand, 1990); variability of methods of scoring red cell–monocyte interaction; and a lack of standardization of methods, e.g. for quantitating the numbers of bound antibody molecules. Not only are fewer IgG3 than IgG1 molecules required for adherence to monocytes, but the rate of interaction between IgG-coated red cells and monocytes is more rapid with IgG3 than with IgG1 (Brojer *et al.* 1989). It has been suggested that the more potent activity of IgG3 compared with IgG1 is due to the relatively long hinge on the IgG3 molecule, leading to greater accessibility to the Fc-receptor binding site (Woof *et al.* 1986; Wiener *et al.* 1987) which, as stated above, is near the hinge on the $C\gamma 2$ domain of IgG.

Whereas about 80% of monocytes have Fc receptors and are capable of forming rosettes, for lymphocytes the number is only about 10%. Moreoever, with lymphocytes the minimum number of IgG3 molecules (monoclonal) for rosetting was 2000 per cell, i.e. four times greater than for monocytes in the same experiments, and no rosetting was found with IgG1 (Merry *et al.* 1988). It should be noted that the number of Fc receptors expressed on a particular cell varies and is increased, for example, under the influence of γ-interferon so that it is uncertain how closely these estimates obtained by experiments *in vitro* indicate events *in vivo*.

Phagocytosis. Using polyclonal anti-D, a phagocytosis assay with monocytes was found to be no more sensitive than a rosette assay, the minimum numbers of IgG molecules per red cell for a positive result being 150–640 for IgG3 and 1230–4020 for IgG1 (Zupanska *et al.* 1987). In several other investigations, using both polyclonal and monoclonal anti-D, IgG3 antibodies have been found to be more active than IgG1 (Douglas *et al.* 1985; Hadley *et al.* 1989; Kumpel *et al.* 1989b) although in one study all of seven examples of IgG1 were more effective than seven examples of IgG3 in mediating phagocytosis (Wiener *et al.* 1988). The cause of these discrepancies is not clear but it may lie in variations in assay conditions. For example, in one investigation, at low ratios of red cells to monocytes, IgG3 was more active and, at high ratios, IgG1 was more active (Hadley and Kumpel, 1989). When measuring phagocytosis, as opposed to adherence, the use of 5% CO_2 appears to be important to maintain pH at an approximately physiological level; if 5% CO_2 is not used the activity of weak antibodies may be overlooked (Branch and Gallagher, 1985).

Many different assays for antibody activity, based on the ability to mediate rosetting and, or, phagocytosis by monocytes or macrophages have been devised. One essential condition in the tests is to bring antibody-coated red cells and effector cells into close contact, so that either centrifugation must be employed or the monocytes and red cells allowed to come together by simple sedimentation, as in the monocyte-monolayer assay (MMA). There are substantial differences between different laboratories in the way in which the test is done: monocytes may be taken from a single donor or from a pool; they may be fresh or stored; the tests may be read as the proportion of monocytes exhibiting rosetting or as the number of red cells engulfed per monocyte; or both adherence and engulfment may be measured and the result expressed as the total association index (TAI).

Not surprisingly, different degrees of success have been reported in assessing the destructive powers of different antibodies but, in some hands, the test seems capable of being of real practical value (see Chapters 10 and 12).

Antibody-dependent cell-mediated cytotoxicity (ADCC) assays

ADCC assays are carried out either with monocytes or macrophages (ADCC(M) assays) or with K lymphocytes (ADCC(L) assays).

ADCC(M) assay. Human monocytes will lyse anti-D-coated red cells *in vitro* (Kurlander *et al.* 1978). Lysis is brought about by the release of lysosomal enzymes (Fleer *et al.* 1978). An assay that has proved valuable in predicting the severity of Rh D haemolytic disease has been devised in which red cells are labelled with ^{51}Cr, coated with antibody, washed and then incubated with pooled monocytes. Lysis is measured by estimating the ^{51}Cr released into the supernatant (Engelfriet and Ouwehand, 1990).

Red cells coated with IgG1 autoantibodies are lysed only when the number of antibody molecules per cell is well above the number needed for a positive DAT; on the other hand, cells coated with a number of IgG3 molecules too small to give a positive DAT may be lysed in an ADCC(M) assay (Engelfriet *et al.* 1981). Similarly, using monoclonal anti-Ds, IgG3 has been shown to be more effective than IgG1 in mediating lysis (Wiener *et al.* 1988).

ADCC(L) assay. Lymphocytes are capable of lysing antibody-coated red cells by producing 'perforins', substances similar to the terminal components of complement, which produce holes in the red cell membrane (Podack and Konigsberg, 1984).

The ADCC(L) assay differs from the ADCC(M) assay not only in the use of different effector cells but also in using enzyme-treated target cells, after the latter have been prepared, they are incubated with serum and lymphocytes (Urbaniak 1979a, b), although in a variation of the test, enzyme-treated red cells may first be incubated with serum and then with lymphocytes. Only a minority of monoclonal IgG_1 antibodies mediate lysis in the ADCC(L) assay (Armstrong *et al.* 1987; Kumpel *et al.* 1989a, b); three of three monoclonal IgG3 anti-Ds were ineffective (Kumpel *et al.* 1989a) as have been all polyclonal IgG3 anti-Ds tested so far; on the other hand, one monoclonal IgG3 anti-c mediated lysis (Second International Workshop on Red Cell Monoclonal Antibodies, 1990).

Results of the ADCC(L) test carried out on the serum of Rh D-immunized mothers are quite well correlated with the severity of haemolytic disease in the fetus (see Chapter 12).

Chemiluminescence (CL) assay

This assay measures the oxidative 'burst' that accompanies phagocytosis (Descamps-Latscha et al. 1983). Mononuclear cells are incubated at 37°C with pre-sensitized red cells and luminol, and the CL response is monitored for 1 h (Hadley et al. 1988). The results of CL assays, carried out on the serum of Rh D-immunized mothers, have been found to be approximately as well correlated with the severity of haemolytic disease in the fetus as have the results of ADCC(M) assays (Hadley et al. 1991; Report of Nine Collaborating Laboratories, 1991).

The results of CL assays have provided the only evidence so far of synergism between IgG1 and IgG3 antibodies. Using several examples of monoclonal anti-D, the metabolic response of monocytes was greater towards IgG3-coated cells than towards IgG1-coated cells but was greater still towards cells coated with both subclasses (Hadley and Kumpel, 1989).

Role of complement in cellular bioassays

Some red cell alloantibodies react in bioassays only if complement is present. In tests with a phagocytosis assay, the number of examples of anti-Fy^a and anti-Jk^a which gave positive results was about 30% greater if complement was present in the sensitization phase (Branch et al. 1984). In detecting anti-Le^a in the presence of complement, a mononuclear phagocyte assay, using cultured macrophages, was as sensitive as the antiglobulin test (Wiener and Garner, 1985). Two examples of anti-Lan which had been associated with rapid destruction of labelled incompatible red cells in vivo (Nance et al. 1987) and several other antibodies, including examples of anti-Jk^a, -Jk^b and -Vel, gave positive results in a bioassay only if complement was present (Nance et al. 1988).

Comparison of different assays

ADCC assays, like the CL assay, have the advantage that they rely on objective measurement rather than, as with tests for rosetting and phagocytosis, on visual inspection.

All these tests have been used in attempts to estimate the ability of antibodies to cause red cell destruction in vivo in two circumstances: first, when a patient requires transfusion and his or her serum contains a warm-reacting alloantibody of doubtful clinical significance, reacting with all red cells tested; and second, when a woman is pregnant with a fetus believed to have haemolytic disease and an estimate is needed of the destructive power of the antibody concerned. Results obtained in these two circumstances are described respectively in Chapters 10 and 12. In performing any particular bioassay, it is essential on each occasion to test a series of dilutions of a standard antibody so as to prepare a calibration curve from which results for the patient's sample can be derived. It is also very informative to undertake 'blind' testing of suitable samples. The results of testing a number of different assays in this way on samples from the mothers of infants with Rh D haemolytic disease have been described (Report from Nine Collaborating Laboratories 1991) and are referred to in Chapter 12.

COMPLEMENT

Complement is the name given to a system of approximately 20 serum proteins which, in response to a stimulus, react with one another sequentially in a cascade reaction: the product of one reaction is the enzyme catalysing the next reaction. The products have potent biological effects: (1) they promote inflammation through chemotaxis and increased vascular permeability; and (2) they cause cell destruction either directly, through activation of the whole complement cascade with the formation of the membrane attack complex (MAC), or indirectly, through a product, C3b, which mediates attachment of coated cells to effector cells, e.g. phagocytes. Activated C3 (C3b) and the MAC both result from activation of either of two pathways, the classical pathway and the alternative pathway, which have structural and functional similarities. It is probable that the alternative pathway was the first to develop during evolution and that the classical pathway evolved from it (Lachmann, 1979). Once activated C3 has been produced by the classical pathway, its production is amplified by the alternative pathway (see below).

Activation of the classical pathway
The components involved in the first phases of activation of the classical pathway are C1 (a complex composed of C1q, C1r and C1s), C2, C3 and C4. All these components are present in plasma in their native unactivated configuration; the concentrations of most components are low although those of C3, C4 and factor B are of the order of 0.1 g/l. Activation consists of the enzymic splitting of the components, which in turn develop proteolytic properties. The components were given numbers before the sequence of events in the cascade was elucidated and the order of activation is C1, 4, 2, 3 followed by C5–9. Activation can be considered in four phases: (1) activation of C1; (2) activation of C42; (3) activation of C3; and (4) activation of C5–9, leading to the formation of the MAC (Fig. 3.9).

Immunoglobulin requirements for activation of the classical pathway
The commonest mode of activation of the classical pathway is through the binding of C1q to the C_H2 domain of IgM or to the C_H2 domain of some IgG1 or IgG3 antibodies. The C1q molecule has six Fc binding sites and, in order to make a firm bond with the Ig complex, at least two of these sites must bind to Ig. In the case of IgG, two antibody molecules must be present on the antigen surface within about 20–30 nm of one another, this being the maximum span of a C1q molecule. In the case of IgM, the mechanism is different; when the molecule is in its planar or 'star' form, (with the $F(ab')_2$ pieces and the $(Fc)_5$ disc in the same plane), there is only a single binding site for C1q on each side of the $(Fc)_5$ disc and C1q cannot bind firmly. However, when combined with antigen, the IgM molecule frequently assumes a staple form with the $F(ab')_2$ at right angles to the $(Fc)_5$ disc (Feinstein *et al.* 1971; see Fig. 3.5). The distortion produced by this movement exposes additional C1q binding sites (Perkins *et al.* 1991)

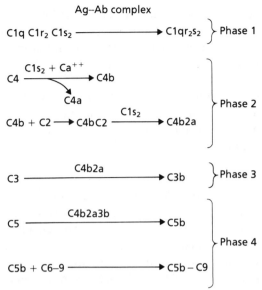

Figure 3.9 Activation of the classical pathway of complement, considered in four phases:
(1) activation of C1; (2) formation of C4b2a (C3 convertase); (3) activation of C3, to form C3b;
and (4) formation of C5b–9, the membrane attack complex. When the rate of formation of C3b is
sufficiently rapid, C4b2a3b catalyses the activation of C5 to C5b and the reaction proceeds to
phase 4 with the formation of transmembrane channels that will increase permeability of the cell
to Na and H_2O, leading to cell lysis.

and a C1q molecule can thus bind to two sites on a single IgM molecule. IgM is thus
considerably more efficient than IgG as an activator of C1 and the binding of a single
IgM molecule to an SRBC can lead to lysis; in contrast, assuming that the red cell has
600 000 antibody-binding sites, about 800 IgG molecules must be bound to provide an
even chance that two will occupy closely adjacent sites and thus activate complement
(Humphrey and Dourmashkin, 1965).

If two IgG antibodies bind to different epitopes on the same antigen, complement
activation is greatly enhanced (Hughes-Jones *et al*. 1984).

When bound to cells, the various subclasses of IgG vary widely in their ability to
bind complement: IgG3 molecules are highly active, IgG1 moderately, IgG2 slightly,
and IgG4 not at all; IgA antibodies do not bind C1. At least one antibody, i.e. anti-Rh
D, bind C1q but nevertheless fails to activate C1 (see Chapter 5).

Phase 1: activation of C1
C1 is a complex composed of two components: (1) C1q, whose function is to bind the
whole C1 molecule to the target; and (2) a tetramer, composed of two C1r and two C1s
molecules ($C1r_2C1s_2$); C1r and C1s are serine proteases present in unactivated C1 in
the proenzyme form. The composition of C1 is thus C1q $C1r_2C1s_2$. The primary event
in activation is the autocatalytic cleavage of C1r which results in the appearance of an
active enzymic site. C1r then cleaves C1s, which in turn becomes an active enzyme,
C1s. Isolated C1 in solution slowly autoactivates, but this does not take place in the
plasma owing to the presence of an inhibitory protein, C1 inhibitor (see below).
Activation of C1q is triggered by antibody binding to antigen (see above). The

mechanism of activation is probably as follows: (1) the C1 inhibitor (C1-Inh) is sterically prevented from gaining access to the C1r molecules: and (2) there is a positive stimulus to activation, the nature of which is not definitely known but may be the provision of optimal conditions for autoactivation of C1 (Hughes-Jones, 1986).

Inhibitor of C1 in serum. Serum normally contains an inhibitor of C1, C1-Inh, which has two functions: (1) it inhibits the autoactivation of native C1 in solution in the plasma by binding weakly to the C1r subcomponent of $C1r_2C1s_2$ tetramer; and (2) it inhibits activated C1r and C1s molecules.

Phase 2: formation of the C3/C5 convertase (C4b2a)

The C3/5 convertase is a bimolecular complex composed of one molecule each of activated C4 and C2. The activation of one C1 complex can generate more than 100 C3/C5 convertases attached to the cell membrane. The C4 molecule is a structural protein which has the dual function of binding to the foreign particle or to the cell surface and to C2, the molecule which carries the active enzyme site. C4 is first split by C1s into the anaphylatoxin C4a, and C4b. The splitting results in the appearance of an active but highly labile thioester bond on C4b which enables it to bind covalently with both -OH and $-NH_2$ groups on the Fc region of Ig in the Ag–Ab complex or to the membrane of the cell itself (red cell, microbe, etc.). In the presence of Mg^{2+}, C2 then becomes attached to the bound C4b and in turn is cleaved by C1s into C2a and C2b. This cleavage results in the appearance of an active site on the C2 molecule; it is this enzyme site (on C2a) which cleaves and activates C3; see review by Hughes-Jones (1986). The C3 convertase, C4b2a is broken down either by a C4 binding protein (C4bp) or by CR1, the cell membrane receptor for C3b, in the presence of Factor I.

Phase 3: the splitting of C3

The initial event in this phase is the splitting of a small polypeptide (C3a, another anaphylatoxin) from the C3 molecule by C4b2a to give C3b. One molecule of C4b2a can generate hundreds of C3b molecules, thus amplifying the cascade even further. C3b carries an active site (identical to that found on C4b) which is highly labile, with a life span of approximately 60 μs, during which time it can diffuse approximately 40 nm (Sim *et al.* 1981). C3b is deposited in clusters on the cell membrane around C4b2a to form the C5 splitting enzyme, C4b2a3b. Activation of complement by blood group antibodies frequently stops at this stage; only C3b can bind to C5 and C3b is very rapidly converted to iC3b (see below). Thus, unless large amounts of C3b are generated, no significant amounts are available for combination with C5, and activation of complement cannot proceed to phase 4. C3b on the cell surface mediates adherence to phagocytic cells through CR1 (see below).

Steps in the degradation of C3 (Fig. 3.10). C3b is cleaved, especially when in solution, by the C3b inactivator, Factor I, using Factor H as co-factor to yield iC3b; *in vitro* this process takes about 1 min (Harrison and Lachmann, 1980). iC3b is further cleaved by Factor I; C3c is split off, leaving only C3dg on the cell surface. In blood, where there are cells carrying CR1 (see p. 134 for a description of complement receptors) which is

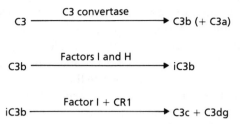

Figure 3.10 Steps in the breakdown of C3; see text.

the co-factor for this cleavage, the reaction is about 50% complete in about 20 min (P.J. Lachmann, personal communication).

Using radiolabelled monoclonal anti-C3c, the rate of cleavage to C3dg was measured after binding C3b to red cells with antibodies of various specificities. The $t_{1/2}$ of cleavage varied from 16 to 48 min. The rate of breakdown of iC3b was correlated directly with the number of CR1 receptors per red cell, reflecting their role as co-factors in the cleavage of iC3b by Factor I (Currie *et al.* 1988).

Another factor regulating the activation of C3 is decay accelerating factor (DAF). DAF is a glycoprotein which dissociates C2a from C4b2a and Bb from C3bBb, thus preventing the formation of C3 convertases of the classical and alternative pathways (Fujita *et al.* 1987). The absence of DAF on the red cells of patients with paroxysmal nocturnal haemoglobulinuria (PNH) probably accounts, in part, for the increased binding of C3 on PNH red cells (Nicholson-Weller *et al.* 1983). For further references see Rosse (1986 and 1989). ('Decay accelerating factor' is now seen to be a misnomer, the term should really be 'C3 activator inhibition factor'.)

Phase 4: formation of the membrane attack complex (MAC)
When C3b is generated rapidly enough and in sufficient numbers, it combines with C4b2a to split C5 into an active molecule C5b and the potent anaphylatoxin C5a. This is the last of the enzymic steps; activated C5b on the membrane binds C6 and then C7, exposing hydrophobic groups on both C6 and C7 with the result that the trimolecular complex C5b67 (which appears on electron microscopy as a rod of length approximately 25–30 nm) is inserted with almost 100% efficiency into the phospholipid membrane of the red cells. C8 then binds to C5b67 and is also partly inserted into the membrane with the result that a small pore is made. The presence of the C5–8 polymer then allows assembly of two or more molecules of the terminal component C9; in the fully developed polymer, up to 10–16 molecules of C9 coalesce to form a tubular structure, which has hydrophobic regions on the outer surface to allow membrane insertion and a hydrophilic region on the inner surface to allow water and solutes to pass freely in and out of the membrane (Podack, 1986). Na^{2+} and H_2O get into the cell, with consequent swelling and lysis.

The lesions in the cell membrane produced by the MAC appear on electron microscopy as holes. With human complement and human red cells, the diameter of the holes is about 10 nm, irrespective of whether the antibody is anti-A, anti-I, biphasic haemolysin (anti-P) or rabbit anti-human red cell (Rosse *et al.* 1966).

In addition to the mechanisms described above, which accelerate the decay of C3 convertase and thus limit the formation of the MAC, there are mechanisms which inhibit the lytic potential of C5b67. C8 binding protein (C8bp) is an intrinsic membrane protein of mol. wt. 65 000 which can bind C8 and thus inhibit the interaction of C5b67 with C8 and C9; C8bp does not accelerate the decay of C3/5 convertases. Thus, C8bp and DAF act synergistically to minimize the self-inflicted damage by complement (Schonermark et al. 1986). Another protein, of mol. wt. 18 000, membrane inhibitor of reactive lysis (MIRL), which is deficient in some PNH cells, also restricts the assembly of the MAC (Holguin et al. 1989).

Biological activity of split fragments
The small peptides split from the native molecules during complement activation, C3a, C5a and to a lesser extent C4a, have important biological functions. They stimulate the respiratory burst associated with the production of oxygen radicals of phagocytic cells, especially neutrophils. These split molecules stimulate the degranulation of mast cells and basophils with liberation of histamine and other vasoactive substances leading to increased vascular permeability, increased smooth muscle contraction and release of lysosomal enzymes from neutrophils. In addition, C5a is a potent neutrophil chemotactic agent, capable of acting directly on endothelial cells of capillaries to induce vasodilatation and increased permeability.

Activation of the alternative pathway (Fig. 3.11)
The series of reactions leading to the activation of C3 which are not mediated by antigen–antibody complexes have been called the 'alternative pathway' of complement activation. Potent stimuli for activation of this pathway are membranes of microorganisms, endotoxins, Ig aggregates, bound IgA, etc.

Six proteins are involved in the alternative pathway; of these, three are concerned with activation (Factors D, B and C3), one with stabilization (properdin, P) and two with inhibition (the enzyme, C3b inactivator or Factor I and its co-factor, H). The function of the alternative pathway is the formation of a C3/C5 convertase, represented as C3bBb, which is different from the classical pathway convertase, C4b2a.

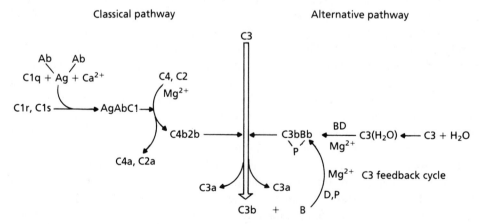

Figure 3.11   Activation of the C3 stage by the classical and alternative pathways.

C3b brings about the destruction of foreign cells (e.g. bacteria) but not of host cells since on them (although not on foreign cells) C3b is continuously degraded to iC3b by the joint action of Factors H and I. On the other hand, bacteria activate and stabilize C3bBb to generate large amounts of C3b on their surface.

In plasma there is a continuous but slow activation of the thioester bond on C3 by H_2O molecules or by plasma proteolytic enzymes to form C3b. This autoactivated molecule reacts with Factor B in the presence of Mg^{2+}; the binding of Factor B results in its modulation so that it is split into Ba and Bb by the action of Factor D, an enzyme always present in an active state at low concentrations (about 1 μg/ml). The resultant molecule, C3bBb, is a C3/C5 convertase which cleaves more C3 molecules to form C3b with activated thioester bonds. These unstable C3b molecules become attached to carbohydrates on cell surfaces and, by combination with Factor B and activation by Factor D, themselves become C3/C5 convertases. These convertase molecules then generate more C3b and the density of C3/C5 convertase molecules on the surface increases exponentially as a result of self-replication and amplification. This process is enhanced by the action of properdin which combines with and stabilizes C3bBb. The end-result is thus both the deposition of large amounts of C3b which, in collaboration with IgG or IgM, brings about phagocytosis, and the activation of C5, with subsequent formation of the MAC and eventual lysis. Due to the action of Factors H and I, the self-replication process does not take place on non-activating surfaces, such as host cells. Factor H reacts with the same binding site on C3b as Factor B and thus inhibits C3bBb formation. Factor I enzymatically cleaves C3b to the inactive form iC3b, using Factor H as co-factor. iC3b is then further degradated by poleolytic enzymes in plasma. The reason why Factors I and H cannot gain access to C3bBb on foreign organisms is not fully understood; the presence of sialic acid on the particle surface would appear to be one of the factors involved in preventing access (Pangburn and Müller-Eberhard, 1984).

Other aspects of complement

Presence of C3d and C4d on normal red cells
As discussed in Chapter 7, small amounts of C3d and C4d are found on normal red cells and larger amounts are found on the red cells in many disease states. As described above, C3 contains an internal thioester bond which undergoes slow spontaneous hydrolysis or activation by trace amounts of proteolytic enzymes. There is a similar internal thioester bond in C4 which, presumably, is also hydrolysed by H_2O (Law *et al.* 1980; Janatova and Tack, 1981). The spontaneous generation of activated C3 and C4 in plasma provides a mechanism for the deposition of complement components on normal red cells.

Complement in the infant
As measured by its power to lyse antibody-coated SRBC the serum of newborn infants has about half the activity of adults (Ewald *et al.* 1961). Estimation of individual components shows that the levels of C1q, C4 and C3 are also about 50% of the adult level; the levels of C5 and C7 are about 70% of the adult level; but that of C9 is only

about 20%. Expressed as a percentage of maternal values the figures are a little lower because the levels of some complement components are higher in pregnant women than in other adults. Adult values of the various complement components are reached within 6–12 months of birth (see review by Adinolfi and Zenthon, 1984).

Species differences in complement activity
The components of complement are so similar in different species that for many purposes they can be interchanged. On the other hand, there are some striking differences in activity, one example of which is that, in bringing about haemolysis, an animal's own complement is often much less effective than that of another species. For example, there are many human alloantibodies which produce little or no haemolysis when incubated *in vitro* with appropriate red cells and with human complement but which are strongly lytic with rabbit complement (Mollison and Thomas, 1959).

    Rabbit complement is used routinely in tissue typing by lymphocytotoxicity tests.

Does complement affect the binding of antibody to red cells?

Possible increase in binding. Evidence that activated C1 can increase the bond between antibody and antigen was provided by Rosse *et al.* (1968). Using a partially purified preparation of C1, containing no detectable C2 or C4, they showed that activated C1 increased the binding of certain examples of human anti-I; EDTA only partially prevented this effect, suggesting the C1q may play some part in the binding of antibody. The observations suggested that only those examples of anti-I with a relatively low binding constant were bound more strongly in the presence of complement, which perhaps explains why Evans *et al.* (1965), using a potent auto-anti-I, found that the rate of association and dissociation of the antibody was unaffected by the presence of complement.

Possible interference with binding. If adult red cells are coated with complement by exposure at 25°C to serum from a patient with cold haemagglutinin disease and are then warmed to 37°C to elute anti-I they are less well agglutinated than control cells by anti-I; there is evidence that the accumulation of complement (now known to be mainly C3dg) on red cells, following exposure to anti-I, interferes with the reactivity of the cells both with anti-I and with complement (Evans *et al.* 1967). Prozones observed when certain group sera are incubated with group A red cells appear to be due to the uptake of complement (Andersen, 1936; Stratton, 1963) which interferes non-specifically with agglutination (Voak, 1972). The uptake of complement on to red cells, mediated by one alloantibody, e.g. anti-Jk[a], may interfere with agglutination produced by another, for instance anti-D, introducing the possibility of misidentification or even of transfusing incompatible red cells (Lown *et al.* 1984).

Anti-complementary activity

Anticoagulants. Ca^{2+} is essential for the integrity of C1 and is therefore needed for the activation of complement by the classical pathway. Mg^{2+} is required for the formation of the C3 convertases of both the classical and alternative pathways, i.e. C4b2a and

C3bBb, respectively. Accordingly, all chelators of Ca^{2+} and Mg^{2+} inhibit C activity; e.g. the addition of 2 mg Na_2 EDTA to 1 ml serum completely blocks the activation of complement.

Heparin is also anti-complementary. According to Strunk and Colten (1976). 2.5 iu heparin per ml will completely inhibit the cleavage of C4 by C1 *in vitro*. Nevertheless, much higher concentrations are required to prevent the uptake of C4 and C3 by antibody-coated cells. For example, if Le(a +) red cells are strongly sensitized with EDTA-treated anti-Le^a serum and then washed, they will still take up complement components from heparinized serum until the amount of heparin exceeds 100 iu/ml (Mollison, 1983, p. 263). Similarly, in lytic tests more than 100 iu/ml are required to reduce the CH_{50} to zero (D.L. Brown, personal communication).

Heating serum to 56°C for 30 min completely inactivates C1 and C2. Heating to 56°C damages C4 to a lesser extent, although after 20 min at 56°C, C4 activity may be reduced to 20% of the initial value (Bier *et al*. 1945; Heidelberger and Mayer, 1948). Factor B of the alternative pathway is inactivated by being heated to 50°C for 20 min.

Stored serum. Anti-complementary properties developing *in vitro* are not well understood. Ehrlich and Sachs (1905), and Bordet (1909) interpreting the work of Gay (1905), suggested that complement might be partly damaged, for example by being heated, and that the altered type of complement ('complementoid') was capable of combining with sensitized cells without producing the usual cell lysis; and that, furthermore, complementoid could block the action of normal complement. Polley and Mollison (1961) showed that the uptake of altered complement on sensitized red cells could be prevented by EDTA; thus if sera containing antibody and 'complementoid' were treated with EDTA and then incubated with red cells, antibody alone was taken up and the sensitized cells, after being washed, would bind complement normally (see p. 348). Polley and Mollison confirmed the observation of Auguste (1934) that, on storage, serum regularly becomes anti-complementary. The alteration in complement occurring on storage may affect principally C4 (M.J. Polley, unpublished observations, 1964).

Complement activation by blood group antibodies

Table 3.8 summarizes the relationship between the blood group specificity of different antibodies and the property of binding complement; in the table and in the following paragraphs almost all references are omitted but they will be found in the following chapters in which the various blood group antibodies are described in more detail.

Haemolysis

Almost all antibodies that will lyse untreated red cells have specificities within the ABO, Lewis, P or Ii systems. Probably all examples of anti-A and anti-B (including anti-A, B in group O serum) will lyse untreated A and B red cells, although when the antibody is weak a high ratio of serum to cells may be required. Anti-H occurring in O$_h$ subjects is lytic. Some examples of anti-Le^a and a very few of anti-Le^b, rare examples of anti-P$_1$, all examples of anti-PP$_1$P^k and anti-P, many of anti-Vel, and potent examples of auto-anti-I and auto-anti-i will also lyse untreated red cells. Occasional examples of

Table 3.8 Complement binding by human red cell antibodies

System	Antibody	Readily detectable haemolysis*	Positive antiglobulin test (anti-complement)
ABO	anti-A ⎫ anti-B ⎬ anti-A,B ⎭	many	many
	anti-A$_1$	none	very few
	anti-HI	none	few
	anti-H[†]	all	all
Lewis	anti-Le^a	some	?all
	anti-Le^b	few	many
P	anti-P$_1$	few	few
	anti-PP$_1$P^k	all	all
	anti-P (auto-)	all‡	all[‡]
	anti-P (allo-)	many	?all
Ii	anti-I ⎱ auto- anti-i ⎰	many	many
Sd	anti-Sd^a	?none	some
Rh	anti-D	none[§]	none[§]
	anti-c, -E, etc.	none	none
K	anti-K	none	many
Fy	anti-Fy^a	none	many
Jk	anti-Jk^a	few	all
MNSs	anti-M, -N	none	none[§]
	anti-S, -s	none	some
Lu	anti-Lu^a, -Lu^b	none	none
Di	anti-Di^a	few	few
Xg	anti-Xg^a	none	many

many = at least 20% of examples; some = more than 10% of examples; few = less than 5% of examples; none = no examples reported although, doubtless, exceptions occur.
* Incubation at 25°C of one volume of a 10% suspension of untreated red cells with two volumes of fresh serum; supernatant examined after 1 h.
[†] In O$_h$ subjects.
[‡] Positive if serum and cells first chilled, then warmed.
[§] Exceptions described.

anti-Jk^a and anti-Di^a will lyse untreated red cells and an example of lytic anti-D has been described.

With enzyme-treated red cells, all the aforementioned antibodies produce more rapid and more extensive lysis than with untreated red cells. Moreover, many examples of antibodies of these specificities which produce no detectable lysis of untreated red cells will readily lyse enzyme-treated red cells; for instance, although only a few examples of anti-Jk^a will lyse untreated red cells, virtually all examples will lyse enzyme-treated red cells.

A few antibodies that fail to lyse red cells with human complement are lytic if rabbit complement is used; examples of antibodies behaving in this way include potent anti-P_1, some examples of anti-K and of -Fy^a, and possibly all examples of anti-Jk^a (Mollison and Thomas, 1959).

Coating with complement components without lysis

Antibodies which, when potent, are lytic (e.g. anti-Le^a), when present in low concentrations bring about the attachment of complement components up to the C3 stage but produce little or no lysis. As explained above, activation of C5, followed by lysis, occurs only when complement is powerfully activated, leading to the generation of large amounts of C3b. Certain antibodies, such as anti-Jk^a, are seldom lytic but invariably activate complement and bind C4 and C3 to the cell surface, as shown by positive reactions with anti-complement sera (e.g. anti-C3d). Antibodies of some other specificities, e.g. anti-K and anti-Fy^a, may or may not activate complement; those examples that do activate complement are not lytic.

CHAPTER 4

ABO, LEWIS, Ii AND P GROUPS

FIGURES

TABLES

The antigens of the ABO, Hh, Lewis, Ii and P groups are synthesized by the sequential addition of sugar residues to a common precursor substance. As a consequence, the systems interact in a number of ways. For example, single molecules may carry specificities determined both by the ABO and the Lewis genes. The various interactions can be understood only by studying the chemistry of the biosynthetic pathways. However, since not all readers may wish to go into so much detail, a relatively simple account of the systems is given first, at a serological and clinical level, and a description of the chemistry of the antigens and of the biosynthetic pathways is given at the end of the chapter.

THE ABO AND Hh SYSTEMS

The ABO blood group system, which was the first human blood group system to be discovered (see Chapter 3), remains the most important in transfusion practice. This is because of the regular occurrence of the antibodies anti-A, anti-B and anti-A,B, reactive at 37°C, in persons whose red cells lack the corresponding antigens (see Table 4.1), so that if transfusions were to be given without regard to the ABO groups, about one-third (in Whites) would be incompatible (see Chapter 3).

The regular presence of anti-A and anti-B is made use of in the routine determination of ABO blood groups; in addition to testing red cells for A and B antigens, the group is checked, in serum or 'reverse' grouping, by testing the serum against red cells of known ABO groups.

Table 4.1   Antigens and antibodies in the ABO system

Group	Subgroup	Antigens on red cells	Antibodies (agglutinins) in serum
O	—	none*	anti-A anti-A$_1$ anti-B anti-A,B[†]
A	A$_1$ A$_2$	A + A$_1$ A	anti-B[‡]
B	—	B	anti-A anti-A$_1$
AB	A$_1$B A$_2$B	A + A$_1$ + B A + B	nil[‡]

* With very rare exceptions human red cells contain the antigen H; the amount of H is influenced by the ABO group: O cells contain most H and A$_1$B cells least (see p. 154).
[†] Inseparable, cross reacting anti-A,B.
[‡] Also anti-A$_1$ in 1–8% of A$_2$ subjects and 22–35% of A$_2$B subjects; anti-HI is found in the serum of occasional A$_1$ and A$_1$B subjects.

Although H and h are encoded by genes, on separate chromosomes from *ABO*, the Hh blood groups system is subsumed in the ABO system, H being a precursor of A and B, and the Hh system is therefore included in this chapter.

Antigens of the ABO system

A brief account of the main phenotypes and genotypes of the ABO system, including the frequency of the common genes in Whites, has been given in the preceding chapter.

ABO phenotypes in different populations

Table 4.2 gives figures for the frequency of ABO phenotypes in selected populations. The figures have been chosen simply to illustrate a few points; e.g. South American Indians all belong to group O; in Australian aborigines only groups O and A_1 are found; in some populations (e.g. Bengalese) the commonest group is B; finally, in some populations (e.g. Lapps) there is a relatively high frequency of A_2.

In Africans (Blacks) B is in general a much stronger antigen than in Europeans (Whites) (Mourant *et al.* 1976) and Blacks have a higher level of *B*-specified enzyme in the serum (Badet *et al.* 1976). For a discussion of the relative frequency of ABO haemolytic disease of the newborn in group A and B infants, and in different ethnic groups, see Chapter 12.

Subgroups of A

A_1 and A_2. In Europeans about 80% of group A individuals belong to subgroup A_1, almost all the rest being A_2. The distinction is most conveniently made by testing red cells with the lectin from *Dolichos biflorus* (Bird, 1952). When diluted appropriately the lectin agglutinates only A_1 cells (but see Table 7.3 on p. 313); if too concentrated an extract is used, some adult A_2 samples, though not adult A_2B or cord A_2 samples, may be agglutinated (see Voak and Lodge, 1968).

The distinction between A_1 and A_2 may be difficult to make in newborn infants: the red cells of some infants who can be clearly shown to be A_1 when they are older may, at the time of birth, fail to react with anti-A_1 reagents. Tests with the anti-H

Table 4.2 Frequencies of ABO groups in a few selected populations (figures from Mourant *et al.* 1976)

Population* (no. tested)	Percentage of various phenotypes						Special characteristics
	O	A_1	A_2	B	A_1B	A_2B	
South American Indians (539)	100	0	0	0	0	0	all O
Vietnamese (220)	45	21.4	0	29.1	4.5	0	no A_2; B commoner than A
Australian aborigines (126)	44.4	55.6	0	0	0	0	no A_2 or B
Germans (100 000)	42.8	32.5	9.4	11.0	3.1	1.1	
Bengalese (241)	22	22.2	1.8	38.2	14.8	0.9	B commonest
Lapps (324)	18.2	36.1	18.5	4.8	6.2	6.2	very high A_2

* The figures are for selected populations and do not necessarily apply to the racial group as a whole.

lectin from *Laburnum alpinum* may be helpful in distinguishing between A_1 and A_2 red cells in the first months of life, A_2 red cells reacting much more strongly than A_1 red cells: the anti-H lectin from *Ulex europaeus* does not discriminate so well (Pawlak and Lopez, 1979). The lectin from *Dolichos biflorus* is better than human anti-A_1 at distinguishing A_1 from A_2 in newborn infants (Race and Sanger, 1975), especially if the cells are enzyme-treated.

Some differences between A_1 and A_2 red cells. As described below, the number of A sites is substantially higher on A_1 than A_2 red cells. Both for A_1 and A_2 cells the number of A sites per red cell varies considerably within the cell population of an individual but this heterogeneity is much greater for A_2 than for A_1 red cells. Using haemocyanin-conjugated anti-immunoglobulin G (IgG) and an IgG fraction of anti-A, anti-A binding was visualized by electron microscopy; on A_2 cells the number of A sites (actually the number of haemocyanin molecules) varied from 4 to 144 per μm^2 and on A_1 cells varied from 121 to 216 per μm^2 (Smalley and Tucker, 1983).

The immunodominant sugar is identical on A_1 and A_2 red cells, namely N-acetylgalactosamine and this has led to the view that the difference between A_1 and A_2 red cells is purely quantitative. It has been estimated that a minimum of $2.5–4 \times 10^5$ A sites per red cell are needed for agglutination by anti-A_1 reagents (Lopez *et al.* 1980). Anti-A_1 is then visualized as an antibody which reacts only with a conformation produced by a certain minimum density of A sites. Studies with monoclonal reagents suggest that although this explanation is correct for the lectin of *Dolichos biflorus* and for at least one monoclonal anti-A_1, it is not correct for one other monoclonal anti-A_1 which recognizes a qualitative difference between A_1 and A_2 (see p. 200).

In any case, the difference between A_1 and A_2 and A_1B and A_2B is not completely clear-cut; there are some individuals who type as A_1 or A_1B with some anti-A_1 reagents and as A_2 or A_2B with others. In addition, there are subjects whose red cells type as A intermediate (A_{int}), reacting more weakly than A_1 red cells with anti-A_1, yet unexpectedly more strongly than A_2 red cells with anti-H (see Race and Sanger, 1975, p. 17).

Anti-A_1 is found in the serum of some A_2 and A_2B subjects (see Table 4.1) but, except in rare individuals in whom the antibody is active at $37°C$, can be ignored in blood transfusion. Hence, there is no need to distinguish A_2 from A_1 donors in routine practice. Perhaps the main importance of A subgroups in clinical medicine is that A_2 infants are protected from haemolytic disease due to anti-A.

A_3 and weaker forms of A. Forms of A even weaker than A_2 are occasionally encountered: A_3 red cells give a characteristic mixed field pattern when tested with anti-A from group B donors, consisting of small agglutinates in a sea of unagglutinated cells (Friedenreich, 1936); with group O serum, agglutination is stronger. About one in 1000 group A bloods belong to subgroup A_3 (Gammelgaard, 1942). The character A_3 was shown by Friedenreich (1936) to be inherited, but some blood samples, which can be shown by family studies to be genetically A_2B, behave as A_3B in grouping tests (Salmon *et al.* 1959c).

Many other weaker forms of A have been described based on: (i) the presence or absence of reactions of the red cells with anti-A, -A$_1$, -H and -A,B; (ii) the presence of anti-A$_1$ in serum; and (iii) the presence of A and H substances in the saliva of ABH secretors. The following list is not comprehensive (see Salmon and Cartron, 1977, for further information).

A$_x$ red cells are agglutinated weakly or not at all by serum from group B donors but are agglutinated by serum from most group O donors (see Race and Sanger, 1975). The frequency of A$_x$ in the French population is 0.0002 (C. Salmon, personal communication, 1986). Anti-A$_1$ is usually present in the serum of A$_x$ people.

A$_m$ red cells are either not agglutinated at all or are agglutinated only very weakly by anti-A in O or B sera, but anti-A can be adsorbed by, and eluted from, the red cells. The saliva of secretors contains a normal amount of A and H. No anti-A$_1$ is present in the serum.

A$_{el}$ red cells are not agglutinated by group B or group O serum but, following incubation with anti-A, anti-A can be eluted from the cells. The saliva of secretors contains H but not A: the serum may contain anti-A$_1$ (Reed and Moore, 1964).

A$_{end}$ cells give a mixed field pattern of agglutination with most group O but with few B sera (Sturgeon et al. 1964). H but not A is found in the saliva of secretors: anti-A$_1$ is present in the serum. The frequency of A$_{end}$ in the French population is 0.0001 (C. Salmon, personal communication, 1986).

Mixtures of A and O red cells, as found in chimeras (or in group A patients transfused with O cells), may at first be mistaken for A$_3$ samples (Dunsford et al. 1953).

Evidence that A subgroups form a single antigenic continuum. In a study in which glutaraldehyde-fixed cells were treated with anti-A (or -A$_1$) and then with anti-IgM conjugated with horse-radish peroxidase, no sharp differences could be found between subgroups of A; e.g. red cells from A$_2$ donors appeared to be a mixture of cells, with a continuous spectrum from heavily labelled cells, like the majority of cells from A$_1$ donors, to non-labelled cells. Red cells from A$_3$ donors were mostly unstained: up to 10% of stained A cells were seen. A$_1$ cells treated with anti-A$_1$ resembled A$_2$ treated with anti-A. The authors concluded that the phenotype in any A subgroup results from the presence of multiple populations of cells differing by the amount of detectable antigen (Reyes et al. 1976). Evidence of an uneven distribution of A sites between the red cells of a single individual was also obtained using an antibody-dependent cytotoxicity assay with monocytes (Bakacs et al. 1988).

Subgroups of B

There is no subgroup of B analogous to subgroup A$_2$ but various types of B cells reacting weakly or not at all with anti-B have been described.

Salmon (1976) suggested that terminology should parallel that of A subgroups and he proposed that the term B$_3$, B$_x$ and B$_{el}$ should be used as follows: B$_3$ cells show a mixed-field agglutination pattern with B in the saliva of secretors (the term B$_3$ was used by Moullec et al. 1955 for a different kind of very weak B in which no B was found in the saliva); B$_x$ shows a weak agglutination pattern and the saliva inhibits the reaction between anti-B and B cells; weak anti-B is found in the serum. B$_{el}$ cells are not agglutinated by anti-B but will absorb anti-B which can subsequently be eluted; H but not B is found in the saliva of secretors.

In detecting weak B antigens, as in detecting weak A antigens, the preparation of an eluate may be helpful in two ways: first, it may be possible to prepare quite a potent eluate from cells which agglutinate only very weakly; in fact it appears that on the whole the weaker the antigen the more potent the eluate (see Celano et al. 1957);

second, an eluate prepared from cells with a very weak antigen (e.g. B_x) may agglutinate the cells even though they are not agglutinated by the whole serum used in making the eluate (Alter and Rosenfield, 1964a).

Competition between A- and B-transferases

A- and B-tranferases act upon the same precursor substance and it is therefore not surprising that subjects who have both an A and B allele show diminished expression both of A and B antigens. Thus, A_1B red cells have less A than A_1 cells and A_2B cells less A than A_2 cells. In certain pedigrees, red cells of genotype A^1B may behave as A_2B, due presumably to an interference with the expression of A^1 by a strong B allele (for references see Alter and Rosenfield, 1964b).

Two separate cases of apparent exclusion of paternity involving Black parents of phenotype group A_2B with A_1 offspring were solved by studies of A-, B- and H-transferases. All group A members carried a normal A^1-transferase; the alleged father was thus not excluded in either case. Group AB individuals showed increased B-transferase activity, possibly accounting for the observed A_2B phenotypes (Fredrick et al. 1985).

A_1B cells react slightly less strongly with anti-B than B cells (Gillespie and Gold, 1960; Sacks and Lennox, 1981).

The weaker reactions of A_1B cells compared with A_1 are more obvious when the lectin from *Dolichos biflorus* is used (Bird, 1959) and the weaker reaction of B in A_1B cells compared with B cells is shown very strikingly with the lectin from *Fomes fomentarius* (Gillespie and Gold, 1960) or from salmon ova (Downie et al. 1977).

Cis AB

Occasionally, an individual passes on both A and B so that, for example, a group AB father and a group O mother have an AB child.

In the *cis* AB phenotype the B antigen is usually very weak so that the phenotype cannot be confused with normal AB. The serum from most *cis* AB individuals contains alloanti-B. It was originally postulated that the phenotype was due to the fact that A and B are not truly allelic but can very rarely be present on the same chromosome. However, from an examination of sera from 13 individuals with *cis* AB phenotype for A- and B-transferase activity, Badet et al. (1978) concluded that there was probably only a single enzyme produced by a mutant gene.

The concept of a mutant gene capable of producing substantial amounts of both A and B became easy to accept following the demonstration by Watkins et al. (1981) that the normal A- and B-specified transferases are very similar and have overlapping functions. The A^1-transferase can, under certain conditions, synthesize group B determinants (Yates and Watkins, 1982) and the B-transferase has the potential to synthesize blood group A-active structures, using the same donor and acceptor substrates as the A-transferase (Yates et al. 1984; Watkins, 1990).

In one family with the *cis* AB phenotype it was shown that the A- and B-enzyme activities were inseparable (Watkins et al. 1981). Similar findings were recorded in two families by Yoshida et al. (1980b) but in another family the A- and B-enzymes were separable (Yoshida et al. 1980a), raising the possibility that not all examples of *cis* AB have the same genetic origin.

B cells reacting with anti-A and A cells reacting with anti-B

Using a very potent monoclonal anti-A, and a saline suspension of red cells, about 1 in 1000 B cells ('B(A)' cells) are agglutinated. Conversely, some A(B) red cells have been demonstrated with a potent monoclonal anti-B (for references see Voak, 1990). With enzyme treatment, all A cells form fragile agglutinates with potent monoclonal anti-B and all B cells react with potent monoclonal anti-A. These findings are explained by the fact that the *A*-transferase has the potential to synthesize B determinants and *vice versa* (see above). B(A) cells come from individuals with strong B-transferases. On the other hand A(B) individuals do not have higher levels of *A*-transferase but have very potent *H*-transferases with abundant H precursor substance which may lead to the formation of some B determinants by the *A*-transferase (see Watkins, 1990). The unusual reactivity of potent monoclonal antibodies can be overcome by dilution of the reagent.

H antigen on red cells

The H determinant is found on all human red cells except those of subjects of phenotype O_h. Since H is a precursor of A and B, A and B subjects have less H than O subjects. The order of reactivity of anti-H with red cells of various ABO groups tends to be $O > A_2 > A_2B > B > A_1 > A_1B$. Exceptions to this order are provided by occasional subjects who are genetically A_1 or A_1B but group as A_2 or A_2B, respectively, because normal synthesis of A is hindered by a deficiency of H (Voak *et al.* 1970). In such 'A_2' or 'A_2B' subjects, H is more weakly expressed than in cells of normal A_1 or A_1B subjects.

Numbers of A, B and H antigen sites on red cells

Estimates of the numbers of sites on the red cells of adults and newborn infants of common ABO phenotypes are shown in Table 4.3. As the table shows, it has been estimated that there are approximately 800 000 A sites on adult A_1 cells and about as many B sites on adult B cells. The only estimate for the number of H sites on the red cells of adults suggests that these are twice as numerous on O cells as are A or B sites on A or B cells. However, this apparent discrepancy is probably due simply to the method of calculation. The numbers of A and B sites are calculated from the numbers of antibody molecules combining with the red cells, on the assumption that one antibody molecule combines with one antigen site. Since in fact there is evidence that the majority of anti-A and anti-B molecules bind to red cells by both their combining sites, the number of A and B sites is presumably approximately twice the number given in the table. On the other hand, the number of H sites was estimated from the number of ^{14}C-labelled GalNAc residues transferred to red cells using *A*-specified enzyme (Schenkel-Brunner, 1980a).

Compared with the red cells of adults, the red cells of newborn infants have about one-third the number of A and B sites.

The numbers of antigen sites on weak A samples from adults were found to be: A_3, 35 000; A_x, 4800; A_{end}, 3500; and A_m, 700 (Cartron, 1976, and other papers in vol. 19, no. 1 of the *Revue française de Transfusion et Immunohématologie*, March 1976).

O_h, A_h and B_h red cells

In subjects of the very rare genotype *hh* (phenotype O_h), no H is made on red cells or in secretions and therefore no A or B can be made either (see section on Biosynthesis).

Table 4.3 Various estimates of the number of A, B and H sites on red cells of different phenotypes from adults and newborn infants

	Sites $\times 10^6$ per red cell	Reference*
A sites[†]		
A_1 adults	0.83	(1)
A_1 adults	0.81–1.17	(2)
A_1 adults	0.85	(3)
newborn	0.25–0.37	(2)
A_2 adults	0.24–0.29	(2)
A_2 adults	0.24	(3)
newborn	0.14	(2)
A_1B adults	0.46–0.85	(2)
newborn	0.22	(2)
A_2B adults	0.14	(2)
B sites[†]		
B adults	0.75	(2)
newborn	0.2–0.32	(4)
A_1B adults	0.43	(2)
H sites		
O adults	1.7	(5)
newborn	0.325	(5)
A, B, AB newborn	0.07	(5)

* (1) Greenbury *et al.* (1963); (2) Economidou *et al.* (1967a); (3) Cartron *et al.* (1974); (4) E.L. Romano (personal communication); (5) Schenkel-Brunner (1980a;b).
[†] Assumes antibody molecule binds to one antigen site; true number of A and B sites may be twice the estimates given.

The serum contains anti-H as well as anti-A and anti-B. The first example of a blood of this kind was found in Bombay (Bhende *et al.* 1952), hence the name 'Bombay', often given to *hh* bloods.

The red cells of almost equally rare 'para-Bombay' bloods, A_h, B_h, O^A_{Hm} and O^B_{Hm}, react very weakly with anti-A and anti-B, respectively, but not at all with the anti-H lectin from *Ulex europaeus*, although weak reactions have been observed with selected anti-H from O_h subjects (see Race and Sanger, 1975, for details and references). A_h and B_h subjects do not secrete ABH whereas the saliva of O^A_{Hm} and O^B_{Hm} subjects contains A and H, or B and H, respectively. The serum from A_h and B_h subjects contains anti-H but the antibody in the serum of O^A_{Hm} and O^B_{Hm} subjects is anti-HI. Although H in 'para-Bombay' subjects cannot be readily detected serologically, its presence has been uncovered by converting B_h cells, using suitable enzymes, into B(–), H(+) cells (Mulet *et al.* 1979).

Development of the A, B and H antigens
A and B can be detected on the red cells of 5- or 6-week-old embryos but even at birth are not fully developed (Kemp, 1930). Red cells of newborn infants also react less strongly than those of adults with anti-H. In tests on ten cord blood samples and ten adult samples, the average scores were as follows: with an extract of *Ulex europaeus*, 11.4 vs 22.6; and with three samples of serum from O_h donors, 19.2 vs 27.6 (Haddad,

1974). The number of A and B sites on the red cells of newborn infants is less than on those of adults (see Table 4.3).

When the reactions of the red cells of group A infants and adults with anti-A sera are compared, only slight differences are found in the agglutination of saline-suspended red cells but larger differences are observed in the indirect antiglobulin test (anti-IgG) and in tests for lysis (Crawford et $al.$ 1953a). In tests with rabbit anti-A, on average, 27% of A_1 cord red cells and 54% of A_1 adult red cells were lysed. The adult figure had almost been reached by the end of the first year of life and had been fully reached by the age of 2–4 years (Grundbacher, 1964).

The red cells of newborn infants who are genetically A_1 react relatively weakly with human anti-A_1 (Witebsky and Engasser, 1949; Crawford et $al.$ 1953a); for the reactions with lectins, see the previous section on subgroups of A. Fetal A_2 red cells behave like adult A_x red cells, that is, they react better with O serum than with B serum (Constantoulakis et $al.$ 1963). The section on Biosynthesis deals with the biochemical differences between adult and fetal group A red cells.

The relative binding of anti-A to adult and cord blood group A red cells, in relation to the serological findings in ABO haemolytic disease of the newborn, is considered in Chapter 12.

Weakening of A, B and H antigens in acute leukaemia

In acute leukaemia the A antigen may be weakened (van Loghem et $al.$ 1957). Sometimes the blood appears to contain a mixture of group A and group O cells (Salmon et $al.$ 1958; Gold et $al.$ 1959) or of A_1 and weak A (Salmon et $al.$ 1959a). In other cases the red cells react weakly with anti-A, even behaving like A_3 or A_m (Salmon et $al.$ 1959a). The latter authors pointed out that in the course of testing some 300 000 blood samples they had encountered 22 weak A samples (ten A_x, four A_m and eight A_3). All the ten A_x samples came from normal subjects but two of the four A_m and two of the eight A_3 came from patients with acute leukaemia.

In a patient with erythroleukaemia, of group B, as shown by B-transferase in the serum, 60% of the cells were not agglutinated by anti-B and appeared to be group O, but were really very weak B: when separated from the normal B cells they would absorb anti-B (Bird et $al.$ 1976c).

ABH antigens may also be lost from carcinomatous tissue cells; see Chapter 3.

Acquired B antigen in A_1 subjects

In the original report of this condition, seven A_1 blood samples were described which reacted weakly with some anti-B sera, giving the appearance of group AB with a weak expression of B. In each case the serum contained normal anti-B. Five of the seven subjects had cancer and six were over 60 years old (Cameron et $al.$ 1959).

In investigating nine similar cases it was found that the number of A sites was inversely related to the amount of B activity and it was suggested that 'acquired B' may result from the action of the bacterial deacetylase which converts N-acetyl-galactosamine to α-galactosamine, which is very similar to galactose, the chief determinant of B (Gerbal et $al.$ 1975). It was further shown that if acquired B cells were acetylated they no longer reacted with anti-B but gained reactivity with an extract of $Dolichos$ $biflorus$. Similarly, normal A_1 cells treated with deacetylase lost some A reactivity but gained B reactivity (Gerbal *et al.* 1976a). Some monoclonal anti-Bs fail to react with acquired B cells and are thus useful in discriminating between normal and acquired B. Another means of discrimination is to adjust the pH of anti-B sera to 6, since the sera will then no longer react with acquired B. A mouse monoclonal antibody specific for the acquired B group, reacting with a distinct epitope resulting from the deacetylation of the blood group A trisaccharide, was reported by Oriol *et al.* (1990). Red cells with acquired B may also show T- or Tk-activation (see Chapter 7), all these changes being produced by enzymes from Gram-negative bacteria commonly associated with carcinoma of the colon or rectum, or with intestinal obstruction.

It has been suggested that the rarity of acquired B may be due to the fact that all A_2 and 95% of A_1 subjects have an antibody which can destroy B-modified cells and that most coliform organisms lack deacetylase (Gerbal *et al.* 1975). The kind of acquired B described above may be called the 'deacetylase-type' and can be made only on A_1 cells. The second type of acquired B which may be called the 'passenger antigen' type is caused by adsorption of B-like bacterial products on to O or A cells but occurs only *in vitro* (Bird, 1977).

Conversion of O cells to A or B
Group O cells (but not O_h) can be converted to A- or B-active red cells by incubation with the appropriate nucleotide sugar and *A*- or *B*-transferase (see p. 199).

Conversion of B cells to O
Treatment of B red cells with an α-galactosidase hydrolyses away the terminal α-glycosidically linked galactose, thus removing group B activity (Harpaz *et al.* 1975). Red cells treated in this way react as group O cells and, after labelling with ^{51}Cr, have been shown to survive normally not only in the group B donor of the cells but also in a group A and a group O subject (Goldstein *et al.* 1982). It should be possible to convert A cells to group O red cells in a similar manner using the appropriate α-N-acetylgalactosaminidase, but the process seems to be more difficult due to internal A repetitive antigenic sites in addition to the terminal A sites in A_1 red cells (see Chemistry section). Full units of 160–196 ml 'enzymatically converted O' packed red blood cells, originally grouped as B, were transfused to group O and B normal volunteers. The converted O cells had a normal survival in the recipients, who showed no increase in the potency of their anti-B, provided that sufficient α-galactosidase had been used. Group O recipients require red cells treated with higher levels of enzyme than group B recipients, i.e. 185–200 U/ml compared with 90 U/ml (Lenny *et al.* 1991).

Secretors and non-secretors of ABH
The fact that A and B substances are present in the saliva of most A and B individuals ('secretors') was first discovered in 1930 by Lehrs and Putkonen (for references to these and other early papers see Wiener, 1943, p. 275). Approximately 80% of subjects are secretors of ABH.

The secretion of H, A and B is controlled by the secretor genes, *Se* and *se*. The term secretor is applied to those persons (genotype *SeSe* or *Sese*) who secrete H with or without A and, or, B and does not take into account the presence of Lewis or other blood group substances in the saliva. Thus the saliva of group O secretors contains H and that of group A secretors contains A and H (Morgan and Watkins, 1948). The 20% of subjects who are classified as 'non-secretors' secrete very small amounts of H and also of A or B according to their ABO group (Hartmann, 1941). It has recently been shown that low levels of H-transferases are present in the submaxillary glands of non-secretors (see section on Biosynthesis).

The amount of A glycoprotein in the saliva of group A secretors follows a log-normal distribution. The amounts of A and H in the saliva appear to vary independently of one another, although there is a significant correlation between the ratio of A to H amongst sibs (Clarke et al. 1960).

H, A and B glycoproteins in saliva are produced predominantly by the submaxillary and sublingual glands (Wolf and Taylor, 1964). The greatest amounts of A glycoprotein were found in saliva from the sublingual and lip mucous glands and there was negligible activity in parotid saliva (Milne and Dawes, 1973).

Group-specific glycoproteins have been found in seminal fluid, tears, sweat, urine, digestive juices, bile, milk, pleural, pericardial and peritoneal fluids, amniotic fluid and in the fluids of hydroceles and ovarian cysts (Wiener, 1943, p. 274). The amounts in different secretions of the same individual vary widely.

A, B and H substances in serum

Moss (1910) showed that group A serum contains a substance which will inhibit the haemolytic properties of an anti-A serum, and Schiff (1924) demonstrated the presence of A substance in group A serum by immunization experiments in rabbits. Aubert et al. (1942a) tested samples from more than 300 subjects and found that the sera of about 50% of group A or AB subjects would inhibit anti-A and that the sera of almost 90% of subjects of group B and AB would inhibit anti-B. Using a radio-immunoassay, A activity was detected in all group A sera tested, with higher levels in A_1 than in A_2, and in secretors than in non-secretors; the highest activity was found in Le(a − b −) secretors (Holburn and Masters, 1974b). ABH substances in serum are glycolipids but their cellular origin is unknown.

A or B substances were found to be present in the serum of almost all group A or B newborn infants examined by Høstrup (1963a), although the concentration was lower than in adults. Denborough et al. (1969) also noted that the amount of A was less in infants with group O mothers than in those with A mothers and suggested that this was due to neutralization of A substance by passively acquired maternal anti-A.

Patients with an increased amount of A or B glycoprotein in their serum have been described: most have had pseudomucinous ovarian cysts, glycoprotein from which is presumed to have entered the blood stream (for references, see previous editions of this book).

Michel (1964) found that the inhibitory power of A in plasma increases on storage: A_1 blood from a secretor was mixed with ACD and stored for 3 weeks. At the end of this time the plasma showed an approximate eight-fold increase in inhibition titre which was not due to haemolysis. The cause of the phenomenon seems to be the shedding of microvesicles from the red cell surface; see Chapter 9.

Serum from group O donors inhibits occasional examples of anti-H, e.g. from an A_1 donor described by Gouge et al. (1977), from an O_h donor described by Voak et al. (1969) and from a B_h donor described by Rouger et al. (1979). Since H in plasma, unlike H on red cells, occurs on glycolipids with type I chains (see p. 195), it seems that most examples of anti-H combine with type II rather than type I structures; all examples tested by Daniels (1984) showed a preference for type II chains. In another study, sera from 'Bombay' subjects were shown to have similar amounts of anti-type I H and anti-type II H, whereas in sera from 'para-Bombay' (A_h and B_h) subjects anti-type I H preponderated (Le Pendu et al. 1986). There is more H in the plasma of O and A_2 subjects than in that of A_1 and A_1B subjects (Rouger et al. 1979).

Uptake of A and B substances by group O red cells in vivo was first described by Renton and Hancock (1962). In five patients of group A or B transfused with group O blood, after some days the O cells became agglutinable by certain group O sera. Similarly, group O red cells exposed *in vitro* to group A glycosphingolipid fractions become agglutinable by anti-A (Tilley et al. 1975).

In chimeric twins of groups O and A it would be expected that in the twin who was genetically A (and a secretor), the 'donor' (group O) cells would have small amounts of A substance on their surface and would be agglutinated by selected O sera. Tests in one such chimeric twin showed this to be the case (Race and Sanger, 1975). In two further blood group chimeras (without evidence of twinning) the group O cells were agglutinated by group O serum (Bird et al. 1976d; Szymanski et al. 1977). Both chimeras were secretors of A and H.

A, B and H substances in amniotic fluid. Soluble A, B and H substances are found in amniotic fluid from about the ninth week of gestation onwards, and are derived from the fetus; according to several authors they are found only when the fetus is a secretor (e.g. Przestwor, 1964; Harper et al. 1971), although according to Høstrup (1964) small amounts of A, B and H substances may be found even when the fetus is a non-secretor. Blood group substances corresponding to the maternal ABO group may be found if care is not taken to exclude cells from the fluid examined.

A, B and H on leucocytes, platelets, other cells and bacteria

Granulocytes. Despite earlier reports to the contrary, it seems that A, B and H cannot be detected on human granulocytes (Dunstan et al. 1985a; Gaidulis et al. 1985).

Lymphocytes. A and B are present on lymphocytes and are detectable by lymphocyto-toxicity tests. These antigens, like Lewis antigens, are acquired from the plasma (Rachkewich et al. 1978; Oriol et al. 1980a;b), and thus are most readily detected on the lymphocytes of individuals whose plasma contains relatively large amounts of A or B glycolipid. For example, in cytotoxicity tests with three group O sera, the strongest reactions were obtained with the lymphocytes of A_1. Le(a – b –) secretors and A_2, Le(a – b –) secretors; the lymphocytes of non-secretors failed to react (Rachkewich et al. 1978).

Platelets. At least part of the A, B and H antigens detectable on platelets are acquired by adsorption of glycolipids from plasma (Kools et al. 1981; Kelton et al. 1982). However, in addition to type I H, representing passively acquired antigen, type II H can also be detected on platelets and is presumably synthesized by the cells themselves (Dunstan *et al.* 1985c). The distribution of ABH antigens on platelets was shown to be heterogeneous by fluorescence flow cytometry (Dunstan and Simpson, 1985). The distribution of ABH on megakaryocytes was also shown to be heterogeneous but the platelets derived from individual megakaryocytes showed uniform ABH expression.

Other cells. The presence of A and B antigens has been demonstrated on epidermal cells, cells of amniotic fluid, sinusoidal cells of the spleen and spermatozoa, as well as in the cell walls of the endothelium of capillaries, veins and arteries. In non-secretors, A and B are demonstrable only in the deeper layers of the gastric mucosa but in secretors they are also demonstrable in glands, goblet cells and secreting surface epithelia (for references see Mollison *et al.* 1987).

The amount of ABH-active glycolipids in parenchymatous organs (liver, spleen, kidney) is about the same as in red cells whereas the amount in glandular tissues (pancreas, gastric mucosa) is larger (see Watkins, 1980). Some cells, such as vascular endothelial and biliary cells, are rich in ABH as well as in HLA antigens, whereas other cells such as the hepatocytes are totally devoid of them. These differences in antigen distribution may be important in graft rejection (Rouger *et al.* 1982b).

In embryos of 5–60 mm crown–rump length, A, B and H have been found on all epithelial cells except those of the central nervous system, and on all endothelial cells (Szulman, 1965).

H-specified transferases have been isolated from kidneys, stomach mucosa, salivary glands and plasma. Two types of enzyme can be isolated depending on the source tissue and on the *HAB* and *Se* genes of an individual, one reacting preferentially with type I and another with type II chains (Le Pendu, 1983; Betteridge and Watkins, 1985; see section on Biosynthesis).

A and B antigens on bacteria. Schiff (1934) first showed unequivocally that a bacterium (*Shigella shigae*) had blood group activity, after growing it in a medium free from blood group substances. Springer *et al.* (1962) tested approximately 300 strains of bacteria and found that about half of them had A, B or H activity.

Antibodies of the ABO system
The common occurrence of naturally occurring antibodies reacting with antigens of the ABO, Hh, Ii, Lewis and P systems indicates that these antigens are widely distributed in nature, e.g. in animals other than humans and in bacteria. The antibodies tend to be IgM cold agglutinins; they activate complement and, when active at 37°C, they are often lytic.

Anti-A and anti-B
If A is absent from a person's red cells, anti-A agglutinins are found in the serum, and if B is absent from a person's red cells the serum contains anti-B agglutinins (see Table 4.1). The titre of the agglutinins varies considerably in different sera and appears to have a log-normal distribution. The titre recorded is affected by the red cell phenotype (e.g. A_1 or A_2), by the concentration of red cells in the final mixture, by the time and temperature of incubation, and by the technique of reading the end-point.

There is usually a wider range of titres for anti-A (e.g. 8–2048) than for anti-B (e.g. 8–256).

In Whites, anti-A titres tend to be higher than anti-B titres, either when comparing group B with group A subjects or when comparing the titres of the two antibodies in group O subjects. The anti-A titre tends to be higher in group O subjects than in group B subjects, although there is little difference between the anti-B titre of group O and group A sera (Thomsen and Kettel, 1929). Ichikawa (1959) confirmed all of these findings except that he found the titre of anti-B to be higher in group O than in group A subjects. In Blacks, anti-A and anti-B titres tend to be higher than in Whites and anti-B titres are almost as high as anti-A titres (Grundbacher, 1976). In a series of Nigerian donors, although anti-A agglutinin titres were higher than those of anti-B, haemolytic activity was more commonly anti-B than anti-A (Worlledge *et al.* 1974). It is possible that the differences in strength and haemolytic characteristics of ABO antibodies are more strongly correlated with environmental factors than with race; a recent study of donors living in the UK failed to show any significant differences between Blacks, Whites and Asians (Redman *et al.* 1990).

Except in AB subjects, complete absence of anti-A and anti-B is very rare in healthy subjects. Race and Sanger (1975) refer to only three cases of missing anti-A or anti-B, for which no cause could be found. Extremely weak anti-B was presumably present in the three healthy group A subjects described by van Loghem *et al.* (1965) since, although no antibody could be detected serologically, the survival of group B cells was shortened: $T_{50}Cr$ 10, 20 and 21 d, compared with 29 ± 3.5 d in normal subjects.

Anti-A and anti-B are often present in very low concentration in patients with hypogammaglobulinaemia and are absent in the rare X-linked Wiskott–Aldrich syndrome. Boys with this syndrome are unable to mount an immune response to polysaccharide antigens and thus have no ABO antibodies; responses to protein antigens are often unimpaired (see Miescher and Müller-Eberhard, 1978). Anti-A and anti-B may also be present in very low concentration in patients immunosuppressed by therapy or disease and in patients undergoing intensive plasma exchange.

In chimeras, the presence of a population of red cells of different ABO group may lead to the absence of the corresponding alloantibody; e.g. in a chimera who is genetically group O but has a population of A cells, anti-A is absent (see Race and Sanger, 1975, p. 526).

Development of anti-A and anti-B
As described in Chapter 3, the only immunoglobulin synthesized in relatively large amounts by the fetus is IgM, and the level of this protein in cord serum is about one-tenth to one-twentieth of that in adult serum.

Anti-A and anti-B present in cord sera are usually IgG and are of maternal origin, but occasionally they are IgM synthesized by the fetus. For example, eight out of 192 unselected infants had an agglutinin in cord serum which could not have been of maternal origin, e.g. anti-B in the cord serum of an infant born to a group B mother (Thomaidis *et al.* 1967). In another series, in 33 selected cases, in all of which it would have been possible to have detected anti-A or anti-B of non-maternal origin, such antibodies were found in seven cases (Chattoraj *et al.* 1968b). In a third series, agglutinins incompatible with maternal red cells were found in eight out of 44 neonatal sera (Toivanen and Hirvonen, 1969).

The production of ABO agglutinins in fetal life appears to be more common in Nigeria: of 50 cord bloods tested using a 'sensitive technique', 40% had IgM anti-A and, or, anti-B which, on the basis of specificity, could not have been of maternal origin (Worlledge *et al.* 1974).

In most infants anti-A and anti-B agglutinins (presumably IgM) produced by the infant can first be demonstrated at 3–6 months (Morville, 1929). In one series of 900 infants, levels at 3 months were 25% as high as those of adults (Godzisz, 1979). In another series, 85% of infants had the expected agglutinins at the age of 6 months (Yliruokanen, 1948). In a series of 150 group O children tested by Fong *et al.* (1974), the median anti-A titre was 4 at 3–6 months, 16 at 6–9 months and 64 at 12–18 months. The maximum value (128) was reached in the fifth year. Anti-B titres tended to lag behind, particularly in the first year of life, so that by the age of 12 months although 30% of O and B children had anti-A titres equal to the adult median value, only 4% of group A children had anti-B titres equal to the median adult level. These findings show that reverse ABO grouping in infants is not worth performing before 6 months of age.

The titre of anti-A and anti-B agglutinins reaches its maximum at the age of 5–10 years (Fig. 4.1), and the level of haemolysins follows a similar pattern, reaching a maximum at 7–8 years. Levels are higher in girls than in boys (Grundbacher, 1967).

In adults, anti-A and anti-B levels fall with increasing age (see Fig. 4.1). Of 181 subjects aged 51–98 years, six had missing agglutinins and in eight the titre was only 1 (Somers and Kuhns, 1972). Similarly in a study on patients aged 65 years or over, in 19 of 59 subjects of groups A, B or O the titre was only 2–4 (Baumgarten *et al.* 1976).

The influence of genetic factors on agglutinin titres is unclear. In one series it was found that the difference between dizygotic twins was no greater than that between

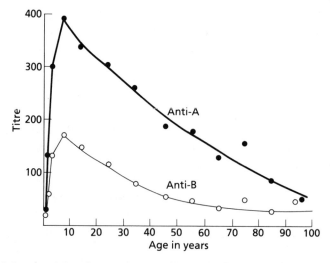

Figure 4.1 Anti-A and anti-B agglutinin titres in group O subjects of different ages (from the data of Thomsen and Kettel, 1929).

monozygotic twins (Nijenhuis and Bratlie, 1962) although in a study by Grundbacher (1976) it was concluded that genetic factors played some part.

Monoclonal anti-A and anti-B from murine hybridomas
Numerous monoclonal anti-A and anti-B have been produced and have proved entirely suitable as blood grouping reagents (see Chapter 8). Anti-H has also been produced (see p. 182). However, some ABO monoclonals cannot be used in absorption/elution tests to classify weak subgroups of A (Zelenski, 1986). Also, inhibition tests have shown that monoclonal anti-A vary according to the source of the A immunogen; an anti-A stimulated by human A substance was inhibited by synthetic A oligosaccharide (Synsorb A) and by synthetic Forssman antigen whereas two anti-A stimulated by bacterial A substance were not inhibited (G. Inglis, personal communication).

IgM, IgG and IgA anti-A and anti-B
In a given serum anti-A may be wholly IgM, or partly IgM and partly IgG (Fudenberg et al. 1959), partly IgM and partly IgA, or may be made of all three immunoglobulins (Kunkel and Rockey, 1963), even in subjects who have had no identifiable stimulus. IgG anti-A and anti-B are found far more commonly in group O than in B or A subjects (Rawson and Abelson, 1960b).

The serological characteristics of IgM anti-A may be studied in a serum which lacks IgG and IgA anti-A; those of IgG anti-A may be studied in a fraction obtained by DEAE-cellulose chromatography; and those of IgA anti-A may be studied either in a serum fraction or in colostrum, in which IgA is the main immunoglobulin.

In mixtures containing IgG and IgM anti-A, the IgM antibody can be inactivated by treatment with 2-mercaptoethanol (2-ME) or dithiothreitol (DTT); see Chapter 3. The serological activity of IgA anti-A is reduced but not destroyed by treatment with 2-ME (for references see Mollison et al. 1987).

IgG subclasses. Of 42 sera containing IgG anti-A and anti-B, obtained from group O mothers of A or B infants, 39 reacted with subclass antisera; of these, one was solely IgG2 and the remaining 38 were all partly IgG2; the other subclasses present were as follows: IgG1 (19); IgG1 + IgG3 (3); IgG1 + IgG3 + IgG4 (12); and IgG1 + IgG4 (4) (Brouwers et al. 1987a).

Complement-binding. Both IgM and IgG anti-A may be haemolytic (Rawson and Abelson, 1960a). Polley et al. (1963) found that all examples of IgG anti-A and about 90% of examples of IgM anti-A were readily haemolytic and that the remaining examples of IgM anti-A would haemolyse cells if the test was made sensitive enough. On the other hand, IgA anti-A is not haemolytic (for references see Mollison et al. 1987). Similar results are obtained if complement binding is detected by the use of specific antiglobulin sera. Thus if IgG, IgM and IgA antibodies are tested at a dilution at which they will agglutinate red cells only weakly, the addition of anti-complement to the washed cells enhances agglutination if the anti-A is IgG or IgM (Polley et al. 1963) but not if it is IgA (Adinolfi et al. 1966).

The minimum number of IgM anti-A molecules which when bound to a group A red cell will activate complement is not known, but on theoretical grounds might be one (see Chapter 3). The minimum number of IgG anti-A molecules for complement binding is expected to be substantial. Romano and Mollison (1975) found that, using an anti-C3c reagent to demonstrate complement binding by the antiglobulin test, a minimum of 14 μg IgG anti-A per ml red cells was required, corresponding to approximately 7000 molecules of anti-A per cell or very approximately 1% of the maximum number which could be bound.

An approximate estimate of the minimum number of IgG anti-A molecules which will cause lysis can be calculated from the data of Ishizaka et al. (1968). Making various assumptions about the equilibrium constant of the antibody and the number of antigen sites, the number of antibody molecules required for lysis is of the order of 30 000 per cell (N.C. Hughes-Jones, personal communication).

Demonstration that all anti-A sera are potentially haemolytic. Three factors are known to influence the haemolysis of group A red cells by a given example of anti-A; first, the time for which the red cells have been stored; second, the ratio of serum to red cells, presumably influencing the number of antibody molecules bound to the red cell; and third, the freshness of the serum, presumably indicating that complement activity is affected even by short periods of storage.

All fresh anti-A sera will lyse group A red cells which have been left as a saline suspension for 1–4 d (Hesser, 1924; Thomsen and Thisted, 1928a). Similarly, group A red cells stored as clotted blood or with oxalate for 1 week or as ACD blood for 3 weeks are more easily lysed than fresh red cells (Chaplin et al. 1956b). Dacie (1949) found that all anti-A sera would lyse even fresh red cells from a (group A) patient with paroxysmal nocturnal haemoglobinuria (PNH).

The importance of the ratio of serum to cells has been noted by many authors. For example, Chaplin et al. (1956b) found that the proportion of anti-A sera which were lytic was much greater when a 2% cell suspension was used rather than a 5% suspension. Polley et al. (1963) found that when the ratio of serum to cells was 20 to 1 (e.g. two volumes of serum to one volume of a 10% suspension of red cells) 58% of group O sera would haemolyse A_1 cells; when the ratio was 40 to 1, 90% were lytic, when 80 to 1, 96% were lytic, and when 200 to 1, all sera were lytic. In demonstrating haemolysis at the ratio of 200 to 1, the technique of release of ^{51}Cr from ^{51}Cr-labelled group A_1 cells was used and this made it relatively easy to detect the 15–30% of haemolysis which occurred. According to Jandl et al. (1957), in order to obtain 100% haemolysis with some sera the ratio of serum to cells must exceed 500 to 1.

Evidence that the freshness of serum is important in revealing haemolysis is as follows: Thomsen and Thisted (1928b) noted that many anti-A and anti-B sera which were not otherwise lytic would produce lysis if they were absolutely fresh (tesed within 2 h of bleeding) and if a very weak (1%) suspension of red cells was used. This observation suggests a parallel with the remarkable anti-Rh D serum 'Ripley' which was often observed to haemolyse suspensions of D-positive red cells when it was freshly taken (Waller and Lawler, 1962) but which after it had been in the post for 3 or 4 d produced no trace of haemolysis even when fresh serum was added (unpublished observations, PLM). Kabat and Mayer (1961, p. 136) refer to the fact that the haemolytic activity of complement deteriorates after 1 or 2 h incubation at 37°C.

Enhancement by specific antiglobulin serum. If a serum fraction containing only IgG anti-A is titrated, the greatest dilution in which the anti-A can be detected by the indirect antiglobulin technique after adding anti-IgG is found to be about five doubling dilutions greater than the dilution which will agglutinate red cells suspended in saline; e.g. a fraction which agglutinates red cells to a titre of 64 will, at a dilution of 2048, sensitize red cells to agglutination by anti-IgG (Polley et al. 1965). The use of anti-IgA increases the titre of IgA anti-A by about two doubling dilutions but anti-IgM scarcely enhances agglutination by IgM anti-A at all (Ishizaka et al. 1965; Adinolfi et al. 1966).

Enhancement of agglutination by serum or plasma. Agglutination produced by IgG anti-A is enhanced in a medium of serum compared with saline (Polley *et al.* 1963). Previously, Boorman *et al.* (1945b) and Witebsky (1948) had observed that immune anti-A sera produced much stronger agglutination in a medium of serum than in saline. Plasma is considerably more effective than serum. When group A red cells were coated with varying amounts of IgG anti-A, the least amount of anti-A detectable by agglutination in plasma was about 0.5 μg/ml cells, which was about the same as when they were tested with antiglobulin serum; however, the least amount detectable by agglutination in serum was 2.2–3.0 μg/ml cells (Romano and Mollison, 1975).

Inhibitory effect of A substance. Witebsky (1948) was the first to observe that immune anti-A is far more difficult to inhibit with A substance than is naturally occurring anti-A. Kochwa *et al.* (1961) showed that as a rule IgM anti-A is more readily inhibited than IgG anti-A. Polley *et al.* (1963) estimated that to obtain an equivalent reduction in agglutinin titre the amount of purified human A substance required to inhibit IgG anti-A was 20 times that required to inhibit IgM anti-A. Occasional examples of IgG anti-A are readily inhibited (Kochwa *et al.* 1961; Polley *et al.* 1963). That IgM anti-A and anti-B are as a rule far more easily inhibited than IgG anti-A and anti-B seems to be due to the fact that, when reacting with A and B glycoproteins in solution, IgM anti-A and anti-B have higher binding constants than corresponding IgG antibodies, presumably because IgM combines multivalently with a single glycoprotein molecule in solution (Holburn and Masters, 1974a).

The amount of A glycoprotein required to inhibit the ability of an immune serum to lyse group A red cells is much less than the amount required to inhibit the ability to agglutinate red cells or to sensitize them to an antiglobulin serum (see Mollison, 1956, p. 186).

In the ease with which it is inhibited by A glycoprotein IgA is intermediate between IgM and IgG anti-A (Rawson and Abelson, 1964; Adinolfi *et al.* 1966).

Thermal optimum. Naturally occurring anti-A and anti-B react more strongly at 4°C than at 37°C. By contrast, immune sera react equally well at 37°C and at 4°C (Wiener, 1941a), or even better at 37°C (Hubinont, 1949). Using 2-ME-treated serum, Voak *et al.* (1973) concluded that IgG anti-A agglutinates untreated or papain-treated red cells as well at 37°C as at 4°C.

Effect of heating. Heating a serum at 56°C for 3 h has no measurable effect on the titre of IgG or IgA anti-A but leads to a distinct fall in IgM anti-A titre (Adinolfi *et al.* 1966).

Anti-A and anti-B in colostrum and saliva. The titre of anti-A and anti-B tends to be higher in colostrum than in plasma from the same woman; alloagglutinins in colostrum are often wholly IgA but some IgM antibody may be present (for references, see Mollison *et al.* 1987).

Anti-A in low concentrations is present in the saliva of most group O and group B subjects (Adinolfi *et al.* 1966). Anti-B is found a little less commonly than anti-A and is less common in group A than in group O subjects (Denborough and Downing, 1969).

Concentration and equilibrium constants of IgM and IgG anti-A and anti-B

Concentrations needed to produce agglutination. Greenbury et al. (1963) concluded that to bring about 50% agglutination of a suspension of group A red cells, only 25 IgM anti-A molecules per cell were required, but for IgG anti-A the number was 20 000. The minimal concentration of anti-A required for agglutination (i.e. at the end-point of a titre) was estimated by Economidou et al. (1967b) to be, for IgG, 0.2 μg/ml and for IgM 0.01 μg/ml; taking into account that the mol. wt. of IgM is five times that of IgG, the agglutinating effect of IgM was thus approximately 100 times as great as that of IgG (for an exception, see p. 129).

Equilibrium constants. Examples both of human and rabbit IgM and IgG anti-A were investigated by Economidou et al. (1967b). Equilibrium constants ranged from 0.6 to 13.0 $\times$ 10^8 l/mol, but on the average were approximately the same for IgM antibodies as for IgG. Monomers prepared from IgM anti-B were tested by Economidou et al. (1967c) and found to have an equilibrium constant 36–170 times lower than that of the whole IgM molecule, providing further support for the idea that native IgM anti-B (and anti-A) is attached to red cells by at least two binding sites. The authors concluded that both with IgM and IgG anti-B more than one antigen–antibody bond must be broken simultaneously to permit dissociation of the antibody. Previously, Greenbury et al. (1965) had concluded that both antigen-binding sites on IgG anti-A are normally attached to adjacent antigen sites on the red cell. Nevertheless, some IgG anti-A molecules must bind univalently to each cell or there would be no agglutination.

The association constant of rabbit IgG anti-A was found to have the following values: with A_1 cells 7.4 $\times$ 10^8 l/mol; with A_1B cells 5.1 $\times$ 10^8 l/mol; and with A_2 cells 2.1 $\times$ 10^8 l/mol. Anti-A was found to dissociate three times more rapidly from A_2 than from A_1 cells (Economidou et al. 1967a).

The binding constant of human IgG anti-A for cord A_1 red cells was found to be 3.3 $\times$ 10^7 l/mol compared with 5.7–8.7 $\times$ 10^7 l/mol for adult A_1 red cells and that for cord A_1B red cells to be 2.1 $\times$ 10^7 l/mol compared with 3.2–7.0 $\times$ 10^7 l/mol for adult A_1B red cells (Economidou, 1966).

Exposure to A and B antigens in early life. Jakobowicz et al. (1959) tested the hypothesis that individuals exposed to A glycoprotein in fetal life might be partially tolerant to A. Adults were given injections of a preparation of tetanus toxoid containing A substance and it appeared that the rise in anti-A titre was greater in individuals with group O mothers than in those with group A mothers.

On the other hand Hraba et al. (1962) could find no influence of the maternal blood group on agglutinin titre in infants aged 6 months, and Kennell and Muschel (1956) found that in 137 group O children the characteristics of anti-A (agglutinin titre, haemolytic activity, etc.) were not influenced by the mother's ABO group.

Crossreacting anti-A,B
Moss (1910) found that absorption with A or B cells could reduce the titre of group O serum against both A and B cells, and Landsteiner and Witt (1926) showed that some of the antibody in group O serum behaved as anti-AB; thus, the eluate made from A

cells previously incubated with group O serum would agglutinate both B and A cells. Similarly, the reaction of group O serum with B cells is inhibited by the saliva of A or B secretors and the reaction with A cells is inhibited by the saliva of B or A secretors.

The best explanation might seem to be that the anti-AB in group O serum is an antibody directed against a structure common to A and B (Owen, 1954). However, this would imply that the crossreacting antibody eluted from group A red cells is the same as that eluted from group B red cells whereas in fact the two appear to be different (Dodd *et al.* 1967). Moreover, crossreacting anti-AB can be completely inhibited either with D-galactose or N-acetylgalactosamine (Holburn, 1976), confirming the structural similarity of the two sugars (see section on Biosynthesis).

Crossreacting anti-A,B can be either IgG or IgM and can probably also be IgA: very little anti-A,B can be demonstrated in the serum of an unimmunized group O subject (Yokoyama and Fudenberg, 1964). Crossreacting anti-A,B increased in concentration in all six group O subjects immunized with blood group substances (Contreras *et al.* 1983a) and it was easier to demonstrate its presence if the cells used for absorption and elution were of a different specificity from that of the glycoprotein used for immunization (Dodd *et al.* 1967; Contreras *et al.* 1983a). The role of anti-A,B in haemolytic disease of the newborn is discussed in Chapter 12.

Crossreacting anti-AB may be cytotoxic for the lymphocytes of group A secretors (for references, see Mollison, 1983, p. 281).

Anti-A$_1$
If serum from a B or O person is absorbed once or twice with A$_2$ cells it will no longer agglutinate A$_2$ cells but will still agglutinate A$_1$ cells. On the other hand if B or O serum is absorbed with A$_1$ cells it will no longer react with A$_1$ or with A$_2$ cells. Accordingly, B (or O) serum is regarded as containing two separate populations of antibody molecules: anti-A reacting both with A$_2$ and with A$_1$ cells, and anti-A$_1$ reacting only with A$_1$ cells. The anti-A$_1$ has a lower thermal range than the anti-A (Friedenreich, 1931). If an excess of A$_2$ cells is used in absorbing group B serum, anti-A$_1$ as well as anti-A may be absorbed (Lattes and Cavazutti, 1924).

When tested at room temperature, anti-A$_1$ was found in 1–2% of A$_2$ bloods and in 25% of A$_2$B bloods by Taylor *et al.* (1942) and in 22% of A$_2$B bloods by Juel (1959). Anti-A$_1$ occurring in A$_2$ and A$_2$B subjects is usually inactive at 37°C. A rather higher incidence of anti-A$_1$ was reported by Speiser *et al.* (1951), namely 7.9% in A$_2$ bloods and 35% in A$_2$B bloods.

According to Speiser (1956), anti-A$_1$ is very rare in infants; one example was found in examining 10 000 blood samples.

As expected, anti-A$_1$ in an A$_2$B serum proved to be wholly IgM but, perhaps surprisingly, anti-A$_1$ separated from group O serum by absorption with A$_2$ cells was found to be wholly IgG (Plischka and Schäfer, 1972). An example of anti-A$_1$ which became active at 37°C after a series of transfusions was partly IgG and partly IgM (Lundberg and McGinniss, 1975).

Two kinds of anti-A$_1$ can be recognized: the first reacts with A$_1$ red cells independently of their Ii group and is inhibited by the saliva of group A secretors. The second is anti-AI; it does not react with A$_1$i cells and is not inhibited by the saliva of group A secretors. In discussing this second type, originally described by Gold (1964),

Romans *et al.* (1980) pointed out that the allo-anti-AI found in the serum of an Ai adult by Tippett *et al.* (1960) behaved as anti-A$_1$. The first type of anti-A$_1$, i.e. reacting independently of Ii group, is the commoner (C.A. Tilley and D.G. Romans, unpublished observations, 1980).

Clinical significance of anti-A$_1$. Most examples of anti-A$_1$ found in A$_2$ or A$_2$B subjects agglutinate A$_1$ cells only up to a temperature of 25°C or so and are of no clinical significance. Antibodies which are active *in vitro* at about 30°C but only dubiously active at 37°C will bring about the destruction of a proportion of A$_1$ cells *in vivo* when a small dose of cells is injected (see Chapter 10). Those antibodies that are only dubiously active at 37°C would almost certainly fail to produce detectable red cell destruction following the transfusion of therapeutic quantities of blood. On the other hand, in several instances in which anti-A$_1$ has been quite clearly active at 37°C, extensive destruction of A$_1$ cells *in vivo* has been recorded (see below). Such cases are extremely rare.

It appears that following the transfusion of A$_1$ cells to patients whose serum contains anti-A$_1$, there is usually no increase in the thermal range of the anti-A$_1$ (see Stratton, 1955a), but a few exceptions have been recorded. Jakobowicz *et al.* (1961) described a patient of subgroup A$_2$, suffering from lymphosarcoma with associated macroglobulinaemia; after transfusion of at least 7 units of A$_1$ blood, anti-A$_1$ with a titre of 4 at 37°C which was very difficult to inhibit with A glycoprotein was found in the serum; the antibody lysed papain-treated but not untreated A$_1$ cells.

Several other examples of the development of anti-A$_1$, active at 37°C, following a series of transfusions, have been described; see e.g. Lundberg and McGinniss (1975). References to haemolytic transfusion reactions due to anti-A$_1$ are given in Chapter 11.

Anti-A$_1$ passively transferred to A$_2$ or A$_2$B recipients by the transfusion of group O blood may cause the destruction of subsequently transfused A$_1$ or A$_1$B red cells; see Chapter 11.

Anti-A$_1$ may develop in the serum of group A$_2$ subjects who have received a tissue graft from a group O donor 1 week or so previously; see Chapter 11.

Anti-A and anti-B as autoantibodies

Anti-A and anti-B are sometimes found as autoantibodies (see Chapter 7). Anti-A or anti-B 'pseudo-autoantibodies' may be found in A, B or AB subjects who have recently received a group O bone marrow or solid organ transplant (see Chapter 11).

Anti-A$_1$ has been found as an autoantibody, reacting weakly at room temperature, in a patient of group A$_1$ without haemolytic anaemia. The auto-anti-A$_1$ reacted with adult A$_1$i red cells and was inhibited by group A secretor saliva (Wright *et al.* 1980).

Anomalous occurrence of anti-A and anti-B. Occasionally, anti-A and anti-B are found in A or B subjects respectively, but not as autoagglutinins, i.e. with a specificity which differs from normal anti-A or anti-B. A few examples of anti-A of this kind have been found in A$_1$ subjects (M. Stroup, personal communication). As mentioned above, the serum from most *cis* AB people contains allo-anti-B.

In a group A$_1$B subject whose serum agglutinated group B red cells, though not her own cells, the B-specified transferase was shown to be abnormal (Yoshida *et al.* 1981b).

Anti-H and anti-HI

'Pure' anti-H is a very uncommon antibody; it is found in subjects of the very rare phenotype O_h as a haemolysin, and as an agglutinin which is almost as active at 37°C as at 0°C. All of three examples tested by Chattoraj et al. (1968a) were found to be IgM but some examples are partly IgG (Moores, 1972; Haddad, 1974). Anti-H may also be found rarely in A_1 subjects (Gouge et al. 1977).

The 'normal incomplete cold antibody' has anti-H specificity and is neutralized by secretor saliva; see Chapter 7.

The name 'anti-H' used to be applied to an alloagglutinin found not uncommonly in sera from A_1 and A_1B donors (see Morgan and Watkins, 1948), but the name was changed to anti-HI after it had been shown that the antibody reacted only with red cells carrying both H and I specificities (Rosenfield et al. 1964a). Anti-HI, like anti-H, reacts most strongly with O red cells and most weakly with A_1B cells. Voak et al. (1968) mentioned that all examples of anti-HI which they had found were in women, most of whom were pregnant. Their findings were made impressive by their mention of the fact that more than 90 000 samples from males were tested each year.

Potent anti-HI is found invariably in the serum of O_{Hm}^A and O_{Hm}^B people.

An example of anti-H (possibly -HI) which in the presence of sodium azide (0.1% w/v) reacted strongly at 37°C, but in the absence of azide reacted only weakly and only in the cold, was encountered by P. Watson (personal communication, 1981). The effect of the azide appeared to be due to some interaction with plasma protein rather than with the red cell membrane. An autoagglutinin enhanced by azide is mentioned in Chapter 7.

Anti-A, -A₁, -B and -H lectins

A highly potent anti-A can be extracted from the albumin gland or the eggs of various species of snail, e.g. *Helix aspersea, Helix hortensis* and *Helix pomatia; Otala lactea* and *Cepaea nemoralis* (for references see Mollison et al. 1987).

Some snail anti-A extracts react equally well with A_1 and A_2 red cells, although others do not (Boyd et al. 1966) and still others react equally well with A_1 and A_2 cells but less strongly with A_2B. The different specificities of the anti-A from different snails can be indicated by referring to them, for example, as anti-A_{HP}, for *Helix pomatia* (Prokop et al. 1968). Anti-A purified from the albumin gland of *H. pomatia* was found to be a fairly homogeneous protein with a mol. wt. of 100 000; from the point of view of specificity, it was more homogeneous than human anti-A (Hammarström and Kabat, 1969). Snail anti-A reactions are enormously enhanced with bromelin-treated red cells. For further information, see Salmon and Cartron (1977).

The reactions of the lectin from *Dolichos biflorus*, with anti-A_1 specificity, have been described earlier. The purified protein consists of two electrophoretically distinguishable isolectins with apparent mol. wts 109 000 and 113 000. The two species showed great similarity in amino acid composition and were indistinguishable in immunodiffusion against specific antisera (for references see Goldstein and Hayes, 1978). The carbohydrate-binding specificity of the purified lectin has been studied in detail by precipitation: A_1 substances were more reactive than A_2 and no reaction was seen with B or O substances (Etzler and Kabat, 1970).

Useful anti-B can be prepared from the fungus *Fomes fomentarius* (Mäkelä et al. 1959).

Reagents with the specificity anti-H can be obtained from three plants: *Ulex europaeus*, *Lotus tetragonolobus* and *Laburnum alpinum*. Most workers use *Ulex* extract as their standard anti-H reagent. Sera from the eel *Anguilla anguilla* are less satisfactory since, although most samples will agglutinate O cells preferentially, many samples are not inhibited by H substance and may have anti-HI specificity (Chessin and McGinniss, 1968).

Immune responses to A and B antigens

Incompatible transfusions
If A blood is injected i.v. into a person of group B or group O, or B blood is injected into a person of group A or group O, the titre of anti-A or anti-B increases after an initial fall due to absorption of antibody (Wiener, 1941a).

Perhaps the first record of such a response is that of Thalheimer (1921). His patient, a boy aged 6 years, received a first transfusion from his father without incident; however, a second transfusion from his father 18 d later produced a severe haemolytic reaction. It was now found that the father was group B and the child group O. Direct matching before the first transfusion had not revealed incompatibility, and it may be presumed that at that time the child had only a low titre of anti-B. Because of the success of the first transfusion, it was considered unnecessary to carry out a direct matching test before the second transfusion, although had the test been repeated the incompatibility would presumably have been obvious.

Rø (1937) studied a group O patient who received 500 ml group A blood. The anti-A titre rose after transfusion and subsequently fell again. In a case described by Mollison and Young (1941b) the patient (group O) received 360 ml group B blood. Eight hours after transfusion the

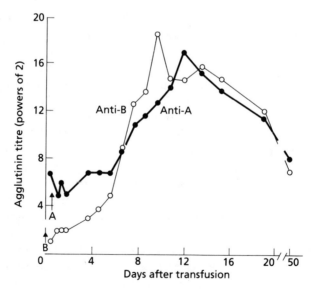

Figure 4.2 Changes in anti-A and anti-B titre (as log$_2$) in a group O patient after the transfusion of 360 ml group B blood (at 'B') and of group A serum (at 'A'). These titrations and those recorded in Fig. 4.3 were performed by the standard technique of making doubling dilutions, using the same unrinsed pipette, and were not checked by making direct dilutions (from the date of Mollison and Young, 1941b).

anti-B titre was only 2 compared with an anti-A titre of 128. After 48 h the anti-B titre started to increase, and between the sixth and tenth days it rose very rapidly to a peak. It then fell slowly and, 3 weeks after transfusion, had still not reached a stable level (see 'Anti-B' in Fig. 4.2).

After the transfusion of incompatible blood the peak titre of anti-A or anti-B is usually reached after about 9–12 d (Boorman *et al.* 1945a) (see also Figs 4.2 and 4.3). Although an increase in agglutinin titre is common after the transfusion of ABO-incompatible blood it is by no means invariable; it was noted in only six of 15 group O subjects after the i.v. injection of 25 ml A_1 or A_2 blood (Wiener *et al.* 1953b).

Although the initial decrease in titre, after the transfusion of ABO-incompatible blood, is associated particularly with the transfusion of large amounts of blood, it was observed in several of the subjects of Wiener *et al.* (1953b) referred to above and has even been noted after the injection of as little as 4 ml of incompatible red cells (see p. 470).

Intramuscular injections of incompatible blood. In a series in which subjects received four to six injections each of 10–15 ml of a 50% suspension of twice-washed red cells, some group O or B subjects who had received A red cells developed powerful anti-A haemolysins although no changes in agglutinin titre were observed (Thomsen, 1930). The development of haemolysins was also noted by Rapoport and Stokes (1937) following i.m. injections of blood.

During an epidemic of poliomyelitis, Rapoport and Stokes carried out an investigation of the prophylactic value of i.m. injections of blood. Sixty millilitres of blood were taken from one or other of a child's parents and injected into the child's buttocks. Among 1341 children, 52 showed a reaction which followed a characteristic pattern: some 6 d after the injection the child

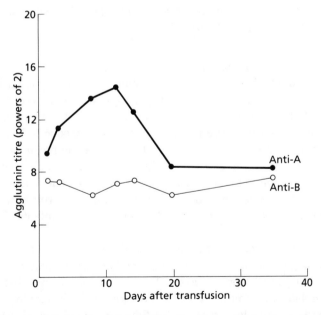

Figure 4.3 Changes in anti-A and anti-B agglutinin titre in a group O patient after the transfusion of 45 ml group A blood (data from Mollison, 1943a).

became acutely ill and febrile; the sites of injection became hot, red and painful. The reaction subsided after 3–4 d. In 17 cases the blood groups of the child and its parents were investigated; in every case the parent's cells were incompatible with the child's serum. In 13 of 17 cases in which the test was made within 4 weeks of injection, the child's serum haemolysed the parent's cells. In one case a child who had had a reaction was given a second injection of blood some months later; in this case the second reaction developed only 28 h after the injection.

Solid organ transplants. Except for bone marrow transplantation, where ABO incompatibility can be dealt with by depleting the donor bone marrow of red cells or by lowering the titre of anti-A and anti-B in the recipient by plasma exchange, organ transplantation across the ABO barrier often leads to vascular or humoral hyperacute graft rejection (Cooper, 1990).

Injections of human blood group substances

The A and B group-specific substances are present in the plasma and serum. Even when the substances cannot be detected serologically, they may provoke an immune response following the transfusion of serum to a suitable recipient (e.g. A to O). The peak of the immune response is usually reached at about 10–15 d after the transfusion (Aubert *et al.* 1942a; see also Figs 4.2 and 4.3). Immune responses to A have also been produced by injecting saliva (Wiener *et al.* 1953a) and urine (Freda *et al.* 1957).

Cryoprecipitates and Factor IX concentrates may also stimulate the production of 'immune' anti-A and anti-B (McShine and Kunst, 1970).

Good immune responses to A or B have been produced by injecting purified preparations of human material from meconium (Sickles and Murdick, 1953) and from pseudomucinous ovarian cysts (Loutit and Morgan, 1946). Using a later, more purified preparation from the latter source, substantial increases in titre and avidity were found, using 1.5 mg doses of the preparation; 0.1 mg appeared to be a suboptimal dose (Polley *et al.* 1963; Contreras *et al.* 1983a).

Alloimmunization by A and B antigens during pregnancy

The term 'ABO-incompatible' may conveniently be used to describe a pregnancy in which the infant's red cells carry A or B and the mother's serum contains the corresponding antibody. Dienst (1905) first observed that, following such pregnancies, after delivery there might be a rise in the mother's anti-A or anti-B agglutinin titre. Jonsson (1936) made a systematic study of ABO-incompatible pregnancies but looked for haemolysins only. Whereas in a control series of group O males the incidence of anti-A or anti-B haemolysins was 3.5%, in a series of recently delivered group O women it was 14.5%. In relation to the group of the infants born to the mothers, the incidence of haemolysins was as follows: O infants, 7.1%; B infants, 20.8%; and A infants, 28.1%.

After delivery, most commonly between 10 and 20 days, there is a rise in the titre of anti-A or anti-B agglutinins in most women who have given birth to an infant of the corresponding ABO group (Boorman *et al.* 1945a). There is evidence that those infants who fail to stimulate an immune response are non-secretors (Smith, 1945). Unlike Boorman *et al.* (1945a) and Hurst *et al.* (1946), Smith frequently noted a rise in the titre of anti-A or anti-B during the last month of pregnancy.

Injections of purified group-specific substances of animal origin
An experiment made by Forssman (1911) revealed the existence of serologically related substances in animals widely separated in the zoological system: the injection of extracts of guinea pig organs into rabbits provoked the formation of lysins active against sheep red cells. Subsequently the name 'Forssman antigen' was used for any substance which would stimulate the formation of sheep haemolysin. The sheep antibody produced in this way is an example of a 'heterophil' antibody; the cardinal feature of such an antibody is that it is produced by an animal in response to contact with an antigen from a different species and is found to react with antigen from another species. It is the antibody which is heterophil, not the antigenic determinant; the antigens are identical or related (Franks and Coombs, 1969).

Human A antigen is closely related to the Forssman antigen; in both, the terminal sugar is N-acetylgalactosamine (Sweeley and Dawson, 1969). A proposed structure of the Forssman antigen (Siddiqui and Hakomori, 1971) is included in the footnote to Fig. 4.4.

In the past, hog A substance and equine AB substance were used for stimulating the production of potent anti-A or anti-B in human volunteers and for neutralizing anti-A and anti-B in group O plasma (Witebsky, 1946) but animal group-specific substances are no longer considered suitable for use in humans.

Injections of vaccines containing hog pepsin. Increases in anti-A or anti-B concentration following the injection of diphtheria or tetanus toxoid are due to the presence of hog pepsin (Christiaens, 1937; Ottensooser and Willenegger, 1938; Moullec, 1947). Tetanus toxoid prepared in a medium free from peptone of animal origin does not cause rises in anti-A or anti-B titre (Hendry and Sickles, 1951).

Injections of pneumococcal or influenza vaccine. Substantial rises in anti-A titre have been found in patients receiving certain batches of pneumococcal vaccine. Although it was at first suggested that this response was due to antigenic similarity between type 14 pneumococcus and blood group A, later studies indicated that the effect was due to A-like substances from culture media tightly bound to the bacterial polysaccharide (Noël, 1981; Siber *et al.* 1982).

Injections of influenza virus vaccine may stimulate anti-A; it seems that this is due to the incorporation of A-like substances present in the cytoplasm of the chick embryo on which the virus is grown (Springer and Tritel, 1962; Springer and Schuster, 1964).

Injections of horse serum. Davidsohn (1938) found that the injection of horse serum might stimulate anti-A and anti-B, and observed that such responses were most pronounced in subjects who developed serum sickness. However, the most important source of A substance in horse anti-tetanus serum is not horse A but hog A substance from the pepsin used in digesting the serum (André *et al.* 1952).

Clinical significance of stimulation of anti-A and anti-B by vaccines, etc.
The practical importance of injections of vaccine containing hog pepsin in rendering group O donors 'dangerous' was shown by Dausset and Vidal (1951); they described six haemolytic reactions following the transfusion of O blood to A recipients; in every

case the donor had received injections of vaccine known to contain hog pepsin. In most cases the donors had received the injections within the previous 3 months, but in two instances it was shown that the immune characteristics of the donor's anti-A persisted for at least 7 years after the last injection.

In a case described in Chapter 11, of a severe haemolytic transfusion reaction in a group A patient following the transfusion of group O blood, 1 month before giving blood the donor had received an injection of anti-tetanus serum prepared by digestion with hog pepsin. It seems logical to conclude that stimulation of anti-A in group O women following the injection of vaccines, etc., containing A-like substances must also lead to the production of potent IgG anti-A and thus increase the risk that any A infants born subsequently will be affected by haemolytic disease of the newborn. In fact, there is virtually no evidence of the magnitude of the risk. One survey suggested that the offspring of women who had received injections of tetanus toxoid during the last trimester of pregnancy had an increased risk of developing ABO haemolytic disease (Gupte and Bhatia, 1980) but the control group was not strictly comparable.

In a study of 11 moderately severe cases of haemolytic disease of the newborn due to ABO incompatibility it was noted that not one of the mothers gave a history of having had injections of bacterial vaccines or toxoids (Crawford et al. 1953a).

Toxocara infection. Emulsified toxocara worms inhibit anti-A and anti-B; infected children commonly have high titres of these antibodies (Heiner and Kevy, 1956; Shrand, 1964).

IgM, IgG and IgA anti-A and anti-B in relation to immune responses
In group B subjects, before and after stimulation with A substance, IgM anti-A predominates. In group O subjects, even before stimulation, some of the anti-A may be IgG; after stimulation IgG anti-A as well as IgM anti-A is produced in most subjects (Abelson and Rawson, 1961; Kochwa et al. 1961).

In five normal B subjects studied by Polley et al. (1963) no IgG anti-A could be detected before antigenic stimulation; after two injections, each of 1.5 mg human A substance, at an interval of 1 week, low titre IgG anti-A was produced in three of the five subjects, but in no case was this antibody readily haemolytic. In four of the five the titre of IgM anti-A increased. Of five O subjects who were stimulated in the same way, three had IgG anti-A before stimulation and all five had IgG anti-A after stimulation. Similarly. Abelson and Rawson (1961) found that whereas in B subjects IgM anti-A predominated in 80% before stimulation and in 90% after stimulation, in O subjects IgG predominated in 48% before stimulation and in 88% after stimulation.

Most sera containing IgA anti-A have come from subjects who have recently received an antigenic stimulus (Kunkel and Rockey, 1963; Ishizaka et al. 1965; Adinolfi et al. 1966), although in a few group O subjects IgA anti-A or anti-B are found before immunization (Contreras et al. 1983a).

Persistence of immune anti-A. Allen and Kabat (1958) found that after an injection of hog A substance or horse A and B substances the peak level of antibody tended to be maintained for many months. There was then a steady fall but even after 12 months the level was still about 50% of the peak. Tovey (1958) found that in blood donors whose serum contained anti-A or anti-B haemolysins, repeated tests during a 2-year period showed that these antibodies persisted in 80% of subjects.

THE LEWIS SYSTEM

The Lewis blood group system differs from most of the other human blood group systems in some important ways. First, it is a system of soluble antigens present in saliva and plasma (Grubb, 1951) and red cells acquire their Lewis phenotype by adsorbing Lewis substances from the plasma (Sneath and Sneath, 1955). Second, the Lewis phenotype of the red cells is influenced by the ABH secretor status (although the Lewis genes and secretor genes are inherited independently); a person who inherits *Le* will have the red cell phenotype Le(a + b −) if they are a non-secretor (*sese*), but the phenotype Le(a − b +) if he is a secretor (*Sese* or *SeSe*) (Grubb, 1951; Ceppellini, 1955). Third, since the products of *ABH* and *Le* share the same precursor substrate, the Lewis phenotype may be modified by the ABO phenotype; e.g. A_1 may decrease the expression of Le^b (Andresen, 1948) and also of Le^a (Cutbush *et al.* 1956). Some examples of the interactions of the *Hh, Sese, ABO* and *Lele* genes are shown in Table 4.4. The biochemical basis of the Lewis system and the relationship between the Lewis and ABH antigens are described in later sections.

The Lewis blood group system shows many resemblances to the J blood group system in cattle and to the R blood group system in sheep. In all three systems the antigens are acquired passively by the red cells from the plasma. Thus, J-negative cells can be transformed into J-positive cells by incubating them with the plasma of J-positive animals (Stormont, 1949), and a similar transformation can be carried out with R-negative cells in sheep (Rendel *et al.* 1954). J is serologically related to the human A antigen (Stormont, 1949), as is R (Neimann-Sørensen *et al.* 1954).

The Lewis groups of adults (see Table 4.5)

The phenotype Le(a − b +)
Subjects with the phenotype Le(a − b +) have the alleles *H, Se* and *Le* and their secretions contain H, Le^a and Le^b glycoproteins (and A or B, if the subject is group A or B).

Table 4.4 Some examples of interactions of the *Hh, Sese, ABO* and *Lele* genes (based on Watkins, 1966).

	Blood group substances	
Alleles*	in secretions	on red cells
H, Se, A, Le	H, A, Le^a, Le^b	H, A, Le^b
H, sese, A, Le	Le^a	H, A, Le^a
H, Se, A, lele	H, A	H, A
H, Se, OO, Le	H, Le^a, Le^b	H, $(Le^a)^†$, Le^b
hh[‡]*, Se, A, Le*	Le^a	Le^a

* The alleles *H, Se, A* (or *B*) and *Le* produce their effect when present in single or in double dose; when the amorphic alleles *h, O, le* and *se* are present in double dose, no detectable effect is produced.
† In some group O (and A_2) subjects who have the alleles *H, Se* and *Le*, some Le^a as well as Le^b can be detected on the red cells (see p. 176).
‡ The *H* gene is necessary for the formation of H, A and Le^b substances (see Fig. 4.6).

Table 4.5 Lewis groups of adults

Red cell phenotype	Genotype	Lewis substance in saliva	H substance in saliva	Frequency in Whites (approx.)
Le(a – b +)	H, Se, Le	$Le^b + Le^a$	+	75
Le(a + b –)	H, sese, Le (very rarely, hh, Se or sese, Le)	Le^a	–	20
Le(a – b –)*	H, Se, lele	—	+	4
Le(a – b –)†	H, sese, lele (very rarely hh, Se or sese, lele)	—	–	1

* Apart from intrinsic type II H, red cells carry type I H (previously called Le^d), taken up from the plasma and also present in the saliva.
† Red cells carry Le^c, taken up from the plasma and also present in the saliva.

The plasma of Le(a – b +) persons contains predominantly Le^b glycosphingolipid but also some Le^a. The amount of Le^a in the saliva of Le(a – b +) subjects is substantially less than in that of Le(a + b –) subjects.

The amount of Le^b-active glycoplipid in the plasma of 35 group O, Le(a – b +) subjects was estimated to be 0.9 μg/ml; no Le^b was present in the plasma of group O, Le(a + b –) and Le(a – b –) subjects. About one-third of the total Le^b-active glycolipid in whole blood was associated with the red cells, the rest being in the plasma (Rohr et al. 1980).

As discussed later on there are two main types of anti-Le^b; anti-Le^{bH} (anti-HLe^b), reacting preferentially with cells carrying Le^b and abundant H (i.e. group O and A_2 Le(a – b +) cells) and anti-Le^{bL}, reacting with Le(b +) cells regardless of ABH groups.

The phenotype Le(a + b +)
The red cells of O and A_2 subjects who have the alleles H, Se and Le react not only with anti-Le^b but also with some examples of anti-Le^a; this latter reaction is usually weak and may be demonstrable only by the indirect antiglobulin test. If the Le(b +) cells are first enzyme-treated, most if not all samples of O and A_2 cells appear to be Le(a + b +); such cells are subject to variable degrees of destruction *in vivo* by anti-Le^a (Cutbush et al. 1956). The reaction between anti-Le^a and group O, Le(a + b +) red cells can be inhibited by Le(a + b –) plasma *in vitro* (Cutbush et al. 1956) and *in vivo* (Mollison et al. 1963).

The phenotype Le(a + b +) has not been found in A_1 adults probably because they make less Le^a substance, as the result of the competition between the A^1- and Le-transferases for substrate. In the family described by Crookston et al. (1970) the Le(a + b +) phenotype was expressed in five members, all O or A_2, of three generations, but not in A_1 members of the family.

The phenotype Le(a + b +) is commoner in adults from Polynesia and Taiwan and perhaps from elsewhere in the Orient. In these subjects, Le^a is relatively strongly expressed but Le^b can be detected only with certain potent anti-Le^b reagents (mainly monoclonal antibodies). The weak expression of Le^b may be explained by the existence of a 'partial secretor' gene and a very low incidence of the non-secretor gene (Henry *et al.* 1990; Lin Chu and Broadberry, 1990).

The phenotype Le(a + b –)
Persons belonging to this phenotype have Le^a substance in their plasma and in their saliva, and their red cells are agglutinated by anti-Le^a. They are non-secretors of ABH.

Great variation is found between the reactions of Le(a + b –) cells from different O donors, as judged by their degree of agglutination in an antiglobulin test after exposure to anti-Le^a at 37°C (Mollison and Cutbush, 1955). Agglutination tests at room temperature apparently fail to detect these differences.

Le(a + b –) red cells do not react with anti-Le^b either *in vitro* or *in vivo*, showing that they have no Le^b antigen. Thus in a patient of group AB, Le(a – b –) with potent anti-Le^b in her serum who was given test injections of O, Le(a – b +) and O, Le(a + b –) red cells, more than 80% of the Le(b +) red cells were destroyed within 6 min of injection but the Le(a + b –) red cells underwent no destruction (Mollison, 1967, p. 274).

The phenotype Le(a – b –)
Subjects of genotype *lele* have red cells of the phenotype Le(a – b –) which react either with anti-Le^c or with anti-type I H (previously anti-Le^d). The genotype *lele* is four to five times commoner in Blacks than in Whites.

Subjects of phenotype Le(a – b –) were previously subdivided into Le(c + d –) or Le(c – d +), according to whether they had Le^c or Le^d in their saliva and plasma. Le^d is type I H and is therefore not a product of *Le* or *le*. For the status of Le^c and Le^d, see section on Chemistry.

Subjects of the genotype *lele* have traces of Le^a in their serum (Holburn, 1973) and saliva (Grubb, 1951; Arcilla and Sturgeon, 1973), and have traces of readily detectable Lewis antigens in tissues such as colon and bladder (Ørntoft *et al.* 1991).

Lewis groups in pregnant women
The agglutinability of red cells by anti-Le^a and anti-Le^b is reduced during pregnancy (Brendemoen, 1952b; Taylor *et al.* 1974). This effect does not seem to be due primarily to the slight decrease in Lewis glycolipid in plasma during pregnancy, but rather to the increased ratio of lipoprotein to red cell mass that occurs during pregnancy and which results in a repartition of glycolipids between plasma and red cells (Hammar *et al.* 1981).

Lewis groups and bladder cancer
The higher frequency of the phenotype Le(a – b –) in patients with cancer of the bladder seems to be due to the conversion of Le-positive to Le-negative with advanced disease. The true Le phenotype can be determined by measuring fucosyltransferase in saliva (Langkilde *et al.* 1990).

The Lewis groups of infants
Cord red cells do not react with anti-Le^b and are not agglutinated by anti-Le^a. However, if the indirect antiglobulin test is used, Le^a can be demonstrated on the red

cells of about 50% of cord blood samples (Cutbush et al. 1956).

The red cells of an infant which is destined to become an Le(a – b +) adult may react successively as Le(a – b –), Le(a + b –) and finally Le(a – b +) during the first 15 months of its life (Cutbush et al. 1956).

The weak reactions of the red cells of newborn infants seem to be due to the very low concentration of Lewis glycolipids in the plasma. The plasma of newborn infants will not 'transform' red cells, although the red cells of newborn infants can be transformed by plasma from adults (Mäkelä and Mäkelä, 1956) or by glycosphingolipid fractions of plasma from adults (Tilley et al. 1975).

The frequency of the Le(a +) phenotype is much higher in infants under the age of 1 year than it is in adults (Andresen, 1947; Jordal and Lyndrup, 1952). In one study, the frequency was 90% at 1–2 months, 45% at 12 months, and 22%, i.e. about the same as in adults, at 2–3 years (Jordal, 1956). Those Le(a + b –) infants who are going to retain this phenotype as adults can be distinguished by their failure to secrete ABH substances.

Discrepant results in testing the red cells of newborn infants with Lewis antisera may well be due to the presence or absence of the antibody anti-Le^x in the test serum, since anti-Le^x reacts with the red cells of 90% of newborn infants (Jordal, 1956), i.e. presumably with all those who have an Le gene, and whose red cells carry a low density of Le antigens (Schenkel-Brunner and Hanfland, 1981).

Uptake of Lewis substances on to red cells

Sneath and Sneath (1955) found that when Le(a + b –) cells were transfused to a Le(a – b +) recipient, the cells adsorbed Le^b substance from the recipient's plasma and then reacted as Le(a + b +). The transformation could also be produced in vitro by incubating Le(a + b –) cells in Le(a – b +) plasma at 35 °C for 24 h. Le(a + b –) or Le(a – b +) cells incubated with Le(a – b –) plasma lost their antigen to the plasma. Nevertheless, Lewis substances on red cells are relatively firmly attached; even after washing Le(a +) cells 20 times in saline they still react just as well with anti-Le^a sera (Cutbush et al. 1956); similarly, Le(a – b –) cells which have taken up Le^a or Le^b from glycosphingolipid fractions are not affected by repeated washing in saline (Tilley et al. 1975). It is now established that there is a continuous exchange of glycosphingolipids between plasma and the red cell membrane (Cooper, 1977).

As already mentioned, Sneath and Sneath (1955) suggested that the red cell might simply adsorb Lewis antigens in vivo and that the Lewis phenotype might depend entirely on uptake of antigens from the plasma. The correctness of this view was confirmed by the findings of Nicholas et al. (1957). These authors described twins displaying red cell chimerism. One twin had 49% O cells and 51% A$_1$ cells. The 'true' genotype of this twin was shown to be OO by the finding of H substance but not A substance in the saliva; all the red cells in this twin behaved as Le(a – b +). In the other twin, 61% of the cells were A$_1$ and 39% O. The saliva of this twin contained Le^a substance but not A or H; all the red cells behaved as Le(a + b –). Thus, red cells of the non-secretor twin behaved as Le(a + b –) in that twin, but as Le(a – b +) in the secretor twin. The red cells from the secretor twin behaved as Le(a – b +) in that twin and as Le(a + b –) in the circulation of the non-secretor twin.

Two other chimeric twins provided evidence that a complex, ALe^b, is present in the plasma of subjects who carry H, Se, A^1 and Le alleles. When such a subject receives O cells, by graft or transfusion, the O cells become coated with ALe^b, these coated cells are agglutinated by anti-A$_1$Le^b (Crookston *et al.* 1970; Swanson *et al.* 1971a). Reactions of anti-A$_1$Le^b with the cells of a chimera can thus indicate the 'true' genotype (Wrobel *et al.* 1974; Bird *et al.* 1976d; Szymanski *et al.* 1977).

Rate of uptake or loss of Lewis substance from red cells in vivo
In a case in which group O, Le(b +) red cells were transfused to an A$_1$,Le(b +) recipient and the O cells were extracted for testing, no uptake of ALe^b substance was found at 48 h; on days 4 and 5 the cells reacted weakly and on days 7 and 11 more strongly with anti-A$_1$Le^b (Crookston *et al.* 1970).

In a case in which the loss rather than the uptake of Lewis substance was investigated, O,Le(b +) red cells were transfused to an A$_1$Le(a – b –) patient and the transfused red cells separated by agglutinating out the patient's cells. The extracted O cells still reacted strongly with anti-Le^b after 48 h but at 7 d gave a scarcely detectable reaction (Mollison *et al.* 1963).

Lewis antigens on leucocytes and platelets
Using a cytotoxicity test, Lewis antigens have been demonstrated on lymphocytes (Dorf *et al.* 1972; Oriol *et al.* 1980b) and, using fluorescence flow-cytometry, have been demonstrated both on lymphocytes (Dunstan, 1986) and on platelets, where their distribution was found to be heterogeneous (Dunstan and Simpson, 1985). Lewis antigens could not be demonstrated on granulocytes or monocytes (Dunstan, 1986).

Antibodies of the Lewis system
Systematic work on the Lewis blood group system stemmed from the discovery by Mourant in 1946 of an antibody which was subsequently given the name anti-Le^a. There is little doubt that isolated examples of anti-Le^a had been encountered by earlier workers. Landsteiner and Levine (1929) described five sera which gave parallel reactions and agglutinated about 16% of samples. The agglutination reactions were 'of a special sort' — a few rather large clumps, but mostly free cells. Parr and Krischner (1932) described an antibody which at 36°C failed to agglutinate red cells but caused slow lysis; Neter (1936) described an antibody which showed agglutinating and haemolysing activity, acting on about 25% of blood samples. Levine and Polayes (1941) also described an antibody which agglutinated 25% of red cell samples at 20°C and caused lysis at 37°C. As described below, anti-Le^a sera react with about 20% of samples in Whites and, unlike most other human blood group antibodies, cause haemolysis *in vitro*.

The second antibody belonging to the Lewis blood group system was discovered by Andresen in 1948 and subsequently named anti-Le^b. Both anti-Le^a and anti-Le^b as well as anti-Le$^{a + b}$ are found mainly in Le(a – b –) people.

Anti-Le^a
Anti-Le^a occurs relatively commonly in human sera. For example, in one series of 17 000 samples tested at room temperature, 57 (0.3%) contained anti-Le^a (Kissmeyer-Nielsen *et al.* 1955). Similarly, of 72 000 Parisians tested, 249 were found to have anti-Le^a, 49 had anti-Le^x (Salmon *et al.* 1984). Anti-Le^a is found only in persons who

are Le(a – b –) and secrete ABH substances (Miller *et al.* 1954b; Pettenkofer and Hoffbauer, 1954). Jordal (1956) examined the sera of 121 adults of this phenotype and found 14 examples of anti-Le^a and nine of anti-X (anti-Le^x, see below). This is an overall frequency of about 20% in Le(a – b –) subjects and would correspond to about 1% in the population as a whole. This figure is significantly higher than figures reported by Kissmeyer-Nielsen *et al.* (1955) and Salmon *et al.* (1984), but the difference may be partially explained by the fact that in Jordal's series a special search was being made for Lewis antibodies.

Donors of anti-Le^a belong more frequently to groups A, B or AB than would be expected in a random distribution (Jordal, 1956; Mollison, 1961b, p. 290). Kissmeyer-Nielsen (1965) found that of 548 donors of Lewis antibodies approximately 30% were group O compared with 44% of group O subjects in a random sample of the population.

A remarkable finding reported by Jordal (1956) was the occurrence of potent anti-Le^a in the cord serum of an infant of group A$_1$; the mother was group A$_1$ Le(a + b –), Le(x +) and her serum did not contain anti-Le^a.

A single example of 'auto-anti-Le^a' has been reported in a multitransfused Le(a – b +) patient with carcinoma of the oesophagus. The patient's own red cells partially adsorbed the antibody (Judd *et al.* 1978).

Anti-Le^b

Anti-Le^b can often be demonstrated as a weak antibody in serum which contains a relatively potent anti-Le^a. Anti-Le^b occurs on its own relatively infrequently; e.g. Pettenkofer and Hoffbauer (1954) tested the sera of 12 000 unselected pregnant or recently delivered women and found 52 examples of anti-Le^a but only two of anti-Le^b (i.e. without anti-Le^a). Most sera which contain a potent anti-Le^b do not contain anti-Le^a.

Subjects who make anti-Le^b without anti-Le^a are usually of the phenotype Le(a – b –) although they may be Le(a + b –), as first reported by Brendemoen (1950). In three further cases the donors were A$_1$, Le(a +), and the antibody was anti-HLe^b (Garratty and Kleinschmidt, 1965; Kornstad, 1969).

Some anti-Le^b sera fail to react with A$_1$ cells while reacting strongly with cells of group O or A$_2$ (Andresen, 1948). There are in fact two kinds of anti-Le^b (Brendemoen, 1950; Ceppellini, 1955; Ceppellini *et al.* 1959; Sneath and Sneath, 1959): (1) those, found more commonly, that are inhibited by the saliva of all ABH secretors (i.e. including those of Le(a – b –) subjects); these anti-Le^b sera, called anti-Le^{bH} (i.e. anti-HLe^b) by Ceppellini *et al.* (1959), react only with O and A$_2$ samples; and (2) those that are not inhibited by the saliva of Le(a – b –) secretors of ABH but are inhibited by the saliva of Le(a – b –) persons. These anti-Le^b sera react with A$_1$ Le(a – b +) samples almost as well as with those of other ABO groups, and were called anti-Le^{bL} (i.e. true anti-Le^b) by Ceppellini *et al.* (1959). Of 72 000 individuals tested in Paris, 29 were found to have anti-Le^{bH} and only two anti-Le^{bL} (Salmon *et al.* 1984).

Anti-Le^{bH} occurring as an autoantibody active only at 4°C with the patient's own red cells or at 18°C with other Le(b +) red cells was described by Giles and Poole (1979).

Anti-A$_1$Le^b and anti-BLe^b

An antibody reacting with A$_1$,Le(b +) red cells but not with A$_2$Le(b +), A$_1$, Le(b –) or O,Le(b +) cells was described by Seaman *et al.* (1968); further cases were reported by Crookston *et al.* (1970) and Gundolf (1973). Anti-A$_1$Le^b and anti-BLe^b have been detected in lymphocytotoxicity tests (Jeannet *et al.* 1972, 1974; Oriol *et al.* 1980a;b). These antibodies react with red cells and lymphocytes which have been exposed *in vivo* or *in vitro* to the plasma of individuals carrying the alleles *H, Se, A^1, Le* (or *H, Se, B, Le*). Such A_1,Le(a – b +) cells may fail to react with anti-Le^b; anti-A_1Le^b thus distinguishes 'pseudo A_1Le(a – b –)' (i.e. some persons with *H, A^1, Le* and *Se* alleles whose cells fail to react with anti-Le^b) from 'true A_1Le(a – b –)' (i.e. persons with the A^1 allele, but without the *Le* allele) (Crookston *et al.* 1970).

Anti-Le^x

This antibody was described (as anti-X) by Andresen and Jordal (1949); it reacted with all blood samples except those of the phenotype Le(a – b –). According to Jordal (1956) anti-Le^x reacts with more than 90% of cord samples and, moreover, reacts almost as well with cord red cells as with adult red cells — a claim upheld by Sturgeon and Arcilla (1970) (see also Arcilla and Sturgeon, 1974).

There is some evidence that the structure with which anti-Le^x reacts is in fact Le^a and that anti-Le^x is capable of reacting with red cells carrying only a very low density of Le^a receptors (Schenkel-Brunner and Hanfland, 1981). The structure named Le^x by Hakomori (1984b) is carried on a fucosylated unbranched type II chain and is not the same as the Le^x detected by the anti-Le^x reagents described originally by Andresen and Jordal (1949).

Anti-Le^c

This antibody reacts with the red cells of Le(a – b –) non-secretors, i.e. from individuals of genotype *lele, sese* and also with those of genotype *lele, hh*; the antibody is inhibited by saliva from individuals of the same genotypes. The first example of anti-Le^c was found in a group O,Le(a – b +) woman (Gunson and Latham, 1972). The second example of anti-Le^c was raised in goats (Graham *et al.* 1977). Le^c is not a product of an allele at the *Lewis* locus (Watkins, 1980) but may be the basic type I chain with no fucose added (see Biosynthesis section).

Anti-Le^d

This antibody reacts with the red cells of Le(a – b –) secretors, i.e. from individuals of genotype *lele, H, Se* (Potapov, 1970); the strongest reactors are of group O or A_2. The structure of the Le^d antigen is type I H (see section on Biosynthesis); hence Le^d cannot be part of the Lewis system.

Other antibodies reacting with Le(a – b –) red cells

Andersen (1958) described an antibody 'Magard' in an A_2,Le(a – b +) subject which reacted only with the red cells of Le(a – b –) secretors who were group A_1 or A_2. Hirsch *et al.* (1975) suggested that Magard is an antibody against type I A, previously termed ALe^d, which is taken up from the plasma by red cells and lymphocytes and which is present in the greatest concentrations in A,Le(a – b –) secretors.

Polyclonal and monoclonal Lewis antibodies produced in animals

Anti-Le^a, -Le^b, -Le^d and -Le^{dH} have been produced after injecting Lewis glycoproteins in different forms into rabbits or goats (for references see Mollison *et al.* 1987, p. 305).

Several laboratories have produced monoclonal Lewis antibodies which have proved suitable as grouping reagents, although a proportion of anti-Le^b have proved to be anti-Le^{bH}. Some monoclonal anti-Le^a and anti-Le^b can be lymphocytotoxic (Mayr *et al.* 1990). Some of the monoclonal Lewis antibodies are available commercially and are more potent than polyclonal reagents.

Monoclonal anti-type I H (-Le^d), -type II H, -type I A and -type I B have also been produced (Knowles *et al.* 1982a; Richert *et al.* 1983; Young *et al.* 1983; see also Hakomori, 1984b).

Serological characteristics of Lewis antibodies

Sera containing anti-Le^a usually agglutinate Le(a +) cells suspended in saline and react more strongly at 4°C and at room temperature than at 37°C. Red cells agglutinated by anti-Le^a have a 'stringy' appearance (Dunsford and Bowley, 1955). In some cases the serum may fail to agglutinate cells at 37°C (Grubb and Morgan, 1949) and occasionally may not agglutinate saline-suspended cells at all and be detectable only by the indirect antiglobulin test, especially if the cells and serum have been incubated at temperatures below 37°C.

Lewis antibodies seem almost always to bind complement. Most examples of anti-Le^a will bring about some lysis of red cells at 37°C (Andresen and Henningsen, 1951; Rosenfield and Vogel, 1951); Le(a +) cells from infants lyse more readily than Le(a +) cells from adults (Cutbush *et al.* 1956). Sera that fail to lyse untreated test cells almost always lyse enzyme-treated cells (Rosenfield and Vogel, 1951).

A very sensitive test for Lewis antibodies is the indirect antiglobulin test using an antiglobulin reagent containing anticomplement. The reactions are enhanced if the test is carried out in a medium of low ionic strength, or using enzyme-treated cells. In detecting anti-Le^a in those occasional samples of fresh serum which are anticomplementary or in samples of stored serum, which are frequently anti-complementary, the two-stage antiglobulin test described in Chapter 8 should be used.

In general, Lewis antibodies, especially anti-Le^{bH}, will react more strongly with group O cells than with A or B cells.

Lewis antibodies and type of immunoglobulin

Potent Lewis antibodies will sensitize red cells to agglutination by anti-IgM but very seldom to agglutination by anti-IgG.

One example of anti-Le^a which appeared to be solely IgG has been reported (Mollison, 1967, pp. 281–3); the antibody bound complement only weakly. An example of anti-Le^b which was solely IgG was found by G. Garratty (personal communication) in a man who said he had never been transfused; the antibody was potent and did not bind complement.

In tests with ^{125}I-labelled Le^a or Le^b substances in solution, IgG anti-Le^a was demonstrated in five of five potent anti-Le^a sera. The IgG anti-Le^a had a significantly lower binding constant than the accompanying IgM anti-Le^a, and the difference was thought to account for the failure to detect IgG anti-Le^a by the indirect antiglobulin test. An IgG concentrate of the anti-Le^a serum, treated with 2-ME to inactivate any IgM antibody present, agglutinated ficin-treated Le(a + b –) red cells (Holburn, 1984) and sensitized red cells to agglutination by anti-IgG (Mollison 1983, p. 310).

Using an enzyme-linked immunosorbent assay, IgG anti-Le^a was demonstrable in 13 of 13 samples from mothers with anti-Le^a and in 12 of 13 of the infants (Spitalnik *et al.* 1985).

Studies with ^{125}I-labelled IgM anti-Le^a

In studies with ^{125}I-labelled IgM anti-Le^a, the maximum number of molecules bound was found to be 4500–7300 per red cell (group O or A). The amounts of Le^a in the plasma and on the red cells of the same individual were not well correlated. The binding constant of intact (i.e. pentameric) IgM antibody molecules was 8.4×10^9 l/mol but that of the monomeric fragments (IgMs) prepared from the antibody was very low. It was concluded that anti-Le^a normally binds multivalently to clusters of Le^a sites on the cell surface, thus accounting both for the good complement-binding properties and the poor agglutinating properties of the antibody. With IgM anti-Le^a an agglutinin titre of 1 corresponded to an antibody concentration of 1.1 μg/ml with 5900 molecules of antibody bound per cell; using a tile test, an indirect antiglobulin titre of 1 with an anti-IgM serum corresponded to an antibody concentration of 0.42 μg/ml, with 500 molecules bound per cell, an indirect antiglobulin titre of 1 with an anti-complement serum corresponded to an antibody concentration of 0.04 μg/ml, with 50 molecules of antibody bound per cell (Holburn, 1973).

Immune responses to Lewis substances

In subjects whose serum already contains Lewis antibodies, significant rises in titre can be produced either by transfusion of Lewis-incompatible blood (Hossaini, 1972) or by the i.m. injection of 5 mg purified Lewis glycoprotein (Holburn, 1973). In a case in which Lewis-incompatible blood and plasma were transfused after giving injections of purified Le^a and Le^b substance, the titre of anti-Le^a rose from 2 to 8000 and that of anti-Le^b from 1 to 250 (Mollison *et al.* 1963) (see Chapter 10).

The appearance of IgG Lewis antibodies in the plasma after massive transfusion, in patients in whom no Lewis antibodies could be detected before transfusion, has been described (Cheng and Lukomskyj, 1989).

Clinical significance of Lewis antibodies

Lewis antibodies are frequently found in subjects who have never been transfused or received any other known antigenic stimulus, and they are therefore regarded as naturally occurring. Lewis antibodies are found more frequently in Blacks, who have a higher frequency of the Le(a – b –) phenotype. In subjects whose serum contains anti-Lewis, the antibody titre may increase considerably after an antigenic stimulus (see above). It seems that in some countries in South East Asia, Lewis antibodies are significantly more potent than in Europe and can cause severe haemolytic transfusion reactions (D. Chandanayingyong, personal communication).

Lewis antibodies are found more commonly in women in the reproductive period (Kissmeyer-Nielsen, 1965). Alloimmunization during pregnancy by fetal Lewis antigens may be the explanation (Pettenkoffer and Hoffbauer, 1954). Lewis antibodies can be made during pregnancy by women carrying a *Le* gene when their Le antigens are depressed.

Lewis antibodies are not known to cause haemolytic disease of the newborn; this outcome is to be expected because Lewis antibodies are predominantly IgM and also because the red cells of newborn infants react only very weakly or not at all with Lewis antibodies.

A group A_1 infant of unknown Lewis status, born to a mother whose serum contained relatively potent IgG anti-Le^b, was found to have a weakly positive direct antiglobulin test and anti-Le^b was eluted from its red cells. The serum bilirubin concentration reached a maximum of 13 mg/dl (221 μmol/l) on the fourth day of life (Bharucha et al. 1981). There was no clinical or haematological evidence of a haemolytic process.

Lewis antibodies, particularly anti-Le^a, can cause rapid destruction of small volumes of injected washed incompatible red cells but, for reasons discussed in Chapter 10, very rarely cause haemolytic transfusion reactions. The only risk arises if Le(a +) red cells of group O, which have more Lewis antigens than A or B cells, are selected for a patient whose serum contains potent anti-Le^a; in these circumstances Le(a –) red cells should be transfused. When screening patients of group A, B or AB whose serum contains Lewis antibodies, the antibodies will react with Lewis-positive cells in the panel since these cells are group O. However, when donor red cells of the patient's ABO group are crossmatched, most samples will be found to be compatible since Lewis antigens are more weakly expressed on A, B and AB cells than on O cells (see also section on Chemistry). In these circumstances, compatible red cells untyped for Lewis can be transfused in the knowledge that they will survive normally.

From a study of a relatively small number of cases it was concluded that Lewis antibodies might play a role in the rejection of renal grafts (Oriol et al. 1978). A larger series showed that the graft survival difference between Le(a – b –) and Lewis-positive recipients was not significant, although when both Lewis and HLA groups were taken into account the correlation was better than with HLA alone (quoted by Salmon et al. 1984). In a prospective study involving 70 donor–recipient pairs of cadaveric renal allografts, no significant differences in 1-year graft survival were found between Le-matched and Le-mismatched pairs (Posner et al. 1986).

THE Ii ANTIGENS AND ANTIBODIES

Antigens

Antigens on red cells
I and i are carbohydrate antigens present on red cells as glycoproteins or glycolipids (see Feizi, 1980a; Gardas, 1983). The red cells of almost all healthy adults have I determinants (Wiener et al. 1956; Jenkins et al, 1960b; Tippett et al. 1960) and lesser numbers of i determinants (Marsh and Jenkins, 1960). I and i cannot, therefore, be determined by the alleles of a single gene, and thus I and i are classified as a 'collection' of antigens rather than as a blood group system. Very rare normal adults of phenotype i have little or no I antigen and may have anti-I in their serum (Jenkins et al. 1960b).

Red cells that fail completely to react with anti-I are very rare; they are classed as i_1 and usually come from White persons; i_2 red cells that have a small amount of I (and a large amount of i) are usually from Black persons, and are slightly less rare. The adult i phenotype is inherited (see Race and Sanger, 1975).

Cord red cells react weakly with anti-I and strongly with anti-i (Marsh and Jenkins, 1960) and are classed as i_{cord}. During the first 18 months of life the red cells gradually come to react strongly with anti-I and weakly with anti-i (Marsh, 1961). This phenotype (strong I, weak i) is retained by healthy persons throughout life (Burnie, 1973).

Among adults, there is a wide normal range of reactivity of the red cells with anti-i and with anti-I (both auto- and allo-anti-I). Hillman and Giblett (1965) showed that the i reactivity of the red cells of normal subjects could be increased by repeated phlebotomy and suggested that there was an inverse relationship between i reactivity and marrow transit time. There is evidence that as red cells age in the circulation they become progressively less reactive with anti-i (Testa et al. 1981).

I^T was described by Booth et al. (1966). The antigen was strong on cord red cells, weaker with normal adult cells and weaker still with adult i cells; because the antigen appeared to be best expressed during the transition from i to I, the name I^T was chosen. With anti-I^T, fetal cells react more strongly than cord cells and the description 'transitional' for the antigen may not, therefore, be entirely appropriate (Garratty et al. 1972).

The number of I and i sites on red cells
Estimates of the number of I sites on adult cells have varied from 5×10^5 (normal red cells, Evans et al. 1965b; (paroxysmal nocturnal haemoglobinuria) red cells, Rosse et al. 1966) to 1×10^5 with one example of anti-I and half this number with another (Doinel et al. 1976), and an even lower number, 0.3×10^5, with yet another (Olesen, 1966). The number of i sites on cord red cells was found to be between 0.2 and 0.65×10^5 (Doinel et al. 1976).

I on red cells of other species
The I antigen has been found on the red cells of many species, e.g. rabbit, sheep, cattle and kangaroo (Curtain, 1969).

I in saliva and milk
Only a minority of anti-I agglutinins are strongly inhibitable by saliva, milk and extracts of stroma from O I red cells (Feizi and Marsh, 1970). Inhibition studies have emphasized the heterogeneity of anti-I sera since, for example, the glycoprotein from milk inhibited only two of 21 anti-I sera (Feizi et al. 1971). The amount of I in secretions is not correlated with that on red cells, indicating that the two may be under separate genetic control (Salmon et al. 1984).

I and i in plasma
Samples of plasma from all of 39 adults, after treatment with 2-ME to inactivate any anti-I present, inhibited one example of anti-I. There was no relationship between the amounts of I and i in the plasma of the different samples (Rouger et al. 1979).

Ii antigens on leucocytes and platelets
The presence of I and i on leucocytes can be demonstrated in agglutination tests (Lalezari

and Murphy, 1967), or in cytotoxicity tests (Lalezari, 1970). Three examples of potent anti-i and one of anti-I were shown to be lymphocytotoxic at 25 °C (Shumak *et al*. 1971). I was more weakly expressed on cord lymphocytes than on adult lymphocytes, but i was almost as strongly expressed on adult lymphocytes as on cord lymphocytes.

Anti-I and anti-i kill both T and B peripheral lymphocytes and about one-third of monocytes and granulocyes (Pruzanski *et al*. 1975).

I antigens on platelets show a heterogeneous distribution when tested by flow-cytometry (Dunstan and Simpson, 1985).

Changes in Ii antigens in disease
An increased agglutinability by anti-i was found with the red cells of all patients with thalassaemia major tested (excluding those recently transfused) and with the cells of some patients with hypoplastic anaemia, sideroblastic anaemia, megaloblastic anaemia, chronic haemolytic states and acute leukaemia (Giblett and Crookston, 1964; Cooper *et al*. 1968). The red cells of patients with hereditary erythroblastic multinucle-arity with a positive acidifed serum (HEMPAS) test give a very high agglutination score with anti-i and are usually susceptible to lysis both by anti-i and by anti-I (Crookston *et al*. 1969a). The lysis of HEMPAS cells by anti-I appears to be due to increased uptake of antibody by the cells (Lewis *et al*. 1970) and to an increased sensitivity to complement (Crookston *et al*. 1969b).

The amount of I antigen on the red cells of patients with leukaemia has been found to be decreased by some (Jenkins *et al*. 1956b; McGinniss *et al*. 1964) and unchanged by others (Ducos *et al*. 1965). The discrepancy may be explained by the differences in specificity of different anti-I, and by the types of leukaemia studied.

The amount of i on lymphocytes of patients with chronic lymphocytic leukaemia is greatly reduced even in the early stages of the disease, whereas the amount is normal on the blasts of patients with acute lymphocytic leukaemia and on the lymphocytes of some patients with lymphosarcoma cell leukaemia (Shumak *et al*. 1979).

Schmidt *et al*. (1965) showed that red cells treated with extracts of mycoplasma (PPLO) were less well agglutinated by anti-I; the relationship of mycoplasma to I specificity is discussed briefly in Chapter 7.

In the Japanese population, the genes coding for i and for autosomal recessive congenital cataracts are linked (see Page *et al*. 1987).

Anti-I and anti-i

Anti-I was first described as a potent cold autoagglutinin in the serum of a patient with acquired haemolytic anaemia (Wiener *et al*. 1956) and later, as a weak cold autoagglu-tinin in the serum of most normal subjects (Tippett *et al*. 1960). The monoclonal antibody found in patients with cold haemagglutinin disease has anti-I specificity in the vast majority of cases; compared with auto-anti-I found in normal subjects, the antibody has a far higher titre (usually much greater than 1000 at 4 °C), and has a much wider thermal range, often reacting at 30 °C or more. Auto-anti-I is described in more detail in Chapter 7.

Anti-I is found as an alloagglutinin, acting best at 4 °C (titre 16–32) and sometimes at room temperature, in the serum of most i subjects (Jenkins *et al*. 1960b; Tippett *et al.* 1960). One example was examined further by Polley *et al.* (1962) and Adinolfi *et al.* (1962). The serum was found to agglutinate red cells at temperatures up to 30°C; in tests carried out strictly at 37°C the serum did not produce agglutination but it sensitized the cells to agglutination by anti-IgM and, provided that complement was present, it also sensitized them to agglutination by anti-complement. This anti-I was found to be solely IgM.

The foregoing properties are typical of auto-anti-I (see Chapter 7) although, in general, polyclonal anti-I alloagglutinins are more consistent in their reaction pattern with I-active glycolipids than monoclonal anti-I autoagglutinins. This difference may reflect the fact that potent auto-anti-I is produced under pathological conditions (Gardas, 1983).

In one i subject with allo-anti-I, normal red cells were cleared within 15 min whereas red cells from the subject's daughter, which also behaved serologically as normal I cells, survived almost normally (Chaplin *et al.* 1986).

Two examples of murine monoclonal anti-I have been described (Messeter and Johnson, 1990).

Anti-i was first described by Marsh and Jenkins (1960) as a cold autoagglutinin in the serum of a patient with reticulosis; auto-anti-i is not uncommon in the serum of patients with infectious mononucleosis (see Chapter 7). No example of allo-anti-i has been described.

The difficulty of classifying potent cold autoagglutinins as anti-I or anti-i was emphasized by a study of 13 such sera by Cooper and Brown (1973). The ratio of antibody removed by cord cells to that removed by adult cells varied from 2.4 : 0.0, i.e. there was a spectrum from those sera which clearly had anti-i specificity to those which were clearly anti-I, with many in between which reacted slightly more strongly with cord cells than with adult cells or *vice versa*.

Anti-I^T, occurring as a warm IgG alloantibody in a White subject with Hodgkin's disease, was described by Garratty *et al.* (1972).

Anti-HI, -AI, -BI, Hi, Bi, -P_1I, -$P_1$$I^T$ and -HILe^b

Of this list of antibodies which react only with red cells carrying I (or i) and a second antigen, anti-HI is the commonest. Antibodies with this specificity often cause problems when pre-transfusion tests are carried out at room temperature. Most patients who make anti-HI are group A_1; when the patient's serum is screened against a panel of group O red cells, it will be found to contain an antibody (i.e. anti-HI) but when it is crossmatched with A_1 red cells, the result will be negative. Of the others, anti-AI was described by Tippett *et al.* (1960), anti-BI by Tegoli *et al.* (1967b), anti-Hi by Bird and Wingham (1977a), anti-Bi by Pinkerton *et al.* (1977), anti-P_1I by Issitt *et al.* (1968), anti-$P_1$$I^T$ by Booth (1970), and anti-HILe^b by Tegoli *et al.* (1971).

Anti-P_1I and -$P_1$$I^T$ are only slightly inhibited by hydatid cyst fluid, in contrast with anti-P_1 which is readily inhibited.

Anti-HILe^b was found to agglutinate only red cells which were O,I,Le(a – b +) or A_2,I,Le(a – b +). The antibody (which can also be described as anti-ILe^{bH}) was inhibited by saliva containing I, H and Le^b but was not inhibited by serum from the donor of the saliva.

THE P SYSTEM AND RELATED ANTIGENS

The P blood group system was discovered by Landsteiner and Levine (1927) by testing immune sera prepared by injecting human red cells into rabbits.

The terminology of this 'system' is particularly confusing, partly because some of the antigens belong to a blood group system and others to a collection and the system and the collection interact (see below), and partly because the antigen discovered by Landsteiner and Levine is now called P_1 and the name P is given to an antigen which is closely related but is not part of the same system as P_1.

Antigens (Table 4.6)
Almost all individuals are either P_1 (about 75% of the English population) or P_2; P_2 subjects frequently have anti-P_1 in their serum as a cold agglutinin which is only occasionally active at 20°C or higher. Among P_1 subjects there is considerable variation in the strength of the P_1 antigen and this variation is inherited (Henningsen, 1952).

When measured by fluorescence flow cytometry, the distribution of P and P_1 antigens on red cells was shown to be heterogeneous, the amounts varying from cell to cell within a given red cell population (see Dunstan, 1986). P and P_1 antigens were found on platelets and their distribution was also heterogeneous (Dunstan *et al.* 1985b). P_1 and P are present on lymphocytes and fibroblasts. P^k is present on fibroblasts of normal P_1 and P_2 people (Fellous *et al.* 1974).

Almost all P_1 and P_2 individuals have the antigen P on their red cells. Very rarely, P is lacking and such individuals either have the P^k antigen, or P_1 and P^k, or neither on their red cells; in the latter subjects, of phenotype p, the serum contains anti-PP_1P^k (originally described as anti-Tj^a by Levine *et al.* 1951a).

The nomenclature used so far for the P groups implies that all the antigens are determined by alleles at a single locus whereas it is now clear that the antigens are determined by at least two independent genetic systems (see section on the Chemistry of the P antigens). Hence, the ISBT Working Party on Terminology of Red Cell Antigens has decided that P_1 and P_2 form the P system and the rest of the antigens, P, P^k and LKE form the Globoside collection, number 209 (Lewis *et al.* 1990).

Table 4.6   Antigens and antibodies related to the P system

Frequency* (%)	Phenotype	Antigens on red cells	Antibodies in serum
75	P_1	P_1P $(P^k)^†$	none
25	P_2	P $(P^k)^†$	anti-P_1 [‡]
very rare	⎧ $P_1{}^k$	P_1P^k	anti-P
	⎨ $P_2{}^k$	P^k	anti-P
	⎩ p	none	anti-PP_1P^k

* Frequency in the English population.
† P^k has been detected on P_1 and P_2 cells (Tippett, 1975; Naiki and Marcus, 1979), although this antigen is not detected routinely on such cells.
‡ Not present in all P_2 subjects.

Echinococcus cyst fluid. A potent example of anti-P_1, active at 37°C, was reported by Merritt and Hardy (1955) in a patient with hydatid disease of the lung. The fact that the stimulus for anti-P_1 production came from scolices in hydatid cyst fluid was first appreciated by Cameron and Staveley (1957), who found that the cyst fluid specifically inhibited the antibody; however, they found only two examples of anti-P_1 among 132 patients with hydatid disease, of whom about 27 were expected to be P_2.

Bovine liver flukes. In an outbreak of bovine liver fluke disease (fascioliasis), of five P_2 subjects all had powerful anti-P_1 in their serum (Bevan *et al.* 1970). In another series, 12 of 13 P_2 patients with fascioliasis had anti-P_1 levels above the reference range; by contrast, anti-P_1 was detectable in only ten of 20 P_2 patients with hydatid disease, and only five patients had anti-P_1 levels above the reference range (Ben-Ismail *et al.* 1980).

Clonorchiasis. In South-East Asia infestation with *Clonorchis sinensis* is common. In a study of refugees from Kampochea and Laos in whom the frequency of the phenotype P_2 happens to be as high as 80%, it was found that about 50% of P_2 subjects had an IgM anti-P_1 active at room temperature (Petit *et al.* 1981).

Pigeon protein. Pigeon red cells and serum contain an antigen similar to, but not identical with, human P_1 (Brocteur *et al.* 1975). In pigeon breeders who are P_2 there is an increased incidence of anti-P_1 (Radermecker *et al.* 1975).

Antibodies (see Table 4.6)

Anti-P_1
Henningsen (1949b) found that anti-P agglutinins (now called anti-P_1) were present in the serum of approximately two of three unselected P_2 individuals; the agglutinins were usually very weak and were active only at low temperatures. In pregnant P_2 women the frequency of anti-P_1 was almost 90% but no evidence was obtained that this was connected with alloimmunization in pregnancy. Moreover, some of the most potent anti-P_1 sera came from men who had never had injections or transfusions of blood.

Relatively few examples of anti-P_1 will agglutinate red cells at 25°C and fewer still are active at 37°C. Those sera that agglutinate cells at or near 37°C may fix complement as shown by an indirect antiglobulin test and by the lysis of ficin-treated cells (Cutbush and Mollison, 1958).

In most patients whose serum contains anti-P_1 no increase in anti-P_1 titre is observed following the i.v. injection of P_1 red cells, even when the anti-P_1 is active at 37°C before injection (unpublished observations, PLM), although the development of anti-P_1 after a series of transfusions has been described (Wiener and Unger, 1944).

The only really clear-cut immediate haemolytic transfusion reaction due to anti-P_1 seems to be that reported by Moureau (1945). A patient with acquired haemolytic anaemia became increasingly jaundiced after the transfusion of P_1 blood and was found to have an anti-P_1 agglutinin with a titre of 32 at 37°C; *in vitro*, the addition of guinea pig serum resulted in the lysis of P_1 cells by the patient's serum. Anti-P_1 was undoubtedly responsible for a delayed haemolytic transfusion reaction, characterized by a fall in packed cell volume (PCV) and a substantial rise in serum bilirubin concentration, in a patient described by DiNapoli *et al.* (1977); the patient's plasma contained a potent lytic IgG anti-P_1 active over a wide thermal range. In another case, haemoglobinuria occurring on the second day after massive transfusion was attributed to red cell destruction by anti-P_1 (Chandeysson *et al.* 1981) but this conclusion has been questioned (Mollison, 1983, p. 317).

The effect of anti-P_1 on the survival of small volumes of transfused P_1 red cells is described in Chapter 10.

Production of anti-P_1 in animals

Anti-P_1 has been produced in rabbits by injecting human (P_2) or rabbit red cells tanned and coated with Echinococcus cyst fluid (Levine *et al.* 1958) and by injecting pig hydatid cyst fluid alone into goats (Kerde *et al.* 1960).

Two murine monoclonal anti-P_1, both IgM, reacting in high dilution at 4°C were obtained from hybridomas after immunization of mice with turtle-dove ovomucoid, which carries the immunodominant trisaccharide of the P_1 antigen (Bailly *et al.* 1986).

Anti-PP_1P^k (anti-Tj^a)

Anti-PP_1P^k is found only in subjects of the very rare phenotype p. According to Race and Sanger (1975, p. 154), the frequency of the p phenotype is 5.8 per million in most parts of the world (and slightly greater in parts of north Sweden). Most anti-PP_1P^k contain separable antibody specificities but in some sera it is not possible to isolate anti-P^k by absorption of anti-PP_1P^k with P_1 cells.

Anti-PP_1P^k is not present at birth in the serum of p infants but develops early in life without exposure to foreign red cells (Obregon and McKeever, 1980).

Anti-PP_1P^k is associated with abortion early in pregnancy (Levine and Koch, 1954). Although some women found to have the antibody in their serum have a history of several live births without any abortions (Race and Sanger, 1975, p. 170), the overall frequency of abortion is highly suggestive of a causal relationship. Among p women with anti-PP_1P^k in their serum, abortions are no commoner when the partner is P_1 than when he is P_2 (Sanger and Tippett, 1979). Moreover, some examples of anti-PP_1P^k, at least, react as well with P_2 cells as with P_1 cells (Levene, 1979). The effect of anti-PP_1P^k on the fetus seems to be closely related to the IgG subclass of the antibody (see below) and to the presence of the P antigen in the placenta (Hansson *et al.* 1988). Haemolytic disease of the newborn due to anti-PP_1P^k is mentioned in Chapter 12.

Anti-PP_1P^k is haemolytic *in vitro* and is capable of causing rapid destruction of transfused red cells. In the first subject (Mrs 'Jay') in whom the antibody was found, a test injection of 25 ml incompatible blood was followed by an immediate severe reaction with haemoglobinaemia. Subsequently the antibody titre rose from 8 to 512 (Levine *et al.* 1951a).

'Anti-Tj^a-like'

Vos *et al.* (1964) described a 'haemolytic activity' with anti-Tj^a (anti-PP_1P^k) specificity found at one time or another in 89% of pregnant 'habitual aborters'. The activity might be present one week and absent the next, or even disappear within 9 h. The haemolytic activity has been found only during pregnancy (Vos, 1965). *In vitro*, the serum lyses the patient's own washed red cells at 37°C; haemolysis is not complement dependent (Vos, 1966) nor does the haemolytic factor appear to be an immunoglobulin; serum heated to 56°C for 30 min is no longer haemolytic and does not regain its activity after the addition of fresh normal serum (Vos *et al.* 1964). This strange activity found in the serum of habitual aborters living in Perth, Australia, has not been found in habitual aborters in the USA or Canada (Vos *et al.* 1964).

Anti-P found in all P^k people

Anti-P differs from anti-PP_1P^k in not reacting with $P_1{}^k$ or $P_2{}^k$ cells. However, this kind of anti-P behaves serologically like anti-PP_1P^k, that is to say as an agglutinin at room temperature and as a haemolysin at 37°C. In contrast, anti-P occurring as an autoantibody behaves as a biphasic haemolysin (Donath–Landsteiner antibody), producing lysis only when allowed to act first at a relatively low temperature and subsequently at a higher temperature (see Chapter 7). The P^k phenotype is even rarer than p (Race and Sanger, 1975).

'Anti-p'

Three examples of an antibody reacting preferentially with p cells have been described but, for reasons given later, the designation anti-p for these antibodies is inappropriate.

Immunoglobulin classes and IgG subclasses of antibodies of the P system and globoside collection

Examples of potent anti-P_1 and of anti-PP_1P^k which appeared to be solely IgM have been descirbed (Adinolfi *et al.* 1962; Polley *et al.* 1962). However, anti-PP_1P^k, as mentioned above, may be partly IgG, predominantly IgG, or wholly IgG (Wurzel *et al.* 1971; Lopez *et al.* 1983).

In a study of 29 pp subjects, anti-P or anti-P^k was detected in every case. Almost all the antibodies were partly IgM and partly IgG, the latter being almost solely IgG3. Of the 29 subjects, 17 were parous women; of these 17, three had had only normal pregnancies and in two of these no IgG3 anti-P or anti-P^k was found. All of the remaining women had had one or more spontaneous abortions and 13 of these 14 had IgG3 antibodies, suggesting a causal relationship between anti-PP_1P^k of IgG3 subclass and abortions (Söderström *et al.* 1985). In a smaller series, a relationship was found between early abortions and cytotoxic IgG anti-P^k (Lopez *et al.* 1983). Biphasic haemolysins are always IgG. An exceptional case of anti-P found in a patient with cold haemagglutinin disease was IgM; see Chapter 7.

BIOSYNTHESIS OF THE P, HAB* (ABH), Ii AND LEWIS ANTIGENS

As mentioned at the beginning of this chapter, the antigens of all these blood group systems are synthesized by the sequential addition of sugar residues to a common precursor substance. Since the antigenic determinants are carbohydrates and not

---

* The sequence HAB, rather than ABH, is used in this section since, in biosynthesis, the formation of H precedes that of A and B (Watkins and Morgan, 1959).

proteins, they cannot be the direct gene products. The gene products are glycosyl-transferases which transfer a specific sugar to a specific oligosaccharide chain.

On red cells the oligosaccharide chain may be bound by D-glucose through sphingosine to fatty acid moieties, in which case the blood group substance is a glycosphingolipid (or glycolipid). More commonly, the oligosaccharide chain is bound to a peptide chain, usually through N-acetyl-D-glucosamine to asparagine and the blood group substance is then a glycoprotein. In glycoproteins in secretions the oligosaccharide chains are bound through N-acetyl-D-galactosamine to serine or threonine. HAB, Lewis and P antigens in plasma are carried on glycosphingolipids and the oligosaccharide chain is bound by D-glucose to ceramide.

The P system is discussed first because the P genes act early in the biosynthetic pathway (see Fig. 4.6 on p. 198).

Chemistry of the P antigens

As stated above, the terminology used so far is confusing because it implies that all the P antigens belong to the same system. However, as Fig. 4.4 shows, two biosynthetic pathways are involved, one leading to the production of P^k and P and the other to the production of P_1. The relevant transferases have not been identified.

P is present on the red cells of almost all individuals; in those rare subjects who lack the P gene, trihexosylceramide cannot be converted to globoside and so P^k is found on the red cells. Since the P^1 gene is independent of the P gene, P^k subjects may be P_1^k or P_2^k.

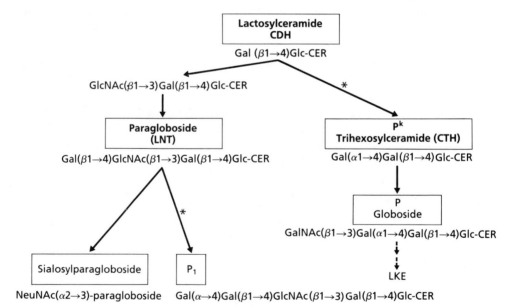

Figure 4.4 Biosynthetic pathways of the P^k, P and P_1 glycolipid antigens (adapted from Watkins, 1980). Abbreviations: Gal, D-galactose; Glc, D-glucose; GalNAc, N-acetyl-D-galactosamine; GlcNAc, N-acetyl-D-glucosamine; NeuNAc, N-acetylneuraminic acid; CER (ceramide), N-acylsphingosine. The Forssman antigen is globoside with a terminal αGalNAc linked to the βGalNac. *An α-galactosyl-transferase is required for the synthesis of P^k and P_1 antigens from different precursors.

P is assumed to code for the transferase which converts P^k to P by adding N-acetylgalactosamine to trihexosylceramide (Marcus *et al.* 1981). It is also assumed that P^k codes for the α-galactosyltransferase which synthesizes trihexosylceramide; hence *P* and P^k are not alleles.

Since P_1 and P^k possess the same terminal non-reducing disaccharides Gal($\alpha1\rightarrow4$)Galβ (see Fig. 4.4), the nature of the P_1-specified transferase poses a problem. One possibility is that it codes for the α-galactosyltransferase which can use paragloboside but not lactosylceramide as an acceptor and that it is not an allele of P^k. A second possibility is that P_1 codes for a protein which interacts with the P^k-transferase and alters its acceptor specificity so that it can use both lactosylceramide and paragloboside as substrates (Marcus *et al.* 1981). A third possibility is that P^k and P_1 are alleles that code for different α-galactosyltransferases; P_1 can use either lactosylceramide or paragloboside, but P^k can use only lactosylceramide (Graham and Williams, 1978).

P, P^k and P_1 antigens on red cells are on glycosphingolipids (Marcus *et al.* 1981). P (globoside) and P^k (trihexosylceramide) also occur in plasma as glycosphingolipids. Antigens of the P system have not been found in secretions.

It has been shown that the terminal disaccharide Gal($\alpha1\rightarrow4$)Galβ shared by P_1 and P^k is a receptor on epithelial cells for one of the adhesins of most strains of uropathogenic *Escherichia coli*. Strains with adhesins specific for this disaccharide agglutinate red cells from individuals of blood groups P_1, P_2 and P^k but not p (Källenius *et al.* 1981; Leffler and Svanborg-Edén, 1981; Lomberg *et al.* 1986).

LKE and its proposed biosynthetic relationship to P

The Luke antigen was discovered by finding that the serum of a patient with Hodgkin's lymphoma agglutinated all red cells tested except those of the rare p or P^k phenotypes and about 2% of P+ samples (Tippett *et al.* 1965). Three more Luke antibodies have been described, all of no clinical significance; the fourth example showed that the Luke-negative phenotype has recessive inheritance and that its incidence in the west of Scotland is 0.0017 (Bruce *et al.* 1988).

A murine monoclonal antibody was found to react with the same antigen as that detected by the Luke serum and this antigen was named LKE (Luke erythocyte antigen). The monoclonal antibody is inhibited by the terminal trisaccharide of the globoseries ganglioside: NeuAc ($\alpha2\rightarrow3$)Gal($\beta1\rightarrow3$)GalNAc($\beta1\rightarrow3$)Gal($\alpha1\rightarrow4$)Gal($\beta1\rightarrow4$)Glc-CER, which represents the addition of two sugars, galactose and N-acetylneuraminic acid to globoside or P (see Fig. 4.4). However, no such glycosphingolipid has been isolated from the red cell membrane. LKE-negative people are supposed to lack the terminal neuraminic acid and possibly also the galactose added to globoside. Since P+, LKE-negative individuals have stronger expression of P^k, it has been postulated that the terminal neuraminic acid of the hypothetical LKE structure could be replaced by galactose in such individuals, giving rise to a Gal–Gal–globoside structure which could react with anti-P^k (see Tippett, 1986).

Inhibition studies

Anti-P_1 is inhibited by sheep hydatid cyst fluid (Cameron and Staveley, 1957). The inhibiting substance is a glycoprotein with a terminal trisaccharide (Cory *et al.* 1974) which has the same structure (Gal(α1→4)Gal(β1→4)GlcNAc) as the terminal trisaccharide of the P$_1$ glycolipid isolated from red cells (Naiki *et al.* 1975). Anti-P$_1$ is highly specific for the terminal trisaccharide and is not inhibited by the terminal disaccharide shared with P^k (see Watkins, 1982). Egg whites from pigeons and turtle doves are powerful inhibitors of anti-P$_1$ (François-Gérard *et al.* 1980).

Anti-P^k is obtained either by absorption of anti-PP$_1$P^k with globoside or by absorption of some anti-PP$_1$P^k with P$_1$ red cells. Potent monoclonal anti-P^k have been produced in mice (Tippett, 1986; Messeter and Johnson, 1990). Anti-P^k is inhibited by both hydatid cyst fluid and trihexosylceramide isolated from red cells. The inhibition of anti-P^k and of anti-P$_1$ by hydatid cyst fluid is not surprising since both P^k and P$_1$ have the same terminal disaccharide (Gal(α1→4)Gal).

Anti-P, whether occurring as an autoantibody (biphasic haemolysin) or as an alloantibody in P$_1$^{k} and P$_2$^{k} individuals, is inhibited by globoside (Naiki and Marcus, 1975; Marcus *et al.* 1976; Watkins and Morgan, 1976). The first example of monoclonal anti-P was described by von dem Borne *et al.* (1986d).

Many examples of anti-P, whether allo- or autoantibodies, are also inhibited by Forssman glycosphingolipid, indicating that P antibodies represent a heterogeneous response to globoside and Forssman glycolipids, present in many animal tissues, as well as to crossreacting microbial antigens (Marcus *et al.* 1981).

'Anti-p'. Three examples have been described of a cold agglutinin which reacts best with p red cells, less well with P$_2$ cells and only very weakly with P$_1$ cells (Engelfriet *et al.* 1972a; Metaxas *et al.* 1975; Issitt *et al.* 1976b). The antibody is inhibited by sialosylparagloboside (Schwarting *et al.* 1977) and more strongly inhibited by glycolipids containing the same terminal structure as sialosylparagloboside (see Fig. 4.4) but with two or three repeating Gal(β1→4) GlcNAc units (Marcus *et al.* 1981). These latter compounds also inhibited two examples of anti-Gd (see Chapter 7).

Sialosylparagloboside is expected to accumulate in pp people due to blocking of the synthesis of globoside and trihexosylceramide (see Fig. 4.4) which would lead to accumulation of paragloboside, which would then be available for other biosynthetic pathways (Schwarting *et al.* 1977).

Chemistry of HAB, Ii and Lewis antigens

Secretions and plasma
The HAB and Lewis antigens in secretions and plasma are determined by the interaction of the *Hh*, *Sese*, *ABO* and *Lele* genes. All subjects, except for those of the very rare Bombay types, express ABH antigens on their red cells, but only those with an *Se* gene (80% in Whites) have H in secretions; thus *Se* is conventionally regarded as a regulator gene (see Table 4.4 on p. 175). Subjects with red cells deficient in H can be either secretors or non-secretors of H. The products of the *H*, *A*, *B* and *Le* alleles are glycosyltransferases which transfer the immunodominant sugar for H, A, B or Lewis specificity to an acceptor chain on glycoproteins or glycolipids (see Table 4.7 and Fig. 4.5).

Table 4.7 Products of *H(Se)*, *Le*, *A* and *B* genes (after Morgan and Watkins, 1969)

Genes	Gene product	Sugar attached by enzyme	Terminal structure of oligosaccharide chain	Serological specificity
			Gal(β,1→3)GlcNAc-R	*
H(Se)	$\alpha1$→2-L-fucosyl-transferase (1)	Fuc	Gal($\beta1$→3)GlcNAc-R | ($\alpha1$→2) Fuc	H[†]
Le	$\alpha1$→4-L-fucosyl-transferase (2)	Fuc	Gal($\beta1$→3)GlcNAc-R | ($\alpha1$→4) Fuc	Le^a
H(Se) and *Le*	α-L-fucosyl-transferases (1 and 2)	Fuc	Gal($\beta1$→3)GlcNAc-R | ($\alpha1$→2) | ($\alpha1$→4) Fuc Fuc	Le^b
A	α-N-acetyl-D-galactosaminyl-transferase	GalNAc	GalNAc($\alpha1$→3)Gal($\beta1$→3)GlcNAc-R | ($\alpha1$→2) Fuc	A
B	α-D-galactosyltransferase	Gal	Gal($\alpha1$→3)Gal($\beta1$→3)GlcNAc-R | ($\alpha1$→2) Fuc	B

* Type 1 chain or Le^c; [†] Type 1 H is Le^d in plasma.
Abbreviations: Gal, D-galactose; GlcNAc, N-acetyl-D-glucosamine; Fuc, fucose; GalNAc, N-acetyl-D-galactosamine; R, remainder of chain. In type 2 chains, the α Fuc–βGlcNAc linkage is 1→3 and the antigenic structures corresponding to Le^a, Le^b, Le^c and Le^{d}d are Le^x, Le^y, I and H (Oriol *et al.* 1986).

Conventionally it is postulated that the product of the structural gene *H* is a single $\alpha2$-L-fucosyltransferase which in the presence of the *Se* gene in secretions and the Z gene in red cells, adds L-fucose in $\alpha1$→2 linkage to the terminal β-galactose in either a type 1 oligosaccharide chain or a type 2 chain (Watkins, 1980; see Fig. 4.5). In red cells, the HAB-active glycolipids and glycoproteins are carried on type 2 chains only, whereas in serum the HAB-active glycolipids are carried on type 1 chains. Neverthe-less, both type 1 and type 2 chains may occur as branches on a single glycoprotein molecule (see Watkins, 1980).

Based on the difference in the second positions of the terminal β-galactose in type 1 and 2 chains, the existence of two $\alpha2$-L-fucosyltransferases coded by two different structural genes has been proposed: *H* encoding for the transferase on red cells and working preferentially on type 2 chains, and *Se* encoding for the transferase in secretions and working preferentially on type 1 chains (Oriol *et al.* 1986). Studies on several H-deficient families have confirmed that *H* and *Se* were segregating; and it was also shown that *H* and *Se* are closely linked on chromosome 19. Thus the idea of two structural genes may be the right one (see Oriol, 1990); it gains further support from the recent cloning of the gene encoding for the *H* transferase (Rajan *et al.* 1989; see section on cloning at the end of this chapter).

The *A*-transferase adds N-acetyl-D-galactosamine in $\alpha1$→3 linkage to the terminal D-galactose of H; the *B*-transferase adds D-galactose in $\alpha1$→3 linkage to H. The product

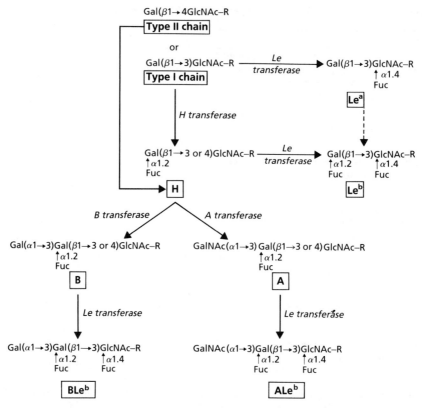

Figure 4.5 Biochemical pathways for the synthesis of H, A, B, Le^a, Le^b, ALe^b and BLe^b structures on type I chains in glycoproteins and glycolipids. The *Le*-specified transferase cannot add fucose to type II chains. R = rest of the molecule. The pathway from Le^a to Le^b represented by the dotted line has not been proven to exist (adapted from Watkins, 1980).

of the *Le* gene is an α-L-fucosyltransferase which adds L-fucose in $\alpha1\rightarrow4$ to the subterminal *N*-acetyl-D-glucosamine of a type I acceptor. Since several glycosyl transferases may use the same precursor substance, competition for substrate occurs frequently.

The *Le*-transferase adds L-fucose to an unsubstituted type 1 (or type 2) acceptor to form Le^a (or Le^x), to H to form Le^b, to A to form ALe^b and to B to form BLe^b (Fig. 4.5); hence, the same structural gene *Le* codes for the expression of both Le^a and Le^b antigens. The addition of L-fucose to *N*-acetyl-D-glucosamine would act as a chain-stopper; once L-fucose is added, no other sugar can be added to the chain (Kobata *et al.* 1968). Therefore, it is generally accepted that Le^a cannot be converted to Le^b.

Type 2 isomers of Le^a and Le^b are referred to as Le^x and Le^y. Le^x results from the transfer of the $\alpha1\rightarrow3$ fucose residue to the βGlcNAc of the type 2 precursor chain, and the Le^y antigen from the transfer of the $\alpha1\rightarrow2$ and $\alpha1\rightarrow3$ fucose residues to the same type 2 precursor chain. Three types of α3-fucosyltransferase, capable of adding fucose in $\alpha1\rightarrow3$ linkage to the subterminal βGlcNAc of type 2 chains, have been described by Oriol (1990). In exocrine secretions this transferase could be encoded by the *Le* gene, in the same way as the α4-fucosyltransferase (Oriol, 1990), or by a different gene called X (Watkins, 1990), leading to the formation of Le^x in unsubstituted type 2 chains and to Le^y in type 2 H.

In an individual with H, Se, A, B and Le genes, not all of the acceptor is converted to A or B, or to Le^b; thus, the secretions and plasma of such an individual will contain some acceptor and H as well as A, B and Le^b. In addition, some Le^a will be present since, even in the presence of H (and Se), the Le-transferase converts some type I acceptor to Le^a.

A similar series of interactions may occur between type 2 H, A and B structures and the X (or Le) gene specified α_3-fucosyltransferase.

The structures of I and i antigens are considered below in the section on red cells.

The HAB and Lewis antigens occur in plasma as glycosphingolipids (Marcus and Cass, 1969; Tilley et al. 1975). The presence of Lewis antigens on red cells and the presence of Lewis and A antigens on lymphocytes depend entirely on the plasma environment (Sneath and Sneath, 1955; Rachkewich et al. 1978). The amount of A (and B) antigen in plasma is determined by the A subgroup, the secretor genes and the Lewis phenotype. There is more A in the plasma of an A_1 secretor than in an A_2 secretor; there is more A in an A_1 secretor than in an A_1 non-secretor; and there is more A in a secretor who is A_1,Le(a – b –) than in a secretor who is A_1,Le(a – b +) (Tilley et al. 1975). The amount of A in plasma probably depends on competition between the A- and Le-transferases for the H acceptor, i.e. in the absence of Le, more H can be converted to A.

Since Le^a, Le^b and ALe^b are type I chains, H, A and B glycosphingolipids in plasma must also be type I. Evidence that H is present in plasma as a type I chain was provided by experiments with 'anti-Le^d', i.e. anti-type I H (Handfland and Graham, 1981).

In Fig. 4.6, the biosynthetic relationship of the glycolipid H, A and B antigens in plasma is compared with those on red cells. Type I, H and A and B antigens are not synthesized by red cell precursors but can be passively adsorbed from plasma. These structures (H type I, A type I and B type I) were previously termed Le^d, ALe^d and BLe^d (see below). The new terms are logical because neither the le gene nor the Le gene is involved in the production of these antigens. H, A and B antigens synthesized by red cell precursors are type II.

Ulex europaeus and several murine monoclonal anti-H react well with red cells because they are specific for H type II (Handfland and Graham, 1981; Young et al. 1981; Knowles et al. 1982a).

Le^c occurs in plasma as a glycosphingolipid and is adsorbed on to red cells. The structure of the Le^c determinant is unfucosylated type 1 precursor chain βGal1$\rightarrow$3 βGlcNAc1–R (Hirsch and Graham, 1980; Oriol, 1990). Anti-Le^c reacts with samples from se/se, le/le individuals (Le Pendu et al. 1982). Monofucosylation of type 1 chains in Se, le/le individuals leads to H type 1 or Le^d antigen: Fucα1$\rightarrow$2 Galβ1$\rightarrow$3 GlcNAcβ1–R (Oriol, 1990). Only 11 subjects lacking the serum α_3-fucosyltransferase have been described; they were all Le(a – b – c – d –), suggesting that the locus for this enzyme is either closely linked to the locus for the Le-transferase or that both enzymes share a common regulator (Greenwell et al. 1986; Oriol, 1990).

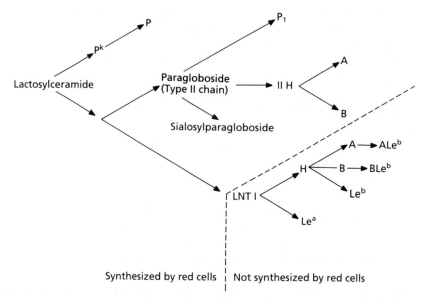

Figure 4.6 Biosynthesis of P, HAB and Lewis antigens. Structures within the area indicated by the broken line are present in plasma: they are not made by the red cells. Details of these pathways and structures can be seen in Figs 4.4 and 4.5 and Table 4.7. Abbreviations: I, type I chain; II H, type II H chain; LNT, lacto-*N*-tetraose or basic type I chain = Gal(β1→3) GlcNAc(β1→3) Gal(β1→4) Glc-CER.

As discussed above, it is clear that Le^c (and Le^d) are not products of the *Le* gene.

The i antigen occurs in plasma as glycoprotein (Cooper and Brown, 1973).

Transferases in serum
The fact that *H*-, *A*- and *B*-transferases are present in serum has facilitated kinetic studies in large numbers of donors of common phenotypes, as well as the assay of these transferases in donors with rare phenotypes. The *H*-transferase in serum, unlike the *H*-transferase in secretions, is present in secretors and in non-secretors; it is present in the serum of all donors with an *H* gene. Thus the *H*-transferase in serum is made by cells which resemble red cell precursors in that the production of the *H* transferase is not under the control of the *Se* gene. (See pp. 195 and 200, for the alternative hypothesis that *Se* and *H* are structural genes.) The hypothesis that the O$_h$ phenotype results from a lack of the *H* gene was confirmed when it was shown that the serum of O$_h$ individuals lacks the *H*-transferase (Schenkel-Brunner *et al.* 1972; Munro and Schachter, 1973).

The α-L-fucosyltransferase specified by the *Le* gene is present in saliva and milk but has not been found in serum.

The *A*- and *B*-transferases, like the *H*-transferase, are present in the serum of non-secretors as well as in the serum of secretors. As expected, the serum of O$_h$ individuals who have an *A* (or *B*) gene contains *A*- (or *B*-) transferase (Race and Watkins, 1972a).

The major site of synthesis of the *H*-, *A*- and *B*-transferases in serum is unknown.

Studies in chimeric twins have shown that the haemopoietic tissue contributes about 20% of the A-transferase in serum (Schachter *et al.* 1971; Wrobel *et al.* 1974).

The level of A^1-transferase in serum (and presumably the level of B-transferase) is affected by pregnancy. The level of A^1-transferase in pregnant A_1 women is less than one-half the level in non-pregnant A_1 adults (Schachter *et al.* 1971; Tilley *et al.* 1978a). Although the red cells of group A_1 newborn infants have fewer A_1 antigen sites than the red cells of group A_1 adults (Economidou *et al.* 1967a), the level of A^1-transferase in the serum of newborn infants is much higher than the level in non-pregnant A_1 adults (Tilley *et al.* 1978a).

The relatively small number of B sites on the red cells of newborn infants is due presumably to lack of precursor. When group O red cells from newborn infants are incubated with uridine diphosphate-galactose and B-specified enzyme, the number of B sites generated is about one-quarter of the number generated on adult group O cells (Romano *et al.* 1978).

A^1- and A^2-transferases in serum differ qualitatively as well as quantitatively. The level of A-transferase in the serum of A_2 donors was found to be only about 10% of the level in A_1 donors. Moreover, the A_1- and A_2-transferases differed in their pH optima, cation requirements and Michaelis constants (Schachter *et al.* 1971, 1973). In a donor of the genotype A^1A^2, the A^1- and A^2-transferases in serum can be separated using isoelectric focusing (Topping and Watkins, 1975).

As mentioned above, the A^1- and A^2-transferases have the same specificity. However, since the A^2-transferase is less efficient than the A^1-transferase, there are fewer A sites on A_2 red cells than on A_1 red cells.

Conversion of O red cells to A or B cells. In the presence of the appropriate nucleotide sugar and the A- (or B-) transferase, group O red cells are readily converted to A- (or B-) active red cells (Schenkel-Brunner and Tuppy, 1969; Race and Watkins, 1972b); O_h red cells are not converted (Race and Watkins, 1972b).

Group O red cells have been used to demonstrate the presence of B-transferase in saliva; the transferase was present both in secretors and non-secretors (Kogure and Furukawa, 1976).

Examples of the value of estimating A- and B-transferases in plasma. Confirmation of the theory that the O_h phenotype results from an absence of the H gene was obtained by showing that in O_h subjects the H-transferase is absent but the plasma contains A- and B-transferases appropriate to the true ABO genotype (Race and Watkins, 1972a).

Studies of plasma A-specified enzymes indicate that A_3 is heterogeneous, as are A_m and A_x (see review by Watkins, 1980).

Studies of A- and B-transferases in the plasma of subjects of the rare phenotype 'cis AB' have shown that some examples, at least, are due to the presence of a mutant gene (see p. 153). Such studies can also be used to determine the true ABO genotype of twin chimeras and to diagnose dispermic chimerism (see Watkins *et al.* 1980).

HAB, Ii and Lewis antigens in secretions
All these antigens occur in secretions, e.g. saliva, as glycoproteins. The frequency of

non-secretors of HAB is significantly increased in patients with infections due to *Candida albicans*, meningococci or pneumococci (Blackwell *et al.* 1986). When pneumococci and *Haemophilus influenzae* are incubated with milk glycocompounds, known to contain HAB antigens, their attachment to epithelial cells decreases considerably (Andersson *et al.* 1986). Two mechanisms have been proposed by which glycoproteins in secretions might influence the adherence of micro-organisms to epithelial cells: (1) A, B or H substances in saliva of secretors inhibits binding of the yeast or bacterium to epithelial cells; and (2) the Le^a antigen in secretions recognizes an adhesin on the surface of the micro-organism and subsequently binds to the epithelium along with the attached microbe (see Blackwell *et al.* 1986).

Expression of H antigen in epithelia and secretions depends on the inheritance of the *Se* allele of the secretor gene. Although it was formerly considered that *Se* was a regulator gene, it has been proposed that it is a second structural gene encoding a tissue specific α2-fucosyltransferase (Oriol *et al.* 1986). Hence, the *H* gene would encode the α2-fucosyltransferase expressed in red cells and acting preferentially on type 2 chains, and the *Se* gene would encode the α2-fucosyltransferase expressed in saliva and acting preferentially on type 1 chains (Oriol, 1990).

HAB, Ii and Lewis antigens on red cells

HAB. A, B and H antigen sites on red cells are found partly on glycolipids (about 5% on simple glycolipids and 10–15% on polyglycosyl ceramides) but mainly on glycoproteins, most (70%) being on band 3, the main integral protein of the red cell membrane; the final 10% of sites are found on sialic acid-rich glycoproteins (Wilczynska *et al.* 1980; Schenkel-Brunner, 1980a; Finne, 1980; Karhi and Gahmberg, 1980).

A_1 *and* A_2. As discussed above, the A^2-transferase is less efficient than the A^1-transferase and it is therefore to be expected that in A_2 subjects fewer H structures will be converted to A structures, and that there will be fewer A sites and more H sites on A_2 red cells than on A_1 cells. Because the A^2-transferase is less efficient it is to be expected that on highly branched glycolipids and glycoproteins there will be fewer A determinants in close proximity to each other in the macromolecules isolated from the red cells and secretions of A_2 persons than in the macromolecules from A_1 persons.

According to Hakomori *et al.* (1977) four types of short-chain blood group glycolipids with A activity can be isolated from red cell membranes. The first two (A^a-2 and A^b-2) are relatively short chains with unbranched structures whereas the second two (A^c and A^d) are longer and branched. The branched A structures (A^c and A^d) are the major A antigens in adult red cells and are virtually absent from cord and fetal red cells (Watanabe and Hakomori, 1976). A_1 and A_2 cells both have short-chain glycolipids, although in different amounts, but A^c and A^d chains are preferentially expressed on A_1 cells. Studies with monoclonal anti-A indicate that one kind of monoclonal antibody (like the lectin from *Dolichos biflorus*) reacts only with the short-chain unbranched structures and not with longer chains or with A^c and A^d structures. It thus seems that these anti-A_1 reagents differentiate between A_1 and A_2 on the basis of quantitative, non-structural features (Furukawa *et al.* 1985). On the other hand, there is another kind of anti-A_1 monoclonal which reacts with type 3 chain A which is essentially a repetitive A epitope attached to a type II chain. Thus the distinction between A_1 and A_2 made by this second kind of monoclonal is based on the preferential expression of type 3 A chains on extended or branched structures of glycolipids on A_1 red cells (Clausen *et al.* 1985). The essential qualitative difference between A_1 and A_2 could be ascribed to the ability of the A^1-transferase, and the inability of the A^2-transferase to convert type 3 H chains of glycolipids to type 3 A chains (Clausen *et al.* 1985). It thus seems that whether the difference between A_1 and A_2 is regarded as qualitative or quantitative depends on the properties of the reagents used to distinguish between the two cell types (Furukawa *et al.* 1985).

Competitive inhibition assays, using different ^{125}I-labelled monoclonal murine anti-A, have shown that antibodies which are better agglutinators of A_2B cells with weakly expressed A are bound in substantially greater quantities than the poorer agglutinators (Lubenko, 1985; Lubenko and Ivanyi, 1986). The better agglutinating antibodies recognize the terminal trisaccharide common to all A molecules; the poorer agglutinators bind to a narrower range of A-like structures wherein the A trisaccharide is linked to Gal or GalNAc, rather than to GlcNAc (Gane *et al.* 1987a). In addition, competitive inhibition assays using both types of murine monoclonal anti-A have shown that most human hyperimmune polyclonal anti-A or anti-A,B sera react preferentially with the trisaccharide common to all A epitopes; some recognize the restricted A-active tetrasaccharides while the occasional serum reacts with a third, as yet uncharacterized, blood group A structure (Lubenko and Savage, 1990).

The work of Hakomori's group relates to short-chain glycolipids; the relative contribution of the predominating highly branched glycoconjugates on the red cell membrane to the serological distinction between A_1 and A_2 antigens is unknown.

I and i. The i specificity is determined by a straight polylactosamine chain containing repeating Gal($\beta1\rightarrow4$)GlcNAc($\beta1\rightarrow3$) sequences, attached to ceramide or protein (R below). The development of I is dependent on the presence of a branching enzyme, controlled by a gene Z, which adds a branch by $\beta1\rightarrow6$ linkage to the middle galactose of the unbranched i-active structure, as shown in the structure below; up to five branches can be added per chain (see review by Hakomori, 1981).

i: Gal($\beta1\rightarrow4$)GlcNAc($\beta1\rightarrow3$)Gal($\beta1\rightarrow4$)GlcNAc($\beta1\rightarrow3$)Gal($\beta1\rightarrow4$)Glc-R

I: Gal($\beta1\rightarrow4$)GlcNAc($\beta1\rightarrow3$)Gal($\beta1\rightarrow4$)GlcNAc($\beta1\rightarrow3$)Gal($\beta1\rightarrow4$)Glc-R

                  /   ($\beta1\rightarrow6$)

Gal($\beta1\rightarrow4$)GlcNAc

These structures may carry, on their non-reducing end, other antigenic determinants such as ABH, Lewis and P_1.

The combined action of $\beta1\rightarrow3$ GlcNAc-transferase and $\beta1\rightarrow4$ Gal-transferase is required for the biosynthesis of i antigenic structures (Piller and Cartron, 1983). The *I* gene can be considered to be a structural gene encoding the $\beta6$-N-acetylglucosaminyl-transferase responsible for the branching. However, up to now, there is no evidence for the expression of this enzyme in differentiation (Watkins, 1990).

It seems that the heterogeneity of anti-I depends upon recognition of different parts of the above structure. Using analogues of the branched glycolipid on red cells, Feizi *et al.* (1979) found three patterns of reaction: some examples of anti-I recognized the $1\rightarrow4$, $1\rightarrow6$ branch; others recognized the $1\rightarrow4$, $1\rightarrow3$ sequence in the presence of branching; and others required both branches to be intact. However, it seems clear that the immunodominant group of the I antigen is GlcNAc linked $1\rightarrow6$ to a galactose; substitution of the 3 position of this galactose is necessary for the expression of the I activity with most anti-I sera, but not for all. Substitution of other positions of the GlcNAc sequence will either depress or enhance I activity and this effect will be different for different examples of anti-I.

In general, ABH determinants of red cells are carried on branched type II chains linked to lipids (ceramide) or to intrinsic membrane glycoproteins (band 3 and band 4.5, see Chapter 3) in adults, while red cells of the fetus and newborn have unbranched type II molecules. The Ii determinants available for reactivity with anti-I and anti-i can be regarded as uncompleted ABH-active chains (Childs *et al.* 1978; Feizi *et al.* 1979; Watanabe *et al.* 1979; for review see Hakomori, 1981, 1984b). The process of branching through GlcNAc ($\beta1\rightarrow6$) linkage is related to the ontogenic development of red cells, and the total quantity of type II chains increases during differentiation of erythroblasts or erythrocytes (Hakomori, 1984b).

Lewis. As shown in Fig. 4.5, *in vitro*, the *Le*-specified transferase can use only type I chains as acceptors to join L-fucose to the C-4 position of the subterminal N-acetylglucosamine. Since red cells only synthesize type II chains where the C-4 position of the subterminal N-acetylglucosamine is occupied by the terminal β-galactosyl residue, it is not possible to form Le^a or Le^b structures on these chains. Hence, the Lewis antigens present on the red cells are derived solely from the plasma by adsorption of glycosphingolipids (see Watkins, 1980). Group O,Le(a – b –) red cells become agglutinable by anti-Le^b when as few as 400 molecules of Le^b-active glycolipid per red cell have been adsorbed but larger quantities of Le^a-active glycolipids are needed to convert the same O,Le(a – b –) cells into O,Le(a + b –) cells (Hanfland, 1978).

ABO, H and Lewis antigens in tissues and tumours

Monoclonal antibodies have contributed to the detection of these antigens in tissues and to the determination of the various type of groupings at the non-reducing end of carrier oligosaccharide chains to which antigenic determinants are attached. These oligosaccharide chains may be part of glycolipids or glycoproteins. Thus, considerable diversity of A and B structures may be generated in tissues. In addition to the type 1 and type 2 disaccharide endings present on red cells and in plasma, three other endings are found in naturally occurring molecules: type 3 (βGal1$\rightarrow$3 αGalNAc-R), type 4 (βGal1$\rightarrow$3 βGalNAc-R) and type 6 (βGal1$\rightarrow$4 βGlc-R). The type 3 disaccharide is also the basis for the repetitive A epitope of A$_1$ antigens described by Clausen (1985) as glycosphingolipids, and in tissues it is joined directly to serine or threonine in the peptide backbone. In type 4, βGalNAc is joined to a galactosyl residue in glycolipids. Type 6 constitutes the lactose-based free oligosaccharides found in milk and urine. The monofucosylated and difucosylated Lewis structures have been described only on type 1 and type 2 chains. Type 5 (βGal1$\rightarrow$3 βGal-R) has not been described yet in human tissues but has been synthesized in the laboratory (Oriol, 1990; Watkins, 1990).

Aberrant expression of ABO, H and Lewis antigens in tumours

As discussed in Chapter 3, neoplastic change may be accompanied by changes in cell surface antigens, with loss of antigenic expression in some types of carcinoma and appearance of new antigens (neoantigens) in others. In carcinoma of the bladder, deletion of A and B antigens occurs frequently; the loss of A activity is associated with a failure of expression of the *A*-transferase with the consequent accumulation of Le^b due to the fucosylation of the excess H antigen formed. On the other hand, although the A antigen is not normally expressed in the adult distal colon, in group A patients with carcinoma of the colon A is 'neo-expressed'. In normal distal colon, the levels of *H*-transferase are very low, but in colonic tumour there is a significant elevation of this enzyme, allowing synthesis of H which leads to the neo-expression of A (for references see Watkins, 1990).

Cloning of *A*, *B* and *H*

Until recently, cloning the genes for the *A*- and *B*-transferases was hampered by the inability to isolate the transferases in large quantities. However, the *A* gene specified transferase, in soluble form, has been isolated from human lung tissues and part of its amino acid sequence determined. Based on this partial sequence, appropriate clones were identified in a complementary DNA (cDNA) library constructed from a human stomach cancer cell line with high levels of A antigen, after screening the library with a radiolabelled fragment of the transferase cDNA, amplified by polymerase chain reaction (PCR). A coding region of 1062 nucleotide base pairs, encoding a protein of 41 kDa, was sequenced. Using this *A*-transferase probe, DNAs from cell lines of different ABO groups were cloned and sequenced. Thus, the nucleotide sequence differences between *A*, *B* and *O* genes were determined. A difference in four nucleotides leading to four amino acid changes (residues 176, 235, 266 and 268) was found between *A* and *B* cDNAs. In contrast, cDNA clones from group O cell lines all had a single nucleotide deletion in the coding region close to the *N*-terminus (residue 258), indicating that the lack of transferase activity in group O individuals is due to a shift in the reading frame. Thus the lack of functional transferases in group O subjects is due, not to a failure of expression, but to the translation of an entirely different protein which does not crossreact with *A*- or *B*-transferases (Yamamoto *et al.* 1990a). The sequence differences between *A*, *B* and *O* in cDNA were shown to be also present in genomic DNA (Yamamoto *et al.* 1990b). It was predicted that a few amino acid substitutions, in addition to those distinguishing the *A* and *B* alleles, could be responsible for A and B subgroups. In fact, compared with A^1, A^2 has been found to have only a single base deletion (Yamamoto, 1991).

The *H* gene has also been isolated recently by expressing a human α-L-fucosyltransferase in transfected mouse cells (Rajan *et al.* 1989). However, the genetic basis for the Hh polymorphism has not yet been established.

CHAPTER 5

THE Rh BLOOD GROUP SYSTEM (AND LW)

The clinical importance of the Rh blood group system stems from the fact that the antigen D of the system is highly immunogenic: if a unit of D-positive blood is transfused to a D-negative recipient, the recipient forms anti-D in some 90% of cases and thereafter cannot safely be transfused with D-positive red cells. Moreover, if a D-negative woman becomes pregnant with a D-positive (ABO-compatible) infant, the passage of red cells across the placenta from fetus to mother induces primary immunization to D in about one in six cases, unless the mother receives anti-D Ig. In a subsequent pregnancy with a D-positive infant, secondary immunization may be induced, leading to haemolytic disease in the infant. Rh is also involved in the specificity of the warm autoantibodies of autoimmune haemolytic anaemia.

In this chapter, the antigens and antibodies of the Rh system, and of the closely related LW system, are considered, together with immune responses to transfused red cells carrying foreign Rh alloantigens and the suppression of the response to D by passively administered anti-D. Immunization to D and other Rh antigens during pregnancy is considered in Chapter 12.

Rh ANTIGENS: NOMENCLATURE

Fisher's scheme

According to the theory put forward by R.A. Fisher in 1943 (see Race, 1944), the Rh system is composed of three closely linked allelic genes, each with two alleles, C and c, D and d, and E and e. A person inherits a set of alleles of the three Rh genes from each parent, for example CDe from one parent and cde from the other. These sets of alleles of closely linked genes are known as haplotypes; the commonest of them are listed in Table 5.1.

It was originally expected that each allele would be found to determine a corresponding antigen but only C, c, D, E and e have been recognized and it is presumed that d is amorphic.

Recent work, using Southern blot analysis, suggests that there may be only two Rh genes, one determining D and one determining C, c, E and e. D-negative individuals were found to have only the gene determining C, c, E and e with no allelic counterpart of D (Colin *et al.* 1991).

Relative importance of D

D is by far the most immunogenic of the Rh antigens, being at least 20 times more immunogenic than c, the next most potent Rh antigen. In most clinical situations in which alloimmunization to blood group antigens is a possibility, D is the only Rh antigen taken into account, so that in clinical practice 'Rh positive' is commonly taken to mean 'D positive' unless otherwise specified. Nevertheless, due to the widespread use of immunoprophylaxis with anti-D, the frequency of anti-D in comparison with

Table 5.1 Frequency of common Rh haplotypes

Short symbol*	CDE nomenclature	Frequency [†]
R^1	CDe	0.4076
r	cde	0.3886
R^2	cDE	0.1411
R^0	cDe	0.0257
R^{1w}	C^wDe	0.0129
r''	cdE	0.0119
r'	Cde	0.0098
R^z	CDE	rarer
r^y	CdE	

* The symbols are based partly on those originally introduced by Wiener (1949b) and partly on those introduced by Race (1944). Regardless of superscript, R implies that the gene determines D, and r that it does not.

[†] These frequencies, for an English population, are taken from Race *et al.* (1948a).

other Rh antibodies has greatly declined in the past 20 years. In the opinion of the authors, the time has come to discontinue the use of Rh and anti-Rh as synonyms for D and anti-D, and in this edition the more specific terms have been used throughout.

Wiener's scheme

Wiener (1951a) proposed that the inheritance of Rh antigens is determined by a single gene with multiple alleles. For example, the inheritance of CDe is determined by the allele R^1 of a single Rh gene rather than by alleles of the three separate genes Cc, Dd and Ee. In Wiener's notation, separate terms are used for an agglutinogen, i.e. the whole complex of antigens determined by the gene, and for factors, i.e. each separately reacting part of the antigenic structure. To illustrate the difference between this system and that of CDE, in the following example the CDE terms are given in brackets: the allele R^1 determines the agglutinogen Rh_1 (CDe) and this has multiple factors, which include: Rh_0(D), rh'(C), hr"(e) and rh_i(Ce). The main objection to the terminology is that it is less explicit than the CDE terminology. Whereas the complex CDe obviously contains the antigen e, it is not obvious that Rh_1 contains hr".

A World Health Organization (WHO) expert committee on biological standardization has recommended that in the interest of simplicity and uniformity, Fisher's nomenclature should be universally adopted (WHO, 1977). Meanwhile, the demonstration that C and c are carried on a different polypeptide from D, and that E and e are probably on a third polypeptide (see below) has greatly strengthened the scientific case for Fisher's scheme. On the other hand, a criticism of CDE terminology is that it is deceptively simple, implying, for example, that CDe contains only C, D and e and combined products such as Ce, whereas it may in fact contain others (Wiener, 1958). Because of the shortcomings of Fisher's scheme, albeit only when dealing with Rh at an advanced level, a third terminology has been proposed.

A numerical nomenclature

Rosenfield et al. (1962) started from the position that the terms should be 'free of bias and divorced from speculative implications' and that the 'usage in the past of a genetical format for designating what are basically patterns of serological reactions now appears to have been unwise'. As an example of the difficulties which had been reached they pointed out that the allele cD – , i.e. an allele without derminants for E or e, nevertheless determines ce (a 'joint' product, see later) and should thus be regarded as determined by a gene 'c without E'. The system proposed was essentially a description of the reactions of red cells with particular antisera, which gave equal importance to positive and negative findings. D is Rh1 and anti-D is anti-Rh1, etc.; see Table 5.2, which also gives the equivalent terms for Rh antigens in the CDE and Rh–Hr nomenclatures. A sample which reacts with anti-Rh1 and anti-Rh2, but fails to react with anti-Rh3 is described as Rh: 1, 2, – 3. In the paper of Rosenfield et al. 21 Rh antigens or qualitatively different reactions were recognized; as Table 5.2 shows, the number has now more than doubled (Lewis et al. 1990). Rh 9, 10, 11, 20, 22, 23, 28, 30, 32, 33, 35, 36, 37, 40, 42, 43, 45 and 47 are found in fewer than 1% of Whites; Rh 17, 18, 29, 34, 38, 39, 44, 46 and 48 are found in more than 99%.

Wiener's symbols, particularly those shown in Table 5.1 (Rh–Hr), are still used to some extent and some of the numbers, e.g. Rh 29 are used for lack of more convenient

Table 5.2   Rh antigens in three nomenclatures

No.	CDE	Rh–Hr	No.	CDE	Rh–Hr	No.	CDE	Rh–Hr
1	D	Rh_0	17	†	Hr_0	33	¶	
2	C	rh′	18	†	Hr	34	Bas	Hr^B
3	E	rh″	19	—	hr^s	35	1114 ‖	—
4	c	hr′	20	VS, e^s	—	36	Be^a	—
5	e	hr″	21	C^G	—	37	Evans	—
6	f, ce	hr	22	CE	—	38	Duclos	—
7	Ce	rh_i	23	Wiel, D^w	—	39	C-like	Hr_0-like
8	C^w	rh^{w1}	24	E^T	—	40	Tar	—
9	C^x	rh^x	25	$LW^‡$	—	41	Ce-like	rh_i-like
10	V, ce^s	hr^v	26	Deal, c-like	—	42	Ce^s	hr^H-like
11	E^w	rh^{w2}	27	cE	—	43	Crawford	—
12	G	rh^G	28	—	hr^H	44	Nou	—
13	*	Rh^A	29	'Total Rh'	—	45	Riv	—
14	*	Rh^B	30	Go^a	—	46	Sec	—
15	*	Rh^C	31	e-like	hr^B	47	Dav	—
16	*	Rh^D	32	§		48	JAL	—

* Corresponds to part of the D mosaic present in some D-positive people who make anti-D.
† High frequency antigens reacting with antibodies made by –D–/–D– subjects.
‡ No longer regarded as part of the Rh system.
§ Low incidence antigen determined by $\bar{\bar{R}}^N$.
¶ Low incidence antigen determined by R_0^{Har}.
‖ (C) D (e) cells positive with 1114 antibody.

alternatives. In general, though, the CDE terms have been found to be the best and are used almost exclusively in the rest of this chapter.

Molecular biology of Rh antigens

If intact red cells are labelled with ^{125}I and the cell membranes are then examined by electrophoresis followed by autoradiography, a diffuse but strongly labelled band of approximately 28–32 kD is observed. On adding anti-D, this band is specifically immunoprecipitated (Gahmberg, 1982; Moore et al. 1982). Anti-c and anti-E immuno-precipitate similar bands from c-positive and E-positive red cells (Moore et al. 1982). These 'Rh polypeptides', unlike all other known blood group antigens, completely lack carbohydrate. The serological activity of Rh antigens depends on the presence of phospholipid (Green, 1968; Hughes-Jones et al. 1975). Although it has been shown that palmitic acid is covalently linked to Rh polypeptides, it is not known whether the palmitylation of Rh polypeptides is important in their primary antigenic reactivity (DeVetten and Agre, 1988; Agre and Cartron, 1991). There is indirect evidence that Rh polypeptides are linked to the red cell skeleton (Ridgwell et al. 1984).

The D polypeptide (31.9 kD) is different from the C/c and E/e polypeptides (33.1 kD) (Moore and Green, 1987; Bloy et al. 1988). Although C/c and E/e are very similar, C/c, D and E/e appear to be three distinct proteins (Blanchard et al. 1988; Hughes-Jones et al. 1988). As previously noted by Edgington (1971), there is no steric hindrance between the binding of anti-c, -D and -E (Hughes-Jones et al. 1988).

Cloning of Rh polypeptides leads to the conclusion that Rh has a mobility of 45.5 kD; the mobility of 32 kD deduced from sodium dodecyl sulphate-polyacrylamide gel electrophoresis (SDS-PAGE) may be due to increased binding of SDS (Agre and Cartron, 1991). Analysis of complementary DNA (cDNA) sequencing predicts that most of the Rh polypeptides are deeply buried within the phospholipid bilayer of the red cell membrane (Cherif-Zahar *et al.* 1990). Modelling suggests 13 bilayer spanning domains with the N-terminus in the cytoplasm and the C-terminus facing outwards (Agre and Cartron, 1991).

Observations with polyclonal anti-D, -c and -E (Moore and Green, 1987) and with murine monoclonal antibodies (Gardner *et al.* 1991) indicate that Rh blood group antigens are associated with a complex of two groups of related polypeptides, one of mol. wt. 30 000 and one of mol. wt. 45 000–100 000. There are $1–2 \times 10^5$ copies of this complex per red cell (Gardner *et al.* 1991). The protein of mol. wt. 45 000–100 000 is a glycoprotein carrying ABH but not Rh determinants. This protein, like Rh polypeptides, LW and several other distinct glycoproteins is lacking in Rh_{null} red cells (see reviews by Anstee, 1990; Agre and Cartron, 1991).

Phylogeny of Rh
Studies on non-human primates suggest that, during evolution, the C epitope was the first to appear, followed by D; thus, only C is found in gibbons whereas both D and c are found in higher apes. E and e are found only in humans (Wiener *et al.* 1964). E and c have several oligopeptides in common (Blanchard *et al.* 1988). The most reasonable explanation of these findings is that D and Ee arose by gene duplication (Hughes-Jones *et al.* 1988) and is consistent with the early suggestion of Fisher and Race (1946) that the order of Rh genes is DCE. On the other hand, if there are only two Rh genes (*D* and *CcEe*), D and Ee cannot both have arisen by gene duplication from C (Agre and Cartron, 1991).

Rh phenotypes
The completeness with which the Rh phenotype can be determined depends on the antisera available; if anti-c is available but not anti-C, samples can be classified as c-positive (i.e. cc or Cc) and c-negative (i.e. CC). If anti-C is also available, Cc can be distinguished from cc.

A convenient notation for Rh phenotypes is that introduced by Mourant (1949). Suppose a sample is tested with anti-C, anti-c, anti-D and anti-E and gives positive reactions with all four antisera, the phenotype is written CcDE. If positive reactions are obtained with anti-C, anti-c and anti-D, but the reaction with anti-E is negative, the phenotype is written as CcDee, since an absence of E implies a double dose of e. This notation is occasionally misleading; e.g. although a negative reaction with anti-E usually implies that the cells are *ee*, they may be $e^s e$. Perhaps a more important objection to the notation is that it is very clumsy in speech; for this reason, the short symbols shown in Table 5.1 are often used although when so used they refer only to probable phenotypes. For example, use of the term $R_1 r$ implies that the genotype is $R^1 r$ (*CDe/cde*) and that the phenotype is CcD(d)ee. However, the genotype may be $R^1 R^0$ (*CDe/cDe*) and the phenotype is then CcDDee.

One of the advantages of the numbered nomenclature is that the sera used in testing a sample are always indicated. Thus the description Rh: $-1, -2, -3$ indicates that the sample does not react with anti-D, anti-C and anti-E.

Determination of probable Rh genotype

When a woman has anti-D in her serum it is desirable to know whether her partner is homozygous or heterozygous for the gene determining D, i.e. whether he is *DD* or *Dd*. If he is *DD* he can father only D-positive infants but if he is *Dd* there will be a 50% chance that any child which he fathers will be D negative and so be unaffected by anti-D in the woman's plasma. Routine serological tests do not distinguish reliably between red cells with a single and double dose of D, and indeed there is an overlap between the numbers of antigen sites on the cells of heterozygotes and homozygotes (see below). With some antibodies, e.g. anti-c, -C^w, -E, -e and -ce (Race and Sanger, 1975) discrimination between heterozygotes and homozygotes is better. If relatives of the partner are available, it may be possible to establish his D genotype (i.e. *DD* or *Dd*), with certainty. For example, if either of his parents is negative he must be *Dd*. When relatives are not available, and since there is no anti-d serum, the genotype will have to be guessed by determining the Rh phenotype as completely as possible and then calculating the probabilities. For example, suppose the Rh phenotype is CcDee, the genotype is likely to be either *CDe/cde* or *CDe/cDe*. The frequencies of these two Rh genotypes in an unselected English population are approximately 32% and 2% respectively. Therefore, the chances are 16 : 1 that the genotype is *CDe/cde*. On the other hand, when the person tested is the father of an infant with haemolytic disease of the newborn, since in most cases he has then handed on *D* twice in succession, he is a selected person and the probability that he is *Dd* rather than *DD* is only about 4 : 1. The chance that he is *DD* increases with the number of D-positive infants which he fathers. Evidently, if a man of the phenotype CcDee fathers a D-negative child he must have the genotype *Dd*.

The commonest Rh genotypes and phenotypes

From a knowledge of the gene frequencies in any blood group system, the genotype (or phenotype) frequencies can readily be calculated. As Table 5.1 shows, the commonest Rh haplotypes in an English population are *CDe* and *cde*. Thus the commonest three Rh genotypes are *CDe/cde*, with a frequency of 2 × (0.4076 × 0.3886) = 0.32, or 32%; *CDe/CDe* with a frequency of (0.4076 × 0.4076) = 0.16, or 16%; and *cde/cde*, with a frequency of (0.3886 × 0.3886) = 0.15, or 15% (D negatives include *Cde/cde*, *CdE/cde*, etc., and total 17%).

The overall frequency of the phenotype CcDee is 34.89%; the frequencies of the next commonest phenotypes in order are: CCDee 18.51%; ccddee 15.10%; CcDEe 13.34%; and ccDEe 12.67%. These together account for approximately 95% of the total Rh phenotypes of English people (figures derived from Table V of Race, in MRC, 1954).

The frequency of the different Rh antigens varies widely in different parts of the world. For example, the frequency of D negatives varies from 20–40% in Basques to 0–1% in Japanese, Chinese, Burmese, Melanesians, Maoris, American Indians and Eskimos (Mourant *et al.* 1976).

Effect of Rh phenotype on number of D sites per red cell

Masouredis (1960), using ^{131}I-labelled anti-D, found that C-positive red cells from *DD* donors took up 1.6 times as much anti-D as those from *Dd* donors, and that C-positive, D-positive cells took up only 0.7 times as much anti-D as C-negative, D-positive cells.

Similarly, Evans *et al.* (1963b) found that red cells with a double dose of D took up more anti-D than those with a single dose, and that when C was present as well as D the uptake by D was diminished.

Rochna and Hughes-Jones (1965), using purified ^{125}I-labelled anti-IgG, estimated the number of available antigen sites on intact red cells of different phenotypes. For D, the results were as follows (donor's probable genotypes in parentheses):

CcDee	(*CDe/cde*)	9900–14 600
ccDee	(*cDe/cde*)	12 000–20 000
ccDEe	(*cDE/cde*)	14 000–16 000
CCDee	(*CDe/CDe*)	14 500–19 300
CcDEe	(*CDe/cDE*)	23 000–31 000
ccDEE	(*cDE/cDE*)	15 800–33 300

Similarly, the number of D sites on cells of the probable genotype *CDe/CDe* was estimated to be 17 000 by Edgington (1971) and on *cDE/cDE* cells to be 27 900 by Masouredis *et al.* (1976). The latter authors used a method depending upon electron microscopy of stroma from D-sensitized cells treated with ferritin-conjugated anti-immunoglobulin G (IgG) and suggested that their estimates might be too low.

Although DD subjects could not be distinguished from Dd subjects in a random population, in families in which haemolytic disease of the newborn had occured investigated by Masouredis *et al.* (1967), the red cells of heterozygous fathers took up the same amount of anti-D as those of their offspring, whereas those of homozygous fathers took up almost twice as much.

Four examples of –D–/–D– red cells tested by Hughes-Jones *et al.* (1971a) were found to have between 110 000 and 202 000 D sites per cell. A sample of ·D·/·D· cells tested by Contreras *et al.* (1979a) was found to have 56 000 sites per cell.

Numbers of c, e, and E antigen sites per red cell
The findings of Hughes-Jones *et al.* (1971a) were as follows:

c sites: cc red cells, 70 000–85 000
         cC red cells, 37 000–53 000
e sites: ee red cells, 18 200–24 000
         eE red cells, 13 400–14 500

E sites. A great variation was found according to the source of anti-E and the phenotype of the red cells, and results varied from only 450 to as many as 25 600 sites per cell.

Substantially different estimates were reported by Masouredis *et al.* (1976). Using the method described above, the number of c sites on *cde/cde* red cells was found to be 31 500 and on *cDE/cDE* cells, 24 000. The number of e sites on *CDe/c^{w}De* cells was 20 000 and of E sites, 27 500 on *cDE/cDE* and 17 900 on *cDE/cde* cells. The authors pointed out that for various reasons these estimates might be too low.

Distribution of Rh antigen sites on the red cell surface
Antigen sites on the red cell surface can be visualized by first treating the red cells with

specific antibodies (e.g. anti-D), then with ferritin-labelled anti-IgG and finally examining the cells by electron microscopy. The distribution of D antigen sites appears to be random (Nicolson *et al.* 1971), a conclusion reinforced by studies on the binding of C1q to bound anti-D (see pp. 223–224).

It seems that E, e, C and c sites cannot be very close to D sites since the uptake of F(ab') anti-D is not interfered with by IgG anti-E, -e, -C or -c (Edgington, 1975). Similarly, using ^{125}I-labelled monoclonal antibodies, no steric hindrance to binding was found between anti-D, -c and -E, although anti-D inhibited the uptake of anti-G (Hughes-Jones *et al.* 1988).

Weak D (D^u)

A weakly reacting form of D was described as D^u (Stratton, 1946) and came to be considered as a definable phenotype. In fact, there is no hard and fast line between D and D^u, D^u red cells being merely ones with a relatively small number of D antigen sites and are evidently D positive. Accordingly, there is no such thing as a D^u test, i.e. one that will distinguish between D and D^u; a red cell sample that fails to react with anti-D in one test may react with it in another. In the past, the terms low-grade and high-grade D^u have been used to describe relatively weakly and relatively strongly reacting samples of D-positive red cells with a weak expression of D. Without estimates of the number of D antigen sites on the samples, the terms are almost meaningless but are used here when they have been used in published work.

The original kind of D^u was shown to be inherited (Stratton, 1946; Race *et al.* 1948b). However, most 'high-grade' D^u samples are due to an interaction between *Cde* and normal *D* in the subject's other Rh haplotype, e.g. red cells from a person of genotype *CDe/Cde* often react weakly with anti-D (Ceppellini *et al.* 1955). The number of D antigen sites on cells classified as CD^ue/cD^uE was found to be 540 per cell; four siblings classified as CD^ue/cde had 340–470 sites per cell, and two siblings classified as CD^ue/cde had 110–174 sites per cell, supporting the idea that *C* in *cis* (i.e. on the same chromosome) may weaken the expression of *D* (Bush *et al.* 1974). On the other hand, *E* in *cis* enhances the expression of *D*.

Red cells from donors should be tested for D using two potent agglutinating anti-D sera and a sensitive automated method. In a survey in which 15 000 samples from donors were tested in the Groupamatic, using potent anti-CD and anti-DE, the frequency of 'D^u', i.e. samples which were classified as D negative in the Groupamatic but which reacted with anti-D in the antiglobulin test, was 0.23% (Contreras and Knight, 1989).

Although D^u is a convenient term for weakly reacting D, its use should really be abandoned since, as already discussed, it has no agreed definition. Moreover, some, but not all, monoclonal IgM anti-D reagents agglutinate saline-suspended very weak D red cells, previously classified as D^u, so that with the use of monoclonal reagents disagreements about the classification of samples as D^u will become more frequent. The description 'weak D' is therefore to be preferred to D^u.

Clinical significance of very weakly reacting D

Two questions can be asked about very weakly reacting D red cells: (1) can they, if transfused to a D-negative subject, induce immunization to D?; and (2) are they destroyed at an accelerated rate in a subject with anti-D in the plasma?

Very few observations have been made and, in these, it is not known how weakly reacting the cells were; in particular, information about the number of D sites on the red cells concerned is not available. Nevertheless, one can say with confidence that weakly reacting D is much less immunogenic than normal D (see p. 230). As for accelerated destruction of D^u red cells by anti-D, there seem to be very few observations to discuss: a report of a haemolytic transfusion reaction due to the transfusion of D^u blood to a D-immunized subject (Diamond and Allen, 1949) and at least five cases of haemolytic disease of the newborn in D^u infants—one was described by Mollison and Cutbush (1949c) and two more by Stern (1960) who referred to an additional two in the literature. It is notable that no similar cases have been published in the last 30 years and it seems safe to conclude that the samples concerned would nowadays be regarded as within the normal range of D. In summary, very weakly reacting D red cells are poorly immunogenic and are probably not susceptible to rapid destruction by anti-D. Accordingly, if the very weakly reacting D red cells of a donor are misclassified as D negative, and transfused to a D-negative subject it is very unlikely that harm will result. If the red cells come from a pregnant or recently delivered woman, misclassification of the sample may result in a dose of anti-D Ig being given unnecessarily but this will be harmless. Similarly, if a patient with weakly reacting D cells is misclassified as D negative and transfused with D-negative red cells, no harm will result.

Partial D (D variants; categories of D)

The D antigen has at least eight epitopes, all of which are present on the red cells of most D-positive subjects (see below). Partial D is the best description for red cells which lack one or more of these epitopes; subjects with partial D may make an antibody against the epitopes which are missing (Tippett and Lomas, 1991). In the first study which recognized the existence of missing epitopes, the red cells were described as Rh variants; originally, three, Rh^A, Rh^B and Rh^C were defined (Unger and Wiener, 1959) and a fourth (Rh^D) was soon added (Sacks et al. 1959). The collection of original sera defining these four variants is no longer available.

In the second classification, D-positive subjects who have made anti-D are divided into seven categories (Tippett and Sanger, 1962, 1977; Lomas et al. 1986). Antibodies made by different members of the same category may not be identical but, by definition, red cells and sera of members of the same category are mutually compatible.

Classification by categories is likely to fall out of use and to be replaced by a system in which partial D antigens are classified according to the D epitopes which they carry (Tippett and Lomas, 1991). Testing with anti-D monoclonals has already shown that red cells which lack at least one D epitope are relatively common (P. Tippett, personal communication).

Category I: abandoned.

Category II: very rare. The red cells react with all anti-D sera tested except anti-D made by category II people.

Category III: the serum used in identifying this category is the original anti-Rh^D of Sacks et al. (1959). Most subjects in this category are Blacks and are then ccDee, VS + , V – ; some have been G negative. The four category III Whites found so far have been C + , VS – .

Category IV: mainly Blacks. The cells fail to react with anti-D made by category IV subjects and react weakly with the original category III anti-D. Anti-Go^a, reacting with a low-frequency Rh antigen, subdivides this category into Go(a +), mainly Blacks with an enhanced expression of D, and Go(a –), found only in Whites with normal expression of D. Anti-Go^a has caused haemolytic disease of the newborn.

Category V: the cells of all members fail to react with the original anti-Rh^C made by some category VI people and fail to react with the anti-D made by category III, category IV and, of course, category V people. The cells from most propositi react with anti-D^w, an antibody to a Rh low-frequency antigen. Anti-D^w and anti-Go^a are thought to be specific antibodies reacting with the missing parts of the D antigen.

Category VI: this is the most frequently detected of the categories. The cells fail to react with anti-D made by subjects in all the other categories except some in category IV, and react with only about 35% of anti-D made by D-negative subjects. The vast majority of subjects in category VI have been Whites and have had the genotype *CDe/cde* (Tippett and Sanger, 1977). Although category VI is sometimes equated with Rh^B it should not be, since Rh^B was originally described as part of normal D and should therefore react with virtually all normal anti-D sera. Moreover, some red cells of category VI are Rh^{abcd} and some are Rh^{abcd}. Using a monoclonal anti-D (H 26), the frequency of category VI in donors in Bristol (England) was estimated to be 1 per 5000, or 5% of subjects classified as D^u (Leader *et al.* 1990)

Category VII: the red cells of two D-positive women who have made this antibody carry the low-frequency antigen Target (Tar); the anti-D in their serum reacts with most D-positive samples but has a specificity different from the anti-D made by subjects in categories I–VI (Lomas *et al.* 1986). Most monoclonal anti-Ds react with category VII cells.

Many examples of partial D react more weakly with polyclonal anti-D than do normal D and were formerly described as D^u variants; less than 10% of weakly reacting D samples are partial D (personal observations, MC). When tested with polyclonal anti-D, weakly reacting partial D cannot be distinguished from weakly reacting D which has no missing epitopes, although the difference is of potential clinical significance.

Most D-positive subjects who form anti-D either belong to category VI or cannot be classified because their red cells react too weakly. For example, of 22 D-positive patients with anti-D found in several British transfusion centres, seven belonged to category VI and one to category IV; the remainder reacted too weakly to be classified (personal communications from seven directors of centres).

Since most D-positive subjects who make anti-D belong to category VI a very good guess as to whether a donor is weak D or partial D (i.e. category VI) can be made by testing the red cells with a polyclonal anti-D reagent known to react with category VI samples and with a monoclonal anti-D known not to react. Most hyperimmune polyclonal anti-D sera react with category VI cells. On the other hand, the vast majority of monoclonal anti-Ds fail to react with category VI cells although they do react with most weak Ds. As already mentioned, most D-positive subjects who form anti-D belong to category VI. Patients, particularly females, should be typed with two anti-Ds that fail to react with category VI cells; they will come to no harm if typed as D negative.

Haemolytic disease of the newborn due to anti-D made by D-positive (usually category VI) mothers is referred to in Chapter 12.

Table 5.3 Epitopes of D detected on partial D cells of different categories (see text)

Epitope	Category of D						
	III	IVa	IVb	Va	Vc	VI	VII
epD1	+	−	−	−	−	−	+
epD2	+	−	−	+	−	−	+
epD3	+	−	−	+	−	+	+
epD4	+	+	−	+	−	+	+
epD5	+	+	+	−	+	−	+
epD6/7	+	+	+	+	+	−	+
epD8	+	+	+	+	+	−	−

Epitopes of D (see Table 5.3)

Using monoclonal anti-Ds, eight epitopes of D have been recognized and named epD1–8 (Tippett, 1990). Only two of the epitopes (epD3 and epD4) are present on category VI cells whereas all eight are present on the red cells of category III. Of the 29 monoclonals tested, 18 reacted with epD6 and epD7, suggesting that the predominant antibodies in polyclonal antisera are those recognizing these epitopes. Epitopes 6 and 7 could be distinguished only by competitive binding assays (Gorick *et al.* 1988). The finding that category VI lacks five epitopes (including epD6 and epD7) may explain the observation that category VI is the one that most frequently fails to react with polyclonal anti-D (Lomas *et al.* 1989; Tippett, 1990).

Using bivalent 7S subunits obtained from seven purified IgM monoclonal anti-Ds, it was found that the number of sites detected per *CDe/cDE* red cell varied from 9400 to 28 500. These findings were taken to indicate that a number of different epitopes on the D antigen were being recognized. There was competition between IgG and IgM antibodies for binding to the red cells, indicating that both classes of antibody were recognizing epitopes on the same D polypeptide (Hughes-Jones *et al.* 1990).

Antigens of the Rh system other than C, c, D, E and e

G

Almost all red cells which carry D and all cells which carry C also carry an antigen G (Allen and Tippett, 1958). Amongst the findings which this observation helps to explain is that about 30% of D-negative subjects who are deliberately immunized with ccDee red cells make an antibody which reacts with C-positive, D-negative red cells, the explanation being that the donor cells elicit the formation of anti-G which, as implied above, reacts with all C-positive red cells.

Very rarely, a sample may be D positive but G negative (Stout *et al.* 1963) or C and D negative but G positive, when it is called r^G (Race and Sanger, 1975, p. 202). The number of G sites on red cells of various Rh phenotypes was estimated by Skov (1976), using an eluate made from G-positive *cdE/cde* cells previously incubated with ^{125}I-labelled IgG anti-CD. Estimates of the number of sites on some of the cells tested were as follows: *CDe/cDE*, 9900–12 200; *Cde/Cde*, 8200–9700; *cDE/cDE* 3600–5800.

Anti-G can also be made in the absence of $r^G r$ cells by eluting anti-CD from Cde/cde cells and then re-eluting from cDe cells. However, not all non-hyperimmune anti-CD sera contain anti-G (Issitt and Tessel, 1981).

C^w

This antigen was originally regarded as a product of C^w, a gene producing C^w and C (Callender and Race, 1946). It is now known that it can also be produced by a gene that produces C^w and c (Sachs et al. 1978). C-positive, C^w-negative subjects can form anti-C^w as a result of transfusion with C^w blood or pregnancies with C^w fetuses. In a few cases, anti-C^w has caused haemolytic transfusion reactions and haemolytic disease of the newborn (e.g. Lawler and van Loghem, 1947). The antigen C^w is rare, occurring in fewer than 2% of Whites.

C^G

This antigen is a component of cells carrying r^G which reacts with only some anti-C sera (Rosenfield et al. 1962). There is no specific anti-C^G serum, only anti-CC^G, and C^G is difficult to define (Race and Sanger 1975). On the other hand, in the USA, the term anti-C^G is used for those anti-C sera that react with r^G cells (Issitt, 1985) even though it is admitted that pure anti-C^G is difficult to isolate from anti-CC^G (Rosenfield et al. 1962).

'Joint products' of the CDE genes

Ce. Rosenfield and Haber (1958) described an antibody reacting with a product of C and e in cis. A large number of anti-C sera contain separable anti-Ce (or -rh_i) which reacts with cells of the genotype cDE/Cde but not with those of CDE/cde.

ce or f. When c and e are in cis, they determine a compound antigen ce(f); for example, ce is determined by CDE/cde but not by CDe/cDE (Rosenfield et al. 1953). Anti-ce can distinguish between CDE/cde and CDe/cDE.

CE and cE. Antibodies to these compound antigens have also been found (see Race and Sanger, 1975).

V (ce^s) is an antigen found in about 27% of Blacks in New York and 40% of West Africans but only very rarely in Whites (de Natale et al. 1955).

Other Rh antigens are listed in Table 5.2.

Red cells lacking some expected Rh antigens

–D– is a very rare haplotype which determines D without C, c, E or e (Race et al. 1951).

–D–/–D– red cells appear to have an abnormally large amount of D antigen as judged by their agglutination in a saline medium by most sera containing incomplete anti-D. As mentioned above, –D–/–D– cells have an increased number of D sites. The amount of lysis produced by the complement-binding anti-D serum 'Ripley' (Waller and Lawler, 1962) was found to be 50–70% for –D–/–D– cells compared with not more than 5% for cells of common Rh phenotypes (Polley, 1964).

$\cdot D\cdot$ is another very rare haplotype which also determines D without C, c, E or e. $\cdot D\cdot$ (but not $-D-$) produces a low-incidence antigen 'Evans' (Contreras *et al.* 1978). $\cdot D\cdot / \cdot D\cdot$ cells have more D sites than cDE/cDE cells but less than $-D-/-D-$ cells. They react with sera from alloimmunized $-D-/-D-$ subjects.

$cD-$ is a haplotype which determines increased D, decreased c and some f (Tate *et al.* 1960). Not all $cD-$ haplotypes express f (Race and Sanger, 1975).

C^wD-/C^wD- was described by Gunson and Donohue (1957).

Rh_{null}

A sample of blood which completely failed to react with all Rh antibodies was described by Vos *et al.* (1961) and given the name Rh_{null} by R. Ceppellini (cited by Levine *et al.* 1964). A second example was described by Levine *et al.* (1964); in this case, the parents and one offspring had normal Rh phenotypes although the Rh antigens had diminished reactivity; the authors suggested that the Rh_{null} phenotype was due to the operation of a suppressor gene (X^0r) in double dose, and that the relatives with diminished Rh reactivity were heterozygous for the suppressor gene.

A family in which the Rh_{null} phenotype was apparently the result not of a suppressor gene but rather of an amorphic Rh haplotype (in double dose) was described by Ishimori and Hasekura (1967). This kind may be called the amorph type of Rh-null to distinguish it from the 'regulator' type described above (Race and Sanger, 1975, p. 220).

Rh_{null} cells lack not only Rh polypeptides but also various glycoproteins associated with Rh (see p. 208). In addition to lacking Rh antigens, Rh_{null} cells lack LW, Fy5 and Duclos and have a marked depression of U and, to a lesser extent, Ss; glycophorin B levels are approximately 30% of normal (Dahr *et al.* 1987).

Rh_{null} red cells exhibit spherocytosis and stomatocytosis and have a diminished life span, associated with a mild haemolytic state (Schmidt and Vos, 1967; Sturgeon, 1970). The red cells have an increased content of HbF and react more strongly with anti-i; the cells also have an increased osmotic fragility and an increased Na^+-K^+ pump activity (Lauf and Joiner, 1976); the increased osmotic fragility is probably due to a decrease in the area of the red cell membrane (Ballas *et al.* 1984).

In Rh_{null} subjects the commonest antibody formed in response to transfusion or pregnancy reacts with all cell except Rh_{null} and is called anti-Rh29.

Rh_{mod}, originally described by Chown *et al.* (1972), may be due to an incomplete suppression of the development of Rh antigens by a variant of the regulator gene responsible for one of the two types of Rh_{null} (Tippett, 1972). Rh_{mod} cells have very greatly weakened Rh antigens and, like Rh_{null} cells, have a reduced life span (Chown *et al.* 1972) and bind anti-U, -S and -s only weakly.

Transient weakening of Rh antigens in autoimmune haemolytic anaemia was observed in an infant; when recovery occurred and the direct antiglobulin test became negative, the antigens became normally reactive (Issitt *et al.* 1983).

Absence of D from tissues other than red cells

D has not been demonstrated in secretions or in any tissues other than red cells (for references see Mollison, 1983, p. 343; see also Dunstan *et al.* 1984; Dunstan, 1986).

It seems that Rh expression appears very early during haematopoietic differentiation, even before commitment to erythroid and megakaryocytic lineages, but that antigen density on pluripotent cells is very low. After commitment, Rh expression behaves as a differentiation marker, increasing progressively during erythroid differentiation (Cherif-Zahar *et al.* 1990).

LW

Although LW is a blood group system genetically independent from Rh, for convenience it is considered here. The first example of anti-LW was obtained by injecting rhesus monkey red cells into rabbits and guinea pigs (Landsteiner and Wiener, 1940; 1941). The resulting antisera, after partial absorption with certain samples of human red cells (later described as D negative) reacted only weakly with the same cells but reacted strongly with other samples (later described as D positive). Althoughfor a time it appeared that the antibody produced was identical with human anti-D it was later shown to be directed against a different specificity to which the name LW (Landsteiner/ Wiener) was given (Levine *et al.* 1963b).

The first evidence that anti-LW was different from anti-D was produced by Fisk and Foord (1942) when they showed that anti-rhesus sera (i.e. anti-LW produced in guinea pigs) reacted equally strongly with D-negative and D-positive cord blood red cells. Other evidence soon followed: it was found that the injection of extracts of D-negative red cells into guinea pigs induced the formation of an antibody which, although it was not the same as anti-D, resembled it (Murray and Clark, 1952; Levine *et al.* 1961a); this antibody was later indentified as anti-LW.

The first two examples of anti-LW ('anti-D like') in humans were identified by Race and Sanger in 1955 (Race and Sanger, 1975, p. 228); the antibodies gave the same reactions as the animal sera and were later shown to give negative reactions with Rh$_{null}$ cells. The cells of one of the antibody makers and her brothers were then tested by Levine and found to be negative with the guinea pig anti-LW (Levine *et al.* 1963b). A distinction can easily be made between anti-D and anti-LW with the use of pronase which, unlike other proteolytic enzymes, destroys LW (Lomas and Tippett, 1985).

LW genes are inherited independently of Rh genes (Tippett, 1963; Swanson and Matson, 1964), although evidently there is a close phenotypic relationship between the *LW* and *Rh* gene products. This closeness was illustrated by showing that the injection of Rh$_{null}$ red cells into guinea pigs failed to produce anti-LW (Levine *et al.* 1962). *LW* has been assigned to chromosome 19 whereas *Rh* is located on chromosome 1 (see Chapter 3), lending further support to the idea that the two systems are inherited independently.

LW is a glycoprotein which is distinctly different from Rh D. It is not a glycosylated form of Rh protein nor is Rh a precursor of LW (Bloy *et al.* 1990).

LW antigens may disappear temporarily from the cells of LW-positive people who can then transiently make anti-LW. The number of LW sites on D-positive red cells was found to be 4400 and on D-negative cells to be 2835–3620 (Mallinson *et al.* 1986).

Subdivisions of LW. After the discovery of an antibody, now named anti-LW^b but originally anti-Ne^a (Sistonen *et al.* 1981), the following scheme was suggested: the commonest type of LW-negative red cells are termed LW (a – b +) and the antibody made by subjects with this phenotype is anti-LW^a. The antibody which gives anti-thetical reactions, mentioned above, is anti-LW^b and is made by LW(a – b +) subjects. The antigen LW^b (originally called Ne^a) is found in about 6% of Finns but in fewer than 1% of other Europeans. A single subject with LW (a – b –) red cells has been described who made an antibody, anti-LW^{ab}, reacting with both LW(a + b –) and LW(a – b +) red cells (Sistonen and Tippett, 1982).

All the LW antibodies described above react more strongly with D-positive than with D-negative red cells and fail to react with Rh$_{null}$ cells. Auto-anti-LW is mentioned on pp. 237 and 302.

Observations on the effect of LW antibodies on the survival of incompatible red cells are described in Chapter 10.

Rh ANTIBODIES

In this section the specificities of Rh antibodies are briefly considered together with some of their serological characteristics; Rh immunization by transfusion and pregnancy is considered in later sections.

Naturally occurring Rh antibodies

Anti-D
When the sera of normal D-negative subjects are screened in an AutoAnalyzer, using a low-ionic-strength method, cold-reacting IgG anti-D is found in occasional samples. In one series the frequency was 2.8% in D-negative pregnant women and 3% in males (Perrault and Högman, 1972). In another series the frequency was substantially lower, namely 0.16% in pregnant women and 0.15% in blood donors; in this series the antibodies were detected in the AutoAnalyzer but identified using a manual polybrene test; cold-reacting anti-D could be demonstrated in cord serum and on the red cells of newborn D-positive infants born to mothers whose serum contained the antibody (Nordhagen and Kornstad, 1984).

Of four males with cold-reacting anti-D who were given repeated injections of D-positive red cells, two formed immune anti-D; when ^{51}Cr-labelled D-positive red cells were injected into the two subjects who had failed to form anti-D, a diminished survival time was found in one but a strictly normal survival in the other (Lee *et al.* 1984).

Rarely, anti-D detectable by the indirect antiglobulin test at 37°C is found in previously unimmunized subjects; in two men described by Contreras *et al.* (1987) the antibodies were mainly IgG in one case and wholly IgG in the other; a small dose of D-positive red cells was destroyed at an accelerated rate in both cases (50–99% destruction in the first 24 h). In the same series there was one subject with anti-D detectable at 37°C only with enzyme-treated cells in whom the survival of D-positive cells was normal.

Rh antibodies other than anti-D

Anti-E is found not infrequently in patients who have not been transfused or been pregnant. Often the antibody can be detected only by the agglutination of enzyme-treated cells; at one centre 60 of 146 examples of anti-E found in pregnant women were of this kind (Harrison, 1970). The highest incidence was in primigravidae whose partners were no more frequently E positive than in a random sample of the population. In the whole series, only 60% of partners were E-positive, reinforcing the conclusion that most examples of anti-E encountered in pregnant women are naturally occurring.

In the course of screening sera from more than 200 000 individuals (prospective recipients of transfusion, antenatal patients, etc.), Kissmeyer-Nielsen (1965) found the incidence of anti-E in D-positive subjects to be over 0.1%. Most of the antibodies were very weak, however, and the detection of so many was perhaps partly due to the use of papain-treated *cdE/cdE* cells; only 20% were reactive by the indirect antiglobulin technique. Of 218 examples of anti-E detected in a single year by Dybkjaer (1967) using papain-treated *cdE/cdE* cells from a single donor, only 14% gave a positive indirect antiglobulin reaction. Twenty-one per cent of the subjects had never had a previous transfusion or pregnancy.

Some examples of naturally occurring anti-E are detectable by the indirect antiglobulin test at 37°C. In two such cases E-positive red cells were destroyed at an accelerated rate although in another subject in whom anti-E could be detected (at 37°C) only with enzyme-treated cells, the survival of E-positive cells was normal. All three examples of anti-E were wholly, or mainly, IgG (Contreras *et al.* 1987).

Examples of naturally occurring anti-C, -C^w and -C^x have been described (for references, see previous editions of this book). The antibodies have been agglutinins tending to react more strongly at 20°C than at 37°C, and to react more strongly with enzyme-treated red cells; one anti-C was shown to be IgM. Other examples of antibodies within the Rh system which may be naturally occurring are anti-Rh 30 and anti-Rh 32. A very low incidence of cold-reacting Rh antibodies with specificities other than anti-D was reported by Nordhagen and Kornstad (1984).

Cold-reacting auto-anti-LW

In screening 45 000 blood samples in the AutoAnalyzer using a low-ionic-strength polybrene method, ten examples of auto-anti-LW were found. The sera reacted as well at 18°C as at lower temperatures but did not react at 31–35°C. The titre, as determined in the AutoAnalyzer in eight of the cases, was 8 or less. Three sera were fractionated by DEAE-cellulose chromatography; two of the antibodies appeared to be solely IgG and one to be partly IgM and partly IgG. The cold anti-LW was found to be less positively charged than the bulk of the IgG, unlike immune IgG anti-LW which resembled IgG anti-D in being more positively charged (Perrault, 1973a).

Immune Rh antibodies

Since it has long been a routine practice to transfuse D-negative subjects only with D-negative blood, the formation of anti-D as a consequence of transfusion is now uncommon. When an antibody within the Rh system is formed as a consequence of transfusion, it is quite likely to be of a different specificity, such as anti-c, since c is not normally taken into account when selecting blood for transfusion (unless, of course, the recipient is known to have formed anti-c). By contrast, in women immunized to Rh antigens by pregnancy, anti-D was, until the introduction of immunoprophylaxis in about 1970, easily the commonest antibody to be found. At one American centre, of immune antibodies within the Rh system found in pregnant women, 94% were anti-D (Giblett, 1964). At an English centre the figure (for 1970) was substantially lower, namely 82% (L.A.D. Tovey, personal communication), possibly because examples of non-immune anti-E were included among the Rh antibodies. At this latter centre the figure for anti-D, as a percentage of all Rh antibodies found in pregnant women, had fallen to 35% by 1989 (G.J. Dovey, personal communication).

Of sera containing anti-D about 30% will also react with C-positive, D-negative red cells and about 2% will react with E-positive, D-negative red cells (Medical Research Council, 1954).

In tests on 50 single donor sera containing anti-CD or anti-CDE, 37 were found to react with r^G red cells, at first suggesting that these sera contained anti-G. However, after sequential elutions from Ccddee and ccDee cells, only three of the original sera contained potent anti-G and a further 12 contained weak anti-G. The reactions of many of the original sera with r^G red cells were presumed to be due to the presence of anti-C^G (Issitt and Tessel, 1981; see also above).

In sera from immunized patients who have formed Rh antibodies other than anti-D, the antibodies most commonly found are anti-c and anti-E; anti-c reacts with approximately 80% of random samples from Whites and anti-E with approximately 30%. Figures for the prevalence of these antibodies are given in Chapter 3.

Anti-ce is present in most sera containing anti-c and in most sera containing anti-e. Anti-CE is sometimes found with anti-D (Race and Sanger, 1968, p. 164) or with anti-C (Dunsford, 1962).

Anti-C without anti-D is rare. As mentioned above, C appears to be contained within the broader specificity of G; since D-positive subjects are almost invariably G-positive, they will not regard G as foreign. However, even in D-negative subjects C, in the absence of D, is poorly immunogenic (see below). In sera containing 'incomplete' anti-D, anti-C is not uncommonly present as an agglutinin (IgM); such sera are often used as anti-C reagents in blood grouping. The finding of anti-C in a C^w-positive person (Leonard et al. 1976) is very rare indeed. Most anti-C sera are mixtures of anti-C and anti-Ce.

Anti-V and anti-VS (e^s) react with corresponding antigens found most commonly in Blacks. 'Anti-non-D' (Rh 17) is made by –D–, C^wD–, cD– and ·D· subjects (Contreras et al. 1979a). 'Anti-total Rh' (Rh 29) is made by some Rh_{null} subjects.

Because of the outstanding importance of anti-D, this antibody has been far more thoroughly studied than any other antibodies of the Rh system and the following sections deal exclusively with it. Immune responses to Rh antigens other than D are discussed later.

Characteristics of anti-D

Most examples of anti-D are IgG and, in a medium of saline, unless present in high concentration will not agglutinate untreated D-positive red cells but can be detected using a colloid medium, polybrene or enzyme-treated red cells, or by the indirect antiglobulin test.

A minority of anti-D sera contain some IgM antibody, almost always accompanied by IgG antibody; provided the IgM antibody is present in sufficient concentration these sera agglutinate red cells suspended in saline. Occasional anti-D sera contain some IgA antibody but, in all examples encountered so far, antibody of this Ig class has occurred as a minor component in a serum containing predominantly IgG antibody.

IgM anti-D. As mentioned above, sera that contain a sufficient amount of IgM anti-D agglutinate untreated D-positive red cells suspended in saline. The properties of purified IgM anti-D were investigated by Holburn *et al.* (1971b). When the preparation was diluted in recalcified plasma rather than in saline, the titre was enhanced about four-fold; this effect was obtained, using as a medium recalcified plasma diluted up to 1 in 32 (Holburn *et al.* 1971a). The reactions of the purified IgM anti-D were only slightly enhanced (× 4) when enzyme-treated red cells were used but even so, several examples of IgM anti-D have been described which could be detected only by the agglutination of enzyme-treated red cells (Dodd and Wilkinson, 1964; van der Giessen *et al.* 1964).

The fact that an antibody can be detected with enzyme-treated red cells but not with the indirect antiglobulin test does not by itself indicate that it is IgM. In low concentration, IgG anti-D is far more readily detected by a test with enzyme-treated red cells than by the indirect antiglobulin test unless the latter is modified for maximum sensitivity by using an increased ratio of serum to cells or by using a low-ionic-strength medium.

In the early stages of Rh D immunization, it is common to be able to detect anti-D only by a test with enzyme-treated red cells. Clearly, this finding gives no indication of the Ig class of the antibody. A positive result with enzyme-treated cells is usually soon followed by a positive indirect antiglobulin test due to a reaction with anti-IgG. According to Davey *et al.* (1969), IgG and IgA antibodies are formed first, followed by IgM.

The number of IgM molecules that can be taken up by a particular sample of D-positive red cells is considerably smaller than the number of IgG anti-D molecules that can be taken up by the same sample. For instance, a particular sample of *CDe/cde* red cells would take up about 31 000 IgG molecules per cell but only 11 500 molecules of IgM anti-D (Holburn *et al.* 1971b). Some monoclonal IgM anti-Ds have made excellent blood grouping reagents (see Chapter 8).

IgG anti-D. If undiluted anti-D serum containing incomplete, i.e. IgG, antibody is mixed with D-positive red cells suspended in saline, agglutination is sometimes observed (Wiener *et al.* 1947); occasionally, with potent IgG anti-D, agglutination may be observed even when the serum is diluted in saline as much as 1 in 100 (personal observations, MC).

Although, apart from the exceptions just mentioned, IgG anti-D in a medium of saline will not agglutinate untreated D-positive red cells of 'normal' phenotype, some examples will agglutinate red cells which are heterozygous for the very rare haplotype −D− and most examples will agglutinate −D−/−D− cells (Race and Sanger, 1975, p. 214).

IgG anti-D will agglutinate red cells in a variety of colloid media, e.g. 20–30% bovine albumin will agglutinate enzyme-treated cells suspended in saline and will sensitize red cells to agglutination by an anti-IgG serum.

IgG subclasses and anti-D. IgG Rh antibody molecules are predominantly of the subclasses IgG1 and IgG3 (Natvig and Kunkel, 1968) although they may be partly IgG4 (Frame *et al.* 1970) or partly IgG2 (Abramson and Schur, 1972). In testing the serum of 96 RhD-immunized male volunteers, IgG1 anti-D was present in all cases with, or without, anti-D of other subclasses. Thus, in many cases IgG3 anti-D was present, in eight cases moderately potent IgG2, and in three cases moderately potent IgG4 anti-D (personal observations, CPE). An example of anti-D which was wholly or mainly IgG2 has been described. The donor had been immunized many years previously and the antibody concentration was only 1 *μg*/ml (Dugoujon *et al.* 1989).

In demonstrating the presence of different IgG subclasses amongst anti-D molecules it is important to use red cells with a 'strong' D antigen (ccDDEE rather than ccDee or CcDee) as otherwise minor subclass components may be overlooked (personal observations, CPE). It may sometimes be helpful to fractionate sera on DEAE-cellulose before testing them. For example, an anti-D found to be partly IgG4 by Frame *et al.* (1970) was tested by Erna van Loghem (personal communication) who found the IgG4 component difficult to demonstrate in whole serum but readily demonstrable in a fraction relatively rich in IgG4.

In women immunized by pregnancy it is common to find that anti-D is composed predominantly of a single subclass; on the other hand, most subjects who have been hyperimmunized by repeated injections of D-positive cells have both IgG1 and IgG3 anti-D (Devey and Voak, 1974). The findings in another series were similar, anti-D being composed of more than one IgG subclass more commonly in immunized male volunteers than in women immunized by pregnancy (personal observations, CPE).

The different effects produced by IgG1 and IgG3 anti-D in monocyte assays *in vitro* and in causing red cell destruction *in vivo* are referred to in Chapters 3, 10 and 12.

Different IgG subclass composition of anti-D in individual donors and in immunoglobulin preparations from pooled donations. After incubating D-positive red cells with anti-D sera, the amounts of IgG1 and IgG3 anti-D bound to the cells can be determined using monoclonal anti-IgG1 and anti-IgG3 in a procedure involving flow cytometry. Using sera from 12 hyperimmunized subjects, the mean amount of IgG3 bound was 16% of the total (Shaw *et al.* 1988). In another series, an almost indentical figure (17%) was obtained, with a range of 0–60% (Gorick and Hughes-Jones, 1991). In this second investigation, 17 IgG anti-D preparations for immunoprophylaxis were also tested and, unexpectedly, found to deposit less IgG3 on red cells: the mean was 8% of the total, with a range of 1–18%. It was suggested that certain methods of IgG production may result in preferential loss of IgG3.

Anti-D in relation to Gm allotypes. In those subjects who make anti-D and who are heterozygous for G1m(f) and G1m(a) there is a preferential production of anti-D molecules bearing G1m(a) (Litwin, 1973). Gm allotypes are described in Chapter 13.

In a case described by Natvig (1965) an example of anti-D examined in 1957 contained both G3m(b) and G1m(f) molecules but in a sample taken from the subject 8 years later the antibody carried only G1m(f) molecules.

IgA anti-D can be demonstrated by the antiglobulin test, using a suitably diluted anti-IgA, in some sera which contain at least moderately potent IgG anti-D. Although many sera containing IgA anti-D do not agglutinate D-positive red cells in saline, one example containing IgA anti-D with a titre of 128 agglutinated saline-suspended red cells after centrifugation (unpublished observations, PLM). Fractionation of plasma from this later sample confirmed that the agglutinating activity was present in the IgA but not in the IgM fraction (W. Pollack, personal communication).

The production of IgA anti-D seems to be associated with hyperimmunization. In one case, following boosting of an already immunized subject, the titre of IgG anti-D rose first and IgA anti-D became detectable only some months later (Adinolfi *et al.* 1966). Estimates of the frequency with which IgA anti-D is found in hyperimmunized subjects vary. In one series, of 52 sera with IgG anti-D titres of 1024 or more, 50 gave positive results with one anti-IgA serum and 47 gave positive results with another (J. James and M.G. Davey, personal communication). In another series, of 11 hyper-immunized donors, IgA anti-D was found in six, with IgG anti-D concentrations varying from 29 to 75 μg/ml but no IgA anti-D could be demonstrated in the remaining five donors, including one with an IgG anti-D concentration of 272 μg/ml. No discrepancies were found between tests made with two different anti-IgA sera (Mollison, 1973, p. 351). In another series of hyperimmunized subjects, IgA anti-D was detected in 14 of 19 (Morell *et al.* 1973).

Failure of anti-D to activate complement
The vast majority of anti-D sera do not activate complement. If untreated red cells, or cells treated with a proteolytic enzyme, are incubated with fresh serum containing potent incomplete anti-D, no lysis is observed, even using a sensitive benzidine method (Mollison, 1956, p. 217). Similarly, in testing red cells sensitized with anti-D, positive results with anti-complement have scarcely ever been reported; the most fully studied example came from a donor 'Ripley': freshly taken serum lysed D-positive red cells (Waller and Lawler, 1962); the serum also sensitized D-positive red cells to agglutination by anti-C4 and anti-C3 as well as by anti-IgG (Harboe *et al.* 1963). D-positive red cells take up twice as much antibody when incubated with 'Ripley' as when incubated with a normal anti-D serum (N.C. Hughes-Jones, personal communication).

A mysterious example of a complement-binding anti-D was described by Ayland *et al.* (1978). The donor had a weakly reacting partial D and the anti-D was therefore of restricted specificity; although the antibody was not potent it sensitized red cells to agglutination by anti-complement as well as by anti-IgG.

The usual explanation for the failure of almost all examples of anti-D to bind complement is that the D sites are too far apart on the red cell surface. As discussed in Chapter 3, two IgG molecules must be present on the red cell surface within the maximum span (20–30 nm) of a C1q molecule if C1q is to be bound. When there are 10 000 D antigen molecules per red cell and if the molecules are uniformly distributed on the red cell surface, the average distance between two molecules may be about

0.13 μm or 130 nm (Mollison, 1983, p. 337). On the average then, two bound IgG molecules will be too far apart to activate complement. On the other hand, if the antigen sites are randomly distributed a certain fraction of the sites will be within the span of a C1q molecule so that, particularly when red cells are heavily coated with anti-D, the binding of a certain number of C1q molecules is expected. Using ^{125}I-labelled C1q and ^{131}I-labelled IgG anti-D, it has been shown that in fact C1q molecules can bind to anti-D on the red cell surface; the number of C1q molecules bound is relatively low (about 100 per cell) when the number of anti-D molecules per cell is 10 000, but when the number of anti-D molecules per cell rises to 20 000, approximately 600 C1q molecules per cell are bound. In experiments in which D-positive red cells were very heavily coated with anti-D as many as 1600 C1q molecules per cell were bound (Hughes-Jones and Ghosh, 1981). Nevertheless, when purified labelled C1 is added to red cells coated with anti-D, C1r and C1s are not activated, as shown by absence of cleavage (N.C. Hughes-Jones, personal communication).

It is at first sight perplexing that although the abundance of K antigen molecules is even lower than that of D molecules, some examples of anti-K activate complement. The explanation might be that more than one anti-K molecule can bind to a K antigen, thus bringing two or more IgG molecules into close apposition. In contrast, there is evidence that the D antigenic site which contains the various D epitopes is so small that only a single molecule of anti-D can be bound (Lomas *et al.* 1989).

Rosse (1968) found that whereas C1 was not fixed by a single Rh antibody it might be fixed by a combination of Rh antibodies of different specificities, e.g. anti-D, anti-c and anti-e. Moreover, when red cells from a patient with paroxysmal nocturnal haemoglobinuria (PNH) were exposed to such a combination of antibodies in the presence of complement, they were lysed. Although these observations seem to make the point decisively, they must now be reinterpreted. The lysis of PNH red cells observed by Rosse was probably not due to activation of complement by Rh antibodies of different specificities acting in concert, but may have been due to activation of complement by IgG aggregates, as pointed out by Freedman *et al.* (1980). The latter authors provided further evidence—using radiolabelled antiglobulin sera—that Rh antibodies do not activate complement.

Published work on the failure of anti-Rh to activate complement has been concerned exclusively with IgG antibodies although it has been found that IgM but not IgG anti-D will lyse glutathione-treated D-positive red cells (F. Stratton and V.I. Rawlinson, personal communication); it is not known whether this reaction is complement dependent.

Quantitation of Rh antibodies

Methods of estimating the concentration of anti-D are described in Chapter 8. The approximate minimum concentrations of anti-D detectable by different techniques are as follows: AutoAnalyzer, 0.01 μg/ml; 'Spin' indirect antiglobulin test, 0.02 μg/ml; two-stage papain test, 0.01 μg/ml; manual polybrene test, 0.001 μg/ml.

The maximum concentration of IgG anti-D found in serum is about 1000 μg/ml. The lowest concentration of IgM anti-D detectable in a medium of saline is about 0.03 μg/ml (Holburn *et al.* 1971b), although in a medium of recalcified plasma a concentration of 0.008 μg/ml can be detected (Holburn *et al.* 1971a,b).

Equilibrium constants of Rh antibodies

Hughes-Jones *et al.* (1963a) demonstrated the heterogeneity of equilibrium constants both among examples of antibodies of the same specificity from different donors and within the population of antibody molecules of a particular specificity from a single donor (see also Hughes-Jones *et al.* 1964a).

Hughes-Jones (1967) studied 24 examples of IgG anti-D and found that the equilibrium constant varied from 2×10^7 to 3×10^9 l/mol, with an average of approximately 2×10^8 l/mol. The equilibrium constants of some other IgG antibodies are as follows: anti-E, 4×10^8 l/mol; anti-e, 2.5×10^8 l/mol and anti-c, 3.2–5.6×10^7 l/mol (Hughes-Jones *et al.* 1971a). In anti-D immunoglobulin prepared from pooled plasma, as expected, the range is less: 18 of 25 preparations tested by Hughes-Jones and Gardner (1970) had equilibrium constants within the range 2×10^8 to 4×10^8 l/mol.

Holburn *et al.* (1971b) found that the equilibrium constant of one example of purified IgM anti-D was 1.7×10^9 l/mol, which was ten times greater than that of IgG anti-D isolated from the same serum.

The affinity constants of monoclonal IgG anti-D have been found to be in the same range as those of polyclonal IgG anti-D (Gorick *et al.* 1988; Thompson and Hughes-Jones, 1990). IgM anti-D monoclonals have slightly lower affinity constants (Thompson and Hughes-Jones, 1990).

Rh D IMMUNIZATION BY TRANSFUSION

The response to large amounts of D-positive red cells

When a relatively large amount of D-positive red cells (200 ml or more) is transfused to D-negative subjects, within 2–5 months anti-D can be detected in the plasma of more than 80% of the recipients. In almost all those D-negative subjects who fail to make serologically detectable anti-D after a first relatively large transfusion of D-positive red cells, further injections of D-positive red cells fail to elicit the formation of anti-Rh (see section below on responders and non-responders).

Evidence that more than 80% of D-negative subjects will make serologically detectable anti-D after a single transfusion of D-positive red cells is as follows. Pollack *et al.* (1971b) found that, within 6 months of receiving 500 ml D-positive blood, 18 of 22 D-negative subjects developed anti-D; none of the remaining four subjects made anti-D within 14 d of a further injection of D-positive red cells, although in two of the subjects the D-positive cells were cleared rapidly (Bowman, 1976). In another series in which D-negative subjects received 200 ml red cells, previously stored in the frozen state, 24 of 28 produced anti-D within 6 months (average time 120 d); two of the remaining four produced anti-D after a further injection of D-positive red cells (Urbaniak and Robertson, 1981). The overall incidence of primary Rh D immunization following an injection of about 200 ml of D-positive red cells in these two series seems therefore to have been as high as 92% (46 of 50).

In a follow up of D-negative patients who had received an average of 19.4 units of D-positive blood during open heart surgery, anti-D was detected in 19 of 20 cases (Cook and Rush, 1974), but this report is made a little less impressive by the fact that in seven of the subjects the antibody was detected only in tests with enzyme-treated cells and in two of these seven the antibody was detectable only on a single occasion and could not be detected subsequently.

The response to small amounts of D-positive red cells

Following a single injection of 0.5–1.0 ml D-positive red cells, in many series anti-D has been detected in less than 50% of the recipients; see Table 5.5 on p. 230. The table also shows that if a second injection of D-positive red cells is given at 6 months to the subjects without detectable anti-D, some of them form readily detectable antibody within a few weeks, indicating that the original injection of D-positive cells evoked primary immunization.

Krevans *et al.* (1964) showed that, 6 weeks after giving a first injection of D-positive red cells to D-negative subjects, although anti-D was not detectable in the plasma, a second injection of D-positive red cells might be rapidly cleared from the circulation. In subjects showing this rapid clearance anti-D became detectable in the plasma later (see also Woodrow *et al.* 1969). Similar observations were made by Mollison *et al.* (1969). Of 13 D-negative subjects injected with 1 ml CcDEe red cells, only two formed anti-D within the following 6 months but when a second injection of red cells was given to the other 11 subjects five showed reduced survival of D-positive cells at 7–10 d and four of these subjects cleared virtually all the D-positive cells from their circulation within 30 d (Fig. 5.1). These four subjects formed readily detectable anti-D within about 1 month of the second injection.

The fact that a D-negative subject can be primarily immunized to D without having

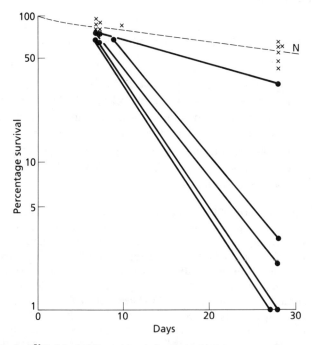

Figure 5.1 Survival of ^{51}Cr-labelled D-positive red cells in 11 D-negative subjects, each of whom had received an injection of 1 ml D-positive red cells 6 months previously. In five subjects (●) survival was below normal at 7–10 d and subsequently; all these subjects formed anti-D. Two other subjects (not shown) developed serologically demonstrable anti-D a few months after their first injection. In the remaining six subjects (×) the survival of D-positive red cells was normal and, despite further injections of D-positive red cells, anti-D was never formed (data from Mollison *et al.* 1969). N = normal survival of ^{51}Cr-labelled red cells.

serologically detectable anti-D in the plasma was first recognized by Nevanlinna (1953) who described the condition as 'sensibilization'. As just described, sensibilization is observed more commonly after the injection of small doses of D-positive cells than of large ones; it is observed commonly in women primarily immunized by a pregnancy.

Responders and non-responders

As already mentioned, of D-negative subjects transfused with 200 ml D-positive red cells, about 15% fail to make anti-D within the following few months; about half of these subjects fail to make anti-D after further injections of D-positive red cells and are termed non-responders.

The terms responder and non-responder were originally used by Levine et al. (1963c) to describe the ability, or inability, of particular strains of guinea pigs to produce antibodies against hapten–polylysine conjugates, a characteristic which they showed was under genetic control (see also Chapter 3). There must be a strong presumption that responsiveness to Rh D is genetically determined although this has not been demonstrated. No consistent differences between the HLA groups of responders and non-responders have been found, Although a non-significant increase of DRw6 in responders has been reported by two groups (see Darke et al. 1983), in another series no differences in HLA groups were found between high and low responders to Rh D (Teesdale et al. 1988).

When small amounts of D-positive red cells are injected into D-negative subjects and the subjects are subsequently given a second small injection of D-positive red cells, the cells may survive normally on both occasions. When this occurs, the subject invariably fails to form anti-D even when further injections of small amounts of D-positive red cells are given (Krevans et al. 1964; Mollison et al. 1969; Woodrow et al. 1969; Samson and Mollison, 1975; Contreras and Mollison, 1981). The survival of D-positive red cells continues to be normal even after a series of injections has been given; some examples are shown in Table 5.4. These subjects are clearly non-responders to small amounts of D-positive red cells. However, since the frequency of non-responders seems to be significantly higher when small amounts of D-positive red cells are given, it seems likely that there are intermediate grades of responder. The

Table 5.4 Repeatedly normal survival of D-positive red cells in two D-negative subjects ('non-responders')

| Subjects | Injection of D-positive red cells | | Cr survival at 28 d (%) |
	No.	Date	
Mor	2nd	Oct. 1967	58.5
	5th	Jan. 1969	62
	7th	Dec. 1969	54
Slo	2nd	Oct. 1967	42
	5th	Jan. 1969	46
	7th	Dec. 1969	51

First injections given March 1967; all injections were of 1 ml red cells except the third and fourth which were 0.2 ml. Sixth injections given with an i.v. dose of IgM anti-Rh (from Mollison et al. 1970 and Holburn et al. 1971a, supplemented by unpublished observations, PLM).

probability that this concept is correct is reinforced by the observation that the proportion of responders can almost certainly be increased by giving a very small amount of IgG anti-D together with a small dose of D-positive red cells; see later.

Poor responders
Although most D-negative responders produce serologically detectable anti-D after two injections of D-positive red cells, given at an interval of 3–6 months, a few do not; such subjects can be classified as responders or non-responders only if the survival of D-positive red cells is measured or if several further injections of D-positive cells are given. Details of one such case are shown in Fig. 5.2.

Two similar cases were encountered in a long-term follow-up of the 'series I' of Archer *et al.* (1969) in which subjects received 10 ml D-positive blood initially, followed by 5 ml every 5 weeks. Of 124 subjects, 73 developed anti-D within 18 months. In two further subjects who received regular injections for about 1 year and then, after a further year, two small injections in one case and one small injection followed by a 3-unit transfusion in the other, anti-D was detected for the first time 2.5 years after the start of the experiment; in both cases the antibody was present in relatively low titre.

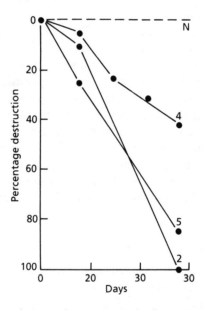

Figure 5.2 Results of Cr survival tests with D-positive red cells in a 'poor responder'. In order to express the extent of red cell destruction due to antibody, results on any particular day (*n*) have been expressed as

$$100 - \left(\frac{\text{Observed Cr survival, day } n}{\text{Expected Cr survival, day } n} \right) \times 100$$

so that if survival had been normal, a horizontal line (N) would have been obtained. The serial number of each injection of red cells is shown against the appropriate curve. Injection 2 was given 6 months after injection 1; injection 3 (not shown) was given 5 months later; injection 4, 3 months after that; and injection 5, after a further 5 months. Anti-D was detected for the first time approximately 2 months after the fourth injection (from Mollison *et al.* 1970).

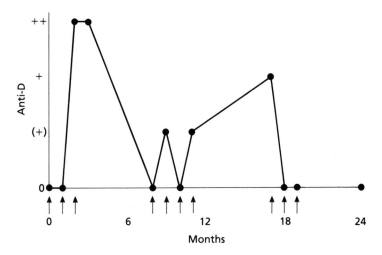

Figure 5.3 Disappearance of anti-D from the serum despite repeated injections (↑) of D-positive cells (data kindly supplied by T. Gibson). The amount of anti-D detectable by a test with papainized red cells is shown on an arbitrary scale.

A few subjects produce a trace of anti-D after a few injections of D-positive cells but no increase in antibody level occurs after further injections. The antibody may even become undetectable (Fig. 5.3).

Subjects who take a long time to produce anti-D tend to produce low-titre antibody; in subjects in whom anti-D was first detected only 12 months or more after a first injection of red cells, the titre reached a maximum of 128 or less in eight of 18 cases; in contrast, in 116 subjects who produced anti-D within 9 months of their first injection, the titre eventually reached 512 or more in every case (Fletcher *et al.* 1971).

Similarly, Lehane (1967) found that in D-negative subjects in whom antibody was first detected only after three or more injections of D-positive cells, the titre never exceeded 8, whereas in those subjects who formed detectable anti-D after a single injection of cells, titres of 128 or more were reached in all cases.

Effect of donor's Rh genotype
Table 5.5 shows that of 41 subjects injected with 1 ml *CDe/cde* red cells, eight (20%) made anti-D within 6 months of the first injection and a total of 15 (37%) made anti-D after two injections. By contrast, of 24 subjects receiving 1 ml *CDe/cDE* or *cDE/cDE* red cells, nine (38%) made anti-D within 6 months of the first injection and a total of 15 (63%) made anti-D after two injections. Again, among subjects receiving approximately 1 ml blood at monthly intervals, after 1 year only 30% of those injected with *CDe/cde* red cells but 84% of those injected with *cDE/cde* red cells had detectable anti-D in their plasma. The data set out in Table 5.5 cannot be considered to establish decisively that red cells of the probable Rh genotype *CDe/cde* are less immunogenic than red cells of other Rh genotypes because the studies were not carried out in a properly controlled fashion; e.g. the sensitivity of serological tests may have varied, the subjects may not have been strictly comparable, etc. Nevertheless, they supply suggestive evidence of

Table 5.5 Formation of anti-D after injections of 1 ml red cells of different Rh genotypes

Donors	Recipients			
		No. with anti-D		
Probable Rh genotype	Total no.	Within 6 months of 1st injection	Within a few weeks of 2nd injection	Reference
CDE/cde	10	1	4	Mollison et al. (1969)
CDe/cde	31	7	11	Woodrow et al. (1975)
CDe/cDE	12	5	9	Samson & Mollison (1975)
cDE/cDE	12	4	6	Contreras & Mollison (1981)
CDe/cde	20*		6	{ B. Bevan, personal
cDE/cde	19*		16	{ communication

* These subjects received an initial injection of 2 ml whole blood, then two further injections of 1.5 ml whole blood at monthly intervals; after a 4-month rest, three further injections of 1.5 ml blood were given at monthly intervals. The other subjects in the table received two injections of red cells at an interval of about 6 months.

the poor immunogenicity of *CDe/cde* red cells when given in small volumes. It should be noted that *CDe/cde* red cells, when transfused in relatively large volumes, do not appear to be less immunogenic than those of other genotypes; see the results of Pollack *et al.* (1971b) referred to above.

Immunogenicity of weak D (D^u) red cells
There have been two reports of the formation of anti-D in D-negative subjects after repeated injections of red cells originally believed to be Ccddee but later recognized as D^u. In both, injections of Ccddee cells were given twice weekly. In the first case, anti-C was detected after 13 injections and anti-D after 17 (van Loghem, 1947). The donor was then found to be 'low on the scale of grades of D^u antigens' (R.R. Race, in a footnote to the same paper). In the second report, three of four subjects made anti-D after 7, 11 and 18 injections, respectively (Ruffie and Carrière, 1951). Nevertheless, in a follow-up of 45 D-negative subjects who had been transfused with weakly reacting D (D^u) red cells (68 transfusions, 50 of ccD^{u}E and 18 of ccD^{u}ee blood), none developed anti-D although one developed anti-E and one developed anti-K. In 34 of the recipients, D-positive red cells could be detected for up to 100 days after transfusion (Schmidt *et al.* 1962b). The transfused red cells were described as low-grade D^u and the frequency of such cells in the relevant donor population was 0.4%. Among the 45 recipients there were 15 who were receiving drugs (6-mercaptopurine or steroids) known to suppress immune responses, but even if these 15 are excluded the failure of 30 D-negative subjects to develop anti-D after transfusion suggests that weak D (D^u) is far less immunogenic than normal D. This conclusion is reinforced by the fact that the development of anti-D after the transfusion of apparently D-negative red cells, i.e. later shown to be weakly reacting D-positive, has never been reported, leaving aside the experiments on deliberate immunization described above.

Only a single case has been described in which partial D red cells (actually D^{Va}) stimulated the production of normal, although very weak, anti-D (Mayne *et al.* 1990b).

The minimum dose of D-positive red cells for primary immunization
Ideally, one would like to have dose–response curves for a range of doses of D-positive red cells of different phenotype, plotted against the amount of antibody produced: (1) after a single stimulus; and (2) after secondary stimulation. It would then, for example, be possible to estimate the probability of primary immunization following a dose of red cells of a given size. Unfortunately, very few observations have been made with doses less than 0.5 ml. In the series of Zipursky *et al.* (1965) five injections each of 0.1 ml D-positive cord blood (approximately 0.05 ml red cells) of unstated Rh phenotype were given at 6-weekly intervals to D-negative subjects. Four of 15 formed anti-D. In the series of Jakobowicz *et al.* (1972) injections of 0.01 ml blood (about 0.005 ml red cells) of phenotype R_2r were given at 2-weekly intervals to eight D-negative subjects. Six of the subjects were parous women and only the data for the two male subjects can be used to decide whether such a dose can induce primary immunization. Of the two, one formed anti-D after six injections, i.e. after a total of about 0.03 ml red cells. Two other men were given injections of about 0.05 red cells at 2-week intervals and one of these formed anti-D after ten injections, equivalent to a total of 0.5 ml red cells. These findings, though valuable, clearly do not go very far in defining the minimum dose of D-positive red cells that will induce primary immunization in most responders.

Earliest time at which anti-D can be detected
In a series in which 22 D-negative subjects were transfused with a unit of D-positive blood, all still had detectable D-positive red cells in their circulation at 1 month; 2 months after transfusion, nine of the subjects had detectable anti-D in their serum, and at 3 months, 16; anti-D was detected for the first time at 4 months in one subject and at 5 months in another (Pollack *et al.* 1971b).

In a series reported by Gunson *et al.* (1970a) of six subjects receiving 5 ml *cDE/cDE* red cells, one had detectable anti-D at 37 d, although in four other responding subjects antibody was first detected at 63–119 d.

In another series in which 12 subjects were injected with 1 ml *cDE/cDE* red cells, and in which the subjects were tested at 2-weekly intervals, the earliest time at which anti-D was detected was 4 weeks; all four subjects who made serologically detectable anti-D after the first injection had detectable antibody in their plasma by the end of 10 weeks (Contreras and Mollison, 1981).

In previously unimmunized D-negative subjects anti-D cannot be produced more rapidly by giving a series of injections of D-positive red cells rather than a single injection. For example, among 121 subjects given an initial injection of 5 ml positive blood, followed by 2 ml every 5 weeks, eight formed anti-D within 10 weeks, and 27 within 15 weeks (Archer *et al.* 1969).

Apparent discrepancies between different series in the earliest time at which antibody is detected are doubtless due partly to differences in the sensitivity of testing.

Production of anti-D within a few weeks of a first stimulus was observed by Gunson *et al.* (1971), after the injection of specially treated D-positive red cells. The cells were incubated in a low-ionic-strength medium at 37°C and at the time of injection reacted strongly with anti-C4, -C3 and -C5. No observations were made on the rate of disappearance of the cells after injection into D-negative volunteers. Of seven subjects, one first developed anti-D at 15 d and five others developed antibody between 41 and 71 d after injection. It was considered that the time before the appearance of antibody was not significantly shorter than that observed following the injection of untreated cells (see above).

Influence of ABO incompatibility on primary Rh D immunization

The effect of ABO incompatibility in protection against Rh D immunization was first discovered from an analysis of the ABO groups of the parents of infants with D haemolytic disease (see p. 557) and was first demonstrated experimentally by Stern *et al.* (1956). These investigators gave from two to ten intravenous injections of D-positive red cells at intervals of 6–10 weeks (sometimes 5 months). The amounts injected were at first 5 ml, then 2.5 ml. If anti-D developed, only one further injection of 1 ml was given. Only one adverse reaction was noted (flushing of the face and faintness), and this was in a subject receiving ABO-incompatible cells. Of 17 subjects injected with ABO-compatible cells, ten developed anti-D; in five subjects the titre rose to between 16 and 128, and reached from 256 to 512 in the remainder. By contrast, anti-D developed in only two of 22 subjects receiving ABO-incompatible D-positive cells, and the titre was only 2–8. In one of these two cases seven further injections of D-positive cells failed to produce any increase in titre.

In a later study (Stern *et al.* 1961), the series was extended slightly and the total figures for the production of anti-D became: after ABO-compatible D-positive cells, 17 of 24 (anti-D titre 16 or more); after ABO-incompatible cells, five of 32 (anti-D titre 8 or less in four of five subjects). Ten subjects who failed to form anti-D after receiving ABO-incompatible D-positive cells were subsequently injected with ABO-compatible D-positive cells and four produced anti-D.

ABO incompatibility also protects against immunization to c and other red cell antigens; see Chapter 3 for references.

Effect of cytotoxic drugs on primary immunization to D

Of 19 D-negative patients who were transfused with many units of D-positive red cells during liver or heart transplant surgery, only three made anti-D, in each case at 11–15 d. In two of these three, the response was assumed to be secondary (both were women with previous pregnancies); in the third, the response was possibly primary. Of the remaining 16 patients, not one made anti-D within the following 2.5–51 months; 13 of the 16 were followed for more than 11.5 months. The low rate of primary immunization was assumed to be due to immunosuppressive therapy with cyclosporine and corticosteroids (Ramsey *et al.* 1989b).

Secondary Rh D immunization

In subjects who had been primarily immunized to D by being given a first injection of 1 ml D-positive red cells but at 6 months had made no detectable anti-D, a second injection of D-positive red cells at that time often produced a relatively slow and weak secondary response. In six such subjects, who had been given two doses of 1 ml D-positive red cells at an interval of 6 months, anti-D was first detected in four at 2–5 weeks and in two more at 10–20 weeks after a second injection; in no case did the antibody concentration exceed 0.3 μg/ml (Samson and Mollison, 1975; Contreras and Mollison, 1981). On the other hand, when anti-D was made after a first injection of

1 ml D-positive red cells and a second injection was given at 6 months, antibody levels rose rapidly and in one case reached a level of 92 μg/ml (Samson and Mollison, 1975).

In subjects immunized to D by transfusion or pregnancy some years previously, with low levels of anti-D in the plasma, the injection of 0.2–2.0 ml D-positive red cells often produced a maximal or near-maximal increase in anti-D concentration within 3 weeks; in nine of 30 subjects, the level rose from less than 4 μg/ml to more than 40 μg/ml (Holburn et al. 1970).

In another series in which six out of ten subjects had pre-injection levels of 4 μg or less and in which eight of the ten subjects received only one injection of about 0.5 ml of R_0r cells (two injections in the other two cases), the average antibody level reached 112 μg/ml, sometimes within 2 weeks and in all cases by 4 months (J. Bowman, personal communication). In other subjects, antibody levels may continue to rise for many months when injections are given at intervals of 5–8 weeks (Archer et al. 1971).

In the series of Holburn et al. (1970) about 50% of subjects eventually reached anti-D levels greater than 40 μg/ml; when no further injections were given, there was a progressive decline in antibody concentration; e.g. in five subjects, the values fell to 50% of the maximum in 5–13 months. A more rapid initial fall was noted by Gunson et al. (1974), titres falling to 50% of their maximum value in 11–40 d in some subjects although not until 100 d in others. On the other hand, some subjects maintain anti-D concentrations above 50 μg/ml for 1–2 years without further injections of red cells (unpublished observations, MC).

Antibody concentrations tend to be higher in restimulated subjects than in women immunized by pregnancy; Moore and Hughes-Jones (1970) found that 96% of restimulated donors but only 7% of naturally immunized women had anti-D levels of 21 μg/ml or more; 42% of the restimulated donors had levels of 101 μg/ml or more.

In a case referred to in Chapter 11, in which a subject with a faint trace of anti-D (0.004 μg/ml) was transfused with 4 units D-positive blood and developed a delayed haemolytic transfusion reaction, the anti-D concentration on day 9 was estimated to be 512 μg/ml.

In the secondary response it is common for saline agglutinins to be formed in addition to incomplete antibodies. For example, in one series before restimulation only four of 30 Rh D-immunized subjects had anti-D saline agglutinins but after stimulation the proportion was 20 of 30; in ten cases the agglutinin titre exceeded 4 (Holburn et al. 1970). In another series in which male donors who had been immunized some years previously were restimulated, about 1 week after reinjection most had agglutinin titres vs. saline-suspended red cells of 16–128 (Gibson, 1979). Similarly, in a series of about 100 women immunized by previous pregnancy the injection of 1 ml D-positive red cells provoked the appearance of anti-D agglutinins in 30% of cases (Hočevar and Glonar, 1972). The agglutination of saline-suspended cells by the serum of reimmunized subjects appears to be due to IgG anti-D since the property is not diminished by treatment of the serum with dithiothreitol (unpublished observations, MC).

In stimulating secondary responses, R_1r cells seem to be as effective as R_2R_2 cells (Gunson et al. 1974) and i.m. injections of D-positive cells as effective as i.v. injections (personal observations, PLM), although after i.m. injection the peak titre may be reached as late as 28 d compared with 7–14 d after i.v. injection (Gunson et al. 1974).

Persistence of antibodies

Anti-D can sometimes be detected in the serum a very long time after the last known stimulus; in a case mentioned by Stratton (1955b) the antibody was found in a woman 38 years after her last pregnancy. In cases in which anti-D can no longer be demonstrated serologically, a transfusion given 20 years or so after the last known stimulus may evoke a powerful secondary response leading to a delayed haemolytic transfusion reaction (see Chapter 11).

Because immunization to D persists indefinitely, D-negative blood should always be used for transfusion to D-negative women, even when the menopause has been reached and there is no history of pregnancy. One must always consider the possibility that the patient has been immunized by a pregnancy which she does not choose to reveal or by an abortion of which she is unaware.

Whereas, in subjects immunized to Rh D, incomplete antibodies may persist for very long periods, complete ('saline') agglutinins disappear comparatively rapidly: in women found to have saline agglutinins shortly after their last pregnancy, the titre was found to decline very rapidly during the following 12 months, so that at the end of this time only one-third of the women had a saline agglutinin titre of 8 or more, and after 4 years less than a tenth of the women had a saline agglutinin titre of 8 or more. In women whose serum contained incomplete anti-D the rate of decline was much slower; 6 years after the last pregnancy incomplete antibody could still be demonstrated in 460 of 478 cases (Ward, 1957; see also Hopkins, 1969a).

Rarely, anti-D saline agglutinins are demonstrable in subjects who have not received an antigenic stimulus for 10 years or more; in one such case, the antibody (titre 5000) was shown to be IgM (unpublished observations, MC). In a single case, in which anti-D had been shown to be partly IgA as well as partly IgG, the titre of IgA anti-D actually rose over a period of 12 years after the last known stimulus (unpublished observations, PLM).

Cyclical fluctuations in anti-D level were observed by Rubinstein (1972): daily samples were taken from eight female and two male Rh D-immunized subjects for several weeks; all samples were tested at the same time. In six out of the ten subjects values fell for 3–5 d, then rose more rapidly so that the total cycle from one low point to another was exactly 7 d. The difference between the highest and the lowest levels was 25–30%.

Rh D immunization by red cells present as contaminants

Platelet concentrates

In a retrospective study of 102 D-negative patients, all of whom had diseases associated with impaired immunological reactivity (mainly acute leukaemia), and all of whom were receiving immunosuppressive drugs, who received numerous units of platelets from D-positive donors, within an average of about 8 months from the first platelet transfusion eight patients (7.8%) developed anti-D. It was estimated that each platelet concentrate contained approximately 0.37 ml red cells (Goldfinger and McGinniss, 1971). In another series, of patients with a variety of malignancies, only two of 115 developed anti-D (Lichtiger and Hester, 1986).

When platelet concentrates from D-positive donors are transfused to D-negative women who have not yet reached the menopause, an injection of anti-D immunoglobulin should be given to suppress primary Rh D immunization. Such an injection is not expected to impair the survival of platelets from D-positive donors, since platelets do not carry Rh antigens.

Plasma transfusion
Liquid-stored plasma may contain small numbers of red cells, and plasma transfusions have been shown to be capable of causing both primary and secondary responses to red cell alloantigens. In one case, primary immunization was observed in a patient with systemic lupus erythematosus who had received liquid-stored plasma from 104 D-positive donors during the course of several plasma exchanges. It was estimated that between 0.1 and 0.5 ml D-positive red cells were introduced; anti-D was found in the plasma 6 weeks after the last plasma exchange (McBride *et al.* 1978). In another case, the transfusion of a single unit of liquid-stored plasma from a D-positive donor apparently induced primary immunization, although red cell counts on other units of similarly prepared plasma suggested that each unit contained not more than about 0.05 ml packed red cells; in four further cases, the transfusion of a small number of units of stored plasma induced secondary responses, in two cases to D, and in two to Fy^a (K.L. Burnie and R.M. Barr, personal communication).

It is possible that traces of stroma in frozen plasma from D-positive donors can stimulate a secondary response to D (Barclay *et al.* 1980).

Renal transplantation
Anti-D developed in a D-negative male 3 months after the transplantation of a cadaver kidney from a D-positive donor, despite the fact that the kidney had been immediately perfused with saline after removal from the donor (Kenwright *et al.* 1976). Two further cases of the development of anti-D after renal transplantation were encountered by K.L. Burnie and R.M. Barr (personal communication).

Bone grafts
In two women of child-bearing age bone allografts appear to have been the cause of Rh D immunization. One of the women was ccD^uee and made anti-D; 13 years after receiving the graft her first infant was born with haemolytic disease (Hill *et al.* 1974). The second woman was D-negative and made anti-C and anti-G which were detected on routine antibody screening after a blood donation (Johnson *et al.* 1985).

Contaminated syringes
Cases have been reported in which young women have been immunized to D by sharing syringes for the i.v. injection of 'hard' drugs. In one reported by Vontver (1973), the patient received an injection of cocaine to which blood from her sexual partner had deliberately been added in a 'ritualistic mingling'. She received further injections from shared syringes, contaminated with her partner's blood, over the next few months; 11 months from the time of the first injection she had an anti-D titre of 1000.

In a case reported by McVerry *et al.* (1977), a young woman was immunized by sharing a syringe for i.v. morphine injections with her sexual partner and with other people. The partner was not only R_1R_2 but K positive and the patient developed not only potent anti-D but also anti-K.

Immunization to Rh antigens other than D

G, C and E

The formation of anti-G, anti-C and (far less frequently) anti-E in subjects immunized to D is relatively common, but the formation of these antibodies in subjects who are D positive and therefore do not form anti-D is very rare. Presumably, this difference is simply an example of the augmenting effect of strong antigens on weak antigens, discussed on p. 117.

The formation of anti-G (at first mistaken for anti-D) after the transfusion of Ccddee blood to a ccddee recipient has been reported only once (Smith *et al.* 1977).

Anti-C alone, i.e. without anti-D, is rare. Some evidence of the low immunogenicity of C is as follows. In one series in which either C-negative or E-negative, D-positive recipients were given frequent i.v. injections of C-positive or E-positive red cells over a period of 1–1.5 years, not one of the 32 subjects formed the desired antibody (Jones *et al.* 1954). In a study in which 74 C-negative, D-negative subjects were transfused with one or more units of C-positive, D-negative blood (and in some cases also with E-positive, D-negative blood) only two formed anti-C. Of 66 C-negative, D-positive patients transfused with 136 units of C-positive blood, none made antibody (Schorr *et al.* 1971). In four ccddee subjects reported by Huestis (1971) who had been transfused with 2, 4, 7 and 17 units of Cde blood respectively, none made anti-C.

Anti-E is much commoner than anti-C but, as explained above, is often naturally occurring. Immune anti-E is uncommon. In the series of Schorr *et al.* (1971) none of 47 E-negative, D-negative patients transfused with a total of 89 units E-positive blood made anti-E. Of 44 E-negative, D-positive patients transfused with 71 units E-positive blood, only one made anti-E.

Issitt (1979) reviewing data from the literature, and comparing them with his own experience in Cincinnati, showed that the frequency with which anti-C and anti-E were found in D-negative subjects was virtually the same whether they were transfused with D-negative blood which was also C negative and E negative, or with D-negative blood which was either C positive or E positive. With either practice, the frequency of anti-C was about 1 in 10 000 and of anti-E about 1 in 1000. Moreover, of four examples of anti-C and 44 examples of anti-E detected in Cincinnati every example was found in a D-positive patient.

C^w

van Loghem *et al.* (1949) gave twice-weekly injections of 0.5 ml C^w blood to three volunteers. After 21 injections one of these recipients produced anti-C^w.

c

In an attempt to produce anti-c, Wiener (1949) gave repeated injections of ccddee blood to 19 CCDDee individuals; not one produced antibody. However, Jones *et al.* (1954a) succeeded in producing anti-c in two out of nine volunteers who were given repeated injections of c-positive blood over a period of 10 months.

After anti-D, anti-c is (in Whites) the most important Rh antibody from the clinical point of view. Although anti-E is commoner than anti-c, as mentioned above anti-E is frequently a naturally occurring antibody; on the other hand, anti-c (like anti-e) is found only as an immune antibody. Anti-c is relatively often involved in delayed haemolytic transfusion reactions and in haemolytic disease of the newborn.

e

Jones et al. (1954a) gave repeated injections of e-positive blood to a volunteer of the probable genotype cDE/cDE. After 6 years anti-e was found for the first time. van Loghem et al. (1953a) gave injections of e-positive blood to three cDE/cDE recipients. Eight injections of 0.5 of cde/cde blood were given at weekly intervals; after 2 months' rest, weekly injections were begun again. After the third injection immune antibodies were found in one of the three recipients; seven more injections were given in an attempt to increase the strength of the antibody. The serum was now found to contain not only anti-e (titre 8) but also anti-K (titre 4) and anti-Fy^a (titre 2).

Development of a positive direct antiglobulin test (DAT) following Rh D immunization

Positive direct antiglobulin test following secondary immunization
As described in Chapters 3 and 11, the DAT may become positive following secondary immunization. The positive DAT persists long after the stimulating red cells have been cleared from the circulation. Two examples are as follows: in a D-negative patient who developed potent anti-D after a transfusion of 4000 ml D-positive red cells the DAT was positive at 6 months though negative at 1 year. It is probably not relevant that, after the transfusion, the patient was given 7000 μg anti-D in the hope of suppressing Rh D immunization before it was realized that she was already primarily immunized (Beard et al. 1971).

In a patient of group Rh^d who had developed anti-Rh^D, D-positive red cells were transfused and rapidly destroyed. The DAT was positive at 4 d and more strongly positive 4 months later; the reaction was weaker at 6 months and negative at 7 months (Lalezari et al. 1975a).

Anti-LW developing in subjects who are transiently LW negative
Chown et al. (1971) observed that in two D-negative, LW-positive pregnant women anti-LW developed as well as anti-D. At this time the patients' red cells behaved as LW negative. One of the two patients now developed a positive DAT and the anti-LW could no longer be demonstrated in the plasma. Ten weeks later the patient was clearly LW positive. The authors postulated that the anti-LW was responsible for the positive DAT and they further suggested that the anti-LW was probably produced only when the patient was functionally LW negative and was therefore not really an autoantibody. From the time when the patient became LW positive again the antibody was like a passively acquired incompatible antibody. A very similar case was reported by Giles and Lundsgaard (1967). A D-negative woman was found to have developed anti-D 3 weeks before her first delivery. In addition her plasma reacted with all D-negative samples. Just before delivery her DAT became positive. It was still positive 6 months

later but was negative at 1 year. The patient's cells were LW negative at the time of delivery but positive 1 year later. At the time of delivery the serum contained anti-LW as well as anti-CD but at 1 year only anti-CD.

Anti-LW may also develop transiently in D-positive patients who have a chronic, often terminal, illness, possibly with some underlying immunological disorder. These subjects do not develop anti-D (Perkins *et al.* 1977; Giles, 1980).

D-negative subjects of undetermined LW status
In a series in which male D-negative subjects were immunized to provide anti-D for immunoprophylaxis it was found that pooled plasma obtained from them reacted weakly with bromelin-treated D-negative cells. Samples from 11 of 18 subjects when tested separately showed the same reaction and the red cells of two more subjects gave a positive DAT. Five months later all reactions had become negative and no clinical signs of red cell destruction were observed at any time (Cook, 1971). Although the specificity of the autoantibody was anti-LW (P. Tippett, personal communication) the LW status of the subjects during the period when the DAT was positive was not determined. In several other series this phenomenon has been looked for but not found (e.g. Contreras and Mollison 1981; 1983).

Association with intensive plasma exchange
In two women described by Isbister *et al.* (1977), both of whom had had previous infants with hydrops fetalis, intensive plasma exchange was carried out in a subsequent pregnancy between about the 11th and 24th weeks. The total amount of plasma exchanged in this period was about 95 litres. In one of the two cases, despite this treatment, the antibody titre rose from 512 at 17 weeks to about 60 000 at 24 weeks and in both cases the mothers had a stillbirth at about the 25th week, in one case following an intra-uterine transfusion. In both women, at the conclusion of the course of plasma exchange, it was found that the patient's red cells had acquired a positive DAT and that the plasma reacted with D-negative red cells. An IgG antibody of apparent specificity anti-G was eluted from the red cells. In one of the patients who was followed up for a year the DAT remained positive, but there were no signs of a haemolytic process. The reaction of the patient's own red cells with anti-LW was not determined.

Auto-anti-D in a D-positive subject with weak D
In the first case of this kind to be reported a man with the phenotype CCD^uEe and a 'very low grade' D (D^{abcd}) developed anti-D and anti-c following transfusion, and also developed a positive DAT. The strength of this reaction varied directly with the amount of anti-D in his serum at any particular time; anti-D could be eluted from his red cells (Chown *et al.* 1963).

A positive DAT in a D-positive subject following a massive dose of anti-D
In an experiment described by Mohn *et al.* (1964), plasma containing potent anti-CD was transfused to an R_2R_2 subject, producing a severe haemolytic episode. Between 70 and 229 d after the transfusion an eluate prepared from the recipient's red cells contained specific anti-E and this eluate reacted with the recipient's pre-transfusion red cells. The authors concluded that an autoantibody had been produced, possibly due to an alteration to the Rh site by an interaction of transfused anti-CD with the D antigen.

SUPPRESSION OF PRIMARY Rh D IMMUNIZATION
BY PASSIVELY ADMINISTERED ANTI-D

(For a general discussion of the suppression of primary immunization by passively administered antibody, see Chapter 3.)

Early work
The first experiments showing that passively administered anti-D could interfere with primary Rh D immunization were performed by Stern *et al.* (1961) who found that if D-positive red cells were coated *in vitro* with anti-D before being injected into D-negative subjects, there might be no antibody response. Of 16 subjects given a course of injections (in most cases five) of coated D-positive cells, not one produced anti-D; ten of the subjects were later given injections of uncoated D-positive cells and five produced anti-D. These experiments were not pursued further and it was left to others to consider the possibility that Rh D immunization which would otherwise occur as a result of pregnancy could be suppressed by a timely injection of anti-D.

In a brief report of a meeting of the Liverpool Medical Institution, Finn (1960) was quoted as saying '. . . It might be possible to destroy any fetal red cells found in the maternal circulation following delivery by means of a suitable antibody. If successful, this would prevent the development of erythroblastosis, so mimicking the natural protection afforded by ABO incompatibility.'

The Liverpool group at first assumed that treatment would have to be given during pregnancy; accordingly, their first experiments were made with IgM antibody since, following injection into the mother's circulation, this type of antibody would not cross the placenta to cause harm to the fetus (Finn *et al.* 1961). At much the same time, Freda and Gorman (1962) referred to experiments which they had started in male volunteers, and discussed the possibility that it might be necessary, in treating pregnant women, to use either 19S antibody or 3.5S fragments of antibody, neither of which was expected to cross the placenta.

Suppression of Rh D immunization by 'incomplete' (IgG) anti-D was demonstrated by Clarke *et al.* (1963) and also by Freda *et al.* (1964; 1966), who were the first to use an immunoglobulin concentrate of IgG anti-D, given intramuscularly. Shortly afterwards, it was realized that transplacental haemorrhage occurred chiefly at the time of delivery and both groups showed that anti-D given soon after delivery, would suppress Rh D immunization which would otherwise have occurred (Combined study, 1966; Pollack *et al.* 1968b).

In the present chapter, the suppression of Rh D immunization following the i.v. injection of D-positive red cells is discussed; the suppression of Rh D immunization which would otherwise follow pregnancy is discussed in the chapter on haemolytic disease of the newborn (Chapter 12).

Minimum amount of IgG anti-D which will suppress immunization

Intramuscular administration of anti-D
Although there is relatively little evidence about the minimum amount of IgG anti-D required to suppress Rh D immunization when different volumes of D-positive red cells

are injected, and although it seems quite possible that the amount varies with different preparations of anti-D immunoglobulin, the rule of thumb that 20 μg anti-D per ml D-positive red cells is sufficient to suppress Rh D immunization is a very useful one. Some of the evidence on which this rule is based is as follows.

Less than 10 ml red cells. A dose of 50 μg anti-D appears to be sufficient to suppress Rh D immunization completely when 2.5 ml *cDE/cDE* red cells (approximately 5 ml blood) are injected. Of 39 treated subjects who received the anti-D 72 h after the D-positive cells and who received a second injection of 0.1 ml D-positive cells at 6 months (without anti-D), none had anti-D in their serum 2 weeks later. In control subjects who received the same doses of D-positive cells but no anti-D, 11 of 36 made anti-D during the 6 months after the first injection of red cells and three more made anti-D within 2 weeks of the second injection (Crispen, 1976).

In an earlier series it was reported that when 40 μg anti-D were injected with 2.0–2.5 ml red cells, i.e. approximately 18 μg anti D per ml cells, immunization was not suppressed (Pollack *et al.* 1968a). However, it seems not unlikely that the dose of anti-D given was overestimated; the same anti-D preparation produced apparent augmentation of the immune response at an approximate dosage of 4.5 μg antibody per ml cells, which is substantially higher than later estimates of the probable augmenting dose (see below). The estimates in the series of Pollack *et al.* were made very shortly after the method for quantitating anti-D was first described.

A dose of 10 μg anti-D per ml red cells (5 μg anti-Rh with 0.5 ml *cDE/cDE* red cells) failed to suppress Rh D immunization (Gunson *et al.* 1971). In another series, in which 5 μg anti-D were given with 1 ml *cDE/cDE* red cells, there was suggestive evidence of partial suppression of primary immunization (Contreras and Mollison, 1981).

10–40 ml red cells. Bartsch (1972) gave 260 μg IgG anti-D with about 12 ml D-positive red cells to ten subjects and with about 25 ml to ten others. No anti-D could be detected at 6–9 months in any subject. Between 6 and 30 months after the first injection of red cells, 2.5 ml red cells were injected, followed by a further injection of 260 μg anti-D. (This second injection of anti-D was given to suppress primary Rh D immunization and was not expected to interfere with secondary immunization.) No subjects formed anti-D.

In easily the most valuable experiment yet described on defining the dose of anti-D required to suppress Rh D immunization, a fixed amount of IgG anti-D, namely 267 μg, was given to groups of D-negative subjects who received doses of D-positive red cells varying from 11.6 to 37.5 ml. Control subjects received the same dose of red cells without anti-D. All the subjects were given a challenge dose of 0.2 ml whole blood at 6 months and tested 1 week later. Of the controls, 49 of 86 (57%) formed anti-D. There was suggestive but not decisive evidence of a relation between the dose of D-positive red cells and the incidence of Rh D immunization. From the results in the treated group (Table 5.6), it was concluded that 267 μg of this particular preparation of anti-D was completely effective against about 13 ml red cells and was partially effective against larger amounts (Pollack *et al.* 1971a).

Sooner or later, an attempt is likely to be made to repeat this experiment but using monoclonal anti-D. It is therefore worth pointing out that, at least after primary

Table 5.6 An estimate of the maximum amount of D-positive red cells against which a fixed amount of anti-D will protect from immunization (from Pollack *et al.* 1971a)

	Average amount of red cells (ml) injected					
	11.6	13.4	18.1	21.2	30.1	37.5
	Proportions immunized					
Treated	0/19	0/18	3/18	2/8	4/12	6/17
Control	7/16	6/12	11/19	5/8	7/11	13/20

Treated subjects received 267 μg anti-D intramuscularly; control subjects received 'inert' immunoglobulin.
The totals for the numbers immunized are for subjects who developed detectable anti-D either 6 months after the first injection of cells or 1 week after that, after having received a challenge dose of 0.2 ml D-positive red cells.

immunization with 1 ml red cells, if subjects are tested only 1 week after a second dose of D-positive red cells, given 6 months after the first, there is a serious risk of failing to detect some secondary responses (see p. 232).

200 ml red cells. In an experiment in which 22 D-negative subjects were transfused with 500 ml blood, eight were given 14.6 μg anti-D per ml cells and 14 received 20 μg per ml cells. None of the 22 subjects formed anti-D within 5 months (Pollack *et al.* 1971b). When challenged with a small dose of D-positive cells at 5 months, many of the subjects showed accelerated clearance (Bowman, 1976) but this was probably due to the persistence of a small amount of the passively administered anti-D.

Intravenous administration of IgG anti-D
As described on pp. 471 and 670, following the i.m. administration of anti-D the maximum level in the plasma is reached only after about 48 h. Moreover, the maximum concentration reached is equivalent to only about 40% of the level expected if the anti-D were injected i.v. If the suppression of Rh D immunization is related to the degree of antibody coating of red cells at the time of clearance the amount of anti-D required for suppression when given i.v. should be less than half the amount required when given i.m.

The only direct evidence of the superiority of the i.v. route in suppressing Rh D immunization comes from an experiment described by Jouvenceaux (1971). D-negative subjects were given 5 ml *cDE/cDE* blood with an injection of 15 μg anti-D, given either i.m. or i.v. At 5 months, when none of the subjects had formed antibody, a second injection of *cDE/cDE* blood (2 ml) was given. Five months later anti-D was present in four of six subjects who had received the anti-D i.m., but in none of eight subjects who had received anti-D i.v. The probability of getting such a difference by chance is only 0.015.

In D-negative women who have inadvertently been transfused with D-positive blood, and particularly when more than 1 unit has been transfused, it is advantageous to give the anti-D immunoglobulin i.v., mainly to avoid the discomfort of injecting large amounts of the material i.m., but also because the dose needed for suppression when

Table 5.7   Administration of anti-D immunoglobulin i.v. to four D-negative women inadvertently transfused with D-positive blood

D-positive blood transfused (units)	Anti-D (μg)		Time to clear D-positive red cells (days)	Reaction	Follow-up
	total given	per ml red cells			
1	3000	15	6	nil	no anti-D at 6 and 12 months
2	5625	14	3	nil	no anti-D at 4 years
2	4000	10	2	haemoglobinuria	no anti-D after 2nd D-positive pregnancy
3	7750	13	8	pyrexia	no anti-D at 8 months

given i.v. is probably smaller. Table 5.7 shows some results in four cases (Mollison, 1983, p. 385). The results of the serological follow-up suggest, but do not prove, that a dose of 10–15 μg anti-D per ml red cells, given i.v., is sufficient to prevent primary Rh D immunization when 1 or more units of D-positive blood are transfused.

The effect of delayed administration of anti-D
In an experiment described by Samson and Mollison (1975), D-negative volunteers were given 1 ml ^{51}Cr-labelled, D-positive red cells, followed 13 d later by an i.m. injection of 100 μg anti-D. Control subjects received only D-positive cells. At 6 months, five of 12 control subjects but no treated subjects had anti-D in their serum. Both treated and control subjects were now given second injections of 1 ml labelled D-positive red cells. After a further 6 months a third injection of labelled D-positive red cells was given to those subjects in the treated group in whom the survival of the second injection had been normal. From these experiments it was concluded that Rh D immunization was completely suppressed in half of the responders in the treated group; that is to say, in these subjects the survival of the second injection was normal but that of a third injection was grossly curtailed and followed by the production of anti-D.

Can Rh D immunization be switched off once it has been initiated?
In a series of pregnant D-negative women in whom anti-D was detected only with enzyme-treated red cells, the injection of anti-D immunoglobulin failed to prevent the development of a progressive increase in anti-D concentration. Moreover, in some women injected with anti-D immunoglobulin at a time when they had no detectable antibody, immunization subsequently developed, suggesting that once primary Rh D immunization has been initiated the process cannot be reversed by passively administered antibody (Bowman and Pollock, 1984).

Failure of passively administered anti-D to affect secondary responses
In one experiment with randomized controls, in subjects with relatively low concentrations of IgG anti-D in their plasma the i.m. injection of 500 μg anti-D failed to modify the response to 0.3 ml red cells (De Silva et al. 1985).

Possible augmentation by passive antibody

Rh D immunization facilitated by small amounts of 'passive' IgG anti-D?
There is suggestive evidence that when D-positive red cells are injected with a relatively small dose of IgG anti-D into D-negative subjects, the probability of Rh D immunization is increased. This effect was first noted in experiments in which a fixed amount of red cells (approximately 2.25 ml) was injected i.v. together with varying amounts of anti-D (1–40 μg) i.m. As judged by the formation of anti-D within 3 months, subjects receiving 10 μg anti-D (at an approximate ratio of 4.5 μg anti-D per ml red cells) had an increased chance of responding, i.e. eight of 11 made anti-D compared with one of six receiving no anti-D and with seven of 25 who received either 1 μg or 20 μg anti-Rh (Pollack *et al.* 1968a).

These results, though suggestive, were not statistically significant. In two later studies the administration of a small dose of IgG anti-D with D-positive red cells has also resulted in a suggestive increase in the proportion of responders:
1   In a trial carried out at five different centres, 83 of 113 (73%) subjects injected with 7 ml red cells and 10 μg anti-D (1.4 μg anti-D per ml red cells) became immunized compared with 53 of 98 (54%) of subjects receiving only 7 ml red cells (W.Q. Ascari, personal communication, 1984). Although these results are very suggestive of augmentation, the data were somewhat heterogeneous.
2   Subjects who were injected with 0.8 ml red cells and 1 μg anti-D: nine of 13 subjects made anti-D within 6 months and two more made anti-D after a second injection of red cells (Contreras and Mollison, 1983). These results were compared with those observed earlier in subjects given 1 ml red cells alone from the same donor; amongst these subjects four of 12 made anti-D after a single injection of red cells and two more after a second injection. Apart from the fact that this was not a strictly controlled experiment, the difference observed between the numbers making anti-D after a first stimulus (nine of 13 vs. four of 12) was only just significant ($P < 0.05$). Nevertheless, the dose (1.25 μg anti-D per ml red cells) which produced suggestive augmentation was very close to that used in Ascari's study. In both studies the dose that appeared to produce an increase in the proportion of responders was appreciably lower than that (4.5 μg/ml cells) found by Pollack *et al.* (1968a) to be augmenting but, as discussed above, it is possible that the anti-D content of the preparation used by Pollack *et al.* may have been overestimated. In another series in which D-negative subjects were given 1 ml D-positive cells with 5 μg anti-D there was mild suppression of the immune response as judged by the anti-D concentration of plasma after a second injection of red cells, viz. a mean of 0.55 μg/ml compared with 8.6 μg/ml in a control series (Contreras and Mollison, 1981).

Effect of IgM anti-D
As described in Chapter 3, there is convincing evidence, derived from animal experiments, that passively administered IgM antibody can augment immunization. It is probable that all the IgM antibodies which have been shown to have this effect are capable of activating complement and it is very doubtful whether the same effect can be produced by a non-complement-binding IgM antibody such as anti-D. As discussed in Chapter 10, evidence that IgM anti-D alone can destroy red cells is very meagre. If it cannot mediate red cell–macrophage interaction, it is doubtful whether it can affect immunization.

In an often-quoted experiment, of 11 D-negative volunteers who were given two i.v. injections of D-positive red cells alone, only one became immunized, whereas of 13 who were given two i.v. injections of cells with an i.v. dose of plasma containing agglutinating anti-D, eight became immunized (Clarke *et al.* 1963). This result certainly suggests that the effect of the agglutinating anti-D was to increase the probability of Rh D immunization, but this may not be the correct interpretation. It is possible that the effect was due instead to the relatively small amount of IgG anti-D which was present in the plasma (in addition to the IgM anti-D).

Experiments with purified IgM anti-D appeared to show that the antibody could clear D-positive red cells (Holburn *et al.* 1971a) but it has subsequently been pointed out that the anti-D preparation may have contained enough IgG antibody to have produced the effect (Mollison, 1986). Accordingly, it now seems unsafe to draw conclusions from these results about the possible augmenting effect of IgM anti-D.

In another experiment, D-negative volunteers injected with D-positive red cells weakly agglutinated by being mixed with plasma containing IgM anti-D formed anti-D after a mean interval of 5.4 weeks compared with 10.75 weeks in subjects injected with untreated D-positive red cells (Lee *et al.* 1977). Three points may be made: the difference in time interval between the two groups was not significant; earlier formation of antibody after immunization is not a recognized effect of immune augmentation; and, if an effect was produced, it could have been due to the presence of small amounts of IgG anti-D in the plasma used for agglutinating the D-positive red cells.

Treatment of inadvertent D-positive transfusion

In any D-negative woman who is not already immunized to Rh D, and who may have further children, the inadvertent transfusion of D-positive blood should be treated by the administration of a suitable dose of anti-D. In D-negative post-menopausal women or in men who have been transfused with D-positive blood, it does not seem worth trying to suppress Rh D immunization; first, because the consequences to the subject of becoming immunized are not likely to be serious, and second, because treatment with large amounts of anti-D can produce unpleasant effects.

When the decision is taken to try to suppress Rh D immunization in a subject whose circulation contains large amounts of red cells, various questions arise: How much anti-D should be given? Should it be given in a single dose or in divided doses, and by what route should it be given? When anti-D is given i.m. the total dose should be about 25 μg/ml red cells (WHO, 1971). When it is given i.v. it is probable that a lesser dose will suffice, i.e. 10–15 μg/ml red cells. The main advantage of i.v. injection is that it avoids a large and therefore painful i.m. injection. However, the chance of transmitting infection when certain immunoglobulin preparations are given i.v. may be higher than when given i.m. (see Chapter 16). When anti-D is injected i.m., to minimize pain the dose should not all be injected into the same site. However, there is no need to separate the doses in time, since the material is absorbed slowly from the site of injection and the peak concentration in the plasma is not reached for about 48 h. On the other hand, when anti-D is injected i.v. several different types of reaction may be produced, two of which may be caused by injecting too much anti-D within a given period. First, there may be rapid red cell destruction resulting in shivering and fever as in patients described by Huchet *et al.* (1970); in two cases of massive transplacental haemorrhage equivalent to about 75 ml red cells, 600 μg of anti-D were injected i.v. resulting in clearance of the red cells with a $t_{1/2}$ of about 85 min. Second, haemoglobinuria may develop; see Table 5.7 and Chapter 11.

Apart from reactions due to red cell destruction, the i.v. injection of anti-D immunoglobulin may cause immediate, hypersensitivity-type reactions. These may be due to the activation of complement by aggregated IgG in the preparation or, very rarely, to an interaction between IgA in the immunoglobulin preparation and anti-IgA in the recipient's plasma.

Although the i.v. injection of IgG is potentially hazardous, very low reaction rates have been observed following the i.v. injection of anti-D immunoglobulin purified on DEAE-Sephadex (see Chapter 12). In practice, when large amounts of immunoglobulin are being administered at one time, it seems wise to give a dose of hydrocortisone (100 mg i.v.) immediately before the injection of anti-D immunoglobulin. To avoid reactions due to the rapid destruction of large volumes of D-positive cells, it is suggested that the initial dose of anti-D should be limited to about 5 μg per ml D-positive red cells and should be administered, diluted in saline, over a period of 1 h. In the cases recorded in Table 5.7, the anti-D immunoglobulin was always given in divided doses, no more than 2500 μg being given on a single occasion. Provided that no adverse reaction develops after the first injection of anti-D, a further dose of 5 μg/ml red cells may be given after 12 h. Thereafter, rosetting tests should be made to see that the D-positive cells are being cleared reasonably rapidly from the circulation. If all the cells have not been cleared after 2–3 d, a further dose of anti-D should be given.

Preliminary exchange transfusion with D-negative red cells
In D-negative subjects who have been transfused with very large volumes of D-positive red cells, the dose of anti-D needed for the suppression of primary Rh D immunization can be greatly reduced by carrying out a preliminary exchange transfusion with D-negative blood. This manoeuvre is particularly worthwhile in D-negative infants who have inadvertently been transfused with D-positive blood. If an exchange transfusion is now given with D-negative blood, the amount of D-positive red cells remaining in the circulation can be reduced to an amount of the order of 5 or 10 ml (a formula for calculating the amount is given in Chapter 1). It will then be necessary to give only a relatively small dose of anti-D immunoglobulin to ensure that primary Rh D immunization is suppressed. It should be added that evidence of the frequency with which newborn infants become immunized to red cell antigens by transfusion is meagre.

Failure of D antigen, given orally, to induce tolerance
As described in Chapter 3, antigen given orally may induce tolerance; however, there is no evidence that tolerance can be induced to Rh D in this way. In an experiment in male volunteers the administration of D antigen daily by mouth for 2 weeks had no apparent effect on subsequent Rh D immunization, the percentage of subjects forming anti-D after a single i.v. injection of D-positive red cells being virtually the same as in a control group (Barnes *et al* 1987).

CHAPTER 6
OTHER RED CELL ANTIGENS

In this chapter, various other red cell antigens are described in the order in which they were given the status of 'systems'. Then, a list is given of 'collections' of antigens (see below), followed by a description of other high and low frequency antigens.

Corresponding antibodies, both naturally occurring and immune, are also described but only brief notes are included about their clinical significance, which is considered in more detail in Chapters 7, 10, 11 and 12.

THE KELL (K) AND Kx (Xk) SYSTEMS

Antigens
A list of the antigens of the Kell system is given in Table 6.1. K (K1) is by far the most important from a clinical point of view since the corresponding antibody is involved in haemolytic transfusion reactions and in haemolytic disease of the newborn more frequently than any other antibody outside the Rh system.

Nine per cent of the English population are K (K1) positive, having the genotype *KK* or *Kk*; the frequency of *K* is 0.046 and that of *k*, 0.954. In Blacks, *K* is even rarer and less than 0.1% are *KK*. (Throughout this chapter, whenever possible, frequencies of alleles are taken from Race and Sanger, 1975.)

Three other sets of alleles are closely linked to *K* and *k* but only two of these sets, *Kp*^{a}, *Kp*^{b} and *Kp*^{c}, and *Js*^{a} and *Js*^{b}, are known to be clinically important. In Whites, *Kp*^{b} and

Table 6.1 Notations and frequencies of antigens in the Kell blood group system (slightly modified from Marsh and Redman, 1990)

Notation			Antigen
Name	Letter	Number	frequency (%)
Kell	K	K1	9.0
Cellano	k	K2	99.8
Penny	Kp^a	K3	2.0
Rautenberg	Kp^b	K4	>99.9
Peltz (K$_0$)	Ku	K5	>99.9
Sutter	Js^a	K6	< 1.0 in Whites
			19.5 in Blacks
Matthews	Js^b	K7	>99.9 in Whites
			99.9 in Blacks
	Kw	K8	5.0
Claas	KL	K9	>99.9
Karhula	Ul^a	K10	2.6 in Finns
			> 0.1 in others
Côté		K11	>99.9
Bockman		K12	>99.9
Sgro		K13	>99.9
Santini		K14	>99.9
	Kx*	K15	>99.9
	k-like	K16	99.8
Weeks	Wk^a	K17	0.3
Marshall		K18	>99.9
Sublett		K19	>99.9
	Km	K20	>99.9
Levay	Kp^c	K21	< 0.1
Ikar		K22	>99.9
Centauro	Cent	K23	< 0.1
Callois	Cls	K24	< 2.0

* Kx does not belong to the Kell system but to the *Xk* system.

Js^b have a very high frequency. Although *Js^a* is rare in Whites, it is not uncommon in Blacks. In the extremely rare null phenotype K$_0$ none of the seven antigens mentioned above is present on red cells, although larger than normal amounts of Kx are present.

The antigen Kx is expressed most strongly in red cells which lack Kell antigens, i.e. K$_0$ red cells. Similarly, red cells treated with 2-aminoethylisothiouronium bromide (AET), to destroy Kell antigens and produce artificial K$_0$ red cells, have a high expression of Kx (Advani *et al.* 1982).

Kx is probably determined by an X-borne gene, X^1k, although it is possible that *Xk* (the gene determining the McLeod phenotype, see below) is a regulator of both *Kx* and *Kell*; when Kx is not expressed, as in the McLeod phenotype, Kell antigenic activity is diminished. Although the biochemical relationship between Kx and K is unknown, the two proteins on which these antigens are carried are known to be different (Marsh and Redman, 1990).

In the numerical notation, phenotypes are designated according to reactions with particular antibodies; e.g. a sample reacting negatively with anti-K is designated K: – 1; if the sample has also reacted positively with anti-k, it is designated K: – 1,2.

Relationship between Kell groups and chronic granulomatous disease (CGD)
Some patients with X-linked CGD have red cells with greatly weakened Kell antigens
(Giblett *et al.* 1971) and no Kx (Marsh *et al.* 1975); such cells are said to be of the
McLeod phenotype. The majority of patients with X-linked CGD have red cells of
common Kell types with a normal amount of Kx (P. Tippett, personal communication).
A third type of patient has McLeod red cells but has normal leucocytes and does not
have CGD.

In patients with the McLeod syndrome about 30% of the red cells exhibit acanthocytosis with decreased permeability to water and an associated haemolytic anaemia
(Taswell *et al.* 1976; Wimer *et al.* 1977; Symmans *et al.* 1979). All of 11 patients with the
McLeod syndrome, but without CGD, were found to have high levels of serum creatine
phosphokinase and evidence of muscle cell changes; patients with the McLeod syndrome and CGD have either normal or raised levels of the enzyme (Marsh *et al.* 1981).

Numbers of K and k antigen sites
Using ^{125}I-labelled anti-K the average number of K antigen sites was found to be 6100
on *KK* red cells and 3500 on *Kk* cells (Hughes-Jones and Gardner, 1971). Fairly similar
figures, namely between 2300 and 5900 sites on *Kk* cells, were found using ferritin-
labelled anti-IgG (Masouredis *et al.* 1980a); the number of k sites, both on *Kk* and *kk*
cells, was found to be 2000–5000.

Using an ^{125}I-labelled Kell-related monoclonal antibody which agglutinates all cells
except K_0 and AET-treated cells and which only weakly agglutinates McLeod cells,
the number of binding sites per red cell was estimated to be 2500–5900. However, the
same number of sites was estimated for K_0 and for McLeod cells, indicating that the
Kell-related protein might not be absent from these cells but present in an abnormal
form for which the antibody has a low affinity (Merry *et al.* 1984a).

The major antigens of the Kell system are absent from platelets (Dunstan *et al.*
1984).

Molecular biology and chemistry of Kell antigens
The protein which carries Kell (K1) has a mol. wt. of 93 000. The antigens k, Kp^b, Ku
and Js^b, together with the high frequency antigens K12, 14, 18, 19, 22 and 23, are
also carried on a 93-kD protein which may be identical to the glycoprotein carrying
K1. Knowledge derived from cloning of the *Kell* gene indicates that the protein has 732
amino acids, 665 of which are extracellular, and that there are 16 cysteines,
suggesting that the external part of the molecule is highly folded, in agreement with its
sensitivity to reducing agents. There are six glycosylation sites. The molecule has
striking similarities to neutral endopeptidase (Lee *et al.* 1991). It is not known whether
differences in oligosaccharides or in amino acid sequences of the Kell glycoprotein or
both are responsible for the differences between the various antigens of the Kell
system.

Treatment of red cells with a reagent 'ZZAP', containing 0.1 mol/l dithiothreitol
(DTT) and 0.1% papain, inactivates Kell antigens (Branch and Petz, 1980). Treatment
of red cells with DTT at very low concentrations (2 mmol/l) denatures Js^a and Js^b
whereas much higher concentrations (100–200 mmol/l) are required for the denaturation of K, k, Kp^a, Kp^b and Ku. These results suggest that at least two disulphide bonds
are required for maintenance of Kell antigenic integrity and that Js^a and Js^b are either

located on a different molecule from that carrying the other Kell antigens, or are on the same molecule but at an antigenic site dependent on more labile disulphide bonds (Branch *et al.* 1983). On the other hand, treatment with 2 mmol/l DTT enhances the expression of Kx on normal red cells and results in the expression of Kx on McLeod cells, although in lower amounts than on normal cells (Branch *et al.* 1985).

K_0 red cells, occurring naturally or produced by treating red cells of common groups with AET (see above), may be useful in demonstrating that antibodies are or are not recognizing antigens within the Kell blood group system and may also be useful in recognizing antibodies outside the Kell system when these are present together with Kell antibodies (Advani *et al.* 1982). However, some antigens outside the Kell system are also inactivated by AET, and antigens or antibodies should not be ascribed to the Kell system on the sole basis of the reactions of antibodies with AET-treated cells.

Kell antigens are inactivated after the combined treatment of red cells with trypsin and chymotrypsin; treatment with either of these enzymes separately enhances the expression of Kell antigens (Judson and Anstee, 1977).

The membranes of acanthocytic red cells of McLeod phenotype have a normal phospholipid composition and distribution but a markedly enhanced transbilayer mobility of phosphatidylcholine (Kuypers *et al.* 1985).

Red cells can acquire K-like antigens; the red cells of a K-negative patient with *Streptococcus faecium* septicaemia were shown to react with anti-K. K-negative red cells became agglutinable by anti-K when treated *in vitro* with the streptococcus isolated from the patient. Jk (b –) cells also became agglutinable by anti-Jk[b] when this organism was disrupted and used to treat the cells (McGinniss *et al.* 1984).

Kell antigens on other cells. Using immunofluorescence flow cytometry, K and k antigens were not detected on lymphocytes, monocytes or granulocytes (Dunstan, 1986a) or on platelets (Dunstan *et al.* 1984).

Antibodies of the Kell and Xk systems

Anti-K
Naturally occurring anti-K is rare. Although an example which was IgG has been described (Mollison 1967, p. 344), most examples of non-immune anti-k are IgM, usually reacting best at room temperature and, in some cases, first found after an illness and disappearing following the patient's recovery (Tegoli *et al.* 1967a; Kanel *et al.* 1978; Marsh *et al.* 1978; Judd *et al.* 1981). In the case described by Marsh *et al.* (1978), the antigenic stimulus was an infection with an uncommon strain of *Escherichia coli* 0 125 : B15. A cell-free filtrate of a culture of the organisms inhibited the anti-K (and the anti-A) in the serum of the patient, who was a newborn infant. Both the anti-K and the anti-A had disappeared by the time the infant was 3 months old. The patient described by Kanel *et al.* (1978) had pulmonary lesions suggestive of tuberculosis but no organisms were indentified; the patient of Tegoli *et al.* (1967a) also had tuberculosis.

It has been shown that some strains of *Campylobacter jejuni* and *Campylobacter coli*, major aetiological agents of gastrointestinal infections in humans, carry surface sites reactive with anti-K (Wong *et al.* 1985).

Outside the ABO and Rh systems, anti-K is the commonest immune red cell antibody, accounting for almost two-thirds of non-Rh immune red cell alloantibodies (see Table 3.6, p. 112). An estimate of the frequency with which it is formed in K-negative subjects transfused with at least 1 unit K-positive blood was made by Kornstad and Heistö (1957). In a series of 130 such subjects, 53 were tested at 4–12 months and five had anti-K; of the remaining 77 subjects, tested at 13–37 months, only one had anti-K. The authors concluded that the probability that a K-negative subject transfused with a unit of K-positive blood would develop anti-K was about 1 in 10. If this estimate were correct, K would be eight times less immunogenic than D, but it may be even less immunogenic than this.

Other evidence of the immunogenicity of K comes from two series of experiments: in the first, three spaced injections of K-positive red cells were given to 16 subjects, at least ten of whom were K negative; none formed anti-K (Wiener et al. 1955). In the second, a series of injections of K-positive, D-positive red cells was given to 31 K-negative, D-negative subjects (F.M. Roberts, personal communication). Of the 19 subjects who failed to form anti-D, none formed anti-K. Of the 12 who formed anti-D, six formed anti-K but it is well known that subjects who make anti-D have a greatly increased chance of making antibodies to other antigens carried by the immunizing D-positive red cells (see pp. 116–117).

Opportunities for alloimmunization to K as a result of pregnancy are relatively common but, assuming that K is ten times less immunogenic than D, it can be shown that the incidence of haemolytic disease of the newborn due to anti-K in second pregnancies would be expected to be only about 1 in 3500 (Mollison, 1983, p. 405).

Among 13 000 pregnant women tested by E.R. Giblett (personal communication) anti-K was found in 13, an incidence of 1 in 1000, but most of the women whose serum contained anti-K gave a history of a previous blood transfusion.

In screening samples for anti-K, *Kk* red cells are almost always used; since some samples of anti-K can be detected only with *KK* red cells, the estimates given above for the frequency of anti-K must be too low.

The woman in whose serum anti-K was first discovered (Coombs et al. 1946) had been transfused previously with blood from her husband (information not in the original paper), as had the woman investigated by Chown (1949) who emphasized the moral 'never transfuse a woman with her husband's blood'.

Anti-k
Anti-k was first found in the serum of a recently delivered woman whose infant was mildly affected with haemolytic disease of the newborn (Levine et al. 1949). The rarity of the antibody can be partly accounted for by the fact that only three in 1000 White subjects are k-negative (i.e. *KK*).

A mouse monoclonal anti-k has been described (Sonneborn et al. 1983).

Other antibodies of the K system and antibodies of the Xk system
Anti-Kp^a, anti-Kp^b, anti-Js^a and anti-Js^b are all rare. Anti-Ku deserves special mention because it reacts with all samples except those of the phenotype K_0 and is found only in K_0 subjects (Corcoran et al. 1961). Anti-KL found in patients with the McLeod syndrome is a mixture of anti-Kx and anti-Km. Anti-KL is found only after transfusion.

Anti-Km reacts with all samples except K_0 and Kx negative; anti-Kx, on the other hand, reacts strongly with K_0 red cells, which possess greatly increased amounts of Kx (Marsh et al. 1975). Anti-Kx can cause rapid destruction of Kx-positive red cells, associated with haemoglobinuria, but does not interfere with the successful transfusion of granulocytes (Taswell et al. 1976), implying an absence of Kx from such cells.

The original example of anti-Kp^a appeared to be naturally occurring (Allen and Lewis, 1957); this antibody and anti-Kp^b occur as autoantibodies (see Chapter 7); the other antibodies mentioned in this section have been described only as immune alloantibodies.

A mouse monoclonal antibody reacting with all cells tested except K_0 and giving weak reactions with McLeod red cells was reported by Parsons et al. (1982). Specificities of other murine monoclonals reported since include anti-K2 and anti-K14 (Nichols et al. 1987a) and anti-Kp^{bc} (Parsons et al. 1991).

Serological characteristics of immune anti-K and anti-k

Anti-K and anti-k are usually IgG. Kell antibodies were found to be solely IgG1 in seven of eight and 12 of 14 cases, respectively (Engelfriet, 1978; Hardman and Beck, 1981). As with anti-D, sera containing only IgG anti-K may, when undiluted, agglutinate saline-suspended cells. Many examples of IgG anti-K activate complement but only to the C3 stage, and are non-lytic.

Anti-K may be IgM but only the most potent examples agglutinate red cells suspended in saline; weaker examples sensitize red cells to agglutination by anti-IgM. Two examples of IgM anti-K examined by Polley (1964) gave stronger indirect antiglobulin reactions with anti-complement than with anti-IgM.

Anti-K tends to react poorly in low-ionic-strength solution (LISS) and may be relatively difficult to detect when the LISS indirect antiglobulin test (IAT), or the low-ionic strength polybrene method, with or without the IAT, are used and in the AutoAnalyzer (see Chapter 8).

Studies with ^{125}I-labelled anti-K

The equilibrium constants of several examples of IgG anti-K ranged from 0.6 to 4.5 $\times$ 10^{10} l/mol, figures which are 100 times greater than those found with IgG anti-D, indicating that, if anti-K binds monovalently, its intrinsic affinity for K must be much higher than that of anti-D for D. The concentration of anti-K corresponding to an indirect antiglobulin titre of 1 is about the same as for anti-D (Hughes-Jones and Gardner, 1971).

Clinical aspects

Anti-K and much less frequently anti-k and anti-Kp^a can cause severe haemolytic transfusion reactions and severe haemolytic disease of the newborn. Anti-Js^a and anti-Js^b have rarely been reported to cause mild or moderate haemolytic disease of the newborn, and anti-Ku has once been reported as causing disease severe enough to need transfusion (for references, see Vengelen-Tyler, 1984). Anti-K has several times been the cause of haemolytic transfusion reactions due to interdonor incompatibility (see Chapter 11 and West et al. 1986). Antibodies of the Kell system, particularly anti-Kp^b, may be found as autoantibodies in autoimmune haemolytic anaemia; there may be concomitant depression of the patient's own Kell antigens (see Chapter 7).

Acquired transient depression of Kell antigens with red cells resembling those of the McLeod phenotype was seen in a young patient with autoimmune thrombo-cytopenic purpura who developed a transient antibody to a high incidence Kell antigen (Vengelen-Tyler *et al.* 1987).

THE DUFFY (Fy) SYSTEM

The red cells of about 66% of the English population are Fy(a +), belonging to the genotype Fy^aFy^a or Fy^aFy^b, the remainder being Fy^bFy^b (Cutbush *et al.* 1950).

In Whites, the genes Fy^a and Fy^b have frequencies of 0.425 and 0.557, respectively; a further gene, Fy^x, which makes a weak form of Fy^b, has a frequency of 0.016. In Whites, the frequency of the gene *Fy*, which produces neither Fy^a nor Fy^b, is only 0.002 but in Blacks in the USA is about 0.7. In parts of tropical Africa the frequency of *Fy* is 1.0, all the native inhabitants having the phenotype Fy(a – b –) (Mourant *et al.* 1976).

The *Fy* locus is on chromosome 1; it was the first to be assigned to an autosome in humans (Donahue *et al.* 1968).

Further antigens, Fy3, Fy4, Fy5, have been described; the last is of particular interest since 'it may be formed by the interaction of the Rh and Duffy gene products' (Colledge *et al.* 1973).

Fy^a and Fy^b sites on red cells and nature of the Fy^a and Fy^b antigens
The number of Fy^a sites on Fy^aFy^a red cells and of Fy^b sites on Fy^bFy^b red cells was estimated to be 17 000; the number of Fy^a sites on Fy^aFy^b was estimated to be 6900 (Masouredis *et al.* 1980b). Using an immunoaffinity technique for isolating antigens in the form of soluble antigen–antibody complexes, Moore (1983) showed that the Fy^a and Fy^b antigens are associated with membrane components of apparent mol. wt. 40 000. However, since Fy^a and Fy^b antigens are present on Rh_{null} cells, known to be LW(a –), the relationship between Duffy and LW remains unknown. By immunoblot-ting of red cell ghosts using a potent anti-Fy^a, Hadley *et al.* (1984) were able to locate the Fy^a antigen on a protein of 35 000–43 000 mol. wt. migrating between bands 5 and 6. The Fy^a antigen is destroyed by crude preparations of proteolytic enzymes though not by crystalline trypsin (or neuraminidase); it is destroyed by chymotrypsin (Morton, 1962; Judson and Anstee, 1977). Fy3, 4 and 5 are not destroyed by papain. Inactivation of Fy^a by proteases and neuraminidase and the binding of the Fy^a-carrying protein to concanavalin A and wheatgerm agglutinin indicates that it is a glycoprotein (Hadley *et al.* 1986). Treatment of membrane components with endoglycosidase F (Endo F) sharpened the diffuse band, carrying Fy^a activity, obtained by immunoblotting to a band of 26 000 mol. wt.; it was concluded that the Fy^a protein is heavily glycosylated, with 40–50% of its mass consisting of N-glycosidically linked oligosacchar-ides (Tanner *et al.* 1988).

Fy^a and Fy^b tend to elute from red cells stored in a low pH low-ionic-strength medium, leading to the appearance of substances with specific inhibitory activity for anti-Fy^a or anti-Fy^b in the supernatant fluid. Duffy antigens also elute from red cells after prolonged storage, or mixing, in saline at pH 7.0 (Williams *et al.* 1981).

Fy antigens on other cells. Using a sensitive radioimmunoassay, Fy antigens were shown to be absent from platelets (Dunstan *et al.* 1984). Using immunofluorescence flow cytometry. Fy^a, Fy^b and Fy5 were not detected on lymphocytes, monocytes or granulocytes (Dunstan, 1986a).

Duffy groups and malaria

Fy(a – b –) subjects are protected from infection by *Plasmodium vivax* (Miller *et al.* 1986), although Fy^a and Fy^b are not themselves the receptors for *P. vivax* (Mason *et al.* 1977; see also review by Valko, 1988).

A recently described antigen, Fy6, defined by a murine monoclonal antibody reacting with most human red cells except those of the phenotype Fy(a – b –), is responsible for the susceptibility of red cells to penetration by *P. vivax*. In non-human primates, the presence of Fy6 is associated with susceptibility of red cells to penetration by *P. vivax*, regardless of the presence of the Fy antigens. Invasion of red cells of some of these primates by *P. knowlesi* is not associated with the presence of Fy6 (Nichols *et al.* 1987b). Evidence that the Fy6 determinant, or a closely related epitope on the Duffy glycoprotein, acts as a ligand for the invasion of human red cells by merozoites of *P. vivax* was provided by a study using an *in-vitro* culture system: human and non-human primate red cells of various Fy phenotypes were incubated with *P. vivax* merozoites and anti-Fy6 (Barnwell *et al.* 1989).

For *P. falciparum* infection, there is no association with Duffy groups, so that Blacks are as susceptible as Whites. There appear to be two sites for invasion of red cells by this parasite, one dependent on sialic acid (see review by Valko, 1988) and one which is sialic acid independent and which may be on glycophorin C (Pasvol *et al.* 1984).

Antibodies of the Duffy system

Anti-Fy^a

This antibody occurs about three times less frequently than anti-K (see Table 3.6, p. 112). Only one example of naturally occurring anti-Fy^a has been described (Rosenfield *et al.* 1950). Most examples of anti-Fy^a are IgG; about 50% activate complement up to C3.

Anti-Fy^a (and -Fy^b) are predominantly IgG1; in three series they were solely of this subclass in six of seven, 12 of 14 and 11 of 16 cases, respectively (Engelfriet, 1978; Hardman and Beck, 1981; Szymanski *et al.* 1982). In the last of these series, three anti-Fy^a had an IgG2 component and four were partly IgM; two anti-Fy^b were entirely IgG1.

Despite the susceptibility of Fy^a to damage by proteolytic enzymes, anti-Fy^a can readily be detected in the AutoAnalyzer using bromelin-treated red cells (Rosenfield *et al.* 1964b).

Occasionally, anti-Fy^a agglutinates Fy(a +) red cells suspended in saline and may react with Fy(a + b –) cells more strongly than with Fy(a + b +) cells (Race *et al.* 1953). Sometimes, in a subject in whose serum anti-Fy^a can be detected only by the IAT, following antigenic stimulation anti-Fy^a agglutinating activity develops. Two such examples were described in the second edition of this book (Mollison, 1956, p. 242). A similar phenomenon occurs with anti-D (see p. 233) and anti-K. Some anti-Fy^a fail to react in manual polybrene and polybrene-antiglobulin tests (Malde *et al.* 1986).

Fy^a is significantly more immunogenic in Fy(a – b +) Whites than it is in Fy(a – b –) Blacks. In two series, of 25 and 130 patients with anti-Fy^a, four and 11, respectively, were Fy(a – b –) Blacks (Kosanke 1983; Vengelen-Tyler, 1983); in the second series, none of 11 patients with anti-Fy^b was Black.

Anti-Fy^b
Anti-Fy^b is much rarer than anti-Fy^a; a few examples agglutinate red cells suspended in saline. An example of naturally occurring anti-Fy^b reacting by the indirect anti-globulin technique was described by Issitt (1985).

Anti-Fy3, -Fy4 and -Fy5
Anti-Fy3 reacts with all human red cells except those of the phenotype Fy(a – b –) (Albrey *et al.* 1971). Since the latter phenotype is approximately 100 000 times commoner in Blacks than in Whites, it is very surprising that of the five examples of anti-Fy3 which had been reported up to 1981 only three were in Blacks (Oberdorfer *et al* 1974; Molthan and Crawford, 1978; Oakes *et al.* 1978).

Anti-Fy4 reacts with all Fy(a – b –) cells from Blacks and with most Fy(a + b –) and Fy(a – b +) cells from Blacks, i.e. of presumed genotypes *Fy^{a}Fy* and *Fy^{b}Fy*, respectively.

Anti-Fy5 reacts with most red cells except with Fy(a – b –) cells from Blacks, with Rh$_{null}$ cells (Colledge *et al.* 1973) or with cells carrying variant forms of the e antigen regardless of their Fy status (Meredith, 1985).

Both anti-Fy4 and anti-Fy5 are extremely rare.

Clinical aspects
Duffy antibodies seldom cause severe haemolytic transfusion reactions; they only occasionally cause haemolytic disease of the newborn which is then usually mild.

Fy antibodies have been implicated in delayed haemolytic transfusion reactions in multitransfused Black patients with sickle cell disease. Of five patients with anti-Fy3 or anti-Fy5, four had evidence of delayed haemolytic transfusion reactions; anti-Fy^a preceded the appearance of anti-Fy3 or anti-Fy5 (Vengelen-Tyler, 1985). In another series, five Fy(a – b – 3 –) patients with sickle cell disease experienced delayed haemolytic transfusion reactions or failed to show the desired HbA increment after transfusion; they all had anti-Fy^a and other alloantibodies in the serum (Le Pennec *et al.* 1987).

Mimicking anti-Fy^b has been found in autoimmune haemolytic anaemia (see Chapter 7).

THE KIDD (Jk) SYSTEM

About 76% of Whites possess the Jk^a antigen; 26% have the genotype *Jk^{a}Jk^a*, phenotype Jk(a + b –), and 50% have the genotype *Jk^{a}Jk^b*, phenotype Jk(a + b +). The remaining 24% have the genotype *Jk^{b}Jk^b*, phenotype Jk(a – b +). Gene frequencies in Whites: *Jk^a*, 0.514; *Jk^b*, 0.486. The number of Jk^a sites on *Jk^{a}Jk^a* red cells has been estimated to be 14 000 per red cell (Masouredis *et al.* 1980b).

The type Jk (a – b –) was first recognized in a Filipino (Pinkerton *et al.* 1959) and several reports of Jk (a – b –) subjects, mainly in the Far East, have been described (see Race and Sanger, 1975, pp. 366–7). Only three Jk (a – b –) Caucasian propositi have been reported (Habibi *et al.* 1976; Klarkowski, 1984; Sistonen, 1984), the latter was a female with four Jk (a – b –) sibs. Two different genetic backgrounds seem to be responsible for the Jk (a – b –) phenotype: a silent recessive gene *Jk* (Race and Sanger, 1975) or a dominant inhibitor of the expression of Kidd antigens (Okubo *et al.* 1986).

Whereas normal red cells, when exposed to 2 mol/l urea, rapidly become swollen and spherocytic before lysing, Jk (a – b –) red cells exhibit shrinkage and crenation and lyse relatively slowly (Heaton and McLoughlin, 1982). Urea, 2 mol/l, penetrates the membrane of the red cells of all Jk phenotypes but selectively blocks the entrance of water to Jk (a – b –) cells (Edwards-Moulds and Kasschau, 1986). This unusual behaviour of Jk (a – b –) red cells in 2 mol/l urea was used in screening 638 460 Osaka blood donors; 14 Jk (a – b –) were found. Polyacrylamide gel electrophoresis in the absence of SDS, on the membranes of the Jk (a – b –) red cells revealed an unusual protein of very approximate mol. wt. 67 000 (Okubo *et al.* 1986).

Kidd antigens were found to be absent from platelets when using a sensitive radioimmunoassay (Dunstan *et al.* 1984) and from lymphocytes, monocytes and granulocytes when using immunofluorescence flow cytometry (Dunstan, 1986a).

Antibodies
The first example of anti-Jk^a was discovered in the serum of a woman who had given birth to an infant with haemolytic disease of the newborn (Allen *et al.* 1951). Anti-Jk^b is rarer than anti-Jk^a, and is usually found in sera that contain other immune blood group antibodies. The antibody anti-Jk^{a}Jk^b (i.e. inseparable), also known as anti-Jk3, was found in the serum of the Jk (a – b –) patient described by Pinkerton *et al.* (1959). Several examples have been found since, mainly in Polynesians or Chinese people. A naturally occurring example was described by Arcara *et al.* (1969).

Anti-Jk^a and anti-Jk^b invariably bind complement and may give stronger reactions in the IAT with anti-C3 than with anti-IgG. In identifying anti-Jk^a a dosage effect is common with all tests, so that positive results may be obtained only with *Jk^{a}Jk^a* cells. Anti-Jk^a may lyse ficin-treated red cells, and characteristically shows a striking dosage effect, so that lysis of *Jk^{a}Jk^a* cells may be 100% but that of *Jk^{a}Jk^b* cells only 25% (Haber and Rosenfield, 1957).

Anti-Jk^a (and anti-Jk^b) are usually IgG but may be IgM. Of 15 examples of anti-Jk^a tested by Polley *et al.* (1962) using specific antiglobulin sera, 12 were IgG, two IgM and one a mixture of IgG and IgM. One anti-Jk^b, selected because it failed to sensitize red cells to agglutination by anti-IgG, sensitized them to anti-IgM; fractionation of this serum on DEAE-cellulose confirmed that the antibody was wholly IgM. Occasionally, anti-Jk^a sera agglutinate red cells suspended in saline, but most examples of IgM anti-Jk^a and anti-Jk^b do not.

Naturally occurring antibodies within the Kidd system have not been described.

Anti-Jk^a and anti-Jk^b were found to be predominantly IgG3 in three of three cases (Engelfriet, 1978), and a mixture of IgG1 and IgG3 in 16 of 17 cases (Hardman and Beck, 1981). In the latter series, in contrast with Fy antibodies, Jk^a antibodies were found to be very heterogeneous: of ten examples, seven were found to have an IgG3 component and two of these were solely IgG3; seven were partly IgG1, six partly IgG2, three had an IgG4 component: five had an IgM component.

Three IgM human monoclonal anti-Jk^b and one IgM anti-Jk^a have been produced from the Epstein–Barr virus (EBV) transformed lymphocytes of immunized donors. The antibodies are specific and agglutinate cells, even of phenotype Jk (a + b +), in saline after an immediate spin (Thompson *et al.* 1991).

Clinical aspects
It is not uncommon for Kidd antibodies to become undetectable within a few months of first being detected. Anti-Jk^a is a relatively common cause of haemolytic transfusion reactions, particularly of the delayed type; it only very rarely causes haemolytic disease of the newborn. Anti-Jk^a has occasionally been found as an autoantibody in autoimmune haemolytic anaemia (see Chapter 7). A transient auto-anti-Jk^b was apparently stimulated by proteus urinary tract infection; Jk (b –) red cells pre-incubated with *Proteus mirabilis* became agglutinable by anti-Jk^b (McGinniss *et al.* 1979).

Temporary suppression of Jk^a was observed in a patient of phenotype Jk (a + b –), in association with the development of anti-Jk^{a}Jk^b (anti-Jk3); the antibody appeared to be responsible for a haemolytic reaction following the transfusion of Jk (a + b –) blood (Issitt *et al.* 1990b).

THE MNSs SYSTEM

Antigens
The antigens M and N were discovered by injecting human red cells into rabbits, absorbing the resulting immune serum with one sample of human cells and showing that it would still react with other samples (Landsteiner and Levine, 1927).

M and *N* are alleles giving rise to three genotypes, *MM, MN* and *NN*, with frequencies in Whites of about 28%, 50% and 22%, respectively. The corresponding phenotypes are written M + N – , M + N + and M – N + . When tested with most anti-M, M + N – red cells react more strongly than M + N + cells. Red cells of the phenotype M + N – show some reaction with anti-N except when they come from a subject who is S negative, s negative, because the Ss glycoprotein also carries the amino-terminal determinant with N specificity, sometimes written 'N' (see below).

As described in more detail below, in the section on the chemistry of MN and Ss blood group systems, M and N are carried on glycophorin A (MN glycoprotein) and the antigens S and s are carried on glycophorin B (Ss glycoprotein). The inheritance of S and s is closely associated with that of M and N, i.e. the *Ss* locus is very close to the *MN* locus. The antigen S is found about twice as frequently in *MM* as in *NN* subjects (Sanger *et al.* 1948). Among Whites about 55% are S positive and 89% are s positive (Race and Sanger, 1975). Haplotype frequencies in Britain are as follows: *MS*, 0.247; *Ms*, 0.283; *NS*, 0.080; *Ns*, 0.390.

Rare genetic variants associated with MN *and* Ss
There are many rare genetic variants associated with the MNSs blood group system. Some of these variants behave as alleles of *M* and *N*, e.g. *M^g*. Others are due to: (1)

complete absence of MN glycoprotein, as in some types of En (a –) red cells; (2) complete absence of MN and Ss glycoproteins, as in the extremely rare genotype M^kM^k; (3) complete absence of the Ss glycoprotein, as in subjects with red cells of the phenotype S – s – ; (4) mutant forms of the MN glycoprotein, as in Mi. (Miltenberger) I, Mi.II, Mi.VII and Mi.VIII; (5) abnormal forms of the Ss glycoprotein, as in Mi.III; or (6) hybrid molecules composed of a part of the MN glycoprotein linked to a part of the Ss glycoprotein, e.g. Mi.V, Dantu, St^a.

There are also low frequency antigens, e.g. M^v, Ri^a, which may be inherited with M or N. Corresponding antibodies have occasionally been the cause of clinically significant red cell destruction (see below).

M^g does not react either with anti-M or anti-N, and for this reason can be the cause of serious errors in interpreting the MNSs results in paternity testing. For example, a child born to an M^gM father (typing as M + N –) and an MN mother might be M^gN (typing as M – N +) and thus seem to be from a different father. With anti-M, M^gM cells react as if they had a single dose, rather than a double dose, of M which should provide a warning that the cells are unusual.

En (a –). There are at least two kinds of En (a –) red cells: (1) the kind originally described by Furuhjelm *et al.* (1969) in which there is a total absence of the MN glycoprotein but a normal Ss glycoprotein and therefore some trypsin-resistant 'N' activity; and (2) the kind described by Darnborough *et al.* (1969), En (UK), now considered to be probably *En M^k* in which there is a total lack of N and 'N' but a weak trypsin-resistant M; it has been shown that this represents a hybrid molecule of a normal M-active MN glycoprotein amino-terminal with the carboxy-terminal from a normal S-active Ss glycoprotein i.e. an $\alpha\delta$ hybrid (Dahr *et al.* 1978).

Flow cytometric analyses with monoclonal antibodies to glycophorin A support the suggestion that En (UK) represents a hybrid of glycophorins A and B (Langlois *et al.* 1985). Both kinds of En (a –) red cells have a greatly reduced sialic acid content and electrophoretic mobility (Furuhjelm *et al.* 1969). The red cells (if Rh D positive) are agglutinated in saline by IgG anti-D.

Sialic acid deficiency *per se* does not seem to affect red cell survival since the En (a –) condition is not associated wih a haemolytic anaemia (Darnborough *et al.* 1969). Moreover, Tn red cells, which are also sialic acid deficient, may survive normally (see Chapter 7). On the other hand, sialic acid deficiency of red cells induced experimentally with neuraminidase in animals is associated with gross shortening of red cell survival (Jancik and Schauer, 1974; Durocher *et al.* 1975).

Anstee (1981) pointed out that the use of the terms En^a antigen and anti-En^a is inappropriate since what is being observed is the inherited deficiency of glycophorin A and the antibody response of glycophorin A-deficient individuals to the surface of normal cells.

M^k is regarded as a silent allele resulting, in homozygotes, in the absence of MN and Ss antigens. Two M^kM^k individuals investigated by Tokunaga *et al.* (1979) had red cells which completely lacked the MN and Ss glycoproteins and had a sialic acid content between 25% and 31% of normal; both subjects were normal haematologically. Three other M^kM^k propositi have been found: one was a Black child, one a Japanese woman and the third, a Turkish woman (Leak, 1990).

$S - s -$. This phenotype is found mainly in Blacks; it has been found in one Indian family but not yet in Whites. About 16% of $S - s -$ subjects have the antigen U.

U. The U antigen is found in all Whites who have S or s and is found in about 16% of $S - s -$ subjects.

On Rh_{null} cells the Ss and U antigens may be difficult to detect (Schmidt *et al.* 1967), especially when using the IAT. The amount of glycophorin B was found to be reduced to one-third in Rh_{null} cells and it has been suggested that, during biosynthesis, the Rh protein (or proteins) forms a complex with glycophorin B facilitating its incorporation into the red cell membrane (Dahr *et al.* 1987).

The Miltenberger (Mi.) series of antigens, e.g. Vw, Mur, are examples of low-incidence antigens reacting with relatively common alloantibodies, e.g. anti-Vw (Cleghorn, 1966; Giles, 1982). The antigens are inherited together with particular MNSs haplotypes. For a recent review of the chemistry of the antigens, see Dahr (1992).

An MN phenotype associated with a positive antiglobulin test. Red cells with an inherited abnormality characterized by very weak M or N antigens and a positive direct antiglobulin test (with no signs of haemolytic anaemia in the donor) have been described (Jakobowicz *et al.* 1949; Jensen and Freiesleben, 1962). In one case cited by Race and Sanger (1975, p. 106) the cells of a mother and son had a positive direct antiglobulin test (DAT) but had normal M reactions. There is something odd about the positive antiglobulin reactions because the red cells do not react with anti-IgG (Jensen and Freiesleben, 1962) nor with anti-IgA or anti-C3 (Jeannet *et al.* 1964). The latter authors found that anti-IgM was needed for a positive reaction, but anti-IgM does not seem likely to have been present in the antiglobulin sera found by Race and Sanger (1975, p. 472) to give positive reactions.

Numbers of S, s and U antigen sites

The number of available s sites on *ss* red cells was found to be approximately 12 000 and of available U sites on U-positive red cells to be about 17 000 (Masouredis *et al.* 1980b). These numbers are clearly far less than the number of potential sites; it has been estimated that each red cell has about 2.5×10^5 copies of glycophorin B and, incidentally, about 1×10^6 copies of glycophorin A (see review by Anstee *et al.* 1982).

MNSs antigens on other cells. M, N, S, s and U antigens were not detected on lymphocytes, monocytes or granulocytes by immunofluorescence flow cytometry (Dunstan, 1986a). Using a sensitive radioimmunoassay, MNSs antigens could not be detected on platelets (Simpson *et al.* 1987).

Glycophorin A, MN antigens and probably glycophorins B and C have been detected on renal capillary endothelium (Hawkins *et al.* 1985).

Chemistry of the MN and Ss antigens (Fig. 6.1)

As described above, MN and Ss antigens are found respectively on glycophorin A and B of the red cell membrane. Glycophorin A (α-sialoglycoprotein, MN glycoprotein) is composed of 131 amino acids and 16 oligosaccharide chains, 15 of which are O-glycosidically linked to threonine or serine residues (Tomita and Marchesi, 1975) and one, N-glycosidically linked. Studies with endo-β-N-acetylglucosaminidase F

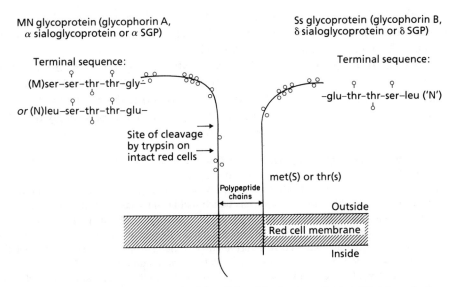

MN glycoprotein (glycophorin A,
  α sialoglycoprotein or α SGP)

Ss glycoprotein (glycophorin B,
  δ sialoglycoprotein or δ SGP)

Terminal sequence:

(M)ser–ser–thr–thr–gly–

or (N)leu–ser–thr–thr–glu–

Terminal sequence:

–glu–thr–thr–ser–leu ('N')

Site of cleavage
by trypsin on
intact red cells

met(S) or thr(s)

Polypeptide
chains

Outside

Red cell membrane

Inside

Figure 6.1 Diagrammatic representation of the MN and Ss glycoproteins (modified from Anstee, 1980). 0 = alkali-labile oligosaccharides.

(Endo F) have confirmed the presence of an N-glycosidically linked oligosaccharide on glycophorin A and its absence from glycophorin B or Ss glycoprotein (Tanner *et al.* 1987).

The only difference between M and N is that the polypeptide chain determining M has the terminal sequence: ser-ser-thr-thr-gly- and that the chain determining N has the terminal sequence: leu-ser-thr-thr-glu- (Wasniowska *et al.* 1977). Some examples of anti-M react with the 'ser' region of the determinant and others with the 'gly' region (Nichols *et al.* 1985).

The content of alkali-labile (i.e. O-linked) oligosaccharides is the same in M and N. That part of the MN glycoprotein which carries M or N specificities is cleaved from the intact red cell by treatment with proteolytic enzymes other than chymotrypsin; accordingly, enzyme treatment 'destroys' the M and N antigens on glycophorin A although 'N' on glycophorin B is trypsin resistant (Judson and Anstee, 1977).

In M^g, determined by an allele at the *MN* locus, the terminal amino acid sequence is the same as that of N, except that asparagine is substituted for threonine in position 4, so that the terminal sequence is leu-ser-thr-asn-glu-. A further difference between M^g and N is that in the former the serine and threonine in positions 2 and 3 are not glycosylated. The absence of glycoside residues contributes to the difference in specificity, emphasizing the importance of the glycosidic residues in determining the specificity of MN groups. In M^c the terminal amino acid sequence is ser-ser-thr-thr-glu; the amino acid residues at positions 2, 3 and 4 are glycosylated as in M and N. Accordingly, the only difference between M^c and M is the substitution of glu for gly in position 5, and the only difference between M^c and N is the substitution of ser for leu in position 1. This finding suggests that the alleles which code for these two forms of MN protein have evolved from a common ancestral gene (Furthmayr *et al.* 1981).

S and s are carried on glycophorin B and differ from one another in a single amino acid substitution, i.e. at position 29 there is a methionine in S and a threonine in s

(Dahr *et al.* 1980b). The Ss glycoprotein on intact red cells is not affected by trypsin treatment but is inactivated by pronase and by high concentration of chymotrypsin (Judson and Anstee, 1977) and by bromelin, ficin and papain.

The first 26 residues of the Ss and the N-specific MN glycoproteins are identical (Dahr *et al.* 1980a), thus explaining the fact that red cells of M + N – subjects, unless they are S – s – , react with anti-N. Nevertheless, with anti-N the reactions of 'N' (see p. 256) and N are not identical: with anti-N, *MM* red cells react less strongly than *MN* red cells, which in turn react less strongly than *NN* red cells.

It seems that oligosaccharides (sialic acid residues) attached to terminal amino acids of the MN glycoprotein, as well as the amino acids themselves, are involved in M and N specificity (Uhlenbruck *et al.* 1976). In investigations reported by Judd *et al.* (1979a) nine of 27 examples of anti-M reacted more weakly with M + red cells which had been treated with neuraminidase, i.e. which had had sialic acid removed. The other 18 examples of anti-M reacted just as well with neuraminidase-treated cells, indicating that in these cases MN specificity was not determined by sialic acid, although it may have been determined by other carbohydrate structures. Of five examples of anti-Vw, four reacted more strongly with neuraminidase-treated red cells, suggesting that sialic acid residues were interfering with the fit of the antibody. The authors pointed out that with the methods they were using only 40–80% of sialic acid was released by neuraminidase treatment, but even with a method which released 95% of sialic acid some antibodies continued to react with the red cells.

Evidence that specific sialic acid structures are important in MN specificity was also provided by Sadler *et al.* (1979). Red cells were treated with neuraminidase to remove sialic acid, then resialated with different sialyltransferases. Although the MN phenotype was never changed by this process, the reactivity of cells with different antisera varied according to which sialyl transferase was used.

Antibodies of the MNSs system

Anti-M
In adults, anti-M is a relatively common naturally occurring antibody reacting optimally at 4°C and weakly or not at all at 37°C. In a case described by Crowley *et al.* (1957) an apparently naturally occurring example had a titre of 64 at 4°C and 25°C, and a titre of 8 at 37°C.

In screening 45 000 blood samples in an AutoAnalyzer using a low-ionic-strength polybrene method against *MN* and *NN* cells, 62 examples of anti-M were found in M-negative individuals (Perrault, 1973b). However, *NN* cells were sometimes used and *MM* cells were never used, so the prevalence of anti-M detectable by this technique, in M subjects, must be substantially greater than 1%. The prevalence of naturally occurring anti-M in all donors, detectable in micro-plates with saline-suspended M + N – or M + N + cells at room temperature is one in 2500 and one in 5000, respectively (A. Lubenko, personal communication).

Anti-M is distinctly commoner in infants than in adults (Strahl *et al.* 1955), a conclusion supported by findings at the Hospital for Sick Children in Toronto. Over a 2-year period, 14 examples of anti-M, agglutinating red cells at room temperature by manual methods, were found among 362 irregular antibodies, most of which were naturally occurring agglutinins such as anti-P_1; i.e. of agglutinins active at room temperature, approximately 4% were anti-M. These findings may be compared with those at the Toronto General Hospital where only adults were tested. Over a 2-year period, 12 examples of anti-M were found among 1157 antibodies which agglutinated red cells at room temperature, i.e. approximately 1% were anti-M.

The development of anti-M in Rh D-immunized subjects following a series of boosting injections has been reported (Wiener, 1950; Teesdale *et al.* 1991). In the latter publication, anti-M developed in three of 25 NN subjects but in two of the three the antibody was very weak and reactive only at room temperature.

Although almost all examples of anti-M occur in M – N + subjects, a few have been found in M + N + subjects (Konugres *et al.* 1966: Schmidt and Taswell, 1969; Howard and Picoff, 1972). In these cases the anti-M was not an autoantibody and may have been directed at some part of the M antigen which the subject lacked. Anti-M occurring as an autoantibody in M + N + subjects has also been described (Fletcher and Zmijewski, 1970; Tegoli *et al.* 1970; Perrault, 1973b).

Using IgG and IgM human anti-M in an enzyme-linked antiglobulin test, M – M + as well as M + M – cells bound significant amounts of immunoglobulin showing that, using non-agglutinating techniques, human anti-M recognizes determinants shared by the M and N antigens (Blumberg *et al.* 1982).

Anti-M detectable only at reduced pH. Some examples of anti-M can be detected only after the serum has been acidified. Twenty-one such examples were found in testing the plasma of 1000 group N donors (Beattie and Zuelzer, 1965). The presence of anti-M should be suspected when an agglutinin is found in the plasma of an ACD (or CPD) sample from a donor in whose unacidified serum no abnormal antibodies can be detected.

Anti-M reacting only with glucose-treated red cells was described by Reid *et al.* (1981). The antibody agglutinated M-positive red cells which had been incubated in 2% glucose for a minimum of 2 h at 37 °C or for substantially longer periods at low temperatures. It also agglutinated red cells from patients with diabetes mellitus. The antibody was first detected when the patient's serum was tested against a commercial panel of red cells suspended in a glucose-containing medium. Red cells which had become agglutinable following glycosylation could be rendered unagglutinable by incubation in saline. The anti-M activity was totally inhibited by adding an equal volume of 1% glucose to the serum. Fourteen other examples of human anti-M were not inhibited by glucose. The anti-M agglutinin described by Morel *et al.* (1981) had a slightly different specificity because it reacted with red cells incubated either with glucose or galactose and was inhibited by 2% glucose, mannose or maltose.

Anti-M$_1$ is found as an additional specificity in about one in three sera containing anti-M; it has only rarely been found on its own. M$_1$ is commoner in Blacks than in Whites (Race and Sanger, 1975).

Immunoglobulin class of anti-M. As might have been expected, an example of naturally occurring anti-M investigated by Adinolfi *et al.* (1962) was shown to be IgM. Similarly, of some ten examples of human anti-M investigated by P. Rubinstein (personal communication) all were at least partly IgM. Nevertheless, naturally occurring anti-M may be IgG: a single case in which anti-M was solely IgG was described by Mollison (1977a, p. 332). Of a series of 45 cases described by Smith and Beck (1977), anti-M was at least partly IgG in 34, being solely IgM in the remainder.

Most anti-M react more strongly in albumin than in saline; one example associated with haemolytic disease of the newborn reacted as well at 37°C as at 4°C (Stone and Marsh, 1959) and was subsequently shown to be IgG (Adinolfi et al. 1962).

Apart from one case of allo-anti-M (see p. 449) and one of auto-anti-N (see below), no examples of anti-M or anti-N have been shown to bind complement using ordinary serological methods. However, in an investigation with ^{125}I-labelled anti-C3d, a small amount of complement appeared to be bound by one example of IgM anti-M, although not by two examples of IgG anti-M (Freedman et al. 1980).

Murine monoclonal antibodies to M and N have been reported (e.g. Fraser et al. 1982; 1985) and are available as blood grouping reagents. Some examples of anti-M have had titres as high as 10 000 with M red cells and have reacted with N cells although only with titres of about 50 (Nichols et al. 1985).

The reactions of monoclonal anti-M and anti-N, like those of some polyclonal anti-M (see above), are greatly affected by pH. Testing the pH dependency of MN monoclonals is important because, in some instances, the specificity of agglutination reactions can be greatly improved by selection of the proper pH (Lisowska, 1987).

Other non-human sources of anti-M and of M

Good anti-M sera can be produced in rabbits; for a method see Menolasino et al. (1954). The anti-M lectin prepared from the seeds of *Iberis amara* (candytuft) does not seem to be a useful reagent.

One strain of pyelonephritogenic *E. coli* was found to have M-specificity (Väisänen et al. 1982). The haemagglutinating activity of certain influenza viruses can be inhibited by glycophorin A (see Dahr, 1986).

Allo-anti-N

Anti-N is rarer than anti-M; in a series of 86 000 patients tested in Toronto (excluding patients on renal dialysis, see below), only two examples were found (B. Croucher, personal communication).

The demonstration that the Ss glycoprotein carries 'N' antigen (see above) explains the old observation that at temperatures of 23°C or lower anti-N will agglutinate M + cells (Hirsch et al. 1957) and also that anti-N will agglutinate trypsin-treated M + cells, since the 'N' antigen on Ss glycoprotein is not destroyed by trypsin.

As expected, anti-N does not react with M + N − , S − s − red cells. Similarly, potent anti-N is found almost exclusively in S − s − subjects (Telischi et al. 1976); examples were described by Francis and Hatcher (1966) and Issitt and Issitt (1975).

Anti-N reacting only with glucose-treated red cells was found in three different sera by Morel et al. (1975). The reactions were inhibited by adding glucose to the serum. Glucose-dependent anti-N requires a determinant resulting from the reaction of glucose with the N-terminal amino acid glycophorin A, but no sialic acid, for binding (Morel et al. 1981; W. Dahr, unpublished observations, cited by Dahr et al. 1981b).

Although naturally occurring anti-N is typically an IgM cold agglutinin, inactive above a temperature of 20–25°C, one naturally occurring IgG anti-N was encountered by Eloise R. Giblett (personal communication).

In screening 45 000 blood samples against M – N + (or M + N +) cells in the AutoAnalyzer, using a low-ionic-strength polybrene method, low titre anti-N not detectable by manual methods was found in six M + N + subjects and in one M + N – subject; a more potent example was found in one M – N + subject (Perrault, 1973b). The last example was remarkable in that it was IgG and could be detected by manual methods only by using a 10–20% cell suspension, no agglutination being obtained with a 2% cell suspension. The antibody was active at 4°C but not at 12°C or at higher temperatures.

It is very rare for anti-N to be formed as an immune antibody. The first example was described by Callender and Race (1946). IgG anti-N developing after multiple transfusions in a subject of phenotype M + N – S – s – U – was described by Ballas et al. (1985).

Anti-Nf developing in patients on chronic haemodialysis

Patients undergoing regular haemodialysis, irrespective of their MN phenotype, may develop anti-N, usually active at 20°C as well as 4°C but never active at 37°C (Howell and Perkins, 1972). The speculation of Howell and Perkins that the stimulus for anti-N production might come from small amounts of red cells left in dialysis equipment previously sterilized by formaldehyde treatment has been fully confirmed; the specificity developed is described as Nf. Exposure of M + N – red cells to 0.06% formaldehyde induces Nf specificity after only 30 s at 37°C; at room temperature exposure to a concentration as low as 0.002% is sufficient to induce Nf specificity in 20 h (Gorst et al. 1977). In a series described by Fassbinder et al. (1978) anti-Nf was found in 68 of 325 patients on renal dialysis. In all the 68 cases a formaldehyde-sterilized dialyser had been used. No example of anti-Nf was found amongst 73 patients in whom a non-formaldehyde-sterilized dialyser was used.

Although anti-Nf, being inactive at 37°C, is not expected to destroy transfused red cells, a case has been described in which the antibody appeared to be responsible for the rejection of a chilled transplanted kidney. When a second kidney from the same cadaver was perfused with warm saline before transplantation, grafting was successful (Belzer et al. 1971).

Anti-N lectins

Anti-N is present in the seeds of *Vicia graminea* (Ottensooser and Silberschmidt, 1953), and also in the seeds of *Bauhinea purpurea* var. *alba* (Boyd et al. 1958). Of the two, the lectin of *Vicia graminea* is the more potent.

The anti-N lectin from *Vicia graminea* reacts not only with N + red cells but also with neuraminidase-treated red cells of all MN phenotypes; however the lectin does not have T specificity (Rolih and Issitt. 1978). The receptor with which the lectin reacts is known as N_{vg}.

A lectin from *Moluccella laevis* apparently carrying anti-A and anti-N on the same molecule was described by Bird and Wingham (1970a). The activity against A and N is inhibited both by D-galactose (related to N specificity) and by *N*-acetylgalactosamine (related to A specificity). The lectin also reacts strongly with T and Tn cells (Bird, 1978a).

Anti-N lectin from *Vicia graminea* reacts with both normal N and 'formaldehyde N' red cells but the lectin from *Moluccella laevis* reacts only with normal N (of group B or O subjects) (Bird and Wingham, 1977b).

Anti-S, anti-s, anti-U

Anti-S has occasionally been found as a naturally occurring antibody (e.g. Constantoulis *et al.* 1955), but is more commonly found as an immune antibody in patients who have received many transfusions.

Some examples of 'incomplete' anti-S can be detected much more readily by incubating serum and red cells at room temperature rather than at 37 °C (Lalezari *et al.* 1973, see below). Although most examples of 'immune' anti-S are incomplete IgG antibodies, two examples behaving as saline agglutinins investigated by Adinolfi *et al.* (1962) were found to be IgM.

Antibodies to low frequency antigens are commonly found in anti-S sera; of nine anti-S investigated with a collection of S-negative rare cells, seven were found to react with one or more cells and two sera contained 15 specificities each (A. Lubenko and MC, personal observations).

Anti-s is rare; it may be IgG or IgM.

In tests in an AutoAnalyzer, Lalezari *et al.* (1973) noted that all of seven examples of anti-s and one of anti-U (all IgG) reacted more strongly at low temperatures. Similarly, using IAT, three examples of anti-s and one of anti-S gave stronger reactions at low temperatures, whereas examples of anti-D, -K and -Fy^a reacted more strongly at 37 °C (cf. p. 334–345).

Anti-U is also rare; as a rule it is a non-complement-binding IgG antibody (Issitt, 1981). The antibody is found exclusively in Blacks. There are two kinds of anti-U, one reacting with about 1.25% of Blacks and one with about 0.25%, i.e. 1% of Blacks have a U variant antigen (see Issitt, 1990). Anti-U is occasionally encountered in frequently transfused patients with sickle cell disease.

Anti-S and anti-U were found to be IgG1 with or without other subclasses in 13 of 17 examples tested. On the other hand, anti-s was found to be solely IgG3 in four of five cases (Hardman and Beck, 1981).

Other antibodies of the MNSs system

Anti-Vw and anti-M^g each has a frequency of 1–2% and most commonly occurs as an agglutinin reacting more strongly at room temperature than at 37 °C.

Anti-Vw, which reacts only with Miltenberger class I cells (Mi.I), occasionally develops immune characteristics and its specificity then broadens to become anti-Mi^a (reacting with Mi.I, II, III, IV and VI cells) (T.E. Cleghorn, personal communication).

'Anti-En^a'

As mentioned above, there is no such antigen as En^a although subjects who lack glycophorin A ('En (a –)') may make a spectrum of antibodies, 'anti-En^a', which are directed against different portions of the glycophorin A molecule (Pavone *et al.* 1981; Vengelen-Tyler *et al.* 1981). Anti-En^a has only once been found as a naturally occurring antibody (Taliano *et al.* 1980), the other examples having been found following transfusion or pregnancy.

The term 'auto-anti-En^a has been used to describe a heterogeneous group of related but not identical specificities, several of which recognize different portions of the MN sialoglycoprotein (Pavone *et al.* 1981). Auto-anti-En^a is found in certain patients with the warm antibody type of autoimmune haemolytic anaemia.

Clinical aspects

The main antibodies of the MNSs system have all been recorded as rare causes of haemolytic transfusion reactions or of causing the destruction of a small dose of labelled red cells: anti-M (Wiener, 1950; see also Chapter 10), anti-N (Ballas *et al.* 1985), anti-S (Mollison and Cutbush, 1949) and anti-s (Fudenberg and Allen, 1957). Anti-U can cause immediate haemolytic transfusion reactions (Wiener *et al.* 1953c) and delayed haemolyic reactions (e.g. Meltz *et al.* 1971), particularly in frequently transfused patients with sickle cell disease (Davies *et al.* 1986).

Antibodies to low frequency antigens such as Vw are of negligible importance in blood transfusion because of the rarity of the corresponding antigen. One of the very few haemolytic transfusion reactions associated with antibodies to low frequency antigens occurred in a patient who happened to be transfused more than once with blood from the same donor—a carrier of the low frequency antigen Kamhuber (Speiser *et al.* 1966), later shown to be identical with FAR (Giles, 1977). Antibodies to the low frequency antigens of the MNSs system have almost all been discovered in the serum of women whose infants have been affected with haemolytic disease of the newborn. Whereas in blood transfusion the chance of receiving more than one unit carrying one of these antigens is very low when random blood donors are used, in women who have several children by a man who carries one of the antigens the chance of alloimmunization is obviously far higher.

Cold-reacting anti-N and warm-reacting anti-U have been found as autoantibodies (see Chapter 7).

THE LUTHERAN (Lu) SYSTEM

The first example of an antibody revealing the existence of this system was found by Callender *et al.* (1945b) in a patient who had had two blood transfusions.

About 8% of Whites are Lu (a +). Almost all of these have the genotype Lu^aLu^b, the overall frequency of the genotype Lu^aLu^a being only 0.15%. Virtually all other subjects (approximately 92% of the population) have the phenotype Lu (a – b +) (gene frequencies: Lu^a, 0.039; Lu^b, 0.961). Very rarely, subjects have the phenotype Lu (a – b –) (Crawford *et al.* 1961). The first example to be detected was found to be due to a dominant inhibitor gene, *In (Lu)*, but other examples may be due to a double dose of a recessive gene *Lu* or to an X-borne recessive inhibitor, *XS2*, of expression of the Lu antigens; *XS1* is the common allele permitting expression of Lu (see review by Crawford, 1988). *In (Lu)* also inhibits the production of P_1, i, Au^a, In^b and the high incidence antigen, AnWj. Thus, antibodies which fail to react with Lu (a – b –) samples may not always belong to the Lutheran system.

With anti-Lu^b, Lu (a – b +) samples from newborn infants react more weakly than those from adults (Kissmeyer-Nielsen, 1960) and Lu (a + b +) samples from newborn infants react very weakly indeed (Greenwalt et al. 1967).

Lutheran antigens have been found only on red cells. Using a sensitive radioimmuno-assay, the main Lu antigens could not be detected on platelets (Dunstan et al. 1984) and, using immunofluorescence flow cytometry, Lu^b could not be detected on lympho-cytes, monocytes or granulocytes (Dunstan, 1986a).

The antigens Au^a and Au^b were included in the list of collections of antigens by Lewis et al. (1990) but have subsequently been shown to be part of the Lutheran system. The antigens, which are not present on Lu$_{null}$ cells, have been renamed Lu18 and Lu19 (Daniels et al. 1991); they are present in approximately 80% and 50% of Whites, respectively.

Chemistry of Lutheran antigens

Lu^b activity has been detected in human red cell gangliosides, most of which contain the lactoneotetraosyl structure, as found in P$_1$ and Ii. The inhibitor type of Lu (a – b –) may therefore result from the action of a glycosyltransferase that adds an extraneous sugar to the backbone structure shared by the Lu, P$_1$, i and Au antigens (Marcus et al. 1981) as well as by AnWj, In^a and In^b.

Using a murine monoclonal anti-Lu^b, two glycoproteins, of mol. wt. 78 000 and 85 000 carrying Lu^b activity have been identified. Expression of Lu^b was shown to depend on the presence of one or more N-glycosidically-linked oligosaccharides and on the presence of disulphide bonding. Trypsin-treated Lu (b +) red cells were not agglutinated by the monoclonal antibody (Parsons et al. 1987). There may be different Lu^b specificities, one unaffected by AET treatment (Advani et al. 1982) or by DTT treatment (Branch et al. 1983) and one affected by AET treatment (Advani et al. 1982; Telen et al. 1983) and by DTT treatment (Parsons et al. 1987). Perhaps, some anti-Lu^b recognize the relevant carbohydrate structure only in a particular peptide environ-ment. A similar heterogeneity has been reported for T (Hoppner et al. 1985).

Using a murine monoclonal anti-Lu^b the number of Lu^b sites per red cell was estimated to be about 2000–4000 on Lu^{b}Lu^a cells and 1000–2000 on Lu^{a}Lu^b cells (Merry et al. 1987).

The Lu^a antigen is destroyed by trypsin, chymotrypsin and pronase (Judson and Anstee, 1977).

Antibodies of the Lutheran system

Anti-Lu^a

This antibody usually occurs as an agglutinin, reacting more strongly at room temperature than at 37°C. Typically, although large agglutinates are formed, many cells are unagglutinated (Callender and Race, 1946). Anti-Lu^a is most commonly IgM but may be IgG or a mixture of IgM and IgG, and may also be partly IgA. Of 19 examples, only three failed to agglutinate red cells suspended in saline and these three appeared to be solely IgG; of the remaining 16, at least nine were partly IgG and at least two partly IgA, as judged by the fact that agglutinating titres were enhanced by anti-IgG or anti-IgA respectively (A. Lubenko, personal communication).

In a deliberate search for anti-Lu^a, only three examples were found in more than 18 000 donors (Greenwalt and Sasaki, 1957). Attempts to stimulate the formation of the antibody by injecting Lu (a +) red cells have given apparently conflicting results. In one series, two of eight patients developed anti-Lu^a 2–4 weeks after the transfusion of a single unit of blood, although the antibody was detectable only transiently (Mainwaring and Pickles, 1948). In another, in which four injections of relatively small amounts of blood were given at 3-monthly intervals to 12 subjects, none formed antibody (Race and Sanger, 1954, p. 208). Perhaps the apparent discrepancy is explained by the fact that large amounts of red cells are required to induce immunization to Lu^a.

Anti-Lu^b

The first example of this antibody was found in a Lu (a + b –) woman who had never been transfused but had had three previous pregnancies (Cutbush and Chanarin, 1956). Anti-Lu^b is rare, as expected from the rarity of the Lu (a + b –) phenotype; all examples have been found in patients who have either been pregnant or have been transfused.

Most examples of anti-Lu^b appear to be mixtures of IgM and IgG. In one laboratory, 14 of 16 examples agglutinated red cells in saline, the remaining two being solely IgG; of the 14 agglutinins all were enhanced by anti-IgG but only four were enhanced by anti-IgA (A. Lubenko, personal observations). In another laboratory, all examples were at least partly IgG although some may have been partly IgM; none were IgA (W.L. Marsh, personal communication).

Of 11 IgG anti-Lu^b, all were believed to be at least partly IgG4 (Hardman and Beck, 1981). However, since most anti-Lu^b are agglutinins and since IgG subclasses cannot be determined reliably on DTT-treated sera, the finding is difficult to confirm.

Anti Lu^{a,b} (anti-Lu3)

An antibody with this specificity in which the anti-Lu^a and anti-Lu^b activities were inseparable was found by Darnborough et al. (1963) in a woman of the rare phenotype Lu (a – b –). The antibody may have been immune since it was absent from the woman's serum before she had a transfusion 13 years previously and was also absent during a pregnancy which she had had 6 years previously. This, and subsequently described examples of anti-Lu^{a,b} reacted more strongly by IAT than by agglutination tests. The antibody seems to be made by subjects of the recessive type and not by those of the dominant type of Lu (a – b –).

Other Lutheran antibodies

Many other antibodies against high frequency antigens, e.g. anti-Lu4, etc., have been described; all fail to react with Lu (a – b –) red cells but react with the red cells of other rare Lutheran phenotypes; according to Race and Sanger (1975, p. 272), some of the antigens recognized are certainly part of the Lutheran system, but the evidence for others is less substantial.

Two monoclonal antibodies detecting high frequency antigens absent from red cells of the dominant type of Lu (a – b –) were described by Knowles et al. (1982b).

Clinical aspects
Anti-Lu^a has not been clearly incriminated as a cause of increased red cell destruction; anti-Lu^b has very rarely caused a delayed haemolytic transfusion reaction but is not known to have caused haemolytic disease of the newborn. (Lu^b is weakly expressed at birth). Destruction of small volumes of incompatible red cells by anti-Lu^b and anti-Lu6 is described in Chapter 10.

THE Di, Yt, Xg, Sc, Do, Co, Ch/Rg, Ge AND Cr SYSTEMS

Diego (Di)
The antibody revealing the existence of the antigen Di^a was found in a woman whose infant was affected with haemolytic disease of the newborn (Layrisse *et al.* 1955); the family was of mixed native Venezuelan and White race. It was subsequently found that all of 1000 samples from White donors were Di(a–) whereas about 36% of samples from certain South American Indians were Di(a+) (Levine *et al.* 1956; Layrisse *et al.* 1955). The antigen was found in 5–15% of Japanese and Chinese people (Layrisse and Arends, 1966) but the frequency among the Chinese in Taiwan has been reported to be only 3.2% (Lin-Chu *et al.* 1991). Surprisingly, Di^a is found in about 0.5% of Poles (Kusnierz-Alejska and Bochenek, 1992). Anti-Di^a may be naturally occurring (Race and Sanger, 1975); an IgG naturally occurring anti-Di^a was found to have a titre of 128 (Steffey, 1983).

The number of Di^b sites on *Di^{b}Di^b* red cells was estimated to be 19 000 per cell by Masouredis *et al.* (1980b). Di^b was not detected on lymphocytes, monocytes or granulocytes (Dunstan, 1986a).

The first two examples of anti-Di^b were described by Thompson *et al.* (1967). Both antibodies could be detected only by IAT and, apparently, their reactions were not enhanced by complement. One subject had had a transfusion 20 years previously and had then had several normal infants.

Clinical aspects
The first of the two subjects mentioned above had a delayed haemolytic transfusion reaction after a second transfusion. In one case, a non-complement-binding IgG anti-Di^a of subclasses IgG1 and IgG3 caused haemolytic disease of the newborn (Alves de Lima *et al.* 1982); anti-Di^b either fails to cause haemolytic disease (e.g. Habash *et al.* 1991) or causes only mild disease (Lin-Chu *et al.* 1991).

Cartwright (Yt)
Yt^a is a very common antigen, being found on the red cells of all but two per 1000 Whites; gene frequencies: *Yt^a*, 0.959; *Yt^b*, 0.041 (Race and Sanger, 1975, p. 379). About 8% of Whites are Yt(b+).

The Yt^a antigen is completely denatured after treating the red cells with 200 mmol/l DTT, showing that at least one disulphide bond is needed to maintain a protein tertiary or quaternary structure responsible for antigen integrity (Branch *et al.* 1983). Immune precipitation of radioiodinated red cells with anti-Yt^a and anti-Yt^b yielded components of mol. wt. 160 000 under non-reducing conditions and of 72 000 under reducing conditions in 10% w/v acrylamide gels. Bands of similar mobility were obtained with monoclonal anti-acetylcholinesterase (AChE-1 and AChE-2). Immune precipitates obtained with anti-Yt^a and anti-Yt^b contained 30% and 50% AChE activity, respectively. These findings suggest that the Yt^a and Yt^b antigens are located on erythrocyte AChE (Spring and Anstee, 1991).

Yt^a was found to be absent from lymphocytes, monocytes and granulocytes (Dunstan, 1986).

The first example of anti-Yt^a was found in a subject who had received several transfusions (Eaton et al. 1956). Many further examples have been reported, either in subjects who have been transfused or have been pregnant; naturally occurring anti-Yt^a has not been described. The original example of anti-Yt^a did not react with papain-treated red cells, but of 14 examples tested by Vengelen-Tyler and Morel (1983) six reacted with papain- or ficin-treated red cells.

Anti-Yt^a may be partly IgG (Bergvalds et al. 1965) or wholly IgG (Bettigole et al. 1968; Göbel et al. 1974). Some examples bind complement, e.g. the case of Bettigole et al. (1968); others do not, e.g. the examples described by Göbel et al. (1974) and by Ballas and Sherwood (1977). Of four of 14 examples of anti-Yt^a which could be typed with subclass antisera, all were solely IgG$_4$ (Vengelen-Tyler and Morel, 1983). Of 16 examples examined by Pierce et al. (1980), 13 could be typed and of these two were solely IgG4 and three partly IgG4; 11 were partly IgG1 but none was IgG3.

Anti-Yt^b was described by Giles and Metaxas (1964).

Clinical aspects
Some examples of anti-Yt^a can cause red cell destruction but others cannot (see Chapter 10). The antibody is not known to have caused a haemolytic transfusion reaction or haemolytic disease of the newborn.

Xg
The great interest of this blood group system lies in the fact that the relevant genes are carried on the X chromosome so that males have only one gene for this system instead of the pair of genes which they have for all the other known blood group systems. Up to the present only one antigen, determined by the gene Xg^a, has been described. An allele, Xg, which may be amorphic, is postulated.

X-inactivation or 'Lyonization' is the phenomenon occurring in very early embryonic life in which one of the two X chromosomes (maternal or paternal) is inactivated in a given cell and in all the subsequent progeny of that cell (Lyon, 1972; see also Race and Sanger 1975). However, the Xg locus is not subject to inactivation since it has been shown that Xg^a can produce Xg^a antigen in heterozygous women when Xg^a is carried on the 'inactive' chromosome. Hence, in humans lyonization does not apply to all loci on the 'inactive' X chromosome (for references see Race and Sanger, 1975).

Females may be Xg^aXg^a, Xg^aXg or $XgXg$ but males can only be Xg^a or Xg. Thus males who are Xg (a +) pass on Xg^a to all their daughters but cannot transmit any Xg genes to their sons; the mating of an Xg (a +) man with an Xg (a –) woman must produce all Xg (a +) daughters and Xg (a –) sons. The frequency of the phenotype Xg (a +) is about 89% in females and 67% in males (Race and Sanger, 1968, p. 523).

Gene frequencies: Xg^a 0.659; Xg, 0.341. In males these are also the genotype and phenotype frequencies; in females genotype frequencies are: Xg^aXg^a, 0.434; Xg^aXg, 0.450; $XgXg$, 0.116.

The Xg^a antigen is inactivated by treatment with proteases (Habibi *et al.* 1979).

The first example of anti-Xg^a (Mann *et al.* 1962) was found in a man who had been transfused repeatedly, as was the second (Cook *et al.* 1963) and the third (Sausais *et al.* 1964). The antibodies could be detected only by IAT; the first two examples sensitized red cells to agglutination by anti-complement as well as anti-IgG; the third was not tested with specific anti-complement but there was evidence that it did not bind complement (Sausais *et al.* 1964). A potent example of a complement-binding anti-Xg^a was found to be of IgG1 and IgG2 subclasses (Devenish *et al.* 1986). An example of anti-Xg^a capable of agglutinating red cells suspended in saline was described by Metaxas and Metaxas-Bühler (1970).

A successful attempt at producing anti-Xg^a was described by Shepherd *et al.* (1969). A man who had received one previous transfusion without forming any red cell allo-antibodies was given weekly intradermal injections of mixed leucocytes and red cells. After the third injection a weak red cell antibody developed and after two further injections the antibody was identifiable as anti-Xg^a. After a rest and two further injections the titre of the antibody reached 32. A second subject failed to develop anti-Xg^a.

Up to 1986, 36 examples of anti-Xg^a were known to Ruth Sanger (personal communication) and at least ten of these were naturally occurring.

Clinical aspects
One example of anti-Xg^a has been shown not to cause red cell destruction (Sausais *et al.* 1964). Anti-Xg^a has never been incriminated as a cause of a haemolytic transfusion reaction or haemolytic disease of the newborn; it has once been described as an autoantibody.

Scianna (Sc)
Sc1 was originally described as a very high frequency antigen, Sm (Schmidt *et al.* 1962a), and Sc2 as a very low frequency antigen, Bu^a (Anderson *et al.* 1963a) before it was realized that *Sc^1* and *Sc^2* were alleles. The frequency of Sc:2 subjects in northern Europe is about 1% whereas the frequency of Sc: – 1 subjects is about 0.01%. Gene frequencies: *Sc^1*, 0.992; *Sc^2*, 0.008. Sc1 is absent from lymphocytes, monocytes and granulocytes (Dunstan, 1986a).

Sc1 and Sc2 are carried on a red cell membrane glycoprotein of 60 000 kD. Intact disulphide bonds are necessary for full expression of the antigens and the presence of one or more complex *N*-glycans is needed for the expression of Sc2 (Spring *et al.* 1990).

There is only a little evidence about the immunogenicity of Sc2. The original example of anti-Sc2 (which was detectable by IAT) was found in a man who had been transfused on a single occasion with 3 units of blood. In a series described by Seyfried *et al.* (1966), amongst 14 Sc: – 2 subjects injected with Sc2 red cells four made anti-Sc2. The experience of one of us (PLM) suggests that Sc2 is very much less immunogenic than D: of 19 D-negative, Sc: – 2 subjects given two or more injections from a D-positive, Sc:2 donor, eight formed anti-D and only one of these also made anti-Sc2. Of the 11 who failed to make anti-D, none made anti-Sc2.

The phenotype Sc: – 1, – 2 is very rare, although a cluster of eight subjects with this phenotype was found in Papua New Guinea (Woodfield *et al.* 1986). Sc: – 1, – 2 subjects can make anti-Sc3, reacting with all except Sc: – 1, – 2 red cells (Nason *et al.*

1980). An example of IgG anti-Sc3 was found in a transfused thalassaemic child; the antibody disappeared after splenectomy and was not stimulated by transfusion with Sc:1, – 2 blood (Woodfield *et al.* 1986). Naturally occurring antibodies within the Sc system have not been described.

Clinical aspects
Alloantibodies of this system have not been incriminated as a cause of increased red cell destruction. One example of anti-Sc1 composed of IgG3, detected in a pregnant woman, led to a positive DAT in the infant but not to haemolytic disease of the newborn (Kaye *et al.* 1990). Anti-Sc1 has been found as an autoantibody in a healthy donor (McDowell *et al.* 1986) and, possibly, in a patient with Evans-like syndrome (Steane *et al.* 1982a).

Dombrock (Do)

Approximately 66% of northern Europeans are Do (a +) and 82% are Do (b +). Gene frequencies: Do^a, 0.42; Do^b, 0.58. The antibody anti-Do^a, defining this system, was discovered in a woman who had been immunized by transfusion. The antibody gave a positive IAT only with certain anti-IgG sera; stronger reactions were obtained when enzyme-treated red cells were used; the antibody did not bind complement. Anti-Do^b was described by Molthan *et al.* (1973). No examples of naturally occurring antibodies within this system have been described.

Clinical aspects
The antibodies of this system are rare and usually weak; however, anti-Do^a has caused immediate haemolytic transfusion reactions (Judd and Steiner, 1991) and anti-Do^b has been the cause of both immediate and delayed haemolytic reactions (Moheng *et al.* 1985; Halverson *et al.* 1989).

Colton (Co)

About 99.8% of Whites are Co (a +) and about 8% are Co (b +). Gene frequencies: Co^a, 0.959; Co^b, 0.041. There is a hint that Blacks in the USA may have a lower incidence of Co (a –) (Race and Sanger, 1975, p. 391). The antibody which revealed the Colton system was described by Heistö *et al.* (1967); three examples of anti-Co^a were described, all probably immune in origin and one, at least, IgG. An immune anti-Co^b was shown to be IgG, unable to fix complement and reacting best with enzyme-treated red cells (Dzik and Blank, 1986). Anti-Co^b was described by Giles *et al.* (1970). Anti-$Co^{a,b}$ was found by Rogers *et al.* (1974) in the serum of a woman whose cells were Co (a – b –). The Co^a antigen was not detected on lymphocytes, monocytes or granulocytes (Dunstan, 1986a).

Clinical aspects
Anti-Co^a is not known to have caused a haemolytic transfusion reaction. It has been the cause of a positive DAT in an infant without signs of haemolytic disease (McIntyre *et al.* 1976). The anti-Co^b described above (Dzik and Blank, 1986) was shown to cause accelerated destruction of Co (b +) cells. A delayed haemolytic transfusion reaction due to anti-Co^b has been described; see Chapter 11.

Chido/Rodgers (Ch/Rg)

Ch and Rg are antigenic determinants on the complement C4 component (O'Neill *et al.* 1978) and are thus antigens of plasma adsorbed on to red cells. Rg and Ch determinants can be demonstrated on a tryptic C4d fragment (Tilley *et al.* 1978b). The antigenic determinants of C4 are very stable in plasma or stored serum and can be used in haemagglutination inhibition assays with human anti-Ch and anti-Rg reagents. *Chido, Rodgers* and *HLA* are closely linked in chromosome 6 (Middleton *et al.* 1974; Giles *et al.* 1976). Rg-negative individuals are almost always HLA-A1-B8-DR3 (Giles *et al.* 1976; James *et al.* 1976). Red cells normally carry only small amounts of C4d passively adsorbed from plasma and it is therefore not surprising that reactions of anti-Ch and anti-Rg with normal red cells are usually weak. Conversely, if red cells and serum are incubated at low ionic strength, e.g. by adding ACD blood to a relatively large volume of 10% sucrose, which causes large amounts of C4 (and C3) to be deposited on the red cell surface, the resulting cells are strongly agglutinated by anti-Ch and anti-Rg provided that the corresponding antigens are present in the plasma (Tilley *et al.* 1978b). The reactions of anti-Ch and anti-Rg with Ch-positive and Rg-positive red cells are inhibited by the addition of Ch-positive and Rg-positive plasma respectively (Swanson *et al.* 1971b; Middleton and Crookston, 1972; Longster and Giles, 1976). Depending on the inhibitory capacity of plasma, individuals can be classified as total, partial or non-inhibitors for either Ch or Rg. Partial inhibition of anti-Ch or anti-Rg is an inherited, qualitative characteristic (for details see Nordhagen *et al.* 1980; Giles, 1985a). Two Rg and six Ch determinants, all of high frequency, as well as a lower frequency (20%) determinant WH, have been defined by haemagglutination inhibition tests (Giles, 1989).

In patients with cold haemagglutinin disease the red cells carry increased amounts of C4d and therefore react strongly with anti-Ch and anti-Rg when both Ch and Rg are present in the patient's plasma (Tilley *et al.* 1978b).

All normal individuals are either Ch positive and, or, Rg positive: 95% are Ch + Rg +, 3% are Ch + Rg – and 2% are Ch – Rg + (Middleton and Crookston, 1972; Longster and Giles, 1976); C4 null individuals are Ch – Rg – (O'Neil *et al.* 1978).

The C4 polymorphism is controlled by two genes, *C4A* and *C4B*, which are thought to have arisen by duplication. Most of the polymorphism is located on the α-chain within the C4d fragment. There is an electrophoretic polymorphism of C4 with 13 C4A and 22 C4B allotypes. A strong association has been found between C4A allotypes and Rg, and between C4B and Ch, but this association is not complete (Giles, 1989).

Anti-Ch and anti-Rg are found only as immune antibodies, in the plasma of Ch- or Rg-negative subjects. Anti-Ch is found twice as commonly as anti-Rg (Giles, 1985b). Neither anti-Ch nor anti-Rg can cause red cell destruction. Of four anti-Ch tested in an automated antiglobulin test, all had a strong IgG4 component and three were partly IgG2; one was partly IgG1 and partly IgM (Szymanski *et al.* 1982).

Two mouse monoclonal anti-C4d reagents were found to have specificities related to Rg:1 and Ch:1 rather than C4A and C4B (see Giles, 1989).

Gerbich (Ge)

There are seven antigens in the Ge system, Ge2, Ge3, Ge4, Ge5 (Wb), Ge6 (Ls[a]), Ge7 (An[a]) and Ge8 (Dh[a]) (Lewis *et al.* 1991), which are carried on β and

γ sialoglycoproteins (glycophorins C and D). β and γ sialoglycoproteins (SGP) have an identical COOH terminal sequence for about 100 amino acids. It has been suggested that γ SGP is coded for by the same gene which encodes β SGP but probably results from an alternative site of initiation of translation of messenger RNA (mRNA), produced by a single locus (GYPC) on chromosome 2 (Cartron *et al.* 1990). Three different types of the Ge-negative phenotype occur; all three are characterized by absence of normal β and γ SGP. The differences between them are determined by absence of the one or more of the four exons of the gene for β SGP. In one of the three Ge-negative phenotypes ('Leach'), some of the red cells are elliptocytes (for references see review by Reid, 1989).

Although Ge-negative subjects are excessively rare amongst Whites, they are common in some parts of Papua New Guinea (Booth and McLoughlin, 1972). The first three examples of anti-Ge, all of which came from pregnant or recently delivered women, were described by Rosenfield *et al.* (1960). All were incomplete antibodies and could be revealed only by IAT. The infants born to all three women had a positive DAT but no evidence of haemolytic disease. Of 15 examples of anti-Ge reviewed by McLoughlin and Rogers (1970), six were immune and nine naturally occurring; one of the latter, encountered in a previously untransfused male, agglutinated red cells at room temperature and had an indirect antiglobulin titre of 64.

Anti-Ge has not been known to cause a haemolytic transfusion reaction although an IgG1 example which gave positive reactions in a monocyte bioassay caused mild haemolytic disease of the newborn (Sacks *et al.* 1985). Of ten other examples of anti-Ge which could be typed with subclass antisera, nine were solely IgG1 (Vengelen-Tyler and Morel, 1983).

Anti-Ge has been described as an autoantibody involved in autoimmune haemolytic anaemia. In the third case to be reported the antibody was IgA (Göttsche *et al.* 1990).

Murine monoclonal anti-Ge has been described (Rouger *et al.* 1983; Anstee *et al.* 1984). These antibodies react with determinants on β SGP and, although not true anti-Ge, distinguish between Ge positives and negatives in agglutination tests.

The Ge antigen has not been detected on granulocytes (Gaidulis *et al.* 1985), or on lymphocytes or monocytes (Dunstan, 1986a).

Cromer (Cr)

The antigens Cr^a, Tc^a, Tc^b, Tc^c, Dr^a, WES^a, WES^b, Es^a, UMC and IFC are phenotypically related (i.e. Cromer-related) and are all carried on the decay accelerating factor (DAF; see Chapter 3); they have recently been recognized as forming a blood group system (Lewis *et al.* 1991). Three of the antigens (Tc^b, Tc^c and WES^a) are of low frequency and the remaining seven of high frequency. All ten antigens are destroyed by chymotrypsin but not by other proteolytic enzymes. The null phenotype, Inab, is devoid of all Cromer-related antigens. Inab cells are DAF deficient and are significantly more susceptible than normal cells to lysis by complement, either by haemolytic antibody or in the sucrose lysis test (see Daniels, 1989). None of the four Inab individuals reported so far has shown signs of increased red cell destruction although such signs are characteristic of individuals with PNH whose red cells lack not only DAF but also several other molecules of the family of glycoproteins, all of which are anchored to the cell membrane through glycosylated phosphatidylinositol molecules (Rosse, 1989). Inab-negative individuals can make anti-IFC, which reacts with all except Inab cells. Several monoclonal antibodies have been found to react with all cells tested except Inab; the antibodies react weakly with Dr (a –) cells (Spring et al. 1987).

Antibodies to Cromer-related antigens are mostly IgG and predominantly IgG1. The first example of anti-Cr^a (Stroup and McCreary, 1975), like all subsequently recognized examples, was found in a Black person. In two cases, anti-Cr^a caused only dubious destruction of a test dose of incompatible red cells: in the first the $T_{50}Cr$ was 14 d but the subject had rheumatoid arthritis (Smith et al. 1983); in the second, Cr survival at 96 h was 73%; survival was not followed further and the subject was transfused uneventfully 2 months later with Cr (a +) red cells (Ross and McCall, 1985). In a third case, more than 40% of a test dose of Cr (a +) cells was destroyed within 4 h (McSwain and Robins, 1988).

In a patient who had formed an antibody against the Cromer-related antigen Tc^a, the survival at 24 h of a test dose of incompatible red cells was probably within normal limits and a monocyte monolayer assay (MMA) was normal; at this time the antibody was a mixture of IgG2 and IgG4, although some years previously it had also been partly IgG1 and the results of an MMA had been well above normal limits (Anderson et al. 1991a).

COLLECTIONS OF ANTIGENS

This term has been introduced to describe specificities that are connected in one of the following ways (Lewis et al. 1990): (1) serological, i.e. dosage results supporting a genetic relationship; or altered expression of some, if not all, of the antigens in certain phenotypes; or antigen absence in apparent 'null' phenotypes; (2) biochemical, i.e. studies of epitope structures; and (3) genetic, i.e. family or population studies.

In the collections described below, the name is followed by the symbol in brackets.

Indian (In)
The In^a antigen was discovered by Badakere et al. (1973). Soon after, its frequency in various communities in Bombay was found to be between 2.3% and 4.5%, with a gene frequency for In^a of 0.0371 and for In (i.e. not In^a) of 0.9629 (Badakere et al. 1974). The antibody to the high incidence antigen Salis was shown to be antithetical to anti-In^a and Salis became In^b (Giles, 1975). Amongst Asians living in the UK, In^a has a frequency of 0.02 and In^b of 0.98; no example of In^a was found in English blood donors (Longster et al. 1981).

Anti-In^a was found together with anti-D in the serum of a blood donor from Bombay and subsequently in many of the anti-Rh D sera produced by commercial firms in Bombay. These antibodies reacted in saline and antiglobulin techniques but not with enzyme-treated cells.

The original anti-Salis and anti-In^b sera, found in pregnant Asians living in the UK, reacted by the antiglobulin technique but not with enzyme-treated cells. Although these antibodies were IgG, no cases of haemolytic disease of the newborn or of a positive DAT on cord cells have been reported. One example of anti-In^b from a pregnant women gave weak results in an ADCC assay and inconclusive results with

IgG isotyping sera; the infant showed no signs of haemolytic disease (S.F. Garner, personal communication).

The In antigens are located on CDw44, a ubiquitous glycoprotein of mol. wt. 80 000. Expression of the antigens is weakened in the *In(Lu)* type of Lu (a – b –) cells (Spring *et al.* 1988).

Cost (Cs)

This collection includes the antigens Cs^a, Cs^b, York (Yk^a), Knops (Kn^a and Kn^b), McCoy (McC^a) and Sl^a. The reactions given with corresponding antibodies are weak although the sera may have titres of 64 or more, for which reason the antibodies were in the past referred to as 'high-titre, low avidity' (HTLA) antibodies. The term HTLA is best avoided because not all the antibodies of these specificities have high titres and not all react weakly, and in any case the term 'low avidity' is imprecise. Of the antibodies, anti-Yk^a and anti-McC^a are much commoner than the others. For evidence that these antibodies do not bring about red cell destruction *in vivo*, see Chapter 10.

Kn and McC are carried on the complement receptor CR1 (Rao *et al.* 1991).

Gregory (Gy)

There are two antigens in this collection, Gy^a and Hy, with frequencies of >99% and >95%, respectively. The corresponding antibodies are weakly reacting, non-complement-binding IgGs. Examples of anti-Gy^a have been found in women who have been pregnant but whose infants have not had haemolytic disease (Swanson *et al.* 1967), probably because Gy^a (like Hy) is poorly expressed on red cells in the newborn (Moulds *et al.* 1975). Anti-Gy^a has caused severe transfusion reactions, though without definite evidence of increased red cell destruction (Moulds *et al.* 1975). One definite haemolytic reaction due to anti-Hy has been reported (Beattie and Castillo, 1975) and the antibody has been shown to cause accelerated destruction of a small dose of incompatible red cells (Hsu *et al.* 1975).

Er

Er^a has a frequency of more than 99% and Er^b one of less than 1%. Anti-Er^a failed to cause a delayed haemolytic transfusion reaction in one case and failed to cause haemolytic disease of the newborn in another (Daniels *et al.* 1982).

I, i

These antigens are described in Chapter 4.

P, P^k LKE (globoside collection)

These three antigens were formerly considered to belong to the P system but are now recognized to be determined by genes independent of P_1. For convenience they are discussed in Chapter 4.

Wright (Wr)

There are two antigens in this collection, Wr^a and Wr. Wr^b is situated in the α-helical region of glycophorin A at a point very close to the red cell membrane (Ridgwell *et al.* 1983). Subjects who lack glycophorin A, i.e. En (a –) and M^kM^k, and those who have only hybrid SGPs in the membrane, i.e. Mi.V/Mi.V and Mi.V/M^k, are Wr(a −) as well as Wr(b −), suggesting that Wr^a is also carried on glycophorin A. Based on serological dosage tests, Wr^a and Wr^b have an antithetical relationship, suggesting that they may be determined by alleles (Wren and Issitt, 1988). On the other hand, glycophorin A from En (a +), Wr(a + b −) red cells has an amino acid sequence identical to that of glycophorin A from Wr(b +) cells. The expression of Wr^b requires band 3, as well as glycophorin A, for its expression (Telen and Chasis, 1990). Whether Wr^a has the same requirement is unknown.

Wr^a is present in about one in 1000 blood samples in England (Dunsford, 1954; Cleghorn, 1960). The corresponding antibody, anti-Wr^a, was first found in the serum of a woman who had given birth to two infants affected with haemolytic disease of the newborn; the antibody could be detected only by IAT (Holman, 1953). According to Dunsford (1954) the antibody is commoner than the antigen and can be detected in approximately one in 100 blood samples. It is often found in males who have never been transfused. For some unexplained reason, anti-Wr^a is often found in the serum of patients who have formed other blood group antibodies and very often found in the serum of patients with autoimmune haemolytic anaemia (T.E. Cleghorn, personal communication).

Naturally ocurring anti-Wr^a often agglutinates red cells in saline, reacting more strongly at room temperature than at 37°C, but is frequently incomplete. Of 44 examples of anti-Wr^a, 16 were solely IgM, nine were partly IgM and 19 were solely IgG (Lubenko and Contreras, 1992).

Anti-Wr^a was solely IgG_1 in nine of nine examples tested by Hardman and Beck (1981). Anti-Wr^b was described by Adams et al. (1971). The antibody has also been found, as a separable specificity, together with anti-En^a, in the serum of two En (a −) subjects who were also Wr(a − b −) (Pavone et al. 1978).

Clinical aspects
Anti-Wr^a has been shown experimentally to cause red cell destruction and is also known to have caused haemolytic transfusion reactions (van Loghem et al. 1955a; Metaxas and Metaxas-Bühler, 1963) and haemolytic disease of the newborn (Holman, 1953).

The first example of anti-Wr^b was an alloantibody (Adams et al. 1971) and several other Wr^b alloantibodies have been described; see, for example, Judd et al. (1983). Warm autoantibodies in AIHA sometimes have Wr^b specificity (see Chapter 7).

OTHER ANTIGENS WITH A VERY HIGH OR VERY LOW INCIDENCE

Antigens with a very high incidence
Many antigens that occur on the red cells of almost all human subjects and that belong to one of the systems (H, Rh29, LW, k, Kp^b, Lu^b, Yt^a and Sc1) or collections (I, P) of antigens have already been discussed. Further antigens, not known to be related to any others, and in most cases found in more than 999 of every 1000 individuals (Sd^a and MER2 are exceptions), are described here.

If a patient in need of a blood transfusion is found to have an antibody reacting with a high incidence antigen, the specificity should be identified, as it may then be possible to find an antigen-negative blood for transfusion from a panel of donors of rare groups (e.g. WHO, American Red Cross) or a bank of frozen red cells (American Red Cross, Council of Europe). A simpler way of searching for compatible red cells is to test siblings and close relatives.

Vel

Of the first two examples of anti-Vel described, one was an agglutinating antibody and the other haemolytic (Sussman and Miller, 1952; Levine et al. 1955). An example described by Levine et al. (1961b) was also haemolytic and had apparently been formed as an immune response to transfusion. A later transfusion provoked a rigor, lumbar pain and anuria. Six relatives of the propositus were also Vel-negative (Ve(a –)); none of them had anti-Vel in their serum. Anti-Vel may be partly IgG but has not been associated with haemolytic disease of the newborn (Stiller et al. 1990).

Anti-Vel has twice been found as an autoantibody (Szalóky and van der Hart, 1971; Herron et al. 1979).

The Vel antigen was not detected on lymphocytes, monocytes or granulocytes (Dunstan, 1986a).

Sid (Sd^a) and Cad

About 91% of English people have Sd (a +) red cells. Anti-Sd^a, when mixed with Sd (a +) cells, gives a characteristic pattern of agglutination with compact agglutinates in a sea of unagglutinated cells. Only about 1% of samples react strongly; about 80% show distinct small agglutinates and about 10% react very weakly with only occasional tiny agglutinates (Pickles and Morton, 1977). Sd^a is not demonstrable on cord blood red cells and begins to be detectable only at about the age of 10 weeks. In pregnancy there is a weakening of the Sd^a antigen (Pickles and Morton, 1977).

The Sd^a antigen is present in most secretions, with the greatest concentration in urine. Approximately half of the Sd (a +) people with Sd (a –) red cells secrete Sd^a in the urine (Morton et al. 1970), i.e. 96% of English people are Sd (a +).

In urine, the Sd^a determinants are on Tamm–Horsfall glycoprotein, carrying 1–2% terminal N-acetylgalactosamine linked $\beta1{\rightarrow}4$ to Gal. In Sd (a –) subjects, GalNAc is virtually absent from this glycoprotein (Soh et al. 1980).

Anti-Sd^a. Of the 4% of people who are Sd (a –), about one-half (i.e. about 2% of the population) have demonstrable anti-Sd^a in their serum (Morton et al. 1970). Similarly, Renton et al. (1967) gave a figure of 1%; the antibody is generally IgM. Most examples of anti-Sd^a react with saline suspensions of red cells at 20°C and 37°C, and may fix complement. The antibody can also be detected with enzyme-treated cells (occasional sera, when fresh, haemolyse enzyme-treated cells), and by the antiglobulin test (Pickles and Morton, 1977).

Anti-Sd^a is of no clinical significance although one example caused some destruction of a sample of red cells with a very strongly expressed Sd^a antigen (see Chapter 10).

Cad is an antigen of very low frequency associated with polyagglutinability (Cazal *et al.* 1968), due to the presence of anti-Cad in almost all samples of human serum (Gerbal *et al.* 1976b). Since Cad red cells react very strongly with anti-Sd^a, some believe that Cad may simply be a very strong form of Sd^a (Sanger *et al.* 1971). Both gangliosides and glycophorins carrying the Cad antigen inhibit human anti-Sd^a and it is possible that trace amounts of Cad ganglioside are present in Sd (a +) subjects (Blanchard *et al.* 1985).

Cad red cells, even when group O, are agglutinated by an extract of *Dolichos biflorus* (Cazal *et al.* 1968). Anti-Cad is present as a separate specificity in *Dolichos* extract, which is not removed by absorbing the extract with A$_1$ red cells. On the other hand, both anti-Cad and anti-A$_1$ are inhibited by N-acetylgalactosamine, and Cad red cells are also agglutinated by snail anti-A (Cazal *et al.* 1971).

Possible relation of Sd^a and Cad antigens to the ABO system. Sd^a is found in secretions, is not fully developed at birth, and may be weakened in pregnancy (cf. Lewis); anti-Sd^a is found as a naturally occurring agglutinin.

A pentasaccharide ending in N-acetylgalactosamine, like the A determinant, was isolated from glycophorins A and B and from gangliosides in Cad red cells, and found to carry Cad and Sd^a specificities; the terminal trisaccharide, GalNAc $\beta(1\rightarrow4)$ [NeuAc$\alpha(2\rightarrow3)$] Gal, was found to be the same as that isolated from Tamm-Horsfall glycoprotein in the urine of Sd (a +) subjects. The Cad specificity on red cell membranes is carried on both sialoglycoproteins and on a novel ganglioside which consists of sialosylparagloboside with a GalNAc residue added to the majority of O-linked oligosaccharides. The ganglioside binds to *Helix pomatia* lectin. The red cell component carrying the Sd^a determinant has not been identified (Blanchard *et al.* 1983; 1985; Gillard *et al.* 1988).

AnWj (Anton or Wj)
AnWj is an antigen of high frequency defined originally by autoantibodies and, more recently, by monoclonal antibodies (Poole and Giles, 1982; Marsh and Johnson, 1985). The antigen is present on all red cells except cord cells and cells from subjects carrying *In (Lu)*, the dominant inhibitor of Lutheran and other antigens (see section on Lutheran). Only two AnWj-negative subjects with normal Lu antigens and with allo-anti-AnWj have been described; one patient had a transient loss of the antigen (Mannessier *et al.* 1986); the other was a 55-year-old patient with a neurological disease (Harris *et al.* 1986). The allo-anti-Wj described by Harris *et al.* (1986) was a mixture of IgG1, weak IgG3, IgM and IgA; it fixed complement and reacted equally well with untreated and with papain-treated red cells.

AnWj has been shown to be a red cell receptor for *Haemophilus influenzae*, the main agent for bacterial meningitis in infants (van Alphen *et al.* 1986).

Other high-incidence antigens are as follows: Lan, At^a, Jo^a, Jr^a, Ok^a, JMH, Emm, MER2 and Duclos (Lewis *et al.* 1991). Anti-Lan has been shown to destroy test doses of incompatible red cells (Clancey *et al.* 1972; Lampe *et al.* 1979; Judd *et al.* 1984) and to cause haemolytic disease of the newborn (Smith *et al.* 1969); anti-At^a is known not to have caused haemolytic disease of the newborn in many cases where the opportunity existed and there is no evidence about the clinical significance of anti-Jo^a (see Issitt, 1985, pp. 400 and 405). In addition to the phenotypic association between Jo^a and the Gy^a/Hy collection, there is recent evidence that Jo^a is carried on the same glycoprotein as Gy^a and Hy (Spring, 1991). Anti-Jr^a can cause red cell destruction (Kendall, 1976) but causes only mild haemolytic disease of the newborn (Nakajima and Ito, 1978; Toy *et al.* 1981); the only known example of anti-Ok^a caused rapid destruction of a test dose of incompatible red cells (Morel and Hamilton, 1979); anti-JMH (found mainly in old people) failed to destroy red cells in three different patients (Sabo *et al.* 1978) and was at least partly IgG4 in 14 cases (Tregellas *et al.* 1980).

Antigens with a very low incidence

Low frequency antigens are genetically or serologically associated with various blood group systems, e.g. C^x and Evans to the Rh system; He, Vw to the MNSs system; Lu14 to the Lutheran system, or with various collections, e.g. In^a with the In collection (see Lubenko and Contreras, 1989). Outside the systems and collections, 36 'private' antigens with a frequency of less than one in 400 Caucasians (the 700 series) were recognized in 1990 (Lewis *et al.* 1991). Some low frequency antigens have frequencies greater than one in 400 in certain non-Caucasian populations or even in isolated Caucasian populations. The list is as follows: By, Chr^a, Sw^a, Bi, Bx^a, Tr^a, Bp^a, Wu, Jn^a, Rd, To^a, Pt^a, Re^a, Je^a, Mo^a, Hey, Fr^a, Rb^a, Li^a, Vg^a, Wd^a, Os^a, Hg^a, NFLD, Milne, RASM, SW1, Ol^a, JFV, Kg, BOW, Jones, FPTT, HJK, HOFM and ELO.

Some low frequency antigens stimulate the production of maternal antibodies, leading to a positive DAT in the fetus or to haemolytic disease of the newborn. In general, low frequency antigens are unimportant in blood transfusion since it is so easy to find compatible donors for patients with the corresponding antibodies. On the other hand, the antibodies tend to be present in sera used for blood grouping since such sera may be derived from hyperimmunized donors in whom antibodies to low frequency antigens are often present (see below). Anti-E and anti-S sera are notorious for having antibodies to low-frequency antigens, but even polyclonal anti-A and anti-B may have them. The presence of these unwanted antibodies may have serious consequences; for example, anti-Wr^a in an anti-Rh D reagent might lead to a D-negative, Wr(a +) woman being misgrouped as D positive. Of course, problems of this kind do not arise when monoclonal reagents are used.

In sera from patients with autoimmune haemolytic anaemia, it is not uncommon to find antibodies to several low frequency antigens. Cleghorn (1960) noted that anti-Sw^a, -Wr^a and -By, as well as -Vw, -Mi^a, -M^g and -C^x, might be present. In another series, one or more antibodies to low frequency antigens were found in 30% of patients with autoimmune haemolytic anaemia (Salmon and Holmberg, 1971).

Antibodies to low frequency antigens were found more commonly in D-negative donors hyperimmunized to RhD than in control subjects, suggesting that such antibodies may be made when the immune system is stimulated by alloantigens as well as by autoantigens (Contreras *et al.* 1979b). Multiple antibodies to low frequency antigens are also not uncommon in normal donors. One donor was found to have as many as 27 such antibodies and many other normal donors to have between six and 15 (personal observations, MC).

HLA ANTIGENS DETECTABLE ON RED CELLS

HLA antigens were first demonstrated on reticulocytes by showing that these cells, but not mature red cells, would adsorb cytotoxic antibodies (Harris and Zervas, 1969). The presence of HLA antigens on reticulocytes was confirmed by Silvestre *et al.* (1970) using fluorescein-labelled anti-HLA. The distribution of sites appeared to be similar to that found on lymphocytes.

The first observations indicating that HLA antigens were also, in all probability, demonstrable on mature red cells were made by Rosenfield *et al.* (1967a). Using the AutoAnalyzer, agglutinins for red cells were demonstrated in all of 26 sera containing leucocyte antibodies, although in only two instances was the red cell agglutinin of the same specificity as the leucocyte antibody. The first leucocyte antigen to be demonstrated unequivocally on the red cells was HLA-B7. Seaman *et al.* (1967) showed that when blood grouping tests were carried out in an AutoAnalyzer, one of these antigens, Bg^a, could be recognized on the red cells of 30% of subjects, a much higher incidence than that observed with manual tests. The Oxford workers next showed that Bg^a was present on leucocytes as well as on red cells and was intimately related to HLA-B7, probably being a part of this compound antigen (Morton *et al.* 1969). Bg^b (much less common in Whites than Bg^a) was shown to correspond with HLA-B17 and Bg^c with HLA-A28 (Morton *et al.* 1971). Subsequent work showed that red cells carrying Bg^c also reacted with anti-HLA-A2, a not unexpected observation since the antigens A2 and A28 are known to crossreact (Norhagen and Ørjasaeter, 1974).

When monoclonal antibodies to common determinants of HLA class I and class II molecules were used by radioimmunoassay or flow cytometry, it was shown that red cells from approximately 50% of blood donors bound antibodies to HLA-A, B and C but not to DR; subjects with HLA-B7 consistently expressed HLA antigens on red cells but the expression of HLA on cells of HLA-B7-negative donors did not correlate with that of any other recognizable antigen (Rivera and Scornik, 1986). The same authors showed that expression of HLA antigens on red cells was unaffected by freezing or by storage at 4°C for 21 d. However, HLA class I antigens can be removed from the red cell membrane by chloroquine treatment (Swanson and Sastamoinen, 1985); the procedure may be useful in identifying antibodies or grouping red cells when using sera containing Bg antibodies.

Of the HLA antigens regularly present on red cells, A28 and B7 are the most strongly expressed, followed by B8 and B17 (Nordhagen, 1978). HLA-A10 (Morton *et al.* 1971) as well as A9, B12 and B15 (Nordhagen, 1977) are also sometimes recognizable.

HLA-B17, when expressed on red cells, crossreacts with most anti-HLA-A2/28 sera, an interesting and surprising finding since the antigens concerned are products of different HLA loci (Nordhagen, 1983).

Increased expression of HLA antigens on red cells
A normal donor with strongly expressed HLA antigens on his red cells was described by van der Hart *et al.* (1974). When the red cells were crossmatched with serum containing HLA antibody, the antiglobulin test (anti-IgG only) was strongly positive. The HLA antigens detectable were A2, B7 and BW40. If the red cells were incubated with cytotoxic HLA antibodies of more than one specificity, complement as well as IgG was bound.

Two donors with exceptionally strong HLA reactivity of red cells were described by Nordhagen (1979). In the first donor, with HLA groups A1, 2; B8, 17, all but HLA A1 could be recognized on the red cells by IAT. In the second donor (HLA A2, 11; B5, 40), B5 and B40 were particularly strongly expressed on the red cells. It was suggested that during maturation of red cells an enzymic process may first split off β_2-microglobulin, followed by the rest of HLA, and that this second stage may fail to occur in exceptional individuals. On the other hand, β_2-microglobulin was found on all red cells expressing HLA antigens, using flow cytometry with a monoclonal antibody (Rivera and Scornik, 1986).

In healthy subjects, red cells with strongly expressed HLA antigens must be very rare. In a deliberate search only five examples were discovered over a period of several years (P. Rubinstein, personal communication).

Increased expression of HLA antigen on red cells in disease. Following an attack of infectious mononucleosis the red cells of HLA-B7 patients may show a greatly increased reactivity with the corresponding antibody; the increase is found from about the third week of the illness and thereafter decreases slowly over a period of months or years. The cause of this phenomenon is not yet known. There is no evidence that the less dense, i.e. youngest, red cells in the circulation react any more strongly than the rest (Morton *et al.* 1977).

Bg antigens, i.e. certain HLA-related antigens, are more reactive in patients with leukaemia, lymphoma, polycythaemia, megaloblastic anaemia and haemolytic anaemia; other HLA-related antigens which are of low incidence on the red cells of normal donors are found in much higher incidence in these patients (Morton *et al.* 1980).

Agglutination due to HLA antigens on red cells

Unwanted positive results in crossmatching due to HLA are common because HLA-A28 and B7 are so commonly present on red cells and because the corresponding antibodies are frequently present in sera: anti-HLA-B7 (anti-Bg[a]) has been found in the serum of about 1.5% of the general patient population (Marshall, 1973; Eska and Grindon, 1974) and in more than 10% of multiple transfused patients (personal observations, MC). It is important to ensure that typing sera, particularly polyclonal anti-D, are free of anti-HLA (Pavone and Issitt, 1974).

Clinical aspects

HLA antibodies have both been incriminated as a cause of haemolytic transfusion reactions or of haemolytic disease of the newborn. Some examples, but not others, bring about the accelerated destruction of small volumes of red cells carrying the corresponding antigens (see Chapter 10).

MEMBRANE ABNORMALITIES INVOLVING RED CELL ANTIGENS

Sialic acid deficiency

En (a –) red cells have been described earlier in this chapter; Tn red cells are described in Chapter 7.

An abnormality detected in some Melanesians in Papua New Guinea
In about 15% of Melanesians in coastal areas of Papua New Guinea, the following antigens are depressed: I^T, I^F, LW, C, D, e, Kp^b, S, s, Jk^a, Jk^b, Xg^a, Wr^b, Scl and En^a; the following are not depressed: A_1, I^D, i, MN, P_1, Lu^b, k, Fy^a, Co^a, Vel and Ge. The sialic acid content of the red cells is normal. Some of the subjects have oval red cells. The depressed determinants may all depend for their full expression upon the same membrane component, the synthesis of which is affected. The antigens that are depressed include most of those to which warm antibodies are made (Booth *et al.* 1977).

HEMPAS red cells
Patients with hereditary erythroblastic multinuclearity with a positive acidified serum test (HEMPAS) have red cells which, at 15–20°C, are agglutinated (and lysed) by an IgM antibody present in the serum of most normal subjects. The red cells exhibit various other abnormalities such as a greatly increased reactivity with anti-i and an increased sensitivity to complement (Crookston *et al.* 1969a,b). H is depressed (Bird and Wingham, 1976). For a review, see Crookston and Crookston (1982).

Rh null and Kx-negative (McLeod syndrome)
These different abnormalities, which are both associated with the absence of a normal red cell membrane protein, have been described earlier.

Other abnormalities involving red cell antigens. See Chapter 3.

CHAPTER 7

RED CELL ANTIBODIES AGAINST SELF ANTIGENS, BOUND ANTIGENS AND INDUCED ANTIGENS

In immunohaematology the term autoantibody is used for any antibody which reacts with a corresponding antigen on the subject's own red cells even if the reaction takes place only *in vitro* and whether or not any pathological effects are produced *in vivo*.

The most important antibodies considered in this chapter are those that react with self antigens, intrinsic to red cells. In addition various antibodies that may react with a subject's own red cells are described: these include antibodies against antigens which are normally hidden but may become exposed (e.g. T) as a consequence of the action of bacterial enzymes and antibodies against bound, non-red-cell antigens, e.g. penicillin. Bacterial antigens may be adsorbed on to red cells *in vitro* and the coated red cells may then be agglutinated by sera containing the corresponding bacterial antibodies. The phenomenon does not usually result in autoagglutination but may be a cause of polyagglutinability.

The various antibodies listed in the above paragraph may seem to have little to do with blood transfusion. On the other hand, investigations to detect them have always been carried out in blood transfusion or immunohaematology laboratories, owing to the need to use the same techniques as are used in pre-transfusion testing. Moreover, the antibodies may have to be identified in patients who require blood transfusion.

Red cell autoantibodies
Most red cell autoantibodies can be classified as 'cold' or 'warm'.

Cold antibodies, by definition, are those that react more strongly at 0°C than at higher temperatures. The thermal range of particular cold autoantibodies varies widely; at one extreme there are the harmless cold autoagglutinins found in all normal subjects which are active only up to a temperature of 10–15°C; at the other extreme there are cold autoagglutinins active *in vitro* up to a temperature of 30°C or more which are associated with such harmful effects as blocking of small vessels in the hands and feet on exposure to cold, due to red cell agglutination, and the production of haemolytic anaemia. In between, there are many examples of cold autoagglutinins which are active up to a temperature of 25°C or so, and which are found in association with disease. For instance, many patients with mycoplasma infection transiently develop anti-I in their serum, but usually this antibody is active only at low temperatures and may be regarded as harmless. For cold antibodies the distinction between harmless and harmful depends solely on the maximum temperature at which they are active. Cold autoantibodies which are harmless, because they are active only up to a temperature of about 25°C, may nevertheless be very troublesome in the laboratory, especially if tests are carried out at room temperature or the antiglobulin test is carried out in an albumin-containing solution or in a low-ionic-strength medium.

Warm autoantibodies react as strongly at 37°C, or more strongly at 37°C, than at lower temperatures. These autoantibodies, too, may be classified as harmful or harmless, according to whether or not they are associated with red cell destruction. In these cases the property of harmlessness is clearly not related to thermal range but depends rather on the biological properties of the particular immunoglobulin molecules as well as on the number of antibody molecules that bind to the red cells and therefore also on the number and distribution of the corresponding antigen sites.

Whereas in patients with cold autoagglutinins the bulk of the antibody is in the serum, in patients with warm incomplete autoantibodies most is on the red cells.

HARMLESS COLD AUTOANTIBODIES (see Table 7.1)

Normal cold autoagglutinins
Landsteiner (1903) observed that if the serum of an animal was mixed with its own red cells at a temperature near 0°C, agglutination occurred. He later showed that serum from most human subjects would agglutinate autologous red cells at 0°C (Landsteiner and Levine, 1926).

Table 7.1 Some cold autoantibodies

Description	Specificity	Notes
Harmless		
normal cold autoagglutinins	anti-I	present in all normal sera, occasionally accompanied by anti-i
	anti-Pr, etc.	very rare
normal incomplete cold 'antibody'	anti-H	present in all normal sera, not an immunoglobulin but fixes complement to cells *in vitro*
Harmful		
pathological cold autoagglutinins	anti-I	usual specificity in chronic cold haemagglutinin disease (CHAD); also found transiently after mycoplasma infection
	anti-i	rare alternative to anti-I in CHAD; also sometimes found transiently after infectious mononucleosis
	anti-Pr, etc.	see text
biphasic haemolysins (Donath–Landsteiner antibody)	anti-P	usual specificity in paroxysmal cold haemoglobinuria
	other	very rare

The titre of normal autoagglutinins at 0–2°C does not usually exceed 64 using a tube technique with a 2% cell suspension and reading the results microscopically (Dacie, 1962, p. 460) but is much higher with more sensitive methods, e.g. when using microplates. In about one in four cases the titre of normal cold autoagglutinins is enhanced two- to four-fold if the serum is titrated in 22% bovine serum albumin instead of saline (Haynes and Chaplin, 1971).

Normal cold autoagglutinins almost always have the specificity anti-I (Tippett *et al.* 1960) but occasionally may have other specificities: a mixture of anti-I and anti-i (Jackson *et al.* 1968); anti-I^T (Booth *et al.* 1966); anti-Pr (Garratty *et al.* 1973; Roelcke and Kreft, 1984); anti-A, -B, -A_1I and -BI (for references see Mollison, 1983, p. 292); anti-M and -N (Moores *et al.* 1970; Tegoli *et al.* 1970; Sacher *et al.* 1989). Anti-LW occurring as a cold autoantibody is described in Chapter 5.

Anti-i was found in ten of 47 patients with cirrhosis of the liver, but active only at low temperatures and with a titre of 32 or less in seven of the ten cases (Rubin and Solomon, 1967).

Anti-I cold agglutinins can usually be demonstrated in cord blood (Mollison, 1956, p. 252). They are IgM and presumed to be synthethized by the fetus *in utero* (Adinolfi, 1965b).

An exceptional high-titre cold agglutinin which agglutinated cells at 37°C, but which was not associated with red cell destruction *in vivo*, has been described (Sniecinski *et al.* 1988).

Autoagglutinins inhibited by ionized calcium
Some examples of cold autoagglutinins react only in the absence of ionized calcium.
The first example was described by Parish and Macfarlane (1941) as an autoagglutinin
reacting in citrate but not in saline. Many examples have since been published, most
with anti-HI or anti-H specificity. In all cases agglutination has been inhibited by Ca^{2+}
and has depended on the presence of citrate or EDTA (for references see previous
editions of this book).

An autoagglutinin demonstrable only against borate-suspended red cells, with anti-A
specificity, was described by Strange and Cross (1981).

An autoagglutinin enhanced by sodium azide, with anti-I specificity, was reported by
Reviron *et al.* (1984).

Normal incomplete cold 'antibody' (n.i.c. antibody)
The n.i.c. antibody, which binds complement to red cells at low temperatures (Dacie,
1950; Dacie *et al.* 1957), has anti-H specificity (Crawford *et al.* 1953b) but is not an
immunoglobulin (Adinolfi *et al.* 1963) and, in its properties, has some resemblance to
properdin (Adinolfi, 1965a).

HARMFUL COLD AUTOANTIBODIES (see Table 7.1)

By definition, harmful cold autoantibodies are those associated with haemolytic
anaemia and, or, vascular occlusion on exposure to cold. Autoimmune haemolytic
anaemia (AIHA) is less commonly associated with cold autoantibodies than with warm
ones. In several published series, each of more than 100 cases of AIHA, about 15–20%
have been due to cold autoantibodies (Dausset and Colombani, 1959; Dacie, 1962; van
Loghem *et al.* 1963; Petz and Garratty, 1975). A similar percentage (16%) was found in
a series of 2000 patients with red cell autoantibodies (Engelfriet *et al.* 1982). A slightly
higher percentage (about 35%) was observed in two other series (Vroclans-Deiminas
and Boivin, 1980; Sokol *et al.* 1981).

Harmful cold autoantibodies may be: (1) cold autoagglutinins and haemolysins; or
(2) biphasic haemolysins (Donath–Landsteiner antibodies).

Cold haemagglutinin disease (CHAD) with autoimmune haemolytic anaemia
Two clinical syndromes may be distinguished, one chronic and one transient. In both,
the pathological effects of the autoantibodies — vascular occlusion and accelerated red
cell destruction — are exacerbated when the patient is exposed to cold. Vascular
occlusion is seen particularly in the exposed parts of the body; accelerated red cell
destruction may lead to haemoglobinuria.

The chronic syndromes are nearly always, if not always, associated with IgM
paraproteins (monoclonal) with cold agglutinin activity. Only a small proportion of IgM
paraproteins have cold agglutinin activity, e.g. 11 of 99 in the series of Pruzanski *et al.*
(1974). Of patients in whose serum IgM paraproteins are found, the majority have
chronic lymphocytic leukaemia or some form of lymphoma and a minority have

so-called Waldenström's macroglobulinaemia (Mackenzie and Fudenberg, 1972); intermediate disease states are not uncommon (Tubbs *et al.* 1976). In some of the patients the paraproteinaemia is of the benign kind. Sometimes the cold autoagglutinins are detected before the paraproteinaemia becomes manifest.

In the transient syndromes the cold haemagglutinins are polyclonal. The syndromes occur following infectious diseases, particularly mycoplasma infection and, less commonly, infectious mononucleosis. When the antibodies are active at 30°C or higher there may be an associated immune haemolytic anaemia.

In children, following infectious disease, high titre cold agglutinins are only rarely observed (Habibi *et al.* 1974) although cold antibodies of unspecified titre were found in 13 of 44 children reported by Zupanska *et al.* (1976). Ten of the 13 children had had an infectious disease.

Thermal range of autoantibody
Some examples of pathological cold autoagglutinins have titres of 1×10^6 or more at 0–4°C. At higher temperatures they are markedly less active and often will not agglutinate red cells *in vitro* above a temperature of about 31°C (Dacie, 1962, p. 462). Less commonly, the titre at low temperatures is only moderately increased but the antibody has a very wide thermal range; it should be emphasized that the clinical significance of a cold antibody is determined entirely by its ability to combine with red cells at, or near, body temperature rather than by its titre at some lower temperature.

In two cases the titre of cold autoagglutinins (IgM anti-I) was only 256 at 0°C but 16–32 at 37°C; both patients had moderately severe haemolytic anaemia and one had acrocyanosis (Schreiber *et al.* 1977).

Factors enhancing agglutination
In many cases the titre of cold autoagglutinins is enhanced by using albumin rather than saline as a medium; 22% albumin is distinctly better than 12% (Haynes and Chaplin, 1971). In testing 28 examples of anti-I associated with AIHA, at 30°C 14 failed to agglutinate cells suspended in saline but all 28 agglutinated them in albumin. In tests at 37°C only two examples agglutinated cells suspended in saline but 19 agglutinated cells suspended in albumin (Garratty *et al.* 1977). In some cases it is necessary to use an increased ratio of serum to cells to demonstrate clinically significant cold autoantibodies.

At any given temperature, enzyme-treated red cells take up more cold autoantibody than untreated cells and are agglutinated by potent anti-I up to about 38–40°C (Evans *et al.* 1965).

In studies with ^{131}I-labelled potent cold autoagglutinins maximally sensitized cells took up 8.9 mg antibody per ml red cells, corresponding to rather more than 500 000 molecules per cell (Evans *et al.* 1965). The same authors found that the rate of association and dissociation of anti-I was unaffected by the presence of complement, suggesting that complement did not affect the binding of this antibody. On the other hand, Rosse *et al.* (1968), using the C1 transfer test, found that complement did affect the binding of some examples of anti-I. For example, in the presence of C1, fewer red cells were required to absorb the same amount of antibody (for further discussion see Chapter 3).

Complement binding

When normal red cells are sensitized *in vitro* with fresh serum containing anti-I some cells may be lysed (see below); unlysed cells react with anti-C3c and anti-C4c as well as with anti-C3g, anti-C3d and anti-C4d. On circulating red cells the only C3 and C4 components detectable are C3d and C3g (Lachmann *et al.* 1982; Voak *et al.* 1983), and C4d (and, possibly, C4g). Serum containing potent autoagglutinins is always capable of producing some lysis of normal red cells at 20°C, although it may be necessary to adjust the pH of the serum to 6.8 to produce this effect (Dacie, 1962, p. 468). Potent cold autoagglutinins which are readily lytic may be confused with biphasic haemolysin (Donath–Landsteiner antibody), but the latter antibody is non-agglutinating and almost always has anti-P specificity.

When the possibility of confusion between anti-I and biphasic haemolysin arises, the following comparison is useful in distinguishing between them (H. Chaplin, personal communication): in one test, two samples of serum, one untreated and one acidified to pH 6.8, are incubated continuously (with red cells) at 20–25°C for 1 h and in the other, serum and red cells are first kept at 0°C for 30 min, then at 37°C for 30 min. Biphasic haemolysin gives maximal lysis under these latter conditions and is unaffected by acidification; on the other hand anti-I haemolysins are maximally lytic when incubated continuously at 20–25°C, especially with acidified serum.

At low temperatures the agglutination caused by anti-I is very intense and when agglutination is dispersed some lysis may be observed due, apparently, to mechanical damage during dispersal of the agglutinates (Stats, 1954). Although it has been claimed that potent cold autoagglutinins directly lyse red cells without the aid of complement (Salama *et al.* 1988), the effect may be a laboratory artefact.

Acquired resistance to complement-mediated lysis

When normal red cells are incubated at 20–30°C with anti-I serum and then warmed to 37°C, anti-I is eluted but complement components remain bound to the red cell surface (Harboe, 1964; Evans *et al.* 1965). As described in Chapter 3, bound C3b is very rapidly converted to iC3b which is then cleaved relatively slowly, leaving only C3dg on the cell surface. Normal red cells exposed to anti-I and complement *in vitro* under conditions which are suboptimal for producing lysis become coated with α_{2D} (i.e. C3dg) and become resistant to lysis (Evans *et al.* 1968; de Wit and van Gastel, 1970) and take up little or no β_{1A} (i.e. C3b) upon renewed exposure to anti-I and complement (Engelfriet *et al.* 1972b; see also Jaffe *et al.* 1976).

Red cells made resistant to lysis by anti-I in the way just described are partially protected against lysis by anti-Le^b (Engelfriet *et al.* 1972b) and by anti-Le^a (unpublished observations, MC and PLM). These findings are explained, presumably, by the fact that I and Lewis antigen sites are on the same molecule and thus bring about the accumulation of C3dg molecules on closely similar areas of the red cell membrane. Cells coated with complement by exposure to serum at very low ionic strength are not protected against lysis by anti-I (de Wit and van Gastel, 1970), possibly because the C3dg molecules are dispersed over the red cell surface and thus present in too low concentrations in the critical areas round I sites.

Circulating red cells of patients with CHAD are strongly coated with C3dg and are relatively resistant to red cell destruction. Thus, if a sample of red cells from a patient with CHAD is labelled with ^{51}Cr and reinjected into the circulation, the rate of red cell destruction is uniform and relatively slow. On the other hand, when red cells from a normal donor are injected, some 50% are destroyed in the first hour although subsequently the rate of destruction is far slower (Evans *et al.* 1968); see also below.

The question of transfusion in CHAD is discussed below.

Specificity of cold autoagglutinins associated with autoimmune haemolytic anaemia

Ii. In patients with CHAD the antibody usually has anti-I specificity. In determining specificity, samples from several newborn infants should be used since the red cells of some infants, although reacting predominantly as i may react relatively well with anti-I (Burnie, 1973). Red cells from adults of the very rare phenotype i are also useful in determining specificity. It may be necessary to test the antibody at the upper end of its thermal range (e.g. 30°C) to reveal its preference for adult cells (Burnie, 1973). The patient's own red cells tend to react poorly with his or her own serum, presumably due to interference by complement on the red cells (Evans *et al.* 1968). Nevertheless, the patient's cells react well with other anti-I sera, possibly reflecting the heterogeneity of anti-I (Rosenfield and Jagathambal, 1976) which may lead to differences in the site of binding.

Much less commonly, the antibody in CHAD has anti-i specificity (Marsh and Jenkins, 1960).

Pr(Sp). In a small number of the cases the antibody reacts equally well with adult and cord red cells. The antibody was originally called anti-Sp$_1$, because it was thought to be specific for humans (Marsh and Jenkins, 1968). Later, Pr was chosen to indicate that the antigen is destroyed by proteases (Roelcke and Uhlenbruck, 1970).

Pr antibodies recognize carbohydrate determinants represented by tri- or tetra-saccharides (or both), *O*-glycosidically bound to the *N*-terminal region of glycophorin A, B and C (Dahr *et al.* 1981a). A cold agglutinin, anti-PrM, which recognizes the above saccharides but whose affinity for them is increased ten-fold when they are attached to the M-specific peptide background of glycophorin A, was described by Roelcke *et al.* (1986). Several other subspecificities of Pr, e.g. Pr$_1$, Pr$_2$ etc., have been described (e.g. Roelcke *et al.* 1976). An example of anti-Pr which was completely inhibited by citrate has been described (Green *et al.* 1988b). The effect of citrate on some cold autoagglutinins has been discussed above. Anti-Pr cold agglutinins have been found after rubella (Geisen *et al.* 1975; König *et al.* 1985) and in one patient after varicella. Surprisingly the antibody in the latter case was (IgG κ) (Northhoff *et al.* 1987).

Other specificities. Cold agglutinins of many other specificities may be found in patients with CHAD. Some of the corresponding antigens, such as Vo (Roelcke *et al.* 1984), are related biochemically to Ii and some, e.g. Gd (Roelcke *et al.* 1977), Sa (Roelcke *et al.* 1980), Lud and Fl (Roelcke 1981a,b) to Pr. Rarely the specificity may be anti-A (Parker *et al.* 1978), anti-A$_1$ (Rochant *et al.* 1972; Castella *et al.* 1983), anti-B (Atichartakarn *et al.* 1985) anti-type II H (Uchikawa and Tohyama, 1986), anti-P (von dem Borne *et al.* 1982), anti-M-like (Sangster *et al.* 1979; Chapman *et al.* 1982), anti-D (Longster and Johnson, 1988) or anti-Sd^x, re-named anti-R^x (Marsh *et al.* 1980; Bass *et al.* 1983).

Is it necessary in clinical practice to determine the specificity or the titre
of cold agglutinins?
There is seldom any point in determining the specificity of cold autoagglutinins. The serological diagnosis of CHAD is made by demonstrating the antibody's wide thermal range and does not depend on determining its specificity. In the unlikely event of transfusion being needed for a patient with CHAD there will be an indication for determining specificity only if blood from random donors fails to produce beneficial effects and sufficient ii blood can be obtained. Determination of cold agglutinin titres is not worthwhile as a routine, although an association between a low titre and a response to corticosteroids has been observed; titres are little affected by therapy although exceptions have been reported (see p. 292).

Anti-I and anti-i associated with acute infections
Following infection with *Mycoplasma pneumoniae* there is commonly a transient increase in the titre and thermal range of anti-I cold autoagglutinins. When the thermal range is high enough, the patient may develop an episode of haemolytic anaemia, which may be severe.

The fact that the titre of anti-I is increased following infection with *M. pneumoniae* suggests the possibility of the presence in that organism of I-like antigen. Although intact *M. pneumoniae* do not inhibit anti-I, lipopolysaccharide prepared from these organisms does. Furthermore, *M. pneumoniae* inhibits the cold agglutinins produced in rabbits following an injection of these organisms (Costea *et al.* 1972). It has been suggested that anti-I may arise in *M. pneumoniae* infection in response to a modification of the 'self' antigen I by the micro-organism (Feizi, 1980b). The erythrocyte receptors for mycoplasma are long-chain oligosaccharides of sialic acid joined by α (2–3) linkage to the terminal galactose residues of poly-*N*-acetyllactosamine sequences of Ii antigen type (Loomes *et al.* 1984).

Anti-I in very high titre has been found following infection with *Listeria monocytogenes*, which carries an I-like antigen: the patient had transient haemolytic anaemia (Korn *et al.* 1957). A transient increase in anti-I titre has also been described in a patient with systemic leishmaniasis associated with haemolytic anaemia (Kokkini *et al.* 1984) and following an acute cytomegalovirus infection not clearly associated with haemolytic anaemia (Pien *et al.* 1974).

In infectious mononucleosis, anti-i is frequently present as a transient phenomenon (Jenkins *et al.* 1965a; Rosenfield *et al.* 1965). From a review of published cases. Worllcdgc and Dacie (1969) concluded that anti-i is present in about 50% of patients with infectious mononucleosis: whereas normal sera agglutinate cord red cells only up to a titre of 4 at 4°C, in 14 of 30 sera from patients with infectious mononucleosis, the titre was 16 or more. The antibody was very seldom detectable *in vitro* at a temperature higher than about 24°C. According to the same authors, fewer than 1% of patients with infectious mononucleosis develop a haemolytic syndrome and in these the antibody is active *in vitro* up to a temperature of at least 28°C. Anti-i is completely separable from the Paul–Bunnell antibody.

In investigating a case in which haemolytic anaemia complicated infectious mononucleosis and in which the patient's serum contained a potent cold autoagglutinin, it was discovered that the agglutinin was an IgG–IgM complex. The autoantibody (presumably anti-i) was found to be IgG; the IgM was an anti-IgG antibody. Both the IgG and the IgM antibodies acted most strongly at 4°C (Goldberg and Barnett, 1967).

One subsequent investigation suggested that the serological findings described by Goldberg and Barnett (1967) were the rule in infectious mononucleosis (Capra *et al.* 1969), but observations of others cast doubt on this conclusion. H. Chaplin (personal communication, 1980) tested 20 samples of serum from patients with infectious mononucleosis with haemolytic anaemia without finding a single example of a cold IgG anti-i combined with a cold IgM anti-IgG — although his laboratory subsequently encountered one such case (Gronemeyer *et al.* 1981).

Again, in a patient with infectious mononucleosis complicated by a haemolytic episode, there was no evidence that an anti-IgG was playing any part in serological reactions and anti-i activity was completely abolished by treatment of the serum with 2-mercaptoethanol. The case was remarkable in that the antibody was active *in vitro* at 22°C but not at 32°C, although exposure of red cells to serum at 4°C, followed by warming of the mixture to 37°C, led to 42% lysis, i.e. the antibody, although IgM, behaved serologically like biphasic haemolysin (Burkart and Hsu, 1979).

In one, apparently unique, case anti-N was formed instead of the expected anti-i in a patient with infectious mononucleosis. AIHA was diagnosed 3 weeks after the onset of the patient's illness, at which time there was transient moderately severe haemolytic anaemia. The direct antiglobulin test (DAT) was strongly positive but only with anti-C3 and anti-C4. The patient's red cells were MNSs and the serum contained anti-N (IgM) with a titre of 512 at 4°C, but only 1 at 37°C. Anti-N was eluted from the red cells. One month later the anti-N could no longer be detected and the DAT was only very weakly positive (Bowman *et al.* 1974).

In investigations on patients with massive tropical splenomegaly in Papua New Guinea, Pitney *et al.* (1968) found that anti-i was frequently present in the serum. The sera contained macroglobulin, 16–33% of which was cold agglutinin. The authors commented that the production of anti-i appeared to be associated with hyperplasia of reticuloendothelial tissue.

Persistent anti-I and anti-i cold agglutinins not associated with haemolytic anaemia have also been found in the serum of patients with acquired immune deficiency syndrome (AIDS) or AIDS-related complex (Pruzanski *et al.* 1986). The thermal range of the antibodies was not established.

Red cell transfusion in patients with cold haemagglutin disease
When red cells from a normal (I-positive) donor are transfused to a patient with CHAD due to anti-I, there is a phase of destruction which lasts until the cells have acquired resistance to complement-mediated destruction; during this phase, a proportion of the transfused population is destroyed within minutes; an identical phenomenon is observed with complement-activating alloantibodies (see Chapter 10). In CHAD, therefore, transfusion should be avoided if possible. If a transfusion is judged to be essential, the blood should be pre-warmed, although a more important step is to nurse the patient in a warm room (see below). Red cells from ii adults have been shown to survive normally in patients with CHAD due to anti-I both in the chronic form (van Loghem *et al.* 1963) and in the transient form (Woll *et al.* 1974), but ii donors are seldom available.

Most patients with CHAD are not severely anaemic; if a haemolytic crisis does develop, red cell destruction can usually be arrested by putting the patient in a really warm environment (40°C). In cases in which the cold autoagglutinins have a low titre but a wide thermal range, treatment with corticosteroids has been successful (Lahav et al. 1989). Treatment with α-interferon resulted in a prompt clinical response and a considerable decrease of the titre of the cold agglutinins in a patient with severe CHAD (O'Connor et al. 1989).

Immunoglobulin structure of cold agglutinins

In chronic cold haemagglutin disease most examples of anti-I and anti-i are IgM κ, although a few IgM λ examples have been described (Pruzanski et al. 1974; Roelcke et al. 1974). Of the relatively few examples of anti-Pr, four have been IgA κ and all these have had Pr$_1$ specificity (Angevine et al. 1966; Garratty et al. 1973; Roelcke, 1973; Tonthat et al. 1976); one, which was IgM κ, had Pr$_2$ specificity and another, which was IgM λ, Pr$_3$ (Roelcke et al. 1974; 1976).

IgM cold agglutinins with λ light chains are rarely directed against the I antigen. They are frequently cryoprecipitable and are often found in malignant conditions. Such agglutinins thus differ markedly from cold agglutinins with κ light chains.

Patients with chronic CHAD synthesize IgM at approximately ten times the normal rate; treatment with alkylating agents results in a diminished rate of synthesis (Brown and Cooper, 1970).

Occasionally, cold IgM anti-I is accompanied by a warm IgG autoantibody of the same or another specificity (see below). Examples of anti-I cold agglutinins which appeared to be solely IgG were described by Ambrus and Bajtai (1969) and Mygind and Ahrons (1973), and an example of anti-Pr which was IgG1 κ was described by Dellagi et al. (1981); this antibody had an agglutinin titre of 16 at 4°C and of 1 at 37°C.

The possibility that IgM anti-I is always accompanied by at least traces of IgG and IgA autoantibodies is raised by the finding of Hsu et al. (1974a). Using a PVP-augmented antiglobulin test in the AutoAnalyzer they found that, in patients with typical anti-I cold agglutinins, IgG and IgA could always be detected on the patient's red cells in addition to C3 and C4. Similarly, Ratkin et al. (1973) prepared eluates from 19 sera from patients with cold agglutinin disease and regularly found an excess of IgG and of IgA, both having agglutinating activity of relatively low titre. They interpreted their observations to mean that in patients in whom IgM autoantibodies predominated, autoantibodies of classes IgG and IgA were also regularly present, though in lower titre.

In mycoplasma infection, when a patient develops potent cold autoagglutinins of anti-I specificity as a transient phenomenon the antibody is made of heterogeneous IgM and contains both κ and λ light chains (Costea et al. 1966), although the heterogeneity is restricted (see Feizi, 1977).

Production of cold autoagglutinins following repeated blood transfusions
Rous and Robertson (1918) observed that in rabbits transfused almost daily with the blood of other rabbits, cold autoagglutinins developed in about half the animals. The animals with the most potent agglutinins developed a sudden anaemia, due perhaps to immune clearance of

transfused cells. The agglutinins persisted in the animal's serum long after transfused cells had disappeared. Thus, in one case, 133 d after the last blood transfusion there was still gross autoagglutination on chilling the animal's blood.

Ovary and Spiegelman (1965) gave repeated injections of Hg^A-positive red cells to an Hg^A-negative rabbit: the animal produced not only the expected anti-Hg^A active at 37°C, but also a cold agglutinin.

The production of cold autoagglutinins in humans, following alloimmunization and in association with a delayed haemolytic transfusion reaction, has been observed only occasionally (see Chapter 11).

Cold (biphasic) autohaemolysins

In the syndrome of PCH the patient's serum contains a cold, complement-fixing antibody. This antibody, often referred to as the Donath–Landsteiner antibody after its discoverers, produces haemolysis both *in vitro* and *in vivo* when the blood is first cooled (to allow the binding of antibody) and then warmed (to provide optimal conditions for complement-mediated haemolysis). Because of this behaviour, the antibody is described as a 'biphasic haemolysin'.

Although biphasic haemolysin was originally described in a patient with tertiary syphilis, the majority of cases seen nowadays are associated with viral infections, particularly in children. In one series of 11 cases, only three were definitely syphilitic; of five which were definitely non-syphilitic, one followed measles and one mumps (Worlledge and Rousso, 1965). Biphasic haemolysin may also occur transiently following chickenpox, influenza-like illness and prophylactic immunization with measles vaccine (Bird *et al.* 1976b).

Of 19 patients with biphasic haemolysin reported by Sokol *et al.* (1982; 1984), 17 were children. All patients were non-syphilitic. In ten of the children the biphasic haemolysin developed after an upper respiratory tract infection. The other patients had infections with adenovirus type 2, influenza A virus or *Haemophilus influenzae*; one had chickenpox. The authors stressed the fact that in the acute form which typically occurs in children, the onset of the haemolytic anaemia is sudden, usually with haemoglobinuria, prostration and pallor. In the chronic form haemolysis is only mild; this form occurred in only two patients, one a child and the other an adult. Biphasic haemolysin in an adult patient with pneumonia due to *Klebsiella* was described by Lau *et al.* (1983).

It has been suggested that for the prevalent non-syphilitic form of the syndrome the term Donath–Landsteiner haemolytic anaemia should be used rather than PCH, since the clinical manifestations are rarely paroxysmal, seldom precipitated by cold and not necessarily characterized by haemoglobinuria (Wolach *et al.* 1981).

Several estimates of the relative frequency of biphasic haemolysin in AIHA are available. In one series of 347 cases of AIHA, the antibody was found in six, i.e. fewer than 2% (Petz and Garratty, 1980, p. 54). Similarly, of red cell autoantibodies from 2000 patients, 48 (2.4%) were biphasic haemolysin (Engelfriet *et al.* 1982). On the other hand, the antibody was present in four of 34 (12%) acute cases of AIHA in children in one series (Habibi *et al.* 1974) and in 17 of 42 (40%) cases in another (Sokol *et al.* 1984).

Although maximum haemolysis is observed when red cells are left with biphasic haemolysin and complement in the cold phase, the requirement for complement in the cold phase is not absolute. Thus when red cells are first left at 0°C with EDTA-treated serum containing fairly potent antibody then washed and incubated at 37°C with fresh normal serum, some haemolysis occurs (Polley *et al.* 1962). Similarly, Hinz *et al.* (1961a) found that if PNH red cells were used, haemolysis occurred quite readily when complement was supplied only in the warm phase of the reaction. An experiment described by Dacie (1962, p. 553) shows clearly that the reason why much more haemolysis is found when complement is present in the cold phase of the reaction is that, on warming, antibody very rapidly elutes from the red cells so that at higher temperatures there is usually too little antibody on the cells to activate complement. Hinz *et al.* (1961b) showed that optimal lysis occurred even when only C1 was present with antibody in the cold phase of the reaction; C4 could be present either in the cold or warm phases but C2 and C3 were essential in the warm phase.

False-negative results may be observed due to hypocomplementaemia and it may then be necessary to add fresh normal serum to demonstrate the presence of the biphasic haemolysin (Wolach *et al.* 1981).

In cases in which biphasic haemolysin is associated with syphilis (tertiary or congenital) the antibody is seldom active above 20°C; that is to say, red cells and serum must be cooled to a temperature below 20°C if there is to be haemolysis on subsequent warming. In cases in which the antibody appears transiently in children following infections, the thermal range is greater and the antibody may be active *in vitro* up to a temperature as high as 32°C (see Bird *et al.* 1976b). A monophasic haemolysin acting *in vitro* up to 32°C, in an adult, was described by Ries *et al.* (1971).

As mentioned above, potent cold autoagglutinins which are readily lytic may be confused with biphasic haemolysin, but the latter is usually non-agglutinating, produces substantially more lysis, is IgG rather than IgM, and has anti-P rather than anti-I specificity. A test that helps to distinguish unusually-lytic anti-I from biphasic haemolysin is described on p. 288.

Specificity. Classically, biphasic haemolysin has the specificity anti-P (Levine *et al.* 1963a; Worlledge and Rousso, 1965). Very occasionally, the specificity may be anti-'p' (see Chapter 4).

Biphasic haemolysins with anti-P specificity are inhibited by globoside; some are more strongly inhibited by the Forssman glycolipid, which contains the globoside structure with an additional terminal GalNAc residue, suggesting that the antibodies are probably evoked by Forssman antigens which are widespread in animal tissues and micro-organisms (Schwarting *et al.* 1979).

Occasionally, biphasic haemolysins have a specificity outside the P system: anti-IH (Weiner *et al.* 1964), anti-I (Engelfriet *et al.* 1968b; Bell *et al.* 1973a), anti-i, as described above, or anti-Pr like (Judd *et al.* 1986b). In practice, determination of the specificity of biphasic haemolysins is not helpful in diagnosis. On the other hand, in children with antibodies of wide thermal range and severe red cell destruction, confirmation of anti-P specificity may be helpful in treatment, since transfusion of pp red cells is sometimes very successful (see below).

Immunoglobulin class. Biphasic haemolysin (of specificity anti-P) is composed of IgG (Adinolfi *et al.* 1962; Hinz, 1963). If red cells are incubated at a temperature such as 15°C with fresh serum containing biphasic haemolysin and then washed at room temperature, they react weakly with anti-IgG but strongly with anti-C4 and anti-C3, as expected from the fact that the antibody elutes rapidly as the temperature is raised. During, and for some time after, an attack of haemoglobinuria, the red cells of patients with PCH give a positive DAT. Only complement components (presumably C3d and C4d) can be detected on the red cells.

Red cell transfusion in patients with biphasic haemolysins

Red cell transfusion is seldom required in PCH. When the thermal range of the antibody extends only to 20°C or so *in vitro*, the patient is not severely anaemic. In patients in whom the thermal range extends to 30°C or more, severe anaemia does occur occasionally but in these patients the disease is usually transient and recovery has usually begun before the question of transfusion has to be considered. The successful use of P-negative red cells (from a bank of frozen blood) has been reported (Rausen *et al.* 1975) but unwashed, unwarmed P-positive blood has also been used successfully in three affected children (Wolach *et al.* 1981). In a child with PCH and severe anaemia, who did not respond to transfusion of P-positive blood, the transfusion of P-negative blood resulted in a sustained rise in Hb level (I. Franklin and MC, personal observation).

HARMLESS WARM AUTOANTIBODIES

IgG class of harmless warm antibodies

Since only IgG1 and IgG3 adhere to Fc receptors (see Chapter 3), only autoantibodies of these subclasses are expected to cause red cell destruction. Furthermore, there is evidence that a certain minimum number of IgG1 molecules must be bound per red cell to bring about attachment to phagocytic cells and thus cause destruction (see below). Thus subjects with only a relatively small number of IgG1 molecules bound per red cell or subjects with only IgG2 or IgG4 on their red cells might be expected to have a positive direct antiglobulin test without any signs of red cell destruction.

Positive direct antiglobulin test in apparently normal subjects

The fact that an apparently normal donor has a positive DAT is often first discovered when the donor's red cells are used in crossmatching. Sixty-five cases were found in this way in one region during a period in which one million donations were collected. Assuming that for every ten donors detected one was missed, the frequency of donors with a positive DAT was estimated to be one in 14 000 (Gorst *et al.* 1980). In another prospective survey donors with a positive DAT were discovered either by antiglobulin testing or by noting autoagglutination of a blood sample in an automated or manual test and then doing an antiglobulin test. The frequency of donors with a positive DAT was one in 13 000 (Habibi *et al.* 1980). Although the results of these two surveys look very similar there were apparent differences between the two. In the first there was only C3d (and C4d) on the red cells of 28 of the 65 donors. All donors with a positive

DAT were haematologically normal; of 32 of the donors followed for many years, 31 remained well and only one, with a strongly positive DAT with anti-IgG, developed AIHA (Gorst *et al.* 1980).

In the second series, immunoglobulin was detectable on the red cells in all of 69 cases (IgG in 67, IgM in 2). Ten per cent of the donors had subnormal Hb values; a further 29% had reticulocytosis, with or without hyperbilirubinaemia: 61% appeared to be normal haematologically but when Cr survival studies were carried out in a few of these subjects, results were below normal in about 50% of the cases (Habibi *et al.* 1980). It should be noted that 25% of the donors with a positive DAT were receiving methyldopa, a circumstance which might have debarred them from donation in many countries. In any case it must be said that the evidence presented for a haemolytic state in many of the donors was rather slight. No donor had a reticulocyte count higher than about 4.5% or a bilirubin value higher than 2.2 mg/dl (37 μmol/l). Slightly reduced Cr survival in haematologically normal subjects is difficult to interpret. Finally, in many of the donors who were followed for a period of 1 year or more, haematological findings became normal.

A very much higher frequency of positive DATs in normal donors than that found in the two series mentioned above was reported by Allan and Garratty (1980), namely one in 1000, but the discrepancy may be more apparent than real since over 90% of the reactions were only '1 +' or less.

In 22 of 23 normal donors with IgG on their red cells from the series of Gorst *et al.* (1980), the IgG subclass of the antibody was later investigated. In 20 of the cases it was solely IgG1 and the number of IgG1 molecules per red cell varied from 110 to 950; in the remaining two subjects the red cells were coated only with IgG4 (Stratton *et al.* 1983). In another series of ten subjects five had only IgG1, three IgG4, one IgG2 and one both IgG1 and IgG3 (Allan and Garratty, 1980).

In normal donors with a positive DAT, the specificity of the autoantibody, as in patients with AIHA, is often related to Rh (Issitt *et al.* 1976a; Habibi *et al.* 1980) but may be outside the Rh system, e.g. anti-Jk^a (Holmes *et al.* 1976) and anti-Xg^a (Yokohama and McCoy, 1967).

In normal subjects with IgG on their red cells, the red cells may be agglutinated by anti-complement as well as anti-IgG, although the frequency with which both IgG and complement have been found has varied widely in different series, i.e. 15% (Gorst *et al.* 1980); 44% (Allan and Garratty, 1980); 70% (Issitt *et al.* 1976a).

Positive direct antiglobulin test (IgG) in hypergammaglobulinaemia
An association has been observed between hypergammaglobulinaemia and a positive DAT. Of 50 patients with an increased concentration of IgG in their serum, 25 had a positive DAT without signs of increased red cell destruction. The eluates from the red cells were unreactive (Huh *et al.* 1988). In another study of 20 patients with an increased serum IgG and a positive DAT, there were no signs of increased red cell destruction. These eluates were also unreactive (Heddle *et al.* 1988). In a prospective study of 44 patients with increased serum IgG, the DAT was positive in the three patients with the highest IgG concentrations. The DAT became positive in two other patients who were treated with high-dose intravenous immunoglobulin and, again, the eluates were unreactive (Heddle *et al.* 1988).

C3d (and C4d) alone on red cells

In 40–47% of normal donors with a positive DAT only complement is detected on the red cells (Allan and Garratty, 1980; Gorst *et al.* 1980). C3d can be demonstrated on all normal red cells by using a sufficiently potent anti-C3d serum (Graham *et al.* 1976) and both C3d and C4d can be demonstrated by using the sensitive PVP-augmented antiglobulin test (Rosenfield and Jagathambal, 1978). The presence of these fragments on red cells is taken as evidence of continuing low-grade activation of complement (see Chapter 3). There is no reason to believe that autoantibodies of any kind are responsible for this activation and it is therefore not logical to discuss this subject under the general heading of 'harmless warm autoantibodies', but it is nevertheless convenient.

The amount of C3d on the red cells of normal adults has been estimated by using rabbit IgG anti-C3d and ^{125}I-labelled goat anti-rabbit IgG; in 174 normal adults there were estimated to be between 50 and 200 C3d molecules per red cell, i.e. too few to be detected in the ordinary DAT. There was no difference between males and females and no evidence of any change in the number of molecules per cell over the age range 20–65. There was also no evidence that the number was different in children (Chaplin *et al.* 1981).

Weakly positive DATs due to increased amounts of C3d on the red cells appear to be relatively frequent in subjects who are ill. Dacie and Worlledge (1969) found that 40 out of 489 (8%) of patients in hospital gave weakly positive antiglobulin reactions due to complement. Similarly, Freedman (1979) found that of 100 EDTA samples from hospital patients, taken at random, seven gave positive reactions with anti-C3d and anti-C4d; all seven patients were seriously ill. Again, in 8% of random hospital patients values greater than 230 C3d molecules per cell were found by Chaplin *et al.* (1981), who also noted that in random patients in hospital 33% had values for the numbers of C3d molecules per red cell which were above the range found in more than 90% of healthy adults.

In testing red cells with anti-C3d and anti-C4d, freshly-taken EDTA blood should be used whenever possible since the amounts of C3d and C4d on red cells in ACD blood may increase slightly during brief storage at 4°C (Engelfriet, 1976); after 21 d storage, the increase of C3d and C4d may be two-fold (H. Chaplin, personal communication).

Positive direct antiglobulin test associated with various diseases,
but without signs of increased red cell destruction

Malaria. A positive DAT has been found in 40–50% of West African children with falciparum malaria (Topley *et al.* 1973; Facer *et al.* 1979; Abdalla and Weatherall, 1982). In most cases, only C3d is detected on the red cells but in some both C3d and IgG are present and, in a few, IgG alone. Although in one series there was a relationship between a positive DAT and anaemia (Facer *et al.* 1979); in the others there was not. It was suggested that a positive test might be associated with the development of immunity to malaria (Abdalla and Weatherall, 1982).

Kala-azar. The presence of complement on the red cells of patients with this disorder was reported by Woodruff *et al.* (1972).

Patients on α-methyldopa and other drugs. The development of a positive DAT without any evidence of a haemolytic process is very common in patients taking α-methyldopa and is found occasionally in patients taking a variety of other drugs. The subject is considered in more detail in the section on drug-induced haemolytic anaemia.

Patients with autoimmune haemolytic disease in spontaneous remission without signs of red cell destruction may have a positive DAT (Loutit and Mollison, 1946). In a patient reported by Goldberg and Fudenberg (1968), the red cells were initially agglutinated by anti-IgG and anti-C3; the serum contained an IgM antibody reacting with IgG-coated red cells. After treatment with steroids, the patient went into complete haematological remission and the IgM antibody disappeared from the serum; however, the red cells were still strongly agglutinated by anti-IgG and anti-C3.

In a patient reported by von dem Borne *et al.* (1977), who initially suffered from severe AIHA, a long-lasting remission was induced with steroid therapy and it was then found that the antibody on the patient's cells was predominantly IgG4; the coated red cells induced only weak rosetting with monocytes *in vitro* and it was postulated that there had been a switch in the subclass of the autoantibody, with production of a subclass (IgG$_4$) which was incapable of producing destruction *in vivo*.

HARMFUL WARM AUTOANTIBODIES

As mentioned above, antibodies reacting as well, or better, at 37°C than at lower temperatures are found in about 80% of all cases of AIHA. In the warm antibody type of AIHA the DAT is almost always positive but the indirect test (for antibody in serum) is sometimes negative. Harmful warm autoantibodies are of two kinds: incomplete antibodies and haemolysins.

Incomplete warm autoantibodies

IgG alone has been found in 18.3% (Petz and Garratty, 1975), 36% (Worlledge, 1978) and 64% (Engelfriet *et al.* 1982) of cases.

IgG alone was found invariably in patients with a positive DAT associated with α-methyldopa in two series (Worlledge, 1969; Issitt *et al.* 1976a), although in a third, IgM and complement (C1q), in addition to IgG, were found on the red cells of all patients who developed α-methyldopa-induced haemolytic anaemia (Lalezari *et al.* 1982), results that could not be reproduced by one author (CPE) or by Ben-Izhak *et al.* (1985). The detection of the IgM antibodies appears to depend on the anti-IgM serum used. It has been suggested that if the affinity of the anti-IgM for IgM is much greater than that of the IgM red cell antibodies for the red cell antigen, the IgM antibodies are removed from the red cell in the antiglobulin phase of the test (P. Lalezari, personal communication).

IgG and complement have been found in 64.5% (Petz and Garratty, 1980), 44.4% (Worlledge, 1978) and about 34% (Engelfriet *et al.* 1982) of cases; in the latter series, IgG and complement were found on the red cells of all patients with a combination of IgG incomplete warm autoantibodies and warm haemolysins (see below).

When complement and IgG are found on the red cells of patients with incomplete warm autoantibodies, it does not follow that complement has been fixed by autoantibody. Some of the evidence for this assertion is as follows: (1) neither IgG incomplete warm autoantibodies present in the serum nor those detectable in an eluate from the red cells are capable of fixing complement *in vitro*; (2) in at least 50% of patients with IgA incomplete warm autoantibodies alone, complement is detectable on the red cells; and (3) the frequency with which both IgG and complement are found on the red cells is much higher in patients suffering from a typical immune complex disease such as systemic lupus erythematosus (SLE), than in other cases of the warm type of AIHA. Thus, in SLE, both IgG and complement were found on the red cells in all cases by Chaplin (1973) and Worlledge (1978), in virtually all cases by Petz and Garratty (1980) and in 81% of cases by Engelfriet *et al.* (1982).

IgG subclass of warm incomplete autoantibodies

IgG warm autoantibodies are IgG1 in the vast majority of patients (Engelfriet *et al.* 1982). IgG1 alone was found in 72% of patients and IgG1 together with antibodies of another subclass in 25%. In only 23 of 572 patients was no IgG1 detectable. IgG2 and IgG4 antibodies were found the least frequently. Table 7.2 shows the frequency with which IgG autoantibodies of only one subclass were detected and the relation of the subclass of the autoantibodies to increased red cell destruction.

As already mentioned (see Chapter 3) in subjects whose red cells are coated with IgG, increased red cell destruction is expected only when the IgG belongs to subclasses IgG1 or IgG3 and, in the case of IgG1, only when the number of antibody molecules per red cell exceeds a certain minimum. Red cells coated with amounts of IgG3 too small to be detected by the DAT are still lysed by monocytes, a finding that may explain the fact that in some cases of presumed AIHA the DAT is negative. When red cells are coated with IgG1 there is a clear relationship between the number of molecules per cell and the severity of haemolytic anaemia (van der Meulen *et al.* 1980a; Engelfriet *et al.* 1981).

As mentioned above, in 20 normal donors with a positive DAT with only IgG1 on the red cells, the number of antibody molecules per cell never exceeded 950. On the other hand, in patients with AIHA with only IgG1 on the cells, the number of IgG molecules per cell was 1200 or more (Stratton *et al.* 1983). This finding agrees well with the observation that at least 1180 IgG1 anti-D molecules must be bound per cell for adherence of the cell to monocyte Fc receptors to occur *in vitro* (Zupanska *et al.* 1986).

Table 7.2 Presence or absence of increased red cell destruction in patients with IgG incomplete warm autoantibodies of only one subclass

Number of patients	IgG1	IgG2	IgG3	IgG4	Increased red cell destruction
416	+	−	−	−	75%
4	−	+	−	−	none
13	−	−	+	−	100%
5	−	−	−	+	none
438*					

* 438 of 572 patients with IgG incomplete warm autoantibodies had antibody of only one subclass (unpublished observations, CPE).

Complement alone was found in about 10% of cases in two series (Worlledge, 1978; Petz and Garratty, 1980), although no cases of this kind were found in another series (Issitt *et al.* 1976a). Only complement was found on the red cells of all patients with cold autoagglutinins, biphasic haemolysins or warm haemolysins without the simultaneous presence (see below) of incomplete warm autoantibodies (von dem Borne *et al.* 1969; Engelfriet *et al.* 1982).

As in all patients on whose red cells complement is bound *in vivo*, C3d (actually C3dg, see Chapter 3) is the subcomponent of C3 present on circulating red cells, and similarly C4d (possibly C4dg) is the only subcomponent of C4 present.

IgA. Incomplete warm autoantibodies may be solely IgA (Engelfriet *et al.* 1968a). IgA alone was found in three of 291 cases in one series (Worlledge, 1978), in two of 102 cases in another series (Petz and Garratty, 1980), and in 11 of 1374 patients in a third series (Engelfriet *et al.* 1982). One example of an IgA incomplete autoantibody with Rh specificity (anti-e) has been described (Stratton *et al.* 1972). For optimal conditions for detecting bound IgA in the antiglobulin test, see Chapter 8. In about 50% of patients with IgA autoantibodies, complement as well as IgA can be detected on the red cells.

The clinical course of patients with IgA incomplete warm autoantibodies is very similar to that of patients with IgG antibodies. Although most investigators have failed to detect Fc receptors for IgA on monocytes, it has been shown that IgA-sensitized cells are cytotoxically damaged by monocytes *in vitro* (Clark *et al.* 1984).

IgM incomplete warm autoantibodies occur with about the same frequency as IgA incomplete warm autoantibodies, i.e. in about 1% of patients with incomplete warm autoantibodies. For example, in one series of 1374 patients, 13 had only IgM autoantibody on their cells (always accompanied by complement), 13 had mixed IgG and IgM incomplete warm autoantibodies (and complement), and a single patient had a mixture of IgA and IgM incomplete warm autoantibodies together with complement (Engelfriet *et al.* 1982). The presence of autoantibodies of more than one immunoglobulin class on the red cells is associated with severe haemolytic anaemia (Ben-Izhak *et al.* 1985).

Warm autohaemolysins and agglutinins
Warm autohaemolysins and agglutinins are of two kinds, complete and incomplete.

The complete kind are capable of agglutinating and haemolysing untreated normal red cells suspended in saline. Such autoantibodies were described by Chauffard and Vincent (1909), Dameshek and Schwartz (1938) and Dacie (1954), but are very rare. In one series they were found in only three of 2000 patients with red cell autoantibodies; their presence is associated with very severe intravascular haemolysis which may be directly responsible for the death of the patient (Engelfriet *et al.* 1982).

In a patient described by Dorner *et al.* (1968) with post-traumatic renal cortical necrosis, treated with blood transfusion and dialysis, a potent IgM autoagglutinin developed, reacting more strongly at 37°C than at 4°C. The antibody agglutinated but did not haemolyse normal donor red cells *in vitro* and was associated with only mild haemolytic anaemia. In a case described by Freedman *et al.* (1977), AIHA was associated with a complement-binding IgM agglutinin and haemolysin of specificity anti-I[T], reacting optimally at 37°C.

The incomplete kind react *in vitro* only with enzyme-treated cells, but in some cases weakly sensitize untreated cells to agglutination by an anti-complement serum. Nearly all warm autohaemolysins are of this second type; they are presumably the ones described by Dacie and DeGruchy (1951), although these authors found that when complement was inactivated the serum agglutinated red cells suspended in saline.

The majority of incomplete warm haemolysins react with antigens susceptible to destruction by phospholipase; the rest react with antigens that are hardly, if at all, susceptible; incomplete warm haemolysins show no specificity for Ii or Rh antigens (Wolf and Roelcke, 1989).

Warm haemolysins, which are nearly always IgM, were the only autoantibodies found in 165 of 2000 patients with red cell autoantibodies (Engelfriet *et al.* 1982). When only IgM warm haemolysins, reacting only with enzyme-treated cells *in vitro*, are demonstrable in a patient's serum, red cell survival is only slightly shortened (von dem Borne *et al.* 1969). IgM warm haemolysins also frequently occur together with incomplete warm autoantibodies, e.g. in 138 of the 2000 patients in one series (Engelfriet *et al.* 1982). Complement is found on the red cells of all patients with IgM warm autohaemolysins.

Cold and warm autoantibodies occurring together

Patients with AIHA with both cold and warm autoantibodies in their serum are not as rare as was thought at one time: in one series the combination was recorded in 63 of 865 patients (Sokol *et al.* 1981). In 25 of these patients studied in more detail, in every case IgG and complement were detectable on the red cells and anti-I or anti-i cold autoagglutinins, reactive at 30°C or above, were detectable in the serum. All the cases were severe; 56% were secondary, the commonest associated diseases being SLE and lymphoma (Sokol *et al.* 1983). In another series, a somewhat lower incidence of this kind of AIHA was reported, namely 12 of 144 patients (Shulman *et al.* 1985); again, the haemolytic anaemia was severe in all cases and, again, many cases were secondary to SLE or lymphoma.

A few other cases have been described in which a patient with AIHA has had both IgG and IgM autoantibodies active at 37°C but in which the features have not been exactly the same as in the series described above. In one of these atypical cases both the IgM and the IgG autoantibodies reacted better in the cold but had a wide thermal range, the IgG antibody lysing enzyme-treated cells at 37°C (Moore and Chaplin, 1973). In two other cases both IgM and IgG autoantibodies had anti-I specificity. There were many features which were quite atypical of CHAD; thus, the patients had a very severe haemolytic process unrelated to exposure to cold and responding well to steroids (Freedman and Newlands, 1977). A case with many similarities was reported by Dacie (1967, p. 751).

Negative direct antiglobulin test in autoimmune haemolytic anaemia

A few patients with the clinical picture of AIHA have a negative conventional DAT (Gilliland *et al.* 1971). In many of these cases IgG, IgM or IgA autoantibodies can be demonstrated by more sensitive methods. For example: (1) using either ^{125}I-staphylococcal protein A (SPA) (which does not react with IgG3 antibodies), or a manual direct polybrene test, positive results were obtained in two of 12 cases (Petz and

Branch, 1983); (2) using a radioimmune DAT, small numbers of IgG autoantibodies were detected on the red cells in 16 of 26 cases (Schmitz et al. 1981); and (3) using the two-stage immunoradiometric assay with ^{125}I-SPA for the detection of antibodies, IgG and, or, IgM were detected on the red cells in all of eight cases (Salama et al. 1985). Using a sensitive enzyme-linked DAT, various combinations of immunoglobulins of different classes were detected on the red cells of 22 of 33 patients on whose red cells only complement could be detected with a conventional DAT and on the red cells of a further 16 patients whose red cells failed altogether to react in a conventional DAT. In 16 of these (22 + 16) cases, only IgM was detected (Sokol et al. 1985). Similar results were obtained in a later study (Sokol et al. 1987). In patients with a positive conventional DAT, it is very rare to find IgM alone and it seems doubtful whether autoantibodies were being detected in these two studies. In another series in which a similar test was used, an increased amount of IgG was detected on the red cells of seven of 35 patients with a negative conventional DAT and a possible diagnosis of warm AIHA. In five of the seven patients, the anaemia was corrected by steroid therapy (Gutgsell et al. 1988).

It has been suggested that in cases of AIHA with a negative DAT the autoantibody may be IgG3, since the number of IgG3 molecules per red cell needed for antibody-mediated lysis by monocytes is lower than that required for a positive antiglobulin test (Engelfriet et al. 1981).

Specificity of warm autoantibodies

Rh related
A few warm autoantibodies are specific for one particular Rh antigen such as e (Weiner et al. 1953) or D (Holländer, 1954); others react more strongly with e-positive than with e-negative samples (Dacie and Cutbush, 1954) but the commonest pattern, found by Weiner and Vos (1963) in two-thirds of cases, is to react well with all cells except for those of the type Rh_{null}.

Celano and Levine (1967) concluded that three specificities could be recognized: (1) anti-LW; (2) an antibody reacting with all samples except Rh_{null}; and (3) an antibody reacting with all samples including Rh_{null}.

Weiner and Vos (1963) classified their cases according to whether they reacted only with normal (nl) D-positive cells or also with 'partially deleted' (pdl) Rh-positive cells, e.g. −D−, or with both these types of cell and also with 'deleted' (dl) cells, i.e. Rh_{null}.

Although Weiner and Vos (1963) concluded that all warm autoantibodies had a specificity within the Rh system it remains uncertain whether the specificity of antibodies which react with all cells including Rh_{null} cells ('anti-dl' in their terminology) is related in any way to Rh. Of 50 cases tested by Marsh et al. (1972), three had specificity involving both Rh and U; about 40% of the antibodies in the series had no recognizable specificity, presumably equivalent to anti-dl.

Anti-dl specificity, or 'no recognizable specificity' as some would call it, was found in 23 of 33 cases associated with α-methyldopa and in 23 of 30 normal subjects with a positive DAT by Issitt et al. (1976a).

Leddy and Bakemeier (1967) found a relationship between specificity and complement binding; with one exception, antibodies reacting weakly or not at all with Rh_{null}

cells failed to bind complement whereas 70% of antibodies reacting as well with Rh$_{null}$ cells as with other cells did bind complement. A similar observation was made by Vos *et al.* (1970), namely that those eluates which fixed complement had broad specificities, as evidenced, for example, by the ability to react both with normal red cells and with Rh$_{null}$ cells.

In patients who develop a positive DAT as a result of taking α-methyldopa, with or without haemolytic anaemia, the autoantibodies have the same Rh-like specificity as in idiopathic AIHA (Carstairs *et al.* 1966; Worlledge *et al.* 1966; Garratty and Petz, 1975).

Often, mixtures of specific autoantibodies, e.g. auto-anti-e and autoantibodies with no recognizable specificity, occur together. In such cases the presence of the specific autoantibody may be suspected if the serum is titrated against red cells of different Rh phenotypes. Differential absorptions of the serum with R_1R_1, R_2R_2 and rr red cells confirm the presence of specific autoantibody or reveal a relative specificity (i.e. stronger reactions with red cells carrying certain antigens, e.g. E), when it has not previously been suspected. If the three red cells are properly selected, so as to cover between them the vast majority of important antigens, clinically significant alloantibodies can also be excluded (Wallhermfechtel *et al.* 1984).

When the autoantibody has a specificity resembling that of Rh alloantibodies, red cells which are compatible *in vitro* survive normally, or almost normally, in the recipient's circulation (Holländer, 1954; Ley *et al.* 1958b; Mollison, 1959a; Högman *et al.* 1960). In the example shown in Fig. 7.1, the patient was ccddee with an autoantibody of apparent specificity anti-e. The mean life span of transfused e-positive (CCDee) red cells was about 8 d which was similar to that of the patient's own red cells (see Dacie, 1962, p. 450), whereas the survival of e-negative (ccDEE) red cells was only

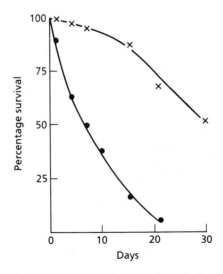

Figure 7.1 Survival, in a ccddee patient with autoimmune haemolytic anaemia, of e + (CCDee) red cells (●), estimated by differential agglutination, and of e – (ccDEE) cells (×), estimated by ^{51}Cr-labelling and corrected for Cr elution. The patient's serum contained an autoantibody reacting preferentially with e + cells. (The legend of this figure as published originally (Mollison, 1959a) stated incorrectly that the e + cells were autologous and were labelled with ^{51}Cr.)

slightly subnormal. For references to further similar cases in which red cell survival has been studied, see Petz and Swisher (1989, pp. 565–7).

Specificity mimicking that of alloantibodies with Rh specificity

A minority of warm autoantibodies at first sight appear to have the specificity of an Rh alloantibody, such as anti-e or -E. For example, an eluate prepared from the red cells of a patient of phenotype CCDee may react more strongly with E-positive than with E-negative cells and thus appear to contain anti-E. However, in about 70% of such cases all antibody activity can be absorbed completely by red cells lacking the corresponding antigen, e.g. CCDee in the present example. The specificity of these autoantibodies seems in fact to be anti-Hr or anti-Hr_0 (Issitt and Pavone, 1978).

The case reported by van 't Veer et al. (1981) in which a negative DAT was found on the red cells of a patient with severe haemolytic anaemia while strong autoanti-bodies of apparent anti-C and anti-e specificity were present in the serum demon-strates that such Rh specificities may be entirely illusory: not only (1) could the autoantibodies be absorbed with C-negative and e-negative cells, respectively, but (2) during the episode in which the DAT was negative and the patient's red cells (CcDee) did not react in vitro with the patient's own autoantibodies, they reacted normally with allo-anti-C and allo-anti-e. The nature of the epitope with which such antibodies react is not known. Neither is it clear why the epitope should be so strongly associated with Rh alloantigens. The case reported by Rand et al. (1978) in which autoantibodies with anti-E specificity were eluted from an E-negative patient's cells clearly demonstrates the mimicking nature of the specificity of the autoantibodies. Not only could the anti-E be absorbed to exhaustion by E-negative cells, but the eluate from the E-negative cells used for absorption contained antibodies that again showed positive reactions only with E-positive cells.

Specificities outside the Rh system

The possible involvement of Wr^b in the specificity of autoantibodies was investigated by Issitt et al. (1976a). Of 64 sera from patients with AIHA, two failed to react with Wr(a + b –) cells and contained only anti-Wr^b; the remaining sera reacted with Wr(a + b –) red cells but, after absorbtion with these cells to remove anti-dl, 32 could be shown to contain anti-Wr^b.

In patients with warm AIHA, autoantibodies with many other specificities are occasionally encountered, e.g. A (Szymanski et al. 1976); K, k and Kp^b in association with weakening of Kell antigens (see below); Kx (Sullivan et al. 1987); Jk^a (van Loghem and van der Hart, 1954; Dausset and Colombani, 1959; Patten et al. 1977; Sander et al. 1987); Jk3 (O'Day, 1987); N (Bowman et al. 1974; Dube et al. 1975; Cohen et al. 1979; Combs et al. 1990); S (Johnson et al. 1978); U (Marsh et al. 1972); Vel (Szaloky and van der Hart 1971; Herron et al. 1979); I^T (Garratty et al. 1974); Ge (Reynolds et al. 1981; Reid et al. 1988; Göttsche et al. 1990; Shulman et al. 1990) and Sd^x (Denegri et al. 1983).

Kell antibodies associated with autoimmune haemolytic anaemia

Several cases have been described in which a patient has developed a postive DAT, usually with overt haemolytic anaemia, and has been found to have autoantibodies of

Kell specificity in the serum associated with weakening of Kell antigens. Seyfried et al. (1972) described a patient with potent anti-Kp^b in his serum; during the period of his acute illness his own red cells reacted with anti-Kp^b only after they had been treated with ficin. Sixteen weeks later, when the patient was better, Kell antigens were of normal strength. Beck et al. (1979) described a patient with similar serological findings but without AIHA.

The frequency of autoantibodies with Kell specificity in patients with warm AIHA was estimated to be about one in 250 by Marsh et al. (1979a).

Autoantibodies mimicking alloantibodies with specificity other than Rh

Autoantibodies may mimic the specificity of anti-K (Garratty et al. 1979; Viggiano et al. 1982); anti-Jk^b plus anti-Jk3 (Ellisor et al. 1983); anti-Kp^b (Manny et al. 1983; Puig et al. 1986) and anti-Fy^b (Issitt et al. 1982; van 't Veer et al. 1984). In all these cases, the patient was negative for the corresponding antigen, the antibodies could be absorbed by red cells negative for the corresponding antigen, and eluates from such cells again showed the mimicking specificity.

Negative direct antiglobulin test despite warm autoantibodies in the serum

A most unusual case was reported by Seyfried et al. (1972) in which, during an episode of severe haemolysis, the DAT on the patient's red cells was negative in spite of the presence of potent autoantibodies in the serum. The antibodies had anti-Kp^b specificity, and weak anti-Kp^b could be eluted from the patient's red cells. The antigens of the Kell system were severely depressed at the time when the DAT was negative, but were of normal strength after recovery. Depression of the LW antigen in three patients with anti-LW in the serum had been reported by Chown et al. (1971), but these patients did not have haemolytic anaemia. Several further cases, similar to the case of Seyfried et al., have been observed in which the autoantibodies have had the following specificities: anti-E (Rand et al. 1978); anti-Rh of undefined specificity (Issitt et al. 1982; Vengelen-Tyler et al. 1983); 'mimicking' anti-C + anti-e (see above) (van 't Veer et al. 1981); anti-En^a (Garratty et al. 1983); anti-Kp^b (Brendel et al. 1985; Puig et al. 1986); specificity for a high frequency antigen in the Kell system (Vengelen-Tyler et al. 1987); anti-Jk^a (Ganly et al. 1988); anti-Jk3 (Issitt et al. 1990) and anti-Fy^a + Fy^b (Harris, 1990). In all the foregoing cases, there was total or severe depression of the antigens against which the autoantibodies were directed. In some cases, although the DAT was negative, an eluate from the patient's red cells contained weak autoantibodies of the same specificity as those in the serum. In some cases the DAT had been positive before the episode of severe haemolysis. In other cases the patient presented with a negative DAT and the antibodies were first thought to be alloantibodies.

In a case reported by Herron et al. (1987) the autoantibodies were found to react much more strongly with old, i.e. relatively dense, red cells than with young cells and it was suggested that the DAT during an episode of severe haemolysis became negative because only young red cells had remained in the circulation.

Red cell transfusion and other therapy for patients with
autoimmune haemolytic anaemia associated with warm autoantibodies

In severe AIHA, transfusion produces only a very transient increase in Hb concentration and carries an increased risk of: (1) inducing the formation of alloantibodies; (2) increasing the potency of the autoantibodies; and (3) inducing haemoglobinuria due to autoantibody-mediated red cell destruction (Chaplin, 1979). Accordingly, even in severely anaemic patients, it is usually best to begin treatment with corticosteroids, following which the Hb concentration usually starts to rise within 7 d (Petz and Garratty, 1980, p. 392). If the effect of corticosteroids is not satisfactory, or if a quicker effect is needed, intravenous immunoglobulin should be given which, in very high doses (e.g. 0.4 g/kg per day) may have a very rapid effect (Mackintyre *et al.* 1985; Newland *et al.* 1986; Argiolu *et al.* 1990). Alternatively, treatment with cyclosporin (4 mg/kg per day) can be tried and may result in a fairly rapid increase in Hb concentration (Hershko *et al.* 1990). Splenectomy is indicated only in patients who have failed to respond to steroids, i.v. Ig and cyclosporin.

Transfusion is indicated only in special circumstances, e.g. if the patient is severely anaemic and is going into cardiac failure, or has neurological signs, or has rapidly progressive anaemia, or is to undergo splenectomy. In most other circumstances it is better to use palliative measures, such as absolute bed-rest, to counteract the decreased tolerance to exercise, whilst monitoring the Hb level.

If transfusions are given, it is important to group the patient's red cells for all clinically significant alloantigens, to facilitate the identification of any alloantibodies which may be produced. In patients who have previously been transfused or have been pregnant, it is also important to try to exclude the presence of alloantibodies which may be masked by the presence of autoantibodies. Either autoabsorption can be used or, if sufficient autologous red cells cannot be obtained, differential absorptions (see Chapter 8). It is helpful to obtain red cells from the patient before the first transfusion is given, and to store these at 4°C or frozen, so as to have cells for autoabsorptions if needed (Petz and Swisher, 1989, p. 564).

When the presence of an alloantibody has been established, antigen-negative red cells must be selected for transfusion; the practice of transfusing 'least incompatible red cells' is not acceptable (see Laine and Beattie, 1985).

In selecting red cells for transfusion, any blood group specificity of incomplete warm autoantibodies should when possible also be taken into account. In Rh D-negative females with auto-anti-e who have not yet reached the menopause, the red cells should, if possible, be e-negative as well as D-negative (i.e. ccddEE). In patients with auto-anti-e, e-negative (EE) red cells may survive better than e-positive cells (see Fig. 7.1) but may stimulate the production of anti-E (Habibi *et al.* 1974).

When transfusing patients with AIHA, packed red cells should be given in just sufficient quantities to raise the Hb to a level that will make it possible for other therapy to be applied. In acute anaemia, oxygen may have to be given. A few patients need regular transfusions despite all other forms of therapy.

As mentioned above, the presence of warm autoantibodies in the serum may make it difficult to detect alloantibodies; the problem is discussed further in Chapter 8.

Haemolytic anaemia in recipients of allografts
Alloantibodies produced by donor lymphocytes in grafted tissue may simulate autoantibodies in the recipient and cause haemolytic anaemia (see pp. 536–537).

ANTIBODIES AGAINST BOUND, OR INDUCED, ANTIGENS

Drug-induced immune haemolytic anaemia

Among cases of acquired immune haemolytic anaemia 18% were due to drugs in the series of Dacie and Worlledge (1969) and 12.4% in the series of Petz and Garratty (1980). The great majority of cases of drug-induced haemolytic anaemia were at one time due to α-methyldopa (Worlledge, 1969) but this drug is now used much less frequently. Cases resulting from other drugs are very rare, penicillin-induced anaemia being the least uncommon (Petz and Garratty, 1980).

There are several ways in which drugs may be responsible for a positive DAT, often associated with immune haemolytic anaemia (see Petz and Garratty, 1980). Of the four described below, number two is the one associated with the greatest number of drugs that can cause a positive DAT:

1 The drug may bind firmly to the red cells; when an antibody is formed against the drug, the drug-coated red cells are destroyed. Penicillin acts in this way and so, occasionally, do drugs of the cephalosporin group and cianidanol.

In about 3% of patients with bacterial endocarditis receiving massive doses of penicillin i.v., a positive DAT develops but AIHA occurs in only a small percentage of these; the first case, associated with the prolonged administration of penicillin in high dosage (20 million units or more daily for weeks), was described by Petz and Fudenberg (1966): the patient's serum contained an IgG penicillin antibody of unusual potency. If it is necessary to continue giving penicillin to patients with AIHA due to penicillin antibodies, transfusions may be required. Normal red cells, since uncoated with penicillin, will appear to be compatible on crossmatching but after transfusion will become coated *in vivo* and destroyed in the same way as the patient's cells.

Although penicillin antibodies are usually IgG they may be partly IgM (Fudenberg and German, 1960) or solely IgM (Bird *et al.* 1975), in which case complement is bound and the red cells are agglutinated by anti-C3. In patients with immune haemolytic anaemia due to penicillin antibody, the antibody can invariably be demonstrated in high titre in the serum, using red cells coated *in vitro* with penicillin (Petz and Garratty, 1980; Petz and Branch, 1985).

IgM or IgG antibodies reactive with penicillin-coated red cells have been found in the serum of about 4% of haematologically normal subjects (Fudenberg and German, 1960).

The benzyl-penicilloyl groups are the most immunogenic of the haptenic groups of penicillin (Garratty and Petz, 1975).

2 The drug does not bind firmly to red cells so that drug-coated cells cannot be prepared. It has been suggested that in these cases, when an antibody is formed against the drug, immune complexes attach to the red cells. The drug antibodies are often IgM and are complement activating. Only complement can be demonstrated on the patient's red cells (Garratty and Petz, 1975). Examples of drugs acting in this way are: quinine, para-amino salicylic acid, sulphonamide, chlorothiazide, tolmetin, rifampicin, probenecid, nomifensine, hydrochlorothiazide and suprofen. Some of these drugs also induce the formation of 'true' red cell autoantibodies in the same patient (see below). In some cases the antibodies are directed against a metabolite of the drug rather than against the drug itself (Salama and Mueller-Eckhardt, 1985; 1987a;b).

The antibodies can then be detected by using urine from subjects who have taken the drug.

Drugs that produce red cell destruction by this mechanism can do so even when given in low doses. The haemolysis disappears within 1–2 d after withdrawing the drug.
3   The drug does not bind firmly to red cells, antibody against the drug is not formed, but IgG autoantibodies are induced. α-methyldopa and levodopa are prime examples of drugs acting in this way. In 15–20% of patients receiving α-methyldopa the DAT becomes positive after 3–6 months of treatment; the development of a positive DAT is dose dependent (Carstairs et al. 1966). Only about 1% of patients receiving the drug develop haemolytic anaemia. It has been suggested that α-methyldopa induces red cell autoantibodies by inhibiting the activity of suppressor lymphocytes (Kirtland et al. 1980), but no effect on suppressor cells could be demonstrated by Garratty et al. (1986). As stated above it has been found that some drugs which do not bind firmly to red cells induce both anti-drug antibodies and red cell autoantibodies: e.g. nomifensine (Martlew, 1986; Salama and Mueller-Eckhardt, 1987b), tolmetin and suprofen (van Dijk et al. 1989).

The inference has been drawn that even when drugs are loosely bound to red cells, they can induce the formation of antibodies against a red cell antigen alone: the fact that in many cases antibodies are formed only when the red cell carries particular alloantigens (see below) has been adduced as supporting evidence (Salama and Mueller Eckhardt, 1987b).
4   The drug may alter the red cell membrane in some way so that proteins are adsorbed non-specifically. Cephalosporin and cisplatin are believed to act in this way as a rule. This mechanism has not been shown to result in haemolytic anaemia.

Effect of red cell antigens on the binding of drug–antibody complexes
In a case in which streptomycin was involved, the drug was apparently bound to the red cell membrane through chemical groups related to M and possibly D (Martinez et al. 1977).

Several similar cases have been reported: three cases in which only Jk (a +) cells were reactive with chlorpropamide (Sosler et al. 1984) or paraben (Judd et al. 1980; Halima et al. 1982a); three cases in which only e-positive red cells were reactive with caprylate (Dube et al. 1977) or glafenin (Ganeval et al. 1978; Goudeman and Salmon, 1980); one case in which 'pdl' was involved in the binding of glafenin (Habibi et al. 1981); and cases in which only E-positive cells were reactive with nomifensine (Salama and Mueller-Eckhardt, 1987a). Finally, several cases have been reported in which only I-positive red cells would react with various drugs, namely rifampicin, nitrofurantoin, dexchlorphenyramine maleate (Duran-Suarez et al. 1981) or thiopental (Habibi et al. 1985).

Treatment of drug-induced haemolytic anaemia
In cases in which antibodies are involved against a drug which binds firmly to the red cell and in cases in which immune complexes are responsible for the destruction of the red cells, stopping the drug is sufficient to arrest the haemolytic process and treatment of the haemolytic anaemia is rarely necessary. In cases in which it is impossible to stop the drug and the patient is anaemic, red cell transfusions should be given. In AIHA induced by α-methyldopa, the drug must be stopped, but red cell destruction may

continue for weeks or months. If treatment is required it is the same as for patients with drug-independent warm AIHA.

In occasional patients, autoantibodies disappear despite continued administration of the drug (Habibi, 1983).

Antibodies against other bound antigens

Fatty acid-dependent agglutinin ('albumin agglutinin')
The serum of a small proportion of people agglutinates red cells suspended in albumin but not those suspended in saline (Weiner *et al.* 1956). Agglutination is found only with caprylate-treated albumin (Golde *et al.* 1969; 1973) and the antibody is in fact directed against sodium caprylate or other fatty acid salts and not against albumin at all (Beck *et al.* 1976b). The term 'fatty acid-dependent agglutinin' is therefore preferable to the previously used 'albumin agglutinin'. Fatty acid-dependent agglutinins may cause false-positive reactions in slide tests in which blood grouping reagents containing albumin are used (Reid *et al.* 1975; Case, 1976) and in the indirect antiglobulin test if albumin is used in the sensitizing phase of the reaction.

Antibiotics
Antibiotics are added to samples of red cells which are distributed commercially for the identification of alloantibodies. Such cells may give false-positive results if antibodies against the relevant antibiotic are present in a sample of serum. In a systematic search for such antibodies, Watson and Joubert (1960) found that six of 1700 routine blood bank serum samples agglutinated chloramphenicol-treated cells. Three examples of an antibody of this kind were found to be IgM and two bound complement (Beattie *et al.* 1976). An IgA antibody agglutinating red cells suspended in 0.1 mg neomycin per ml was described by Hysell *et al.* (1975). Antibodies vs. penicillin-treated red cells are described above.

Acriflavine
Some commercial anti-B-sera have acriflavine added to them as a colouring agent and this may be a cause of false-positive results if anti-acriflavine antibodies are present in a patient's serum, possibly as a result of previous exposure to acriflavine. The antibodies may cause agglutination of normal red cells in the presence of a one in 150 000 dilution of acriflavine (Beattie and Zuelzer, 1968; Beattie *et al.* 1971).

Immune complexes adsorbed to red cells in vitro *in ulcerative colitis*
In occasional patients with ulcerative colitis the DAT on clotted samples is positive but on anticoagulated samples is negative. Allogeneic red cells give a positive indirect antiglobulin test with the patient's serum but a negative test with plasma. It is postulated that the patient's plasma contains an antibody against an activated coagulation factor and that, during clotting, immune complexes form and attach to the red cells (Garratty *et al.* 1980).

Lactose- or glucose-treated red cells
Antibodies have been described which agglutinated any red cells that had been

incubated with lactose (Gray, 1964) or glucose (Lewis *et al.* 1980). In the latter case, red cells from patients with diabetes reacted, although after incubation in saline, the cells were no longer agglutinated. Examples of anti-M and anti-N reacting only with lactose- or glucose-treated red cells are described in the preceding chapter.

Antibody against chemically altered red cells (the LOX antigen)

Red cells exposed to citrate–phosphate–dextrose solution in particular batches of plastic blood packs may acquire a new red cell antigenic determinant 'LOX'. The development of this antigen is probably associated with sterilization of the packs with propylene oxide gas (Bruce and Mitchell, 1981).

POLYAGGLUTINABILITY

Red cells are said to be polyagglutinable when they are agglutinated by almost all samples of normal human serum although never by the patient's own serum. The commonest forms of polyagglutinability are due to exposure, by the action of bacterial enzymes, of antigenic determinants (T, Tk, Th, Tx) which form part of the structure of the normal red cell membrane, but which are usually hidden. Another form of polyagglutinability is believed to be due to somatic mutation leading to the emergence of a line of red cells lacking an enzyme essential for the formation of normal red cell antigens; as a result, a normally hidden antigen, Tn, is exposed. In all the foregoing cases, the red cells are polyagglutinable because antibodies (anti-T, etc.) corresponding to the determinants are present in serum from all normal adults (although not in serum from newborn infants). Further forms of polyagglutinability may be due to the inheritance of an antigen (Cad, NOR or HEMPAS) for which a corresponding antibody is present in almost all normal human sera.

T activation

Exposure of T antigen in vitro

Figure 7.2 shows the postulated structure of the T antigen. As the figure shows, the T determinant is exposed on normal red cells by the removal of N-acetylneuraminic acid from the alkali-labile oligosaccharides linked to sialoglycoproteins (SGPs) (see Chapter 6). T is thus said to be a cryptantigen. The T antigen, normally hidden on human red cells, can be exposed by the action of bacterial or viral neuraminidase.

Anti-T (and anti-Tn, see below), present in the serum of all subjects except infants, are presumably formed as a reaction to T and Tn present in many Gram-negative bacteria and vaccines (Springer *et al.* 1979; Springer and Tegtmeyer, 1981).

Knowledge of T activation stems from the original observation that suspensions of red cells might become agglutinable by ABO-compatible serum after standing for many hours at room temperature, and that this agglutination was associated with infection of the suspension with certain enzyme-producing bacteria (Hübener, 1925; Thomsen, 1927; Friedenreich, 1930). Very many organisms, including pneumococci, strepto-cocci, staphylococci, clostridia, *Escherichia coli*, *Vibrio cholerae* and influenza viruses are capable of producing this effect *in vitro*.

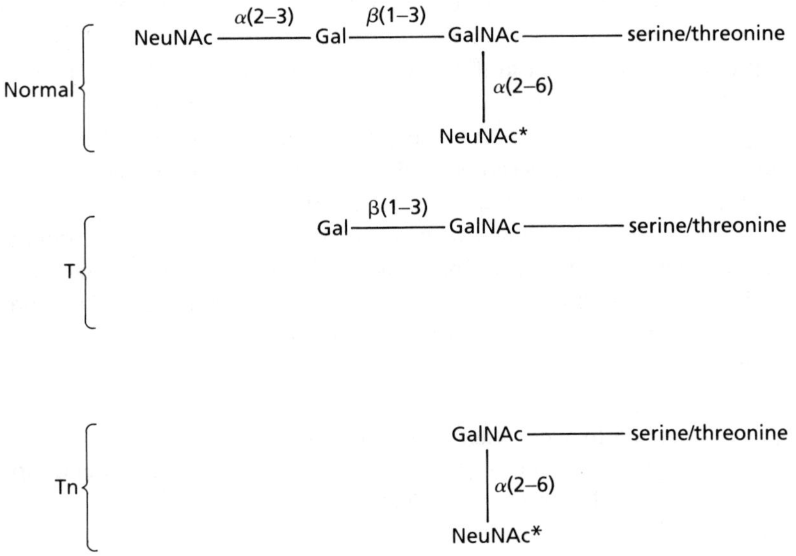

Figure 7.2 Proposed structure of the major O-glycosidically linked oligosaccharides of the sialoglycoproteins in normal, T- and Tn-exposed erythrocyte membranes (modified from Anstee, 1981).
NeuNAc, N-acetylneuraminic acid; Gal, D-galactose; GalNAc, N-acetyl-D-galactosamine.
* It is possible that this NeuNAc residue is present in some but not all Tn structures (P.D. Issitt, personal communication).

Preparation of T-activated red cells. Add 11 mg $CaCl_2$ to 100 ml 0.85% NaCl to provide a solution containing approximately 10 mmol $CaCl_2$/l. Add 0.2 ml of a solution containing 500 units neuraminidase per ml to give an enzyme concentration of 1 unit ml. This solution can be stored at 4°C for 1 year. Wash group O red cells four times in saline and make a 25% suspension of cells in the enzyme solution. Incubate at 37°C for 2–3 h. Remove the supernatant, wash the red cells in saline four times, make a 5% suspension in saline and check for T activation by testing with anti-T lectin (Howard, 1979).

T-activated red cells can be kept for several weeks in Alsever's solution but must be washed thoroughly in saline before being used.

T sites on red cells
Since there are 15 O-glycosidically linked oligosaccharides on each molecule of α-SGP, and probably similar numbers on β- and δ-SGPs, there are many potential T antigen sites on the red cell. There are also T-active structures on red cell membrane components other than SGPs, e.g. on gangliosides (Anstee, 1980).

Activation of T receptor in vivo
T activation may occur *in vivo*. Usually, this polyagglutinability occurs as a transient phenomenon, disappearing within a few weeks or months of the time when it is first observed. The phenomenon is not very common; at a large Blood Transfusion Centre, only 10 cases were observed in 12 years (Stratton and Renton, 1958).

In the past, T activation was almost always detected by finding discrepancies between the results of testing red cells and sera in the course of ABO grouping. Nowadays, since commercially available polyclonal anti-A and anti-B sera do not contain appreciable amounts of anti-T and since monoclonal anti-A and -B are used increasingly, T activation seldom causes trouble in blood grouping.

In many cases the patient has an obvious bacterial infection, but the phenomenon has also been observed in apparently healthy subjects; for a review of some of the earlier reported cases, see Henningsen (1949a). In a case reported by Reepmaker (1952) an organism that was shown to be capable of inducing T transformation was isolated from the patient's urine. Chorpenning and Hayes (1959) made the point that T transformation is not the only kind of polyagglutinability induced by bacterial infection, and that in many reported cases of polyagglutinability it was simply assumed that the change was T transformation.

Similarity of T activation to acquisition of 'B-like' antigen
Certain bacterial enzymes confer B-specificity on red cells as well as rendering them polyagglutinable (Marsh, 1960; see also Chapter 4).

Reactions of T-activated cells
T-activated cells are agglutinated by the sera of most adults but fail to be agglutinated by sera from most newborn infants. The reactions are strongest at room temperature and may be very weak or absent at 37°C. Although the agglutinates may be large, there are many free cells present.

T-activated cells react most strongly with fresh serum and sometimes fail to react with serum which has been stored frozen (Stratton, 1954; Hendry and Simmons, 1955; Chorpenning and Hayes, 1959).

T-activated cells react better with sera containing anti-A than with those that do not (Race and Sanger, 1975, p. 487), probably because of structural similarity between the T and A antigens. The correct ABO group of T-activated cells can usually be determined with commercial anti-A and anti-B reagents, probably because the anti-T has been 'diluted out' and, anyway, if the tests are carried out strictly at 37°C, anti-T is unlikely to interfere. Alternatively, monoclonal anti-A and anti-B, which do not contain anti-T, can be used.

T-activated cells fail to agglutinate in their own serum (the titre of anti-T being low, due presumably to absorption by exposed T) and the cells give a negative direct antiglobulin reaction. At 37°C they are not sensitized to an antiglobulin serum by human sera which agglutinate them at room temperature.

The titre of anti-T varies considerably in samples of serum from different adults. Anti-T agglutinins are usually not present in the serum of newborn infants but are present at or before the age of 2 months (F. Stratton, personal communication). They are distinct from normal cold agglutinins, although they also act more strongly at low temperatures than at 37°C (Lind and McArthur, 1947).

Although cord serum will not agglutinate T-activated red cells, it seems that some IgG anti-T is present which can be demonstrated by radioimmunoassay against purified T antigen or by demonstrating agglutination of T red cells in the presence of polyethylene glycol and gelatin (Kim, 1980).

An anti-T lectin can be extracted from the peanut, *Arachis hypogaea* (Bird, 1964). Fresh raw peanuts may be crushed in a mortar containing a filter paper to absorb fat. One volume of ground peanuts is left with four volumes of saline overnight at 4°C before centrifuging the mixture and harvesting the supernatant (Howard, 1979).

In the first case of T activation *in vivo* to be described, the cells were agglutinated by only 15% of adult sera (Levine and Katzin, 1938). Testing with peanut anti-T lectin is far more sensitive than testing with adult serum. For example, among 26 newborn infants with necrotizing enterocolitis there were nine whose red cells were strongly agglutinated by peanut anti-T lectin (to a titre 512 or more), but only five of the nine samples of red cells reacted with adult serum and then with only 50% of sera (Seger *et al.* 1980).

Reactions of various types of polyagglutinable red cells with different lectins and with polybrene are shown in Table 7.3.

Use of polybrene. Normal red cells (negatively charged) are agglutinated by polybrene (positively charged), but red cells such as T-activated cells which are deficient in sialic acid and thus have a reduced negative charge are not agglutinated. The following method of testing red cells with polybrene is taken from Issitt and Issitt (1975):

A stock solution is made by dissolving polybrene in normal saline to a final concentration of 40 g/l. The stock solution is stored at room temperature in a plastic container. A working solution containing 1 mg polybrene per ml is made by diluting the stock solution 1 in 40 in saline. One drop of working solution is mixed with one drop of a 5% suspension of red cells in a small test tube. Normal cells are used as a control. Agglutination of the normal cells but not of the test cells indicates that the latter are sialic-acid deficient.

The deficiency of red cell sialic acid must exceed about 12% before cells fail to be agglutinated by 0.1 g/dl polybrene in a test tube (E.A. Steane, personal communication, 1978), although with very dilute polybrene solutions (<0.003 g/dl), red cells that have only a 10% reduction in sialic acid are agglutinated (Cartron *et al.* 1978). When polybrene in as high a concentration as 0.6 g/dl is used, prozones are observed, e.g. cells with 30% or more loss of sialic lacid are not agglutinated (Cartron *et al.* 1978).

Table 7.3 Reactions of different kinds of polyagglutinable red cells (based on the publications of G.W.G. Bird and colleagues)

	Arachis hypogaea	*Dolichos biflorus*[*]	*Glycine soja*[†]	GS II[‡]	*Vicia cretica*	*Salvia sclarea*	*Leonurus cardiaca*	Polybrene
T	+	−	+	−	+	−	+[§]	−
Tk	+	−	−	+	−	−	−	+
Th	+	−	−	−	+	−	−	+
Tx	+	−	−	−	−	−	−	+
Tn	−	+	+	−	−	+	−	−
Cad	−	+	+	−	−	−	+	+

[*] Tests with this lectin can be used only when the cells are group O or B.
[†] May not react with weaker examples of Cad.
[‡] *Griffonia simplicifolia II.*
[§] Weak reaction.

A typical case. T-activated cells are usually recognized when discrepancies are found during ABO grouping, as in the following case:

Mrs S. was admitted to hospital with a septic abortion: mixed coliforms and non-haemolytic streptococci were grown from a vaginal swab. Her red cells were strongly agglutinated by anti-A serum and partially agglutinated by anti-B; her serum agglutinated and lysed B cells but failed to agglutinate A cells, suggesting that she really belonged to group A. On further testing, her red cells were found to be agglutinated by four adult AB sera, the reactions being strongest at 4°C and weakest at 37°C; the cells were not agglutinated by several samples of cord blood serum from group A infants.

The patient made a good recovery and 1 week after admission her cells were only very weakly polyagglutinable.

Polyagglutinability, associated with exposure of T receptors (or Tk or Th receptors see below) is frequently observed in neonatal necrotizing enterocolitis (Bird, 1982).

Leucocytes and platelets also become T activated; platelet function is not impaired (Hysell *et al.* 1976).

Haemolytic syndromes due to T activation?
Most patients with T-activated cells do not have an associated haemolytic process. Although several cases have been reported in which such an association has been observed, it is difficult in some of the cases to be sure that T activation has been responsible. The difficulty of incriminating anti-T seems particularly great in infants, in whom anti-T, if present at all, is not strong. Moreover, in many of the cases described the patients have had an infection with *Clostridium perfringens*, an organism notorious for producing violent haemolytic syndromes.

In four cases described by van Loghem (1965) the Hb concentration was between 4.5 and 6.9 g/dl and serum haptoglobin was reduced. Two of the patients showed red cell autoagglutination. In the three cases in which organisms were isolated they were *Clostridium perfringens, Staphylococcus aureus* and pneumococcus. In a patient reported by Moores *et al.* (1975), with a presumed lung infection following a stab wound, there was rapid improvement on treatment with antibiotics but after 7 d there was a sudden deterioration and fall in Hb concentration to 3.4 g/dl and a reticulocytosis of 25%. T activation was demonstrated and anti-T eluted from the patient's red cells. F. Stratton (personal communication) has seen four infants 2 months old or less with T activation, associated with the development of severe anaemia. *E. coli* was implicated in one of the cases. In a child aged 14 months described by Rickard *et al.* (1969) the Hb concentration fell to 3.7 g/dl; the blood film showed spherocytes and Schumm's test was positive.

Further cases were described by Bird and Stephenson (1973) and by Tanaka and Okubo (1977).

The transfusion of normal plasma (containing anti-T) to an infant with polyagglutinable red cells appeared to be the cause of a severe haemolytic transfusion reaction in a case described by van Loghem *et al.* (1955) and in the following case:

Acute intestinal obstruction developed in a girl aged 7 months. After 48 h the Hb concentration was 7.2 g/dl and a transfusion of 90 ml fresh compatible red cells was given; the red cells had been prepared from a unit of blood from which two-thirds of the supernatant plasma had been removed. Immediately after the transfusion haemoglobinaemia and haemoglobinuria developed, followed by renal failure. Laparotomy was then performed and a volvulus with 45 cm of necrotic small intestine was resected. During surgery, 250 ml of 14-day-old blood was given without reaction, but signs of haemolysis persisted. Investigations now showed that the patient's red cells were T activated. The haemolytic transfusion reaction appeared to be due to the small amount of anti-T contained in the supernatant plasma of the red cell concentrate transfused on the third day of the illness (A. Poon, F. Saunders and L. Wakelin, personal communication).

Scepticism about the haemolytic potential of anti-T was expressed by Heddle *et al.* (1977), who found no evidence of significant red cell destruction in three premature infants with T-activated red cells following the transfusion of blood components containing anti-T.

Haemolytic syndromes associated with polyagglutinability have been produced experimentally in guinea pigs following the injection of pneumococcal cultures (Ejby-Poulsen, 1954a,b), and have been shown to occur spontaneously in rabbits in association with enteritis (Evans *et al.* 1963a).

Other kinds of polyagglutinability due to bacterial enzymes or bacteria

Tk activation
This form of polyagglutinability of the red cells is similar to T activation in that it is a transient phenomenon associated with infection. The red cells are agglutinated by the Tk-specific lectin GS II, isolated from *Griffonia simplicifolia* seeds (Bird and Wingham, 1972); they also react with peanut lectin, the reaction being greatly enhanced if the red cells are first treated with papain (Bird and Wingham, 1972).

Tk cells have normal amounts of sialic acid, as indicated by the fact that they are agglutinated by polybrene (see Table 7.3). Further work indicates that Tk is exposed by the action of an endo-β-galactosidase produced by *Bacteroides fragilis* (Inglis *et al.* 1975a,b) or derived from *Escherichia freundii* (Doinel *et al.* 1980) or *Flavobacterium keratolyticus* (Liew *et al.* 1982). Endo-β-galactosidase exposes a terminal N-acetylglucosamine residue on carbohydrate chains of long-chain glycolipids and band 3 glycoproteins (Doinel *et al.* 1980).

T and Tk activation associated with acquired B
In patients with acquired B the red cells often exhibit Tk polyagglutination with or without T activation. In reporting three patients it was pointed out that the changes in each were due to different bacterial enzymes and that, depending on the relative amounts of each of these enzymes, different phenotypes were produced, e.g. in one case T activation might predominate and in another, Tk (Judd *et al.* 1979b; see also Mullard *et al.* 1978; Janot *et al.* 1979).

In Tk polyagglutination H and A red cell antigens are weakened (Inglis *et al.* 1978), as are I and i (Andreu *et al.* 1979).

VA polyagglutination
This condition is considered here for convenience although there is no evidence that it is caused by bacterial enzymes. The condition is characterized by persistent polyagglutination associated with haemolytic anaemia; the red cells are weakly agglutinated by almost all adult sera but only up to a temperature of 18°C. The abnormalities in the

red cells include a slight reduction in sialic acid (3.7%) and a depression of H receptors (Graninger *et al.* 1977a,b). VA accompanied by Tk was reported by Beck *et al.* (1978). VA may represent one end of a Tk spectrum (Bird, 1980).

Th activation

When Th is exposed (Bird *et al.* 1978) the red cells are agglutinated by peanut lectin, extracts from *Vicia cretica* (Bird and Wingham, 1981), *Medicago disciformis* (Bird and Wingham, 1983) and by polybrene, but not by lectins from *Glycine soja*, GS II, *Salvia sclarea* or *Salvia horminum* (Bird *et al.* 1978); see Table 7.3.

In studying 200 paired samples of maternal and cord blood, the incidence of Th activation was found to be much higher in newborn infants (11%) and their mothers (13%) than in blood donors (Wahl *et al.* 1989) in whom the incidence was 1.5% (Herman *et al.* 1987). In none of the cases were the red cells polyagglutinable, which shows that Th activation leads to polyagglutinability only in some cases.

Tx activation

The Tx antigen is exposed on red cells by pneumococcal enzymes (Bird *et al.* 1982). Tx cells are agglutinated by peanut lectin but not by other lectins.

Polyagglutinability due to adsorbed bacteria

Many bacteria or their thermostable products will adhere to red cells (Keogh *et al.* 1948; Jochem, 1958a,b). The red cells will be polyagglutinable when the corresponding antibody is present in most samples of human serum. Antibodies to some bacteria, e.g. *Bacillus cereus*, do not agglutinate red cells coated with the bacteria but sensitize the cells to agglutination by antiglobulin serum (Weeden *et al.* 1960).

Tn red cells

Tn red cells, like T-activated cells, are deficient in sialic acid (Bird *et al.* 1971) and are polyagglutinable (Dausset *et al.* 1959) since anti-Tn, like anti-T, is present in all normal adult sera.

Apart from the fact that T and Tn are quite separate antigenic structures (see Fig. 7.2) Tn polyagglutination differs in three important respects from T polyagglutination or any other polyagglutination associated with infection: first, Tn agglutination is persistent; second, it is associated with haematological abnormalities; and third, affected subjects have two populations of red cells, one normal and one showing the Tn change. The condition (sometimes referred to as persistent mixed field polyagglutination) appears to be due to somatic mutation occurring in stem cells, leading to the emergence of a population of abnormal (Tn) red cells (as originally suggested by Bird *et al.* 1971; 1976a). Data supporting this concept are as follows: in subjects with Tn red cells there are also two populations of platelets, Tn positive and Tn negative (Cartron and Nurden, 1979). Only Tn-positive platelets contain glycoprotein Ib with a modified oligosaccharide chain structure responsible for the expression of Tn antigen (Nurden *et al.* 1982). A similar abnormality is present on Tn-positive granulocytes (Cartron *et al.* 1981). It has also been found that a sizeable fraction of erythrocyte, granulocyte and megakaryocyte colonies grown from the bone marrow of a patient with the Tn syndrome appear to consist exclusively of either Tn-positive or Tn-negative cells, demonstrating the clonal origin of Tn cells (Vainchenker *et al.* 1982). Tn-positive B and T cells can also be demonstrated in patients with the Tn syndrome (Brouet *et al.* 1983) and, finally, expression of the Tn antigen has been demonstrated at a very early stage of differentiation, i.e. in colony forming units (Vainchenker *et al.* 1985).

The relation of the Tn antigen to T is shown in Fig. 7.2. It is postulated that the immunodominant group is the α-linked N-acetylgalactosamine residue, O-glycosidically linked to the polypeptide chain of the red cell SGPs (Dahr *et al.* 1975). The Tn antigen thus results from a deficiency of the galactosyl transferases and sialyl transferases which normally generate the O-glycosidically linked oligosaccharides attached to the red cell SGPs (Anstee, 1981). Deficiency of the appropriate β-3-D-galactosyl transferase (i.e. the T transferase) has in fact been demonstrated in Tn red cell membranes. Furthermore, it has been shown that, in Tn subjects, the normal red cell population, i.e. those red cells with a normal sialic acid content (polybrene positive) have normal or higher than normal β-3-D- and β-4-D-galactosyl transferase activities. The population with a low sialic acid content (polybrene-negative) cells has a selective deficiency in β-3-D-galactosyl transferase but normal or even increased β-4-D-galactosyl transferase activity (Cartron *et al.* 1978).

Although Tn polyagglutination usually persists for long periods, it has been known to disappear in four subjects; two of these disappearances were spontaneous since neither patient was receiving cytotoxic therapy (Bird *et al.* 1976a). Although Tn polyagglutination is usually associated with neutropenia and thrombocytopenia (Gunson *et al.* 1970b; Haynes *et al.* 1970) and may be associated with haemolytic anaemia (Bird *et al.* 1971), it is also found in normal subjects (Myllylä *et al.* 1971; Bird *et al.* 1976c). In a subject investigated by Myllylä *et al.* (1971) it was shown that the survival of the subject's red cells in his own circulation was normal and that no anti-Tn was demonstrable in the serum; when the red cells were injected into the circulation of a normal subject (i.e. with anti-Tn in the plasma) the cells were rapidly destroyed.

When normal red cells are transfused to a subject with Tn polyagglutination the transfused cells do not become Tn-positive (Haynes *et al.* 1970).

Tn red cells are agglutinated by an extract of *Dolichos biflorus* (Gunson *et al.* 1970b) and by snail anti-A but not by purified human anti-A (Bird, 1978b). They are also agglutinated by the lectins from *Salvia sclarea*, *Helix pomatia* and *Glycine soja* (Bird, 1978b).

Tn red cells are best diagnosed by testing with an extract of *Salvia sclarea* (Table 7.3). The lectin must be diluted to avoid non-specific activity but then reacts strongly with Tn cells and not at all with T-activated cells.

Exposure of T and Tn in malignant cells
Immunoreactive T antigen is present in the cytoplasm and on the outer cell membrane of about 90% of the major forms of carcinoma and T lymphoma, as determined by absorption of human anti-T antibodies and immunohistochemistry (Springer *et al.* 1974; 1983). In addition to T, carcinoma cells express Tn antigen. Tn antigen was detected by absorption of human anti-Tn antibody in 46 of 50 primary breast carcinomas and in all six metastases originating from Tn-positive primary carcinomas. Thirteen of 25 (52%) anaplastic carcinomas, but only two of 15 (13%) well-differentiated carcinomas had more Tn than T; one anaplastic carcinoma had neither

antigen. Eighteen of 20 benign breast lesions had no Tn; the two with Tn were premalignant. Tissue from 18 breast carcinomas reacted strongly with anti-Tn (Springer *et al.* 1985). Carcinoma-associated T antigen stimulates profound cellular and humoral immune responses in the patient, early in the disease and throughout its course (Springer *et al.* 1983). Monoclonal anti-T and anti-Tn, which reacted with T- and Tn-positive carcinoma cells, were prepared by Springer *et al.* (1983).

An inherited form, NOR
The red cells of a healthy young male were found to be agglutinable by 75 of 100 ABO-compatible sera; the red cell characteristic, NOR, associated with polyagglutin-ability was shown to be inherited in an apparently dominant manner by four other family members in two generations (Harris *et al.* 1982). The only other inherited characteristics associated with polyagglutinability are Cad and HEMPAS, described in the previous chapter. NOR can be distinguished from Cad by the failure of NOR red cells to react with an extract of *Dolichos biflorus* and can be distinguished from the acquired forms of polyagglutinability, T, Tk, Th and Tn, by the failure of NOR red cells to react either with an extract of *Arachis hypogaea* or of *Salvia sclarea* (Harris *et al.* 1982).

AGGLUTININS FOR OTHER NORMALLY HIDDEN ANTIGENS

Antigens on enzyme-treated red cells
Agglutinins for red cells treated with various enzymes are found in all normal sera; for example, if trypsinized red cells are mixed with normal human serum and incubated for not more than 20 min and then centrifuged they will usually be found to be agglutinated, although if incubation is continued for 1 h only about 1% of samples will still be agglutinated (Rosenfield and Vogel, 1951; Rosenthal and Schwartz, 1951).

If normal serum is heated to 60°C for 2 h the agglutinin, which is IgM (Mellbye, 1966), is inactivated; the heated serum can now be shown to contain a factor 'reversor' which renders cells non-agglutinable by normal serum (Spaet and Ostrom, 1952). 'Reversor' is histidine (Mellbye, 1967).

Although trypsin is adsorbed to red cells during enzyme treatment, the receptor with which the 'trypsin agglutinin' reacts is not trypsin itself but is probably a glycoprotein (Mellbye, 1969a).

According to Mellbye (1969b), agglutinins specific for trypsin-treated, papain-treated, bromelin-treated, neuraminidase-treated and periodate-treated red cells can all be found in normal serum; each agglutinin can be removed only by absorption with the appropriate red cells. The agglutinin for trypsin-treated red cells is the only one found in cord serum and the only one whose reactions are reversed by the addition of histidine.

In testing a very large series of normal samples, a warm haemolysin for papain-treated red cells was found in 0.1%. There was some crossreaction with trypsinized cells but none with bromelin-treated cells. The antibody did not affect the survival of red cells *in vivo* (Bell *et al.* 1973b).

In one series in which the serum of normal donors was tested in the AutoAnalyzer, agglutinins reacting with bromelin-treated red cells were found in 2% of donors (Ranadazzo *et al.* 1973).

Autohaemolysin reacting with trypsinized red cells. Heistö *et al.* (1965) found that the serum of 94 of 961 normal donors would haemolyse the subject's own trypsinized red cells; the haemolysin was twice as common in women as in men and was shown to be inherited; it was not inhibited by trypsin itself.

Antigens demonstrable on stored red cells and on freshly washed cells

A cold agglutinin that would react only with stored red cells was described by Brendemoen (1952a). Red cells became agglutinable after 4–7 d storage at room temperature or 2 d at 37°C or 30 min at 56°C.

Three examples of a similar antibody were described by Jenkins and Marsh (1961). All were in women with severe haemolytic anaemia and all three antibodies were active at 37°C as well as at lower temperatures. Fresh red cells never reacted but became agglutinable after brief enzyme treatment. A further case was described by Stratton *et al.* (1960) and a very thorough study of another case was published by Ozer and Chaplin (1963).

Although enzyme-treated red cells react with the agglutinin and although it is true that enzyme-treatment removes sialic acid from red cells, there is no evidence that the development of the 'special' antigen on stored red cells is related to loss of sialic acid.

An important clue in understanding this mysterious phenomenon was unearthed by Beaumont *et al.* (1976). Their patient had Waldenström's macroglobulinaemia, and a purified monoclonal IgM κ isolated from her serum agglutinated stored human red cells and also precipitated human and animal low density lipoprotein. It appeared that the 'stored red cell antigen' was not completely identical with low density lipoprotein. The authors pointed out that all previously described cases had had clinical evidence of haemolytic anaemia, although there was no definite evidence of this in their own case.

An antibody reacting only with freshly washed red cells was described by Freiesleben and Jensen (1959). The donor's plasma would no longer agglutinate red cells after they had stood at room temperature for periods between 5 min and 4 h after washing (Allan *et al.* 1972). A later example not only agglutinated freshly washed red cells but bound complement to them; washed red cells were found to have a shortened ^{51}Cr survival time (Davey *et al.* 1979).

The changes in the red cell membrane induced by washing in sodium chloride, which renders the cells agglutinable, remain to be determined. It should be added that there is no reason to suppose that the phenomenon is related in any way to an enzyme and that it is included in this section simply for lack of any more convenient place for it.

RED CELL AGGLUTINATION NOT DUE TO ANTIBODIES

Rouleaux formation

If red cells are allowed to sediment in their own plasma, they tend to adhere together in a characteristic way, 'like a pile of coins'. The rate of sedimentation of the red cells depends upon the degree of this tendency to aggregate so that rapid, intense rouleaux formation and a high erythrocyte sedimentation rate (ESR) go hand in hand.

The relation between the ESR and the plasma concentrations of 20 different proteins was determined by Scherer *et al.* (1975). The correlation coefficient was highest with fibrinogen, α-1-acid glycoprotein, α-2-macroglobulin, α-1-antitrypsin, caeruloplasmin and IgM. The best correlation between the concentration of various plasma proteins and ESR was obtained when the molar concentrations of fibrinogen, α-2-macroglobulin and IgM were summed.

Occasional samples of serum with high levels of immunoglobulin, as in myelomatosis, even when diluted with an equal volume of saline, may cause strong rouleaux formation. On the other hand, most samples of human serum, when diluted with an equal volume of saline, will not cause rouleaux formation — a fact that is of great value in distinguishing rouleaux formation from agglutination due to antibodies.

Dextran molecules produce rouleaux formation only when they exceed a certain size (Bull *et al.* 1949). It has been postulated that a monolayer of large dextran molecules serves to increase the distance between cells, so that there is weaker electrical repulsion, and at the same time provides a large absorption area on the cell surface, which provides a bridging force (Chien and Kung-Ming, 1973).

It is often thought that rouleaux formation can be distinguished from true agglutination by simple microscopic examination, but in fact the distinction may be difficult to make. In large rouleaux the cells do not all adhere together in neat piles but tend instead to form large clumps which may easily be mistaken for agglutinates. Conversely, weak agglutination in colloid media can closely resemble rouleaux formation; this may be observed, for example, in the titration of partially neutralized immune anti-A sera against A cells in a medium of serum.

Other causes of non-specific agglutination of red cells

Colloidal silica
When solutions are autoclaved or stored in glass bottles, the solution may become contaminated by colloidal silica, particularly if the solution is alkaline. Colloidal silica is adsorbed by red cells and may be the cause of false-positive serological tests. Red cells suspended in a one in 200 dilution of plasma are completely protected against this effect (see previous editions of this book for references). The potential adverse effects of colloidal silica in serological tests have become of much less importance now that solutions are often stored in plastic rather than glass.

Chromic chloride, etc.
Many other substances cause red cells to agglutinate non-specifically, e.g. multivalent metallic ions such as Cr^{3+} or tannic acid.

Wharton's jelly
Samples of blood contaminated with Wharton's jelly may agglutinate spontaneously (Wiener, 1943, p. 49). Contamination of cord blood with a one in 1000 dilution of the jelly is enough to cause red cell clumping (Flanagan and Mitoma, 1958). The clumping can be dispersed by adding hyaluronidase (Killpack, 1980). The phenomenon is likely to cause trouble only when cord blood is collected by cutting the cord and allowing the blood to drain into the tube. For many reasons this is a very unsatisfactory way of obtaining a sample. A far better way is to take a blood sample with a syringe and needle from the umbilical vein.

CHAPTER 8

DETECTION OF THE REACTION BETWEEN RED CELL ANTIGENS AND ANTIBODIES

The reaction between red cell antigens and corresponding antibodies is most commonly detected by an agglutination test. Red cells suspended in a fluid medium are mixed with serum or plasma and incubated. The red cells are allowed to sediment or are centrifuged and are then examined for agglutination. If no agglutinates are observed, the cells may be washed, mixed with antiglobulin serum, centrifuged and re-examined for agglutination. In practice, the sensitivity of tests is increased in various ways, for example by using special media, e.g. albumin or low-ionic-strength solutions (LISS), or by treating red cells with proteolytic enzymes.

In identifying red cell antigens, the test used depends on the characteristics of the antibodies available. The simplest technique is agglutination in saline and this test can almost always be used when the relevant antibody is IgM. When the antibody is IgG it will usually be necessary to use some slightly more complicated procedure.

The most reliable results for the detection of red cell antibodies are obtained by using a combination of tests; the particular combination adopted in any given laboratory must depend on such factors as the experience of the staff with a particular test, the number of tests to be performed, the time available for their performance and the kind of problems which have to be solved.

The reaction between red cell antigens and antibodies may be detected in various other ways: for example, the antibody may be labelled with a radioisotope such as ^{125}I and the amount of ^{125}I bound to the cells measured; or the antibody may be coupled to an enzyme and the binding of antibody to red cells measured by the amount of colour released from a suitable substrate, as in the enzyme-linked immunosorbent assay (ELISA). Finally, antibody may be bound to a surface and the adherence of cells, carrying the antigen, to the bound antibody measured; methods of this kind are referred to as solid phase systems. Systems in which antibodies or antigens are bound to a surface lend themselves very well to automated measurement.

Until a few years ago all blood grouping tests were done with naturally occurring or immune antibodies (polyclonal) obtained from human or animal blood. Now there is an increasing tendency to use monoclonal antibodies obtained by the culture *in vitro* of hybridomas.

The object of most blood grouping and antibody detection tests in clinical work is to provide completely compatible red cells for transfusion. Accordingly, in most tests only a qualitative answer is required: is a particular antigen or antibody present or absent? Quantitative tests are needed much less frequently.

The detection of a particular antigen on red cells is more straightforward than determining the antibody content of a serum. Even when sera containing polyclonal antibodies are used it is comparatively easy to prepare reagents detecting only a single blood group specificity. On the other hand, to discover the antibody content of a serum it may be necessary to make tests with a large panel of red cells because all red cells carry many antigens and serum often contains antibodies of more than one specificity.

Need to wash red cells
Red cell suspensions used in blood grouping should be washed free of their own plasma. If this is not done clots will form when the red cell suspension, which contains fibrinogen, is mixed with serum, which contains residual thrombin. Other reasons for washing red cells are as follows: (1) plasma tends to cause rouleaux formation which interferes with the interpretation of agglutination tests; (2) plasma contains anticoagulants which are anti-complementary and may thus interfere with the detection of complement binding antibodies; (3) preservative substances added to red cell suspensions, e.g. lactose or neomycin, are occasionally responsible for agglutination due to the presence of a corresponding antibody in the patient's plasma (see Chapter 7); most of the antibodies concerned do not react with red cells washed in saline; (4) with respect to the ABO, Lewis, Chido/Rodgers and Ii antigens the plasma contains blood group substances corresponding to those on the red cells and these substances may inhibit the antibody in the test serum; and (5) plasma may contain so-called albumin

autoagglutinins and may then cause false-positive reactions when whole blood is added to a serum-albumin mixture; see p. 309.

RED CELL ANTIGENS

Quantitative differences between red cells from different donors

Homozygotes and heterozygotes
With respect to some red cell antigens, very big differences in reactivity are found between the cells of homozygotes and heterozygotes. Some examples are as follows: C, c, M, S and Jk^a.

Differences between donors of the same phenotype
The reactivity of red cells from different individuals of the same phenotype is particularly variable with regard to the following antigens: P_1, I, i, Le^a, Le^b, Sd^a, Vel and Ch/Rg.

Differences between newborn infants and adults; see Chapter 3.

Effect of storage on red cell antigens

Storage above 0°C
When red cells are stored at 4°C either as whole blood mixed with CPDA-1 or -2, or with saline-adenine-glucose (SAG) additive for up to 35 or 42 d respectively, there is very little loss of activity of red cell antigens other than M and P_1 (Snyder *et al.* 1983; Myhre *et al.* 1984).

Red cells stored as clotted blood lose their antigenic activity more rapidly than when stored with citrate anticoagulant (Rosenfield *et al.* 1971). Similarly, when blood is collected into plastic bags, if the donor line is not emptied immediately after collection and then refilled with blood mixed with anticoagulant, the clotted blood in the tubing is an unreliable source of red cells for crossmatching tests (Jørgensen, 1964). Furthermore, red cells stored as clotted blood may give false-positive reactions in the antiglobulin test due to uptake of complement components during storage at 4°C.

Reagent red cells may be stored as whole blood with CPD or ACD but more usually they are stored as washed cells in a preservative solution. A modified Alsever's solution, with added inosine (with or without adenine) and with antibiotics is commonly used, permitting satisfactory storage for at least 35 d at 4°C.

Before being suspended in preservative solution, red cells should be freed, as far as possible, from leucocytes. Leucocytes contain proteolytic enzymes which, in the absence of plasma inhibitors, may cause lysis of red cells (Högman *et al.* 1978b). In red cell suspensions stored in LISS in the presence of neomycin, proteolytic enzymes from leucocytes may damage red cell antigens. The damage occurs only when leucocytes are present in combination with LISS and neomycin (Malyska *et al.* 1983). The exact mechanism responsible for the damage is not known, but the authors suggested that aminoglycoside antibiotics promote the release of proteolytic enzymes from leucocytes. Damage to antigens was found to be much more serious with aminoglycoside antibiotics, such as neomycin, than with others (Allan *et al.* 1990). Red cells stored in LISS to which amphotericin B has been added are lysed rapidly, probably due to an increased susceptibility of red cells in LISS for sodium deoxycholate present in the amphotericin solution. However, frozen–thawed red cells can be stored safely for 21 d at 4°C in a LISS solution which does not contain either aminoglycoside antibiotics or amphotericin B (Allan *et al.* 1990). The following solution is advised: glycine, 13.7 g; glucose, 8.5 g; NaCl, 1.9 g; Na_2HPO_4, 0.21 g; $NaH_2PO_4.2H_2O$, 0.23 g; adenine, 0.2 g; inosine, 0.4 g; chloramphenicol, 0.34 g, per litre.

Frozen storage

When red cells were stored at -20°C in a citrate–phosphate–glycerol solution (see Appendix 8) for 1 year the only antigen found to react more weakly was P_1 (Crawford *et al.* 1954). After thawing the frozen cells, glycerol must be removed before the cells can be tested; removal is most conveniently carried out by washing; see Appendix 8.

Unfortunately when red cells are stored at -20°C there may be extensive haemolysis, possibly dependent on the time for which the red cells were stored prior to freezing.

For storage for indefinite periods red cells must be kept at -80°C or lower. One very convenient method is known as 'glycigel'. Tubes containing a glycerol solution mixed with gelatin are kept available in the refrigerator. When red cells for storage are added to one of these tubes and the tube is warmed the glycerol is released slowly as the gelatin melts and cell damage is minimized. The red cells are stored at -80°C or lower and, when wanted, are thawed and washed free from glycerol (Huggins *et al.* 1982; see also Appendix 8).

A very simple method for preparing red cells for frozen storage is to add dextrose or sucrose to them and then add the mixture drop-wise from a syringe into liquid nitrogen (Meryman, 1956). Another method which has proved very satisfactory is the one described by Bronson and McGinniss (1962). Blood mixed with an equal volume of Alsever's solution is mixed with one-tenth its volume of 50% glucose; a metal screen is dipped into the mixture and frozen by immersion in liquid nitrogen. After storage in nitrogen vapour, the blood is thawed by placing the screen in a tube containing 5% glucose in saline at 40°C. The cells are then washed. In washing red cells which have been frozen in this way, better results are obtained if the thawed cells are first washed in a hypertonic solution (Burnie, 1965).

Another simple method for preparing red cells for frozen storage, which is particularly useful when large volumes are needed to provide cell panels, is based on the glycerolization technique used for freezing whole units of blood described by Meryman and Hornblower (1972). For glycerolization the red cells are first shaken vigorously while being mixed with a quarter of the glycerol solution. They are then transferred to the bag in which they are to be frozen and are mixed with the rest of the glycerol. After thawing, the red cells are first washed in a hypertonic solution (12% NaCl) (Högman *et al.* 1986).

FACTORS AFFECTING RED CELL–ANTIBODY INTERACTIONS

Serum vs. plasma

For blood grouping tests serum is to be preferred to plasma, first, because plasma samples may clot when incubated at 37°C and, second, because the detection of some antibodies depends upon complement activation. Anticoagulants such as citrate or EDTA prevent complement activation by chelating calcium; heparin inhibits the splitting of C4 by C1.

Plasma samples have been found to be satisfactory for screening donors using automated instruments (Myhre, 1972) and are, in fact, used for this purpose in most blood transfusion centres.

Storage of sera

If there is no microbial contamination, at 4°C blood grouping sera retain their potency for 1–2 years; when stored at – 20°C, they retain their potency for very many years.

Thiomerosal is a less satisfactory preservative than sodium azide; in a concentration of more than 0.2 g/l it inhibits the action of anti-D sera and tends to cause haemolysis (Simmons and Woods, 1946). Thiomerosal is, however, used in some LISSs in concentrations of 0.1–0.25 g/l.

The use of sodium azide is potentially hazardous. When solutions containing azide are discharged to waste via metal pipes, heavy metal azides, notably of copper or lead, are formed which are readily detonated, explosive compounds. Copper azide is particularly sensitive to mechanical shock. Despite these potential hazards, sodium azide is still added to most commercial blood grouping reagents. Antibiotics such as those used in red cell suspensions may be used as a substitute for azide but the occurrence of corresponding antibodies in human sera (see Chapter 7) may lead to anomalous results.

Colouring agents

Dyes are frequently added to anti-A and anti-B reagents; usually blue is added to anti-A and yellow to anti-B; Patent Blue V (E131) and Ariavit tartrazine (E102) in concentrations of 0.08 g/l are suitable. Although colour is convenient in identifying reagents, it must not be relied on, i.e. the reagent should be identified by reading the label and the use of controls remains essential. A green dye is added to some polyspecific antiglobulin reagents.

Deterioration of complement on storage

When serum with an optimal concentration of complement is required it should be separated from red cells as soon as possible (Fischer *et al.* 1958). On storage of serum at 4°C there is just-detectable deterioration of complement after 24 h and readily detectable deterioration at 1 week (Polley and Mollison, 1961; see also pp. 164 and 336).

Garratty (1970) found that over 60% of normal complement activity was required to avoid the risk of missing weak complement-binding antibodies. In a study of normal sera this level of activity was retained for less than 1 d at 37°C, for 1 d at room temperature, for 2 weeks at 4°C, for 2 months at − 20°C and for at least 3 months at − 55°C or below. Complement deteriorates far less rapidly in the plasma of ACD stored blood than in serum; after 3 weeks at 4°C the average loss of haemolytic activity is only 9%. Stability of complement in citrated plasma may be due to diminished levels of Ca^{2+} and Mg^{2+} (Reich *et al.* 1970).

Serum stored at − 20°C for a few weeks is usually almost as effective as fresh serum as a source of complement in the antiglobulin test (Polley and Mollison, 1961). Sera stored at − 20°C for prolonged periods may become strongly anti-complementary and then the presence in them of antibodies, such as anti-Le^a, may be overlooked if an ordinary 'one-stage' indirect antiglobulin test (IAT) is used (Polley and Mollison, 1961); a method of dealing with this problem is described on p. 348.

Serum stored at − 50°C for 2 months is indistinguishable from fresh serum as a source of complement for antibody detection in antiglobulin tests and in tests for haemolysis (Polley and Mollison, 1961).

Potentiators

The effect of colloids in potentiating agglutination is discussed in Chapter 3. In this chapter some practical aspects of the use of colloids will be considered.

The colloid most widely used as a potentiator of agglutination in manual tests is bovine serum albumin (BSA). It is used in a concentration of 10–20% to enhance agglutination in reagents containing (IgG) antibodies and other potentiators, and in a concentration of 3–8% to enhance agglutination by reagents containing IgM antibodies or reduced and alkylated IgG antibodies.

In 'normal' preparations of BSA, 5–10% of the protein is in the form of dimers or oligomers; the percentage may be deliberately increased to as high as 50% to produce 'polymerized albumin'. In techniques in which red cells are allowed to sediment in albumin, the potentiating effect is greater with preparations containing the largest percentages of dimers and oligomers (Jones *et al.* 1969; Reckel and Harris, 1978; ICSH, 1982).

Polymers such as gum acacia, dextran and polyvinylpyrrolidone (PVP) potentiate agglutination at lower concentrations than BSA but also have a tendency to cause non-specific aggregation. The use of one of these polymers in combination with BSA enables the concentration of albumin to be reduced whilst the rate and strength of agglutination are enhanced. For example, IgG anti-D reagents incorporating a polymer and BSA produce rapid potent agglutination of D-positive cells either on warm slides using whole blood or in tubes with saline suspended cells (Case, 1982). Polyethylene glycol (PEG) is used as a potentiator in the antiglobulin test (see below).

Proteolytic enzymes

As discussed in Chapter 3, treatment of red cells with certain enzymes renders them agglutinable by otherwise non-agglutinating antibodies.

The discovery that enzyme-treated Rh D-positive red cells suspended in saline are agglutinated by otherwise non-agglutinating anti-Rh D was made by chance. In 1946 M.M. Pickles (personal communication) was trying to find out whether there was any connection between T-activated red cells, and antibody-coated cells such as are found in haemolytic disease of the newborn. D-positive and D-negative red cells were included with the various controls which were used. *Cholera vibrio*-treated D-positive red cells but not D-negative red cells were agglutinated by diluted incomplete anti-D (Pickles, 1946). It was soon afterwards discovered that trypsin gave results similar to those with *C. vibrio*-filtrate (Morton and Pickles, 1947).

Several proteolytic enzymes are used in blood grouping tests: trypsin and chymotrypsin, which have a very restricted specificity, and bromelin, ficin and papain, which have a broad specificity for peptide bonds.

Trypsin cleaves peptides which are C-terminal to lysine and arginine whereas chymotrypsin catalyses cleavage primarily after the C-terminal of leucine, methionine, asparagine, glutamine and aromatic amino acids.

Bromelin, ficin and papain are all thiol proteases with a cysteine residue at the active site which must be in its reduced form for activation of the enzyme. Thiol proteases are readily inactivated under normal storage conditions as a result of oxidation of the thiol group of the cysteine or by binding of traces of heavy metal ions to the thiol group. Optimal activation of thiol proteases occurs on simultaneous addition of a thiol reducing agent, such as cysteine, and a heavy metal chelating agent such as EDTA (Kimmel and Smith, 1954). In practice, crude preparations of these three enzymes are normally used, each containing a mixture of different proteolytic enzymes, the proportion and concentration of which may vary from batch to batch. The proteolytic activity, as measured by the hydrolysis of azoalbumin, is correlated with serological activity (Lambert *et al.* 1978; Phillips *et al.* 1984) A lyophilized reference preparation of papain has been made available to all national Reference Laboratories by the ISBT/ICSH working party on enzymes.

Effect of enzymes on particular red cell antigens

In the detection of Rh antibodies, tests with enzyme-treated red cells are extremely sensitive. Giles (1960) found that additional Rh antibodies were often revealed by tests with ficin-treated red cells: e.g. 'pure' anti-D might be found to contain anti-C or anti-E, 'pure' anti-C to contain anti-e and 'pure' anti-E to contain anti-c.

The reactions of anti-P_1 and of Lewis and Kidd antibodies are stronger with enzyme-treated than with untreated red cells and Lewis and Kidd antibodies may lyse enzyme-treated red cells when they will not lyse untreated cells. Other antibodies which react more strongly with enzyme-treated than with untreated cells include anti-I and -i and the antibodies of the Colton and Dombrock systems.

Antigens inactivated or weakened by treatment with certain proteolytic enzymes include Fy^a, Fy^b, M, N, S, s, En^a, Lu^a, Yt^a, Xg^a, Ge, Ch, Rg, JMH, In^b, Yk^a, Tn and Pr. Crude preparations of bromelin, ficin and papain are mixtures of many proteolytic enzymes and these three enzyme preparations weaken most of the above antigens. On the other hand, crystalline trypsin and chymotrypsin have more selective effects: S, s and Fy^a are destroyed by chymotrypsin but not by trypsin, and K is only destroyed when both enzymes are used together; some antigens, e.g. M, N and Lu^a, are destroyed by either enzyme (Judson and Anstee, 1977).

Lu^a and Lu^b were found to be unaffected by treatment with ficin or papain by G. Garratty (personal communication), although variable effects were found by Poole and Giles (1982).

The low frequency antigens of the MNSs system can be classified according to their sensitivity to trypsin treatment. The trypsin-sensitive determinants are located on the MN (α) sialoglycoprotein whereas, the trypsin-insensitive determinants are probably located on the Ss (δ) sialoglycoprotein although they may be located on the MN protein close to the red cell membrane (Giles, 1982).

The reactions of anti-Yt[a] are not diminished by trypsin-treatment of red cells but, in one series, six of six examples failed to react with cells treated with bromelin, chymotrypsin, ficin and papain (Rouger et al. 1982a) and in another series, eight of 14 examples of anti-Yt[a] failed to react with cells treated with ficin and papain (Vengelen-Tyler and Morel, 1979).

The determinants Pr, Tn and T are weakened by treatment with proteolytic enzymes but are not inactivated. Some activity persists because the determinants occur not only on α- and β-sialoglycoproteins, which are split off the red cell membrane by most proteolytic enzymes, but are also carried on δ-sialoglycoprotein, which is not affected by treatment with most proteolytic enzymes (the exception being chymotrypsin).

In some cases, the antigens are damaged only by relatively high concentrations of enzyme. For example, in one investigation destruction of s was not observed until chymotrypsin levels of 132 units/ml were used and even at this level the receptor detected by one example of anti-S was unaffected (Judson and Anstee, 1977). Similarly, although T is not destroyed by concentrations of papain normally used in blood grouping tests (Bird et al. 1971) it is destroyed by 3–4% ficin or papain (Issitt et al. 1972).

Stability of enzymes on storage

Cysteine-activated papain stored at 4°C as a liquid at pH 5.4 loses about 50% of enzyme activity within 2 weeks; most of this loss is due to instability of the activator (M.L. Scott and P.K. Phillips, personal communication). Preparations which have not been cysteine-activated are relatively stable during storage at 4°C (Stapleton and Moore, 1959). Because of the instability of activated enzyme preparations, which may be the cause of false-positive or false-negative results (Holburn and Prior, 1987), many users prepare their own enzyme solutions and store them at – 20°C, at which temperature they may be kept for 6 months. In practice, enzyme preparations are frequently assessed for potency by subjective serological tests.

Liquid enzyme preparations can be stabilized in a form suitable for distribution by reversible inhibition of the enzyme by heavy metal ions; activated enzyme is recovered by the addition of a separately provided activator (M.L. Scott and P.K. Phillips, personal communication). As an activator, cysteine is unsuitable because of its instability; dithiothreitol (DTT) and glutathione are both stable on storage at 4°C but, since DTT added to activated papain destroys Kell antigens (Branch and Petz, 1982) glutathione is preferred.

Enzyme activity can be standardized using azoalbumin as substrate (Scott et al. 1988a). However, there are differences in substrate specificities for bromelin, ficin and papain (Ogasawara and Mazda, 1989). These authors preferred to use casein as substrate because the specific activities of each of these enzymes towards casein were similar. Alternatively enzyme preparations can be standardized using a standard blood grouping reagent, e.g. anti-D which reacts with enzyme-treated cells.

Low ionic strength

As described in Chapter 3, the rate of association of antibody with antigen is very greatly increased by lowering ionic strength. The advantages of using a low-ionic-strength medium are seen chiefly in tests with IgG antibodies (see section on antiglobulin tests below). Nevertheless, it is a fairly common practice to use a low-ionic-strength medium instead of saline for the suspension of red cells. Most workers have found that with anti-A and anti-B results are similar with low-ionic-strength medium and with saline (Elliot *et al.* 1964; Löw and Messeter, 1974; Moore and Mollison, 1976). The reactivity of some cold alloagglutinins is enhanced in a low-ionic-strength medium so that their thermal range becomes wider, e.g. anti-A_1 and anti-P_1 (Mollison, 1983, p. 519); others, e.g. anti-Pr_1 (O'Neill *et al.* 1986), are detectable only in a low-ionic-strength medium. The enhanced activity of cold alloagglutinins may complicate blood grouping and pre-transfusion testing if low-ionic-strength techniques are used in direct agglutination.

Polycations

Protamine and polybrene cause red cells to aggregate. The resulting very close contact allows crosslinking of red cells by IgG antibodies. Non-specific aggregation can be dispersed by the addition of a suitable agent and then only specific agglutinates remain. Manual tests in which a low-ionic-strength medium is used together with protamine have proved very sensitive in detecting alloantibodies. If no agglutination occurs the cells can be washed and antiglobulin serum added as a further step (Rosenfield *et al.* 1979; Lalezari and Jiang, 1980). Details of a manual polybrene test (MPT) are given later.

Reduced and alkylated IgG antibodies

As described in Chapter 3, after mild chemical reduction some IgG incomplete antibodies will agglutinate red cells suspended in saline. Agglutination is greatly enhanced by adding polymerized BSA to a final concentration of 6–8%.

Reagents containing reduced IgG anti-D are used for rapid slide and tube tests and for tests in microplates.

Reduced anti-D needs an incubation time of only 2–5 min at room temperature for the development of optimal reactions whereas polyclonal IgM anti-D usually requires about 15 min at 37°C. On the other hand, reduced anti-D reagents tend not to be very potent.

Monoclonal vs. polyclonal antibodies

Monoclonal antibodies have several advantages over polyclonal antibodies: (1) they provide an unlimited supply of identical material; (2) they are free from unwanted contaminating antibodies, e.g. HLA antibodies or antibodies to low frequency antigens, so that testing and quality control are far simpler; (3) they are free from naturally occurring antibodies such as anti-T so that they do not give false-positive results, e.g. with T-transformed red cells; (4) they are free from viruses of hepatitis and of HIV; and (5) their use avoids the need to immunize and plasmapherese human donors.

Murine monoclonal antibodies have at least two disadvantages: first, as their specificities may apparently vary at different concentrations, tests employing them must be very carefully standardized (McDonald and Gerns, 1986); second, they may give unexpected reactions, e.g. some potent monoclonal anti-As react weakly with some B cells (Voak *et al.* 1987) and some anti-Bs react with A cells. The occurrence of these reactions is known as the B(A) and A(B) phenomenon. Other possible disadvantages of monoclonal antibodies are mentioned in Chapter 3.

Antibodies of only certain specificities can be produced in mice. Some excellent human monoclonals have been produced (see Chapters 3, 4, 5 and 6).

ABO system
Although only selected monoclonal anti-As and anti-Bs are suitable as blood grouping reagents (Rouger and Anstee, 1987; see also Gane *et al.* 1987b), the best monoclonals are superior to polyclonal reagents (Voak, 1991). Some monoclonals are potent reagents for common ABO phenotypes whereas others react well with weak variants; only a few antibodies combine these two properties (Oriol *et al.* 1990) but excellent reagents can be prepared by blending two or more monoclonals (Voak, 1990). Such reagents detect most examples of A_x cells better than previously used polyclonal anti-A,B sera and also reliably detect weak A_2B and A_3B in rapid slide tests. Several anti-A_1B monoclonals which can be used in agglutination tests are now available (Oriol *et al.* 1990).

Rh system
It has not been possible to produce murine anti-D and all monoclonal anti-D reagents at present available are of human origin. Most monoclonal anti-Ds give patterns of reactivity similar to those of polyclonal antisera except that most monoclonals fail to react with cells of the D^{VI} category or with cells of other categories (Rouger and Anstee, 1987; Tippett and Moore, 1990). The ability of different monoclonals to detect weak D and D variants varies with the technique used, weak D being detected more efficiently by antiglobulin techniques than by agglutination of enzyme treated cells. Some reagents detect weak D more efficiently than others (van Rhenen *et al.* 1989; Tippett and Moore, 1990).

Because monoclonal anti-Ds often fail to recognize cells with a partial D antigen, particularly category VI cells, they should be used in parallel with a polyclonal reagent or in a combination shown to react with most D variants. Human monoclonal anti-C, anti-E, anti-c, anti-e and anti-G are now available. One anti-E and one anti-c gave weak reactions with papain-treated E-negative and c-negative cells respectively (Tippett and Moore, 1990).

AGGLUTINATION TESTS

In the agglutination reaction two separate processes may be recognized: first, the uptake of antibody onto the red cells and second, the adherence to one another of the antibody-coated cells. In agglutination tests, the red cells may be allowed to come into contact with one another by sedimentation or the process may be accelerated by the use of centrifugation.

Sedimentation vs. centrifugation
Contact between antibody-coated cells occurs relatively slowly if the red cells are simply left to sediment in a column, e.g. in a test tube; the process can be accelerated by having only a thin layer of cells, as in slide tests, when the cells have only a short

distance to travel before they are all in the same plane. Alternatively, the cell suspension can be centrifuged. In slide tests and in tests in capillary tubes, sedimentation is employed exclusively; when tests are done in test tubes or in the wells of microplates, either sedimentation or centrifugation can be used.

Slide tests

Since water evaporates rapidly from the large surface area, slide tests must be read within 5 min or so; in practice, reagents which produce strong agglutination within 1–2 min are normally used and the tests are employed simply for rapid determination of ABO and Rh D groups. Since the results are read macroscopically, strong cell suspensions (20% or more) should be used to facilitate the detection of agglutination.

Tests in capillary tubes

A method of Rh grouping in capillary tubes was described by Chown (1944) and Chown and Lewis (1946; 1951). Two important advantages of the method were that each test required only 5 μl serum and that results could be read in 15 min. For a review of the many applications of capillary tube tests, see Crawford (1987).

Tests in tubes

Tests in tubes are very widely used. Evaporation is not a problem so that incubation can continue for 1–2 h if desired, although in practice 45 min is usually considered to be long enough. Tubes in racks can easily be placed in a waterbath (at 37°C). The red cells can be allowed to sediment or the tubes can be centrifuged. The tube is then tapped and rolled to resuspend the cells. If no agglutinates are seen with the naked eye the tube can be examined with a hand lens, over a magnifying mirror or under the low power of a microscope. Alternatively, but less conveniently, a drop of cell suspension can be transferred to a slide and examined under a microscope.

Microplate (microtitre plates)

Microplates are clear plastic plates containing, as a rule, 96 wells (8 × 12). With V-shaped wells, very weak cell suspensions (0.03%) can be used, but with U-shaped wells, 1–2% suspensions are optimal. One small volume (e.g. 20 μl) of serum is added to an equal volume of red cell suspension. The plates are centrifuged. As a rule, U wells are agitated and read in a conventional way. V wells are tilted at 75°C to the horizontal for 10 min. Unagglutinated cells stream down the side of the well as a smooth thin line; agglutinated cells remain as a button. The use of microplates has several advantages: the method is very much more sensitive than that of other agglutination systems, primarily because very weak cell suspensions can be used; very small amounts of reagents are needed; titrations are easier with multi-channel pipettes and grades of reactions can be compared. A problem with microplates is that some antibody reagents cannot be used undiluted because their high viscosity causes red cells to adhere to the side of the wells. This problem arises particularly when 'rapid anti-D' reagents and, to a lesser extent, when anti-A and anti-B reagents are used. The problem can be overcome by diluting the reagents with saline. Monoclonal antibodies adhere to the plastic-solid phase and a positive reaction is seen as a monolayer of cells whilst a negative reaction is seen as a button or stream. A semi-automated system is mentioned in a later section. (For a review of the use of microplates, see Blood Transfusion Task Force, 1991.)

Methods using proteolytic enzymes

One-stage vs. two-stage methods

One-stage methods. In a method described by Löw (1955), enzyme (cysteine-activated papain), serum and cells are mixed together, thus allowing enzyme treatment of the cells and the reaction of antigen and antibody to occur simultaneously. Evidently, in such a method an opportunity is provided for the cleavage of Ig molecules by the enzyme. The proteolytic effect of the enzyme is diminished by protease inhibitors in serum (Travis and Salvesen, 1983) but such inhibitors also reduce the effect of enzyme on the red cells. Although one-stage methods are sufficiently sensitive to give reliable results with potent blood grouping reagents, they are unsuitable for antibody detection or determination of specificity with manual techniques.

Two-stage method. In this method, washed red cells are first treated with an enzyme, then washed again and incubated with serum. The method has two substantial advantages over a one-stage method: first, no opportunity is provided for degradation of Ig by enzyme; second, enzyme treatment and red cell–antibody interaction can each be carried out at its optimal pH. For papain and bromelin treatment of red cells the optimal pH is 5.4–5.8, as determined by serological results in a two-stage technique (Scott *et al.* 1987a). The optimal pH for binding of anti-D to red cells is 6.5–8.0 (Hughes-Jones *et al.* 1964a), although the optimum for antibodies of other specificities may be different.

A two-stage papain technique in which washing of the cells after papain treatment is replaced by the addition of a specific papain inhibitor, E-64, has been described by Scott and Phillips (1987). This technique permits optimal enzyme treatment of the red cells while avoiding digestion of immunoglobulins following the addition of serum. It thus combines the sensitivity of two-stage tests with the convenience of one-stage tests. The inhibitor E-64 can also be used for bromelin (Ogasawara and Mazda, 1989).

In automated blood grouping machines, red cells are suspended in enzyme solution and incubated briefly before being mixed with the sera.

A comparison of one-stage and two-stage methods

In a series of six quality assessment exercises in which there were 44 incompatibilities due to antibodies of 15 different specificities the overall error rates for enzyme tests were as follows: one-stage mixing (method of Löw, 1955), 34%; one-stage layering (method of Dodd and Eeles, 1961), 27%; two-stage method, 15% (Holborn and Prior, 1987). In two-stage tests bromelin and papain were equally effective; in one-stage tests bromelin was better than papain, possibly because it retains proteolytic activity better at neutral pH (Scott *et al.* 1988a).

Role of ionic strength

The effects of low ionic strength and of enzyme treatment of cells are not additive (Atchley, 1964; Elliot *et al.* 1964). In external quality assessment surveys the use of low ionic strength was found to have no influence on results obtained with enzyme techniques (Holburn and Prior, 1987).

Optimal period of incubation
When red cells are allowed to sediment, 60 min is optimal but when the mixtures are first centrifuged, incubation for 10 min gives maximum sensitivity (Jørgensen *et al.* 1979). However, most laboratories use a period of 15–30 min and centrifuge at the end of the incubation period.

Agglutination in electrolyte media
Agglutination tests with red cells suspended in normal saline are used in two main circumstances: when reagents containing potent IgM antibodies are available and in crossmatching tests simply to detect ABO incompatibility. Agglutination tests with saline-suspended red cells are also used in a few special circumstances, e.g. in investigations on cold alloagglutinins such as anti-P_1.

Tests in low-ionic-strength saline have been mentioned above.

False-positive results in agglutination tests
The commonest cause is rouleaux formation. Dilution of serum with an equal volume of saline greatly diminishes or completely abolishes rouleaux. Dextran is a potential source of trouble but only high molecular weight preparations (no longer used as plasma substitutes) cause rouleaux formation of untreated red cells. Enzyme-treated red cells may be intensely aggregated even by Dextran 40 (Selwyn *et al.* 1968).

The next commonest cause of false-positive results is the presence of cold auto-agglutinins. These antibodies (usually anti-I) produce strong agglutination up to a temperature of about 25°C, or even sometimes up to 32°C, but are very seldom active at a temperature of 37°C. If red cells and serum are not pre-warmed to 37°C before being mixed, subsequent warming to 37°C may fail to disperse agglutination completely.

When there is difficulty in distinguishing between rouleaux formation and auto-agglutination it is helpful to prepare dilutions of the serum in saline (1 in 2 and 1 in 4) and to incubate these with the subject's own red cells, first at 4°C and then at 37°C. Potent autoagglutinins should react very strongly at 4°C and weakly or not at all at 37°C; furthermore, diluting the serum 1 in 4 should have little or no effect on the degree of agglutination. By contrast rouleaux formation should be more pronounced at 37°C than at 4°C; it should be very much weaker in a 1 in 2 dilution than in undiluted serum and should be completely absent in the 1 in 4 dilution.

Agglutination in macromolecular media
The colloid most widely used for manual tests is BSA.

Spontaneous agglutination of antibody-coated cells in albumin
A problem which arises when albumin is used as a potentiator of agglutination is that red cells sensitized with an autoantibody *in vitro* or *in vivo* may agglutinate sponta-neously in concentrations of albumin as low as 6% (Garratty *et al.* 1984). It is therefore

essential, as a routine, to carry out a control test in which the red cells are mixed with potentiating agent alone. The term potentiating agent is used because some reagents which contain albumin may contain other potentiating agents so that the control used must be one supplied by the manufacturer of the reagent containing everything except the reagent antibody (White *et al.* 1974; Garratty *et al.* 1984).

The manual polybrene test (MPT)

As discussed in a later section, protamine and polybrene are used in certain automated techniques for antibody detection; they are also used in manual tests. In the low-ionic polycation test protamine is used and in the MPT, polybrene. Of these two tests, the most satisfactory appears to be the MPT since it requires fewer manipulations and only a very brief incubation period at room temperature.

One millilitre of a low-ionic-strength medium (dextrose–EDTA) is added to two drops of a 10% cell suspension and two drops of serum; after 1 min at room temperature, two drops of 0.05% polybrene are added, the tubes are spun, and the supernatant is decanted. Two drops of a citrate–dextrose solution are added to disperse polybrene-induced aggregation and the contents of the tube are mixed by gentle rolling. After examining the tube for agglutinates, the red cells can be washed and the antiglobulin test carried out. Since C3 and C4 may bind non-specifically at low ionic strength the antiglobulin reagent should not contain anti-complement (Lalezari and Jiang, 1980).

A modified test in which two drops of serum are mixed with one drop of a 3% suspension of red cells and 0.6 ml of low-ionic-strength medium was used by Ferrer *et al.* (1985). This test was found to be more sensitive than the original test described by Lalezari and Jiang (1980).

For the detection of most antibodies, the MPT was found to be more sensitive than either the standard two-stage enzyme method or the IAT (Fisher, 1983). However, anti-K and anti-Fy^a (particularly the former) are often missed, and may be missed even when the MPT test is followed by a test with antiglobulin serum (Fisher, 1983; Ferrer *et al.* 1985; Malde *et al.* 1986). Using a commercial kit for the MPT, 31 of 47 anti-Ks were not detected and this MPT test was therefore considered to be unsuitable as a primary technique for the detection of alloantibodies (Letendre *et al.* 1987).

For large-scale red cell typing the MPT was found to be as good as routine microplate testing but twice as quick. Antiglobulin serum was needed only for Kell grouping (Etges *et al.* 1982). Satisfactory results were observed in another series although antiglobulin serum was used for testing with anti-Jk^a, -S and -s as well as -K (Anderson and Patel, 1984). The MPT has also been recommended for red cell antibody screening, provided that appropriate positive and negative controls are used (Ferrer *et al.* 1985); the test carried out in microplates was found to be as sensitive as the tube test (Lown and Ivy, 1988).

Mixed field agglutination

This term is used to describe the presence of agglutinated and unagglutinated cells in a red cell suspension treated with an agglutinin. The term is often used to imply that two phenotypically distinct populations of red cells are present, as in mosaics, chimeras, subjects who have been transfused, women whose circulation contains fetal red cells, and subjects some of whose red cells have undergone T or Tn transformation. On the other hand, a similar appearance may be seen in red cell suspensions of a single phenotype, either when the red cells have relatively few antigen sites (e.g. 'weak' varieties of A) or when the agglutinin is of low titre. Lutheran antibodies characteristically produce a mixed field appearance of large agglutinates with many free cells and anti-Sd^a produces small agglutinates in a sea of free cells.

Although mixed field agglutination is included in the present section under the general heading of 'agglutination of red cells suspended in saline', it may be observed in any agglutination reaction, e.g. between antibody-coated red cells and antiglobulin serum. For example, when the direct antiglobulin test (DAT) is performed in a patient who is having a delayed haemolytic transfusion reaction, a mixed field may be observed since (as a rule) only the donor cells are agglutinated.

Again, if an IAT with anti-D is performed on red cells from a D-negative mother whose circulation contains a substantial number of D-positive red cells, due to a TPH from her fetus, a mixed field will be observed and may be misinterpreted as meaning that the mother has a weak D antigen. When a mixed field due to the presence of two phenotypically distinct populations is suspected, there are many tests which can be done to confirm or refute the suspicion. For example, tests may be made with sera containing alloantibodies of various specificities which may reveal that there are two populations of red cells present, differing with respect to many antigens. Alternatively, the agglutinated cells may be separated from the agglutinated cells by differential sedimentation and the agglutinated cells may then be disagglutinated and tested.

An excellent technique for detecting two populations of red cells is the gel test (see p. 351) because one population of cells will remain at the top of the gel (agglutinated) and the other will go to the bottom of the tube (unagglutinated).

TESTS FOR LYSIS OF RED CELLS

Tests for alloantibodies which lyse red cells (haemolysins) are no longer used in blood grouping: first, because, apart from some examples of anti-A and anti-B, most blood group antibodies will not readily lyse red cells and, second, because the lytic property of serum deteriorates rapidly on storage due to the decay of complement. Nevertheless, in some circumstances, it is valuable to know whether or not a serum sample is lytic: (1) if a serum causes specific lysis, it establishes the fact that it contains a complement-binding antibody; (2) if a serum is readily lytic *in vitro* at 37°C, the antibody is likely to cause intravascular lysis of incompatible red cells (although this information would usually be of interest only in a retrospective investigation); (3) in circumstances in which group O blood has to be used for transfusion to group A or B subjects, a screening test for lytic anti-A and anti-B may be the best for detecting really 'dangerous' group O donors see p. 361; (4) if an infant is suspected of having ABO haemolytic disease, the diagnosis is virtually excluded by showing that the mother's serum will not lyse the infant's red cells (Crawford *et al.* 1953a).

Apart from anti-A and anti-B, the commonest lytic antibody encountered is anti-Le^a. Other strongly lytic alloantibodies are all rare, i.e. anti-H (in *hh* – subjects), anti-P, anti-PP$_1$P^k and anti-Vel. Autohaemolysins are described in Chapter 7.

In crossmatching tests, lytic antibodies may be a cause of false-negative results; most of the cells may be lysed and the remainder may be unagglutinated. It is therefore essential to examine the supernatant for lysis before examining the cell button for agglutination, and before washing the cells in the antiglobulin test.

Use of human serum as a source of complement
In testing for haemolysins, it is preferable to use very fresh serum, i.e. serum taken within the previous 2 h (see p. 164), although as a source of complement in the lysis of sensitized sheep red cells, human serum stored at 4°C for up to 1 week is satisfactory (Polley and Mollison, 1961). When stored serum is tested for haemolysins, fresh serum should be added as a source of complement.

In testing for anti-A or anti-B lysins, group O serum from which anti-A and anti-B have been absorbed may be used. In detecting lytic anti-Le^a or anti-Le^b, serum from Le(a – b –) subjects, free from Lewis antibodies, may be used. Alternatively in detecting lysis by Lewis antibodies, a two-stage test may be used and then the Lewis group of the serum used as a source of complement in the second stage is of no importance (Polley and Mollison, 1961).

Use of animal serum as a source of complement; see Chapter 3.

Importance of ratio of serum to cells; see Chapter 4.

Enzyme treatment of cells
Some examples of anti-Le^a, anti-Le^b and anti-Jk^a will lyse untreated red cells; other examples will lyse only enzyme-treated cells.

^{51}Cr release method
The technique of estimating the release of ^{51}Cr from ^{51}Cr-labelled group A$_1$ red cells incubated with anti-A is referred to in Chapter 9. In addition to being convenient for demonstrating very weak haemolysins this method is useful for demonstrating the presence of a very small proportion of A$_1$ red cells in a mixture of A$_1$ and O cells, e.g. in measuring the proportion of A$_1$ cells in blood group chimeras (Booth *et al.* 1957). The method can also be used to estimate the survival of transfused A cells in an O subject (see p. 530 and Appendix 7).

THE ANTIGLOBULIN TEST (COOMBS' TEST)

By definition, non-agglutinating (incomplete) antibodies are those that fail to agglutinate red cells suspended in saline. In the antiglobulin reaction, red cells coated with incomplete antibodies, e.g. IgG anti-Rh, are agglutinated by anti-IgG, which links the IgG molecules on neighbouring red cells. The principle of the test was described by Moreschi (1908) who showed that if rabbit red cells were incubated with a dose of goat anti-rabbit red cell serum too small to produce agglutination, and then washed, they were strongly agglutinated by rabbit anti-goat serum.

The antiglobulin test was rediscovered and introduced into clinical medicine by Coombs *et al.* (1945) who showed that it could be used either to detect incomplete blood group antibodies in serum — the IAT — or to detect the sensitization of red cells *in vivo*, as in haemolytic disease of the newborn (Coombs *et al*. 1946), the so-called DAT.

Most non-agglutinating blood group antibodies are IgG and are detected by an anti-IgG serum. A few IgM antibodies are incomplete, e.g. Lewis antibodies which at 37°C usually fail to agglutinate red cells but may be detectable by the IAT using anti-IgM (Polley *et al*. 1962), although they are best detected with anti-complement.

Blood group antibodies may be partly IgA and may then be detected with anti-IgA (Adinolfi *et al*. 1966).

The fact that an anti-human globulin (AHG) reagent might react with complement components on red cells was first described by Dacie *et al*. (1957) and it was subsequently shown that the main complement components detected were C4 (Jenkins *et al*. 1960a; Pondman *et al*. 1960) and C3 (Harboe *et al*. 1963).

Antibodies required in antiglobulin reagents
As described above, AHG reagents may be used to detect IgM and IgA, as well as IgG antibodies on red cells and may also be used to detect various components of complement.

In considering which antibodies are required in AHG reagents, a distinction must be made between reagents used in detecting alloantibodies by the IAT and those used in diagnosing sensitization *in vivo* by the DAT.

Antiglobulins for indirect tests
In the detection of alloantibodies, using the routine spin antiglobulin test, anti-IgG is clearly essential but anti-IgM is not required. All incomplete IgM antibodies described so far bind complement and can be detected more readily with anti-complement than with anti-IgM, because each bound IgM molecule leads to the binding of many complement molecules. Some blood group antibodies (e.g. anti-A, anti-B, anti-D) may be partly IgA but are then always also partly IgG so that anti-IgG can be used for their detection. A single weak example of anti-K was wholly IgA (Pereira *et al*. 1989).

In detecting alloantibodies by conventional antiglobulin techniques the presence of anti-complement in the AHG reagent often leads to stronger reactions and very occasionally leads to the detection of antibodies which would otherwise be missed (for references see the 8th and earlier editions of this book). When using the conventional spin-antiglobulin test for the detection of alloantibodies the reagent must contain anti-complement. However, when the PEG–IAT is used with either anti-IgG or anti-Ig, or when the low-ionic MPT technique, followed by an IAT with anti-IgG (MPT–IAT) is used, the presence of anti-complement is unnecessary and must even be avoided because it causes false-positive reactions. These sensitive methods are about equally satisfactory; all fail occasionally to detect an antibody.

The optimal anti-complement component or components to be included in AHG reagents has not yet been finally agreed. On theoretical grounds, antibodies against C3 are preferable to those against C4 because, in the activation of complement via the classical pathway, more C3b than C4b is bound to the cell membrane. Moreover, when red cells are stored at 4°C more C4d than C3d is bound (Engelfriet, 1976; Garratty and Petz, 1976), increasing the possibility of 'false-positive' reactions. When C3b is bound to cells it is converted rapidly to iC3b (see Chapter 3); iC3b reacts with anti-C3c, -C3g and -C3d. During incubation at 37°C in the presence of serum, C3c is progressively removed from the cell surface so that after 1–2 h, or less with weak antibodies, the cells may react only weakly with anti-C3c, although still reacting strongly with anti-C3g and anti-C3d. It might seem then that anti-C3g or anti-C3d would be best for detecting bound complement in the IAT but unfortunately C3d (and C4d) are present in small amounts on normal red cells (Graham *et al.* 1976) and these amounts increase on storage (see above) and on incubation in fresh normal serum (Stratton and Rawlinson, 1976; Chaplin and Torke, 1978; Szymanski and Odgren, 1979; Freedman *et al.* 1980). Red cells coated with relatively small amounts of C3dg are agglutinated by relatively high concentrations of anti-C3d or anti-C3g but not by lower concentrations. When using polyclonal antiglobulin sera, false-positive results are not due solely to the detection of C3d (Nsongkla *et al.* 1982) but may be due to the synergistic effect of various antibodies against complement components. Unwanted positive results are less of a problem when using monoclonal AHG reagents although even then anti-C3d may cause trouble (Voak *et al.* 1986a).

In detecting complement binding by alloantibodies in the IAT, the best solution might seem to be to use anti-C3c alone and to limit the period of incubation to less than 30 min, although even polyclonal anti-C3c may cause false-positive reactions if the titre is too high (Voak *et al.* 1986a). On the other hand, because some laboratories use longer periods of incubation, it has been recommended that a suitable concentration (i.e. one incapable of detecting relatively small amounts of bound C3dg) of either anti-C3d (Giles and Engelfriet, 1980) or anti-C3g (Voak *et al.* 1986a) should also be present in AHG reagents. One great advantage of including one or other of these two latter components is that the reagent is then also suitable for the DAT (see below).

Polyspecific reagents containing monoclonal anti-C3 give fewer false-positive reactions than those containing polyclonal anti-C3 (Voak *et al.* 1986a). Potent examples of anti-C3c, anti-C3d and anti-C3g monoclonals have been produced (Pollack, 1980; Barker, 1982; Lachmann *et al.* 1983).

One of the two polyspecific antiglobulin reference reagents, made available by the ISBT and the ICSH, reagent RIIIM, is a blend of polyclonal anti-IgG and monoclonal anti-C3c and anti-C3d. The other reference reagent (R3P) is entirely polyclonal (see Engelfriet and Voak, 1987).

AHG reagents for direct tests
In the detection of autoimmune haemolytic anaemia (AIHA) and drug-induced haemolytic anaemia, using the DAT, anti-IgM is not needed in addition to anti-IgG because IgM autoantibodies are always complement binding and can be detected better with anti-complement. Anti-IgA is needed very rarely because it is very rare for IgA alone to be detectable on the red cells (see Chapter 7). It is simpler to use monospecific anti-IgA to test cells which are negative with a polyspecific reagent than to include anti-IgA in the polyspecific reagent.

The main components of complement found on red cells from patients with AIHA are C3dg and C4d (see Chapter 7). So far, no case of AIHA has been described in which one of these components has been present without the other. Because polyspecific reagents for the IAT contain anti-C3d or anti-C3g, which, although present in restricted amount, will readily detect the large amounts of C3dg found on red cells of patients with AIHA, the same polyspecific reagent can be used for the DAT and the IAT.

Production of antiglobulin reagents
In most laboratories, commercially available AHG reagents are used. For those who wish to produce their own reagents a survey of methods of production is available (Engelfriet *et al.* 1984).

Heteroagglutinins in antiglobulin reagents
When AHG reagents produced in animals are used, heteroagglutinins are a potential source of trouble; methods of dealing with this problem have been described previously (Mollison, 1983, pp. 507–8). If AHG reagents are to be used with enzyme-treated cells, residual heteroagglutinins must be removed by absorption with enzyme-treated cells.

The reaction with bound immunoglobulin
In the IAT, red cells are first incubated with serum to allow the uptake of antibody (and, in some cases, the binding of complement) and are then washed and tested with an AHG reagent.

Reaction between anti-IgG and IgG-coated red cells
Using radio-iodine-labelled antiglobulin serum, the maximum number of anti-IgG molecules that can combine with an anti-D (IgG) molecule on a red cell surface was estimated to be 6–9 by Costea *et al.* (1962) and Rochna and Hughes-Jones (1965). Near-saturation of the antigen sites of an IgG (anti-D) molecule is obtained by having a free equilibrium concentration of 10–15 μg anti-IgG per ml; that is to say, after the uptake by anti-D of the maximum number of anti-IgG molecules, 10–15 μg anti-IgG per ml should remain in solution. With an initial IgG concentration of 15 μg/ml the amount of antibody taken up by sensitized red cells after 4 min is 95% of the final equilibrium value (Rochna and Hughes-Jones, 1965).

Prozones
If an excess of anti-IgG serum is added to a sample of IgG-sensitized red cells agglutination is inhibited. This prozone phenomenon was investigated by van Loghem *et al.* (1950) and considered to be due to the fact that, with antiglobulin in excess, all the IgG molecules attached to the red cells are coated with anti-IgG so that no 'bridges' can be formed by particular anti-IgG molecules reacting with unsaturated IgG molecules on different red cells. An example of a prozone is shown in Table 8.1.

This type of prozone can be eliminated by washing the cells after incubation with AHG; presumably removal of excess unbound AHG facilitates lattice formation by removing competition between bound and unbound AHG molecules (Salama and Muller-Eckhardt, 1982).

Another kind of prozone. In testing serial dilutions of serum containing a blood group antibody, using the IAT with a fixed dilution of AHG serum, the strongest reactions are

Table 8.1 Comparison of optimal dilutions of a particular anti-human globulin serum (Goat, H39), for cells sensitized with an example of anti-Rh (Avg.) and one of anti-Jk^a (Cro.)

Red cells sensitized with the following dilutions of antiserum (as reciprocals)		Dilutions of anti-IgG from Goat (H39) (as reciprocals)						
		50	100	500	1000	5000	10 000	50 000
Anti-Rh (Avg.)	256	+ +	+ + +	+ + +	+ +	+	(+)	–
	512	+ +	+ +	+ + +	+ +	+	–	–
	1024	+	+ +	+ +	+	–	–	
	2048	+	+ +	+ +	+	–	–	–
	4096	–	+	+	+	–	–	–
	8192	–	–	(+)	wk	–	–	–
Anti-Jk^a(Cro.)	2	+	+	(+)	–	–	–	–
	4	+	+	(+)	–	–	–	–
	8	–	(+)	–	–	–	–	–

usually observed with undiluted serum. However, a few cases have been reported in which diluted antibody-containing serum gave stronger reactions (Freiesleben and Knudsen, 1957; Giblett *et al.* 1958).

Optimal concentration of anti-IgG
Using a double antibody radioimmunoassay, the anti-IgG concentration in 19 commercial AHG reagents varied from 1.2 to 12.8 μg/ml. Twenty-one reagents produced by regional transfusion centres (RTC) in the UK showed a somewhat lower range of values. Sixteen of the RTC reagents and the commercial reagents were assessed serologically using a panel of ten weak IgG alloantibodies. The agglutination scores obtained with each dilution of the AHG reagents were summated and compared with the concentrations of anti-IgG. The serological potency of the reagents improved with an increase in anti-IgG concentration, but only up to a concentration of 2–3-μg/ml. (Gardner *et al.* 1983). Although the serological potency of the commercial reagents assessed in the same way showed no relation to anti-IgG concentration, the concentrations were > 2 μg/ml in 17 of the 19 reagents. The conclusion of these studies was that, since there is no apparent correlation between anti-IgG concentrations and serological activity of AHG reagents such reagents must, for the time being, be assessed serologically.

The following procedure has been suggested for assessing the optimal concentration of anti-IgG: strongly sensitized red cells are prepared by incubating a pool of four samples of R_1r red cells with anti-D serum with a titre (IAT) of 512–1024; weakly sensitized cells are prepared by incubating suitable red cells with serial two-fold dilutions of different specificities, particularly anti-D, -K and -Fy^a. Serial dilutions of the AHG reagent are tested with all the samples of sensitized cells. The titre with strongly sensitized cells must be 256–1024; it should not be lower because then negative reactions may occur with weakly sensitized cells and it should not be higher because the reagent may then exhibit a prozone. The reactions with weakly sensitized cells must be comparable to those of the two ISBT/ICSH reference AHG reagents (see above). An important aspect of anti-IgG is its resistance to neutralization by serum which may be left after washing the red cells. The degree of resistance can be tested by adding a range of dilutions of serum to the AHG reagent. The reagent must still agglutinate strongly sensitized red cells after an equal volume of a 1 in 2000 dilution of serum has been added to it (Engelfriet and Voak, 1987).

A single dilution of a particular AHG reagent is usually optimal for detecting almost all examples of anti-D. On the other hand, a lower dilution may be optimal for detecting occasional alloantibodies of other specificities. There is some evidence that aberrant behaviour with anti-IgG sera is related to the specificity of the alloantibody concerned. Specificities which are suspect in this regard are anti-Jk[a] (see Table 8.1), anti-Fy[a] (Pollack et al. 1962) and anti-S, -s, -Xg[a], -Yt[a] and -Vel (Issitt, 1977). It should be emphasized that many alloantibodies of these specificities are best detected with that dilution of AHG reagent which is optimal for detecting anti-D but it may be necessary to compromise by selection of a somewhat lower dilution for normal use.

Because of the heterogeneity of Ig molecules the use of many donors to provide pooled IgG, and the pooling of anti-IgG from many immunized animals, is desirable in producing reagents for routine use.

Relationship between number of bound IgG molecules and reactions with anti-IgG

Using the spin-antiglobulin test the minimum number of IgG anti-D molecules per cell detectable with anti-IgG is between 100 and 150 (Romano et al. 1973; Burkart et al. 1974; Stratton et al. 1983). The minimum detectable number of IgG anti-A and anti-B molecules per red cell bound either to the red cells of adults or newborn infants is also about 150 (Romano et al. 1973). In normal subjects with a negative DAT the number of IgG molecules per red cell was found to be in the range 5–90 (Merry et al. 1982). The findings of Jeje et al. (1984) were almost identical. In both series the average number of IgG molecules per red cell was between 30 and 40.

A correlation exists between agglutination strength and the number of IgG molecules bound per cell in both the DAT and the IAT (Merry et al. 1984b); in the IAT anti-K bound under low-ionic-strength conditions required a greater number of bound molecules for a given agglutination strength than antibodies of other specificities. The number of molecules per cell required for maximal agglutination with anti-IgG is in the range of 500–2000 (Petz and Garratty, 1980; Schmitz et al. 1981; Merry et al. 1984b). As the number of IgG molecules bound per red cell in AIHA frequently exceeds 2000, the strength of agglutination in the DAT is of limited value as an indicator of the degree of antibody sensitization.

In recent external quality assessment surveys in which the majority of participants used spin-antiglobulin tests, more than 97% of participants were able to detect 0.05 μg/ml anti-D in one survey (Holburn and Prior, 1987) and more than 98% were able to detect 0.01 μg/ml in another (Pinkerton et al. 1984).

Inhibition of anti-IgG by IgG in solution

When using an AHG reagent containing about 10 μg anti-IgG per ml, obvious weakening of the reaction between anti-IgG and IgG-coated cells is not likely to occur unless the level of IgG in the suspending medium reaches about 10 μg/ml. Since normal serum contains about 10 mg IgG per ml it must be diluted at least 1000 times during washing of antibody-coated red cells to avoid false-negative results. A better safety margin is a dilution of about 5000.

Suppose that one incubates 0.08 ml (two drops) test serum with 0.04 ml cell suspension, that 4 ml saline is used for each wash and that 0.1 ml supernatant is left with the cells after each wash. A single wash then dilutes the serum only 18-fold, three washes will dilute the original serum almost 6000-fold and will therefore be adequate. Nevertheless, since many commercial AHG reagents appeared to contain much less than 10 μg IgG/ml, it is advisable to wash the red cells four times. The danger of false-negative reactions due to inadequate washing is reduced when two volumes of AHG reagent are used to one volume of washed cell suspension. When cell washing centrifuges are used, correct maintenance of the machines is essential (Voak *et al.* 1986b).

Reactions of anti-IgM

Many IgM antibodies are agglutinins active at 37°C and the reactions of these antibodies are not enhanced by the addition of anti-IgM. However, certain IgM antibodies act as agglutinins only at temperatures up to about 25°C or 30°C, and at 37°C may act as incomplete antibodies and then be demonstrable by the antiglobulin test using anti-IgM. Polley *et al.* (1962) found that the following antibodies behaved in this way: anti-Le^a (eight of eight examples), anti-HI and anti-P$_1$ (single, selected potent examples), and allo-anti-I (from an i donor). In addition to these cold antibodies, Polley *et al.* found a few examples of warm incomplete IgM antibodies that were capable of sensitizing red cells to agglutination by anti-IgM, namely one of three examples of anti-K and three of 15 examples of anti-Jk^a.

The agglutination produced by anti-IgM is weak compared with that produced by anti-IgG, perhaps because of the small number of IgM molecules attached to the red cells. Therefore, when the antibody concerned binds complement it is always easier to detect it by incubating red cells with antibody and complement and then testing the cells with an anti-complement reagent.

Red cells coated only with IgM can be prepared by sensitizing Le(a +) cells with serial dilutions of EDTA-treated serum containing potent anti-Le^a. At some dilution the anti-Le^a fails to agglutinate the cells but sensitizes them to agglutination by anti-IgM. Another method which has been used successfully is to prepare purified IgM anti-D and treat it with 2-mercaptoethanol (2-ME). The treated preparation will fail to agglutinate D-positive red cells but will sensitize them to agglutination by anti-IgM. Anti-Le^a treated with 2-ME will not sensitize Le(a +) red cells to agglutination by anti-IgM because the IgM subunits have a very low affinity (Holburn, 1973).

Reactions of anti-IgA

Anti-A and anti-B are quite commonly partly IgA, as are potent examples of anti-D; Lutheran antibodies may also be partly IgA. Relatively few tests have been made to see whether antibodies of other specificities, e.g. anti-K, are also partly IgA.

Red cell antibodies are seldom made solely of IgA; although a few autoantibodies of this kind have been reported, only a single such alloantibody has been described (see p. 337).

A convenient way of preparing red cells coated with IgA (and also IgG) is simply to take a number of anti-D sera (e.g. ten) from hyperimmunized subjects and use them to sensitize D-positive red cells. Several samples in the batch are likely to sensitize red cells to anti-IgA. The fact that the reactions are not due to contaminating anti-IgG can be confirmed by adding IgG (0.1 g/l) to the anti-IgA serum. An alternative method is to use chromic chloride to couple IgA myeloma protein to red cells; see Chapter 13.

Anti-IgA sera, like anti-IgG, exhibit prozones and usually react optimally at a considerable dilution, such as 1 in 500 (Mollison, 1983, p. 514).

The reaction with bound complement

Unlike anti-IgG reagents, anti-complement reagents produced in animals do not exhibit obvious prozones, although, at least when reading tests on tiles, slight prozoning may be observed. On the other hand, monoclonal anti-C3d reagents, because of their high antibody concentrations, exhibit prominent prozones so that, unless the reagents are adequately diluted, negative reactions may be observed (D. Brazier, personal communication, 1985).

When testing red cells coated with complement components, less washing of the coated cells is required after incubation with serum because of the relatively low concentrations of C3 and C4 in serum (see Mollison, 1983, p. 514). Anti-C3g is not neutralized by serum at all because C3g is not expressed on native C3.

Preparation of complement-coated red cells
For methods see Engelfriet *et al.* (1987).

Quantitation of anti-complement components
In 19 commercial polyspecific AHG reagents, the concentrations of anti-C3b and anti-C3c were found to vary from 0.1 to 1.0 μg/ml. The results suggested that these concentrations were suboptimal, the optimal concentrations being 1–2 μg/ml, i.e. similar to the optimal concentration of anti-IgG in the same assay system. The concentration of anti-C3d in the same reagents varied from 0.05 to 1.0 μg/ml (Gardner *et al.* 1983). In another study, the anti-C3d concentration of 27 of 28 polyspecific antiglobulin reagents appeared to be substantially higher, namely 1.0–3.5 μg/ml (Chaplin and Hoffmann, 1982). It is not known whether the discrepancy is due to a difference in assay procedures or in the materials assayed.

The titre of anti-C3c in the ISBT/ICSH reference antiglobulin reagent which contains monoclonal anti-C3c (reagent RIIIM) is 64 with red cells coated with iC3b and that of reagent R3P which contains polyclonal anti-C3c is 32. To avoid false-positive reactions, titres, particularly with polyclonal anti-C3c, should not be higher. With both the ISBT/ICSH reagents, the titre of anti-C3d with red cells coated with C3d is 2–4 and should not be higher. Otherwise, particularly with polyclonal anti-C3d, false-positive reactions will occur.

Technique of antiglobulin tests

In the IAT red cells are first incubated with serum to allow the uptake of antibody and, in some cases, complement, and are then washed and tested with an AHG reagent. In the direct test the cells are simply washed and tested. The uptake of antibody and complement in the indirect test will be discussed first.

The uptake of antibody

The sensitivity of antibody detection is affected by several variables which determine the rate and extent of antibody uptake.

Effect of the ratio of serum to red cells. The amount of antibody taken up per red cell is at a maximum when the ratio of serum to cells is about 1000 : 1 (Hughes-Jones *et al.* 1964c). Under normal conditions the ratio is much lower. For example, when one volume of serum is incubated with one volume of a 3% suspension of red cells, the ratio of serum to cells is 33 : 1. The effect of lowering the cell concentration from 2.5 to 0.5% is shown in Table 8.2.

Dropper pipettes used for dispensing serum and commercially supplied red cell suspensions were found to deliver between 17 and 43 drops/ml. Moreover, the PCV of the red cell suspensions varied by a factor of 2. When two drops of serum were added to one drop of cell suspension, the ratio of serum to cells varied from 19 : 1 to 70 : 1 (Beattie, 1980).

The titre in the normal-ionic-strength solution (NISS) IAT of most Rh antibodies and of some Kell antibodies was four times higher when four volumes of serum were used instead of one volume with one volume of cell suspension. Similar results were obtained in tests with ficin-treated cells and in low-ionic polycation tests (Ahn *et al.* 1987).

Effect of period of incubation. The time taken for the maximum uptake of antibody depends on the concentrations of antigen and antibody and also on the binding constant of the reaction. Typical figures for incubation at 37°C, with a final concentration of CcDee cells of 2% in 'NISS' and of anti-D, with a binding constant of 10^8 l/mol, of 1 µg/ml are: maximum uptake after 4 h; 40% of this amount after 15 min, 87% after 1 h and 99% after 2 h (N.C. Hughes-Jones, personal communication; see also Hughes-Jones *et al.* 1962). Evidently, the period for which cells and serum are incubated in serological tests is somewhat arbitrary; 30 min is adequate to detect most antibodies, although some weak antibodies need longer incubation (see AABB, 1990); in cases of urgency, shorter periods may be used (see pp. 362–364).

Effect of temperature. In detecting Rh antibodies, incubation at 37°C is optimal (see p. 127). In IATs, scores were never higher at 30°C than at 37°C, not only with Rh

Table 8.2 Effect of: (1) red cell concentration (2.5% vs. 0.5%); and (2) saline vs. LISS as a suspending medium, on the reactions of Fy (a +) cells with anti-Fy^a in the indirect antiglobulin test

Serum dilutions	Cells in saline		Cells in LISS	
	2.5%	0.5%	2.5%	0.5%
1 in 2	½	1½	3	4
1 in 8	0	1	2	3

One volume of diluted serum incubated with one volume of cell suspension for 10 min at 37°C, cells washed and tested with anti-IgG by the spin-antiglobulin technique; strength of agglutination on an arbitrary scale of 0–4.

antibodies but also with those of the Kell, Duffy and Kidd systems. On the other hand, although incubation at 22°C gave lower scores with about 50% of Rh antibodies, it gave the same scores with Kidd antibodies and with 80–90% of Duffy and Kell antibodies. At 10°C scores were as high as at 37°C with 60% of SsU antibodies (Arndt and Garratty, 1988). Many monoclonal Rh antibodies react optimally at room temperature.

Effect of low ionic strength. As discussed above, the uptake of antibody is much more rapid at low ionic strength. With many alloantibodies the titre was found to be increased when red cells were suspended in low-ionic-strength medium but the effect on undiluted serum was not tested (Elliot *et al.* 1964; Hughes-Jones *et al.* 1964c). In view of the observation that red cells exposed to serum at low ionic strength take up complement non-specifically there was for a time reluctance to use a low-ionic-strength medium for routine tests. However, Löw and Messeter (1974) showed that when red cells were suspended in a solution of sodium glycinate containing 0.03 mol/l NaCl, false-positive results were not a problem, and this finding was confirmed by Moore and Mollison (1976). The latter authors gave details of a more convenient method of preparing LISS; incidentally, LISS is prone to growth of bacteria and is best sterilized by filtration. A method of performing IATs using LISS-suspended red cells is as follows:

Red cells are washed twice in saline and then once in LISS; a 3% suspension of red cells in LISS is then prepared. One volume of this suspension is added to an equal volume of serum (drops may be used except with plastic test tubes, for which it is better to use some form of automatic pipette to ensure that the drops of cell suspension and serum are equal in volume). The mixture is incubated at 37°C for 10 min and the red cells are then washed three times; use of LISS for cell washing leads to only slightly stronger reactions than when the cells are washed in saline. Finally, the washed cells are tested with antiglobulin serum in the usual way.

In the technique of Löw and Messeter (1974), ionic strength is reduced by about 20%. In the polybrene technique described by Lalezari and Jiang (1980), ionic strength is reduced by about 80% and the period of incubation, at room temperature, is reduced to 1 min (see p. 334); there is a similar reduction in ionic strength and incubation period in the test of Szymanski and Gandhi (1980).

The chief advantage of suspending red cells in LISS rather than in saline lies in the increased rate of uptake of antibody. Although maximum antibody coating may be observed after a period of incubation as short as 5 min it has been recommended that 10 min incubation should be used as a routine because results are sometimes stronger at 10 min than at 5 min (Moore and Mollison, 1976).

Jørgensen *et al.* (1980) observed that the strength of reaction in a low-ionic-strength antiglobulin technique reached a maximum in 20–40 min and thereafter declined.

The only clinically significant antibody which tends to react less well when incubated with red cells at low ionic strength is anti-K. In investigating a low-ionic-strength additive, three of 16 samples of anti-K failed to react; one was associated with a haemolytic transfusion reaction (Molthan and Strohm, 1981). Some anti-K antibodies were also not detected in the method described by Szymanski and Gandhi (1983).

Using ^{125}I-labelled anti-IgG, Merry *et al.* (1984b) observed an accelerated rate of uptake in LISS of antibodies of several specificities but anti-K antibodies were the exception, less antibody being bound in LISS than in saline. A modification of the low-ionic-strength technique in which improved sensitivity to Kell antibodies was obtained by increasing the ratio of serum to cells to 40 : 1 was described by Voak et al. (1982).

A survey of a large number of anti-K sera showed that there was some variability in behaviour at low ionic strength. Of 195 examples, 189 were detected both in LISS and in saline. Although two examples were not detected in LISS but were detected in saline, there were four which were detected in LISS but not in saline (Dankbar et al. 1986).

A disadvantage of the use of LISS is that occasional serum samples give a positive IAT with all red cells, including the subject's own cells (see e.g. Morel and Vengelen-Tyler, 1979). Red cells suspended in LISS give enhanced reactions with common cold alloantibodies such as anti-A_1 and anti-P_1, but this potential disadvantage can be almost completely overcome by eliminating a room temperature incubation phase and by warming red cells and serum to 37°C before mixing them.

The use of a low-ionic-strength antiglobulin serum in the LISS–IAT was found to increase the sensitivity of the test and, particularly with stored sera, to result in fewer non-specific reactions, compared with the conventional LISS–IAT (Ahn et al. 1987).

Use of albumin. Stroup and MacIlroy (1965) observed that the sensitivity of the IAT could be increased by sensitizing red cells in the presence of albumin rather than saline. Albumin raises the dielectric constant of the medium and the effect is thus similar to the use of a low-ionic-strength medium (Pollack, 1965, supplemented by personal communication).

It has also been suggested that enhancement by albumin in the antiglobulin test may simply be a result of the low ionic strength of albumin solutions (Reckell and Harris, 1978). On the other hand, in a quantitative system with enzyme-linked antiglobulin it was observed that the effects of LISS and of addition of albumin were additive (Leikola and Perkins, 1980b).

Although some workers have confirmed the enhancing effect of albumin in the antiglobulin test (e.g. Cant and Flamand, 1967) others have not (e.g. Fitzsimmons and Morel, 1979). Such discrepancies may be due to the specificities of the antibodies tested. In one study, most Rh antibodies (though not anti-E) were enhanced whereas non-Rh antibodies usually gave weaker reactions when albumin was included (R. Knight, personal communication).

Although albumin enhances the uptake of some alloantibodies it seems to be less effective than the use of a low-ionic-strength medium in accelerating antibody uptake (Moore and Mollison, 1976; I.O. Wen and B.P.L. Moore, personal communication, 1978) and its use adds to the complexity and cost of testing. As emphasized above, the simplest and most effective way of increasing sensitivity is to increase the ratio of serum to cells.

Polyethylene glycol indirect antiglobulin test (PEG–IAT)
PEG, a water-soluble polymer, potentiates red cell–antibody interactions in the anti-globulin test (Nance and Garratty, 1987). A 20% solution of PEG of mol. wt. 4000 was found to be optimal. Of 25 weak antibodies tested, 64% reacted more strongly in the PEG test than in LISS or in the MPT, 28% reacted equally well in all three techniques

and 8% reacted more weakly in the PEG test. It was found that many false-positive reactions occurred if the antiglobulin serum used contained anti-complement.

In another study, 590 unselected sera were tested in the PEG–IAT and in the IAT with BSA (BSA–IAT), using anti-IgG with both (Wenz and Apuzzo, 1989). In seven sera, antibodies which reacted in the BSA, but not in the PEG test were cold antibodies.

These results were confirmed in three investigations. In the first, only some clinically significant antibodies (mainly Rh and Kidd) were detected better in the PEG–IAT, others reacting equally well in the BSA–IAT (Wenz et al. 1990). In the second, reactions of 254 of 363 sera known to contain warm alloantibodies were stronger in the PEG–IAT using polyspecific antiglobulin reagents (de Man and Over-beeke, 1990). Reactions of 100 of the 363 sera were equal in the two tests and those of nine sera were weaker in the PEG–IAT. In 18 of 4685 unselected patient sera, clinically significant antibodies were found only in the PEG–IAT. Only one anti-Le^a serum reacted in the BSA–IAT but not in the PEG–IAT. In the third investigation all samples received in a blood bank in a period of 5 months were tested in the PEG–IAT and a LISS–IAT. Of the 50 antibodies detected, ten reacted only in the PEG–IAT and 14 only in the LISS–IAT. The remaining 26 antibodies were detected in both tests. Only one (anti-Jk^a) of the antibodies detected solely in the LISS–IAT was considered to be of clinical significance, whereas five of the antibodies detected only in the PEG test were considered to be significant. It was concluded that the PEG–IAT is an acceptable technique for routine compatibility testing (Slater et al. 1989).

Clearly the PEG–IAT is more sensitive in detecting warm antibodies than the BSA–IAT, even though anti-IgG or anti-Ig are used in the former and a polyspecific reagent containing anti-complement antibodies in the latter. However, two allo-anti-Vel and one allo-anti-P, which were readily detected in the BSA–IAT using a polyspecific reagent, did not react in the PEG–IAT, presumably because of low affinity of the antibodies (M.A.M. Overbeeke, personal communication). Furthermore, the reactivity of Lutheran antibodies seems to be reduced by PEG (Fisher, 1990).

As mentioned above, the MPT, particularly if it is followed by a test with antiglobulin serum (MPT–IAT), is also more sensitive than the conventional antiglobulin test. In fact it is as sensitive as the PEG–IAT (R. Knight, personal communication). For the antiglobulin test following the MPT, an antiglobulin reagent without anti-complement is used. If either the MPT–IAT or the PEG–IAT replaces the conventional antiglobulin test for the detection of alloantibodies, anti-complement will no longer be required in the antiglobulin reagent.

Use of enzyme-treated cells. Some antibodies which fail to sensitize untreated red cells to agglutination by antiglobulin serum may be detected if enzyme-treated red cells are used (Unger, 1951). The enzyme–antiglobulin method is particularly suitable for detecting anti-Jk^a (van der Hart and van Loghem, 1953). It will also reveal the presence of the antigen Le^a on red cells which by other methods appear to be O Le(a – b +) (Cutbush et al. 1956).

As described below, false-positive results obtained with enzyme-treated cells are sometimes due to the presence of heteroagglutinins in antiglobulin sera. Another potential source of false positives is overtreatment with the enzyme.

The binding of complement

When fresh serum is available and it is not anti-complementary, optimal results are obtained by carrying out the test in exactly the same way as for detecting bound IgG. When testing stored serum in which the complement components may have decayed, fresh normal serum should be added. For example, one volume of fresh normal serum may be added to three volumes of the antibody-containing serum, and the IAT then carried out on the mixture.

Lewis antibodies in the test serum may inadvertently be neutralized by the addition of Lewis substances to the serum, unless Le(a – b –) serum is used as a source of complement. On the other hand when a two-stage test is used, the red cells being incubated first with antibody and then with complement, fresh serum of any Lewis group may be used as a source of complement (Polley and Mollison, 1961).

Two-stage test. Serum which has been stored for any considerable period (several days at 4°C or several weeks at – 20°C) may have become anti-complementary, and better results may then be obtained by the two-stage method of Polley and Mollison (1961). The principle of this method is that the uptake of antibody, but not complement, occurs in the first stage (this is achieved by incubating red cells with EDTA-treated antibody) and that the cells are then washed and, in the second stage, treated with fresh normal serum to allow the uptake of complement.

For a tube technique two volumes of EDTA-treated serum are mixed with one volume of a 3% suspension of cells and incubated at 37°C for 1 h; the cells are then washed three times and incubated with one volume of fresh serum at 37°C for 15 min.

The two-stage test has proved to be highly satisfactory for detecting certain antibodies, but with some examples the results are less good than with a one-stage test (Polley and Mollison, 1961). Presumably much depends on the equilibrium constant of the particular antibody. If the antibody dissociates rapidly, a substantial amount may be eluted from the cells during the many washings required in the test.

'Spin-tube' antiglobulin test

In this test, a weak (3%) suspension of washed sensitized, red cells is mixed with antiglobulin serum in a tube which is then briefly centrifuged, so as to produce a cell button without packing the cells too firmly. The cells are gently resuspended and examined for agglutination either with a hand lens or under the low power of a microscope.

Use of an inverted microscope provides a convenient means of examining the cells microscopically within the tube and avoids the need to transfer the cells to a microscope slide.

Although an immediate spin after adding red cells to antiglobulin serum seems to be optimal for detecting IgG-coated red cells, red cells coated with IgA may be better detected after cells and antiglobulin serum have been in contact for a longer period, e.g. 5–10 min (Sturgeon *et al.* 1979). When the results after an immediate spin are negative, therefore, the tube may be respun after 10 min and read again. C3d reactions may be stronger when cells and antiglobulin serum are incubated before being centrifuged (G. Garratty, personal communication).

Antiglobulin tests in an AutoAnalyzer

The agglutination reactions of antiglobulin sera are greatly increased when the reaction is augmented with K-90 PVP and carried out in the AutoAnalyzer (Burkart et al. 1974). When the PVP-augmented antiglobulin test was used only eight IgG anti-D molecules per cell were required for 5% agglutination and 200 for 50% agglutination, whereas with the manual antiglobulin method 100 molecules per cell were required for a trace of agglutination. When bromelin was added together with PVP it was calculated that only one molecule per cell was required for 5% agglutination and three molecules per cell for 50% agglutination. The sensitivity of the PVP-augmented antiglobulin tests for anti-D, -Jk^a, -Fy^a and -K was 40–200 times greater than that of manual tests. With PVP, but not without, normal cells were specifically agglutinated by anti-IgG, anti-κ, anti-λ, anti-C3, anti-albumin and anti-fibrinogen. C4 and C3, probably as C4d and C3d, have been demonstrated on normal cells by the same method (Rosenfield and Jagathambal, 1978).

Szymanski and Odgren (1984) detected 80 ± 28 C3d molecules per cell on normal fresh red cells by this technique but no C3c; during storage at 4°C there was continuous accumulation of C3d on cells (Szymanski et al. 1984).

Tests in microplates

An antiglobulin test in microplates was first described by Wegmann and Smithies (1966) and found to be suitable for routine use (Crawford et al. 1970). The reliability of the antiglobulin test in microplates for the detection of red cell alloantibodies was confirmed in three large studies (Crawford et al. 1988). Because of the small volume in which the reaction is carried out, the cells should be washed four times (Crawford et al. 1988). Several variations of this technique are used (Gordon and Ross, 1987). Both V- and U-shaped wells can be used and to reduce stickiness the use of saline containing 0.1% BSA and, or, 0.02% Tween 20 for washing the cells is recommended. The advantages of the test are sensitivity and the need for only very small quantities of reagents and cells.

Separation of red cells from serum without washing

A very ingenious method of separating red cells from serum was described by Graham et al. (1982). The method depends on the fact that the specific gravity of red cells is considerably higher than that of serum so that red cells, but not serum, will pass through a medium of intermediate density. In one investigation the amount of serum left with the red cell button was found to correspond to a serum dilution of about 1 in 6000 and the reactions of sensitized cells were only very slightly weaker than when the cells were washed four times in saline (unpublished observations, MC and PLM). As the method makes it possible to separate cells from serum without the risk of aerosol formation, it may be useful for handling serum samples which contain dangerous pathogens.

The antiglobulin test can also be performed without washing the red cells by centrifuging them through a Sephadex gel (see below) or glass micro-beads.

Diluent for antiglobulin reagents

AHG reagents are usually provided at their optimal dilution and for storage at 4°C. A variety of diluents is employed; the following is convenient: 0.1 mol/l NaCl, 0.05 mol/l phosphate pH 7.2, 1 g/l Na$_4$ EDTA 2H$_2$O, 10 g/l BSA and 1 g/l sodium azide. Use of a low-ionic-strength diluent does not appear to enhance reactions of AHG reagents, perhaps because bound IgG antibodies extend beyond the 'ionic cloud' surrounding red cells (Leikola and Perkins, 1980b). Dyes may be added to AHG reagents to provide a means of checking that reagent has been added to tubes. Green is the colour most frequently used for commercial polyspecific reagents and a suitable depth of colour is provided by mixing 0.08 g/l ariavit tartrazine (E102) with 0.02 g/l Patent Blue V(E131).

False-negative results in antiglobulin tests
The most important cause of false-negative results is failure to wash the red cells adequately. To demonstrate that a negative result is not due to neutralization of antiglobulin by residual serum, a drop of D-sensitized red cells should be added. In tube tests, the mixture is spun before being read. An inverted microscope is particularly convenient for this procedure, as the antiglobulin is all retained within the tube. It is particularly important that the D-sensitized red cells are not too strongly sensitized, because strongly sensitized cells may be agglutinated by partially neutralized AHG reagent. The cells should not give stronger reactions than 1 + to 2 + in the IAT (Voak *et al.* 1986b).

Another important cause of false-negative reactions is excessive agitation in reading the test (Voak *et al.* 1986b). The 'tip and roll' procedure, combined with reading under an inverted microscope, or careful transfer of the cell button to a slide with reading under a standard microscope and advised.

Wash solutions should be buffered to pH 7.0–7.4. Failure to detect clinically significant antibodies may be due to the use of wash solutions with pH values below pH 5 or of solutions which have been autoclaved and stored in plastic containers (Bruce *et al.* 1986).

False-positive results in antiglobulin tests
One may distinguish between genuine false-positive results, due to unwanted antibodies in the antiglobulin serum, such as heteroagglutinins (see Chapter 7), and those positive results which are 'true' in that they indicate the presence of globulin on the red cells, but are unwanted, in that they have no obvious clinical significance.

Heteroagglutinins. When heteroagglutinins are present in low concentrations in an AHG reagent, the serum may give false positives with one method but not with another, thus causing confusion. Reagents are only required to be free of heteroagglutinins by the techniques recommended for their use. Accordingly, when using some modification of the antiglobulin test designed to increase sensitivity, e.g. a relatively low concentration of red cells, the AHG reagent should be tested against the same concentration of O, A and B unsensitized red cells to make sure that it does not react.

Agglutinins against enzyme-treated red cells. Three of nine AHG reagents tested by Beck *et al.* (1976a) reacted with enzyme-treated normal red cells, due to residual antispecies antibodies. This observation underlines the need to use suitable controls when testing enzyme-treated red cells with AHG reagents, e.g. when testing C3d cells produced by enzyme-treatment of C3b cells. Under these circumstances the positive reaction may be due to agglutinins for enzyme-treated red cells rather than to anti-C3d (Beck *et al.* 1976a).

Positive direct antiglobulin tests due to anti-red cell antibodies in antilymphocyte globulin
Antilymphocyte globulin (ALG) is commonly prepared in horses and the serum contains antibodies against human red cells. Following the injection of ALG the recipient's red cells acquire a positve DAT within 1–3 d (Lapinid *et al.* 1984; Swanson *et al.* 1984). The reaction between AHG reagent and the horse serum on the patient's red cells can be inhibited by adding diluted horse serum to the AHG reagent without interfering with the reaction between the AHG reagent and any human alloantibodies which may be bound to the patient's red cells (Swanson *et al.* 1984). In the serum of patients injected with ALG, autoantibodies can be detected which usually show no obvious specificity but which occasionally have an Lu-related pattern (Anderson *et al.* 1985b).

Occasionally, a positive DAT in a patient who has been injected with ALG is due to human red cell alloantibody; the alloantibody is derived from the plasma which has been added to the ALG to inhibit horse antibodies against human plasma proteins (Shirey *et al.* 1983).

Administration of ALG may occasionally produce immune red cell destruction; in the case described by Prchal *et al.* (1985) the DAT was negative with AHG reagent but positive with anti-horse immunoglobulin.

Do reticulocytes react with antiglobulin sera?
There are some papers in the literature indicating that reticulocytes are agglutinated by antiglobulin sera (Nelken, 1961; Sutherland *et al.* 1963; Jandl, 1969), and it has been claimed that the reaction is between transferrin attached to reticulocytes and anti-transferrin in the antiglobulin serum (Jandl, 1960). Nevertheless, washed, reticulocyte-rich samples of red cells are often not agglutinated by anti-transferrin serum nor by routine 'broad-spectrum' antiglobulin serum (Mollison, 1959, p. 454). H. Chaplin (personal communication) has not encountered a positive DAT associated with a high reticulocyte count except in patients suspected on other grounds of having a haemolytic anaemia.

The gel test
A new process for the detection of red cell–antibody interactions has recently been described (Lapierre *et al.* 1990). In the test special microtubes filled with a Sephadex gel are used. For the detection of saline agglutinins a neutral gel is used and for the antiglobulin test a gel containing antiglobulin reagent. Gels containing red cell antiserum can also be used. The red cells are centrifuged through the gel. In a negative reaction all cells collect at the bottom of the tube while in a positive reaction the cells are trapped in the gel. The test is said to be easy, sensitive and reproducible. The antiglobulin test can be performed without washing the cells. Advantages of the test are that, after the reaction has occurred, the gels can be kept for at least 24 h, allowing second opinions to be sought, and that photocopies of the tubes can be made.

AUTOMATION OF SEROLOGICAL TESTS

The inducement to use mechanized methods of blood grouping (McNeil *et al.* 1963) came from the hope of introducing greater reliability and of avoiding drudgery. These hopes have been largely realized with the development of machines such as the 16-channel Autogrouper and the Groupamatic, although both these machines are designed for dealing with large numbers of blood samples and are not suitable for hospital laboratories. Automated equipment has proved to be very sensitive in detecting blood group antibodies.

The AutoAnalyzer

A single-channel AutoAnalyzer has been used in the screening of sera for alloanti-bodies. The continuous-flow principle which is used has the following advantages: quantities are measured accurately; agglutinates are never subjected to violent agita-tion; measurement and recording are very precise; and tests are reproducible to within 5% (Allen *et al.* 1963). Two main methods have been used to provide sensitive conditions for antibody detection. In the first, a protease is used together with a polymer, e.g. 0.1% bromelin with 0.25% PVP, K-90 (Rosenfield *et al.* 1964b) or methylcellulose is used instead of PVP (Marsh *et al.* 1968). In the second method, a low-ionic-strength medium is used together with polybrene (Lalezari, 1968).

The disadvantage of the low-ionic-strength method is that it fails to detect some examples of anti-K although none are missed when the bromelin–methylcellulose method is also used (Habibi *et al.* 1973a; Högman *et al.* 1973).

A substantial problem arising from the use of the AutoAnalyzer for screening purposes is that many antibodies detected cannot be identified. For example, Perrault and Högman (1971) found that only 19% of antibodies detected in the AutoAnalyzer could be detected by manual methods. Of the sera that were positive only in the AutoAnalyzer, about one-quarter contained an antibody that could be identified by tests against standard panels, and in half of these the specificity was anti-D. Of the other antibodies detected only in the AutoAnalyzer, some seemed to have anti-HLA specificity and some were autoantibodies. Somewhat similar results were described by Morehead *et al.* (1974). In testing a large series of samples, about 80% had antibodies detectable only in the AutoAnalyzer but the specificity of these antibodies could be determined in only about 30% of cases. The authors concluded that the AutoAnalyzer was not suitable for antibody screening.

The 16-channel Autogrouper (Technicon)

The 16C Autogrouper is a fully automated instrument which reads bar-codes on individual samples, reads the optical density of mixtures containing red cells and serum, interprets the results as positive or negative and feeds the data into a computer. The instrument is designed for use in large centres, for the routine ABO and Rh D grouping of large numbers of samples and for antibody screening.

The Groupamatic system (Kontron)

This instrument was also designed primarily for red cell phenotyping but has since been adapted for a variety of tests. Whereas, in the Autogrouper, samples follow one another consecutively through lengths of plastic tubing, in the Groupamatic, samples are handled discretely in small cups with a period of incubation followed by centrifugation. The instrument is fully automated; it identifies samples and prints out results (Matte, 1971). There are three types of Groupamatic: the Groupamatic 360 which has a processing speed of 340 samples an hour, the Groupamatic 2000 (180 or 240 samples an hour) and the Minigroupamatic (55 samples an hour).

Microplate systems

A semi-automated microplate system for determining ABO and Rh D groups has been described (Bowley *et al.* 1984). In the system a microplate spectrophotometer is linked to a personal computer to interpret and record results. In tests on 20 000 samples, the results of automated reading agreed with those of visual reading in 98% of cases. The 2% of discrepant results were due mainly to reactions of irregular antibodies, e.g. anti-P_1, (Bowley *et al.* 1984).

In another study in which reading was automated, results on 4.6% of 65 269 samples were equivocal, due mainly to weak anti-A and anti-B agglutinins (Hedley *et al.* 1986).

Several commercial systems are now available. The microbank 220 Blood Grouping Systems (Dynatech Laboratories, Chantilly, Virginia, USA) and the Micro Groupamatic (Kontron Instruments) are similar to the system described by Severns *et al.* (1984). The Gamma Micro V system (Gamma Biologicals, Houston, Texas, USA) is a semi-automated system in which microplates containing 21 tear-drop-shaped wells are used (Kutt *et al.* 1988). The Olympus ProGroup System (Olympus, Lake Success, New York, USA) is fully automated. In another fully automated system the wells have concentric rings engraved in their wall. Agglutinated red cells settle evenly on the terraces between the rings whereas non-agglutinated cells fall to the bottom (Gibbons *et al.* 1986). The Standardized Test System-Microtear (Gamma Biologicals) employs a flexible plastic belt containing 84 tear-shaped cuvettes. After incubation the cells are packed tightly by centrifugation. The centrifuge then slows and continues to rotate slowly. At this low centrifugal force, gravity causes the red cells in negative reactions to stream downward, whereas in positive reactions the cells remain packed into a button. Reading is done with an optical scanner. For further information on these systems, see Whitrow and Ross (1990).

Determination of threshold in automated blood grouping tests

Automated microplate blood grouping systems rely on a pair of thresholds to determine whether reactions are positive or negative. The determination of these thresholds is a critical step in the quality control of automated microplate blood grouping. A simple computerized method for automatically setting these thresholds has been described (Severns *et al.* 1989).

Flow cytometry

A flow cytometer provides delivery of a single file of cells or other particles in suspension through a focused laser beam. Signals due to light scattering and, or, emission of fluorescence are available for analysis or may be used as a basis for cell sorting.

Flow cytometry has been used to estimate the survival of transfused red cells, both compatible and incompatible (see Chapters 9 and 10); to detect fetal D-positive cells present in the circulation of an Rh D-negative woman (Chapter 12); to measure the amount of antibody bound to red cells (de Bruin *et al.* 1983); to estimate the amount of antibody on different samples of coated red cells giving maximum agglutination in the antiglobulin test (Nance and Garratty, 1984); and to estimate the density of antigen sites on red cells (Langlois *et al.* 1985; Bockstaele *et al.* 1986; McHugh *et al.* 1987).

Solid-phase systems

Solid-phase techniques for blood grouping and antibody detection were first described by Rosenfield *et al.* (1976). Red cells were attached to the inner surface of plastic tubes to form a monolayer. For the solid-phase antiglobulin test the cells in the monolayer were incubated with serum, washed, and then lysed with water to release Hb and produce a colourless background. After incubation with anti-IgG, a 0.2% suspension of IgG or complement-coated cells was added. In a positive reaction the coated cells were bound to the monolayer.

More recently a series of semi-automated solid-phase red cell adherence assays for ABO and Rh typing, antibody detection and crossmatching have been described (Beck *et al.* 1984; Plapp *et al.* 1984). Another semi-automated system is supplied by Immunocor. The solid phase for ABO cell grouping was prepared by adsorbing monoclonal or affinity-purified human anti-A or anti-B reagents on to microplate wells. Ordinary anti-A or -B sera are unsatisfactory because, since all proteins are adsorbed on to the plastic, the amount of specific antibody adsorbed is relatively low. However, unpurified human reagents can be used if the wells are pre-coated with A or B salivary blood group substances (Beck *et al.* 1985). The solid phase for D grouping consists of wells pre-coated with affinity-purified goat anti-human IgG followed by anti-D purified by absorption and ether elution. Grouping is performed by adding one drop of a 0.5% suspension of bromelin-treated red cells, followed by centrifugation. Positive reactions are characterized by spreading of red cells over the surface of the wells due to adherence to immobilized antibody. Negative reactions are characterized by the formation of discrete cell buttons in the centre of the wells. The solid phase for ABO serum grouping is prepared by immobilizing bromelin-treated group A and B cells in microplate wells previously treated with rabbit anti-human red cell antibody. The cells are lysed and the Hb washed out. The test is performed by adding one volume of serum, incubating for 5 min, removing excess serum, adding one volume of a 0.5% suspension of bromelin-treated A or B cells, centrifuging and reading.

Automated reading is performed at 405 nm using a spectrophotometer (ELISA reader) with the light beam offset to pass 1.5 mm from the centre of the wells in order to avoid the cell button in negative reactions. In tests on 2037 blood donors the results of ABO and D grouping obtained by solid phase showed a 99.6% correlation with results obtained by conventional agglutination techniques. Each discrepancy was recognized by the computer and resolved by visual editing of the results. The problem of occasional errors in reading can be overcome by the use of computer-aided image analysis (Sinor *et al.* 1985).

The solid-phase assay with red cell adherence is also applicable to antibody screening and compatibility testing (Rachel *et al.* 1985a). Red cells are incubated with the patient's serum, washed and then suspended in antiglobulin serum. The suspension is transferred to IgG-coated wells, centrifuged and read visually or photometrically.

A disadvantage of this solid-phase test is that only IgG antibodies are detected and that there is no reaction with anti-complement to facilitate the detection of complement-binding IgG antibodies. This disadvantage can be overcome by coating the plates with AB serum in which complement has been activated with heat-aggregated immunoglobulin to ensure that the AB serum contains a sufficient amount of C3d (Guigner et al. 1988).

In an alternative approach, the detection of haemoglobin peroxidase in adherent cells is used as an indicator system for ABO and D grouping (Moore, 1984). Using this method with wells optimally coated with IgM monoclonal anti-A, anti-B and anti-D, it is possible to group cells without the need for enzyme pre-treatment (Scott, 1991).

A solid-phase system for testing individual samples outside the laboratory has been devised (Plapp et al. 1986). Anti-A or anti-B are bound covalently to individual nylon squares which are then attached to plastic strips to form 'dipsticks'. A drop of blood is added to the dipstick; after 1 min the stick is rinsed with saline; a positive result is indicated by the red colour of adhering cells. From a technical point of view this method seems likely to be more reliable than determining ABO groups on cards on which anti-A and anti-B have previously been dried (Eldon, 1955). Nevertheless, objections to both systems are the same, namely that it is difficult to devise controls which are as reliable as those available when liquid blood group reagents are used and that serum cannot be tested to confirm ABO groups.

QUANTITATION OF RED CELL ANTIBODIES

Antibody titres

The classical method is to determine the titre of a serum, expressed as the reciprocal of the highest dilution of the serum which will produce a detectable reaction with selected red cells. There are several reasons why this method gives only a very approximate indication of antibody concentration. First, the method is unsound in principle since it estimates only the amount of antibody bound to red cells, not the amount of antibody in the serum. At the end-point of the titration, agglutination is caused by the relatively small number of antibody molecules in the serum with the highest affinity, and therefore the proportion of such molecules in the serum has a considerable influence on its titre. As an example, if two sera each contain the same concentration of an antibody but one example has a binding constant ten times higher than the other, then the antibody with the higher binding constant will have a titre approximately ten times greater than the other (Hughes-Jones, 1967). Second, as usually carried out, dilution of the serum is performed in a series of double-dilution steps. This method is inaccurate and, unless special precautions are taken, traces of serum are carried over from one dilution to another. In practice, the titres of anti-D sera determined by a manual method have been found to be poorly correlated with the antibody concentrations of the same sera determined by an isotope method (Hughes-Jones, 1967).

A score is a better estimate of antibody concentration than a titre. To determine a score all positive reactions obtained with serial, doubling dilutions of an antiserum are given a value based on the strength of the reaction, e.g. $++++$ = 10, $+++$ = 8, etc. The sum of these values is the score (see Marsh, 1972).

^{125}I-labelled antiglobulin

Direct labelling of antibody with radio-iodine
When whole serum is labelled with radio-iodine, lipids are labelled in addition to serum proteins. When the labelled serum is incubated with the red cells the lipids exchange rapidly between the serum and cells and mask the specific uptake of antibody (Hughes-Jones and Gardner, 1962). Methods exist for greatly reducing non-specific uptake (Masouredis, 1959; Hughes-Jones and Gardner, 1962; Hughes-Jones et al. 1962) but are too tedious for routine use. Purified IgG is now used for labelling.

Use of radio-iodine-labelled anti-IgG
The use of a labelled antiglobulin serum for assay of anti-D has one great advantage, namely that a given batch of labelled antiglobulin serum can be used to estimate the amount of anti-D in many different human sera, none of which has to be labelled. On the other hand, there is the theoretical objection that the number of antiglobulin molecules which combine with each anti-D molecule may vary from serum to serum.

The labelled antiglobulin method with manual techniques was found to have a coefficient of variation of $\pm 14\%$ (Holburn et al. 1970), although when using an instrument in which the washing of the red cells and the addition of the labelled antiglobulin serum were mechanized, the coefficient of variation was as low as about $\pm 5\%$ (Hughes-Jones et al. 1972).

Hughes-Jones and Stevenson (1968) examined 22 preparations of anti-D immuno-globulin and, using manual techniques, compared direct labelling (i.e. labelling of the immunoglobulin preparation) with the indirect (^{125}I-labelled) antiglobulin method. In 17 of 22 cases the ratio of the estimates made by two methods fell within the range 0.8–1.2, i.e. the estimates were within 20% of one another.

An advantage of the antiglobulin method is that it can be used to estimate concentrations of anti-D as low as 1 μg/ml, whereas the direct labelling technique becomes increasingly inaccurate below 50 μg/ml (Hughes-Jones and Stevenson, 1968).

An assay based on the consumption of anti-IgG by sensitized red cells, the remaining anti-IgG being measured by precipitation with ^{125}I-labelled IgG in the presence of PEG, has been described (van de Winkel et al. 1988). The reproducibility of this technique was found to be excellent.

Enzyme-linked immunosorbent assay
The ELISA technique was adapted by Leikola and Perkins (1980a) for the quantitation of IgG antibody on red cells. Anti-IgG was conjugated to alkaline phosphatase using glutaraldehyde and was calibrated by adding doubling dilutions to tubes containing fixed quantities of IgG; p-nitrophenyl phosphate was added as substrate; the reaction was stopped after 30 min with NaOH and the yellow colour measured at 405 nm.

Similarly, the anti-IgG conjugate was added to antibody-coated red cells followed by substrate and the colour measured. It was found that the test was two to three doubling dilution steps more sensitive than a conventional antiglobulin test and that as little as 5 ng/ml of anti-D could be detected. In a further paper the authors described the use of the enzyme-linked antiglobulin test (ELAT) to study the uptake of antibodies on to red cells suspended in LISS (Leikola and Perkins, 1980b).

ELAT has been used to detect fetal D-positive cells in the circulation of D-negative women; the lowest concentration of D-positive cells which could be detected reliably corresponded to a transplacental haemorrhage of about 6 ml red cells (Riley et al. 1982).

ELATs have also been used to quantitate IgG, IgM, IgA or C3 on the red cells of patients with AIHA (Kiruba and Han, 1988; Sokol et al. 1988).

The AutoAnalyzer
The AutoAnalyzer provides a simple method of quantitating anti-D with fair reproducibility, e.g. with a coefficient of variation of 17% (Judd and Jenkins, 1970). In a study in which 23 laboratories participated, intralaboratory precision varied from 1.5% to 55%, with 61% of the laboratories having a precision better than 20%; interlaboratory means were within 19% of the group mean (Fleetwood and McNeill, 1990). In another study 75% of results were within 25% of the overall mean values (Bowell, 1984). In a comparison with the ^{125}I antiglobulin method, two-thirds of estimates of anti-D made in the AutoAnalyzer agreed to within 24% (Moore and Hughes-Jones, 1970).

Relative sensitivity of different methods of antibody detection

The indirect antiglobulin test
The lowest concentration of IgG anti-D detectable by the standard IAT is about 10 ng/ml; using this test in external quality assessment surveys 98% of unselected participants were able to detect 11 ng/ml (Pinkerton et al. 1984).

ELAT was found to be distinctly more sensitive than the IAT, the lowest concentrations detectable being, respectively, 4 and 10 ng/ml (Postoway et al. 1985).

Other manual methods
Two-stage tests with enzyme-treated cells are generally believed to be more sensitive than the IAT in detecting IgG anti-D, although no evidence in support of this view was obtained in proficiency testing described by Pinkerton et al. (1984).

The manual low-ionic-strength polybrene test is capable of detecting about 1 ng anti-D/ml without an antiglobulin stage (unpublished observations, MC). Although no quantitative studies have been done, it seems that the PEG antiglobulin test is even more sensitive. The titre of ten of 11 alloantibodies was found to be higher in the PEG test than in the polybrene test (Nance and Garratty, 1987).

The AutoAnalyzer
Using the low-ionic-strength polybrene method, or the bromelin–methyl cellulose method, the lowest concentration of IgG anti-D detectable is approximately 2 ng/ml.

Reference preparations

Anti-A, anti-B, anti-A,B and incomplete anti-D and anti-c as well as complete anti-c and anti-E are available as reference preparations from The World Health Organization and can be used for determining minimal acceptable levels of potency.

The anti-D immunoglobulin reference preparation contains 60 μg anti-D; 1 μg is equivalent to 5 iu (Gunson *et al.* 1980). Comparative studies of this preparation, a national standard, two commercial and two national preparations for clinical use showed that the isotope method, manual haemagglutination and the AutoAnalyzer all gave comparable values (Bangham *et al.* 1978). In view of limited supplies of the reference preparation, individual countries and laboratories should set up their own working standards after determining the relation of such standards to the international reference preparation.

Some countries (e.g. the USA) have established their own reference preparations which are supplied to manufacturers, whose reagents must match or exceed the potency of the reference preparations.

The potencies of the international standards and reference preparations are expressed in units. The use of units rather than mass is undoubtedly appropriate when dealing with impure substances or compounds of varying potency but seems far less appropriate when describing the amount of IgG anti-D, which is of known molecular weight. Clearly, it is no more accurate to use units than μg; both are subject to the same errors of measurement. The use of μg has two advantages: first it conveys more information since, for example, it is possible to calculate the number of molecules of antibody attached to red cells under various conditions. Second, whereas when units are used a stable reference preparation is essential, when μg are used the amount of antibody present can be redetermined at any time by a new estimation.

An anti-c reference preparation suitable for use as a standard in quantitating anti-c in the AutoAnalyzer is available (Phillips, 1987).

The two polyspecific reference antiglobulin reagents available from the ISBT and ICSH have been mentioned above.

THE SELECTION OF COMPATIBLE RED CELLS

In selecting compatible blood the normal practice is first to determine the patient's ABO and Rh D groups, second to 'screen' the patient's serum for red cell antibodies other than anti-A and anti-B and, third, having selected blood of the same ABO and Rh D group, to crossmatch the donor's red cells against the recipient's serum. These three steps will be considered in turn.

Determination of the recipient's ABO and Rh D groups

The determination of the ABO groups differs from the determination of other blood groups in two ways. First, the ABO system is by far the most important blood group system in transfusion practice; second, the ABO system is the only one in which the antigens present on the red cells can usually be predicted from a knowledge of the antibodies present in the serum.

The standard method of determining the ABO group of a sample is therefore to test the red cells against anti-A and anti-B and to test the serum against group A and group B red cells. Standard practice includes testing the red cells against anti-A,B to detect weak group A samples which are not agglutinated by anti-A from a group B donor. Nevertheless the use of anti-A,B is not essential in grouping recipients; many anti-A,B reagents fail to detect very weak forms of A and, in any case, recipients with weak group A may be safely transfused with group O blood.

It is usual to test the serum against A_1 rather than A_2 cells, since A_1 cells have more A antigen and thus serve better to detect anti-A. In some subjects of subgroups A_2 and A_2B, the serum contains anti-A_1; if this is active at 37°C, the serum has to be retested to demonstrate that it will not react with A_2 cells.

When speed is essential and when a tube test is used, the mixtures can be centrifuged immediately; alternatively, a slide method may be used.

Similarly, rapid methods of Rh D grouping are available: e.g. a rapid tube or slide test or a method using bromelin-treated red cells. When tests have to be done in a hurry it is more convenient to use blood mixed with an anticoagulant than clotted blood because with the clotted samples there may be delay in separating the clot and obtaining the red cells from the bottom of the tube.

In determining the patient's D group the risk of failing to detect weak D should be ignored. If a recipient with a weak D antigen is misclassified as D-negative and transfused with D-negative blood, no harm will be done. On the other hand, when the IAT is used to detect weak D samples, there is a substantial chance of a false-positive result (see later). Such an error might lead to the subject being transfused with D-positive blood, or, if pregnant or recently delivered, not receiving anti-D immunoglobulin.

If in determining the Rh D group of a donor the IAT is not used to detect weak D, it must be ascertained that the anti-D sera used detect most weak Ds. It has been found that anti-D sera differ very much in their capacity to detect weak D (van Rhenen *et al.* 1989).

In view of the known frequency of errors in ABO and D grouping, due mainly to clerical mistakes, whenever possible results should be confirmed on a second occasion or by a second technician.

Whenever a patient's blood groups are determined, the results should be recorded and filed in the laboratory so that if further samples from the same patient are tested, the file can be examined and the results compared.

Screening tests on the serum of potential recipients

The advantages of screening the serum of potential recipients for the presence of alloantibodies are as follows. First, when the screening test can be carried out well in advance of transfusion and when alloantibodies are detected there will be time to identify the antibody and select compatible units. Second, special red cells can be used for the screening test which have been obtained from donors homozygous for alleles such as *c*, *E*, *Jk^a* and *M*; such red cells react far more strongly than cells from heterozygotes and their use makes it easier to detect a weak alloantibody than when random donors are tested, as in crossmatching. It is virtually impossible to find a single donor who is homozygous for all the relevant alleles and the usual practice is to select two to three donors who between them are homozygous for the most important alleles such as *c* and *Jk^a*. In screening sera for alloantibodies, different samples of red cells should not be pooled since this may lead to failure to detect antibodies (de Silva and Contreras, 1985).

In screening, two techniques should be used: an antiglobulin test, either at normal or low ionic strength, and a second sensitive technique, e.g. the MPT.

In patients who are to undergo operations involving induced hypothermia there is no need to screen the serum at a temperature below 37°C. No convincing account has ever been published of red cell destruction caused, during hypothermia, by a red cell alloantibody active *in vitro* only at a temperature below 37°C.

Antibodies passively transferred by injections of immunoglobulin. D-negative patients receiving injections of anti-D immunoglobulin may, of course, have detectable amounts of anti-D in their plasma for considerable periods after injection. They may also have detectable amounts of antibodies of other specificities if these are present in sufficient concentration in the immunoglobulin. In one such case, passively transferred anti-E, anti-Le[b] and anti-HI, all IgG, were detected in a patient who had received 900 μg anti-D immunoglobulin (Wright *et al.* 1979).

Selection of donor blood (red cells)

In countries where blood is collected at transfusion centres, most hospitals rely entirely on the description on the label of the unit of blood and make no further tests on it. However, when units are issued to patients without compatibility tests, the ABO and D group of the units should be verified before issue. In the USA, the ABO group of all units and the D group of all D-negative units must be verified.

Limitation of the supply of D-negative blood very occasionally makes it necessary to consider giving D-positive blood to D-negative recipients. If the recipient is a male who has not been transfused before, and particularly if the recipient is elderly, the transfusion of D-positive blood is not likely to lead to trouble. Anti-D is not likely to be formed for several weeks after the transfusion, so that if further transfusions are needed within a few days of the first transfusion more D-positive blood can be given (provided that crossmatching is carried out with a sample obtained on the day of transfusion). Although it may sometimes be defensible to give D-positive blood to D-negative males, it must be an absolute rule that D-positive blood is never transfused to a D-negative female who is still capable of child-bearing.

In a D-negative woman who has reached the menopause the transfusion of D-positive blood is much less safe than in a D-negative man because the woman may have been sensitized by pregnancy. Such a case, in which a woman developed a severe delayed haemolytic transfusion reaction after her first transfusion, is described in Chapter 11. Donations for D-negative patients immunized to D must be C negative and E negative as well as D negative because subjects who make anti-D often make anti-C(G) or anti-E as well. However, for D-negative patients who have not made anti-D it is sufficient to give blood which is D negative and the donor red cells need not also be C negative and E negative (cf p. 236).

When alloantibodies active at 37°C, other than anti-A, -B and -D are present, or have been present in the past but are no longer detectable, e.g. anti-Jk[a], red cells lacking the corresponding antigens must be selected for transfusion.

Is it practicable to try to prevent immunization to antigens other than D?

In females who have not yet reached the menopause it seems worth giving serious consideration to the possibility of trying to prevent the formation of anti-K and anti-c. It is relatively easy to avoid using K-positive blood for K-negative recipients but finding c-negative blood for c-negative recipients involves a substantial extra amount of work. Nevertheless, as haemolytic disease of the newborn due to anti-D becomes less common, the possibility of preventing immunization of women by c may seem worth pursuing.

In patients who receive multiple transfusions it is very likely that antibodies will be made to the more immunogenic of the red cell alloantigens which the patients themselves lack. For patients with sickle cell disease or thalassaemia, a case has been made for using red cells matched for Rh antigens and for K (see Chapter 3).

Screening of the donor's plasma

When group O whole blood is transfused to recipients of groups A, B or AB and when the donor's plasma contains potent anti-A,B, a haemolytic reaction may be produced (see Chapters 10 and 11). The risk is diminished when plasma-reduced blood is used and further diminished by the use of red cell concentrates or red cells suspended in additive solutions.

In some hospitals it is the custom to give group O blood (O, D-negative blood for female recipients or for previously transfused males) in grave emergencies without any compatibility tests. When this is done the risk of producing a haemolytic reaction from anti-A or anti-B in the donor's plasma can be greatly reduced by selecting group O donors with low-titre antibodies. A commonly used test is to screen for high-titre anti-A,B using A_1B cells suspended in saline containing AB substance. Donors whose serum give a positive reaction in this test are considered to be dangerous if transfused to patients of groups other than D. This test can be performed in parallel with automated ABO and D grouping. Many transfusion services put a special label on group O units with high-titre anti-A or anti-B, to indicate that these units should be used only for group O recipients.

There is some evidence that a test for anti-A and anti-B lysins might be better than a test for high-titre agglutinins in excluding 'dangerous' group O donors (Grove-Rasmussen *et al.* 1953; Mollison, 1972a, p. 530).

Very few haemolytic reactions due to the presence in the donor's plasma of antibodies other than anti-A and anti-B have been described (see Chapter 11). The increasing use of plasma-reduced blood and red cell concentrates is likely to make such accidents even rarer in the future. In screening the plasma of donors, a relatively simple test, capable of detecting potent antibodies to the most clinically important antigens, is needed. In large donor centres, screening is undertaken on automated machines.

The results of screening the serum of more than 84 000 blood donors during 1975 were described by Giblett (1977). The overall frequency of antibodies was relatively low, i.e. 0.32%, due partly to the fact that the average age of the donors was only about 30 years. Of the antibodies, 68% were anti-D. In the donors with no history of transfusion or pregnancy the frequency of antibodies was 0.04%. It was pointed out that by testing the serum of donors giving a history of previous transfusion or pregnancy, and by also testing the serum of all D-negative donors, only about one in 10 000 sensitized donors would be undetected. In view of the fact that the undetected antibodies would virtually always be of low titre it seems quite unjustified to devote much effort to their detection. Certainly, the use of the antiglobulin test in these circumstances seems very wasteful of time and money (Giblett, 1977).

Crossmatching tests

Ottenberg (1908) was the first to apply Landsteiner's discovery of the blood groups to transfusion practice by testing for lysis and agglutination of donor's red cells by the recipient's serum as a preliminary to transfusion. During the following few years it was found that in over 100 cases in which the patient's serum did not lyse the donor's red cells no haemoglobinuria developed. By contrast, when there was lysis *in vitro* in the 'cross' test (as it was then called — see Ottenberg, 1937), there was always some intravascular lysis in the recipient (Ottenberg and Kaliski, 1913). Crossmatching tests capable of detecting incomplete antibodies became widely used only in the mid-1940s, after the discovery of the effects of suspending red cells in albumin and of using antiglobulin serum. However, a test in which whole citrated blood from donor and recipient was mixed in various proportions, was introduced much earlier by Weil (1915). As pointed out by Rosenfield (1977), the use of this test may have first revealed Rh D antibodies in human sera since the test was positive in five cases of serious reactions following ABO-compatible transfusions described by Unger (1921).

As described above, it is standard practice to screen the serum of potential recipients for red cell alloantibodies. When this has been done, an abbreviated crossmatch procedure can be used, of which the main purpose is to detect ABO incompatibility due, for example, to misidentification of the patient. When preliminary screening has not been done, the test used for crossmatching must be capable of detecting virtually all clinically significant antibodies. In the detection of red cell alloantibodies the IAT is undoubtedly the best single test available. As discussed earlier, the ratio of serum to cells is very important in determining sensitivity; if possible, not less than four volumes of serum should be mixed with one volume of a 2–5% suspension of red cell in isotonic saline. After 3 min at room temperature the tube is centrifuged; the supernatant is examined for lysis and the cells are then resuspended and examined for agglutination. If the test is negative at this stage the tube is incubated at 37°C for at least 30 min; the cells are then washed four times, antiglobulin serum is added, the tube centrifuged once more and the cells examined for agglutination (for further details see earlier section on the antiglobulin test). When the test is carried out at low ionic strength the incubation time can be reduced to 10 min but when low ionic strength is used there is a small risk of failing to detect antibodies of the Kell system (see pp. 345–346).

In patients who are to undergo surgery involving hypothermia, crossmatching tests (like screening tests) should be carried out, as usual, at 37°C.

Advantages of 'grouping and screening' rather than crossmatching when transfusion is unlikely

In many blood transfusion laboratories a great many units of blood (or packed red cells) are crossmatched each day for patients who are most unlikely to require transfusion. In any particular hospital it should be possible to identify those elective surgical procedures in which it is unusual for blood to be transfused and then, in patients undergoing these procedures, simply to group the patient's red cells and screen the serum for abnormal antibodies, i.e. 'type and screen'. The advantage of doing this is that units of blood are not reserved unnecessarily. When many units in a blood bank are held and are not eventually needed for transfusion, the result is almost certain to be that many units of blood go out of date and are wasted.

The foregoing analysis seems to have been put forward first by Henry et al. (1977). As an example they mentioned that, in their own hospital, for 97 consecutive elective cholecystectomies a total of 213 units had been crossmatched but only 5 units had actually been used. They suggested that when the type and screen procedure was used, in the expectation that blood would probably not be needed, and blood was in fact required, it would still usually be possible to perform crossmatching or, in an emergency, to provide blood at once whilst initiating the crossmatch. The fact that the patient's blood had been screened for unexpected antibodies as well as grouped should ensure almost complete transfusion safety (Boral and Henry, 1977).

A useful analysis was provided by Friedman (1979), giving a list of common surgical procedures and the average number of units actually transfused and suggesting how a maximum surgical blood order schedule (MSBOS) could be developed. He considered that a satisfactory order would meet the transfusion requirements of 90% of patients undergoing a particular procedure. Blood order schedules may be refined by identifying subgroups of patients undergoing the same procedure but having different transfusion requirements (Mintz and Sullivan, 1985).

Abbreviated crossmatching

The commonest form of abbreviated crossmatch is simply to mix a saline suspension of donor red cells with recipient's serum in a tube, centrifuge immediately and examine for agglutination, the so-called 'immediate spin'.

The justification for using only an abbreviated crossmatch when the patient's serum has already been screened for antibodies lies in the observation that very few antibodies are detected by rigorous crossmatching that have not been detected by screening. For example, Heistø (1979) reported the results of screening more than 20 000 patients by rather an elaborate technique, involving an IAT with two different cells containing most of the red cell alloantigens and a papain technique against R_1R_2 cells, which revealed alloantibodies in approximately 0.75% of the patients. Only 5030 of the patients became recipients and, in these, compatibility tests revealed previously undetected antibodies in only three cases (0.06%); all three antibodies were very weak. Results reported by Oberman et al. (1978) were similar and led the authors to conclude that if blood which had been carefully screened by the antiglobulin test was subsequently released, after a crossmatch consisting only of an immediate spin, there would have been only about a 0.06% chance that an extremely weak antibody of potential clinical significance would have gone undetected.

The conclusions of Walker (1982) were almost identical. He calculated that the risk that an antibody to a low frequency antigen, missed on screening, might be the cause of incompatibility because it was missed on subsequent abbreviated crossmatching was approximately 0.06% and that such an event would very seldom be of clinical significance because most of the antibodies concerned cause little or no red cell destruction. Although these calculations led Walker (1982) to conclude that there was no need to do an antiglobulin crossmatching test for patients about to undergo surgery who were unlikely to require a blood transfusion, he stated that he would like to retain the antiglobulin test in routine crossmatching procedures for patients who actually needed blood.

In a more recent study, some 47 000 crossmatches were performed for about 17 500 patients, whose serum was also screened for alloantibodies. Of 284 clinically significant antibodies, 30 were detected only during crossmatching, using the IAT. Of the 30 antibodies, 24 were directed to low frequency antigens but were otherwise unidentified; the remaining six had the following specificities: anti-C^w (two cases), -Kp^a, -M, -Mi^a and -Jk^a. In view of the relatively high incidence of antibodies to low frequency antigens detected only by crossmatching, together with the relatively low cost of retaining the antiglobulin test, the authors concluded that the antiglobulin test should be retained for crossmatching (Motschman *et al.* 1985).

Crossmatching in patients having repeated transfusions

In patients who are having blood transfusions every day or two there is a temptation to obtain a large sample of serum and use this for crossmatching for several successive transfusions. One must remember that any one of a series of transfusions may stimulate a secondary response in a previously immunized subject and that the antibody may rapidly increase in titre once it has appeared. In order to minimize the risk of failing to detect newly formed alloantibodies, one should insist on having serum taken not more than 24 h before the next proposed transfusion.

On the other hand, if incompatible red cells are transfused to a patient whose serum contains a weak antibody, all the antibody may be temporarily absorbed so that if the patient requires a further transfusion, serum taken before the first transfusion may be best for crossmatching. Most cases of this kind can be diagnosed by carrying out a DAT on the patient's red cells at the time of the second or later transfusions provided that enough sensitized donor cells are still present.

If a previously identified antibody has been temporarily absorbed, compatible blood may be selected by using a potent example of an antibody of the same specificity. For example, if a patient is known to have had anti-c in their serum but the antibody is no longer detectable, they should receive blood from donors known to be c-negative.

A suggested routine for patients receiving a series of transfusions is to screen the pre-transfusion serum and all subsequent serum samples against red cells containing the common red cell antigens (see above). The pre-transfusion samples of red cells should be taken into a suitable preservative solution and stored at 4°C in case further blood grouping tests are needed; in identifying any antibodies which the patient may form, it is extremely helpful to know the patient's red cell phenotype and it is evidently far easier to determine this on a pre-transfusion sample than on one taken after the patient has received many units of blood.

Compatibility tests in newborn infants

At birth the only alloantibodies present in the sera of most infants are those that have been transferred across the placenta from the mother's circulation. In the occasional cases in which alloagglutinins formed by the infant are present, they are found in only trace amounts. It can be assumed that a sample of red cells compatible with the mother's serum will not cause any immediate untoward effects if transfused to the infant. For example, if the mother is group B and the infant group O, group B red cells transfused at the time of birth will usually be compatible with the infant's serum and are expected to have a normal survival (see cases reported by Jervell, 1924; Wiener, 1943, p. 74; Pickles, 1949; Mollison, 1951, p. 241).

Although the mother's red cells are almost always compatible with her infant's serum at the time of birth, they should not be used when she is Rh D positive and her infant is D negative.

Haemolytic transfusion reactions may occur in infants with undiagnosed hae-molytic disease of the newborn. For example, increased jaundice may follow the transfusion of D-positive blood to an infant with Rh D haemolytic disease. There are special risks in group A or B infants born to group O mothers. In mature infants with ABO haemolytic disease, transfused adult A_1 red cells are destroyed more rapidly than the infant's own red cells and severe jaundice or even haemoglobinuria may result (see Chapter 12). In premature A or B infants born to O mothers, ABO haemolytic disease is believed not to occur because the A and B antigens are so poorly developed. On the other hand, the transfusion of group A or B red cells may be followed by hyperbiliru-binaemia and haemoglobinuria, due to destruction of the donor's red cells by passively acquired IgG anti-A or anti-B (see Chapter 12).

It is suggested that as a routine DAT should be done on the infant's red cells and that when the test is positive the donor's red cells should be matched against the mother's serum, rather than the infant's serum. In group A or B infants born to group O mothers, packed group O red cells should be used for transfusion.

Cases in which all donors seem incompatible

In some circumstances it may be very difficult to find a donor whose red cells do not react with the patient's serum in.vitro.

1 The commonest cause of apparent incompatibility is potent rouleaux formation. If the presence of rouleaux can be confirmed, e.g. by showing that serum diluted with an equal volume of saline does not produce clumping and that the IAT is negative, the red cells can safely be transfused.

2 The next commonest cause of difficulty in finding compatible blood is in patients whose serum contains potent cold autoagglutinins. If the agglutinin is active at a temperature of about 30°C or higher, the patient will probably have a positive DAT (due to complement components on the red cells) and transfused red cells will have a subnormal survival. However, in these circumstances transfusion is not dangerous if the patient is warmed and kept in a warm room. The problem, then, is mainly to avoid overlooking an alloantibody. In performing compatibility tests, the suspension of donor's red cells and the sample of the recipient's serum should be warmed separately to 37°C before being mixed and tests should be read (microscopically) on warm slides. In carrying out the IAT, the cells should be washed in warm saline. If tests are carried out in this way, it should be possible to detect an alloantibody, since the cold autoantibody is unlikely to interfere. If the cold autoantibody is anti-I, it can sometimes

be removed from the patient's serum by absorption at 4°C with the patient's own enzyme-treated red cells or with rabbit red cell stroma.

3 Patients whose serum contains potent warm autoantibodies present more of a problem, since when the IAT is carried out all samples of red cells may be incompatible. Occasionally, by titrating the serum with a selected panel, some definite specificity such as anti-e may be recognized and compatible cells can then be selected. More often, the serum reacts to some extent with all samples of red cells. Under those circumstances there is some possibility that an alloantibody will be overlooked, particularly when the patient has received many previous transfusions.

Some useful advice on the detection of alloantibodies in patients with AIHA was given by Petz and Garratty (1980, p. 366–72). Among the points made by the authors were the following: it is useful to determine the patient's red cell phenotype before embarking on blood transfusion. If the patient's serum reacts with all normal red cells, it may be possible to identify the presence of an alloantibody by noting that the serum reacts more strongly with some panel cells than it does with the patient's cells. An attempt may be made to remove autoantibody from the patient's serum, by absorption with the patient's own red cells, after eluting autoantibody from them. A single absorption at 37°C may be enough to remove a low-titred autoantibody, and four absorptions should suffice for the removal of a potent antibody. Autoantibody can be eluted from the patient's red cells either by the use of chloroquine or of 'ZZAP', which is a mixture of papain and DTT (Branch and Petz, 1982). After absorption the serum is retested. If it no longer reacts with the patient's own cells (from which autoantibody has been eluted) one can conclude that the autoantibody has been removed and tests may be made for alloantibodies in the ordinary way. If the serum still reacts with all red cells it may need further absorptions or, of course, it may contain an alloantibody reacting with a high frequency antigen. When insufficient red cells are available from the patient, donor red cells of known phenotypes can be used for differential absorption (Petz and Garratty, 1980).

The risk that an alloantibody will be present in the serum of a patient with AIHA is of course much greater in patients who have received repeated transfusions. In a series in which alloantibodies were unmasked by a differential absorption procedure, using donor red cells, alloantibodies were found in six of 19 patients who had received more than five previous transfusions; 42% of the alloantibodies were undetectable before absorption (Wallhermfechtel et al. 1984). Using a similar procedure, clinically significant alloantibodies were found in 41 of 109 patients (38%) with warm autoantibodies (Laine and Beattie, 1985), although this very high figure suggests that some of the 'alloantibodies' may really have been autoantibodies with mimicking specificities (see Chapter 7).

When the patient's serum contains an alloantibody reacting with a high frequency antigen, a national or international panel of donors of rare groups may be able to supply compatible blood. Alternatively, the patient's close relatives can be tested since they have a greatly increased chance of being suitable donors.

Should an autocontrol be included in crossmatching tests?
In the past, when a test at room temperature was included in the crossmatch

procedure, testing of the patient's red cells against his or her own serum (autocontrol) was desirable to avoid confusing autoantibodies with alloantibodies. When, as at present, crossmatching is carried out only at 37°C, an IAT carried out as an autocontrol on the patient's own red cells is only dubiously worthwhile. Such a test very seldom detects AIHA (Kaplan and Garratty, 1985) and very seldom detects an alloantibody sensitizing transfused red cells: in a series of almost 800 patients with a positive DAT following transfusion within the preceding 14 d, only six were due to alloantibodies sensitizing transfused red cells and not detectable in the patient's serum (Judd et al. 1986a).

Errors in identifying the donor or recipient

It is well known that most incompatible transfusions result not from failure to detect antibodies but rather from mistakes in identification, such as faulty labelling of samples or confusion between two patients with similar names but different blood groups.

For example, of 22 fatal immediate haemolytic transfusion reactions, all were due to ABO incompatibility and all were caused by clerical errors. The patient most at risk was one of group O, who was unconscious and was in the operating theatre or intensive care unit (Schmidt, 1980a).

Wallace (1977) mentioned that 20 years previously he had made a study of 20 000 recipients of more than 60 000 units, all of which had been crossmatched by standard methods including the IAT. Seven incompatible transfusions were given, six of which were due to ABO incompatibility (the seventh being due to anti-c). Of the six cases of ABO incompatibility, two were due to mislabelling samples from the patient, two to misplacing tubes during laboratory procedures, and two to failure to identify the patient in the operating theatre. In this study, therefore, one in 10 000 units transfused was ABO incompatible and one in 3300 recipients received ABO-incompatible blood, all due to failure to identify patients or blood samples from them. Presumably, the actual frequency with which ABO-incompatible blood was transfused must have been even higher since ABO incompatibility was looked for only in patients who had had a reaction. Even if only about one in 3000 patients received ABO-incompatible blood, the frequency of misidentification must have been about one in 1000, since, when the 'wrong' blood is given, by chance it will be ABO incompatible only one in three times.

Identification of patients and units of blood

Many systems have been described for minimizing the risk of misidentification. The essentials are for patients to be identified in some second way in addition to their name, e.g. by number or date of birth; for the laboratory to enter the details on a label which is securely attached to units of blood found to be compatible for the patient; and for some responsible person to check these details at the bedside against those of the patient who is to receive the blood. The use of wristbands for patients, carrying details of identification, is an important method of avoiding misidentification and it is very important that they should not be removed from patients before surgery as may happen if they are found to be in the way of putting up i.v. lines.

The use of bar-codes, for marking of wrist bands and for the identification of units of blood can further reduce hazards. The bar-codes can be read at the bedside and the information then checked against data entered in the hospital's computer — a system in use at the Mayo Clinic (H.F. Taswell, personal communication).

Another method in use in some countries is to confirm the ABO group of the recipient and of donor units at the bedside. This practice is a legal requirement in France and a recommended practice in Germany but is not completely satisfactory, perhaps because the people carrying out the bedside tests are often relatively inexperienced. Genetet and Mannoni (1978) commented that in their experience the practice had failed to detect gross errors of ABO mismatching either because of faulty technique or because of the 'climat d'urgence'.

Error rates in blood grouping

Proficiency testing schemes have shown how difficult it is to eliminate errors in ABO and Rh D grouping. Results on samples sent to some 2000 laboratories indicated that the average error rate was 0.64% (Myhre *et al.* 1977). In trials carried out in Canada over a 4-year period the frequency of major errors in ABO grouping was between 0.13 and 0.14%; errors in Rh D typing fell from 0.66% to 0.23% over the period (Pinkerton *et al.* 1979; 1981).

Figures for the UK have been similar, i.e. for 1982–83, in ABO grouping 0.12% and in D grouping 0.37% (Holburn and Prior, 1986). Whereas most of the errors in ABO grouping were due to transposition of tubes or errors of interpretation, the majority of errors in D grouping were due to false-positive results. Although some of the false-positive results were due to the presence of contaminating antibodies such as anti-Bg in the anti-D serum, many were due to the inherently high rate of false-positive results obtained in the antiglobulin test (Holburn and Prior, 1986).

Errors in antibody detection

Two kinds of error may be distinguished: those due to technical errors and those inherent in the techniques used. As an example of the first kind one may take the results of quality control exercises in which participants used various techniques.

In a series of eight exercises carried out in the UK in 1983–84 in each of which four to six incompatibilities were included, the percentage of participants who missed at least one incompatibility in the various exercises ranged from 1.7% to 31.1%. In a comparative study carried out in Canada and the UK about 17% of participants failed to detect anti-D at 0.1 iu (0.02 μg) per ml and about 1.5% failed to detect anti-D at 0.25 iu (0.05 μg) per ml (Pinkerton *et al.* 1985).

In surveys in the UK, error rates have been lower with the antiglobulin method than with other methods. Thus, in detecting anti-D at a concentration of 0.05 μg/ml error rates were as follows: antiglobulin test, 2–3%; with an albumin method, 14–21%; and using enzyme-treated cells 27–49% (Holburn and Prior, 1986). Although most laboratories used a one-stage enzyme technique, even two-stage enzyme techniques proved to be less reliable than antiglobulin techniques. Nevertheless, the incidence of false-positive results was significantly higher in the antiglobulin test than in any other technique (Holburn and Prior, 1984; 1986).

As an example of errors in crossmatching which are inherent in the technique, one may consider the problem of detecting ABO incompatibility when abbreviated crossmatching techniques are used. When an immediate spin was used, or a spin after a very short period of incubation, the reaction between A_2B cells and B serum was missed in about 40% of cases although other ABO-incompatible combinations were detected reliably (Berry-Dortch et al. 1985).

Using an immediate spin in 1000 combinations of patients with blood group B and donors with blood group A_2B, incompatibility was detected in only 40% of the cases using a test in saline and in 64.4% using LISS. Incompatibility was also missed sometimes with other combinations (Shulman et al. 1987). These findings do not seem to be very worrying because mis-grouping of A_2B donor units as B is rare.

When the centrifugation step in the immediate spin crossmatch was delayed for 2 min, no agglutination and only weak to moderate lysis was seen in five of 200 crossmatches between group O serum and group A_1 red cells, whereas agglutination did occur when the red cells were suspended in saline containing EDTA (Shulman and Calderon, 1991).

Failure to detect ABO incompatibility may also be due to a prozone effect if the antibodies in the patient's serum are exceptionally strong (Judd et al. 1988).

Using a polybrene method, incompatibility between A_2 and anti-A, and B and anti-B, was missed in a substantial number of cases (Mintz and Anderson, 1985), presumably because IgM antibodies are less reactive in polybrene. In contrast to these findings, when red cells suspended in LISS were incubated with serum at 37°C for 10 min before being spun, only one example of anti-A (and none of anti-B) was missed in the course of testing nearly 3000 sera (Trudeau et al. 1981).

It seems that the most reliable method of all, in looking for ABO incompatibility, is to follow a test for agglutination by the antiglobulin test; the increased sensitivity may be due partly to the longer period for which the red cells are incubated and partly to the potential for detecting bound complement.

Another reason for retaining the antiglobulin test in crossmatching is simply that because in practice there are so many potential sources of error, some redundancy seems desirable. At the same time, it is clear that if the IAT is omitted from crossmatching, in patients in whom no antibodies have been found on screening, the risk of giving incompatible blood will be extremely small.

Omission of crossmatching in desperate cases

These are cases in which the clinician decides that blood must be given at once if the patient's life is to be saved. It must be emphasized that few cases fall into this category, since all but the most severe cases of blood loss can be temporarily treated with transfusions of albumin or infusions of a plasma substitute while compatibility tests are being performed.

If blood must be given without any preliminary tests, group O blood must be used; in addition, if it is to be transfused to a woman who is not known to be D positive, the blood must be D negative.

Tovey (1974) pointed out that if group O, D-negative, K-negative blood is given to recipients who are known to be D negative (or have not been D grouped) and group O, c-negative, K-negative blood is used for patients known to be D positive, the risk of giving incompatible red cells is extremely small.

Identification of antibodies

When an antibody is found on screening, its specificity must be determined, using a suitable panel of red cells, and then blood of a theoretically compatible group selected for crossmatching. If the antibody is first identified there will be a double check on each donor. For example, if the antibody is found to be anti-c, c-negative blood can be obtained either from a transfusion centre or by testing any available units with known anti-c serum. This blood can then be matched directly against the patient's serum. Use of the patient's serum alone for donor selection is inadvisable, because if the anti-c is relatively weak it may fail to detect the antigen on the cells of cC donors.

Use of a panel of red cells

Most red cell alloantibodies can readily be identified by testing them against a suitable panel of red cells.

The fact that weak antibodies of certain specificities may react only with the red cells of homozygous donors or with strongly reacting red cells may cause difficulty in interpreting results. Anti-c, anti-Jk^a and anti-M are examples of antibodies that react more strongly with homozygous cells; anti-P_1, -Sd^a, -Ch, -Kn^a and -Cs^a are examples of antibodies that show a wide spectrum of reactions with red cells from donors whose red cells carry the corresponding antigens.

Specific inhibition

In identifying antibodies it is sometimes helpful to demonstrate that they are specifically inhibited. Some group-specific substances can be obtained from human milk (I), saliva (e.g. Le^a) or urine (e.g. Sd^a); P_1 substance can be obtained from human or sheep hydatid-cyst fluid or pigeon egg-white.

Satisfactory group-specific substances are available commercially (Marsh and Øyen, 1978). Alternatively, specific oligosaccharides (also available commercially) can be used, e.g. group B tetrasaccharide to inhibit anti-B.

Value of knowing the subject's full red cell phenotype

The identification of antibodies is greatly simplified by knowing the full blood groups of the patient.

Concentration of sera

In investigating sera containing weak antibodies it may be helpful to concentrate them. A convenient method is to add polyacrylamidhydrogel ('Lyphogel') which removes water and salts; 1 g removes up to 5 ml water after about 5 h (Wallace and Green, 1983).

Characteristics of antibodies as an aid to identification

Often the behaviour of an antibody *in vitro* provides valuable clues to its identity. Antibodies which agglutinate saline-suspended red cells are likely to belong to the ABO, Ii, Lewis, P or MN systems or to be anti-Sd^a. The Sd^a, Le^a Le^b, P_1, Ch/Rg, Cs^a, Yk^a and Kn^a antigens are much stronger in some samples of cells than in others. Agglutination by anti-Sd^a and anti-Lu^a gives a 'mixed-field' appearance with discrete clusters of red cells in a field of completely unagglutinated cells. Agglutination by Lewis antibodies gives a peculiar 'stringy' appearance.

Antibodies that can be demonstrated by the IAT but not by agglutination in saline are more likely to belong to the Rh, Duffy, Kell and Kidd systems. If reactions are obtained with anti-complement the antibody is virtually certain *not to* belong to the Rh system. Conversely, if no reactions are obtained with anti-complement the antibody cannot belong to the Kidd or Lewis systems, provided that the red cells have been incubated with serum containing complement.

Antibodies that can be demonstrated by the IAT but fail to react with enzyme-treated red cells are most likely to be anti-Fy^a, -Ch/Rg, -JMH, -S, or -Lu^b.

Treatment of serum with dithiothreitol

As described in Chapter 3, treatment of serum with sulphydryl compounds under suitable conditions inactivates IgM but not IgG antibodies. A solution of 20 mmol DTT in saline (15.48 g/l) is commonly used; the solution remains stable for many months at − 20°C. One volume of the solution is mixed with one volume of undiluted serum and left at room temperature for 15 min. Treatment with iodacetamide (IAA), to prevent reassociation of 7S units is unnecessary with whole serum but is indicated with eluates. IAA should be added to a final concentration of 25 mmol/l and the mixture left for 1 h at room temperature before being dialysed against saline overnight at 4°C.

Identification of autoantibodies

In investigations on cold autoagglutinins, blood should be collected into a warm screw-capped container and put into a Thermos flask containing water at 37°C and transferred from there directly into a heated centrifuge. By following this procedure it should be possible to separate serum from a sample which has never been cooled to more than a degree or two below body temperature. If it is necessary to harvest serum from a clotted sample which has been allowed to cool, the sample should be warmed to 37°C for at least 1 h before the serum is separated (Issitt and Jackson, 1968).

Since the specificity of most cold autoagglutinins is anti-I or anti-i, sera should initially be tested against red cells from a normal adult and from a sample of cord blood. The specificity of anti-I and anti-i is often masked unless dilutions of the serum are tested at 20°C or higher with adult and cord cells. When examining cold autoagglutinins, the possibility of other specificities should not be overlooked (e.g. very rarely the specificity of a cold autoagglutinin may be anti-M).

Warm autoantibodies may exhibit clear-cut specificity within the Rh system although as a rule specificity is not very pronounced (see Chapter 7); an eluate prepared from the patient's red cells should be tested against a panel of red cells of known Rh phenotypes including e-negative cells (R$_2$R$_2$).

Isolation of antibodies

Often a serum contains several alloantibodies and it may then be desirable to absorb out or neutralize the unwanted ones or to extract the wanted ones.

Absorption

If only a limited amount of the appropriate red cells is available, more antibody will be removed by two absorptions with half the quantity of red cells than with a single absorption with the whole amount. When the antibody to be removed is haemolytic, the serum should first be heated to 56°C for 30 min to inactivate complement. Alternatively, absorption may be carried out strictly at 0°C.

Absorption of anti-A and anti-B should in any case be carried out at 0–4°C because absorption at 37°C may fail to remove agglutinins active at a lower temperature. Absorption is performed by first washing the red cells three times in saline and then adding an equal volume (or some lesser volume) of packed red cells to the serum and leaving the mixture at 0–4°C for 30 min. The serum is now tested to see if it is capable of agglutinating A_1 red cells and, if so, further absorptions are performed until the serum will no longer react at all. It is desirable to use the least number of absorptions which will suffice, since there is a tendency for the activity of the serum to be slightly reduced by each absorption, due to dilution by saline mixed with packed cells.

Anti-A and anti-B are removed more efficiently if the red cells are enzyme treated. Papain-treated cells are commonly used.

In absorbing cold agglutinins from serum, centrifugation of the sample following absorption at 0°C should preferably be carried out at a similar temperature; if it is necessary to centrifuge the sample at room temperature, efficiency of absorption can be improved by returning the tubes to 0°C for a period before separating the serum (Issitt and Jackson, 1968).

Use of formol-treated red cells. Formol-treated red cells are convenient because they are inagglutinable, do not haemolyse appreciably and can be stored at room temperature for many months, during which period they retain their ability to combine with antibody. The use of formol-treated red cells to absorb anti-A and anti-B was described by Gold *et al.* (1958). Economidou (1966), using radio-iodine-labelled antibody, found that formalin-treated red cells combined with anti-A just as well as fresh red cells.

Use of enzyme-treated cells for absorption. It may be possible to take advantage of the fact that some antigens are destroyed by enzymes. For example, Eaton *et al.* (1956) used enzyme-treated AB, Yt (a +) cells to remove anti-A and anti-B, but not anti-Yt^a, from a serum containing all three antibodies.

Use of immunosorbent columns. A convenient method of removing antibodies from a serum is to pass the serum through a column to which an appropriate oligosaccharide has been attached. For example, anti-B can be removed by passage through a column to which group B tetrasaccharide has been bound. Very satisfactory results have been obtained using purified human A and B substances instead of oligosaccharides (A. Lubenko and S. Gee, personal communication).

Highly purified antibodies may be obtained by elution from columns of CNBr-activated sepharose to which the appropriate antigen has been coupled. For example, purified anti-IgG may be obtained by elution from a column to which purified IgG has been bound. For details of the technique, see Cuatrecasas and Aufinsen (1971).

Neutralization
The use of specific inhibitors for anti-I, anti-P_1, etc. has been described above.

Elution

As described briefly in Chapter 3, antibodies that have been bound specifically to antigens on red cells (or other cells) can be dissociated by heat, changes in pH or treatment with organic solvents.

Heat. In the first method to be described, washed red cells and a small volume of saline are heated to 56°C for 5 min; after centrifugation, antibody is recovered in the pink supernatant (Landsteiner and Miller, 1925). This method has the great advantages of speed and simplicity. It is satisfactory for eluting anti-A and anti-B from red cells, as in the diagnosis of ABO haemolytic disease of the newborn, or for eluting other antibodies which bind more strongly at low temperatures. However, the yield of warm antibodies compares unfavourably with that of other methods. In one study, using ^{131}I-labelled IgG anti-D, only one-third of the amount of antibody originally bound to the red cells was obtained in active form in the eluate (Hughes-Jones *et al.* 1963b).

Freeze–thaw (Lui). A simple method of eluting ABO antibodies consists in freezing washed cells suspended in 5% albumin and then thawing them. After removal of the stroma by centrifugation, the eluate is ready for testing (Eicher *et al.* 1978).

Low pH. In the study referred to above (Hughes-Jones *et al.* 1963b) more than 80% of antibody was recovered from red cell stroma at pH 3.5 but the method described was too cumbersome for routine use.

A method which has been much used is the acid–digitonin method (Kochwa and Rosenfield, 1964). Using a modification of this method (Jenkins and Moore, 1977) which made it suitable for routine use, estimates with ^{125}I-labelled antibody showed that the eluates obtained were slightly less potent than those obtained with the ether method (see below). In another study the method was found to be less reliable than the ether-elution method, no antibody being recovered in the eluate in a small proportion of cases (Steane *et al.* 1982b).

An elution method which involves lowering pH to 3.0 but without lysing red cells was described by Rekvig and Hannestad (1977). Results appeared to be better than with the ether elution method (see below) but only semi-quantitative methods were used. Elution at pH 3.0 from intact red cells was also found to give good results by McKelvey and Edwards (1984).

Although a pH of approximately 3.5 appears to be best for eluting IgG antibodies, elution of IgM antibody is better at pH 10.5, at least with formol treated red cells (J.H. Humphrey, personal communication, 1967).

Organic solvents. A popular method of elution is that of Rubin (1963) using ether, despite the fact that ether is a dangerous substance to work with. In a comparison of methods referred to above, using ^{125}I-labelled anti-D, the method of Rubin was found to yield 70% of the bound antibody provided that incubation at 37°C was continued for not less than 30 min (Hughes-Jones *et al.* 1963b). Using the ELISA method to estimate the amount of antibody recovered, ether elution gave results that were better than those given by many other methods (Gibble *et al.* 1983).

Because of the hazards of using ether, many other solvents have been tested.

Xylene was found to give results at least as good as those obtained with ether (Chan-Shu and Blair, 1979; Bueno *et al.* 1981). Problems with lysis due to xylene in the supernatant can be minimized by adding one volume of 30% BSA to every two drops of eluate before adding red cells (G. Garratty, personal communication).

In a comparison of elution techniques using a quantitative ^{125}I-antiglobulin test, except with a few antibodies (examples of anti-HLA and anti-Jk^a), results were better with xylene than with ether or with heating (Panzer *et al.* 1984a).

Other methods. Treatment of red cells with 'ZZAP' (cysteine-activated papain and DTT) results in complete dissociation of autoantibodies, but MNSs, Duffy and Kell antigens are destroyed (Branch and Petz, 1982).

Treatment of red cells with chloroquine is useful as a preliminary step in determining the phenotype of red cells with a positive DAT. In one study, after treatment for 2 h with chloroquine, 83% of samples which initially had a positive DAT were no longer agglutinated by anti-IgG (Edwards *et al.* 1982).

Effect of phenotype in eluting from red cells

The most strongly binding antibody is obtained from red cells with relatively weak antigens. For example, elution of anti-D from weak D red cells yields antibody which binds very strongly; in contrast, elution from –D– cells yields a very weakly binding antibody, detectable only with enzyme-treated –D– cells (Goodman and Masaitis, 1964).

Concentration of eluates

A satisfactory method is to use pressure dialysis; with this method a relatively large volume of eluate can be concentrated and, since the amount of antibody is expected to be greater when elution is carried out into a large volume, it is satisfactory to elute from one volume of cells into ten volumes of saline. The principle of the method is to place the eluate in a dialysis sac which in turn is placed in a flask provided with a side arm. The flask is now evacuated with a water pump and the vacuum renewed as necessary. The volume may be reduced to approximately 0.5 ml and this residual amount is then dialysed against normal saline for 1 h with stirring.

Matuhasi–Ogata phenomenon

The first description of this phenomenon was published by Matuhasi (1959). When group B, D-negative red cells were incubated with serum containing anti-B and anti-D, an eluate prepared from the cells was found to contain anti-D as well as anti-B. In a following paper, group O, D-negative, Le(a +) red cells were first treated with anti-Le^a, then exposed to anti-B and anti-D; a heat eluate contained anti-B and anti-D as well as anti-Le^a (Matuhasi *et al.* 1960). It was subsequently shown that the phenomenon (1) did not depend on the occurrence of agglutination, and (2) occurred with mixtures of sera each containing a single antibody as well as with a serum containing two or more antibodies (Ogata and Matuhasi, 1962; 1964).

Allen *et al.* (1969) published a thorough study of the Matuhasi–Ogata phenomenon. In 45 cases red cells were incubated with a mixture of antibodies, one incompatible with the cells and one compatible. In 31 cases the titre of the compatible antibody (as well as that of the incompatible antibody) was reduced following incubation; in 11 of the cases the compatible antibody was recovered in an eluate. The authors concluded that probably some 'compatible' antibody was bound in every case. They also concluded that eluates from patients with a positive DAT might well contain alloantibodies as well as autoantibodies. They suggested that the Matuhasi–Ogata phenomenon explained the non-specific loss of antibodies sometimes observed when absorbing sera.

The phenomenon was reinvestigated by Bove *et al.* (1973) using radio-iodine-labelled antibodies and labelled, non-specific IgG. These authors found that the amount of non-specific IgG taken up by red cells was not increased by previous coating of the red cells with specific antibody. They also found that when the IgG taken up non-specifically included a (compatible) red cell alloantibody in relatively high concentration, an eluate subsequently prepared from the red cells contained sufficient of the antibody to be detectable. They concluded that the finding of unexpected antibodies in eluates might be due to non-specific uptake of IgG rather than to the adherence of antibodies to antigen–antibody complexes.

Investigations to determine the serological cause of a haemolytic transfusion reaction

Methods of investigating transfusion reactions are discussed in Chapter 11, and this section deals with tests to be used in obtaining evidence of serological incompatibility.

The first step should be to repeat the ABO and Rh D grouping of donor and recipient, using both pre- and post-transfusion samples from the latter. The sample alleged to have been taken from the patient before transfusion may in fact have come from another individual. A remote possibility is that the donor blood has been wrongly labelled. The next step is to repeat crossmatching.

When pre-transfusion serum is scarce, as it often is, it is best to use post-transfusion serum first and to keep the pre-transfusion serum in reserve.

When repeat crossmatching provides no evidence of incompatibility, despite the fact that the recipient has suffered a severe haemolytic transfusion reaction, the possibility of an interchange of samples must be considered.

In one case, serum alleged to have been taken from a certain group O patient was found to contain anti-B (titre of 64) but no anti-A. The serum contained A substance and had evidently come from a group A patient. Group A blood had been cross-matched with this serum and had been transfused to the group O patient whose name was on the label of the serum specimen (Mollison, 1967, p. 464).

If it becomes clear that incompatible blood has been transfused due to a 'mix-up' of samples, it should be remembered that a second patient may be at risk and immediate steps should be taken to see what is happening to the second patient involved in the mix-up.

The DAT should also be carried out on pre- and post-transfusion samples. If an antibody is found in the recipient's serum but cannot readily be identified, a pre-transfusion sample of the recipient's red cells should be grouped as fully as possible to give some clue to the specificity of the antibody.

The blood group antibodies most frequently involved in haemolytic transfusion reactions, after anti-A, anti-B and anti-D, are anti-c, anti-E, anti-K, anti-Fy[a] and anti-Jk^a in approximately that order and, accordingly, tests to discover whether the patient's red cells carry the corresponding antigens will be very helpful.

If group O blood has been transfused to A, B or AB recipients, it may be helpful to determine the haemolysin and indirect antiglobulin titres of anti-A and anti-B in the donor's plasma. A quantitative differential agglutination test with anti-A (or anti-B) should be carried out to demonstrate the normal survival of group O red cells. The patient's own red cells are expected to give a positive DAT for at least a day or two after the transfusion of incompatible plasma. Other findings are summarized in Chapter 10. Another possibility to consider is that the red cells of one transfused unit have been destroyed by antibody passively transferred from another (see Chapter 11).

When no pre-transfusion sample is available and the patient has been transfused with blood from many donors, it may be difficult to decide which red cells belong to the patient and which are the transfused ones. A method that is sometimes applicable is to test the saliva for ABH substances. The ABO group of a subject can be determined from saliva in 80% of cases. In patients who are too ill to provide a sample of saliva by spitting, sufficient saliva for testing can be obtained by placing a cotton swab under the tongue.

A method of more general application is to separate out the youngest cells in the patient's circulation, since these will be predominantly his or her own. The youngest cells in the circulation can be separated by taking advantage of the fact that they have a lesser density than older cells. When the patient has a high reticulocyte count, relatively crude methods of separation, e.g. high-speed centrifugation (Renton and Hancock, 1964), may suffice. On the other hand, when the reticulocyte count is normal, or only slightly increased, methods that give better separation between reticulocytes and older red cells should be used, e.g. the method of Vettore et al. (1980).

CHAPTER 9

THE TRANSFUSION OF RED CELLS

THE SURVIVAL OF TRANSFUSED RED CELLS

As a rule, transfused red cells survive for long periods in the recipient's circulation, less than 1% of the number transfused being destroyed each day—a fact which goes far to explain the therapeutic success of red cell transfusion.

Estimates of red cell survival are required only rarely in clinical practice, and then usually when trying to resolve a problem of compatibility, for example when serologically compatible red cells have caused a haemolytic transfusion reaction. In research, survival tests continue to be essential in establishing the value of new methods of red cell preservation. For these various purposes, ^{51}Cr is most often used as a red cell label. Nevertheless, because much of our present knowledge about the survival time of transfused red cells, compatible and incompatible, fresh and stored, was obtained by applying the method of differential agglutination (see Appendix 7), this method will first be described, together with results observed when fresh normal compatible red cells are transfused to normal subjects.

Estimation of survival by antigenic differentiation

A method for investigating the fate of red cells after transfusion from one animal to another was first described by Todd and White (1911). This consisted in preparing a serum which, in vitro, would haemolyse the red cells of one bull (Y) but not those of another bull (Z). After transfusing blood from bull Z to bull Y the mixture of cells in a sample from bull Y could be analysed by adding anti-Y serum; the recipient's (Y) cells were haemolysed and the unhaemolysed cells of the donor (Z) were then counted.

Ashby (1919) applied this principle to the investigation of red cell survival in humans. After transfusing group O blood to group A recipients she took blood samples and incubated them with anti-A serum; the A cells were agglutinated, and the group O cells could be counted. Subsequently, differences within other blood group systems were used for the same purpose, e.g. MN (Landsteiner et al. 1928) and Rh (Mollison and Young, 1942; Wiener, 1943).

Differential agglutination can be used in two ways. Either the recipient's red cells can be agglutinated and the donor's red cells recognized by their failure to agglutinate ('indirect' differential agglutination) or the donor's red cells can be agglutinated using a serum which does not react with the recipient's red cells ('direct' differential agglutination; see Dekkers, 1939).

'Indirect' differential agglutination (or haemolysis)

'Indirect' differential agglutination enables the number of surviving red cells to be counted. Provided that highly potent and specific antisera are used and a sufficient number of red cells counted, reliable quantitative estimates can be obtained. When visual counting is used, the method is tedious but cell counting can be carried out instrumentally, using either the AutoAnalyzer (Szymanski et al. 1968) or the Coulter Counter (Valeri et al. 1985).

As mentioned above, Todd and White (1911) used haemolysis rather than agglutination to 'remove' the recipient's red cells. A useful modification, applicable to human blood when the recipient is group A and the donor O, was introduced by Mayer and D'Amaro (1964): having lysed the recipient's A cells the unlysed group O cells are washed and then lysed so that their number can be assessed spectrophotometrically; details are given in Appendix 7. An improvement on this method, in which the mixture of red cells is labelled with ^{51}Cr before lysis so that quantitative estimates can be obtained by radioactive counting, is also described in Appendix 7.

Direct method of differential agglutination

Recognition of the survival of foreign red cells by directly agglutinating them, using a serum which does not react with the recipient's own red cells, is valuable chiefly in the retrospective investigation of suspected incompatibility (see Chapter 11). The method provides only semi-quantitative estimates of survival.

Rosetting tests

These tests, most commonly used for detecting a small number of D-positive red cells in the circulation of a D-negative subject, are described in Chapter 12.

Use of flow cytometry

Using a suitable alloantibody and fluorescein-labelled anti-IgG, red cell populations in a transfused subject can be identified directly, or indirectly, on the basis of antigenic differences.

As an example of direct identification, after transfusing C-positive red cells to a C-negative patient, blood samples from the recipient were treated with anti-C, then with fluorescein-conjugated anti-IgG; the C-positive cells were then quantitated by passage through a flow cytometer (Garratty, 1990). As an example of indirect identification, after injecting 10 ml D-negative red cells to a D-positive patient, and treating samples as above but using anti-D, the non-fluorescent (D-negative) cells were counted (Issitt *et al.* 1990a).

Flow cytometry can also be used to recognize a population of red cells labelled *in vitro* with a dye, PKH-2, which binds to the red cell membrane. The method can detect a labelled population present at a concentration of 0.01% but the dye causes some changes in red cell morphology and studies *in vivo* have yet to be done (Read *et al.* 1991).

Survival of transfused red cells in normal subjects

When compatible red cells are transfused in therapeutic amounts, the number of surviving cells in the recipient's circulation diminishes steadily over a period of 110–120 d (Wiener, 1934; Mollison and Young, 1942; Callender *et al.* 1945a), indicating that all red cells have the same life span. Transfused blood is then presumed to contain cells of all ages, in equal numbers: approximately one-hundredth of the total number are 1 d old, another hundredth 2 d old, and so on. Thus, on each day after transfusion one-hundredth of the number reach the end of their life span and disappear from the circulation.

Callender *et al.* (1947) found that in males the survival curve was linear, from which it may be deduced that there is normally no random destruction of red cells. In females, survival was curvilinear, indicating some random loss. Although menstruation seems the most likely cause of this loss, it was concluded from somewhat complicated mathematical treatment of the data that other factors were involved.

Since there is normally little or no random loss in males, the survival time is determined by donor, rather than recipient, characteristics. In one careful study, red cells from two donors were transfused, in each case to three recipients, and found to have 'potential life spans' (i.e. after correction for any random loss detected) of

114 ($\pm$ 8) and 129 ($\pm$ 5) d respectively (Eadie and Brown, 1955). For other estimates, see later.

Derivation of mean red cell life span from red cell survival curves are described in Appendix 6.

The hypothesis that red cells have a more or less constant life span implies that after a certain period in the circulation the red cells become susceptible to some physiological removal mechanism. Evidence about the possible nature of this mechanism is discussed below.

Methods of separating red cells according to age

Separation by density. A simple method which gives reasonably good separation is centrifugation at 15 000 rev/min at 30°C to enhance red cell deformability, using an angle centrifuge to give better mixing (Murphy, 1973). However, the use of density gradients appears to be essential to enable the cells to float according to their buoyant density (Piomelli *et al.* 1967).

Reticulocytes are less dense than mature red cells (Stephens, 1940), and there is a good deal of evidence suggesting that red cell density increases throughout the life span of red cells. When ^{59}Fe was administered to normal human subjects and blood samples were taken at intervals and centrifuged, the ^{59}Fe was found in increased amounts in the lightest cells for about the first 20 d; the ratio of ^{59}Fe in the top/bottom layers then became approximately 1.0 and was below unity between about 50 and 90 d. After 90 d, due to reutilization, ^{59}Fe began to reappear in the top layer (Borun *et al.* 1957). Similarly, when cohorts of red cells were labelled in rabbits, using glycine-2-C^{14}, and fractions were separated in a discontinuous gradient of bovine serum albumin (BSA), the glycine was found in progressively denser fractions: by day 60, all was in the lowest 50% and most was in the lowest 10%.

When cells were separated by ultracentrifugation without a gradient, the label was concentrated in the top fraction initially but thereafter there was a minimal relation between cell age and position in the centrifuged column (Piomelli *et al.* 1967).

In rabbits, it has been shown that the survival of red cells *in vivo* diminishes with increasing density; for example, the time after injection of labelled cells for Cr survival to fall to 10% varied as follows: top 10% of centrifuged cells, 56 d; unfractionated cells, 42 d; bottom 10% 28 d (Piomelli *et al.* 1978). In the work just quoted, red cells were separated on arabino-galactose; in another study in which red cells were separated by simple centrifugation, Cr survival was also longer (T_{50}Cr 11.2 d) in cells from the top fraction than in unselected cells (T_{50}Cr 9.65 d) and was very much shorter (3.6 d) in cells from the bottom fraction (Gattegno *et al.* 1975).

The densest red cells in human blood have an MCV of 86.7 μ^3, compared with 91.7 μ^3 for unselected cells and 99.3 μ^3 for the lightest cells (Vincenzi and Hinds, 1988).

Despite the foregoing evidence, many investigators have concluded that, apart from the low density of very young red cells, there is no clear relationship between red cell density and age, either using ^{59}Fe (Luthra *et al.* 1979) or both ^{59}Fe and HbA$_{1c}$ (van der Vegt *et al.* 1985a) as age markers. Similarly, using biotin to tag circulating red cells in rabbits, and using avidin to separate cells labelled 50 d previously, the densest fraction was only two to three times enriched in old cells (Dale and Norenberg, 1989).

The most likely explanation for the discrepant views seems to be that the precise method used to separate red cells by density makes a big difference to the results obtained.

Separation by volume. Red cells can be separated by volume, using counter-current centrifugation; the method gives a linear separation by age, with ^{59}Fe and HbA_{1c} as markers. With this method, MCV is found to fall linearly with age, whereas mean corpuscular haemoglobin concentration (MCHC) remains constant, indicating that red cells lose Hb during ageing; the loss of Hb has been estimated to be as high as 25% during the life time of the red cell (van der Vegt, 1985a). Presumably, shedding of Hb-containing vesicles is responsible (Lutz, 1978; Dumaswala and Greenwalt, 1984). Osmotic fragility decreases with ageing due to an increasingly favourable surface area to volume ratio (van de Vegt *et al.* 1985b).

Obtaining old red cells by suppressing erythropoiesis. In animal experiments, populations of old red cells have been obtained by giving transfusions of red cells at 2-weekly intervals from donors of the same inbred strain; by keeping the recipients poly-cythaemic, contamination with reticulocytes was minimal. As ageing progressed, there was a steady reduction in MCV and some loss of Hb from the cells (Ganzoni *et al.* 1971).

Some differences between young and old red cells
Using all of the three methods of separation described above, MCV has been found to diminish steadily with ageing.

The content of some red cell enzymes, e.g hexokinase, is very much higher in reticulocytes than in mature red cells and falls rapidly as the reticulum is lost, although some activity persists throughout the red cell life span (Zimran *et al.* 1988; 1990). With other enzymes, e.g. pyruvate kinase, the loss is slow and progressive throughout the red cell life span.

The densest red cells, with a specific gravity of more than 1.1100, have autologous IgG on their surface which can be eluted by heating to 47°C; the IgG is an autoantibody to terminal galactosyl residues which are normally hidden by sialic acid on red cells. These residues are exposed on the densest red cells and can be exposed on lighter cells by treating the cells with a suitable proteolytic enzyme (Alderman *et al.* 1980; 1981). Only 4% of the circulating red cells have a specific gravity of more than 1.1100 and only these cells gives a positive direct antiglobulin test (Khansari *et al.* 1983). These observations have been interpreted to mean that red cell ageing is associated with progressive loss of cell membrane, leading to exposure of normally hidden structural components ('cryptantigens') for which there are naturally occurring antibodies in the serum, and that the autoantibody-coated red cells are removed by becoming bound to, and subsequently engulfed by, macrophages.

There is also a correlation between increasing red cell density and loss of decay-accelerating factor and C8-binding protein, both of which are deficient in red cells from patients with paroxysmal nocturnal haemoglobinuria, leading to the specu-lation that aged red cells may disintegrate through complement-mediated lysis (Ueda *et al.* 1990). On the other hand, it has been contended that the densest red cells are far from being a pure sample of the oldest cells and that evidence from methods other than density separation is needed before the mechanism by which senescent red cells are removed from the circulation can be established (Beutler, 1988).

Variation in life span within a population of red cells
The hypothesis that in healthy subjects all red cells live for about 110–120 d is doubtless an over-simplification; for one thing, existing data are insufficiently precise to distinguish between a strictly linear disappearance slope and one that is slightly curvilinear, although data obtained both with differential agglutination and with di-isopropyl ^{32}P-phosphofluoridate (DF^{32}P)-labelling suggest that the slope may be very close to linear in most males.

When survival curves are approximately linear a small variation in red cell life span will be revealed by a 'tail' at the end of the curve; see Fig 9.1 for example. If the linear portion of the slope, i.e. up to about 80 d, is extrapolated to the time axis the standard deviation of red cell life span can be deduced by the proportion of red cells surviving at this time (Dornhorst, 1951). Estimates made in this way suggest that the standard deviation of life span may be as short as 6 d in normal subjects (Mollison, 1951, p. 104). Obvious 'tails' can be seen in some published curves (Eadie and Brown, 1955; Szymanski and Valeri, 1968).

The effect of splenectomy on the survival of normal red cells. It is uncertain whether the survival of normal red cells is prolonged in the absence of the spleen. In three patients with 'cryptogenetic splenomegaly', the survival of transfused red cells was normal following splenectomy (McFadzean *et al.* 1958). Similarly, in rabbits, there was no significant difference in ^{51}Cr red cell survival between normal and splenectomized animals (Miescher, 1956b). On the other hand, in splenectomized rats, red cell life span measured with radio-iron was 65 d compared with 59 d in normals; random destruction (0.48%) was the same in the two groups (Belcher and Harriss, 1959).

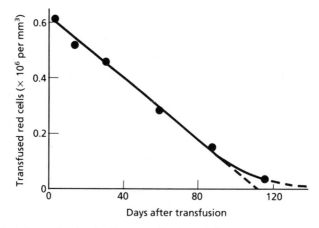

Figure 9.1 Survival of transfused red cells in a male adult. Until elimination of the cells is almost complete the points fall on a slope which may be linear or slightly curvilinear. If the slope is assumed to be linear, mean cell life, estimated by extrapolation of the line to the time axis, is 114 d. The persistence of a few transfused cells beyond 114 d is due to variation in red cell life span (see text).

The survival time of the red cells of newborn infants can be measured by obtaining blood from the placenta of one infant and transfusing it to another infant. In work referred to in the first edition of this book, the results of transfusing placental blood from full-term infants to four anaemic premature infants were described. Each infant also received a transfusion of blood from an adult donor. The survival of the placental red cells was expressed as a percentage of the survival of the adult red cells and the arbitrary assumption was made that the adult red cells were eliminated at the rate of 1% a day. The survival curve of the placental red cells was found to be slightly curvilinear, indicating the presence of a substantial proportion of red cells with a life span less than that of adult red cells. In fact, the mean life span of the red cells of newborn infants must be distinctly less; during the last hundred days of pregnancy the fetus trebles its weight and, presumably, trebles its red cell mass. Accordingly, placental blood must contain an undue proportion of young red cells. If the cells all had a life span of the order of 110 d, the survival curve would be strikingly convex whereas, as mentioned above, it was in fact, found to be slightly concave. The conclusion that red cells produced in late fetal life have a mean life span which is distinctly shorter than that of adult red cells is supported by observations made with ^{51}Cr (see below) and ^{15}N-glycine (Vest *et al.* 1965). From experiments in which cord red cells labelled *in vitro* with DF^{32}P were injected into adults, it was concluded that the mean life span of red cells produced at the end of fetal life is between 45 and 70 d (Bratteby *et al.* 1968a,b).

The effect of plethora

Although it is sometimes tacitly assumed that in subjects rendered plethoric by transfusion there is increased destruction of red cells, there is in fact no evidence of this; in newborn infants with a PCV as high as 0.64 after transfusion the survival of transfused red cells is strictly normal (Mollison, 1943b; 1951, p. 111).

Estimation of survival using ^{51}Cr

Red cells can be labelled with ^{51}Cr by incubating them with radioactive sodium chromate (Gray and Sterling, 1950); the chromate binds predominantly to the β-chains of Hb (Pearson and Vertrees, 1961).

The method of ^{51}Cr-labelling has two great advantages over that of differential agglutination, namely, that the subject's own red cells can be labelled and that the survival of very small volumes (0.1 ml or less) of red cells can be studied; moreover, sites of red cell sequestration can be identified using surface counting, the degree of intravascular haemolysis can be estimated in short-term tests (see Chapter 10), and blood loss in the stools can be estimated. ^{51}Cr liberated from red cells destroyed either within the blood stream or within the mononuclear phagocyte system is not reutilized. Unfortunately, the ^{51}Cr method suffers from a serious disadvantage: survival curves have to be corrected for Cr elution to obtain estimates of true red cell survival.

Cr elutes from red cells at the rate of approximately 1% a day (Ebaugh *et al.* 1953). In addition, during the first 2 or 3 d (mainly during the first 24 h) there is additional loss, so-called 'early loss' (Mollison and Veall, 1955) so that normal Cr survival at 24 h is only about 96% (instead of about 98%) of the 10-min value (see below). The rate at which Cr elutes from red cells is affected by the technique of labelling (Mollison, 1961a; Szymanski and Valeri, 1970).

Two methods of labelling have been shown to give similar results, namely the 'citrate-wash' method (Mollison 1961a; Garby and Mollison, 1971) and an acid–citrate–dextrose (ACD) method in which packed red cells are labelled (Bentley *et al.* 1974). Both these methods have been recommended by ICSH (1971; 1980b) but the

ACD method is more convenient and has therefore been selected as the reference method (ICSH, 1971; see Appendix 2 for details). Table 9.1 gives values for Cr survival obtained using the citrate-wash method. The table also gives factors which convert observed Cr values on any particular day to true red cell survival, assuming that the normal mean life span is 115 d. The results thus corrected for Cr elution are then analysed as described in Appendix 6.

Using the ACD method recommended by ICSH, very similar correction factors were derived. This was a reassuring finding because the factors were derived from a comparison between the results of Cr and DFP labelling, whereas the factors given in Table 9.1 were obtained by comparing Cr results with those expected from normal survival. Furthermore, the figures in Table 9.1 were derived from the survival of allogeneic red cells, whereas those of Bentley et $al.$ were based on autologous red cell survival.

In another recommended method, after incubating ACD or CPD blood with $Na_2{}^{51}CrO_4$, ascorbic acid is added to reduce hexavalent Cr to the trivalent form and thus stop any further uptake, and the whole mixture is then injected. However, after 15 min incubation of red cells with $Na_2{}^{51}CrO_4$ at 37°C, uptake of Cr is virtually arrested even when ascorbic acid is not added, so that the value of adding ascorbic acid is doubtful. The disadvantage of the method, compared with methods in which washed red cells are injected, is that for accurate estimates of red cell volume the amount of ^{51}Cr in the supernatant of the injection suspension must be measured and allowed for. Also, even when only red cell survival is being measured, the amount of

Table 9.1 Mean Cr survival in normal subjects and correction factors which convert the Cr survival into 'true' red cell survival (mean red cell life span 115 d) when the 'citrate-wash' method is used (Garby and Mollison, 1971)*

Day	Cr survival	Correction factor	Day	Cr survival	Correction factor
0	100.0		16	70.7	1.22
1	96.2	1.03	17	69.3	1.23
2	94.0	1.05	18	67.8	1.25
3	92.0	1.06	19	66.3	1.26
4	90.1	1.07	20	64.9	1.27
5	88.2	1.08	21	63.4	1.29
6	86.5	1.10	22	62.0	1.31
7	84.7	1.11	23	60.5	1.32
8	83.1	1.12	24	59.1	1.34
9	81.4	1.13	25	57.6	1.36
10	79.9	1.14	26	56.2	1.38
11	78.3	1.16	27	54.7	1.40
12	76.7	1.17	28	53.3	1.42
13	75.2	1.18	29	51.9	1.45
14	73.7	1.19	30	50.4	1.47
15	72.2	1.20			

* Note that although the $T_{50}Cr$ with this method of labelling is on the average just over 30 d, with some other methods it may be shorter.

The values in the table were reproduced in ICSH (1971). Almost identical values were obtained by Bentley et $al.$ (1974) using the method of labelling described in Appendix 2.

Table 9.2 Relation between $T_{50}Cr$, derived red cell life span and relative rate of red cell destruction (assuming that the rate of Cr elution is normal, i.e. about 1% per day) (from Mollison, 1981)

$T_{50}Cr$ (d)	Mean red cell life span (d)	Rate of red cell destruction
31	115	× 1
23	54*	× 2
18	38*	× 3
14	27*	× 4

* Destruction assumed to be random.

^{51}Cr in the plasma of samples taken within the first 24 h must be estimated. Finally, ascorbate may damage red cells with certain metabolic abnormalities, particularly glucose-6-phosphate dehydrogenate deficiency (Beutler, 1957).

The curvilinear slope of Cr survival in normal subjects cannot be fitted by a simple exponential and the time taken for survival to fall to 50% of its original value should be expressed as the T_{50}, not the $T_{1/2}$.

The mean normal $T_{50}Cr$ is about 31 d and in 95% of healthy subjects falls within the range 25–37 d (Mollison, 1981). When $T_{50}Cr$ is less than 25 d it is best to correct results for Cr elution and deduce mean red cell life span (ICSH, 1971; 1980b), using the method of analysis described in Appendix 6. As Table 9.2 shows, the $T_{50}Cr$ is not a satisfactory index of red cell destruction since it bears no obvious relation to mean red cell life span.

Note that when Cr survival is within normal limits, correction factors should not be applied in the hope of securing a good estimate of true red cell survival. When survival is within normal limits, the daily loss of Cr by elution is approximately equal to the daily loss of red cells and variations in the rate of Cr elution therefore have a relatively large effect on the estimate of true survival.

The rate of Cr elution in healthy subjects was found to vary from 0.70 to 1.55% per day, (mean, 1.0, SD 0.07) by Bentley et al. (1974). In patients with haematological diseases values between 0.6 and 2.3% per day were found by Cline and Berlin (1963a) and between 0.6 and 2.0% by Garby and Mollison (1971). These figures for the variability of elution must somewhat overestimate the true variability since they are derived from a comparison of estimates of Cr and DFP survival and are thus affected by the error of both estimates.

In a wide variety of diseases, estimation of red cell life span based on Cr measurements corrected for elution agree quite well with DFP measurements (Eernisse and van Rood, 1961; Finke et al. 1965; Garby and Mollison, 1971); as expected, though, the Cr method is insensitive in detecting slight increases in red cell destruction (Cline and Berlin, 1963; Finke et al 1965).

Since ^{51}Cr is thought to be bound predominantly to the β-chains of Hb (Pearson and Vertrees, 1961), rates of elution in patients with abnormal β-chains are of special interest. McCurdy (1969) compared Cr and DFP survival in 21 patients with abnormal β-chains (including some with Hb SS, S Thal, AS, SC, CC and AC). With four exceptions, Cr elution had a single component with a mean daily loss of 1.2% which was insignificantly different from that observed in normal subjects. In the four exceptions (four of the nine subjects with Hb SS) there appeared to be an initial rapid component lasting 9–11 d with an elution rate of 4.1–19.5% per day and a later component with a negligible rate of Cr elution.

Binding and elution of Cr

From one study it was concluded that the Cr ion behaves as if it were trapped inside the red cell and bound only weakly to Hb and other ligands such as 2,3-DPG, adenosine triphosphate (ATP) and citrate. It appears that Cr exchanges randomly between these species until it diffuses out of the red cell (Kuehl *et al.* 1981). In an earlier study evidence was obtained that when red cells from ACD blood were labelled as packed red cells rather than as whole citrated blood, the subsequent rate of Cr elution from the red cells was diminished (Mollison, 1961a). It has been shown that the amount of ^{51}Cr bound to Hb and the subsequent rate of elution of Cr from the red cells is different when ACD and CPD are used (Valeri *et al.* 1981a). The amount of ^{51}Cr bound respectively to Hb and low molecular weight compounds varies according to the conditions of labelling, but there does not seem to be any obvious relationship between the patterns of labelling observed *in vitro* and the rate of elution of Cr from red cells *in vivo* (Valeri *et al.* 1981a).

Early loss. There is a great deal of evidence that 'early loss' of Cr is not due to damage to red cells during labelling or washing; the extent of the loss is not related to the dose of Cr used, nor to the number of times the cells have been washed; moreover, the same early loss is observed when red cells are labelled *in vivo* by injecting a small dose of $Na_2^{51}CrO_4$ i.v. (Hughes-Jones and Mollison, 1956). Further evidence was supplied by Kleine and Heimpel (1965) in experiments in which red cells were labelled with $DF^{32}P$ in a donor from whom a sample was taken 48 h later; the cells were now also labelled with ^{51}Cr and it was shown that after injection into a recipient the loss of ^{51}Cr exceeded that of $DF^{32}P$ by about 5% in 24 h. Presumably, 'early loss' is due to the relatively loose binding of a small fraction of ^{51}Cr.

Preferential labelling of young red cells by ^{51}*Cr*

It seems that young cells take up more than their fair share of ^{51}Cr, though how much more is uncertain. According to Walter *et al.* (1962), the most osmotically resistant cells take up 4% more than the average, but according to Valeri *et al.* (1968) the lightest cells (i.e. the top layer of the red cell column of blood mixed with phthalate esters and centrifuged) take up about 16% more than the average.

Toxic effect of chromate on red cells

$Na_2^{51}CrO_4$ is available with a specific activity of 7×10^9 Bq (200 m Ci)/mg. Even when 2 mBq ^{51}Cr are used to label as little as 0.2 ml red cells, the dosage of chromate, expressed as the dose of Cr, will only be about 5 μg/ml red cells. No effect on red cell survival has been noted at doses up to 20 μg Cr/ml cells, although abnormal survival curves have been found when 35 μg Cr/ml cells or more are used (Donohue *et al.* 1955; Hughes-Jones and Mollison, 1956).

The most striking effect of chromate on red cells is the inhibition of glutathione reductase; with a level of chromate corresponding to 20 μg Cr/ml red cells 60% reduction in the level of this enzyme has been observed (Koutras *et al.* 1964). A definite reduction in Cr red cell survival has been observed when the level of glutathione reductase falls to 20% (Ebaugh *et al.* 1964).

Cr survival in the very young and the very old

Red cells of newborn infants. The following values for the $T_{50}Cr$ have been recorded: 20 d (Hollingsworth, 1955); 22.8 d compared with 27.5 for adults (Foconi and Sjölin, 1959); 24 d compared with 30 d for adults (Gilardi and Miescher, 1957); 17.5 d compared with 25 d for adults (Eloise Giblett, unpublished observations, 1955). The $T_{50}Cr$ of red cells from premature infants injected into adults was found to be 15.8 d by Foconi and Sjölin (1959) and to be 16 d by Gilardi and Miesher (1957).

A shorter $T_{50}Cr$ for cord red cells compared with adults is expected since, as mentioned above there is evidence that red cell life span is distinctly shorter in newborn infants.

In children aged 2.5 years or more, Cr survival is the same as in adults (Remenchik et al. 1958).

Cr red cell survival in elderly subjects. Cr red cell survival was found to be normal in five patients aged 70–90 years by Miescher et al. (1958), in ten men and 12 women aged 80–94 years by Woodford-Williams et al. (1962), and in 11 subjects aged 70–90 years by Hurdle and Rosin (1962).

Use of non-radioactive chromium (^{52}Cr)
Human red cells contain about 0.8 μg Cr/l cells; following incubation with $Na_2^{52}CrO_4$, i.e. ordinary non-radioactive sodium chromate, they readily take up large amounts of Cr. Although glutathione reductase is slightly inhibited at Cr levels as low as 2 μg/ml red cells, no effect on red cell survival has been noted at levels up to 20 μg/ml cells (see above). Following the injection of about 20 ml packed red cells labelled with a total of about 40 μg Cr (i.e. 2 μg/ml red cells), in a subject with a total circulating red cell volume of 2 litres, the concentration of Cr is expected to be 20 μg/l cells, i.e. 20 times the normal level. Using Zeeman electrothermal adsorption spectrophotometry, with a graphite furnace attachment, Cr concentrations between 1 and 7 μg/l can be estimated with a coefficient of variation of 4.7% (Heaton et al. 1989c). When red cell volume was estimated using ^{52}Cr, results were similar to those observed with ^{51}Cr-labelled red cells or with estimates deduced from plasma volume; similarly, estimates of the 24 h survival of stored red cells were in essential agreement with those based on ^{51}Cr labelling (Heaton et al. 1989c;d). In another study, in which red cells in 130 ml blood were labelled with a total of 250 μg ^{52}Cr, and results compared with those obtained with ^{51}Cr in the same subjects, the $T_{50}Cr$ values by the two methods were almost identical (Sioufi et al. 1989). Although the idea of using non-radioactive Cr is attractive, the need to use relatively large volumes of red cells, the somewhat elaborate technology, and the relative inaccuracy imply that the method in its present form cannot compete with the use of ^{51}Cr.

Other methods of random labelling of red cells

Use of di-isopropyl phosphofluoridate
DFP binds to cholinesterases in red cells and other cells such as platelets, and also

binds to plasma cholinesterase. DFP has been used to label red cells *in vitro*, using ^{3}H-DFP (Cline and Berlin, 1963b), or DF^{32}P (Bratteby and Wadman, 1968). With the latter, since the maximum amount of DFP which binds irreversibly to red cells is about 0.15 μg/ml cells and since the maximum available specific activity of DF^{32}P is about 400 μCi/mg (14.8 MBq/mg), at least 50 ml red cells must be labelled if not less than 2 μCi (74 kBq) are to be injected. In most experiments, therefore, DF^{32}P has been injected i.v., thus labelling the whole red cell mass (Cohen and Warringa, 1954; Bove and Ebaugh, 1958; Heimpel *et al.* 1964; Bentley *et al.* 1974). Some 4% of the label is lost in the first 24 h but thereafter there is no detectable loss. Some of the loss in the first 24 h may be due to labelling of leucocytes and platelets but almost all the injected DF^{32}P is bound by red cells. Estimates of mean red cell life span using DFP have varied from 99 to 129 d (see Table 9.3).

Use of ^{14}C-cyanate to label red cells *in vitro*

Cyanate binds irreversibly to Hb and in the form of ^{14}C-labelled cyanate can be used to estimate red cell survival. In ten normal subjects red cells from 50 ml blood were labelled and the average mean red cell life span found to be 115 d (Eschbach *et al.* 1977). The slopes were only slightly curvilinear, which is puzzling in view of the evidence that a substantial amount of Hb is lost from surviving red cells (see p. 381).

Biotinylation

Red cells can be coated with biotin and subsequently identified by being bound to avidin. When rabbit red cells were treated in this way, estimates of red cell survival were similar to those obtained with ^{14}C-cyanate (Suzuki and Dale, 1987). The method has been applied to the selective extraction of aged red cells from the circulation of rabbits whose red cells were labelled 50 d beforehand, to investigate the relationship between red cell age and density (Dale and Norenberg, 1990).

In a study in which human red cells were labelled with biotin *in vitro* and then used to estimate red cell volume and survival, in some cases the biotin was rapidly cleared from the circulation — a result apparently associated with the recent consumption of eggs, which are rich in avidin (Cavill *et al.* 1988).

Use of haemoglobin differences between donor and recipient

Restrepo and Chaplin (1962) studied the survival of normal red cells transfused to patients with sickle cell disease or Hb C disease; haemolysates were submitted to starch block electrophoresis and each Hb was then eluted and the amount estimated. The authors pointed out that, like the method of differential agglutination, this method was useful when the decision to estimate red cell survival was made only after transfusion; it could sometimes be used when, because of serological similarities between donor and recipient, differential agglutination was impracticable. Finally, it was sometimes useful in cases in which radio-isotopes were contraindicated.

Methods of labelling a 'cohort' of red cells

By a 'cohort' is meant a population produced over a limited period of time. A cohort of cells can be labelled by giving an injection of radio-iron to normal subjects and taking a blood sample about 5 d later, but an unacceptably large amount of radioactivity has to be used.

Table 9.3 Survival of autologous and allogeneic red cells estimated by several different methods

Reference	Method	Subjects		Method of analysis	Survival or life span (d)
		Sex	No.		
Autologous					
Shemin and Rittenberg (1946)	^{15}N-glycine	M	1	rise and decline of ^{15}N in haem	127
London *et al.* (1949)	^{15}N-glycine	M	1	rise and decline of ^{15}N in haem	120
	^{15}N-glycine	F	1	rise and decline of ^{15}N in haem	109
Cohen and Warringa (1954)	DF^{32}P	F	2	linear fit (least squares)	116, 129
Bove and Ebaugh (1958)	DF^{32}P	not stated	8	linear fit (least squares)	124.6 (SD[‡] 11.0)
Garby (1962)	DF^{32}P	M	6	linear fit (least squares)	122
Bratteby and Wadman (1968)	DF^{32}P	M	4	linear fit (least squares)	99–125
Bentley *et al.* (1974)	DF^{32}P	M / F	12 / 1	linear fit (least squares)	111.2 (SD 20.3)
Berk *et al.* (1970)	Catabolism of bilirubin	M / F	11 / 8	complicated	107 (SD 11) / 94 (SD 11)
Allogeneic					
Wiener (1934)	Differential agglutination	not stated		(semi-quantitative data)	3–4 months
Callender *et al.* (1945)	Differential agglutination	M	3	linear fit	120
Callender *et al.* (1947)	Differential agglutination	M / F	2 / 4	mathematical analysis; average survival and life span* deduced	110–120 / 90–100
Eadie and Brown (1955)	Differential agglutination	M / M	3[†] / 3[†]	mathematical analysis; 'intrinsic life span' deduced	129 (SD 5) / 114 (SD 8)

* Life span, or age at which death rate maximum, 120 d in men and women.
[†] In the series of Eadie and Brown (1955), one male donor gave blood to the first group of three recipients and the second male donor gave blood to the second three recipients. In the other series in which allogeneic red cells were transfused random donors were apparently used.
[‡] Between subjects.

Reticulocytes will take up iron *in vitro* (Walsh *et al.* 1949) and cells labelled in this way have been used successfully to demonstrate the destruction of red cells by alloantibodies and to investigate the subsequent fate of the labelled Hb (Jandl *et al.* 1956).

Use of ^{15}N-labelled glycine

Shemin and Rittenberg (1946) tagged a subject's own red cells by feeding ^{15}N-labelled glycine. The glycine was rapidly incorporated into newly synthesized Hb, although the concentration of labelled nitrogen per unit mass of red cells did not reach its peak for about 25 d after the beginning of the experiment. At about the 80th day the concentration of labelled nitrogen began to decline and then fell steeply. The time separating the mid-point of the rise and the declining portion of the graph was found to be 127 d, and this was taken to be the average life time of the cells.

Although it was originally believed that Hb, and thus ^{15}N, could not be lost from intact red cells, the decrease in labelled haem which began about 60 d after peak values had been reached suggested that label was, in fact, lost (Mollison 1961b, p. 173). There is now direct evidence that red cells lose Hb during their life span (van der Vegt et al. 1985a). Because of the relatively slow incorporation of labelled haem, the loss of label from intact red cells and the reutilization of the label, measurements with ^{15}N-glycine, though providing valuable information about Hb metabolism, do not add anything important to knowledge of the life span of human red cells.

^{14}C-labelled compounds

Berlin et al. (1954) gave i.v. injections of glycine-2-^{14}C to patients with chronic leukaemia to measure red cell life span; the specific activity of CO_2 derived from combustion of extracted Hb was measured in an ionizaton chamber. There was evidence of prolonged uptake and considerable reutilization of ^{14}C, and the method thus appears to be open to the same criticisms as the ^{15}N method.

Use of DF^{32}P

Cline and Berlin (1962) gave unlabelled DFP (0.5 mg/kg) to dogs and produced almost complete (97%) blocking of further uptake of DFP by the circulating red cells; 6–9 d later newly formed red cells were labelled by injecting DF^{32}P. Red cells produced in response to acute blood loss were shown to have a survival time which was distinctly shorter than that of normal young red cells (see also Neuberger and Niven, 1951).

Red cell life span derived from estimation of products of haemoglobin catabolism

The catabolism of 1 mol of haem should result in the excretion of 1 mol of CO and 1 mol of bilirubin; excretion of both products is approximately 6.6 μmol/kg per day (see review by Berk et al. 1970). Measurements of bilirubin turnover were used by Berk et al. to estimate mean red cell life span which was found to be 107 $\pm$ 11 d in 11 normal men and 94 $\pm$ 11 d in eight normal women. The authors suggested that estimates with other labels might give too high values for red cell life span because they overlooked a small amount of random destruction of red cells and were based on the assumption of a linear red cell survival slope.

In a later review of this method it was concluded that mean red cell life span deduced from short-term estimates of bilirubin turnover gave results which were well correlated with estimates made with ^{3}H-DFP or with ^{51}Cr, although it was not suitable for use in any conditions in which there was a marked increase in the fraction of bilirubin turnover not derived from circulating red cells (Berlin and Berk, 1981).

Summary of normal survival of red cells

There are several reasons why generally acceptable values for the mean and range of true red cell survival in normal subjects have not yet been established: the number of studies is not large, many different techniques have been used and, perhaps above all, the data have been interpreted in many different ways. The main difficulty is that the disappearance curve of the red cells is not, as a rule, defined with sufficient precision so that, as a result, it is usually not possible to say whether the points should be fitted by a straight line or a curvilinear slope. Even a minor degree of curvilinearity implies a substantially lower mean survival time (Mills, 1946). Accordingly, if a straight line is fitted to points which really fall on a slightly curvilinear slope, mean cell life is overestimated.

Table 9.3 summarizes some of the available data on the survival of autologous red cells in normal subjects. In most cases the authors have assumed that the data are fitted by a straight line, so that in these cases true mean red cell life span is probably less than the figure given.

Table 9.3 also shows that there is no apparent difference between the survival of allogeneic and autologous red cells. This point is reinforced by data in Table 9.4 which gives estimates for the survival of allogeneic and autologous red cells estimated by ^{51}Cr labelling. All the estimates for allogeneic cells are of the survival of D-positive red cells from one of four donors in selected D-negative recipients who failed to make anti-D after at least two injections of D-positive red cells given at an interval of 5–6 months and were judged to be non-responders (Mollison, 1981). The figure for the survival of autologous red cells is deduced from the data of Bentley et al. (1974).

Rapid destruction of transfused red cells in certain haemolytic anaemias

In all those conditions in which a haemolytic anaemia is due to some extrinsic mechanism rather than to any intrinsic red cell defect, transfused normal red cells are expected to undergo accelerated destruction. Nevertheless, the survival of the transfused red cells may be better or worse than that of the recipient's own red cells.

Reasons why transfused red cells may survive differently from patient's own red cells
There are several possible reasons why, initially, the rate of destruction of transfused red cells may be greater than that of the subject's own cells. First, red cells may vary in

Table 9.4 Survival of allogeneic and autologous red cells labelled with ^{51}Cr (Mollison, 1981)

Donors'	Recipients		Cr survival at 28 d (%)	
Sex (initials)	No.	No. of studies	Mean	SD
*Allogeneic red cells**				
F (M.S.)	18	18	53.4	5.1
F (M.L.)	8	11	58.4	4.4
F (K.B.)	9	18	51.4	4.1
M (H.S.)	14	14	55.2	4.5
Autologous red cells†	13	13	52.5	

* All recipients of allogeneic cells were D-negative 'non-responder' males; for sources of data see text.
† Cr survival at 28 d deduced from the data of Bentley et al. (1974).

their susceptibility to destruction by the haemolytic process; if so, the red cells in the circulation of a subject with an 'extrinsic' haemolytic anaemia will be a selected population, having a higher than average resistance to the haemolytic agent. When red cells from a normal donor are transfused, the rate of destruction will be relatively high initially whilst the most sensitive cells are being destroyed and may thereafter become the same as that of the recipient's own red cells. It is not known whether in practice there are intrinsic differences in average susceptibility to destruction between donor and recipient red cells although it seems likely that there are: the average age of the red cells in a the circulation of a normal donor must necessarily be greater than that of the red cells in a subject with a haemolytic process and old red cells are known to be more susceptible than young red cells to destruction both *in vitro* and *in vivo* by some antibodies, namely haemolytic heteroantibodies (Cruz and Junqueira, 1952; Griggs and Harris 1961; London, 1961; Gower and Davidson, 1963; de Wit and van Gastel, 1969).

In the warm antibody type of autoimmune haemolytic anaemia the survival of transfused red cells may be influenced by the donor's red cell phenotype. In cold haemagglutinin disease the subject's own red cells are relatively resistant to destruction compared with the donor's red cells. These effects are described in Chapter 7.

Unexplained difference between the survival of transfused red cells and of the subject's own red cells; see previous editions of this book.

Diminished survival of transfused red cells in pernicious anaemia

As discussed below, it is seldom necessary to give blood transfusions to patients with untreated pernicious anaemia even when the anaemia is severe. It is therefore not of much practical importance, although it is of considerable interest, that normal red cells have been found to have a diminished survival in patients who have not yet received vitamin B_{12} or have received it not more than 3 d before transfusion (Hamilton *et al.* 1954; 1958; unpublished observations, PLM and P. Crome, 1963).

Diminished survival of transfused red cells in aplastic anaemia

In aplastic anaemia, the survival of the patient's own red cells is usually moderately reduced and this reduction is not due to haemorrhage (Lewis, 1962). In a case reported by Loeb *et al.* (1953) the survival of transfused red cells was moderately reduced, as it was in the case illustrated on p. 425. The reduced survival of the patient's own red cells is presumably due to dyserythropoiesis, but the reduced survival of transfused red cells has not been explained.

Increased red cell destruction in fever

Fever, resulting from the i.v. injection of pyrogen, or the i.m. injection of heated milk, or from external heating, results in an increase in red cell destruction, affecting old red cells more than young ones (Karle, 1969); see also p. 412.

Diminished survival of red cells due to haemorrhage

Loss of blood in the stools. In patients with a low platelet count, poor survival of transfused red cells may be due not to haemolysis but to chronic bleeding into the gastrointestinal tract. If ^{15}Cr-labelled red cells are injected into the circulation, the amount of blood lost in the stools can be measured by estimating their ^{51}Cr content (Roche et al. 1957; Hughes-Jones, 1958a). Correction for blood loss can then be applied so as to discover whether the survival curve, corrected in this way, is normal. According to Hughes-Jones (1958a) the normal daily loss of blood in the stools is about 0.5 ml (or 0.2 ml of red cells); this figure is a little lower than that obtained by Ebaugh and Beekin (1959) who, using a quantitative benzidine method, estimated the daily loss as 2 ml of whole blood.

Loss of blood by venous sampling. Corrections are also needed if substantial amounts of blood are withdrawn during the course of estimating red cell survival. It can be shown that when the amount of blood lost from the circulation is $x\%$ of the blood volume, the corrected survival is given by:

$$\text{Observed survival} \times \frac{100}{(100 - x)}$$

This is the appropriate correction whatever the percentage of surviving cells at the time the sample is taken (Mollison, 1961b, p. 208).

Suppose ^{15}Cr-labelled cells are injected into a subject whose blood volume is 4500 ml. By the 20th day after injection, ten samples each of 15 ml (i.e. total 150 ml or 3.33% of the blood volume) have been withdrawn. The observed ^{15}Cr survival is 55%; corrected survival is:

$$55 \times \left[\frac{100}{(100 - 3.33)} \right], \text{ or } 57\%$$

Hypersplenism

In nine, patients with chronic lymphocytic leukaemia with splenomegaly (average splenic weight approximately 2000 g), the mean $T_{50}Cr$ was 21 d but 1 year after splenectomy was 27 d (Christensen, 1971). Similarly, in three patients with cryptogenetic splenomegaly, the $T_{50}Cr$ was found to be 15–25 d but became normal after splenectomy (McFadzean et al. 1958). In animals, when splenomegaly is induced by implanting percorten, red cell survival is found to be diminished (Miescher, 1956a).

Survival of transfused red cells in haemolytic anaemias
due to an intrinsic red cell defect

In all those haemolytic anaemias which are due to an inherited red cell defect (e.g. hereditary spherocytosis, the haemoglobinopathies and red cell enzyme deficiencies), compatible normal red cells are expected to survive for a normal length of time. For example, the survival of transfused red cells from normal donors is strictly normal in hereditary spherocytosis (Dacie and Mollison, 1943) and in sickle cell anaemia (Callender et al. 1949).

Although normal survival of transfused red cells has also been described in many patients with thalassaemia major (Evans and Duane, 1949; Hamilton et al. 1950) diminished survival has been reported in patients who have been repeatedly transfused. Among 20 children with thalassaemia major who received regular transfusions, many appeared to require transfusion unduly frequently. In six of seven selected cases,

50% of transfused red cells were eliminated in 5–9 d and it was concluded that, although no blood group antibodies could be detected, there must be low grade alloimmunization. After splenectomy, the transfusion requirements were reduced to between one-fifth and one-third (Lichtman et al. 1953). The possible induction of immunological tolerance in children with thalassaemia in whom transfusion is begun early in life is discussed in Chapter 3.

Transfused red cells from healthy donors survive normally in patients with paroxysmal nocturnal haemoglobinuria (Dacie and Firth, 1943; Mollison, 1947).

Estimation of mean red cell life span in haemolytic anaemias; see Appendix 6.

STORAGE OF RED CELLS IN THE LIQUID STATE

History
The first account of the storage of red cells was published by Fleig (1910); 80 ml blood was taken from rabbits and defibrinated. The red cells were washed in isotonic spa water and kept in an ice-box for up to 7 d before being returned to the donor animal. A rise in the red cell count following transfusion suggested that some of the red cells, at least, were viable.

As mentioned in Chapter 1, Weil (1915) also showed that citrated blood stored in an ice-box for several days could be transfused safely to animals. The work of Rous and Turner (1916) was a great step forward. Sugars were tested in the hope that, since red cells were believed to be impermeable to them, they might act like colloids and protect against lysis. Blood taken from one rabbit, stored for up to 12 d in a citrate–sucrose solution and then transfused to another rabbit which had just been bled, prevented the development of anaemia. When human blood was stored, dextrose was found to be marginally better than sucrose in diminishing lysis; accordingly a solution containing dextrose was recommended for the storage of human blood and was soon afterwards used for transfusion (see below). This recommendation must be regarded as having been somewhat fortunate because at the time it was not known that dextrose has a strikingly favourable effect on the metabolism of stored red cells whereas sucrose has not. More than 20 years later it was found that the addition of dextrose to citrated blood decreased the rate of hydrolysis of ester phosphorus during storage (Aylward et al. 1940), and the suggestion was made that dextrose exerted its favourable effects by providing energy for the synthesis of phosphate compounds, particularly DPG and ATP (Maizels, 1941a).

The discoveries of Rous and Turner were put to practical use in the First World War by Robertson (1918). Working with the Allied Expeditionary Forces in Belgium, during a relatively quiet period donors were bled into Rous–Turner solution (500 ml blood were added to 350 ml 3.8% trisodium citrate and 850 ml 5.4% dextrose). After sedimentation had been allowed to occur in an ice-box for 4–5 d the red cells had settled to a volume of 800 or 900 ml, and after 2 weeks or so to 500 ml. After removing the supernatant solution the volume was made up to 1000 ml with 2.5% gelatin in saline. Twenty-two transfusions of this mixture were given to 20 recipients, mainly suffering from severe haemorrhage. The results were apparently as good as those observed with fresh blood. The usual storage time was from 10 to 14 d but some transfusions of red cells stored for up to 26 d were given. Robertson pointed out that the chief advantage of this system was the great convenience of having a stock of blood at hand for busy times, an advantage which remains to this day.

After the end of the First World War interest in the storage of blood seems to have evaporated and it revived only in the 1930s, first in the Soviet Union. For example, Filatov (1937) reported that by the end of 1936 many thousands of transfusions of stored blood had been given in Leningrad and elsewhere. According to Riddell (1939), by about 1937 all large hospitals in Russia were using stored blood almost to the exclusion of fresh blood. Donors attended their local 'Central Institute' where blood was taken and stored and distributed to hospitals as required.

The concept of a blood bank: 'it is obvious that one cannot obtain blood unless one has deposited blood' was formulated by Fantus (1937), who set up the first such bank at Cook County Hospital in Chicago.

The first attempt to supply the transfusion needs of an army in the field seems to have been made during the Spanish Civil War when, between August 1936 and January 1939, stored blood was supplied from a centre in Barcelona. Nine thousand litres of blood were obtained from donors during a period of 2.5 years (Jorda, 1939). Only group O donors were used. Blood was taken into a citrate–glucose solution and six donations, each of about 300 ml, were pooled in a special robust container and stored under a pressure of two atmospheres of air.

The outbreak of the Second World War led to the very rapid setting up of transfusion services equipped to collect and store whole blood on a large scale. At first, citrate alone was used in many services before the value of adding dextrose was rediscovered. A great deal of further work was then done in an attempt to find better preservative solutions. The main advance which resulted from all this work was the discovery of the value of acidifying the citrate–dextrose solution.

Between 1938 and 1942 several papers were published indicating that the rates of efflux of potassium from red cells and of lysis were diminished when blood was stored with an acid diluent (Cotter and McNeal, 1938; Jeanneney and Servantie, 1939; Maizels and Whittaker, 1940; Maizels, 1941b; Wurmser et al. 1942). Nevertheless, no attempt was made to use acidified solutions in clinical practice, mainly because it was thought that they might be harmful. The incentive to test acidified solutions for clinical use arose from the fact that there was one major inconvenience in using solutions of trisodium citrate and dextrose, namely that when they were autoclaved together substantial caramelization occurred, which was thought to be undesirable. It was known that when acidified citrate–dextrose solutions were autoclaved, little or no caramelization occurred, and since it would clearly be simpler to be able to autoclave the entire preservative solution in the blood container rather than having to add autoclaved dextrose separately, a systematic study of ACD solutions was carried out by Loutit et al. (1943). It was found not only that blood stored with these solutions produced minimal effects on the recipients's acid–base balance (in fact they produced a slight alkalosis due to the catabolism of citrate), but that red cell survival after storage was much improved. These findings led to the immediate introduction of an ACD solution as the standard preservative in the UK although ACD came into wider use only after the end of the Second World War.

The work of Rapoport (1947) showed that there was a close association between the ATP content of stored red cells and their viability. Later, Gabrio et al. (1955a) showed that the ATP content of stored red cells could be almost completely restored by incubation with adenosine and that, moreover, restoration of the ATP content was accompanied by an increased post-transfusion survival (Gabrio et al. 1955b). Adenosine was never used in routine transfusion practice because of its toxicity, but a few years later it was discovered that adenine, a far less toxic substance, was also capable, in collaboration with inosine, of 'rejuvenating' stored red cells (Nakao et al. 1960). Furthermore, adenine alone, when added at the beginning of storage would retard the rate of loss of red cell viability (Simon, 1962; Simon et al. 1962).

Until 1967 the role of 2,3-DPG in red cells remained unknown and relatively little attention had been paid to the observation of Valtis and Kennedy (1954) that the oxygen dissociation curve of stored citrated blood is 'shifted to the left' indicating that stored red cells release oxygen to tissues less readily than do fresh red cells. When the role of 2,3-DPG in releasing oxygen from $Hb\ O_2$ was discovered (Benesch and Benesch, 1967; Chanutin and Curnish, 1967), great interest was taken in the 2,3-DPG content of stored red cells. It had already been found that red cell 2,3-DPG was better maintained in a citric acid–citrate–phosphate–dextrose mixture containing less citric acid than the original ACD solution (Gibson et al. 1961) and a new solution 'CPD' came increasingly into use. For the storage of whole blood CPD–adenine is the best available solution. On the other hand, the demand for plasma, to be used mainly for the production of Factor VIII and albumin, has led to the practice of harvesting plasma from blood freshly collected into CPD and resuspending the red cells for storage in a nutrient solution. Saline–adenine–glucose–mannitol has been found to give very satisfactory preservation.

Deleterious changes occurring during storage

Loss of viability

From a practical point of view the most important change occurring in red cells during storage is their progressive loss of viability, i.e. their capacity to survive in the recipient's circulation after transfusion. When blood stored for relatively short periods is transfused, some of the cells are removed from the circulation during the few hours following transfusion and the rest survive normally. With increasing periods of storage the proportion removed in the first 24 h increases (Fig. 9.2) and eventually all the cells become subject to rapid removal. The rate of loss of viability varies greatly according to the preservative solution used, as discussed in a later section.

Although there is an association between the progressive loss of red cell viability during storage and the progressive loss of red cell ATP, it now seems clear that other factors also determine loss of viability.

Depletion of ATP

Fresh red cells contain approximately 3.5 μmol ATP per g Hb (Bensinger et al. 1977; Heaton et al. 1984). During storage there is a fall in ATP content, associated with the following red cell changes (Haradin et al. 1969):

1   A change in shape from discs to spheres.
2   A loss of membrane lipid.
3   A decrease in the critical haemolytic volume (probably related to the loss of membrane lipid).
4   An increase in cellular rigidity.

After 8 weeks' storage as ACD blood, red cells have the appearance of smooth spheres and their ATP content is very low. If the cells are incubated with adenine and inosine at 37°C, the red cells regain their original discoidal shape and their ATP level rises to near-normal. Moreover, the red cells have a 24 h post-transfusion survival of about 90% (Nakao et al. 1962). In blood stored for 4–8 weeks and incubated with adenosine to restore the depleted red cell ATP, there is a very high correlation between the percentage of discoid cells and post-transfusion survival (Haradin et al. 1969).

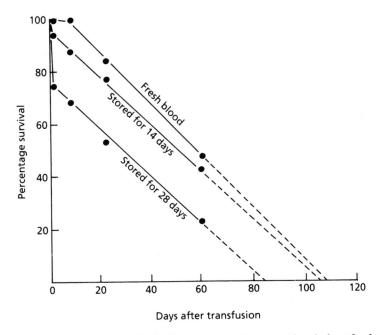

Figure 9.2   Post-transfusion survival of red cells of fresh blood compared with that of red cells stored in acid–citrate–dextrose at 4°C for 14–28 d; when stored red cells are transfused, some leave the circulation in the first 24 h after transfusion but the rest survive well (results obtained by the method of differential agglutination) (slightly revised from Mollison, 1951, p. 13).

The loss of membrane lipid is associated with the formation of microvesicles (Allan *et al.* 1976). These vesicles, which are free of spectrin, can be found in whole blood stored for more than 12 d in CPD and similar vesicles are shed from red cells which have been depleted of ATP by incubation at 37°C in buffered saline (Lutz, 1978). During storage of blood in CPD–adenine over a period of 35 days, the quantity of vesicles in the supernatant plasma and the ratio of lipids to proteins in them increases progressively (Greenwalt *et al.* 1984).

During ATP depletion, changes in red cell shape precede changes in deformability (Feo and Mohandas, 1977). Metabolic depletion leads to dephosphorylation of spectrin and loss of cell deformability (Mohandas *et al.* 1978). Although there is an association between ATP content of stored red cells and their viability, ATP is certainly not the only determinant of viability. Some evidence is as follows: (1) in red cells stored for 7 weeks in ACD, incubation with adenosine restored ATP to normal levels but the post-transfusion survival rate (24 h) was only 68% (Mollison and Robinson, 1959); (2) in one particular donor (R.P., see p. 403), whose red cells survived poorly after 28 d storage in ACD, red cell ATP was no lower than in the stored red cells of other donors (Mishler *et al.* 1979); (3) a study in which red cell ATP was compared with viability showed that a fall from 3.0 to 2.0 μmol/g Hb had little effect on viability, although below about 1.5 μmol/g Hb the relationship was close (Dern *et al.* 1967); and (4) when red cells are stored in a solution of bicarbonate, adenine, glucose, phosphate and mannitol, which maintains high 2,3-DPG levels, but after 42 d, ATP levels as low as 0.34 μmol/g Hb, 87% may be viable (Wood and Beutler, 1967).

A change *in vitro* which is relatively well correlated with survival *in vivo* is red cell deformability. For example, whereas 100% of fresh normal red cells can pass through a pipette of minimal dimension 2.85 μm (thought to be similar to that of the microcirculation in the spleen), after 3 weeks' storage in ACD only about 80% of cells can pass. Discs with a relatively high ratio of surface area to volume are more deformable than spheres and there is a high (0.96) correlation coefficient between survival and the percentage of cells which are discoidal or have a region of central palor (Weed and LaCelle, 1969). The PCV, as determined by the Wintrobe haematocrit, increases progressively during storage but this does not indicate red cell swelling but rather an increase in plasma trapping (J.M. England, personal communication) due, presumably, to increasing rigidity of the cells.

Depletion of 2,3-diphosphoglycerate
The discovery of the central role played by 2,3-DPG in releasing oxygen from Hb in red cells has been described above.

In human red cells DPG and Hb are nearly equimolar. DPG profoundly lowers the affinity of Hb for oxygen at concentrations commonly found in the red cells. One mol of DPG combines with 1 mol of deoxy-Hb to form a complex which has a low oxygen affinity. If DPG is displaced it becomes easier for the Hb molecule to undergo the allosteric transition to the tense (oxy) state with a higher oxygen affinity. ATP has an effect similar to that of DPG, but the concentration of ATP is four to five times lower (Benesch and Benesch, 1969), viz. about 3.5 μmol/g Hb, compared with 13–15 μmol/g Hb for 2,3-DPG (e.g. Bensinger *et al.* 1977).

Valtis and Kennedy (1954) were the first to observe that the oxygen dissociation curve of stored citrated blood was shifted to the left, suggesting that such blood after transfusion would be, at least temporarily, incapable of releasing as large a volume of oxygen to the tissues as fresh blood. They found the changes were nearly maximal after 1 week's storage in ACD and this was confirmed by Gullbring and Ström (1956). It was later found that the changes occur more slowly in a less acid preservative solution, see later.

The logical conclusion that the changes in the oxygen dissociation curve in the red cells of stored blood are due to depletion of DPG was reached by Åkerblom *et al.* (1968) who also showed that the oxygen affinity of stored red cells could be restored to normal by incubation of the red cells with inosine.

Similar results were obtained by Bunn *et al.* (1969b). The parallelism between 2,3-DPG values and the P_{50} values of the oxygen dissociation curve has been confirmed (e.g. Rørth, 1969; Dawson *et al.* 1970; Duhm *et al.* 1971).

2,3-DPG levels in stored red cells can be maintained by adding either dihydroxyacetone (Brake and Deindoerfer, 1973) or 'ascorbate' (Wood and Beutler, 1973) to stored blood. The best effects are obtained when both additives are used together (Wood and Beutler, 1974). The apparent effect of ascorbate is, in fact, due to contaminating oxalate which inhibits pyruvic kinase activity (Beutler *et al.* 1987).

Is the 2,3-diphosphoglycerate level in transfused red cells clinically important?
The fascinating study of Oski *et al.* (1971a) indicates that under some circumstances the level of 2,3-DPG in red cells plays a very important part in dealing with an

increased need for tissue oxygenation. Two subjects were studied, one with red cell hexokinase deficiency and a decreased red cell 2,3-DPG, the other with pyruvate kinase deficiency and an increased red cell 2,3-DPG. Both patients had Hb levels of approximately 10 g/dl. Following vigorous exercise, in the patient with the raised red cell 2,3-DPG, venous oxygen saturation fell to 22.5% (near the critical level) and cardiac output rose by 48%; on the other hand, in the patient with the decreased red cell 2,3-DPG, oxygen saturation fell only to 44.2% and cardiac output doubled.

The clinical significance of DPG levels in stored red cells has proved harder to demonstrate. For example, in an experiment in rats, partial exchange transfusion was carried out using low-DPG blood in one group and normal-DPG blood in the other. A severe acute anaemia, known to be close to the LD_{50} for this type of rat was then produced by haemodilution. Mortality in the two groups did not differ significantly. Analysis of the data indicated that in haemorrhagic shock Hb concentration and the degree of acidosis were more important determinants of survival than the red cell DPG concentration (Arturson and Westman, 1976).

Experiments reported by Collins (1980) suggested that animals can compensate very well for 2,3-DPG-depleted red cells provided that their PCV remains above 0.30.

Rats were exchange-transfused, either with fresh blood or with blood stored in ACD for 14–20 d, and were then bled and transfused with fresh or stored blood with either a high or a low PCV. In animals in which PCV was maintained at over 0.30, survival was the same in those transfused throughout with stored blood as in those transfused with fresh blood. On the other hand, in animals with PCVs of 0.30 or less, the mortality rate was significantly greater in animals transfused with stored blood (Collins, 1980).

Collins (1980) concluded that even complete depletion of red cell 2,3-DPG is probably well tolerated in a moderately stressed patient. On the other hand, anaemia, a limited cardiac reserve and coronary artery insufficiency may provide critical situations in which the level of red cell 2,3-DPG becomes significant, although evidence apart from that for anaemia, discussed above, is scanty.

Some other changes in stored red cells
In blood stored at 4°C the active transport of potassium and sodium across the red cell membrane is almost halted and intracellular and extracellular concentrations tend to come into equilibrium.

Changes which are poorly correlated with the maintenance of viability include changes in osmotic fragility and in the degree of spontaneous lysis.

Changes in osmotic fragility partly reflect the composition of the preservative solution; e.g. red cells stored with sucrose, which does not penetrate the cell membrane, have an increased resistance to lysis by hypotonic saline but, as mentioned above, have a very poor post-transfusion survival. Conversely, red cells stored with a relatively large volume of 5% dextrose are osmotically fragile but have a good post-transfusion survival (Mollison and Young, 1941a; 1942). Although in many other preservative solutions osmotic fragility is negatively correlated with survival *in vitro* (Valeri *et al.* 1965; Dern *et al.* 1966), the correlation is not good enough to make the index valuable in predicting red cell survival.

In stored cells a major part of the increase in osmotic fragility is due to the accumulation of lactate and, to a lesser extent, to the substitution of chloride ion for a diminished cell content of 2,3-DPG. However, in addition to the overall increase in osmotic fragility produced by the increased intercellular osmotically active material, there is a fragile tail of red cells. These cells are the first to be lost following reinjection into the circulation and are presumably a subpopulation which has lost the most membrane during storage and thus has a diminished surface area (Beutler *et al.* 1982).

Spontaneous lysis. Although an increased rate of spontaneous lysis with any preservative solution indicates that viability will be poor, absence of lysis does not indicate that viability will be good. For example, red cells stored for 14 d in a trisodium citrate–sucrose solution show less than 1% haemolysis even though almost all the cells are non-viable (Mollison and Young, 1941a; 1942). Similarly, certain phenothiazine compounds inhibit red cell haemolysis on storage (Halpern *et al.* 1950) but do not increase the post-transfusion survival (Chaplin *et al.* 1952).

Storage antigen. On storage, red cells become agglutinable by a specific antibody; agglutinability appears to be closely related to loss of viability (see Chapter 7).

Reversibility of storage changes
As mentioned above, red cells stored for relatively brief periods show a diminished ATP content and an increase in rigidity and many other changes. Nevertheless, the bulk of red cells stored for relatively short periods survive for long periods in the circulation. Evidently then, many of the changes observed in red cells after storage are reversible. As described in a later section, stored red cells can be 'rejuvenated' by various methods before transfusion. 2,3-DPG levels can be restored by incubation with inosine, phosphate and pyruvate and, following incubation with adenosine or with adenine and inosine, the content of ATP is restored, the original discoidal shape of the cells is regained, the cells regain normal flexibility, and viability is greatly increased. On the other hand, the loss of membrane lipid and the change in critical haemolytic volume of the red cells are not reversible (Haradin *et al.* 1969).

Loss of viability of red cells on storage, seems therefore, to be due to at least two different processes: first, the development of rigidity in the red cell membrane which is reversible *in vitro* by restoring the ATP content of the cells before transfusion; if ATP is not restored *in vitro* and the cells are transfused, viability will be poor since below a certain critical level of ATP red cells lose their capacity of phosphorylating glucose and therefore of deriving energy from it; second, the loss of membrane lipid, which is not reversed by incubation of the red cells with adenosine and which appears at the present time to represent an inevitable deterioration in red cells stored at 4°C. Methods of rejuvenating red cells before transfusion are discussed in a later section.

Changes in the composition of stored red cells following transfusion can be studied after separating donor red cells from samples of the recipient's blood, using the technique of differential agglutination (see Crawford and Mollison, 1955). This method has been used to study the rate at which changes in 2,3-DPG and electrolytes are reversed *in vivo*.

Rate of restoration of red cell 2,3-diphosphoglycerate in vivo. In two studies on red cells stored as blood mixed with ACD and transfused to patients, results were as follows: in the first, in three subjects, at least 25% of the DPG content was restored within 3 h and more than 50% within 24 h; in the second, also in three subjects, about 45% was restored in 4 h and about 66% at 25 h (Beutler and Wood, 1969; Valeri and Hirsch, 1969). In studies in normal volunteers, whose blood had been stored for 35 d with CPD-A1, AS1 or AS3, results were not very different: DPG levels were back to 50% of normal in 7 h and almost to 95% at 72 h (Heaton *et al.* 1989a).

Reversal of electrolyte changes

The concentration of potassium in stored red cells is restored to normal very slowly after transfusion; red cells previously stored in ACD for 15–16 d did not regain a normal content for more than 6 d after transfusion, although their sodium content became normal within 24 h (Valeri and Hirsch, 1969). Similarly, red cells previously stored for 1–3 months at 20°C in a citrate–glycerol mixture did not regain normal potassium values until 4 d after transfusion (Crawford and Mollison, 1955).

Estimation of viability of stored red cells

Although the factors causing loss of red cell viability are now much better understood, no method exists of predicting accurately, from tests *in vitro*, how a given sample of stored red cells will survive in the circulation. Estimation of post-transfusion survival therefore continues to play an essential role in the development of improved methods of red cell preservation.

When red cells which have been stored for a relatively short period are injected into the circulation, some cells are cleared within a few hours but the rest survive normally. With longer storage, the percentage cleared within the first few hours increases progressively and after prolonged storage all the cells are cleared rapidly. In practice, knowledge of the percentage survival at 24 h makes it possible to predict how the whole population will survive and there is therefore no point in making estimates of survival beyond this time.

In view of the fact that, in a population of stored red cells, there are some which are cleared within the mixing time (Fig. 9.3), percentage survival cannot be estimated accurately unless a labelled population of fresh red cells is also injected. True survival can then be determined from an estimation of total circulating red cell volume (RCV) or as a ratio of stored: fresh red blood cell survival. On the other hand, when the proportion of non-viable red cells is relatively small, satisfactory estimates can be made by an extrapolation method (see below), without injecting a second labelled population.

Methods that have been used for estimating the percentage survival of stored red cells have been reviewed elsewhere (Mollison, 1984a). Here, only two methods will be described.

In the double label method, the sample of stored (autologous) cells is labelled with one isotope (^{51}Cr) and a sample of fresh (autologous) red cells is labelled with a second isotope (e.g. ^{99m}Tc). The two lots of labelled red cells are injected as a mixed suspension. RVC is estimated from the ^{99m}Tc values in samples taken at 5–10 min and the percentage survival of the ^{51}Cr-labelled stored cells is calculated from a sample taken at 24 h. This method is the most accurate available. When RCV is estimated simultaneously with two lots of fresh red cells, each labelled with a

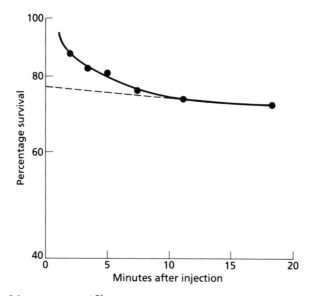

Figure 9.3   Rate of disappearance of ^{51}Cr-labelled stored red cells from the circulation during the 20 min following injection. The red cells were from blood which had been stored for 42 d at 4°C with acid–citrate–dextrose and inosine. The true percentage survival 24 h after injection was about 50%.

Each observation is based on a comparison with the survival of fresh red cells labelled with ^{32}P and injected at the same time. If survival had been based on the ^{51}Cr estimates alone, taking samples from 10 min onwards and extrapolating the estimates to zero time (----) to obtain a figure for apparent 100% survival, 24 h survival would have been estimated as 65% (50/77), instead of 50%.

different isotope, the results agree closely, as expected from the fact that the two lots of cells are injected in the same suspension and that common standards are prepared. Using ^{51}Cr and ^{32}P, the mean value for RCV estimates with the two isotopes differed by less than 0.1% with an SD of 0.9% (Mollison *et al.* 1958). Using ^{51}Cr and ^{99m}Tc, in two series the mean value of estimates with ^{99m}Tc was about 1.2% higher in one small series (Jones and Mollison, 1978) and 0.9% higher in another (Beutler and West, 1984).

As an alternative to using a second red cell label to estimate RCV, ^{125}I has been used to estimate plasma volume (PV) and RCV has then been deduced. This method is far less satisfactory; it has a substantially larger error since: (1) the volumes of labelled plasma and of red cell suspension which are injected are different; (2) different standards are prepared from plasma and from the red cell suspension; and (3) in deducing RCV from PV, a factor has to be assigned for the H_B/H_V ratio (see Appendix 4). Apart from the greater error involved in estimating RCV in this indirect way, ^{125}I has a substantially greater radiotoxicity than ^{99m}Tc.

In the single label method, which is simpler but less accurate than the double red cell label method, a sample of stored red cells is labelled with ^{51}Cr and injected; a series of samples is taken and the values are extrapolated to zero time to obtain an estimate of the 100% survival value. In using this second method it is evident that the first sample must not be taken before mixing is virtually complete and sampling must be confined to a period during which the rate of cell destruction is more or less constant. Mixing is usually not complete for 3–5 min after injection (Strumia *et al.* 1968). In a series in which samples were taken at 2.5-min intervals, the points between 5 and 15 min after injection were well fitted by a single exponential but the 20-min value was above the line, indicating that destruction had slowed by this time. When RCV was estimated by extrapolating a line through the 5–15-min values to zero time the estimates of RCV were within ± 5% of the true value (obtained from the ^{99m}Tc estimate), provided that the 24 h survival was above 70%. When survival was below this, RCV was overestimated by about 25%. For example, in one case the true survival, i.e. estimated from a ^{99m}Tc estimate of RCV, was 13.3%, but if calculated from the RCV determined by extrapolation was 16.9%. This overestimate can either be expressed as 3.6/13.3 × 100, i.e. 27%, or as 16.9 − 13.3, i.e. 3.6%. It has been suggested that the latter figure is the one which is important in practice and that the error of the extrapolation method is therefore not large enough to be important (Beutler and West, 1984). Using this second method of interpreting results, in a series in which the survival rate was always greater than 60% and usually greater than 70%, the single isotope method overestimated survival by only 1–4.3% (Beutler and West, 1985). In another study, in which the 24-h survival rate by a double red cell labelling method averaged 78.2%, survival by the extrapolation method was overestimated by about 3%; when true survival was less than 75%, the overestimate was about 5% (Heaton *et al.* 1989b).

Survival of stored red cells taken from different subjects
In estimating the post-transfusion survival of stored red cells, allowance must be made for the fact that there are significant differences between donors. Dern *et al.* (1966) carried out at least two tests on each of 28 subjects whose blood was stored in ACD for 21 d and found consistent differences between subjects. Whereas the inherent experimental error, including the error of the method, biological variation between tests on the same subject, etc., had an SD of 6.4, the SD of differences between subjects was 6.6. Similar observations have been made by others; for example, C.A. Finch (personal communication, 1955) found that whereas the red cells of most normal donors, after storage in ACD for 3 weeks, had a 24 h survival of 70–85%, those taken from one particular donor regularly had a survival of only 60–65%. Another example is provided by Table 9.5 which shows that the 24 and 48 h survival of subjects 2 and 3 was consistently better than that of subjects 1 and 4. In another series in which red cells from six donors were stored in two different ACD solutions, after 28 d the ranking order of the donors with regard to survival was almost identical. It was particularly striking that one donor had the best survival on both occasions, and one by far the worst; in this latter subject (R.P.) the 24 h survival was 41% and 33% on the two occasions, compared with mean values of 74% and 75% in the other five subjects (Mishler *et al.* 1979). Further investigations on the red cells of R.P. showed that during storage their rate of loss of deformability was substantially greater than in other subjects (Card *et al.* 1983).

In another investigation, donors were selected according to the results of previous measurements of autologous red cell survival after storage. From these previous measurements, nine were predicted to have better than average survival and four, worse than average. Further measurements of the survival of autologous red cells after

Table 9.5 Effect of a preliminary 2 h incubation at 37°C before 28 d storage at 4°C on the subsequent post-transfusion survival of autologous red cells (Mollison, 1961b)

Subject	(A) No preliminary incubation*			(B) Preliminary incubation*		
	Survival (%)[†] at			Survival (%)[†] at		
	10 min	24 h	48 h	10 min	24 h	48 h
1	94	65	67	92	54	53
2	82	79	76	91	74	74
3	94	82	82	87	75	71
4	80	66	66	78	58	59
Mean	87.5	73.0	72.8	87.0	65.3	64.3

For the 24-h figures (A vs. B), $t = 3.68$, $P < 0.05 > 0.01$.
* In order to avoid systematic bias, the red cells of subjects 1 and 2 were stored first by method A, then by method B, and those of subjects 3 and 4 first by method B, and then by method A.
[†] Survival determined by a double labelling method. Fresh red cells labelled with ^{32}P to determine RCV; stored cells labelled with ^{51}Cr; results corrected for Cr elution.

storage showed that observed survival correlated reasonably well ($r = 0.648$) with predicted survival (Myhre *et al.* 1990).

In the above paragraph, autologous rather than allogeneic red cells were used in all series (with the possible exception of that of C.A. Finch) but, as described in the series in the paragraph below, the point is not an important one.

Evidently, in comparing two methods of red cell preservation, it is essential either to use a relatively large number of subjects or, if only a few subjects are used, to compare both methods in the same subject. An example is given in Table 9.5. Note that if method B had been used to store the red cells of subjects 2 and 3 and method A for subjects 1 and 4, the conclusion would have been reached that method B gives a better 24 h survival rate (mean 74.5%) than method A (mean 65.5%) — the very reverse of the probable truth.

The recipient appears to exert a relatively minor effect on the survival of donor red cells. In two different studies, the survival of stored red cells from any particular subject appeared to be the same in the subject's own circulation as in the circulation of a recipient injected with part of the same sample (Dern, 1968; Shields, 1969b; Dern *et al.* 1970).

In subjects with certain diseases, including carcinomatosis, the immediate survival of stored red cells may be better than in relatively normal subjects, e.g. subjects with trauma, although no differences are observed at 24 h; presumably these differences are due to some impairment of the function of the mononuclear phagocyte system (Szymanski and Valeri, 1969).

Differences between young and old red cells
The effect of increasing periods of storage on the post-transfusion survival of red cells calls for some comment. As already mentioned, the survival curve of red cells stored for relatively short periods (under 2 weeks) in a suitable preservative solution is characterized by destruction of up to 10% of the cells within the first 24 h with normal survival of the remainder, i.e. removal of about 1% a day. This finding suggests that the cells rendered non-viable are a random sample of the population and that the remainder are

still capable of normal survival. The idea that young and old red cells are equally susceptible to damage by storage receives support from an observation of Ozer and Chaplin (1963) using an antiserum which agglutinated stored red cells but not fresh red cells; young cells became agglutinable on storage to just the same extent as old red cells.

Red cells stored for 28 d or more (in ACD) show a different survival pattern (Fig. 9.2). About one-quarter are removed in 24 h and the remainder disappear at a rate distinctly faster than 1% a day. This finding suggests that after relatively long periods of storage, young red cells are more affected than old red cells, or alternatively that post-transfusion survival of all the red cells is adversely affected. The experiments of Gabrio and Finch (1954) in dogs showed that after only 20 d storage young red cells were far more severely damaged than old red cells, suggesting that dog red cells show much bigger differences in this respect than do human red cells.

Viability of red cells stored in various media

Trisodium citrate or heparin
In blood stored with trisodium citrate alone, the red cells deteriorate rapidly; after 1 week only about 50% of the cells are viable, and after 2 weeks, almost none (Ross et al. 1947). In blood stored with heparin, red cells deteriorate about as rapidly (Mollison and Young, 1942) but, because it is progressively neutralized by plasma, heparin is even more unsuitable for blood storage than trisodium citrate (see also Chapter 1).

The addition of 3 g dextrose to a unit of blood stored with trisodium citrate enormously improves the maintenance of viability; after storage for 18 d, post-transfusion survival is better than that of red cells stored with trisodium citrate alone for only 1 week (Mollison and Young, 1942).

Citric acid–trisodium citrate–dextrose solutions
In trials of five different solutions with a pH, at room temperature, ranging from 4.59 to 5.66, in which 110 ml solution was added to 420 ml blood, it was found that red cell survival was substantially better than with trisodium citrate–dextrose alone, in which the pH was 5.86 (Loutit et al. 1943).

The first ACD solution to be used routinely, 'disodium citrate–glucose' (Loutit and Mollison, 1943), chosen on the grounds of simplicity and of giving good red cell survival after storage, had a pH of 5.0. More than 20 years later, this pH was shown to be optimal for the long-term preservation of red cell ATP (Beutler and Duron, 1965).

For storage periods up to about 30 d the 24-h survival of red cells stored as blood mixed with ACD decreases linearly with time; thereafter the decrease in viability is a little more rapid. (Dern et al. 1967; Shields, 1968; 1969a,b; 1970; Haradin et al. 1969; Orlina and Josephson, 1969; Dern, 1970; Seidl and Spielmann, 1970; Strumia et al. 1970; Warner, 1970). When blood is stored with CPD (Gibson et al. 1957), which contains relatively less citric acid than ACD (see Appendix 8), viability appears to be lost just a little more slowly. For example, after 21 d storage, Orlina and Josephson (1969) found an average survival of 79.4% for red cells stored in CPD compared with 74.8% for red cells stored in ACD, although in another study survival was approximately 82% both with CPD and ACD (Högman et al. 1974). After 28 d storage, Dern (1970) found the average survival with CPD to be 77% compared with 72% for cells stored with ACD and Warner (1970) found that, with CPD, survival after 28 d storage was 76% in one series and 71.8% in another, whereas with ACD after 21 d storage it was 78%.

Red cell 2,3-DPG is better maintained in CPD than in ACD; at the end of only 1 week most of the 2,3-DPG has been lost from blood stored in ACD, but in blood stored with CPD the level is still appreciable; nevertheless, after 2 weeks, 2,3-DPG may almost have disappeared from CPD blood (see review by Beutler, 1974). The rate of depletion of 2,3-DPG from blood stored with CPD seems to be rather variable. Possibly, factors such as the frequency of mixing (Bensinger et al. 1975) and the permeability of the container to CO_2 may affect the results.

The favourable effect of CPD on DPG levels is due mainly to its higher pH (de Verdier et al. 1964a; Chanutin, 1967a; Beutler et al. 1969; Dawson et al. 1970). The mutase activity of the enzyme which controls the synthesis of 2,3-DPG is favoured by a neutral pH whereas the phosphatase activity of the enzyme, responsible for the breakdown of 2,3-DPG, is favoured by an acid pH (de Verdier et al. 1970). The fact that both mutase and phosphatase activities are carried by a single molecule was demonstrated by Rosa et al. (1975).

Acid–citrate–dextrose with reduced citrate concentration. Partly with the object of diminishing citrate toxicity, a modified ACD solution containing only 1.1 g trisodium citrate/dl instead of 2.2 g/dl, with the same amount of citric acid and dextrose (total citrate 5.1 mmol instead of 7.6 mmol per unit), was devised and tested by Mishler et al. (1978). ATP and 2,3-DPG were found to be just as well maintained after storage as in a solution of the used citrate concentration. Furthermore, red cell viability was as well maintained as with standard ACD after 28 d storage (Mishler et al. 1979). ACD with a reduced citrate concentration is commonly used by some centres for plasmapheresis, cytapheresis and plasma exchange.

Effect of excess of ACD or CPD

During the course of an ordinary donation, the first red cells to be collected are necessarily mixed with an excess of anticoagulant solution. Gibson et al. (1956) labelled the red cells for the first 100 ml blood to be collected into ACD and found that after 28 d storage at 5°C the cells had a post-transfusion survival of 20–32%, whereas the survival of the cells of the whole unit was between 44 and 61%. Similarly, when blood was incubated at 37°C for 30 min with half its volume or more of ACD the survival of the red cells *in vivo* was 50% or less at 24 h (Mayer et al. 1966; 1970).

When a full unit of blood cannot be collected from a donor there is a risk of damage to the red cells, due to the relatively high ratio of anticoagulant solution to blood. From a study in which varying amounts of blood were collected into amounts of ACD or CPD intended for 450 ml blood, and were then stored for 21 d, it was concluded that, with ACD, only collections of 400 g or more should be accepted, although with CPD those of 300 g were satisfactory. With storage periods as long as 35 d red cells of units 'undercollected' into CPDA-1 are actually at an advantage, presumably due to the higher ratio of nutrients to cells; in a carefully controlled study, donations of 275 ml had a mean 24-h survival of 87.7% compared with 78.8% for standard donations of 450 ml (Davey et al. 1984).

Purine nucleosides

Gabrio *et al.* (1955a) showed that the ATP content of stored red cells could be almost completely restored by incubation at 37°C with adenosine for 1 h. Restoration of the ATP content was accompanied by an increased post-transfusion survival: in one experiment red cells were first stored for 21 d in ACD, then incubated for 1 h with adenosine, then stored for a further 21 d at 4°C. Survival was now 87% (average of three cases). Control cells stored for 42 d without intermediate 'rejuvenation' with adenosine had a survival of only 15% (Gabrio *et al.* 1955b).

The addition of adenosine at the beginning of the storage period significantly improves the maintenance of red cell viability. When whole blood was stored without adenosine for 42 d post-transfusion survival fell to 10%, but if adenosine was added at the beginning of the storage period, after 42 d it was 75%. In blood stored with adenosine, post-transfusion survival fell to 50% only after 80–90 d (Gabrio *et al.* 1956). Adenosine is thought to produce its effects by being phosphorylated to adenosine monophosphate (Sahota *et al.* 1980).

Inosine also appeared to be effective in restoring the ATP content of stored red cells (Gabrio and Huennekens, 1955) but it is now thought that the result was due to the contamination of the inosine solution with adenine (Finch, 1985). On the other hand, incubation of red cells with inosine leads to restoration of depleted 2,3-DPG levels; see section on rejuvenation of stored red cells below.

There are potential disadvantages in adding either adenosine or inosine to blood as a routine measure; the toxic effects have been briefly reviewed previously (Mollison, 1961b, p. 23) and may be summarized by saying that although adenosine produces transient hypotension and heart block, these effects would be unlikely to be troublesome in practice when adenosine was added to blood *in vitro* since the compound is rapidly deaminated to inosine. The only probable hazard from inosine is that the catabolism of every mol produces 1 mol uric acid; e.g. 2.5 g inosine yields 1.5 g uric acid (Rubinstein *et al.* 1959). Following the transfusion of 3 units of blood stored with IAG solution (inosine 10 mmol, adenine 0.5 mmol and guanosine 0.5 mmol) there may be considerable rises in serum uric acid (Seidl and Spielmann, 1970).

Adenine

Suggestive evidence of the beneficial effect of adenine was obtained by Nakao *et al.* (1960) when they showed that in blood stored with adenine and inosine, the ATP level in the red cells was higher (and red cell osmotic fragility lower) than in blood stored with inosine alone.

Simon (1962) showed that when adenine in a final concentration of 0.5 μmol/ml was added to ACD blood, after 42 d storage post-transfusion survival was 74% compared with 49% in controls (ACD alone). In another study it was reported that 30 samples from 14 donors had been stored with 0.5–1.0 μmol adenine per ml ACD blood and transfused to 60 recipients and that the average post-transfusion survival of the samples after an average of 43 d was 75% compared with 47% in control samples stored for the same length of time in ACD alone.

Numerous studies have confirmed the beneficial effect of adenine on red cell preservation (de Verdier *et al.* 1964b; Åkerblom *et al.* 1967; Wood and Beutler, 1967; Shields, 1968; 1969a,b; Strumia *et al.* 1970; Warner, 1970). On the average, post-transfusion survival falls to 80% after about 3 weeks in ACD but falls to this level only after 5 weeks in ACD–adenine. Red cells separated from their plasma and mixed with a buffered solution containing adenine and glucose, after storage for 50 d have as good viability (74%) as red cells stored as whole blood mixed with ACD and adenine (Wood and Beutler, 1971).

In ACD blood, the addition of adenine only slightly reduces the rate of spontaneous haemolysis (de Verdier *et al.* 1964a). After 21 d storage in ACD alone, plasma Hb is usually in the range 40–60 mg/100 ml (Chaplin and Chang, 1955); after 35 d in ACD–adenine, the level is about 100 mg/100 ml (de Verdier *et al.* 1964b).

Toxicity of adenine. No adverse clinical reactions attributable to adenine were noted by De Verdier *et al.* (1966) in a series of over 5000 transfusions of blood to which 35 mg (approximately 0.26 mmol) adenine per unit had been added. Åkerblom *et al.* (1967) concluded that the only potential hazard seemed to arise from the formation of the metabolite 2,8-dioxyadenine (DOA), which is poorly soluble and may be deposited in renal tubules.

In practice, it seems that the only patients at risk are those who have really massive transfusions. In one study no impairment of renal function was found in patients who had received approximately 17 units of ACD–adenine blood (Westman, 1972); and in another study, of six patients who had died in the immediate post-operative period, DOA crystals were found in the kidneys in only three of the patients, who had received, respectively, 17, 46 and 95 mg adenine per kg body-weight (Falk *et al.* 1972; Westman, 1974).

CPD–adenine blood (final concentration of adenine 0.25 mmol/l, or approximately 34 mg/l) appears to be safe for exchange transfusion in newborn infants, even when repeated exchange transfusions have to be given (Kreuger, 1976).

A specification for adenine for use in blood preservation together with a description of a standard preparation of at least 99.5% purity was published as a Report of the National Academy of Sciences–National Research Council (1974).

CPD–adenine vs. ACD–adenine

After 4 and 5 weeks' storage the viability of red cells stored in CPD–adenine (final concentration 0.25 mmol/l) is better than in CPD alone, e.g. at 4 weeks, 76% compared with 66% (Åkerblom and Kreuger, 1975). For periods of storage up to 35 d post-transfusion viability is no better maintained in CPD–adenine than in ACD–adenine (Shields, 1968; de Verdier *et al.* 1969; Warner, 1970), although after 42 d, viability is slightly better in CPD–adenine (Warner, 1970).

In a trial in which six different laboratories collaborated, the mean 24-h survival for 50 cases in which red cells were stored as whole blood with CPD–adenine was 79% (SD 10%) (Moore *et al.* 1981). The solution used was CPDA-1, which is the official name for CPD with 25% extra dextrose and with a final concentration of 0.25 mmol/l adenine (see Appendix 8).

The addition of adenine to ACD, to give a final concentration in the blood mixture of 0.5 mmol, hastens the loss of 2,3-DPG (Sugita and Simon, 1965; Beutler *et al.* 1969). In more alkaline media, 2,3-DPG is better maintained (de Verdier *et al* 1964a; Chanutin, 1967b; Beutler *et al.* 1969); if the final concentration of adenine in

CPD–adenine blood is reduced to 0.25 mmol/l, 2,3-DPG falls only very slightly more rapidly than in CPD blood without adenine and ATP is only slightly less well maintained.

In an experimental study, the addition of ascorbate to blood stored in a phosphate–dextrose–adenine solution resulted in good maintenance of DPG values for as long as 5 weeks, with satisfactory maintenance of viability despite reduced ATP levels (Carmen et al. 1988).

Storage of packed red cells

If most of the supernatant plasma is removed from ACD blood and the packed cells are stored, their viability is as well maintained (Ross et al. 1947; Prins and Loos, 1970) or almost as well maintained (Shields, 1969a; 1971) as in whole blood with ACD.

Similarly, after 5 weeks' storage red cells stored as whole blood with CPD–adenine had a mean post-transfusion survival of 78.7%, which was not significantly different from the value of 76.5% for packed red cells from CPD–adenine. Furthermore, red cell 2,3-DPG was the same (30%) in whole blood and in packed cells after 3 weeks' storage (Kreuger et al. 1975).

In another study in which six laboratories collaborated, after 35 d storage in CPDA-1 the mean survival for red cells stored as whole blood was 79% and of red cells stored as a concentrate with a PCV of 0.75 ± 0.05 was 71% (Moore et al. 1981).

When red cells from blood mixed with a CPD–adenine solution (not CPDA-1) were packed to a PCV of 0.70–0.90%, the maintenance of acceptable levels of ATP for a full 42 d was found to depend on doubling the level of dextrose in the anticoagulant solution from 138.7 mmol/l (2.5 g/dl) to 277.5 mmol/l (5 g/dl). If dextrose is doubled, adenine can be decreased to a final concentration of 0.25 mmol/l with maintenance of ATP at more than 2.0 μmol/g Hb (Bensinger et al. 1975). In another study it was also found that beyond 21 d ATP was not quite as well maintained in packed cells from CPD–adenine (final concentration 0.25 mmol/l) as in whole blood, although even after 42 d almost all values were above 40% of the original level. It was concluded that in standard CPD–adenine there is enough dextrose for packed cell storage for 35 d but that in some units the amount may be marginal by 42 d (Dawson et al. 1976).

More detailed studies of the effect of PCV on the maintenance of viability were made by Beutler and West (1979). Red cell concentrates with PCVs of more than 0.80 were found to have consumed all their dextrose by the end of 21 d when they were derived from CPD blood, although when they were derived from a CPD–adenine solution (CPDA-1) adequate dextrose was still left at 21 d, presumably because CPDA-1 contains 1.25 times as much dextrose as CPD. The same authors found that of six CPD units, stored for 21 d as packed cells with a PCV of 0.80 or more, five had a 24-h post-transfusion survival of less than 70%. In one unit stored at a PCV of 0.92, the 24-h survival was 41%. By contrast, of packed cells from seven CPDA-1 units stored for 21 d with a PCV of 0.83–0.96, only those of one (PCV of 0.955) failed to achieve 70% viability. Finally, the authors pointed out that data from ACD packed red cells are not relevant for CPD-packed cells because dextrose consumption is slower in ACD than in CPD due to lower pH and lower phosphate content and that, furthermore, the dextrose concentration is initially slightly higher in ACD units.

Data with regard to adenine in stored packed red cells from CPD–adenine units were supplied by Kreuger and Åkerblom (1980). In two units stored with CPD at PCVs of 0.73 and 0.80, respectively, adenine fell to zero at 2 weeks; after the first 3 weeks ATP levels fell faster than in whole blood. Trials of CPDA-2 (Appendix 8), containing increased concentrations of adenine and dextrose, were reported by Sohmer et al. (1981). After 42 d storage, red cells stored as concentrates with a PCV of 0.75 had a mean 24-h survival of 76.7%, and those with a PCV of 0.85 had a mean survival of 70.6%. It was concluded that CPDA-2 should replace CPDA-1 when red cells were to be stored as concentrates.

Resuspension of red cells in saline–adenine–dextrose solution
The demand for large volumes of fresh plasma for fractionation has led to the practice of storing red cells in electrolyte media.

Red cells resuspended in a medium containing adenine and glucose retain viability very well and in one study were found to have a post-transfusion survival of 80% after 6 weeks' storage (Strauss et al. 1969). If 2,3-DPG levels are to be maintained, the solution must be buffered to prevent the fall in pH which otherwise occurs due to the production of large amounts of lactic acid. Red cells stored in a solution containing bicarbonate, adenine and glucose maintained good levels of 2,3-DPG for 42 d, al-though viability was not so well maintained as with whole blood stored with ACD–adenine. Moreover, satisfactory maintenance of 2,3-DPG was found only when the blood was stored in small bags, probably because such containers permit adequate transpiration of CO_2 (Beutler and Wood, 1972). The problem of the removal of CO_2 produced during storage could be overcome by the development of an internal absorption system, namely granular calcium hydroxide in a small plastic bag, inserted into the blood container. Using this system, and a medium containing bicarbonate adenine, glucose, phosphate and mannitol (BAGPM) it was possible, after 42 d storage, to maintain 2,3-DPG levels at 92% of the original, and ATP at levels of approximately 62%, indicating that viability was probably well maintained (Bensinger et al. 1977).

The clinical value of red cells (freed from buffy coats) stored in a saline–adenine–glucose (SAG) solution was demonstrated in extensive clinical trials in Sweden; it was noted that the final suspensions had less than 20% of the number of micro-aggregates found in whole blood (Högman et al. 1978a). With SAG solution there was an undesirable amount of lysis but this could be prevented by adding mannitol (Beutler, 1979). In further trials, red cells were stored in a modified solution, SAGM (Appendix 8), after separately harvesting platelets, buffy coat and plasma from units of blood. After storage for 5 or 6 weeks the red cell were reinjected into the original donor; viability was estimated by taking seven samples between 5 and 30 min after injection and extrapolating to zero time to obtain the theoretical 100% survival value. After 5 weeks, mean survival was 83.5 (SD 5.3)% and after 42 d was 77.4 (SD 4.7)% (Högman et al. 1983). Similarly, after 42 d storage in SAGM containing twice as much adenine as the original solution, 24-h survival averaged 78.2% (Heaton et al. 1989b).

Tests of a solution containing 60% more adenine and nearly 2.5 times as much glucose (Adsol, Appendix 8) were described by Heaton et al. (1984). The 100% survival value was estimated by taking six samples between 5 and 20 min, plotting the values and extrapolating to zero time. The mean 24-h survival of 20 units after 35 d storage was 86%; there was no significant difference between units with an initial mean PCV of 0.73 and those with an initial PCV of 0.83. Mean survival after 56 d was 71% with five out of ten values between 62% and 69%. After 49 d mean survival was 76%. In another study of the same solution, in which the 100% survival value was calculated from an estimate of plasma volume, mean 24-h survival in ten subjects whose red cells had been stored for 49 d was 57 (SD 9)% (Valeri, 1985). It was suggested that the discrepancy between the results of the two studies was due to the fact that the loss rate of non-viable cells was far higher in the first 5 min than subsequently, i.e. 16% in the first 5 min compared with 4% in the next 25 min. On the other hand, in a third study, in which viability was assessed in ten subjects, first by the extrapolation method and second by using a second red cell label to determine the expected 100% survival value, the estimates made by the two methods differed by only 2.6%, i.e. 75.4% for the extrapolation method and 72.8% for the double red cell label method (Beutler and West, 1985). The results of this third study evidently agree closely with those of Heaton et al. (1984), as do those of one later one, i.e. 79% after 42 d (Moroff et al. 1990).

Effect of mixing red cells during storage

In whole blood stored in plastic bags with CPD or ACD–adenine, the red cells have a significantly better 24 h survival and a higher ATP content and undergo less spontaneous lysis if the blood is mixed daily during storage (Dern et al. 1970). Similarly, red cells stored in SAGM solution (see above) show less spontaneous lysis and shed fewer microvesicles if the suspension is mixed weekly; the effect may be due to dissipation, on mixing, of acid metabolites which collect in the bottom layer of stored red cells (Högman et al. 1987).

'Rejuvenation' of stored red cells

The term 'rejuvenation' as applied to stored red cells has been used in two different senses: first, to describe the restoration of good viability, and second, to describe the restoration of 2,3-DPG levels.

The viability of stored red cells can be greatly increased by incubation with adenosine at 37°C for 1 h before transfusion (Gabrio et al. 1955a,b; Prankerd, 1958; Mollison and Robinson, 1959). A striking effect can also be produced by incubation with adenine and inosine (Nakao et al. 1962).

It is possible not only to restore DPG levels in stored red cells but actually to increase them to supra-normal levels by incubation with inosine, phosphate and pyruvate (MacManus and Borgese, 1961). Pyruvate greatly increases the amount of DPG produced, probably by oxidizing NADH and NAD and thus preventing the inhibition of glyceraldehyde phosphate dehydrogenase caused by NADH (Duhm et al. 1971). In one study it was found that in stored red cells in which the DPG level had fallen from an initial 4200 nmol/ml red cells to 345 nmol/ml, incubation at 37°C for 4 h with final concentrations of 10 mmol/l inosine, 4 mmol/l phosphate and 4 mmol/l pyruvate raised the DPG level to 5980 nmol/ml red cells (Oski et al. 1971b). In another study, incubation at 37°C for 3 h with 10 mmol/l inosine, 10 mmol/l pyruvate and 50 mmol/l inorganic phosphate raised the red cell DPG in fresh and stored ACD blood to four to five times the normal level (Duhm et al. 1971). Similar results were obtained with CPD–adenine and ACD–adenine, although at 4°C the rise in DPG was less pronounced (Åkerblom and Ericson, 1971).

A phosphate–inosine–glucose–pyruvate solution has been used to restore DPG levels of red cells after liquid storage and before freezing (Valeri and Zaroulis, 1972).

Effect of storage temperature on maintenance of red cell viability

Blood is commonly stored at a temperature of about 4°C but the reasons for the choice of this temperature are not obvious. Perhaps the most likely explanation is that the intention has always been simply to keep blood as cold as possible without allowing it to freeze. In fact, blood mixed with ACD solution freezes at about – 0.5°C and may be supercooled to – 3°C and maintained indefinitely at that temperature without freezing (Strumia, 1954a).

It might, therefore, appear that a temperature in the region of, say, 0 to 2°C ought to be used, rather than 4°C. It is rather surprising that so few attempts have been made to discover the optimal temperature for red cell preservation.

Strumia (1954b) claimed that provided a low dextrose concentration was used, storage at 1–2°C was superior to storage at 4–6°C. This conclusion was based on observations of the recipient's bilirubin concentration after transfusion, and the data provide no quantitative information on the relative survival of red cells stored at these two temperatures.

Hughes-Jones (1958b) made a careful study of the effect on preservation of storage at temperatures between – 10°C and + 10°C. He used the same medium for storage at all temperatures, namely, a solution containing citrate–phosphate–dextrose and glycerol. The blood of each of a small group of volunteers was stored in turn at four different temperatures, namely: – 10, – 2, + 4 and + 10°C; storage of red cells from the same donor at different temperatures was an important point because, as mentioned above, considerable differences are found between donors, and if comparisons based on small numbers are to be valid each donor must serve as his own control. The mean post-transfusion (24 h) survival after 34 d storage was: – 10°C, 80%; – 2°C, 78%; + 4°C, 63%; and + 10°C, 52%.

In a study in which ACD blood was stored at temperatures between 4°C and 25°C some 24 h survival values were as follows: after 21 d at 4°C, 81%; after 12 d at 10°C, 74%; after 10 d at 15°C, 59%; after 5 d at 20°C, 45%; and after 1 d at 25°C, 60% (Strauss and Raderecht, 1974).

A period of only 24 h at 22°C has a relatively small effect. Shields (1970) compared the survival of red cells kept at 4°C throughout with that of cells warmed to 22°C for 24 h prior to transfusion. After storage in ACD for various periods, the figures were as follows (unwarmed results first): after 7 d, 92% vs. 87%; after 21 d, 84% vs. 78%; and after 28 d, 75% vs. 62%. A period of 6–7 h at room temperature before storage at 4°C for 21–22 d has a negligible effect on ATP levels, compared with those of samples refrigerated promptly after taking, results in only a slight lowering of 2,3-DPG levels (see below) and has little or no adverse effect on post-transfusion survival (Chapman *et al.* 1977; Avoy *et al.* 1978). As expected from the foregoing results, when blood was held at ambient temperature for 8 h before being stored at 4°C with Adsol for 42 d, 24-h survival was virtually the same as when it was held for only 6 h (Moroff *et al.* 1990).

At 37°C, red cells in ACD blood deteriorate rapidly: the DPG level falls to 20% in 5 h; after 24 h only 30% of the cells are viable; and after 48 h virtually none (Jandl and

Tomlinson, 1958). Even if blood is incubated at 37°C for only 2 h immediately after taking it from the donor and is then stored for 28 d, red cell survival is significantly diminished compared with the survival of red cells from the same donor stored for the same period but without 2 h incubation (see Table 9.5).

Karle (1969) compared the effect of 8-h incubation at 38°C and 41.5°C, respectively, on the subsequent survival of rabbit red cells. The red cells kept at 38°C had a normal survival at 4.5 h and a $T_{50}Cr$ of about 10 d. The cells kept at 41.5°C underwent 20% destruction in the first hour after transfusion and had a 60% survival at 4.5 h; the remaining cells had a $T_{50}Cr$ of about 8.5 d.

Effect of delayed cooling on 2,3-diphosphoglycerate in red cells

Prompt cooling to below 15°C prevents the loss of DPG from red cells. Blood taken freshly (into bottles) has a temperature of 30°C, but within 2 h of putting single bottles (or bags) into a ventilated coldroom the temperature of the blood has fallen below 15°C (Prins and Loos, 1970).

Estimates of the fall in 2,3-DPG in CPD or CPD–Adsol blood kept at ambient temperature of 6–8 h are as follows: after 6 h, 13% (Avoy et al. 1978) and 27% (Moroff et al. 1990), and after 8 h, 43% (Moroff et al. 1990).

Effect of plasticizers on stored red cells

Di (2-ethylhexyl) phthalate (DEHP)

As described in Chapter 15, the plasticizer phthalate leaches into blood during storage. The plastic is taken up by the red cell membrane and has the effect of diminishing the rate of progressive lysis of the red cells and of enhancing resistance to hypotonic lysis (Rock et al. 1983b; Estep et al. 1984; Horowitz et al. 1984). In a convincing experiment it was shown that the addition of phthalate to stored blood also has the effect of substantially slowing the rate of loss of viability of the red cells whether they are stored in plastic or glass containers (Aubuchon et al. 1984).

For a brief discussion of the toxicity of phthalates, see Chapter 15.

Butyryl-n-trihexyl citrate (BTHC)

Because of the potential toxicity of phthalates, a new type of plastic, PL-2209, incorporating BTHC, a plasticizer that is less toxic than DEHP, has been tested. Like DEHP, BTHC reduces red cell lysis during storage, although to a lesser extent. Red cell viability is as well maintained with either plastic (Buchholz et al. 1989; Högman et al. 1991c).

Effect of irradiation of red cells, stored either beforehand or subsequently

One effect of irradiation on red cells which are subsequently stored is to cause an increased loss of potassium (Hillyer et al. 1991). Within 48 h, the potassium concentration in the supernatant of red cell suspensions previously irradiated is about 30 mmol/l (Ramirez et al. 1987). The increased plasma potassium should be taken into account when transfusing premature infants (see p. 427). As plasma potassium rises, plasma sodium falls, suggesting damage to the sodium pump; in plasma-reduced blood irradiated with 15 Gy, plasma potassium reaches about 75 mmol/l after 10 d storage, compared with about 40 mmol/l in unirradiated controls (Dinning *et al.* 1991). Other effects are an increased rate of lysis and a slightly increased rate of loss of ATP and of DPG (Moore and Ledford, 1975), together with a fall in pH, suggesting a minor decrease in viability (Hillyer *et al.* 1991). In the only study of the effect on survival *in vivo*, red cells were irradiated with 4000 cGy after storage for 21 d, and then transfused; irradiation caused a small increase in plasma Hb but 24-h survival was not significantly different from that observed with unirradiated units (Button *et al.* 1981). The study was not rigorously controlled and a small deleterious effect cannot be excluded.

STORAGE OF RED CELLS IN THE FROZEN STATE

Satisfactory storage of red cells in the frozen state became possible when it was discovered that these cells, mixed with glycerol, could be frozen and thawed without damage (Smith, 1950). It was soon shown that rabbit red cells, after being freed from glycerol by dialysis, were capable of survival *in vivo* (Sloviter, 1951) and that human red cells, previously frozen to $-79\,°C$ in glycerol would survive well in humans (Mollison and Sloviter, 1951).

Red cells must be freed from glycerol before being transfused, and unfortunately it has proved to be difficult to develop simple and inexpensive methods for doing this. This difficulty has been chiefly responsible for the rather small use which is made of storage in the frozen state. Nevertheless, prolonged storage is invaluable in some circumstances, as will be described later.

Effects of freezing

The damaging effects of freezing are related to the rate of cooling: if tissues can be cooled within a few seconds to a temperature at which virtually all the water is frozen, severe damage can be avoided. Luyet and Gehenio (1940) showed that if frog cells were subjected to ultra-rapid cooling and thawing they could be recovered intact.

Florio *et al.* (1943) showed that if a small volume of citrated blood was mixed with an equal volume of 20% glucose and immediately frozen, on thawing there was only 2–3% lysis. A similar approach was followed by Meryman (1956) who mixed red cells with glucose and then sprayed them into liquid nitrogen. The resulting droplets were kept at the temperature of liquid nitrogen ($-196\,°C$) and subsequently thawed by being dropped into warm saline. This process has been used for the storage of small volumes of red cells for serological test.

De Verdier *et al.* (1963) carried out experiments to discover whether the red cells which lysed during the rapid freezing and thawing of blood (method of Meryman (1956), see above), were a random selection of the population. They gave radio-iron to normal subjects and bled them at various times in the next 3 months to obtain a population of red cells of different ages. It was concluded that young red cells are a little more resistant (see also Valeri and McCallum, 1965) and that 50% of the lysis is related to cell age, the remaining 50% being random.

When a solution freezes, pure ice forms and the remaining liquid becomes hypertonic. Lovelock (1953a) showed that many of the damaging effects of freezing upon tissues are those expected from exposure of the tissues to a hypertonic solution followed (on thawing) by exposure to an isotonic solution. Lovelock considered that it was the concentration of salts that was responsible for cell injury. However, later work suggests that, at slow rates of freezing, it is the loss of intracellular water and the associated reduction in cell volume, rather than the absolute concentration of solutes, that is directly responsible for injury (Meryman, 1971). The mechanism of damage seems to be either intracellular dehydration or stress to the cell membrane (see Meryman, 1989).

It is believed that at high rates of freezing, damage is due to the formation of intracellular ice rather than to the effects of hypertonicity (Mazur et al. 1972).

Substances that protect against damage by freezing

Substances which, when added to blood, decrease haemolysis after freezing and thawing include dextrose, lactose, sucrose, albumin, HES, PVP (polyvinylpyrrolidone) and dextran. However, whereas the low mol. wt. substances diminish the number of cells which lyse, the higher mol. wt. substances (albumin, HES, PVP and dextran) decrease the amount of Hb liberated from the individual cell without appreciably decreasing the number of damaged cells. The extent to which dextran decreases the lysis of red cells during freezing and thawing thus underestimates the real extent of damage (Zade-Oppen, 1968). Similarly, with PVP, post-transfusion haemoglobinuria after the transfusion of frozen red cells is a problem (see later). It is believed that PVP seals defects in red cell membranes and that these defects become apparent when the PVP is washed away in the circulation (Williams, 1976).

With all the substances mentioned in the foregoing paragraph, the rates of freezing and thawing must be very rapid if lysis is to be avoided. In contrast, when glycerol is used slow freezing and thawing give excellent results. The effect of glycerol is probably due to the fact that it limits ice formation and provides a liquid phase in which salts are distributed as cooling proceeds so that excessive hypertonicity is avoided (Lovelock, 1953b). Glycerol is most effective in protecting those cells (e.g. human red cells) into which it permeates fairly rapidly.

Use of glycerol

In 1949 it was discovered by a fortunate accident that glycerol would protect spermatozoa against the otherwise lethal effects of freezing (Polge et al. 1949) and soon afterwards it was found that red cells could also be protected (Smith, 1950). The following description of the way in which the protective effect of glycerol was discovered is based on published accounts (Sloviter, 1976; Parkes, 1985), supplemented by a personal communication from C. Polge.

In 1948 a group under A.S. Parkes was attempting to preserve spermatozoa in the frozen state; fructose was added because it is the principal metabolic substrate for sperm and is present in moderately high concentration in seminal fluid—but it did not work. C. Polge joined the group and decided to try again. He obtained from a cold room a bottle labelled 'laevulose' (another name for fructose) which contained a solution that had been made some weeks earlier. Spermatozoa were suspended in this solution and, after freezing and thawing, were found to be actively motile. In a freshly prepared solution of laevulose, after freezing and thawing, all sperm were non-motile. It was suggested that the solution might need to be aged but, after being aged, a new batch did not work. Meanwhile, almost all of the original bottle of 'laevulose' had been used up.

The remaining amount of 'laevulose' was then given to an organic chemist who soon found that no reducing sugar was present but that there was a lot of protein; the presence of glycerol was discovered when some of the solution was passed through a Bunsen burner flame and gave off the characteristic odour of acrolein. In the coldroom a bottle of laevulose labelled 'albumin-glycerol' (a solution used for histological preparations) was found. It was presumed that labels had become detached in the coldroom and had been stuck back on the wrong bottles.

Rate of freezing and optimal glycerol concentration

When red cells are frozen slowly, e.g. over a period of 30–60 min, they must be mixed with sufficient glycerol to give a final concentration of 4.5 mol/l (approximately 40% w/v) if haemolysis is to be completely prevented (Hughes-Jones et al. 1957a). On the other hand, when freezing is relatively rapid, as when the blood–glycerol mixture in a thin-walled metal container is plunged into liquid nitrogen, the final concentration of glycerol need be only 20% w/v (Pert et al. 1963). In the process developed by Krijnen et al. (1964), using the same concentration of glycerol, the blood reaches 0°C only after about 8 min, but cooling is then very rapid (about 2°C/s).

When red cells are to be frozen only to – 20°C, a final glycerol concentration of 3.0 mol/l is sufficient to prevent lysis. If the dextrose concentration is raised to about 220 mmol/l, the glycerol concentration can be reduced to about 1.4 mol/1 (see below).

Addition of glycerol to red cells and storage at low temperature

If solutions containing more than about 50% (w/v) glycerol are added to blood, some haemolysis results. The addition of 50% (w/v) glycerol in citrate to an equal volume of blood will give a final concentration of approximately 30% (w/v) in the fluid phase of the mixture, because the glycerol mixes not only with the plasma but also with the water space in the red cells, amounting to about 65% of their volume; if a final concentration exceeding 30% (w/v) glycerol is to be attained it is best to add the glycerol in stages (for an example, see Hughes-Jones et al. 1957a).

Storage temperature and maintenance of viability

Red cells mixed with a glycerol–citrate–phosphate solution and stored at – 20°C deteriorate only very slowly; after 3 months' storage the post-transfusion survival is only slightly less than that of fresh cells (Chaplin et al. 1954). Even after 18 months' storage more than 50% of the red cells are still viable (Hughes-Jones et al. 1957a). With a glycerol–dextrose–adenine–phosphate solution, 24-h survival after 10 months' storage was found to be more than 85% (Meryman and Hornblower, 1978).

At lower storage temperatures, deterioration is further slowed. At temperatures in the range – 40°C to – 50°C there does not seem to be any definite falling off in red cell survival over a period of up to 1 year or more (Chaplin et al. 1957; Hughes-Jones et al. 1957a), although Chaplin et al. (1957) deduced that after 5 years' storage at this temperature, post-transfusion survival would have fallen to 70%.

Storage at – 79°C (achieved by adding solid CO_2 to a bath of alcohol) was used in some of the earlier experiments with glycerol-treated red cells and shown to give satisfactory preservation (Mollison *et al.* 1952; Brown and Hardin, 1953). After a period of storage as long as 21 months at this temperature, post-transfusion survival may be as good as after storage for only a few weeks (Chaplin *et al.* 1956a).

Haynes *et al.* (1960) stored glycerolized red cells at $-80°C$ to $-120°C$ and found no evidence of deterioration with time; the two samples stored for the longest periods (36 and 44 months) had a post-transfusion survival of about 95%. Similarly, cells stored for up to 7 years at $-80°C$ and then stored at $4°C$ for 48 h showed approximately 90% survival at 24 h (Valeri *et al.* 1970). Storage for up to 21 years at $-80°C$ was reported by Valeri *et al.* (1989). Mean 24-h survival with various methods was 80–85%.

Methods suitable for routine use

Storage at $-20°C$
If the concentration of dextrose is increased to about 0.2 mol/l in a mixture of red cells, dextrose and glycerol, the glycerol concentration can be reduced to about 1.4 mol/l in the final mixture and still permit freezing to $-20°C$ and subsequent thawing without lysis. After a single wash in a solution containing mannitol and a relatively high concentration of dextrose, the red cells can be resuspended in a buffered, glycerol-free solution containing dextrose and adenine and stored at $4-6°C$ for up to 35 d. The whole process is carried out in a closed system, using special interconnected bags. In tests in ten subjects, red cells stored at $-20°C$ for 56 d, followed by storage at $4-6°C$ for 14–21 d, mean 24-h survival was 75.5%; recovery *in vitro* was 96% (Lovric and Klarkowski, 1989).

Storage at $-80°C$
The advantage of using a high glycerol concentration (4.0 mol/l or more) is that not only can freezing be slow but subsequent storage can be at a temperature as high as $-65°C$ ($-80°C$ is usually preferred), so that mechanical refrigeration can be used. Moreover, the frozen red cells can be transported in solid CO_2 ('dry ice', temperature $-80°C$).

Glycerol can be added to red cells in their original plastic packs (Valeri *et al.* 1981b); a minor modification of this method is described in Appendix 8. Although plastic blood containers of standard design can be used with this process, polyolefin is preferred to polyvinylchloride because with it there is less lysis during freezing and the containers are less brittle at $-80°C$. The standard method of deglycerolization after thawing is to dilute the thawed, glycerolized blood with 12% sodium chloride and, after allowing the mixture to equilibrate for 5 min, to wash the red cells with 3 litres saline. The cells are finally resuspended in 0.9% saline with 0.2% dextrose.

Storage at $-120°C$ or less
The only advantage of this method is that the final glycerol concentration can be as low as 2.25 mol/l (as in the method described by Krijnen *et al.* 1970). The disadvantages are that special containers must be used for freezing and storage and, because the temperature must not be allowed to rise above $-120°C$, the containers must in practice be stored in and transported in liquid nitrogen ($-196°C$).

Removal of glycerol from red cells
If red cells which have been stored with glycerol are to be transfused, their glycerol content must be reduced to about 1–2% or they will haemolyse on contact with plasma, owing to the fact that water can enter the cells more rapidly than glycerol can leave them. The number of washes needed can be substantially reduced by first exposing the red cells to a hypertonic solution of a non-penetrating substance such as citrate which causes the cells to shrink and lose much of the glycerol so that they can subsequently be washed in saline with little haemolysis (Lovelock, 1952).

In the method of Meryman and Hornblower (1972) 12% NaCl is added to a red cell glycerol mixture, followed, after 3 min by a relatively large volume of 1.6% NaCl. Thereafter the cells can be washed in a suitable blood processor, e.g. a Haemonetics, which uses disposable centrifuge bowls. Other machines which also use disposable equipment and provide for the automated continuous washing cells are the Elutra-matic (Orlina *et al.* 1972) and IBM cell processors. Wash solutions suitable for use with all of these machines are described by Valeri (1975).

Losses of red cells during processing
The disadvantage of freezing processes is that they involve small losses of red cells at various stages which, when added together, may become substantial. Valeri (1974) estimated these losses after varying periods of storage before and after freezing. When red cells were frozen at $-80°C$ in 40% w/v glycerol, then thawed, processed and transfused within 4 h, 86–92% of the original number of red cells was available for transfusion.

The concept of 'therapeutic effectiveness' was introduced by Valeri and Runck (1969) to take account of losses *in vitro* and *in vivo*. The index of therapeutic effectiveness (ITE) is simply the recovery *in vitro*, i.e. the number of red cells available for transfusion as a percentage of the number in the original unit, multiplied by the percentage survival *in vivo* at 24 h. Calculation of this index emphasizes that figures for post-transfusion survival alone give too optimistic a picture of the value of freezing as a means of preservation. For example, in the work of Valeri *et al.* (1989), quoted above, survival *in vivo* after storage for up to 21 years was 80–85%, but the ITE were 70–75%.

Storage of red cells before freezing
Red cells which are to be frozen in glycerol can first be kept as ACD blood for up to 7 d without any adverse effect on their ultimate survival (Valeri, 1965b).

Red cells stored at 4°C for as long as 42 d in a nutrient-additive solution 'AS-3', then frozen in glycerol and stored for 8 weeks, had an *in vitro* recovery of 81% and a 24-h survival of 78%, giving an ITE of 63% (Rathbun *et al.* 1989).

Rejuvenation of stored red cells followed by freezing
Red cells which had been stored as packed cells for 23 d were incubated at 37°C for 1 h with a solution containing pyruvate, inosine, glucose, phosphate and adenine. The cells were then mixed with glycerol and stored at $-80°C$ for up to 12 months. After thawing and washing they were transfused to anaemic patients. Such red cells had a 24-h survival of approximately 82% compared with 71% for cells which had not been

incubated with the 'rejuvenation' solution before being frozen. The rejuvenated red cells had a normal 2,3-DPG content whereas the unrejuvenated cells had almost no 2,3-DPG (Valeri and Zaroulis, 1972).

Storage of red cells after freezing

Red cells that have been thawed and deglycerolized by washing in electrolyte solutions and then resuspended in their own plasma can be kept at 4°C for up to 21 d and still have a post-transfusion survival of about 70% (Valeri, 1976a).

Storage of the deglycerolized red cells in Adsol was found to give better results than storage in dextrose–saline. After 10 d, the mean 24-h survival was 90% and the mean *in vitro* recovery 85.5%, giving an ITE of 77% (Ross *et al.* 1989).

Use of substances other than glycerol

Dimethylsulphoxide is as effective as glycerol in protecting cells against damage by freezing but has no clear advantage over it (for reference, see Mollison *et al.* 1987, p. 156).

PVP is potentially advantageous because it does not permeate red cells and therefore the cells can be transfused after thawing, without first having to be washed. Unfortunately, the process involves substantial lysis, post-transfusion survival is only about 70% (Morrison *et al.* 1968), and it is not certain that PVP is harmless.

Indications for the use of frozen red cells

The main advantage of storing blood in the frozen state is that the red cells can be kept for an indefinite period so that, for example, it becomes possible to accumulate a collection of bloods of rare red cell phenotypes. Accordingly, when a patient is encountered with one or more alloantibodies reacting singly or in combination with most human blood samples, it may be possible to find in the frozen red cell bank sufficient compatible units to supply the patient's needs. The alternative of trying to find suitable donors, willing to be bled at short notice, is likely to be far more difficult.

A particular problem arises when U-negative or Fy(a – b –) red cells are wanted. Many donors with these phenotypes have Hb AS and it is difficult to deglycerolize red cells from sickle cell trait donors, since hypertonic solutions cannot be used (Meryman and Hornblower, 1976). In fact, cell washers cannot be used for red cells from sickle cell trait donors. Incidentally, it is in practice a waste of time to try to freeze red cells from Hb SS donors.

Frozen (and washed) red cells have the advantage of being virtually free from plasma, leucocytes and platelets; see p. 684.

When autologous red cells have been collected but, for one reason or another have to be kept for more than a few weeks, freezing is the only appropriate method of preservation. As mentioned later, frozen red cells may be useful in paediatric practice, e.g. when a premature infant requires a series of transfusions.

If the freezing of red cells and their subsequent processing could be made simple enough and cheap enough there would be the great advantage of being able to accumulate stocks of red cells of common groups and thus to avoid the periodic shortages of supply that occur when blood is stored in the liquid state. So far, due to the cost, very few transfusion centres have felt able to use frozen red cells in this way. One estimate is that the cost of units stored in the frozen state is three times greater than that of units stored in the liquid state (Chaplin, 1984). However, this estimate refers to storage at $-80°C$ in a high glycerol concentration; storage at $-20°C$ in a low glycerol concentration should prove less costly.

THE TRANSFUSION OF RED CELLS IN ANAEMIA

The treatment of acute haemorrhage has been considered in Chapter 2. The present chapter deals only with patients who have a more or less normal blood volume.

Physiological compensations for anaemia

In anaemia the reduced capacity of the blood to carry oxygen is compensated for by (a) an increase in cardiac output and (b) an increase in the 2,3-DPG content of the red cells which causes a shift to the right in the oxygen dissociation curve, the effect of which is that at a given degree of oxygen saturation of the Hb, oxygen is more readily given up to the tissues. As an example, assuming that the oxygenation in the lungs is normal and that a capillary Po_2 of 30 mm Hg has to be maintained, an equal amount of O_2 can be released from 8.4 g Hb when the oxygen dissociation curve is shifted to the right (P_{50} 32 mm Hg) as from 14.0 g Hb when the oxygen dissociation curve is normal, i.e. P_{50} 27 mm Hg; see Högman (1971).

Despite the compensatory change in the oxygen dissociation curve, since the amount of oxygen delivered to the tissues = cardiac output × arterial oxygen content, and since the latter is diminished in anaemia, the anaemic patient can maintain the supply of oxygen to the tissues only by increasing cardiac output and thus diminishing the cardiac reserve. Accordingly, if transfusion is considered for a chronically anaemic patient, the advantage of raising the arterial oxygen content has to be weighed against the hazards of overloading an already hyperkinetic circulation.

Effect of transfusion on the circulation

Normovolaemic subjects

In subjects with a previously stable blood volume, rapid transfusion produces a transient rise in venous pressure, but venous pressure falls to normal as soon as the transfusion is stopped, even though blood volume may remain above normal for many hours after this. For example, in one normal subject the transfusion of 1600 ml serum in 14 min produced a considerable increase in plasma volume, as shown by a fall in Hb concentration of 23.5%. Venous pressure rose from 0 to 10.5 cm H_2O during the transfusion; 14 min after the end of the transfusion venous pressure (measured in an antecubital vein) was only 1 cm, although the Hb concentration was still 20% below the pre-transfusion level (Sharpey-Schäfer and Wallace, 1942b).

After large rapid transfusions of serum or blood, vital capacity is diminished showing that part of the added fluid is accommodated in the blood vessels of the lungs. However, the degree of reduction in vital capacity accounts for only a part of the additional volume and doubtless the larger veins and subpapillary venous plexus also accommodate extra fluid (Loutit *et al.* 1942; Sharpey-Schäfer and Wallace 1942b).

Rate of extrusion of plasma from the circulation. In cats transfused in less than 1 h with an amount of plasma equal to their initial plasma volume, at 24 h plasma volume was back to its original value (Florely and Jenings, 1941). Similarly, in human subjects with a stable blood volume transfused with 700–2100 ml serum in 7–27 min, in most instances plasma volume was only slightly above its initial value at 1 h, although in a few subjects readjustment took more than 24 h (Sharpey-Schäfer and Wallace, 1942a).

Rate of readjustment of blood volume after transfusion

Relatively few observations have been made on the rate of readjustment of blood volume after transfusions of red cell suspensions or whole blood. In four patients transfused with approximately 500 ml of concentrated red cell suspensions in 20–40 min, Hb concentration, PCV and donor red cell concentration were all about 10% greater in the 24 and 48 h samples than in the sample taken 5 min after transfusion. These observations indicate that blood volume was temporarily increased by an amount approximately equal to the volume transfused. In eight further cases an average of 1010 ml citrated blood was transfused in periods varying from 20 to 85 min, and samples were taken in the same way. Again, the estimates at 24 and 48 h all showed a rise in values of about 10% compared with the immediate post-transfusion sample (Mollison, 1947). Notice that these figures do not refer to the total change in values produced by transfusion but to the shift in values following the end of transfusion.

Because some subjects take as long as 24 h to readjust blood volume, the effects of the transfusion of large amounts of blood must always be carefully monitored, particularly in those patients whose venous pressure is already raised before transfusion has begun.

Rate of readjustment of blood volume in newborn infants

An infant weighing 3.5 kg has at the moment of birth about 270 ml blood in its body and about another 120 ml in the placental circulation. Provided that the cord is not tied until about 5 min after birth most of the blood in the placenta is transferred to the infant. During the following 3–4 h the amount of plasma lost from the circulation is greater than the amount transferred from the placenta, so that plasma volume actually shrinks slightly (Mollison et al. 1950; Usher et al. 1963); more than 70 ml plasma may leave the circulation in the first 30 min after birth (Usher et al. 1963).

In a previous edition of this book an example was given of the rapid readjustment of blood volume in a 5-week-old infant transfused in 20 min with 75 ml citrated blood. Readjustment of blood volume was virtually complete by the time a sample was taken 5 min after transfusion (Mollison, 1961b, p. 129)

Diminished control of blood volume in renal insufficiency

If transfusions are given to patients with diminished renal function, the resulting increase in blood volume is far more prolonged than in normal subjects. Because of this prolonged expansion of blood volume the Hb concentration may fail to rise during the day or two following a transfusion and this may lead to a suspicion that the transfused red cells have been eliminated. Figures 9.4 and 9.5 show some findings in a case of this kind (Mollison 1961b, p. 52). As Fig. 9.4 shows, the patient's Hb concentration failed to rise following transfusion of red cells from 2 units of blood

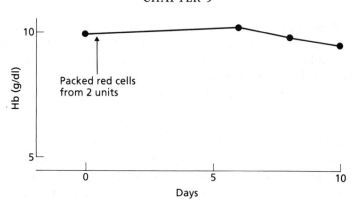

Figure 9.4 Failure of the haemoglobin (Hb) concentration to rise materially following transfusion, in a patient with chronic renal insufficiency. Transfused red cells were shown to survive normally (Fig. 9.5), and the failure of the Hb concentration to rise was evidently due to very slow readjustment of blood volume.

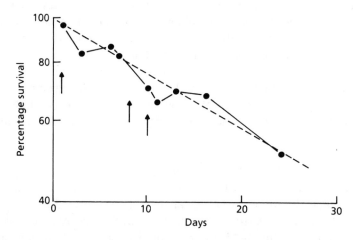

Figure 9.5 Red cell survival (^{51}Cr) in a patient with chronic renal insufficiency (see Fig. 9.4). Following each transfusion (↑), the concentration of labelled red cells was depressed for several days due to slow readjustment of blood volume.

(1 unit = 420 ml blood with 120 ml ACD). Four weeks later a further transfusion of red cells from 1 unit of blood was given and at the same time 10 ml of the red cells were labelled with ^{51}Cr and injected. The red cells were eliminated at the normal rate (Fig. 9.5), although the individual estimates of survival did not fall on a smooth curve, presumably due to the gross fluctuations in blood volume produced by further transfusions during the observation period.

The failure of subjects with impaired renal function to correct blood volume promptly after transfusion was demonstrated by Hillman (1964). In two subjects with renal failure, one of whom was completely anuric, 525 ml stored, pooled plasma was transfused. Two hours later, the increase in blood volume still amounted to 90% of the volume of plasma transfused, whereas in normal subjects the figure was approximately 60%. It was shown that the increase in plasma volume persisted for at least 5 h.

Post-transfusion rise in Hb concentration in patients with splenomegaly

In patients with gross splenomegaly, the transfusion of a given quantity of blood produces a far smaller increase in Hb concentration than in patients with a normal spleen. Huber *et al.* (1964) supplied the following figures: in patients without a major degree of splenomegaly (spleen palpable no more than 5 cm below the costal margin, or not palpable at all), the transfusion of 1 unit whole blood (approximately 180 ml red cells) increased Hb concentration by 0.9 ± 0.12 g/dl; in subjects with splenomegaly the increase was 0.6 ± 0.16 g/dl.

It has been shown that when the spleen weighs more than 750 g it contains 13–66% of the total red cell mass (Motulsky *et al.* 1958; Strumia *et al.* 1962).

Rate of transfusion in subjects with a normal circulation

In subjects who have no degree of circulatory failure there is no harm in producing some temporary increase in blood volume. It has to be remembered that for many patients transfusion is an ordeal which they wish to get through as quickly as possible. It is perfectly safe in the ordinary way to transfuse 1000 ml citrated blood within a period of 2 or 3 h. With giving sets which deliver about 15 drops/min, a rate of 120 drops/min will correspond to giving a unit of blood in 1 h. Since in practice it is difficult to maintain steady drip rates when blood is simply being given by gravity, other methods of checking the rate of transfusion are sometimes helpful. For example, the bag of blood can be hung on a spring balance and the weight noted at the time when transfusion is started; at any subsequent time the amount of blood given can be readily determined.

Transfusion in severe anaemia

In severe anaemia the risk of overloading the circulation can be minimized by: (a) restricting the rate of transfusion to about 1 ml/kg body-weight per hour (Marriott and Kekwick, 1940); (b) using packed red cells rather than whole blood; and (c) taking various measures to reduce the right atrial pressure; e.g. propping the patient up in a sitting position (Sharpey-Schäfer, 1945). Central venous pressure should be recorded continuously in any patient who is regarded as being at risk from overloading. In view of the need to keep a close watch on the patient, transfusions should not normally be allowed to continue at night unless the patient has special nursing care. The administration of a diuretic (e.g. frusemide, initial dose 40 mg) is an essential pre-transfusion measure in all patients whose extracellular fluid volume may be increased, e.g. those in any degree of cardiac or renal failure.

Frusemide must always be given as a separate i.v. injection and not added to the blood which is being transfused: first, for the general reason that it is undesirable to add anything whatsoever to blood which is being transfused, and second, for the particular reason that frusemide is haemolytic, although not as haemolytic as ethacrynic acid (Dunn, 1970).

Circulatory overloading

Overloading produces a rise in central venous pressure, an increase in the amount of blood in the pulmonary blood vessels and a diminution in lung compliance. This may produce the symptoms of headache, tightness in the chest and dyspnoea; a dry cough is common. If these warning signs are neglected, pulmonary oedema soon develops and crepitations can be heard over the dependent parts of the lungs. If dyspnoea develops and the jugular venous pressure is found to be raised, the transfusion should be stopped at once and if the patient is recumbent he or she should be propped up. If a dose of frusemide has not been given recently a further dose should be given. Any signs of circulatory overloading developing during transfusion must be treated as a grave matter. If pulmonary oedema persists despite the above measures, the patient should be treated by positive pressure ventilation.

An occasional consequence of transfusion in patients with nephritis is the occurrence of attacks of hypertensive encephalopathy.

Hypertension, convulsions, severe headache and cerebral haemorrhage have been reported in patients with sickle cell disease or thalassaemia, following successive transfusions over a short period of time (Royal and Seeler, 1978; Wasi *et al.* 1978).

Effect of transfusion on red cell production
Whereas anaemia stimulates erythropoiesis, plethora depresses it.

Robertson (1917) gave repeated transfusions to normal rabbits and showed that the reticulocyte count started to diminish as plethora developed; in established plethora, reticulocytes almost disappeared from the blood. Boycott and Oakley (1933) confirmed these observations and showed that the reticulocyte count of animals could also be diminished by placing them in an atmosphere containing 65% oxygen. Similarly, in humans, the continuous administration of oxygen reduces the output of reticulocytes from the bone marrow (Tinsley *et al.* 1949).

Pace *et al.* (1947) gave transfusions of 1000 ml red cells to a series of normal subjects and, on average, raised the PCV from 0.465 to 0.585. Forty days later the PCV had returned to the pre-transfusion level (Fig. 9.6, upper curve); if red cell production had remained normal the PCV would have remained above the pre-transfusion level for 110–120 d. Further evidence of suppression of red cell production was provided by a fall in the reticulocyte count following transfusion. In children with severe thalassaemia, regular transfusions suppress marrow activity and permit normal bone growth.

Deductions about survival of transfused red cells based on
changes in PCV following transfusion
It was once thought that the survival time of red cells could be deduced by producing a plethora, either by transfusion or by transient exposure to low oxygen tension, and then noting the time taken for Hb concentration to return to its normal level. However, this method gives a correct result only if red cell production remains approximately constant, as it may when already depressed (Fig. 9.6, lower curve). If production diminishes, the time for which the Hb concentration remains elevated is much less than the mean life span of the red cells (Fig 9.6, upper curve). If red cell production were to cease altogether after transfusion, the population of red cells would diminish in a linear fashion, reaching zero at about 115 d. Reference to the upper curve in Fig. 9.6 shows that if the initial slope of the curve immediately after transfusing is prolonged to the time axis it does in fact intersect it at about 120 d, suggesting that production was temporarily arrested following transfusion.

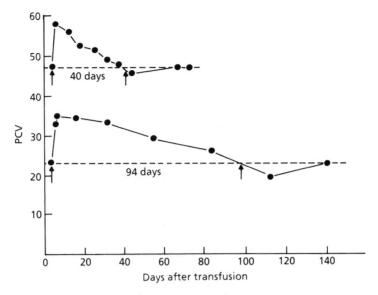

Figure 9.6 Changes in packed cell volume (PCV) following transfusion. Upper curve: a group of normal subjects (data from Pace *et al.* 1947). Lower curve: a single subject with chronic nephritis. In both curves the arrows mark the departure from, and return to, a base line (from Mollison, 1954).

Figure 9.7 shows some observations in a patient with aplastic anaemia. The slope of fall of the PCV, if extrapolated, would have reached zero 50 d after transfusion; thus it could have been concluded that the average red cell life span was 50 d or less. Estimates of survival of the patient's own red cells and of transfused red cells showed that the life span was in fact about 50 d.

As a rough guide, then, if the changes in PCV or Hb concentration following transfusion are plotted, and the initial slope, when extrapolated, intersects the time axis at 115 d or more, it does not prove that survival is normal; but if the time axis is intersected at some earlier time, such as 50 d, it can safely be concluded that the survival of the transfused red cells is reduced.

Transfusion in intermittent blood loss

Anaemia due to recurrent haemorrhage
Patients who have become anaemic as a result of recurrent haemorrhage should be transfused unless it is reasonably certain that there will be no further haemorrhage. For example, patients who have recently had haematemesis and whose Hb concentration is as low as about 70 g/l should be transfused since any further fall in Hb may precipitate circulatory failure and then make transfusion particularly hazardous.

Anaemia due to repeated blood sampling
The amount of blood lost due to sampling for diagnostic tests may be substantial.

In premature infants in intensive care units, the amount of blood removed for tests of

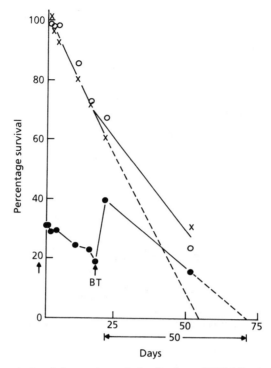

Figure 9.7 Red cell survival and changes in packed cell volume (PCV) following transfusion in a patient with aplastic anaemia. x, Survival of patient's own red cells: ○, survival of transfused red cells. The survival results are similar and extrapolation of the initial slope of the curve gives an estimate of mean life span of approximately 50 d. ●, PCV. After each blood transfusion (BT) PCV fell steadily; if the slope is extrapolated it cuts the base line after about 50 d.

various kinds is such that the infants must be transfused regularly if severe anaemia is to be avoided; see section below.

In adults whose entire hospital stay was in general wards the total blood loss in sampling averaged 175 ml in one study. In the same study patients who spent all or part of their time in intensive care units had an average loss in sampling of 762 ml; the loss in patients with arterial lines was 944 ml (four samples a day). In about 50% of patients transfused during their hospital stay, losses from phlebotomy contributed to the transfusion requirement, i.e. in those patients from whom the equivalent of more than 1 unit of red cells had been withdrawn (Smoller and Kruskall, 1986).

Red cell transfusions in premature infants
It has been estimated that 90% of all transfusions in newborn infants are given to replace losses arising from blood sampling (Lenes and Sacher, 1981). As an example of the quantities involved, in 59 premature infants with birth-weights of less than 1500 g, a mean of 22.9 ml packed red cells was lost during the first 6 weeks of life; 26% of the infants had a cumulative loss that exceeded their red cell mass at birth (Nexo *et al.* 1981). The usual practice is to give red cell transfusions when 5–10% of the estimated total blood volume has been removed (Strauss *et al.* 1990).

Other presently accepted indications for red cell transfusions in newborn infants are to keep the PCV above 0.40 during respiratory distress or in managing symptomatic congenital heart disease, and to treat congestive cardiac failure and episodes of severe apnoea, although few good clinical studies have been done (Strauss *et al.* 1990). Transfusing otherwise well premature infants simply to maintain Hb levels above 100 g/l was found to confer no benefit (Blank *et al.* 1984).

It is usual to transfuse packed red cells (PCV 0.65) in relatively small amounts e.g. 10 ml/kg, given in 3–4 h. In order to economize in blood, donations can be taken into 'pedipacks'. A pedipack consists of a main pack containing enough anticoagulant for 250 ml blood and three attached, initially empty, packs into which convenient amounts of anticoagulated blood from the main pack can be transferred. Thus, when an infant needs several transfusions over a relatively short period of time, blood from the same donor can be used. This arrangement has several advantages: blood is economized, since a single donation will provide for a number of transfusions and, similarly, the need for special testing of donors, e.g. for anti-cytomegalovirus (CMV), is minimized; since the main pack is designed for a donation of 250 ml, donors weighing less than 50 kg can be used or, if the donor is heavier than this, he or she can be recalled after 2–3 weeks for a further donation of 250 ml into a pedipack. As an alternative, aliquots of blood from the same donor can be frozen and thawed, one at a time, as needed. Again, this system minimizes the number of donors to which the infant is exposed; in addition, exposure to leucocytes is minimal, thus reducing the risks of HLA immunization and of infection by cell-borne viruses (e.g. CMV); in addition, red cells with a virtually normal biochemical composition are provided.

The practice of using 'walking donors', i.e. donors whose blood can be taken freshly, on any number of occasions, for transfusion to one or more infants, has been generally condemned: testing is often inadequate, records tend to be unsatisfactory, and there are practical difficulties associated with the taking of blood by syringe (Oberman, 1974).

When liquid-stored blood is used, it is usual to limit the storage period to 7 d, with the intention of transfusing red cells with a more or less normal content of 2,3-DPG. It is thought to be adequate to use standard, rather than special microaggregate, filters.

Although it is not regarded as necessary to irradiate blood components given to mature infants, irradiation, using a minimum dose of 15 Gy, is advised for all components to be transfused to infants *in utero* and to all newborn infants of birth-weight less than 1200 g (Strauss *et al.* 1990). As described earlier in this chapter, when red cells are stored after irradiation, the rate of loss of potassium is increased. Blood or red cells which have been irradiated should not be stored for more than a few days if they are to be transfused to premature infants; alternatively, if stored for longer they should be washed manually and resuspended in fresh frozen plasma (Rivet *et al.* 1989).

Transfusion in chronic anaemia
When there is continuous severe underproduction of red cells, as in aplastic anaemia, or production of red cells with a greatly diminished life span, as in thalassaemia major, regular transfusion may be essential.

Transfusion requirements when red cell production is negligible
Assuming that in a normal adult mean red cell life span is 115 d and mean red cell

volume (male) is 30 ml/kg, normal daily red cell production is 30/115 ml red cells/kg per day or approximately 0.26 ml red cells/kg per day. Thus in a male weighing 70 kg mean red cell production is approximately 18 ml red cells per day. To maintain an Hb concentration of two-thirds normal (100 g/l) would require only 12 ml red cells per day.

In considering the transfusion requirements of a patient with complete failure of red cell production it must be remembered that the above calculations refer to red cells which have a mean life expectancy of 115 d. By contrast red cells taken from the circulation are of all ages and have an average life expectancy of 115/2 or 57.7 d. Thus the daily requirement of transfused red cells to maintain an Hb concentration of 100 g/l in a 70-kg adult male who is making no red cells at all is approximately 12×2 or 24 ml/d. If a unit of stored blood contains 200 ml red cells and, allowing for some wastage from red cells rendered non-viable by storage and from red cells left in the blood container, an average of almost 1 unit a week will have to be transfused. Even more will be needed when the survival of transfused red cells is reduced.

Thalassaemia
A common practice in treating children with thalassaemia major is to try to maintain the Hb concentration at a level sufficient to damp down the overactivity of the bone marrow. In one study a comparison was made of a regimen of 'hypertransfusion' in which washed, frozen, packed red cells were transfused every 4–5 weeks to maintain the PCV above 0.27 with a regimen of 'super-transfusion' in which the PCV was maintained at a level above 0.35. It was found that the introduction of super-transfusion was accompanied by an initial increase in the red cell requirement, but after 1–4 months all patients maintained a PCV of over 0.35 on a transfusion schedule which was identical to that of hypertransfusion. As predicted, it was shown that this developement was due to a mean decrease in blood volume of about 20% following super-transfusion. In turn, there was a significant decrease in erythropoiesis (Propper *et al.* 1980).

Avoidance of transfusion in chronic renal failure; use of erythropoietin
Before recombinant human erythropoietin became available, some 25% of patients on dialysis for end-stage renal disease needed red cell transfusions; treatment with erythropoietin avoids the need for transfusion in at least 97% of patients (Mohini, 1989). To avoid various circulatory complications, the PCV should not be allowed to rise too rapidly and blood pressure should be monitored carefully (Groopman *et al.* 1989). For further discussion and recommended doses, see Chapter 14.

Transfusion of younger-than-average red cells ('neocytes')
Using a cell separator it is possible to collect a selected population of red cells which are younger than average ('neocytes'). The $T_{50}Cr$ of such cells is appreciably longer than that of unfractionated cells, e.g. 43.8 d compared with 27.8 d (Propper *et al.* 1980), and 47.4 d (for neocytes with an estimated mean cell age of 30 d) compared with 29.5 d for unfractionated red cells (Corash *et al.* 1981). Similarly, using fractions obtained with an IBM-2991 cell washer the red cell half-life, after correction for Cr elution, was found to be 43.9 d for the younger fractions and 34.7 d for the older

fractions (Bracey *et al.* 1983). In another study, also using the IBM-2991 cell washer, the top 50% of the cells had a $T_{50}Cr$ of 40 and 42 d in two patients compared with 29 d for unselected cells (Graziano *et al.* 1982). In one patient who received the top 30% of the cells the $T_{50}Cr$ was 56 d, a very high value considering that if all the cells had had an age of only 1 d the $T_{50}Cr$ would not have been expected to have been longer than 70 d (the $T_{1/2}$ of Cr elution). In measurements made with DFP, and thus giving estimates of true life span, red cells were taken from the upper and lower halves of packed red cells of a unit of blood, after spinning for an additional 30 min. ^{14}C-DFP and ^{3}H-DFP were used to label the cells *in vitro*. Linear slopes of disappearance were observed and mean life spans were approximately 120 d for cells from the upper half and just over 80 d for cells from the lower half (see Sharon and Honig, 1991).

When neocytes were used for transfusion to children with thalassaemia it was found that the intervals between transfusions could be increased. On the other hand, although the use of neocytes makes it possible to transfuse smaller amounts of red cells or to give transfusions less frequently and still maintain the same PCV, the method is extravagant in time and money. In fact, the costs are comparable to those of leucocyte collection (Propper *et al.* 1980). In a prospective double-blind trial, the results of using younger-than-average red cells were compared with those of using unselected red cells in the treatment of transfusion-dependent patients with thalassaemia major. The younger-than-average red cells were obtained by centrifuging blood at 3000 rev/min for 15 min in an IBM-2991 cell washer and collecting the least dense 50% of the cells. The reticulocyte counts of these 'young red cells' were on the average 2.5 times higher than those in the original units. In the patients receiving young red cells there was a slight reduction in blood consumption but no reduction in the fall of Hb between transfusions or any increase in the interval between transfusions. It was concluded that any reduction in the rate of iron loading brought about by using young red cells (prepared in this particular way) did not justify the expense, time and work involved (Marcus *et al.* 1985). This conclusion seems unlikely to be overthrown by the contention that neocyte-enriched blood can be prepared more cheaply by simple centrifugation, since two to three times as many donors are needed to produce a neocyte-enriched unit as an ordinary unit (Hogan *et al.* 1986; Simon *et al.* 1989).

Exchange transfusion in treating anaemia
Indications for exchange transfusion are discussed very briefly in Chapter 1. Here only the problem of exchange transfusion in sickle cell disease will be discussed.

Exchange transfusion in sickle cell disease
Exchange transfusion is used in Hb SC and SD diseases and in sickle β-thalassaemia as well as in SS disease. The objects are to increase the concentration of red cells containing Hb A and to decrease the concentration of abnormal sickle cells and thus to diminish blood viscosity and improve the microcirculation. When the proportion of cells that can sickle is reduced to 50% or less, therapeutic benefits are achieved. In order to reduce the proportion of sickleable cells in a short time, without increasing the PCV to unacceptable levels, exchange transfusion must be performed (Klein, 1982). If the pre-transfusion PCV is very low, it is advisable to increase it only moderately,

bearing in mind that high PCVs increase the risk of blocking the microcirculation (Milner, 1982). Since it is undesirable to put a tourniquet on the arm for more than a brief period, it is important to choose a large vein and to induce vasodilatation by warming the patient thoroughly before beginning. Alternatively, a catheter may be passed up the vein for some distance to ensure a good flow. Packed donor red cells, previously passed through a white-cell depletion filter, should be mixed with the patient's own plasma and platelets before transfusion.

The progress of the exchange can be monitored by measuring the proportions of Hb A and S and the patient's total Hb concentration. Exchange transfusion has advantages over simple transfusion: the patient's short-lived sickle cells are removed with a consequent decrease in iron load, blood viscosity is more effectively lowered, risks of circulatory overload are diminished and PCV is not raised to an unacceptably high level. In sickle cell disease, exchange transfusion has been used to prevent recurrence of central nervous system infarction (Sarnaik et al. 1979; Williams et al. 1980) and to treat priapism, recurrent severe vaso-occlusive crises unresponsive to conventional therapy, refractory ankle ulcers, severe pneumonia, meningitis, aplastic crises, severe episodes of red cell destruction and splenic sequestration crises (Weatherall and Clegg, 1981; Milner, 1982).

The majority view is that in the management of sickle cell disease, chronic transfusion therapy, with the sole object either of correcting low haemoglobin levels or of preventing crises, is contraindicated (Milner, 1982; Charache, 1983), mainly because of the risk of red cell alloimmunization, which may hinder future transfusions (Orlina et al. 1978; Coles et al. 1981; Davies et al. 1986). Other risks are those of thrombosis of peripheral veins and of problems of venous access (Charache and Moyer, 1982). Furthermore, delayed haemolytic transfusion reactions seem to be particularly common in patients with sickle cell disease (see Chapter 11).

Exchange transfusion prior to surgery. If a general anaesthetic needs to be administered to a patient with SS disease, it is obviously important to avoid the development of very low oxygen tensions in the blood. Evidently, the risk of sickling can be avoided by carrying out pre-operative transfusion (Morrison et al. 1978; Fullerton et al. 1981). Nevertheless in one review it was concluded that the advantages of partial exchange transfusion before surgery did not outweigh the risks (Searle, 1973). Moreover, the risks of severe sickling crises are evidently small. Homi et al. (1979), from an experience of giving anaesthetics to 200 patients with sickle cell disease, concluded that clinically uneventful anaesthesia was associated with minimal morbidity and mortality. Approximately 70% of the patients underwent operation without blood transfusion. It seems, then, that partial exchange transfusion before surgery in a patient with SS disease is indicated only when there is a special risk that tissue hypoxia may develop in the peri-operative period. Red cell exchange transfusion has proved to be beneficial in patients with proliferative SC retinopathy undergoing surgery for retinal detachment (Brazier et al. 1986). The exchange decreases the risk of vaso-occlusive sickling and improves the blood flow in the anterior segment.

Exchange transfusion in pregnancy. There is no general agreement regarding the prophylaxis of complications of pregnancy by exchange transfusion in women with Hb SS or SC disease (Cunningham and Pritchard, 1979; Milner, 1982; Charache, 1983).

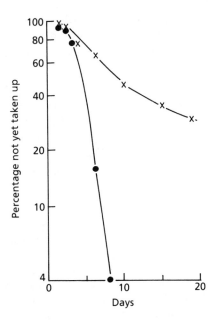

Figure 9.8 Rate of appearance of ^{51}Cr-labelled red cells in the circulating blood after injecting the cells intraperitoneally into an infant.

For convenience, the 'percentage not taken up' has been plotted. For example, when 20% of the injected red cells have appeared in the circulating blood, the point is plotted as 80% 'not yet taken up'. x, Uptake after injecting 1 ml labelled red cells; ●, uptake after injecting 20 ml of labelled red cells.

Some recommend routine exchange transfusion to maintain the Hb A level above 20% (Morrison *et al.* 1980); others recommend it only for patients with severe anaemia or acute complications (Milner, 1982).

Transfusion by routes other than intravenously

Uptake of red cells injected intraperitoneally
Hunter (1884) gave large i.p. transfusions of rabbit blood to other rabbits, and showed that the recipient's red cell count was raised for approximately 21 d. Similar observation were made by Sansby (1925), who concluded that the injected red cells reached the circulation and survived for a considerable period.

Hahn *et al.* (1944) gave i.p. injections of red cells tagged with radio-iron to dogs. They showed that the red cells moved promptly into the circulation via the lymphatics. Nevertheless, uptake was not complete 1 week after the injections.

In humans, quantitative estimates have been made using ^{51}Cr-labelled red cells. Pritchard and Weisman (1957) found that labelled cells appeared in the circulation within 24 h and reached a maximum at 3–11 d. In two patients reported previously there was a lag of about 24 h before any appreciable number of cells appeared in the circulation. In the first patient (a child aged 1 week with severe spina bifida) an injection of 1 ml red cells was taken up very slowly, but when 20 ml red cells were injected 50% of the cells were taken up in 5 d and uptake was almost complete in 8 d (Fig. 9.8). In a second case, a child with thalassaemia major weighing 18 kg, following an i.p.

transfusion of 350 ml citrated blood, more than 50% of the cells were taken up into the circulation by the fourth day after transfusion (Mollison, 1961b, p. 119).

The use of the i.p. route for intra-uterine transfusion is discussed in Chapter 12.

Intramuscular injection

When red cells are injected i.m. only very small amounts reach the circulation. In experiments in rabbits 5 ml of a 40% suspension of ^{51}Cr-labelled red cells were injected i.m. into three or four different sites and samples were taken over the following 2 weeks. The maximum radioactivity in samples of washed red cells never exceeded 0.5% of the injected dose in one case and 0.2% in the other (Mollison, 1961b, p. 123).

Transfusion of red cell suspensions in anaemia

Transfusions of washed red cells were given as early as 1902 by Hédon. At that time it was generally accepted that the transfusion of defibrinated blood was highly dangerous and Hédon decided to try the effect of washing the red cells and giving them as a suspension. He used both rabbits and dogs and showed that when an animal was exsanguinated to the point at which it was extremely unlikely to recover with infusions of saline alone it could be rapidly restored by being transfused with red cells in saline. He even tried the effect of packed red cells; in a rabbit bled of 145 ml over a period of 2 h and with apparently terminal convulsions, the rapid injection of packed red cells from 100 ml blood from another rabbit, suspended to a total volume of 66 ml in saline, produced some immediate improvement with apparent complete recovery at 48 h.

In the 1930s, workers in the Soviet Union became interested in transfusing plasma rather than whole blood in treating haemorrhage and disorders of coagulation; plasma, separated from red cells, was stored for periods of up to 1 month (Filatov and Kartasevskij, 1935). There is a reference to the use of separated red cells for transfusion (Filatov and Kartasevskij, 1934), although the present authors have not succeeded in seeing the paper.

Red cell concentrates

Castellanos (1937) seems to have been the first to use concentrated suspensions of red cells rather than whole blood for transfusion in humans. The use of such suspensions is logical whenever it is important to introduce red cells into a patient's circulation with the least possible disturbance of blood volume. In fact, the widespread use of packed red cells was initially determined by other considerations. In the Second World War plasma was collected on a large scale. It was mainly the hope of salvaging the red cells that were otherwise being wasted that led to clinical trials of the red cell residues (MacQuaide and Mollison, 1940; Cooksey and Horwitz, 1944). An incidental advantage of using packed red cells rather than whole blood is the reduction in the rate of reactions. In an early series it was noted that severe febrile reactions were three times less common with packed red cells (McQuaide and Mollison, 1940); in retrospect, this reduction was probably due to the practice of removing as much as possible of the buffy coat in preparing the packed red cells (see Chapter 15).

Red cell concentrates are preferable to whole blood in transfusing patients with severe anaemia. The PCV of concentrates varies widely according to the method of preparation: according to Chaplin (1969), sedimented cells usually have a PCV of 0.65–0.70, 30% of the original plasma and all the original leucocytes and platelets; centrifuged cells have a PCV of 0.80 and 15% of the original plasma; centrifuged cells with the buffy coat squeezed off have a PCV of more than 0.90, 5–10% of the plasma, less than 30% of the platelets and less than 10% of the leucocytes. Prins and Loos (1970) also noted that the PCV of centrifuged red cells might be as high as 0.90; addition of about one-third the volume of saline lowered the PCV to 0.70 and reduced the relative viscosity from about 5 times to only 1.3 times that of whole blood.

Washed suspensions of red cells are not needed very often. The main indications are as follows:

1 Patients who have had, or are likely to have, reactions to the transfusion of plasma proteins, e.g. patients with class-specific anti-IgA (where donors lacking IgA are not available) or patients with subclass-specific anti-IgA. In patients with anti-IgA, very thorough washing (six times) is needed (see Chapter 15).

2 Patients who have had severe allergic transfusion reactions for which no cause can be found.

3 Patients with T-activated red cells who require transfusion; see Chapter 7.

4 Very occasional patients with severe autoimmune haemolytic anaemia due to haemolysins in whom the supply of complement in transfused plasma may exacerbate red cell destruction.

Washed red cells are used by some for intra-uterine transfusions, i.e. for transfusions given via the fetal peritoneal cavity and also for transfusions given directly into umbilical cord vessels of the fetus *in utero*.

Frozen and thawed red cells; see Chapter 15.

RED CELL INCOMPATIBILITY
IN VIVO

FIGURES

TABLES

Transfused cells are regarded as incompatible if their survival in the recipient's circulation is curtailed by antibodies. The realization that transfusions are inevitably incompatible if donor and recipient belong to different species was made only by degrees.

Transfusion of animal red cells to humans

The first person to give a transfusion to a human being was Professor J. Denis who, with the help of a surgeon Mr C. Emmerez, gave transfusions of lamb's blood or calf's blood to five different patients. His most famous, and last, recipient was a man (Mauroy) with an 'inveterate phrensy, occasioned by a disgrace he had received in some Amours'. Denis hoped that 'the calf's blood by its mildness and freshness might possibly allay the heat and ebulition of his blood'. The first two transfusions given to him apparently relieved his mania, although following the second his arm became hot, his pulse rose, sweat burst out over his forehead, he complained of pain in his kidneys and he was sick at the stomach and the next day passed black urine. After this transfusion the patient became so much better that plans for a further transfusion were temporarily abandoned (Denis, 1667–8). However, at the insistence of the patient's wife a third transfusion was attempted early in 1668. There were technical difficulties and only a few drops of blood were extracted from the patient and probably no blood at all transfused. Nevertheless, the patient died the same night. The case came before the Court at Châtelet on 27 April 1668 and the cause of death was examined; it was concluded that the patient's wife had been putting arsenic in his broth (for further details see Jeanneney and Ringenbach, 1940; Hall and Boas Hall, 1967; Keynes, 1949; 1967). Although the transfusion probably had nothing to do with the patient's death, the episode was seized on by the opponents of transfusion who succeeded in having the operation banned.

Work by Blundell (1824), indicating the need to use a donor of the same species, has been referred to in an earlier chapter. Blundell's work was fully confirmed by Ponfick (1875) who showed that if the red cells of a donor of another species were transfused they underwent rapid intravascular lysis. Ponfick also showed that when the red cells of a donor of one species were mixed *in vitro*, with the serum of another, haemolysis occurred.

Despite Blundell's earlier work, during the last quarter of the nineteenth century an enthusiasm for transfusion and difficulty in recruiting human donors led to a considerable vogue for giving transfusions of lamb's blood (Gesellius, 1874; Hasse, 1874). Not all physicians were impressed, particularly as when lamb's blood was used except in very small quantities an invariable result was the escape via the kidneys of Hb (Fagge and Pye-Smith, 1891); a current witticism was that for a transfusion three sheep were needed, the donor, the recipient and the doctor (Zimmerman and Howell, 1932).

Transfusions between members of the same species
The first studies of red cell survival following transfusion between members of the same species (bulls) were described by Todd and White (1911) in animals which had not previously been transfused. In fact, all the donor red cells were eliminated within a few days, presumably due to the presence of naturally occurring antibodies. Ashby (1919), who used a similar technique to study red cell survival following transfusions between humans, found prolonged survival, due evidently to the fact that she transfused only ABO-compatible red cells.

Scope of this chapter
The present chapter is concerned mainly with experimental studies of the survival *in vivo* of small amounts of incompatible red cells and with theoretical deductions from the results. The following chapter deals with the clinical effects of the accidental transfusion of relatively large amounts of incompatible blood.

Some of the factors that affect the rate and site of destruction are as follows: the characteristics of the antibody, namely binding constant, Ig class and IgG subclass, ability to activate complement, thermal range and plasma concentration; the characteristics of the antigen, namely abundance of sites on the cell surface and association with complement activation (both related to antigen specificity); the number of red cells transfused; the presence of the relevant antigen in the plasma; and the phagocytic activity of the mononuclear phagocyte system (MPS). In analysing the effects of these variables, tests with volumes of red cells as small as 1 ml or less have proved very helpful. The injection of such amounts practically never produces untoward symptoms in the recipient; as a rule, causes virtually no immediate change in the concentration of antibody; and does not tax the capacity of the MPS system. Accordingly, the main factors determining the rate of red cell destruction are the various characteristics of the antibody, including its concentration. The characteristics of the antigen also affect the result but this source of variability can be eliminated by using red cells from a single donor or can be minimized by using red cells of a particular phenotype or 'grade' of antigen.

In the present chapter, the results of tests with small volumes of red cells will be considered first from a qualitative point of view, that is to say from the point of view of the patterns of red cell destruction observed, and second from the quantitative point of view, using evidence derived from investigations in which the amounts of antibody and antigen involved have been determined. The situation met with in clinical practice, in which relatively large numbers of incompatible red cells are transfused, will then be discussed.

Estimation of survival of incompatible red cells
When incompatible red cells are transfused accidentally, as a rule the only way of studying their survival is by application of some serological method. For example, if by chance the donor red cells are group N and the recipient is group M, differential agglutination with anti-M will provide estimates of the survival of the inagglutinable group N donor red cells; if the donor is Rh D positive and the recipient D negative, the donor red cells can be recognized by direct agglutination with anti-D or, if the recipient

has formed anti-D, the surviving red cells can be recognized by the direct antiglobulin test (DAT). If a flow cytometer is available, quantitative estimates can be made whenever there is an antigenic difference between the red cells of the donor and the recipient and suitable antisera are available.

In experiments in which incompatible red cells are deliberately transfused, various labels can be used; e.g. in studying the response of D-negative recipients to D-positive red cells, cord red cells can be transfused and their survival determined by making counts by the acid-elution method. However, the method of most general application and greatest precision is that of labelling with ^{51}Cr.

The following pages describe experiments to determine the relation between the serological characteristics of antibodies and the effects that they produce *in vivo*. The scope of tests with small volumes of incompatible red cells in ordinary transfusion practice has been discussed briefly elsewhere (Mollison, 1981) and a method of carrying out such tests is described on the following page and on pp. 479–480. In clinical practice, tests are indicated only when it is uncertain whether or not the injected red cells will survive normally. When increased destruction is expected and tests are being carried out simply with the intention of increasing knowledge, prior approval should, of course, be sought from the appropriate ethical committee and the subject's informed consent obtained.

Labelling of incompatible red cells

Labelling with radionuclides remains the best method since the survival of amounts less than 1 ml can be estimated accurately. Although flow cytometry can be used in some circumstances, the need to inject about 10 ml red cells (Garratty, 1990; Issitt *et al.* 1990a) is a disadvantage. If the method can be made more sensitive, it may eventually become the method of choice. Almost all the results discussed in the present chapter were obtained using ^{51}Cr which, when survival is to be followed for more than a very short period (a few hours), remains the best label. With Cr, loss of label from red cells is slow, i.e. about 3% in the first 24 h with only about 1% per day thereafter (see Chapter 9); the $T_{1/2}$ of radioactive decay is 27.7 d which allows studies over a period of weeks, if necessary. In contrast, when red cells are labelled with ^{99m}Tc about 4% of the label is lost from the red cells during the first hour; the rate of loss over the next 2 or 3 h is probably similar, but thereafter the rate slows and the loss in the first 24 h is about 30%. The rate of loss of indium (^{111}In or ^{113m}In) appears to be 3–5% during the first 15 min after injection and approximately 15% in the first 24 h. ^{99m}Tc and ^{111}In appear to be suitable for detecting substantial destruction occurring in the first few hours after injection but ^{51}Cr must be used if small amounts of destruction are to be detected reliably or if survival is to be followed for longer periods. For further details and references, see Appendix 2.

Use of ^{51}*Cr.* A dose of 0.2–0.5 μCi (7–18 kBq)/kg may be used, e.g. 12–30 μCi in a 60-kg adult. Using ^{51}Cr with a specific activity of 100 μCi/μg, a maximum of 0.3 μg Cr will be added; thus, even when the amount of red cells injected is as small as 0.3 ml the amount of Cr (1 μg/ml red cells) will be well below the level that is likely to produce any interference whatever with the survival of the red cells.

In the usual circumstance in which tests with small numbers of donor red cells will be made, namely when there is doubt as to whether survival will be normal, it is convenient to use 1 ml red cells. In a few other circumstances it is advisable to use smaller amounts; e.g. in patients whose serum contains potent incomplete antibodies, a dose of 0.5 ml red cells is suggested, since occasionally amounts as small as 1 ml have been known to provoke shivering and fever; in subjects whose serum contains haemolytic antibodies, tests should be made with caution and no more than 0.1–0.2 ml red cells should be injected.

When there is little chance of early rapid destruction of donor red cells it is sufficient to obtain a sample from the recipient 3 min after the injection of the cells and to take this value as 100% survival. In most normal subjects, mixing is at least 98% complete by 3 min (Strumia *et al.* 1958; Mollison, 1959d; see Fig. 10.1) and appreciable destruction of injected red cells within the mixing period is found only with relatively potent antibodies; an example is given in Fig. 10.2. If it is considered that there is any chance of such early destruction an estimate of the patient's red cell volume will be required and this is best obtained by labelling a sample of the patient's own red cells either with ^{99m}Tc or ^{111}In and injecting these labelled red cells and the ^{51}Cr-labelled donor red cells as a single suspension.

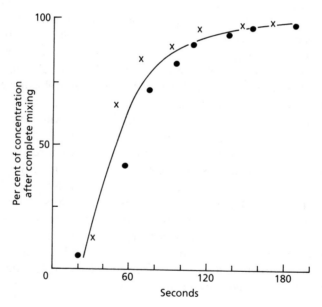

Figure 10.1   The rate of appearance of labelled red cells in samples taken from one superficial arm vein after injecting the cells into a vein in the other arm.

Two different samples of the subject's own red cells were injected, labelled with ^{51}Cr (●) and ^{32}P (×) respectively. One sample was injected about 30 s after the other but in each case the times are expressed as seconds from the mid-point of injection to the mid-point of the sample. '100%' = the concentration attained after complete mixing, based on samples taken 10–20 min after injection (from Mollison, 1959d).

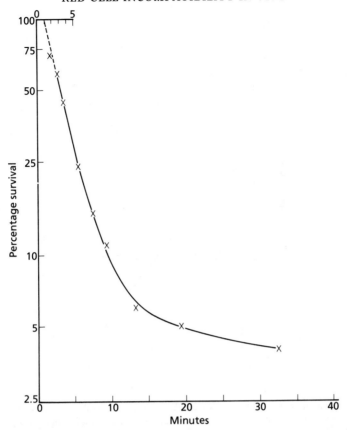

Figure 10.2 Survival *in vivo* of a sample of red cells from an Fy(a +) donor; the cells were labelled with ^{51}Cr, incubated with purified IgG anti-Fy^a and with complement, and reinjected into the donor. Red cell volume was determined by simultaneous injection of another sample of the donor's red cells labelled with ^{32}P but otherwise untreated. Mixing was probably incomplete at 2 min; a line drawn through estimates of survival at 2.8, 3.7 ad 5.6 min cuts the time axis at about 1 min after the mid-point of injection. The initial rate of destruction has a $T_{1/2}$ of 2 min; the rate of destruction starts to slow 5–10 min after injection of the cells (data from Mollison, 1962, case 3b).

QUALITATIVE ASPECTS OF RED CELL DESTRUCTION BY ALLOANTIBODIES

As described in Chapter 3, red cells are not directly damaged by antibodies. The attachment of antibodies leads to destruction in one of two ways; either complement is activated leading to damage to the red cell surface by C8–9 followed by lysis; or the red cells, coated with antibody or complement (C3b), or with both antibody and C3b, become attached to a phagocyte, leading to loss of membrane, lysis or engulfment.

Predominantly intravascular destruction

With rare exceptions, the only antibodies that produce intravascular lysis of the majority of the red cells transfused are those that are readily lytic *in vitro*. The commonest antibodies of this kind are, of course, anti-A, anti-B and anti-A,B. As Fig. 10.3 shows, within 2 min of injecting ABO-incompatible red cells, the plasma may

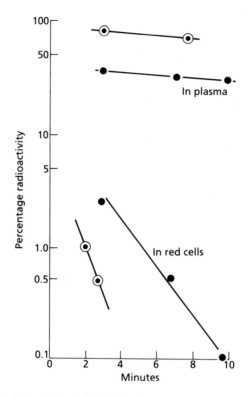

Figure 10.3 Intravascular haemolysis of ^{51}Cr-labelled ABO-incompatible red cells. ⊙ B cells injected into a group A recipient. ● A$_2$ cells injected into a group O recipient (data from Cutbush and Mollison, 1958).

contain Hb equivalent to 90% of the amount contained in the injected intact red cells (see also Jandl *et al.* 1957; Cutbush and Mollison, 1958).

When ABO-incompatible red cells are injected which, *in vitro*, are only weakly lysed by the recipient's serum, either because the antibody or the antigen is relatively weak, less than half the injected red cells may be lysed intravascularly. Figure 10.3 shows an example in which, following the transfusion of a small volume of A$_2$ red cells to a group O recipient, only 40% of the Hb was found in the plasma immediately after injection.

When the anti-A or anti-B in the recipient's plasma is only very weakly lytic so that lysis is observed *in vitro* only when the ratio of serum to cells exceeds about 500 : 1, destruction of the transfused cells may be predominantly extravascular with only 10% of the injected radioactivity being found in the plasma (Jandl *et al.* 1957).

When destruction by anti-A and anti-B is very rapid, 99.9% of the cells may be lysed or phagocytosed within 10 min (Fig. 10.3). When destruction is slower, some cells may survive for relatively long periods having, presumably, acquired resistance to complement-mediated destruction (see below).

Certain other antibodies, particularly anti-PP$_1$P^k and anti-Vel which are readily haemolytic *in vitro*, are undoubtedly capable of causing predominantly intravascular lysis of incompatible red cells but no quantitative data have been published.

Many examples of anti-Le^a and rare examples of anti-Le^b lyse red cell *in vitro* but as a rule the lysis is relatively slow. Accordingly, when small amounts of incompatible red cells are injected, the cells may be cleared by the MPS before there has been time for haemolysis to occur. If relatively large amounts of incompatible red cells are transfused, some intravascular haemolysis may be observed (see p. 520). Exceptionally potent Lewis antibodies may produce some intravascular haemolysis even when small amounts of incompatible red cells are injected.

In the case reported by Mollison *et al.* (1963) at a time when the titre of anti-Le^b in the patient's serum was approximately 100, 0.5 ml of ^{51}Cr-labelled Le(b +) red cells were injected. A sample taken 4 min later contained 60% of surviving cells with 13% of the injected radioactivity in the plasma; the sample at 13 min contained 16% of surviving cells and 7% of the injected radioactivity in the plasma. The discrepancy in the amounts of Hb in the two plasma samples suggested the possibility that the haemolysis might have occurred, partially at least, *in vitro*, after the samples had been withdrawn, and this emphasizes the need to separate cells from plasma promptly when making observations of this kind.

Erythrophagocytosis accompanying lysis by anti-A and anti-B

As mentioned above, not all ABO-incompatible red cells are lysed in the plasma. Presumably, most of the remainder are engulfed by cells of the MPS but some are engulfed by neutrophils, so that erythrophagocytosis is observed in films of peripheral blood (Hopkins, 1910; Ottenberg, 1911). Gross leucopenia may be produced by the injection of as little as 10 ml of ABO-incompatible red cells; see p. 501.

Predominantly extravascular destruction

All antibodies except those that are readily haemolytic *in vitro* bring about extravascular destruction of red cells, chiefly in the liver and spleen. The maximum rate of disappearance of red cells from the blood stream corresponds to the clearance of rather more than one-third of the blood per minute (Mollison, 1962); that is, k, the fractional rate of red cell clearance, = approximately 0.35 min^{-1}

$$\text{Since } k = \frac{\log_e 2}{T_{1/2}\,(\text{min})}, \quad T_{1/2} = \frac{0.693}{0.35} = 1.9\,\text{min.}$$

When clearance occurs with a $T_{1/2}$ of the order of 2 min, it can be shown by surface counting that approximately 75% of the cells have been sequestered in the liver and approximately 10% in the spleen (Mollison and Hughes-Jones, 1958).

Antibodies that fail to activate complement, e.g. anti-Rh D, bring about destruction predominantly in the spleen (Jandl, 1955; Mollison and Cutbush, 1955; Jandl *et al.* 1957). In predominantly splenic destruction the maximum rate of clearance observed corresponds to a $T_{1/2}$ of approximately 20 min (k = approximately 0.035/min); more than 90% of the cells are removed in the spleen (Hughes-Jones *et al.* 1957b). Under these circumstances, the rate of clearance of red cells is limited by the rate of blood flow through the spleen.

Since the blood flow through the liver is approximately ten times greater than that through spleen, it is evident that antibodies such as incomplete anti-D must be very inefficient in bringing about red cell destruction in the liver. In fact, in splenectomized subjects, red cells heavily coated with anti-D are cleared with a $T_{1/2}$ of the order of

3–5 h, indicating that, on a weight basis, the liver is about 100 times less efficient than the spleen at removing D-sensitized red cells from the circulation (Crome and Mollison, 1964).

It has been suggested that, in the spleen, because the packed cell volume (PCV) of the blood is higher, plasma IgG competes with bound IgG antibodies for Fc receptors on macrophages far less successfully than it does in the liver (Engelfriet *et al.* 1981). By contrast, the adherence of complement-coated cells is not inhibited by plasma and therefore the cells bind to macrophages just as well in the liver as they do in the spleen. The synergistic effect of C3b and IgG in binding coated red cells to macrophages is discussed briefly on p. 135.

Before describing the patterns of red cell destruction associated with particular human alloantibodies, some other features of extravascular destruction of incompatible red cells will be discussed.

Delay ('lag') before the onset of extravascular destruction
When the percentage survival of incompatible red cells is plotted against the time after their injection into the circulation there is an apparent 'lag' before destruction begins. The most obvious explanation is that accelerated destruction cannot begin until the cells have taken up sufficient antibody, but this is only part of the story because, even if the cells are previously sensitized by antibodies *in vitro* or rendered non-viable by storage, there is still an apparent delay before the onset of destruction. In a series of measurements with such 'altered' red cells this delay was found to be 1.35 min, SD 0.45 (Mollison, 1962). The most likely explanation for this 'lag' is as follows: the circulation time through the portal circulation is slower than that through the rest of the body so that the time taken for cells to pass from the point of injection to the sampling point (arm vein) may be of the order of 1–2 min. Accordingly, a blood sample taken from an arm vein less than 1 min after the injection of incompatible cells will not include any cells that have been through the portal circulation and thus it will appear that there has so far been no clearance of cells from the circulation (Mollison, 1962).

After the injection of incompatible red cells, which must take up antibody before becoming susceptible to rapid clearance by the MPS, a somewhat longer lag is observed. In ten cases in which the antibody concerned was capable of agglutinating red cells suspended in saline, the mean apparent delay was 2.20 min, SD 0.75; and in 12 cases in which the antibody was incomplete and complement-binding, the mean delay was 4.0 min, SD 1.5 (Mollison, 1962). Obvious examples of lags are provided by several figures in this chapter, e.g. Figs 10.5, 10.6 and 10.7.

When the concentration of antibodies in the serum is very low, very long lags may be observed. For example, in a D-negative subject injected 24 h previously, i.m., with 1 μg anti-D, following the injection of 0.3 ml D-positive red cells i.v., there was a delay of about 5 d before the onset of the maximal rate of red cell destruction (Mollison and Hughes-Jones, 1967). A similarly long delay was observed by Schneider and Preisler (1966) after injecting small amounts of low-titre anti-D and D-positive red cells into D-negative subjects. The delay is due partly to the time taken for the uptake of IgG into the circulation and partly to the time taken for antigen and antibody to come into equilibrium at very low concentrations (Mollison and Hughes-Jones, 1967).

Release of some Hb into the circulation in predominantly extravascular destruction
Jandl *et al.* (1957) found that when D-positive red cells were injected into subjects whose plasma contained anti-D, or when D-positive red cells were incubated with anti-D *in vitro* and then reinjected, haemoglobinaemia developed within a few minutes of the injection and increased steadily to reach a peak 2 or 3 h after the injection.

Personal observations have shown that when amounts of ^{51}Cr-labelled, anti-D-coated red cells of less than 1 ml are injected and the rate of clearance of the cells is approximately 0.035/min, the maximum amount of radioactivity in the plasma is usually 2–5%, reached about 1–2 h after injection (Fig. 10.4). Allowing for the fact that ^{51}Cr and Hb are being cleared steadily throughout this period, the amount released probably corresponds to about 10% of the number of red cells injected.

Jandl *et al.* (1957) found that in subjects injected with approximately 10 ml red cells, the maximum plasma Hb concentration did not as a rule exceed 6% of the amount injected in the red cells, although in one subject injected with a larger volume of red cells (about 20 ml) the plasma Hb concentration reached the equivalent of 12%

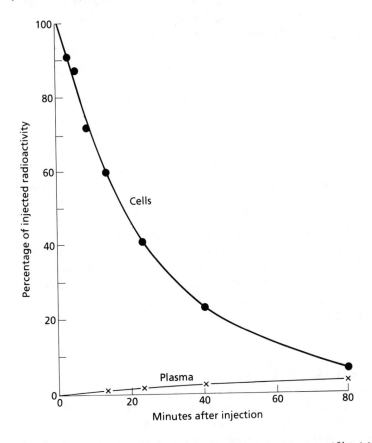

Figure 10.4 Radioactivity found in red cells and plasma following the injection of ^{51}Cr-labelled D-sensitized red cells. A small amount of radioactivity appears in the plasma about 10 min after the injection and reaches a maximum after about 1 h. This radioactivity in the plasma represents Hb liberated into the circulation (from Mollison, 1959d).

of the amount injected in the red cells. Presumably when amounts of this order are injected the capacity of the MPS to clear the Hb–haptoglobin complex is taxed and clearance is slowed so that the level tends to build up in the plasma.

Haemoglobinaemia associated with predominantly extravasular destruction is thought to be due primarily to lysis of red cells by lysosomal enzymes released by macrophages following contact of the antibody-coated cell with the macrophage. Thus, the process is thought to be the same as that observed in antibody-dependent cell-mediated cytotoxicity tests *in vitro*.

Relation between antibody characteristics and patterns of red cell destruction

Those antibodies, whether IgM or IgG , which activate complement but which cause either no lysis *in vitro* or only slow lysis characteristically bring about destruction of red cells mainly in the liver. Initially, destruction is rapid with a $T_{1/2}$ of a few minutes, but after 5–20 min (most commonly 5–10 min) destruction slows abruptly. When the antibody is IgM, destruction is virtually arrested but when it is IgG, destruction continues, although at a reduced rate (Mollison, 1989). These patterns do not indicate that there are two populations of red cells, one susceptible and one insusceptible to rapid destruction. Rather, they are due to the fact that initially the whole population is susceptible to rapid destruction and that then destruction slows, as C3b on the red cells is inactivated. Accordingly, the initial rate of destruction is obtained by extrapolating the tangent to the initial slope to the time axis, rather than by subtracting the 'slow component' (see Fig. 10.9 b below). The method of analysis of this type of disappearance curve in previous editions of this book was incorrect.

Those IgG antibodies which do not activate complement, e.g. anti-D, some examples of anti-K and -Fy^a etc., characteristically bring about destruction in the spleen, often with no measurable destruction in the liver. Destruction produced by immune non-complement-binding IgG antibodies is characteristically described by a single exponential, even when the rate of destruction is very slow. On the other hand, some naturally occurring, non-complement-binding IgG antibodies (anti-D, anti-E) bring about curves described by at least two components (pp. 458–459).

Although evidence reviewed in previous editions of this book appeared to indicate that non-complement-binding IgM antibodies could cause red cell destruction, a reappraisal of the data has led to the conclusion that they do not.

The following sections contain examples of destruction by the various kinds of antibody described above.

Complement-binding IgM antibodies

These alloantibodies, the commonest of which are anti-A, -B, -A$_1$,-HI, -P$_1$ -Le^a and -Le^b, are for the most part naturally occurring. Of this list, only anti-A and anti-B are often strongly lytic *in vitro* and *in vivo*. Lewis antibodies may cause slow lysis *in vitro* but only very rarely cause intravascular haemolysis. Anti-A$_1$, -HI and -P$_1$ are almost never lytic *in vitro*; rare examples activate complement to the C3 stage and when active at 37°C may be capable of destroying small volumes of incompatible red cells *in vivo*.

Some examples of the patterns of destruction produced by complement-binding IgM antibodies are as follows.

Anti-A and anti-B

As described above, anti-A and anti-B commonly bring about the intravascular destruction of a proportion of injected incompatible red cells (see Fig. 10.3).

In subjects with hypogammaglobulinaemia, who often have very low levels of anti-A and anti-B in their serum, destruction may be almost entirely extravascular. Destruction may be relatively rapid with an initial rate corresponding to a $T_{1/2}$ of a few min, with some slowing apparent after 10–20 min (Chaplin, 1959); or 50% may be removed with a $T_{1/2}$ of a few min with much slower removal ($T_{1/2}$ 1.5 d) of the remainder (van Loghem et al. 1965). In some cases there is no evidence of initial hepatic destruction, as in a case in which destruction was predominantly splenic with a $T_{1/2}$ of 12 h (van Loghem et al. 1965); presumably, in such cases, complement activation is too weak to influence the mode of destruction. In still other cases, survival is only slightly subnormal with a $T_{50}Cr$ (see p. 385) of 9–15 d. Similarly, in three healthy group A subjects without serologically detectable anti-B the $T_{50}Cr$ was 10–21 d (van Loghem et al. 1965). In these various cases, it is possible that destruction was influenced by an IgG component of antibody.

The effect of low concentrations of anti-B has also been investigated by injecting small volumes of B cells and of anti-B serum into a patient of group A with hypogammaglobulinaemia in whom group B cells had previously been found to have a $T_{50}Cr$ of 9–15 d; with varying amounts of anti-B the rate of destruction ranged from 1% to 14% per min (Jandl and Kaplan, 1960). It can be inferred from the data that slowing of destruction occurred after 6–21 min when 20–90% of the cells had been destroyed.

Experiments in which cells have been sensitized *in vitro* with anti-A or anti-B and then injected into the circulation of either healthy subjects or subjects with complement deficiency are described below in the section on sequestration and release of injected red cells.

Anti-Le^a and anti-Le^b

Most examples of anti-Le^a give a positive indirect antiglobulin test (IAT) (with anti-complement) at 37°C and cause some destruction *in vivo* of a small dose of Le(a +) red cells. With potent anti-Le^a the initial rate of clearance may have a $T_{1/2}$ as short as 1.9 min. When clearance occurs at this rate and when the 'lag' between the time of injection and the onset of destruction is as short as about 2 min, 10 min after injection survival will be about 5%. Unless observations are continued for longer than this, slowing of destruction may not be appreciated but, as Fig. 10.5 shows, slowing may be detectable by about 20 min when survival may have fallen to about 3%. With less potent examples of Lewis antibodies, slowing of destruction at 10–20 min is usually easy to detect (Mollison and Cutbush, 1955; Cutbush et al. 1956; Cutbush and Mollison, 1958; Mollison, 1959c; Mollison et al. 1963); see Fig. 10.5.

When group O, Le(b +) red cells were injected into the circulation of a group A subject whose plasma contained potent anti-Le^a, 20–50% of the transfused red cells were destroyed owing to the fact that in such subjects the red cells carry a small amount of Le^a substance (Cutbush et al. 1956); see Figs 10.5 and 10.6.

Only some examples of anti-Le^b react at 37°C with cells of the same ABO group as the recipient. With those that do, the pattern of destruction is the same as with anti-Le^a. For example, in one case in which a patient's plasma contained unusually potent anti-Le^b, clearly reactive at 37°C *in vitro*, the initial rate of destruction of group O, Le(a – b +) red cells had a $T_{1/2}$ of 4.5 min; destruction slowed abruptly after about 10 min and 44% of the cells were still present in the circulation at 6 h (Mollison, 1959c).

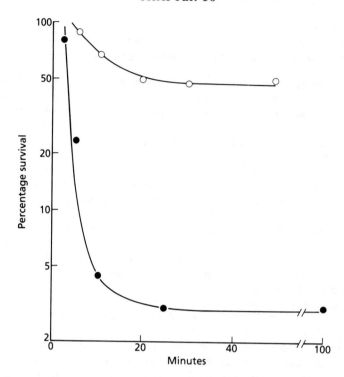

Figure 10.5 Clearance due to complement-binding IgM antibody (anti-Le^a) (from Mollison, 1986).
O—O 1 ml Le(a + b +) red cells injected into a subject whose plasma contained anti-Le^a. After a delay of 3 min, 50% of the cells are cleared rapidly, the initial rate of destruction having a $T_{1/2}$ of about 9 min; the rate of clearance starts to diminish within 10 min of injection and percentage survival is the same at 50 min as at 20 min (data from Cutbush *et al.* 1956).
●—● 1 ml Le(a + b –) red cells injected into the same subject; after a delay of about 2.3 min, 95% of the cells are cleared with a $T_{1/2}$ of 2 min; the rate of clearance starts to diminish within 10 min of injection and percentage survival is the same at 100 min as at 24 min (observations during first 10 min only published by Mollison and Cutbush, 1955).

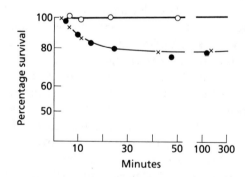

Figure 10.6 Survival of Le(b +) red cells from a group O donor, labelled with ^{32}P on one occasion (●) and with ^{51}Cr on another (×) and of Le(b +) red cells from a group A$_1$ donor (O) in a patient whose serum contained anti-Le^a. The partial destruction of the O red cells is due to the fact that they carry some Le^a antigen (from Cutbush *et al.* 1956).

In five cases in which anti-Le^b was active only at 30°C or less, survival of a small volume of Le(b +) red cells was normal at 24 h; in three others in which anti-Le^b was active at 37°C, 24-h survival ranged from 6% to 58%; in each of the three cases a two-component survival curve was observed (Davey *et al.* 1982).

Anti-A$_1$ -HI and -P$_1$
Most examples of these antibodies are not active *in vitro* above a temperature of about 25°C and are then incapable of causing destruction of injected red cells. In cases in which the antibody has reacted *in vitro* at 37°C, or has given definite reactions only up to 30–34°C, with dubious reactivity at 37°C, there has been some hepatic destruction initially with slowing after 10 min and with only slightly subnormal survival thereafter.

Figure 10.7 shows the patterns of destruction of small amounts of A$_1$ red cells in a patient with an anti-A$_1$ which was weakly active at 37°C. Initially, cells are cleared with a $T_{1/2}$ of a few minutes but within 10 min of injection of the cells the rate of destruction has slowed and after 20 min destruction is almost arrested.

Anti-HI. An example of destruction due to anti-HI is shown in Fig. 10.8; in this case, the antibody was clearly active at 37°C *in vitro* and group O red cells were cleared initially with a $T_{1/2}$ of 4 min; destruction slowed after about 10 min and thereafter was virtually arrested.

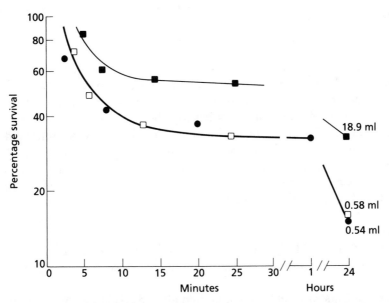

Figure 10.7 Destruction of two different amounts of A$_1$ red cells in the circulation of a patient whose serum contained anti-A$_1$ weakly active at 37°C by the indirect antiglobulin test (complement only). After the injection of about 0.55 ml (two different tests on successive days), about 65% of the cells were destroyed within 30 min. Two days later, after the injection of 18.9 ml cells, only about 45% of the cells were destroyed in the first 30 min (data from Mollison *et al.* 1978).

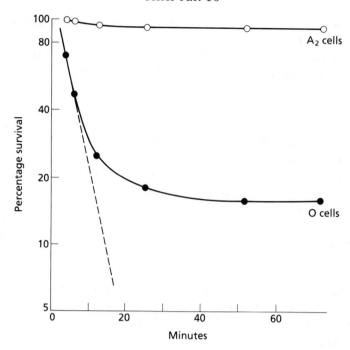

Figure 10.8 Survival of group O and group A_2 red cells in a patient whose serum contained anti-HI, acting *in vitro* as a saline agglutinin up to a temperature of approximately 30°C and behaving at 37°C as an incomplete complement-binding antibody detectable by the indirect antiglobulin test. The A_2 red cells underwent no significant destruction, but more than 80% of the O red cells were rapidly removed from the circulation; the initial rate of destruction (extrapolated as – – –) has a half-time of 3.5 min (from Mollison, 1959d).

Anti-P_1. A close relationship has been observed between thermal range *in vitro* and destruction of a 1 ml dose *in vivo*. For example, in a case in which the antibody was very weakly active at 31°C *in vitro* there was no destruction whatever in the 40 min following injections of 1 ml cells (unpublished observations). In a case in which, at 37°C, the antibody only doubtfully agglutinated red cells but weakly sensitized them to agglutination by an anti-complement reagent there was 20% destruction in the first 20 min with virtually normal survival thereafter. In a further case in which, at 37°C, there was weak agglutination and a definitely positive reaction with anti-complement, 50% of the cells were destroyed in 20 min (see Fig. 10.9).

Auto-anti-I
This antibody is considered here because the pattern of destruction of injected I-positive red cells is indistinguishable from that produced by the foregoing alloantibodies.

In three patients with cold haemagglutinin disease (CHAD) with potent auto-anti-I, following the injection of a small dose of ^{51}Cr-labelled I-positive red cells a two-component curve was observed, 30–60% of the cells being removed in 40–120 min with much slower removal of the remaining cells, i.e. $T_{1/2}$ 5–10 d (Evans *et al.* 1968).

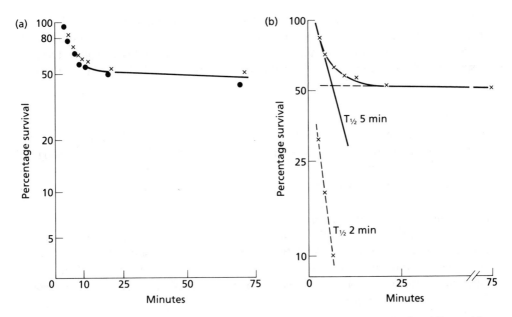

Figure 10.9   Destruction of P_1-positive red cells in a patient whose serum contained anti-P_1, weakly active at 37°C (see text).

(a) P_1-positive red cells labelled with ^{32}P were injected as an ice-cold suspension (●) and red cells from the same donor labelled with ^{51}Cr were injected as a warm (39°C) suspension (×) immediately afterwards. The temperature of the suspension at the time of injection did not appear to influence the survival (from Mollison and Cutbush, 1955). (b) Deduction of the initial rate of destruction of the warm suspension from (a). If it is (wrongly) assumed that there are two subpopulations of red cells, one susceptible to rapid destruction and one insusceptible, the half-time of clearance of the susceptible population, plotted as the difference between the observed points and the extrapolated 'slow' component, is estimated to be 2 min; if it is (correctly) assumed that all cells are initially susceptible, the initial rate of destruction is estimated to have a half-time of 5 min (from Mollison, 1989).

In a case in which detailed observations were made over the first 35 min, destruction started to slow 5–10 min after injection of the red cells and was very slow after 20 min, by which time about one-third of the cells had been destroyed (Mollison, 1985).

Anti-M
This antibody is usually regarded as non-complement binding but one example which appeared to bind complement has been described (patient D.S. of Cutbush and Mollison, 1958). *In vitro*, the serum would not agglutinate *MM* cells above a temperature of 34°C and would not agglutinate *MN* cells above a temperature of 31°C; however, at 37°C the serum did very weakly sensitize *MM* but not *MN* cells to an anti-complement serum. Serological activity was demonstrated only in an IgM fraction of the serum (Adinolfi *et al.* 1962). *In vivo*, about 65% of *MM* cells were removed rapidly, the initial rate of destruction having a $T_{1/2}$ of approximately 4 min; the rate of destruction slowed after about 10 min. *MN* cells were removed very much more slowly, about 50% of the cells being removed with a $T_{1/2}$ of 4.5 d. About 10 d after

injection of *MN* cells the rate of destruction slowed but subsequent analysis of the case suggests that this may have been due to a fall in concentration of serum anti-M consequent upon a further injection of *MM* cells at this time (Mollison, 1986). The slow destruction of *MN* cells may conceivably have been due to IgG anti-M in otherwise undetectable concentration.

Anti-Sd*ᵃ*

As described in Chapter 6, this antibody is IgM and complement binding. In the only example in which the survival of a small dose of incompatible red cells ('strong' Sd (a +)) has been studied, 50% of the cells were removed with a $T_{1/2}$ of 2 d, the rest being removed much more slowly (Petermans and Cole-Dergent, 1970).

Effect of temperature of injected red cells

In a subject with anti-P_1 weakly reactive *in vitro* at 37°C (Fig. 10.9) and in another with anti-M reactive *in vitro* at 34°C though not at 37°C (Mollison, 1959b), one sample of labelled incompatible red cells was warmed to 37°C and one, labelled with a different isotope, was cooled in ice-water; following injection, there was no detectable difference between the survival curves.

Effect of hypothermia on cold alloantibodies

Since almost all cold alloantibodies are IgM and complement binding it seems appropriate to consider at this point their clinical significance in patients undergoing artificial hypothermia. For many years now, in a large number of hospitals, blood has not been crossmatched at a temperature below 37°C for patients having operations involving hypothermia. It can be inferred that those cold alloantibodies which are inactive at 37°C but are active at some lower temperature such as 25°C or 30°C do not cause clinically significant red cell destruction when the patient is cooled. Although it is possible that there is some destruction by the cold alloantibody, it is difficult to make accurate observations of red cell survival because in the circumstances haemorrhage and transfusion disturb blood volume. One approach to this problem is to inject two labelled suspensions of red cells, one susceptible and one insusceptible to destruction, and to see whether the ratio of the two populations changes during hypothermia. In a case investigated in this way, no evidence of destruction by anti-P_1 was observed when the patient was cooled but some destruction had occurred before cooling so that the cells had presumably become resistant to complement-mediated destruction.

The patient, who was to undergo cardiac bypass, was P_1 negative with anti-P_1, weakly active at 37°C. During the early part of the operation, an injection of a mixture of ^{32}P-labelled P_1-negative and ^{51}Cr-labelled P_1-positive red cells was given; 25% of the P_1-positive red cells were destroyed but, then, destruction was virtually arrested. Thirty minutes later, the patient was cooled to 27–30°C for 20 min; no change in the ratio of the two labelled populations was observed (for further details, see previous editions of this book).

Complement-binding IgG antibodies

As described in Chapter 6, IgG antibodies of certain specificities, e.g. anti-K, -Fy*ᵃ* and

-Yt[a], only sometimes bind complement whereas those of other specificities, e.g. anti-Jk[a] and -Jk[b], always do so. Results observed with complement-binding IgG antibodies have been as follows:

Anti-K

In one subject *Kk* cells had a curvilinear slope of destruction; the initial rate had a $T_{1/2}$ of less than 20 min but by 1–2 h the $T_{1/2}$ was more than 1 h; surface counting showed that in the initial phase destruction occurred mainly in the liver, and in the later phase mainly in the spleen (Hughes-Jones *et al.* 1957b) . When *KK* cells were injected the initial rate of clearance had a $T_{1/2}$ of 6 min and destruction slowed about 20 min after injection (see Fig. 10.10). In a further case, about 80% of the cells were removed with an initial $T_{1/2}$ of 6 min; after about 30 min the $T_{1/2}$ had lengthened to about 30 min (Cutbush and Mollison, 1958, case 16).

Anti-Fy[a]

One example was studied extensively; in the subject (R.D.) in whom anti-Fy[a] was first identified, Fy (a +) cells showed a two-component curve of destruction; the initial rate of destruction had a $T_{1/2}$ of 4 min but after 15 min, by which time 90% of the cells had been cleared, destruction became very much slower (Cutbush and Mollison, 1958, case 18). In tests in which Fy (a +) cells were sensitized *in vitro* with purified anti-Fy[a] from R.D., up to 90% of the cells were cleared with a $T_{1/2}$ which could be as short as

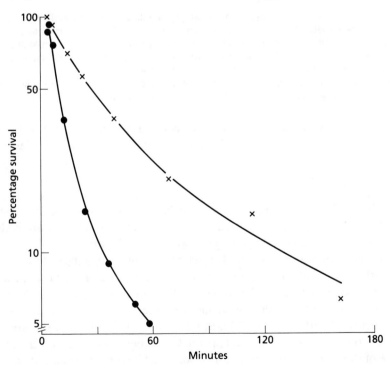

Figure 10.10 Destruction, by a complement-binding example of anti-K, of 1 ml doses of K-positive red cells.

●—●, *KK* cells (not previously published); x — x, *Kk* cells (Hughes-Jones *et al.* 1957b).

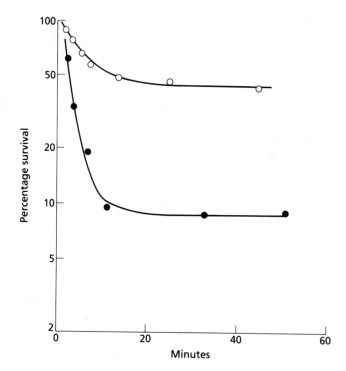

Figure 10.11 Clearance due to complement-binding IgG antibody (anti-Fy^a). Red cells (1 ml) of two Fy (a +) donors were coated *in vitro* with different amounts of anti-Fy^a and returned to each donor's circulation. The anti-Fy^a was a purified IgG fraction from a donor, R.D. (figure from Mollison, 1986).

After a delay of about 1 min, clearance begins with an initial $T_{1/2}$ of 8 min, but slows abruptly after about 10 min (Mollison, 1962, case 6a; rate of clearance recalculated).

After a delay of about 1.2 min, clearance begins with an initial $T_{1/2}$ of 2 min, but slows abruptly after about 10 min (Mollison, 1962, case 5; rate of clearance recalculated).

2.5 min (Cutbush and Mollison, 1958). Destruction slowed abruptly about 10 min after injection of the red cells (Fig. 10.11). The results of quantitative tests are described in a later section.

Anti-Jk^a and anti-Jk^b

Surprisingly, in the few examples that have been investigated, the two-component curves which are characteristic of destruction by complement-binding antibodies have not been observed. In one case, Jk^{a}Jk^a cells were cleared with a $T_{1/2}$ of 4 min, 99% of cells being removed within 30 min of injection. In the same subject Jk^{a}Jk^b cells were cleared with a $T_{1/2}$ of about 80 min and no slowing was observed during the 60 min after injection for which survival was followed (Cutbush and Mollison, 1958). In two other cases substantially slower destruction was observed: with an example of anti-Jk^a, cells were cleared with a $T_{1/2}$ of 75 min (Fudenberg and Allen, 1957), and with an example of anti-Jk^b, destruction also appeared to be described by a single exponential, with 90% of the cells being cleared in a period of 24 h (Howard *et al.* 1982a).

Anti-Yt^a

In a patient with a complement-binding IgG example of this antibody, approximately

85% of Yt (a +) cells were cleared within 12 min, the remainder being cleared much more slowly (Bettigole *et al.* 1968).

Acquired resistance to complement-mediated destruction

In almost all the curves of destruction described above due to complement-binding antibodies, whether IgM or IgG, there is a common feature: destruction is initially rapid, with a $T_{1/2}$ of a few minutes, indicating hepatic destruction, but after an interval which may be as short as 5 min or as long as 60 min (most commonly about 10 min) destruction slows abruptly. There is much evidence to indicate that the slowing of destruction is due to the cleavage of C3b, leaving on the red cell surface the complex C3dg which does not mediate red cell destruction.

Acquired resistance of red cells to destruction by alloantibodies was described by Möller (1964; 1965) in mice. The effect could be produced both *in vitro* and *in vivo* and depended on specific antibody and on some host factor. All cells were susceptible to lysis by undiluted serum but if the cells were incubated with diluted antibody-containing serum and with undiluted complement they became resistant to lysis. When H-2 incompatible red cells were transfused from one strain of mice to another, some of the cells were rapidly eliminated but the rest survived normally, despite the production of humoral antibody directed against the transfused cells. A similar effect was demonstrated in CHAD by Evans *et al.* (1967; 1968). Transfused red cells underwent rapid destruction initially but, within an hour, destruction slowed and the remaining cells were destroyed far more slowly. Donor red cells could be made relatively resistant to destruction by exposure to CHAD serum *in vitro* under conditions which were unfavourable for lysis; resistance to destruction was associated with the accumulation of complement on the red cells. Similar observations were reported by Engelfriet *et al.* (1972b) who discussed the possibility that the accumulation of α_{2D} (C3dg) on the red cell membrane might block the attachment of further C3 molecules; see also Jaffe *et al.* (1976).

Further work confirmed that the presence of functionally active C3 on the red cells was essential for hepatic sequestration and that cells coated with C3d (or C3dg) alone were not cleared from the circulation. Presumably, the active forms of C3 are C3b and iC3b, for both of which products there are receptors on phagocytic cells (Fearon, 1984); the inactive product, found on the red cells of patients with CHAD is C3dg (Lachmann *et al.* 1983).

Acquired resistance of transfused ABO-incompatible red cells to destruction was strongly suggested by observations published by Akeroyd and O'Brien (1958). After the transfusion of group AB cells to a group A patient, some surviving cells could be demonstrated after 6 weeks even though the recipient's serum contained an anti-B lysin. The fact that these cells had become resistant to destruction was implied by the observation that, when a new sample of AB cells was injected, 90% of the cells were removed from the circulation within 45 min.

Acquired resistance to destruction presumably indicates the presence on the red cells of C3dg around the sites of antibody attachment. It has been shown that 85–95% of bound C3d disappears from circulating red cells in 5–8 d (Chaplin *et al.* 1983). It therefore seems that destruction depending on complement activation should be able to continue, although at a greatly reduced rate. It would also be expected that the slowing of the rate of destruction, observed some 10 min after injection of red cells into the circulation, would be much less with IgG than with IgM antibodies, since, whereas IgG alone can cause destruction, IgM antibodies are dependent on complement activation. The difference between the effects produced by IgG and IgM complement-binding antibodies is shown by examples given above. For example, with IgG anti-K, after the initial rapid phase of destruction, the subsequent phase (with KK cells) continued with a $T_{1/2}$ of 30 min. In contrast, in destruction by IgM anti-P_1, after the initial phase of rapid destruction the rate became too small to measure. For further examples, see Mollison (1989).

Sequestration and release of complement-coated red cells

When red cells are sensitized *in vitro* with a complement-binding antibody, or with complement alone, a proportion of the injected population is rapidly cleared but some or all of the red cells slowly return to the circulation. The initial disappearance is presumably due to the attachment of the iC3b-coated red cell to a macrophage. When iC3b is cleaved, leaving only C3dg on the red cell, the cell is released back into the circulation.

This temporary trapping followed by the release of complement-coated red cells has been demonstrated in various experiments:

1 When a sample of red cells from a group B subject was incubated with anti-B and then reinjected into the circulation, 26% of the cells were removed almost immediately but returned to the circulation during the next 2 h (Jandl *et al.* 1957).

2 When the red cells of a patient with CHAD were exposed to their own serum at 4°C *in vitro* and then reinjected, about 40% were removed in 15 min; more than half the cells returned to the circulation within 60 min and most within 24 h (Lewis *et al.* 1960).

3 In experiments in which red cells were coated with complement alone by exposure to their own serum at low ionic strength, following reinjection into the circulation 25–40% were sequestered; some cells returned within 60 min and almost all within 24 h (Mollison, 1965).

4 In C6-deficient rabbits, when red cells were coated *in vitro* with human anti-I and then reinjected, so that they bound C4, C3 (and C5), 45–95% were sequestered but most of the cells returned to the circulation in 2–3 h (Brown *et al.* 1970). For further observations see Schreiber and Frank (1972) and Atkinson and Frank (1974a).

5 When group A or B cells were coated *in vitro* with relatively small amounts of purified anti-A or anti-B (20 IgM molecules per coated cell), after reinjection into the circulation about 30% disappeared within the first 12 min but almost all reappeared within the next 3 h. As the degree of coating with antibody increased, so the proportion of cells that reappeared in the circulation after initial sequestration diminished. In two subjects with low levels of C2 and C4, cells coated with moderate amounts of IgM antibody had a normal survival. The authors concluded that IgM molecules alone were incapable of bringing about accelerated destruction and that red cell destruction depended entirely on complement fixation (Atkinson and Frank. 1974a)

Rate of cleavage of C3b in vitro and in vivo

In vitro, the conversion of C3b to iC3b takes about 1 min; in blood, where there are cells carrying CR1, the co-factor (with I) for the reaction, the further cleavage of the molecule, which splits off C3c and leaves only C3dg on the cell surface has a $T_{1/2}$ of about 20 min (see Chapter 3). This estimate of the rate of cleavage is very approximately consistent with the observation that the rate of destruction of complement-coated red cells may slow within 5–10 min of their injection into the circulation. On the other hand, it does not agree well with the observation that the release of temporarily sequestered complement-coated red cells takes about 2–3 h (see above). The reason for the discrepancy is unknown.

Role of IgM and of complement in producing irreversible sequestration
When incompatible red cells are injected into a subject with a complement-binding antibody which appears to be solely IgM, a proportion of the red cells is rapidly cleared and these cells do not return to the circulation. On the other hand, as described above, when red cells are sensitized *in vitro* with an IgM complement-binding antibody, many of the cells that are initially sequestered later return to the circulation. IgM antibody alone does not cause red cell destruction (see above and see also below) and complement alone seems normally to be almost ineffective. An apparent exception is provided by the phagocytosis by neutrophils of yeast particles coated only with C3b (Forslid *et al.* 1985) but this is only an enhancing effect since neutrophils phagocytose yeast particles not coated with complement. Although C3b seems to be involved primarily in bringing about attachment to macrophages rather than in promoting ingestion (Mantovani *et al.* 1977), macrophages activated by a lymphokine show C3b-receptor-dependent phagocytosis (Griffin and Mullinax, 1977). The enhanced activity of macrophages in infection is mentioned in Chapter 3.

The effect of IgM in phagocytosis seems either to be to collaborate in some unspecified way with complement or to bring about the binding of amounts of complement greater than can be bound without the help of antibody.

Non-complement-binding IgM antibodies
In previous editions of this book several examples of destruction by IgM antibodies which seemed to be non-complement binding were described. Re-examination of the evidence has cast doubt on the interpretation of the data (Mollison, 1986). In brief, the example of anti-M which produced rapid destruction of *MM* red cells should not have been described as non-complement binding, nor should the IgM fraction of the rabbit alloantibody anti-Hg^A. It remains to consider the examples of IgM Rh antibodies which appear to have been responsible for red cell destruction. As described in Chapter 5, the great majority of Rh antibodies which have been examined have been incapable of activating complement. In one series of experiments, various amounts of a purified IgM fraction of anti-D were injected, together with 1 ml D-positive red cells, into D-negative volunteers. Accelerated red cell destruction was observed and the fastest rate of clearance was found in the subject injected with the largest amount (150 μg) of IgM anti-D. In this subject red cells were cleared with a $T_{1/2}$ of 11 h and the rate of destruction slowed after about 12 h. It now seems probable that this effect was due to contamination of the preparation with a small amount of IgG anti-D and that the test — immunoelectrophoresis — which failed to reveal any IgG in the IgM preparation, failed to detect a few μg of IgG anti-D which would have been enough, when given i.v., to have caused the clearance of D-positive cells that was observed. Slowing of

CHAPTER 10

destruction at about 12 h might well have been due to the fall in the serum level of IgG anti-D due to equilibrium of injected IgG with the extravascular compartment (Mollison, 1986). Rapid destruction of c-positive red cells in a subject whose serum contained IgM anti-c is now thought to have been caused by IgG anti-c in the subject's serum; see below.

Non-complement-binding IgG antibodies

Virtually all examples of IgG anti-D and some examples of IgG anti-K, anti-S and anti-Fy[a] fail to bind complement. Antibodies of this kind bring about red cell destruction predominantly in the spleen (Jandl, 1955; Mollison and Cutbush, 1955; Hughes-Jones et al. 1957b; Jandl et al. 1957; Cutbush and Mollison, 1958; Crome and Mollison, 1964; see Fig. 10.12).

As discussed in a later section, with antibodies of most of the specificities mentioned above, the number of molecules of IgG bound per cell cannot exceed about 25 000, due to the relatively small numbers of corresponding antigen sites. On the other hand, with anti-c, due to the greater number of c sites, a theoretical maximum of about 80 000 molecules of anti-c per red cell can be bound. In retrospect, this fact is thought to explain the relatively rapid clearance of c-positive red cells in a subject whose serum contained both IgM and IgG anti-c. In this subject, cc red cells were cleared with a $T_{1/2}$ of 2.8 min, indicating clearance of 70% of the blood at a single passage through the liver (Fig. 10.13), a finding originally believed to indicate clearance by IgM anti-c (Cutbush and Mollison, 1958). The subsequent recognition that the

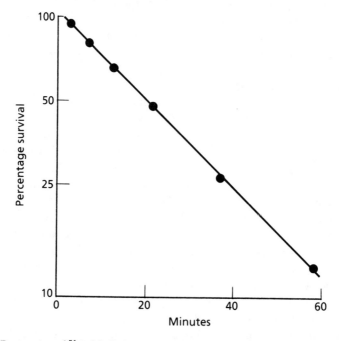

Figure 10.12 Destruction of ^{51}Cr-labelled Kk red cells in subject with non-complement-binding anti-K; the points are fitted by a single exponential with a $T_{1/2}$ of 19 min. After the cells had been cleared from the circulation, virtually all the ^{51}Cr was localized in the area of the spleen (Hughes-Jones et al. 1957, case 3).

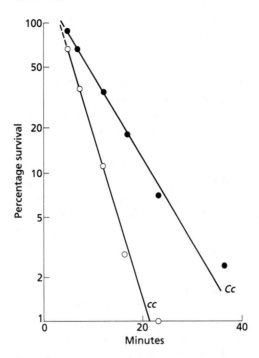

Figure 10.13 Clearance of c-positive red cells in a subject whose serum contained both IgG and IgM anti-c. *cc* cells (○—○) were cleared with a $T_{1/2}$ of 2.8 min, and *cC* cells with a $T_{1/2}$ of 5.6 min (data from Cutbush and Mollison, 1958).

serum also contained relatively potent IgG anti-c, and the subsequent finding that c sites were more abundant than D sites, led to the reinterpretation of the data (Mollison, 1989). It was calculated that the number of anti-c molecules bound per cell might have been 57 000 (N.C. Hughes-Jones, personal communication).

The degree of coating with IgG needed to produce complete clearance of coated red cells at a single passage through the spleen and the degree needed to produce some clearance by the liver are discussed below, in the section beginning on p. 466.

The fact that red cells coated with anti-D are removed from the circulation predominantly in the spleen can be turned to advantage. First, scanning with a gamma camera following the injection of D-sensitized red cells can be used to locate splenic tissue when this is in aberrant position, e.g. on top of the uterus (Mollison, 1979, p. 504). Second, the presence of a splenunculus, as in a patient with hereditary spherocytosis who relapses following splenectomy, can be demonstrated (Mackenzie *et al.* 1962). Third, estimation of the rate of clearance of D-positive red cells coated with an amount of anti-D which would normally give clearance at a single passage through the spleen can be used to determine whether splenic size or splenic blood flow are abnormal. For example, in a patient with hereditary spherocytosis with a spleen later shown at operation to weigh 395 g, D-sensitized red cells were cleared with a $T_{1/2}$ of just over 8 min compared with the normal $T_{1/2}$ of about 18–22 min (Mollison, 1970). Again, in a subject with a normal-sized spleen, suspected of having been damaged at a previous operation, D-sensitized red cells were cleared with a $T_{1/2}$ of 60 min, strongly suggesting that the spleen was infarcted with a much reduced blood flow, a finding confirmed at operation (Mollison, 1979, p. 504). Finally, in subjects in whom the MPS is partially blocked by immune complexes, as in lupus erythematosus, clearance of D-sensitized red cells is much slower than in normal subjects (Frank *et al.* 1979).

Similarly, in adults with AITP injected with 1–1.5 g IgG/kg body-weight, the rate of clearance of D-sensitized red cells was slowed (Fehr *et al.* 1982).

In splenectomized subjects, D-positive red cells coated with an amount of anti-D which, in a subject with a spleen, would bring about clearance at a maximal or almost maximal rate, are cleared with a $T_{1/2}$ of about 5 h (Jandl *et al.* 1957; Crome and Mollison, 1964; Brown, 1983). Red cells which are more heavily coated with anti-D may be removed with a $T_{1/2}$ as short as 90–160 min (Crome and Mollison, 1964; Brown, 1983).

As mentioned earlier in the chapter it is believed that the destruction in the liver of red cells carrying only moderate amounts of IgG is partially inhibited because plasma IgG blocks Fc receptor sites on the macrophages. On the other hand, when the number of IgG molecules bound to red cells exceeds a certain value (which is different for IgG1 and IgG3), IgG in the plasma no longer blocks binding of antibody-coated cells to Fc receptor sites (Engelfriet *et al.* 1981).

Naturally occurring Rh antibodies
The survival of small volumes of incompatible red cells has been studied in a few subjects with naturally occurring anti-E or anti-D; although, in the past, naturally occurring Rh antibodies have been assumed to be solely IgM, recent investigations using more sensitive tests indicate that the antibodies are partly IgG, at least in many instances.

Anti-E is the commonest naturally occuring Rh antibody but its effect on the survival of E-positive red cells has been studied in only a very few cases. In the subject described by Vogt *et al.* (1958), the survival curve had an interesting shape, about one-quarter of the cells being cleared with a $T_{1/2}$ of 20 min and the rest with a $T_{1/2}$ of several hours. This example of anti-E cannot properly be regarded as naturally occurring since the subject had received transfusions of E-positive blood 52 and 41 d respectively before the test was carried out. On the other hand, in the series described by Jensen *et al.* (1965) there was one subject who had not previously been transfused and in whom survival of E-positive red cells was only slightly subnormal ($T_{50}Cr$, 19.5 d).

In a small series studied by Contreras *et al.* (1987) survival was normal in one case but was definitely reduced in two: in one of these, approximately two-thirds of the cells were removed with a $T_{1/2}$ of a few hours and the rest with a $T_{1/2}$ of almost 5 d. In the other, 25% of cells were cleared in 24 h. The antibodies were at least partly IgG.

Anti-D. As described in Chapter 5, the kind of naturally occurring anti-D found on screening in the AutoAnalyzer and by no other method is IgG and cold reacting. In one subject with an antibody of this kind, $T_{50}Cr$ was 19 d, i.e. only slightly reduced (Perrault and Högman, 1972). Strictly normal survival was found in one case by Lee *et al.* (1984). In another series, of three examples of apparently naturally occurring anti-D in males, survival was virtually normal in one but was greatly reduced in the remaining two. In one of these about 75% of the cells were removed with a $T_{1/2}$ of a few hours, the remainder being removed with a $T_{1/2}$ of approximately 6 d. In the remaining case all the cells were removed with a $T_{1/2}$ of 2 h but this subject had an indirect antiglobulin titre of 2 (Contreras *et al.* 1987).

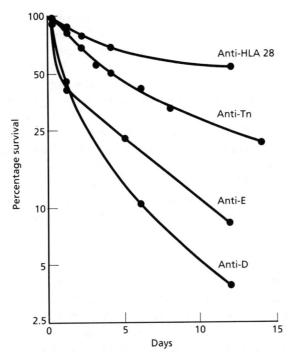

Figure 10.14 Curves with more than one component, associated with destruction by antibodies believed to be non-complement-activating.

Anti-HLA-28: survival of red cells on which HLA-28 was very strongly expressed, in a patient whose serum contained anti-HLA-28 (Nordhagen and Aas, 1978).

Anti-Tn: survival of red cells from a patient with Tn transformation in a normal subject, i.e. with anti-Tn (Myllylla *et al.* 1971).

Anti-E and anti-D: survival of E-positive and D-positve red cells, respectively, in subjects whose serum contained naturally occurring anti-E and anti-D (Contreras *et al.* 1987).

In summary, almost normal, or normal, survival has been found in some subjects with naturally occurring anti-E or anti-D but definitely reduced survival has been found in others. A puzzling feature of these latter cases has been the two-component curves of survival, with slowing occurring as a rule some hours after injection of red cells into the circulation; see Fig. 10.14.

Destruction by other non-complement-binding IgG antibodies
In tests with small volumes of incompatible red cells, destruction by the following antibodies has also been demonstrated:

Anti-Lu^b. Lu (a + b +) red cells: (i) antibody weakly reactive at 37°C: 15% of cells removed in first hour, remainder much more slowly (Cutbush and Mollison, 1958); (ii) antibody titre 256 at 37°C: 54% of cells removed in 8 d (Tilley *et al.* 1977). Lu (a − b +) red cells: (i) antibody weakly reactive at 37°C: 70% of cells removed with $T_{1/2}$ 15 min, remainder much more slowly (Cutbush and Mollison, 1958); (ii) antibody titre 32 at 37°C: cells removed with $T_{1/2}$ 5 h (Peters *et al.* 1978). All the foregoing antibodies were at least partly IgG but may have been partly IgM and, or, partly IgA.

Anti-Yt^a. Accelerated destruction has been reported in several cases (Gobel *et al.* 1974; Ballas and Sherwood, 1977; Silvergleid *et al.* 1978; Davey and Simpkins, 1981). Non-destructive examples of anti-Yt^a are mentioned below.

Other specificities. Destruction by examples of the following IgG antibodies has been described: anti-N; $T_{1/2}$ 0.9 d (Ballas *et al.* 1985); anti-Do^a: $T_{1/2}$ 1.5–3 h (Swanson *et al.* 1965; Polesky and Swanson, 1966); anti-Co^b: $T_{1/2}$ (initially) 4 d (Dzik and Blank, 1986); anti-Wr^a (?partly IgG): $T_{1/2}$ 80 min (Cutbush and Mollison, 1958); anti-Hy: two-component curve with half-times of 3.5 and 15 d, respectively (Beattie and Castillo, 1975); anti-Jr^a: $T_{1/2}$ 80 min (Kendall, 1979); anti-Ok^a: 90% clearance in 3 h (Morel and Hamilton, 1979); anti-In^b, $T_{1/2}$ about 36 h (Ferguson and Gaal, 1988); an IgG1 anti-Lu6, 80% destruction in 1 h; results with ⁵¹Cr and flow cytometry agreed closely (Issitt *et al.* 1990a). A few other cases of the destruction of test doses of red cells by rare antibodies are described in Chapter 6.

Non-destructive antibodies

Antibodies not expected to cause red cell destruction are: (1) those that are active only at temperatures below 37°C; (2) those that are active at 37°C but are solely IgM and do not bind complement; and (3) those that are IgG but are confined to subclasses IgG2 or IgG4, or are IgG1 but present only in low concentration (see pp. 296 and 299).

Since in many cases IgG subclass has not been determined and it is in any case at present impossible to determine the IgG subclass of all antibodies, particularly those present in low concentration, it is often a matter for speculation whether a particular IgG antibody will, or will not, cause red cell destruction.

The following antibodies, though active *in vitro* at 37°C, and though shown to be, or presumed to be, IgG, have failed to bring about red cell destruction or have produced only dubious destruction:

Anti-LW

In two patients whose serum contained anti-LW, a small dose (2–10 ml) of incompatible red cells had a normal survival at 1 h and a slightly subnormal or normal survival at 20 h (78–90%). In both patients 4 units of LW-positive blood were transfused without incident (Cummings *et al.* 1984; Chaplin *et al.* 1985). In a further case there was no evidence that anti-LW destroyed transfused red cells (Tregellas *et al.* 1978). On the other hand, in the first patient in whom anti-LW^b was detected, the antibody (IgG) brought about clearance of a test dose of LW(a – b +) red cells with a $T_{1/2}$ of 2.5 h (Sistonen *et al.* 1981).

Anti-Lu^a

In a patient whose plasma contained relatively potent anti-Lu^a, active at 37°C, ⁵¹Cr-labelled Lu (a +) red cells (approximately 10 ml) were considered to have a normal survival (Greendyke and Chorpenning, 1962). Perhaps the antibody was solely IgM (non-complement binding) or IgG4.

Anti-Yt^a

Examples which appeared to be incapable of destroying red cells were described by

Eaton *et al.* (1956) and by Dobbs *et al.* (1968). In the latter case, ^{51}Cr-labelled Yt (a +) red cells were shown to have a strictly normal survival. In another case mentioned in the seventh edition of this book Yt (a +) red cells had a strictly normal survival at 24 h in a patient whose serum contained IgG anti-Yt^a. As described earlier, several other examples of anti-Yt^a have been shown to cause accelerated destruction of Yt (a +) red cells.

Anti-Xg^a

In one case, in which the titre of the antibody (IgG, apparently non-complement binding) was 8–16, a small volume of Xg (a +) red cells survived normally (Sausais *et al.* 1964). The authors pointed out that it was probable that an example (IgG, complement-binding) described earlier (Cook *et al.* 1963) had also failed to cause destruction.

Anti-Yk^a and anti-Cs^a

Normal survival of Yk (a +) red cells in a patient whose plasma contained anti-Yk^a with a titre of more than 1000 by the IAT was reported by Tilley *et al.* (1977). Apparently normal survival (reported as $T_{1/2}$Cr 21.5 d) of strongly Cs^a-positive cells in a patient whose plasma contained anti-Cs^a was reported by Shore and Steane (1977). For further examples, see Issitt (1985).

Anti-McC^a, -Kn^a and -JMH

In two patients with anti-McC^a, and in single patients with each of the other antibodies listed, an initial test using ^{51}Cr-labelled incompatible red cells showed survival of at least 85% at 1 h. Within 24 h a second injection of red cells was given followed by transfusion of a unit of the same red cells and survival was followed for periods of 9–20 d. T_{50}Cr was strictly normal in the subject with anti-Kn^a but appeared to be somewhat reduced (12–15 d) in the remaining four cases (Baldwin *et al.* 1985). However, the fact that blood stored for approximately 2 weeks was used in two cases and that the patients had diseases which might have shortened the survival of transfused red cells makes it difficult to say whether the antibodies caused any destruction or not. In three further cases in which the serum contained anti-Kn^a the survival of positively reacting red cells was normal at 1 h (Silvergleid *et al.* 1978). In three subjects with anti-JMH, ^{51}Cr-labelled JMH-positive red cells survived normally; in these and in seven other subjects, 'least incompatible blood' was transfused without untoward reactions (Sabo *et al.* 1978).

Anti-HLA ('anti-Bg')

Several examples of normal or almost normal survival of Bg (+) red cells have been described in the circulation of patients with corresponding antibodies (Perkins, 1975; Silvergleid *et al.* 1978). Although, in the series of Panzer *et al.* (1984b) it was concluded that anti-HLA caused accelerated destruction in six of six cases, according to the interpretation of the present authors survival was probably normal in four of the cases (their cases 3–6).

In analysing their Cr survival curves, Panzer *et al.* (1984) calculated mean life span using the method recommended by ICSH (1980b). However, this method was meant to be applied to the survival of autologous, not potentially incompatible red cells. When the red cell survival curve has more than one component, the method proposed by ICSH (1980b) is not applicable. The Cr survival curves published by Panzer *et al.* show that $T_{50}Cr$ in their cases 3–6 was approximately 24–30 d, i.e. probably within normal limits.

Definitely increased destruction, by anti-HLA, of red cells with strongly expressed HLA antigens has been described in a few cases. When red cells from the donor described by van der Hart *et al.* (1974)—see Chapter 6—were injected into a patient with an incompatible cytotoxic HLA antibody, a two-component curve of elimination was observed, about 60% of the cells being removed with a $T_{1/2}$ of about 100 min and the rest with a $T_{1/2}$ of 20 h. A two-component curve of elimination was also observed when red cells with very strongly expressed HLA-28 were injected into a patient whose serum contained anti-HLA-28: 20% of the cells were removed with a $T_{1/2}$ of 1.5 d, the rest having a more or less normal survival (Nordhagen and Aas, 1978; see Fig. 10.14). Similarly, the data published by Panzer *et al.* (1984b), relating to their cases 1 and 2, show about 25% destruction in the first 24 h, with more or less normal survival of the remaining cells, although the data were not interpreted in this way by Panzer *et al.*

Anti-Chido and anti-Rodgers

Small volumes of ^{51}Cr-labelled Ch (+) red cells have been shown to survive normally in subjects with anti-Ch (Moore *et al.* 1975; Tilley *et al.* 1975; Silvergleid *et al.* 1978).

Even if anti-Ch and anti-Rg were capable of causing red cell destruction, they would not be expected to cause haemolytic transfusion reactions except when washed red cells were transfused, because the antigens are present in the plasma as well as on the red cells and thus neutralize the antibodies. Accounts of the uneventful transfusion of Ch (+) blood to patients with potent anti-Ch have been published (Harris *et al.* 1967; Nordhagen and Aas, 1979).

Relation between results of cellular bioassays and destruction *in vivo*

On the whole, a good correlation has been found between the results of monocyte or macrophage monolayer tests and evidence of destruction *in vivo*. In the first series to be described, 25 antibodies (anti-Yt^a, -Jr^a, -Ch, -JMH, etc.) which had failed to cause haemolytic transfusion reactions or haemolytic disease of the newborn gave low values in the assay, whereas two which had caused either a haemolytic transfusion reaction or had rapidly destroyed ^{51}Cr-labelled red cells gave high values (Schanfield *et al.* 1981). In another series, six antibodies (all anti-Yt^a, -Ge or -Lan) which had not caused haemolytic reactions after the transfusion of incompatible red cells or (in two cases) had not rapidly destroyed ^{51}Cr-labelled red cells gave a negative monocyte monolayer assay, whereas five antibodies (anti-Yt^a, -Ge or -Lan) which had rapidly destroyed labelled red cells gave positive results. Two of these five were anti-Lan, and these gave positive results only when fresh serum was used for the assay (Nance *et al.* 1987).

In one series, four patients with anti-McC^a, -JMH or -Hy^a were found to give negative macrophage assays but apparently destroyed incompatible red cells at an accelerated rate; the survival rate of labelled cells was 89–95% at 1 h but the $T_{50}Cr$ was 12–15 d (Baldwin *et al.* 1985). There must be some hesitation in accepting these findings as evidence of antibody-mediated destruction: some patients had chronic bleeding and others were transfused during the study period.

Apart from these relatively extensive studies, there have been many reports of single cases: an example of anti-Cr^a which brought about more than 4% destruction of a small volume of incompatible red cells in 4 h gave a clearly positive result in a monocyte monolayer test (McSwain and Robins, 1988); on the other hand, an example of anti-Lu12 which destroyed 50% of a small dose of incompatible red cells *in vivo*, did not react in a mononuclear assay (Shirey *et al.* 1988).

In a patient who had formed an antibody against the Cromer-related antigen Tc^a, the survival at 24 h of a test dose of incompatible red cells was probably within normal limits and an MMA was normal; at this time the antibody was a mixture of IgG2 and IgG4, although some years previously it had also been partly IgG1 and an MMA had been well above normal limits (Anderson *et al.* 1991).

Using a test for monocyte phagocytosis (see Chapter 3), a negative result was obtained with an example of an IgG1 monoclonal anti-D which failed to destroy D-positive red cells *in vivo* (Crawford *et al.* 1988); and using a test for adherence to, and phagocytosis by, monocytes and an ADCC(M) assay (see Chapter 3), positive results were obtained with two monoclonal anti-Ds, one IgG1 and one IgG3 (Wiener *et al.* 1988), which were subsequently shown to produce accelerated clearance of D-positive red cells *in vivo* (Thomson *et al.* 1990). The same two monoclonal antibodies gave moderately strong results when tested 'blind' in a number of bioassays with monocytes, although they gave only weak reactions in an ADCC(L) assay (Report from Nine Collaborating Laboratories, 1990).

Although bioassays have not yet been demonstrated to predict the speed and extent of red cell destruction produced by particular antibodies, they do seem to be able to distinguish between those antibodies that produce accelerated destruction of red cells and those that do not. Bioassays should, therefore, prove valuable as an adjunct to crossmatching, when the recipient has an antibody of dubious clinical significance, although, so far, they do not seem to have been used in this way. Of course, like serological tests, bioassays cannot be expected to predict cases in which the recipient is primarily immunized to a red cell antigen and may therefore develop a delayed haemolytic transfusion reaction if transfused.

Effect of antigen content of red cells

In earlier sections several examples have been given of differences in the rate of destruction of two samples of red cells depending on their antigen content. The purpose of this section is to bring these observations together and to add a few additional ones.

Subgroups of A

There are a number of clinical observations which indicate that A$_1$ red cells are more rapidly destroyed than A$_2$ red cells when injected into recipients of group O. For example, Wiener *et al.* (1953b) injected 30–40 ml A$_1$ or A$_2$ blood, dilute in saline, to group O recipients over a period of 1 h. In all of five subjects injected with A$_1$ blood, haemoglobinaemia (80–100 mg/dl) was observed and three of the five recipients developed reactions. In five subjects injected with A$_2$ blood no haemoglobinaemia was observed and no reactions developed.

In another group O subject, when 0.5 ml A_1 red cells was injected, a sample taken 3 min after injection contained only 0.5% of the injected cells and 54% of the injected radioactivity was free in the plasma. When 0.5 ml A_2 red cells was injected into the same subject a sample taken 3 min after injection contained 2.5% of the injected red cells and only 38% of the injected radioactivity was free in the plasma (Mollison, 1959d). The rather small difference between the amount of intravascular destruction in the two cases was thought to be due to the fact that the A_2 donor was a relatively 'high grade A_2', i.e. a relatively strong reactor.

Further evidence of the relative insusceptibility of A_2 cells is provided by cases in which an A_2 or A_2B recipient is transfused with A_1 or A_1B blood and then with group O blood containing potent anti-A, when it is found that the A_1 or A_1B red cells are destroyed preferentially (see p. 506).

In a case described by Hartmann (1957) an A_2B patient was transfused with three bottles of A_1B blood during an operation followed by one bottle of group O blood; 'haematuria' was observed. During the next 24 h two more bottles of group O blood were transfused, and after each bottle 'haematuria' was noted. The anti-A titres of the donors were relatively low (64–128). Two months later the patient's circulation contained A_2B and O cells but no A_1B. Anti-A_1 was present but had disappeared after a further month.

Although red cells with a weak A antigen are relatively insusceptible to damage by anti-A, a haemolytic reaction following the transfusion of A_x blood has been reported in a patient whose serum contained potent anti-A; the pre-transfusion titre was 1000 vs. A_1 cells and 8 vs. A_x cells (Schmidt et al. 1959).

B red cells in newborn infants
Although the A and B antigens are considerably weaker in newborn infants than in adults, in experiments in which 1 ml group B cord red cells was injected into group A mothers whose anti-B titre never exceeded 32, all the red cells were destroyed within 20 min and usually within 5 min, mainly by intravascular lysis (see Sieg et al. 1970).

Differences in the P_1 and Lewis antigens
It is well known that there are considerable differences between the 'strength' of P_1 antigen in different P_1-positive blood samples; these differences observed in tests in vitro are correlated with the amount of red cell destruction in vivo. For example, in a patient whose serum contained a strong anti-P_1, the red cells of one P_1-positive donor were injected and the proportion destroyed rapidly was 49% and 51% on two different occasions. In between these two tests the red cells of another P_1-positive donor, whose red cells reacted a little more strongly in vitro, were injected and 60% were destroyed rapidly in vivo.

Another example of the relationship between the strength of reactivity in vitro and the proportion of red cells destroyed rapidly in vivo is provided by tests made in a patient whose serum contained anti-Le^a. In this patient the red cells of adult donors of the phenotype Le (a + b –) were removed with a $T_{1/2}$ of approximately 2 min whereas those of infant donors of the phenotype Le (a + b +) were removed with a $T_{1/2}$ of 3–5 min (Cutbush et al. 1956). In the same subject, as mentioned above, red cells from adult donors of the phenotype O,Le (b +), which carry small amounts of Le^a antigen on their surface, underwent partial destruction.

Differences between red cells from homozygotes and heterozygotes

An example of the slightly more rapid destruction of *cc* red cells compared with *Cc* by anti-c, is shown in Fig. 10.13. Considerably more rapid destruction of *Jk^{a}Jk^a* red cells than of *Jk^{a}Jk^b*, cells by anti-Jk^a and a very big difference between the rate of destruction of *MM* and *MN* cells, was described by Cutbush and Mollison (1958).

Survival curves with more than one component

As discussed above, acquired resistance to complement-mediated destruction seems to be the commonest cause of survival curves with two components. There are only a few examples of two-component survival curves which seem not to be due to acquired resistance to complement-mediated destruction:

1 *Destruction by anti-Tn.* When red cells from a patient with 'mixed field polyagglutin-ability', only 50% of whose red cells were agglutinated by anti-Tn, were injected into a normal subject, almost half the cells disappeared within a few days, the rest having a longer, although still subnormal, survival (Myllylä *et al.* 1971); see Fig. 10.14.

2 *Destruction by anti-B* of a selected population of 'inagglutinable group B red cells'. A large volume of group B red cells was treated with group O serum containing potent anti-B. The unagglutinated cells were separated and treated with a fresh lot of the same group O serum. The process was repeated until a suspension of cells was obtained which was free from agglutinates and was inagglutinable by the anti-B serum. The selected cells were now injected into the group O donor of the potent anti-B and were destroyed far more slowly than an unselected population of group B cells injected into the same donor. After injection of the selected cells there was the usual slowing in the rate of destruction 10–20 min after injection; some 13% of the red cells were left in the circulation at 24 h and the subsequent survival of these could not be described by a single exponential (Winkelstein and Mollison, 1965).

3 *Destruction by anti-Hy.* Just under 50% of the cells had a $T_{1/2}$ of 2–3.5 d and the rest had a $T_{1/2}$ of 15 d; the antibody was IgG and apparently non-complement binding (Hsu *et al.* 1975).

4 *Destruction by anti-HLA.* As mentioned above, destruction has been observed in a few cases and, in these, two-component curves have been observed, often with slowing of the rate of destruction only after 1 d; for an example see Fig. 10.14.

5 *Destruction by anti-Lu^b.* In one case, destruction of Lu (a – b +) red cells was associated with a multicomponent clearance curve (Cutbush and Mollison, 1958), although in two other cases destruction could be described by single exponentials (Tilley *et al.* 1977; Peters *et al.* 1978).

6 *Destruction by anti-Yt^a.* In a case described by Davey and Simpkins (1981) 20% of the cells were removed in the first 30 min, the remaining cells having a $T_{1/2}$ of about 4 d.

7 *Destruction by naturally occurring Rh antibodies (IgG).* As described above, two-component survival curves associated with naturally occurring anti-E and anti-D have been observed. In some cases some cells were cleared with a $T_{1/2}$ of several hours and the remainder with a $T_{1/2}$ of several days; for examples, see Fig. 10.14.

In considering the above results, heterogeneity of antigen seems a likely explanation for nos 1, 2, 3 and 4 and overlooked complement-activation a possible cause for no. 5 (case 1) and no. 6. No explanation whatever can be offered for no. 7.

QUANTITATIVE ASPECTS OF THE DESTRUCTION OF TRANSFUSED RED CELLS BY ALLOANTIBODIES

When small amounts of red cells are transfused, the rate of red cell destruction by any particular antibody is determined by the number of antibody molecules combined with each cell. This number is affected by many factors: the concentration of antigen, which depends not only on the number of red cells but on the number of antigen sites per cell; the concentration of antibody in the plasma; and the equilibrium constant of the reaction between antigen and antibody and its degree of heterogeneity.

When a large volume of incompatible red cells is transfused, the cells are destroyed more slowly than when a small volume is transfused. Two independent factors determine this difference; first, since the amount of antibody in the recipient's plasma is limited, the amount taken up by each incompatible red cell diminishes as the number of transfused cells increases (in principle, antibody-mediated red cell destruction may be limited by complement but there are very few circumstances in which this limitation appears to be of practical importance); second, the number of red cells that can be removed by the MPS in unit time is limited. In some circumstances the amount of antibody bound by various amounts of red cells can be calculated or even directly measured. On the other hand, there is rather little information about the functional capacity of the MPS and the way in which it is affected by the 'load' of antibody-coated red cells.

This rather complicated situation will be dealt with by first reviewing experiments in which the destruction of small numbers of red cells by known amounts of antibody has been studied. Then the limited capacity of the MPS will be considered, and finally the situation actually met with in clinical practice will be described, in which both the limited amount of antibody and the limited capacity of the MPS decrease the rate of red cell destruction.

Relation between number of antibody molecules per cell and rate of clearance

The relation between the average number of antibody molecules on each red cell and the rate of red cell clearance can be determined, or estimated, in three types of experiment: first, red cells can be sensitized with antibody *in vitro* before being reinjected into the circulation; second, incompatible red cells can be injected into the circulation of a subject whose plasma happens to contain the corresponding antibody; and third, a known amount of antibody and of red cells can be injected into a suitable subject.

When red cells are sensitized with antibody *in vitro*, the amount of antibody on the cells can be determined either by using a labelled antibody or by using a labelled antiglobulin serum; when antigen and antibody come into equilibrium only *in vivo*, the amount of antibody on the cells can be calculated if the concentration and equilibrium constant of the antibody are known, together with the number of incompatible red cells taking part in the reaction and the volume within which the reaction is taking place. Further details are given below.

Injections of red cells coated in vitro *with antibody*

Red cells coated in vitro *with non-complement-binding antibody.* In studying the relation between the degree of antibody coating and the rate of red cell destruction, there are two advantages in using red cells sensitized *in vitro*: first, the subject's own red cells can be sensitized, and second, the amount of antibody on the red cells at the time of injection can be measured directly. The main disadvantage of using red cells sensitized *in vitro* is that, after reinjection of the red cells into the circulation, the antibody dissociates progressively from the cells, so that the initial rate of destruction, obtained by drawing a tangent to the initial slope, has to be determined for comparison with the degree of antibody coating. In practice, it is easy to find antibodies with a relatively slow rate of dissociation so that for periods up to about 1 h the rate of red cell destruction approximates to a single exponential (Cutbush and Mollison, 1958; Mollison 1959d; Crome and Mollison, 1964; Mollison *et al.* 1965).

Figure 10.15 shows experiments carried out with a single example of anti-D; there is a fairly close relation between the degree of antibody coating and the rate of clearance.

In Fig. 10.16, results in three of the cases shown in Fig. 10.15 have been replotted so as to show tangents to the initial slopes, which give the initial rates of red cell destruction. Coating with 28.4 μg anti-D/ml red cells (10 400 antibody molecules per

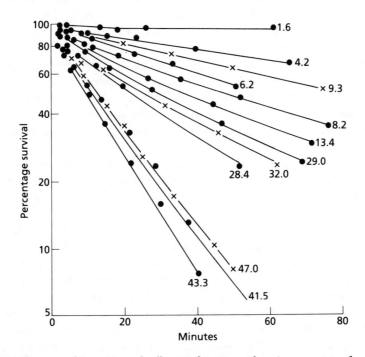

Figure 10.15 Clearance of D-positive red cells coated *in vitro* with various amounts of a particular anti-D (donor Avg.). Purified IgG, prepared from this donor's serum, was used to coat the cells. The figures against each slope are the estimates of the amount of antibody on the red cells at the time of injection as μg antibody per ml red cells. In three cases (×) the estimates were made with labelled antiglobulin serum and in the remainder were made using labelled anti-D (from Mollison *et al.* 1965).

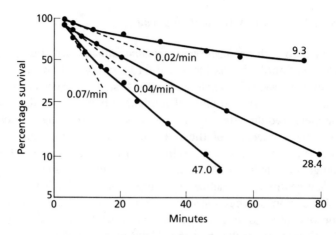

Figure 10.16 Clearance of D-positive red cells coated with different amounts of anti-D; the figures against each curve indicate the amount of anti-D on the cells, as μg/ml red cells, at the time of injection. Three of the cases from Fig. 10.15 have been replotted to show the slight curvilinearity of the slopes (due to elution of about 25% of the antibody during the first hour after injection). The initial rates of destruction are estimated by drawing tangents (–––––) to the initial slopes (slightly modified from Mollison, 1989).

cell) gives an initial rate of 0.04/min, i.e. at the upper limit for clearance solely in the spleen, whereas coating with 47.0 μg anti-D/ml (17 000 antibody molecules per cell) gives clearance with an initial rate of 0.07/min, indicating substantial clearance in the liver as well as in the spleen.

Since the maximum number of D sites on red cells of common phenotypes is about 25 000, the maximum number of anti-D molecules with which red cells can be coated is approximately 20 000; in one experiment in which red cells were thought to have been maximally coated with anti-D, the initial rate of clearance had a $T_{1/2}$ of 5.6 min, corresponding to clearance of about 35% of the blood at each passage through the liver (Mollison, 1989).

As discussed earlier, because c sites are approximately three times as numerous as D sites it is possible for red cells to bind about 60 000 molecules of IgG anti-c per cell, and then as many as 70% of the cells are cleared at a single passage through the liver.

Effect of IgG subclass of anti-D on rate of clearance. The experiments illustrated in Figs 10.15 and 10.16 were carried out with antibody derived from a single donor, Avg. Using a recently devised assay with monoclonal anti-IgG1 and anti-IgG3, it has been found that on D-positive red cells incubated with Avg. about one-quarter of the IgG molecules are IgG3, the rest being IgG1. Tests on other polyclonal anti-D sera have shown that with about three of four sera, less than 20% of the molecules bound to red cells are IgG3, so that Avg. contains more than the average proportion. With preparations of pooled IgG anti-D used for immunoprophylaxis, a smaller proportion of the anti-D molecules bound are IgG3 (Gorick and Hughes-Jones, 1991; see Chapter 5). As discussed below, there is some evidence that, as measured by the amount of antibody required to produce a given rate of clearance, Avg. is more effective than pooled IgG anti-D.

In experiments with two monoclonal anti-Ds, one IgG3 and one IgG1, the IgG3 appeared to be slightly more effective than Avg. and the IgG1 to be less effective than Avg. (Thomson *et al.* 1990).

Rate of clearance affected by recipient differences and by red cell differences. Autologous red cells of different subjects, coated with a certain number of molecules of a particular anti-D, may be cleared at very different rates (Williams *et al.* 1985; Thomson *et al.* 1990). Furthermore, the red cells of a single donor, coated with approximately the same amount of antibody (2500 molecules per red cell), were cleared with half-times ranging from 26 to 81 min in different subjects (Williams *et al.* 1985). These variations may reflect differences in MPS function between different individuals.

Red cells sensitized in vitro *with a complement-binding IgG antibody.* Some quantitative experiments with an immunoglobulin preparation containing complement-binding anti-Fy^a were reported by Mollison *et al.* (1965). The amount of antibody required for a maximal rate of clearance ($T_{1/2}$ of the order of 2 min) was found to be 5–9 μg/ml red cells; an example is shown in Fig. 10.17.

Injection of incompatible red cells

When incompatible red cells are injected, the amount of antibody on the cells cannot as a rule be estimated directly but can be calculated as follows.

Estimation of amount of antibody combined with red cells at equilibrium in vivo. The following data are needed:

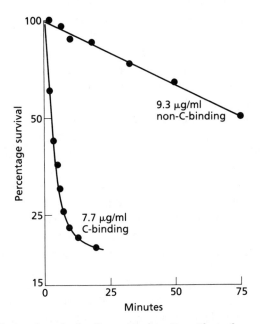

Figure 10.17   Rate of destruction of red cells sensitized *in vitro* with similar amounts of a C-binding antibody (an example of anti-Fy^a) and of a non-C-binding antibody (anti-D) (data from Mollison *et al.* 1965).

1   *The molar concentration of antigen*
    (a) The number of red cells transfused.
    (b) The number of antigen sites per red cell.
    (c) The number of molecules in 1 mole (Avogadro's number).
    (d) The space within which red cells and antibody equilibrate.
2   *The molar concentration of antibody*
    (a) The plasma antibody concentration.
    (b) The molecular weight of the antibody.
3   *The equilibrium constant of the antibody* (K_0) *and its heterogeneity index* (a).

The fraction of antibody bound to the red cells at equilibrium is given by:

$$\frac{(Kc)^a}{1 + (Kc)^a}$$

where c is the concentration of free antigen at equilibrium, K is the equilibrium constant, and a is the heterogeneity index.

In previous editions of this book (e.g. Mollison *et al.* 1987, pp. 554–555), examples were given of detailed calculations applied to a case described by Chaplin (1959). It was pointed out that A and B red cells, because of the large number of antigen sites per cell, can bind very large amounts of antibody so that antibody concentration can be detectably diminished by the transfusion of as little as 4 ml red cells. On the other hand, because Rh D sites are some 40 times less numerous than A and B, D-positive red cells can absorb relatively small amounts of anti-D.

Experiments with passively administered antibody compatible with recipient's red cells, together with a small dose of red cells incompatible with the antibody
In this type of experiment, antibody, preferably as an IgG concentrate, is injected i.m. or i.v. into a subject whose red cells lack the corresponding antigen and incompatible red cells are then injected i.v. For example, in a D-negative subject, anti-D is injected, followed by a small dose of D-positive red cells. The advantage of this type of experiment is that, in some circumstances at least, antigen and antibody come into equilibrium. The concentration of antigen is known fairly accurately from the amount of red cells injected and the number of antigen sites per red cell, as is the recipient's plasma volume (either calculated from red cell volume or deduced from height and body weight); the concentration of antibody is known from the amount injected and the known relation between plasma volume and total IgG distribution space. Accordingly, if the equilibrium constant of the antibody and its degree of heterogeneity have been estimated, and if it is assumed that equilibrium between antigen and antibody has been attained, the amount of antibody bound to the red cells can be calculated.

Unfortunately, in experiments which have been done so far, antibody has usually been injected i.m. either at the same time as the red cells or not more than 24 h previously. Following i.m. injection, the plasma level of antibody does not reach a maximum for about 48 h and is only about 70% of its maximum at 24 h (see Table 10.1). Accordingly, reasonably accurate estimates of the amount of antibody on the red cells can be made only when the rate of destruction is slow in relation to the time required for uptake from the site of injection. For example, in one series of experiments, anti-D immunoglobulin from a single immunized donor (Avg.) was injected into D-negative subjects in doses ranging from 1 to 1000 μg, given i.m. either at the same time or 24 h before 0.3 ml red cells was injected i.v. (Mollison and Hughes-Jones,

Table 10.1 Plasma levels of anti-D expected after i.m. and i.v. injection of 100 μg antibody

| Time | Plasma anti-D concentration (μg/ml) | |
	i.m.	i.v.
5 min	0	0.033
3 h	0.002	0.032
9 h	0.005	0.029
1 d	0.010	0.024
3 d	0.015	0.015
5 d	0.014	0.012

From Smith *et al.* (1972).

1967). When 250–1000 μg anti-D was injected at the same time as the red cells there was a delay of 2–5 h before the onset of red cell destruction but then clearance was rapid ($T_{1/2}$ 2.5 h or less). Under these circumstances the amount of antibody on the cells cannot be calculated.

On the other hand, when 1 μg anti-D was injected i.m. 24 h before injecting 0.3 ml red cells i.v. a maximum rate of red cell destruction was reached at 5–7 d and could thereafter be described by a single exponential with a $T_{1/2}$ of 2.7 d. Assuming that equilibrium between antigen and antibody was reached 1 week after injection, and using the method of calculation described above, it can be calculated that about 1% of the antibody was bound, corresponding to about ten molecules per cell. Incidentally, there was no detectable destruction of the injected red cells at 48 h, i.e. 72 h after injecting the antibody, and it was concluded that the delay in the onset of destruction was due to the time required for antigen and antibody to come into equilibrium at these very low concentrations (Mollison and Hughes-Jones, 1967).

In other experiments in which 1 μg IgG anti-D was injected i.m. and 0.8 ml D-positive red cells i.v., widely varying rates of destruction were observed; in the example shown in Fig. 10.18, the rate of destruction (i.e. after correcting the observations for elution of Cr) has a $T_{1/2}$ of about 5 d. As the figure shows, the rate of destruction appears to remain constant over the period of about 6 weeks, during which time observations were made. This finding is hard to explain in view of the fact that IgG has a half-life of approximately 3 weeks.

Difference between i.m. and i.v. injection. As Table 10.1 shows, when a given dose of anti-D is injected, the maximum plasma concentration when the i.v. route is used is about 2.5 times greater than when the i.m. route is used and, moreover, following i.m. injection the maximum plasma concentration is reached only after about 48 h. It is not surprising that when D-positive red cells are injected at the same time as anti-D, clearance is very much more rapid when the i.v. route is used. In a comparison made by Jouvenceaux *et al.* (1969) in which 300 μg anti-D were injected together with 0.5 ml red cells, the cells were cleared in 6 h when anti-D was given i.v. but only after 48 h when anti-D was injected i.m. Some comparisons made by Huchet *et al.* (1970) with larger amounts of red cells are described below.

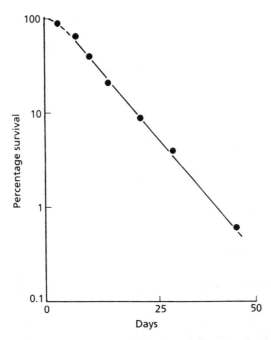

Figure 10.18 Clearance of a small dose (0.8 ml) of D-positve red cells, in an unimmunized D-negative subject, by passively administered IgG anti-D (1 μg) injected i.m. After an initial delay (see text), the rate of clearance becomes constant and remains so for at least 42 d (data from Contreras and Mollison, 1983).

Differences between IgG antibodies (non-complement-binding) in producing clearance
Since IgG antibodies are composed of different subclasses, which vary in their ability to bring about red cell destruction, it is not surprising that the relation between antibody concentration and the rate of clearance is variable. For example, in three cases in which the survival of 1 ml incompatible red cells was measured, the relation between indirect antiglobulin titre and the rate of clearance (as a $T_{1/2}$) was as follows: anti-D, titre 2, $T_{1/2}$ 1.5 h; anti-E, titre 2. $T_{1/2}$ 3.5 d; anti-c, titre 8, $T_{1/2}$ 6 d (Mollison, 1972a, p. 499).

Another example of large differences in biological effectiveness between antibodies of similar concentration was as follows: in two cases in which anti-D could only just be detected, using a sensitive version of the IAT capable of detecting as little as about 2 ng antibody per ml, 1 ml of D-positive red cells was cleared in less than 24 h in one instance but in about 30 d in the other (Mollison *et al.* 1970). In another series of experiments, using anti-D from a single donor (Avg.), the injection of 12.5 μg (expected to produce a plasma concentration at 48 h of about 2 ng/ml) brought about clearance of a 0.3 ml dose of red cells with a $T_{1/2}$ of 24 h (Mollison and Hughes-Jones, 1967).

Other evidence of the relative effectiveness of anti-D from Avg. is as follows: when a very small dose (less than 1 ml) of D-positive red cells was injected i.m. together with 1 μg anti-D (Avg.) i.m. into a D-negative subject, the red cells were cleared with a half-time of 53 h (Mollison and Hughes-Jones, 1967), but with a similar dose of D-positive red cells and pooled anti-D from many donors, the mean red cell survival time in 13 recipients was 24 d (Contreras and Mollison, 1983). As described above, on D-positive red cells incubated with serum Avg., about one-third of the antibody molecules are IgG_3, although it is still uncertain whether this finding explains the fact that anti-D from Avg. appears to be relatively effective in bringing about red cell destruction.

Experiments with passively administered antibody incompatible with the recipient's red cells
See end of chapter.

The destruction of relatively large volumes of incompatible red cells
In the present section some examples are given of the rates of red cell destruction observed after incompatible transfusions. When destruction is predominantly intravascular, its rate and extent are limited only by the supply of antibody and complement.

Since anti-A and anti-B are often partly IgG as well as partly IgM, the relation between the anti-A and anti-B antibody concentration and the amount of haemolysis produced are expected to be variable.

When destruction is due to anti-D, the rate of destruction is affected by the number of antibody molecules bound per cell, by the subclass of the antibody and by the capacity of the MPS.

The capacity of the mononuclear phagocyte system
When red cell destruction depends on phagocytes, the rate of destruction must be limited by the number and activity of the relevant phagocytic cells. This limitation must apply to the destruction both of non-viable stored red cells and of antibody-coated cells, even though the mechanism of destruction in the two cases are believed to be different.

Experiments with non-viable stored red cells in rabbits showed that whereas 100% of a 0.1 ml dose was cleared very rapidly (see Fig. 10.19), only 60% of a 3.1 ml dose was cleared within the first few minutes after injection. From these and other experiments it was concluded that in rabbits injected with non-viable stored red cells up to about 2 ml red cells per kg could be removed within 8 min (Hughes-Jones and Mollison, 1963).

Partial blockage of the capacity for 'immediate removal' is also shown by Fig. 10.19; the second 0.1 ml dose given after an intervening injection of 3.1 ml non-viable red cells is cleared very much more slowly than the first dose of 0.1 ml.

In humans it has also been shown that the rate of clearance of non-viable stored red cells varies inversely with the dose: when the dose of cells was approximately 0.25 ml/kg, half of the cells were removed in 30 min, but when the dose was approximately 1.5 ml/kg, clearance of half the cells took more than 3 h (Noyes *et al.* 1960).

Estimation of the maximum capacity of the MPS is complicated by the fact that destruction sometimes occurs predominantly in the spleen, which contains only a small part of the whole MPS. Thus, the rate at which large numbers of D-positive red cells are destroyed is likely to be determined chiefly by the capacity of the spleen,

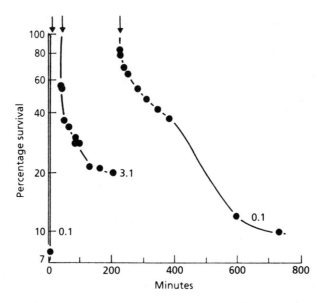

Figure 10.19 Survival in the rabbit of three successive doses (0.1, 3.1 and 0.1 ml) of red cells rendered non-viable by storage at 37°C for 44 h. The first dose of 0.1 ml was completely cleared from the circulation within a few minutes. Following the injection of 3.1 ml of cells, only a proportion was cleared rapidly, and when the final dose of 0.1 ml was given most of the cellls were cleared relatively slowly (from Hughes-Jones and Mollison, 1963).

whereas the rate at which large numbers of stored red cells are destroyed may be determined by the capacity of the whole MPS. This distinction is not absolute, since red cells heavily coated with anti-D are destroyed partly in the liver and, conversely, when stored red cells are injected, part of the non-viable population may be removed only in the spleen.

Table 10.2 contrasts the rate of clearance of large and small amounts of red cells calculated to have been coated with similar amounts of anti-D. As the table shows, when cells were coated with approximately 8 μg/ml, 160 ml red cells were cleared

Table 10.2 Clearance of large and small amounts of D-positive red cells coated with similar amounts of anti-D

	Red cells		
Reference	ml	μg anti-D per ml	Clearance $T_{1/2}$ (h)
Eklund and			
Nevanlinna (1971)	160	8.1	14
Mollison *et al.* (1965)	1	8.0	1 h
Hughes-Jones and			
Mollison (1968)	400	1.6	72
Huchet *et al.* (1970)	5.1	2.0	3.7

* Value given by Mollison *et al.* (1965) determined directly; other values calculated as described in text.

with a $T_{1/2}$ of 14 h and 12 ml with a $T_{1/2}$ of 1 h. When cells were coated with 1.6–2.0 μg/ml, 400 ml red cells were cleared with a $T_{1/2}$ of the order of 72 h and 5.1 ml with a $T_{1/2}$ of 3.7 h.

In the examples given above, when anti-D was injected i.v. it was assumed that the reaction took place within a space equal to the plasma volume, taken to be 3000 ml. When anti-D was injected i.m. 48 h before the red cells were injected, and when the red cells were subsequently cleared with a $T_{1/2}$ of 12 h or less, the amount of anti-D in the plasma was deduced from the figures given in Table 10.1 and it was again assumed that the reaction took place within a volume of 3000 ml. However, when the anti-D was injected i.m. and destruction took place with a half-time measured in days, it was assumed that red cells and anti-D came into equilibrium within a space equal to twice the plasma volume.

An estimate of the maximum capacity to remove D-incompatible red cells is provided by an experiment reported by Mohn *et al.* (1961). After the injection of a large volume of very potent anti-D into a D-positive volunteer, the average rate of red cell destruction may be calculated to have been approximately 0.15 ml/kg per hour, although the maximum rate was probably about 0.25 ml/kg per hour (420 ml red cells destroyed in 24 h in a man who may have weighed 70 kg).

In experiments in rabbits with phenylhydrazine-damaged red cells, it was estimated that the maximum rate of removal of the cells from the circulation was approximately 0.5 ml/kg per hour (Hughes-Jones and Mollison, 1963).

Destruction of relatively large volumes of ABO-incompatible red cells
When the recipient's plasma contains potent anti-A and anti-B, the red cells (approximately 200 ml) of a unit of blood may be destroyed by intravascular lysis within 1 h or, perhaps, within minutes (see Chapter 11).

When the titre of anti-A, or anti-B is low, all detectable antibody may be removed by the transfusion of an amount of red cells as small as 4 ml (Chaplin, 1959). Even when the antibody titre is considerably greater, the titre may be appreciably reduced by the transfusion of relatively small amounts of blood. For example, in one series of observations the transfusion of 25 ml A_1 blood reduced the titre against A_1 cells from 32 to 2; in another case in the same series the transfusion of 40 ml A_2 blood reduced the titre against A_2 from 8 to 1 (Wiener *et al.* 1953b).

After the transfusion of therapeutic quantities of blood, alloagglutinins may become temporarily undetectable and the transfused red cells survive normally until there has been an anamnestic response and sufficient antibody has been produced to bring about accelerated red cell destruction. It previous editions of this book an example was given of a case in which, following the transfusion of 1000 ml citrated group B blood to a group A patient with an anti-B titre of 32, group B red cells survived normally for about 4 d after transfusion but were then all eliminated within a few days as the anti-B reappeared (Mollison, 1972a, p. 504). A case in which 7.5 units group A blood were transfused to a group O recipient and eliminated over a period of about 6 d, with minimal signs of red cell destruction, is described in Chapter 11. A rather similar case, in which 3 units of group A blood were transfused to a group O patient and cleared progressively over about 4 d without any clinical signs of red cell destruction was described by Buchholz and Bove (1975).

Following the transfusion of ABO-incompatible blood, particularly when the recipient's pre-transfusion plasma contains only low-titre anti-A or anti-B, surviving incompatible red cells may be found for days or even weeks after the transfusion. Presumably, such cells are coated with C3dg and are thus insusceptible to complement-mediated destruction.

An elderly group O woman with carcinoma of the lung was inadvertently transfused with 600 ml B blood. Haemoglobinuria was noted but there were no other untoward signs. Examination of a saline suspension of red cells taken from the patient on the following day showed the presence of small agglutinates which were identified as surviving B red cells (Mollison, 1943a, case 4).

The case of Akeroyd and O'Brien (1958), in which some group AB surviving cells were found for 6 weeks after transfusion despite a haemolysin titre of 4 in the recipient's serum, has been described above. A very similar case was observed by M. Metaxas (personal communication, 1964); a group O patient was transfused with 8 units A blood on the day after an operation. Some jaundice was noted clinically but there were no other abnormal signs. Four days after blood transfusion the anti-A titre was 4; by the eighth day it was 128 and the antibody was now capable of causing some lysis of A cells *in vitro*. During this period and subsequently, the serum haptoglobin concentration remained normal. Group A cells could easily be detected in the circulation up to 25 d after transfusion.

Similar results have been observed in dogs, particularly when the transfused red cells contain a 'weak' antigen (see Swisher and Young, 1954).

Complement as a limiting factor in red cell destruction. If fresh human serum is absorbed with an equal volume of red cells sensitized with a complement-binding antibody, it is found that about five successive absorptions are required to remove all complement activity from the fresh serum (unpublished observations, PLM). Although the amount of complement removed by different antibodies doubtless varies widely, the conclusion is that in most situations antibody rather than complement is likely to be the limiting factor determining the destruction of incompatible red cells, except possibly in a patient whose serum complement level is already low before transfusion and in infants with haemolytic disease of the newborn due to ABO incompatibility (see Chapter 12).

In haemolytic anaemia due to auto-anti-I, in which the level of serum complement may in fact be diminished, complement may be a limiting factor in red cell destruction. Evans *et al.* (1968) observed that the transfusion of washed red cells regularly reduced the complement titre. They found that when two transfusions of red cells were given within a day or two of one another, the second lot survived better than the first, and they discussed the possibility that this might be due to a reduction in serum complement levels. It had previously been found that in some patients the transfusion of fresh normal plasma might produce an increase in the rate of the patient's own red cells, apparently by supplying complement (Evans *et al.* 1965).

Experimental work in dogs indicating that the rapid destruction of red cells occurs only so long as both antibody and complement are available in the recipient's plasma was reported by Christian *et al.* (1951).

Destruction of relatively large volumes of Rh D-positive red cells
Information on the rate of destruction of relatively large amounts of D-positive red cells by anti-D is available from several different sources: first, inadvertent transfusions of

D-positive blood to subjects who are already immunized to Rh D; second, inadvertent transfusions of D-positive blood to D-negative subjects who are not already immunized to Rh D, but who are given a dose of anti-D in the hope of suppressing primary immunization; third, experimental transfusions of large amounts of D-positive red cells together with large doses of anti-D to D-negative subjects to determine the conditions under which Rh D immunization is suppressed; fourth, the administration of large doses of anti-D to D-negative women who are found to have relatively large amounts of D-positive fetal red cells in their circulation after delivery; and finally, the experimental administration of potent anti-D to D-positive volunteers. This last category is considered in a later section, but the others will be considered here.

Transfusions of D-positive blood to D-immunized subjects. Figure 10.20 shows the survival of therapeutic quantities of D-positive red cells in three cases.

In case A, the plasma contained potent anti-D and the rate of destruction of red cells following the transfusion of 4 units D-positive blood was of the order of 200–300 ml red cells a day, that is to say, almost maximal for destruction by anti-D (see above).

Following the transfusion of relatively large amounts of D-positive red cells to subjects whose serum contains potent anti-D, a considerable number of surviving D-positive red cells are usually found for at least 24 h after the transfusion. It is also

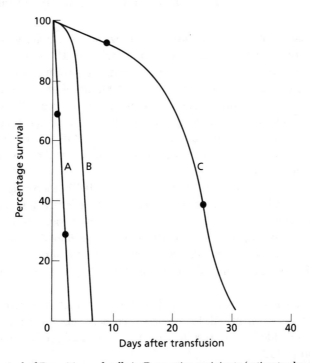

Figure 10.20 Survival of D-positive red cells in D-negative recipients (estimates by differential agglutination). Case A: potent anti-D present at time of transfusion: 4 units transfused. Case B: very weak anti-D present at time of transfusion; delayed haemolytic transfusion reaction (curve diagrammatic). Case C: no anti-D present at time of transfusion but present by day 39.

usual to find free anti-D, as expected from the rather poor absorbing capacity of D-positive red cells for anti-D due to their relatively small number of D antigen sites.

Suppose a patient's serum has an anti-D concentration of 10 μg/ml, corresponding approximately to an indirect antiglobulin titre of 500. If plasma volume is taken as 3000 ml, there will be 3×10^4 μg anti-D in the plasma. If 2 units D-positive red cells are transfused containing 400 ml red cells, and supposing that 30 μg anti-D are taken up by each ml of red cells to give approximately maximal saturation, then the total amount of anti-D absorbed would be 1.2×10^4 μg, or only about half of the total amount in the plasma.

'Case B' shown in Fig. 10.20 is hypothetical in the sense that it is based on a number of cases (see Mollison, 1983, p. 604). When the patient's serum contains only a trace of anti-D at the time of transfusion, it is usual for the antibody titre to increase very rapidly so that signs of increased red cell destruction become apparent on about the fourth or fifth day after transfusion and the circulation may be completely cleared of incompatible cells by the seventh day. Further details of this kind of case are given in the following chapter.

Finally, Fig. 10.20 shows an example of a case (C) in which primary Rh D immunization developed following transfusion. As the figure shows, survival was subnormal at 28 d and at some time between then and 39 d had fallen to zero, by which time anti-D was detectable in the serum. (The transfusion was given 20 d before the patient was delivered of her first infant, so that it is possible, though unlikely, in this case that primary immunization had already been induced by fetal red cells.)

Inadvertent transfusion of D-positive blood to D-negative subjects followed by injections of anti-D. In a case described by Hughes-Jones and Mollison (1968), a D-negative woman who had been inadvertently transfused with 2 units D-positive blood (approximately 400 ml red cells) was given an i.m. injection of 1000 μg of anti-D; the red cells were cleared with a $T_{1/2}$ of approximately 3 d. Assuming that the red cells equilibrated with the antibody available in the whole IgG space, it was calculated that approximately two-thirds of the amount of injected antibody was bound to the red cells, corresponding to occupancy of about 5% of the antigen sites, equivalent to 1.6 μg anti-D per ml red cells (see Table 10.2).

In a case described by Eklund and Nevanlinna (1971) following the inadvertent transfusion of 400 ml D-positive blood (160 ml red cells) to a D-negative woman, plasma containing about 2500 μg anti-D was transfused i.v. over the course of 2 h. The transfusion was then stopped because the patient developed severe shivering and fever. The rate of clearance was estimated to have a $T_{1/2}$ of approximately 14 h. It can be calculated that at equilibrium there was about 7.3 μg anti-D per ml red cells (see Table 10.2).

In Chapter 5 some details are given of four cases in which between 1 and 3 units of D-positive blood were transfused, following which between 3000 and 7750 μg anti-D were given i.v. in divided doses, resulting in clearance of all the red cells within 2–8 d; see Table 5.7 on p. 242.

Injections of anti-D following massive transplacental haemorrhage (TPH). Massive TPH is quite arbitrarily defined here as the presence in the mother's circulation of more than about 10 ml fetal red cells, as found in about two per 1000 of recently delivered women (see Chapter 12).

In this section, a few examples are given of the rates of clearance of D-positive red cells which have been observed after giving various amounts of anti-D.

Intramuscular injections of anti-D. In a case in which a mother's circulation was estimated to contain 60 ml fetal red cells, an injection of 500 μg anti-D brought about clearance with a $T_{1/2}$ of 5–6 d (Hughes-Jones and Mollison, 1968). A similar rate of clearance was observed in a case in which a TPH of an estimated 175 ml red cells was treated with a dose of 500 μg anti-D (de Wit and Borst-Eilers, 1968).

Distinctly more rapid clearance, with removal of all D-positive cells within 5 d, was observed in one case in which a TPH of 75 ml red cells was treated with 1500 μg anti-D (C.D. de Wit and E. Borst-Eilers, personal communication) and in another in which a TPH of about 85 ml red cells was treated with 1000 μg anti-D (Woodrow *et al.* 1968).

In two cases described by Huchet *et al.* (1970) in which the size of TPH was estimated to be equivalent to 28 and 43 ml red cells, respectively, two successive i.m. injections each of 600 μg were given at an interval of 1–3 d; the cells were not completely cleared for 5–7 d. As pointed out on p. 671 many injections which are intended to be made into muscle are in fact made into fat and when this is done the time taken for IgG to reach the plasma is substantially longer.

Intravenous injections of anti-D. Huchet *et al.* (1970) emphasized the very much more rapid clearance of red cells following i.v. injection by contrasting the two cases just described, in which the anti-D was given i.m., with two further cases in which, although the size of TPH was greater (equivalent to 60 and 88 ml red cells, respectively), a single i.v. injection of 600 μg of anti-D resulted in clearance with a $T_{1/2}$ of the order of 85 min. It can be calculated that in these two cases, at equilibrium, there would have been about 5 μg anti-D on each ml red cells. The rate of clearance seems more rapid than expected since a 1 ml dose of red cells, coated *in vitro* with about 4 μg anti-D per ml, was found to be cleared with a $T_{1/2}$ of 2.0 h (Mollison *et al.* 1965).

Interpretation of tests made with small numbers of incompatible red cells
When the results of serological tests are difficult to interpret, it is helpful to estimate the survival of small volumes of ^{51}Cr-labelled red cells from potential donors. The following procedure is suggested.

Method
Since it is likely that potential recipients will require at least 2 units red cells, it is suggested that approximately 1 ml citrated blood should be taken from each of two potential donor-units and pooled and the red cells labelled with ^{51}Cr. Since tests will usually be carried out in circumstances in which early rapid destruction of injected red cells is highly unlikely, the procedure described on p. 438 will usually be appropriate: the first sample is taken at 3 min and the concentration of donor red cells in this sample is taken to represent 100% survival; as an absolute minimum two further samples are taken, at 10 and 60 min after injection, respectively. The plasma of these

two latter samples must be counted as well as samples of whole blood, the purpose being to detect any substantial degree of intravascular destruction. When survival is normal, and when the samples are counted to a statistical accuracy of $\pm$ 1%, the 60-min value should be at least 97%. Because of random errors, destruction must be at least 5% before there is 95% chance that the 60 min value will be less than 97% (Mollison, 1981). Evidently, the chance of detecting only a slight increase in the rate of red cell destruction is greatly improved by taking samples over a longer period. When 5% is the least amount of destruction which can be detected reliably, by taking a sample at 5 h, a rate of destruction of only 1% per hour can be detected.

When it is considered possible that there will be early rapid destruction of injected red cells, i.e. within the mixing period, a double red cell labelling method must be used if accurate estimates of survival are to be obtained.

The shape of the survival curve during the first 60 min gives some indication of the likelihood of an immune response. When there is a two-component curve with much slower destruction between 10 and 60 min than between 3 and 10 min it can be deduced that the antibody is complement binding and that the surviving cells have acquired resistance to complement-mediated destruction. Some complement binding antibodies are IgM and cold-reacting and, with this type of antibody, there is often no immune response. Other complement-binding antibodies may be IgM or IgG and are warm-reacting; with these, an immune response is usually observed. Similarly, when the curve of red cell destruction is a single exponential the antibody concerned will probably be a non-complement-binding IgG and the injection of incompatible red cells is almost certain to be followed by an immune response.

If, after carrying out a test with a small volume of incompatible red cells, it is decided that because of the small amount of red cell destruction observed it would be safe to give a large volume of incompatible red cells, the chance of a delayed haemolytic transfusion reaction will obviously depend on the immune response provoked by the transfusion.

A note of the recommendations of ICSH (1980b) for determining
red cell survival using ^{51}Cr
The document published by a panel of the International Committee on Standardization in Haematology (ICSH, 1980b) was chiefly concerned with the conduct of red cell survival tests in patients suspected of having a haemolytic process. The recommendations included methods of labelling with ^{51}Cr, time of taking blood samples, corrections for Cr elution and analysis of the resulting corrected red cell survival curves. These methods were never intended to be applied to investigating the survival of red cells from a potentially incompatible donor, and separate recommendations were given for the use of ^{51}Cr-labelled red cells as a test for compatibility. It was suggested that, for this purpose, approximately 0.5 ml red cells should be labelled and that blood samples should be taken 3, 10 and 60 min after injection. These recommendations have been widely ignored by authors claiming to have followed the method proposed by ICSH. For example, in testing for compatibility *in vivo*, some authors have used the methods devised for estimating the survival of autologous red cells. These methods are wholly inappropriate when the survival curve has more than one component (see pp. 461– 462 for an example). Many others have injected 10 ml or so of red cells instead of

0.5 ml. Although, from a practical point of view, the precise amount of cells injected is not very important, the test is often done partly to add to scientific knowledge and because of this it seems desirable to keep to the ICSH recommendation and to give approximately 0.5 ml donor red cells. Another common practice is to take the first sample from the recipient 10 or even 30 min after injecting the incompatible cells. The recommendation to take the first sample at 3 min was based on the observation that there is an apparent lag of about 2.5 min before destruction begins, except when destruction is extremely rapid (see Fig. 10.2). Since, in most cases, mixing is almost complete by 3 min, a sample taken at this time can be used as the 100% survival value with relatively little error (see Mollison, 1989, for examples). If the first sample is not taken for 10 min or more after injection the major component of destruction may be missed when destruction is brought about by complement-activating antibodies, since the rate of destruction may be rapid for the first 10 min and then slow abruptly.

Difference between the survival of large and small volumes of incompatible red cells
When the recipient's serum contains a low concentration of antibody the survival of a large amount of incompatible red cells may be much better than that of a smaller amount. Observations in a patient of subgroup A_2 with anti-A_1 weakly active at 37°C in her serum are shown in Fig. 10.7 (p. 447). When 0.5 ml red cells were injected, approximately 65% of the cells were removed from the circulation within 30 min. When 18.9 ml red cells were injected only about 45% were destroyed within 30 min, and the titre of anti-A_1 fell appreciably. One week later when a unit of A_1 red cells was transfused, survival was virtually normal but the titre of anti-A_1 appeared to have fallen spontaneously by this time so that if a whole unit had been transfused at the outset there might have been measurable destruction. However, by extrapolation from the difference between the survival of 0.5 and 18.9 ml red cells, it seems safe to conclude that the amount of destruction of a unit or more of red cells would have been less than 20% and might have been too small to have been measurable.

A case in which there was an even greater difference between the survival of a small and a large amount of red cells transfused to a patient with a very low concentration of anti-B was described by Chaplin (1959). When 4 ml were transfused, all the cells were destroyed within minutes but the survival of a unit of red cells was almost normal.

Clearance of large vs. small amounts of incompatible red cells in rabbits
The difference between the rate of clearance of small and of large amounts of incompatible red cells in rabbits is relatively small at high antibody concentrations but relatively large at low antibody concentrations. For example, when sufficient IgG anti-Hg^A was injected into an Hg (A –) rabbit to give an indirect antiglobulin titre of 256 and the time taken for the destruction of 50% of a dose of Hg (A +) red cells was estimated, it was found that for a 1.0 ml/kg dose of red cells the time was 18 min and for a 0.01 ml/kg dose, 7 min. However, when the titre was only 16, the times were 102 h and 18 min, respectively. With IgM antibodies the greatest amount of antibody injected gave a titre of only 2 and this level was associated with a clearance $T_{1/2}$ of 2.5 min when a 0.01 ml/kg dose of Hg (A +) red cells was injected. With a 1 ml/kg dose, only one-third of the cells were cleared within the first hour after injection and one-third of the cells were still present in the circulation at 72 h (Burton and Mollison, 1968).

Attempts to inhibit the destruction of incompatible red cells

At least three approaches can be envisaged: specific inhibition of particular antibodies by injecting blood group-specific substances; inhibition of complement activity; and interference with the activity of the MPS. All these three have been tried but unequivocal success has been achieved only with the first.

Injections of soluble group-specific substances

The only blood group substances available in a purified form are A, B, Le^a and Le^b. The injection of a sufficient amount of these substances would be expected to neutralize all circulating antibody so that, temporarily, red cells of a theoretically incompatible group would survive normally in the circulation. In the case of anti-A and anti-B the effect would not be expected to be long lived since an immune response would usually follow; it might then become impossible to suppress antibody completely and the incompatible red cells would thus undergo accelerated destruction.

In the case of anti-Le^a and anti-Le^b the position is more promising for two reasons: first, Lewis antibodies are mainly IgM and, like IgM anti-A and anti-B, are readily inhibited. In fact, Lewis antibodies are much easier to inhibit since they are usually far weaker than most examples of anti-A and anti-B. (When anti-A and anti-B are IgG they are very much more difficult to inhibit than when they are IgM.) Second, after transfusion to an Le (a – b –) subject, Le (a +) and Le (b +) red cells lose their Lewis antigens and become Le (a – b –). Since this transformation occurs within a few days of transfusion, the red cells are likely to have become Le (a – b –) by the time that Lewis antibodies have appeared in high concentration in the recipient's plasma (if a secondary immune response has been induced).

The suggestion that Le^a substance in transfused plasma might play a decisive part in preventing haemolytic transfusion reactions from anti-Le^a was first put forward by Brendemoen and Aas (1952) who had observed a haemolytic reaction in a subject transfused with packed red cells from O,Le (a +) blood.

In a case described by Mollison *et al.* (1963) anti-Le^a and anti-Le^b were suppressed by the injection of Lewis substances to allow the successful transfusion of Le (b +) blood (see Figs 10.21 and 10.22). Although in this case potent purified Lewis substances were used for suppression, preliminary observations with the transfusion of relatively small amounts of Le (a + b –) plasma had shown that plasma alone could not only suppress all detectable antibody but allow the subsequent normal survival of Le (a + b –) red cells (see Fig. 10.21).

The subject was group B, Le (a – b –) and his serum contained anti-Le^a and anti-Le^b. He was due to undergo an operation, involving cardiac bypass, for which the blood of large numbers of donors was expected to be needed. In order to avoid the difficulty of finding sufficient group B,Le (a – b –) donors it was decided to attempt to suppress the Lewis antibodies and to use Le (b +) donors. Pre-operative tests of the survival of Le (a +) and Le (b +) red cells before and after the transfusion of Le (a +) plasma and injection of purified Le^b substance are shown in Fig. 10.21.

Immediately before operation, a further injection of purified Le^b substance was given. During the operation and the following 36 h the patient lost a considerable amount of blood and a total of 34 units Le (a – b +) blood and 13 units Le (a – b –) blood was transfused; there was no evidence that the haemorrhage was related to incompatibility.

As Fig. 10.22 shows, within 48 h after the end of the blood transfusion, anti-Le^a and anti-Le^b had reappeared in the patient's circulation. There were still no signs whatever of a haemolytic

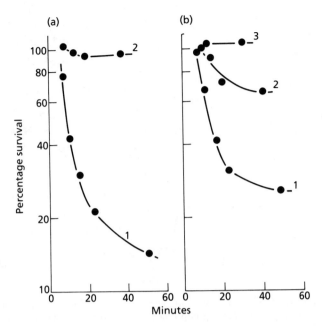

Figure 10.21 Survival of 0.5 ml amounts of group O,Le (a + b –) red cells (a) and of group O,Le (b +) red cells (b), before (1) and after (2) the transfusion of 200 ml Le (a + b –) plasma. After the second test an i.v. injection of 0.4 ml of a 1% solution of purified Le^b substance was given and the survival of group O,Le (b +) red cells estimated once more (3) (from Mollison *et al.* 1963).

reaction and it was now shown that the transfused red cells were reacting only very weakly with anti-Le^b. Within a few days the cells were phenotypically Le (a – b –).

In a second case, of an A_1,Le (a – b –) woman whose serum contained a relatively strong anti-Le^b and a weak anti-Le^a, a preliminary test showed that within 30 min of injection approximately 60% of A_2,Le (b +) cells and 10% of A_1,Le (b +) red cells were destroyed. Following a transfusion of 250 ml of EDTA-plasma from the A_2,Le (b +) donor a second injection of A_2,Le (b +) red cells was given and underwent no destruction within the following 30 min. Le (b +) blood was transfused without incident (unpublished observations).

Other cases in which Lewis antibodies were suppressed by the transfusion of plasma alone and in which several units of Le (a +) or Le (b +) blood were subsequently transfused without a clinical reaction were described by Hossaini (1972), Pelosi *et al.* (1974), Andorka *et al.* (1974) and Athkambhira and Chiewsilp (1978). In one case, a relatively potent anti-Le^b was not completely suppressed by the transfusion of about 800 ml group A,Le (b +) plasma (Morel *et al.* 1978, supplemented by personal communication).

In summary, the relatively small amount of trouble caused by Lewis antibodies in blood transfusion seems to be due partly to the effect of Lewis substances in the donor's plasma in suppressing corresponding antibodies in the recipient's plasma and partly to the chameleon-like behaviour of red cells which within a few days of transfusion assume the phenotype of the recipient.

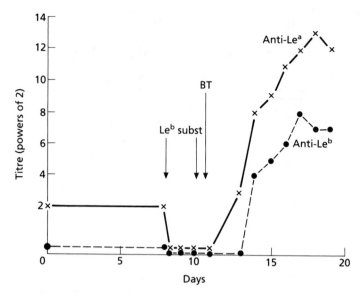

Figure 10.22 Changes in the titre of Lewis antibodies in a group B,Le (a – b –) subject before and after the transfusion of large amounts of group B,Le (b +) blood (B.T.). The transfusion was preceded by the injection of two doses of Le^b substance, one given immediately before transfusion and one given 48 h beforehand (from Mollision *et al.* 1963).

The addition of soluble A and B substances to group O plasma to produce partial inhibition of anti-A and anti-B is described below.

Inhibition of complement activity

The effect of heparin. As described in Chapter 3, heparin prevents the activation of complement *in vitro* only at concentrations of the order of 100 iu/ml, but lower concentrations than this may have some inhibitory effect on red cell destruction *in vivo*. For example, Cooper and Brown (1971) found that 69 iu/ml was effective in inhibiting relatively slow destruction by anti-I in rabbits although 28 iu/ml was ineffective. Observations reported by Rosenfield *et al.* (1967b) suggested that concentrations as low as about 20 iu/ml might prevent the destruction of antibody-coated red cells in rats.

The use of C1-esterase inhibitor has been considered as a therapeutic measure in autoimmune haemolytic anaemia (AIHA) with warm haemolysins (see Chapter 7) and has potential value in preventing destruction by complement-binding alloantibodies, particularly those which are IgM.

Intravenously injected immunoglobulin (i.v. Ig) inhibits the uptake of complement on to target cells: (a) in guinea pigs treated with 600 mg Ig/kg per day i.v. for 2 d, clearance of IgM-sensitized guinea pig red cells, which is wholly complement dependent, was reduced, although the effect was relatively small, e.g. at 90 min, survival of injected red cells was about 60% compared with about 45% in control animals (Basta *et al.*

1989a); (b) in guinea pigs given a single slow infusion of 1800 mg IgG/kg i.v., 3 h before being subjected to Forssman shock, survival was prolonged and, or, death prevented, an effect believed to have been due to suppression of C3 fragment uptake on to target cells (Basta *et al.* 1989b). Further work indicated that i.v. Ig is an effective inhibitor of the deposition of C4b and C3b on to target cells (Basta *et al.* 1991).

Interference with the activity of the mononuclear phagocyte system
Two methods have been tried, the injection of corticosteroids to reduce monocyte activity and the injection of IgG to compete with bound antibody for Fc-receptor sites.

The effect of corticosteroids. In AIHA the administration of corticosteroids results in a slowing of red cell destruction within a few days. The most important effect of corticosteroids is to decrease the amount of lysosomal enzymes released following contact between antibody-coated cells and phagocytes (Fleer *et al.* 1978).

In animal experiments administration of large doses of corticosteroids has been shown to interfere with the sequestration of antibody-coated red cells in rats and guinea pigs (Kaplan and Jandl, 1961; Atkinson and Frank, 1974b). Only a few observations have been made in humans: in eight subjects given 1–3 ml ^{51}Cr-labelled ABO-incompatible cells, the administration of 90 mg prednisolone 30 min before and at the same time as the injection of incompatible cells failed to prevent the rapid i.v. destruction of the cells (Hewitt *et al.* 1961). This result is not surprising since the destruction of ABO-incompatible cells by potent antibodies is predominantly intravascular and macrophages are not involved. On the other hand, suggestive evidence of a small diminution of the rate of clearance of D-sensitized red cells was observed in six patients with rheumatoid arthritis after 5 days of corticosteroid therapy (Mollison, 1962a).

Intravenously injected IgG (i.v. Ig) has been used with apparent success in a case in which anti-Kp^b was involved (Kohan *et al.* 1991).

A man aged 50 with rectal cancer, who had been transfused during surgery with 2 units blood, was found to have an unexpectedly low PCV (0.10). Following the transfusion of 50 ml packed red cells he developed a severe febrile reaction accompanied by intense lumbar pain. His serum was found to contain anti-Kp^b. He was started on a regimen of 400 mg IgG/kg per day i.v. (together with 500 mg hydrocortisone). After 24 h he was transfused uneventfully with 2 units Kp (b +) blood and the PCV rose to 0.18.

DESTRUCTION OF TRANSFUSED RED CELLS WITHOUT SEROLOGICALLY DEMONSTRABLE ANTIBODIES

The cases to be considered fall into two classes: those in which at some stage of the investigation the antibody is in fact detected so that its specificity and characteristics are known and those in which no antibody can ever be demonstrated *in vitro* so that its presence is simply inferred.

Antibody demonstrable at some stage
In delayed haemolytic transfusion reactions, antibody may be detected for the first

time after the onset of red cell destruction, as described in the following chapter. In the
past, cases have also been described in which antibodies have previously been found
but have since become undetectable and in which small amounts of theoretically
incompatible red cells have been rapidly destroyed (Fudenberg and Allen, 1957;
Chaplin and Cassell, 1962). In one case, after the transfusion of a unit, there was an
immediate haemolytic reaction (Fudenberg and Allen, 1957). Now that more sensitive
tests for antibody detection have been introduced, cases of this kind are very rare.

Accelerated destruction of transfused red cells during primary immunization
In primary Rh D immunization, accelerated clearance of D-positive red cells can often
be observed before anti-D can be detected.

    The survival of a first injection of 1 ml D-positive red cells in previously unimmu-
nized D-negative subjects has been studied in two series. In the first, R_1R_2 red cells
were injected and in the second, R_2R_2 cells; in both, the red cells were labelled with
^{51}Cr and samples were taken weekly after injection. Subjects who failed to form anti-D
within 6 months of a first injection were given a second injection of labelled cells
(Samson and Mollison, 1975; Contreras and Mollison, 1981). Taking the two series
together, nine subjects formed anti-D after the first injection and six more after a
second injection. Amongst these 15 responders, there were four subjects with normal
survival at 28 d but who nevertheless made anti-D within 6 months. Conversely, there
were five subjects who eliminated virtually all the injected red cells within 28 d of a
first injection but who formed serologically detectable anti-D only after a second
injection.

    Further information about the time of onset of accelerated destruction during
primary immunization can be obtained from the paper by Woodrow *et al.* (1969).
Repeated injections of ^{51}Cr-labelled D-positive red cells from 5–10 ml blood were given
to 11 D-negative subjects and followed for 7 d in each instance; the intervals between
injections varied but were most often 4–9 weeks. Seven subjects formed anti-D and in
three of these subnormal survival was noted 10–23 weeks before anti-D could be
detected.

Accelerated destruction during secondary immunization
In the two series referred to above, in which two injections of ^{51}Cr-labelled D-positive
red cells were given to D-negative subjects at an interval of 6 months, there were six
subjects who formed serologically detectable anti-D only after the second injection; in
four of these, survival was clearly subnormal at 7 d, indicating that anti-D was present
at the time of the second injection, even though it became detectable only later.

    The effect on the survival of transfused red cells of a developing secondary response
is illustrated in Figs 11.5–11.7 in Chapter 11.

Antibody never demonstrable despite shortened survival of transfused red cells
In subjects whose own red cells have a normal survival, shortened survival of
transfused red cells in the absence of demonstrable alloantibodies is uncommon when
therapeutic quantities of red cells are transfused but relatively common when small
volumes of red cells (less than 10 ml) are transfused. There may be an initial phase of
normal survival lasting for 10 d or more, followed by a phase of accelerated destruc-

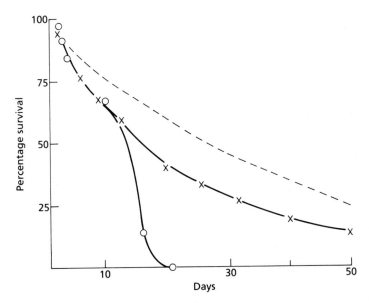

Figure 10.23 Survival of ^{51}Cr-labelled red cells from two newborn infants following injection into a normal adult. Small samples of blood were taken from two infants, the first aged 35 h and the second aged 50 h. The samples were mixed with acid–citrate–dextrose and then labelled with ^{51}Cr in the usual way. O—O Cr survival of red cells from the first infant; 2 ml red cells were labelled. ×—×, Cr survival of red cells from the second infant; 8 ml red cells were labelled. The interval between the two injections was 34 d. The dotted line shows the normal Cr survival curve observed when red cells from normal adults are labelled with ^{51}Cr in the same way (Eloise R. Giblett, unpublished observations).

tion, suggesting that the transfusion has induced an immune response; this type of curve has been called a 'collapse' curve (Mollison, 1961b, p. 484); an example is shown in Fig. 10.23. Alternatively, there may be random destruction from the time of transfusion onwards, suggesting that the recipient is already immunized.

Although survival curves can often be classified as showing either normal survival followed by collapse, or random destruction throughout, in some cases, due to insufficient data, survival has simply to be categorized as subnormal.

It is convenient to consider results observed with large and small volumes of red cells separately, mainly because subnormal survival in the absence of demonstrable antibodies is much less common when large amounts of red cells are transfused.

Subnormal survival of therapeutic amounts of transfused red cells
in the absence of demonstrable antibodies
In three of 35 recipients of red cells stored in an acid–citrate–glucose solution, the rate of destruction was initially average but all the cells were eliminated within 40–60 d; further investigation suggested that some kind of incompatibility was involved (Loutit *et al.* 1943; Mollison, 1951, p. 107). Some similar cases were encountered in studying the survival of frozen red cells.

In one patient (a recently delivered woman), the survival of a therapeutic quantity of previously frozen red cells was zero at 6 weeks. The red cells of the same donor, injected on two subsequent occasions 3 years later was again grossly subnormal (see

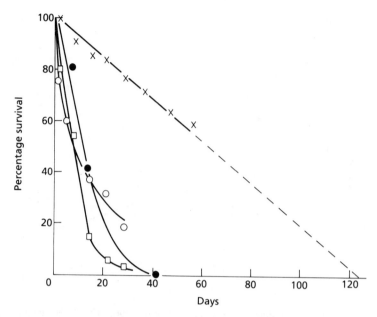

Figure 10.24 Accelerated red cell destruction in the absence of serologically demonstrable alloantibodies, in a recipient I.S. ●—●, Survival of previously frozen red cells from a normal donor (L.F.), estimated by differential agglutination. ○—○ and □—□, Survival of L.F.'s red cells on two subsequent occasions, estimated with ^{51}Cr. x — x Survival of L.F.'s ^{51}Cr-labelled red cells in her own circulation. All ^{51}Cr estimates corrected for Cr elution. For red cell phenotyping, see text (from Mollison, 1959d).

Fig. 10.24). Red cell phenotyping of donor and recipient showed that incompatibility could not have been due to anti-D, -c, -C, -e, -K, -Fy^a, -Jk^a, -Jk^b, -S or -s; anti-E was a possibility, particularly because the red cells of another E-positive donor survived poorly and the red cells of one E-negative donor had an only slightly subnormal survival, which might have been due to the recipient's menorrhagia. Nevertheless, repeated attempts to demonstrate anti-E in the recipient's serum were unsuccessful (Mollison, 1959d, patient I.S.).

More rapid destruction of transfused red cells without demonstrable antibodies was reported by Jandl and Greenberg (1957); in one case after a first transfusion the cells survived normally for 11 d but by the 17th day had all been eliminated. The same recipient was transfused with blood from three other donors and in each instance destruction of red cells began immediately after transfusion and was complete within 5–10 d. On the other hand, the red cells of a fifth donor survived normally. In the second case the survival of transfused red cells was progressively shortened with each transfusion, although on each occasion survival was normal for a short period before the phase of accelerated destruction began. No antibodies could be demonstrated in either of these two cases.

Even more rapid destruction was observed by Stewart and Mollison (1959) in a patient who had developed haemoglobinuria following the transfusion of apparently compatible blood. As Fig. 10.25 shows, transfused red cells were eliminated within 24 h.

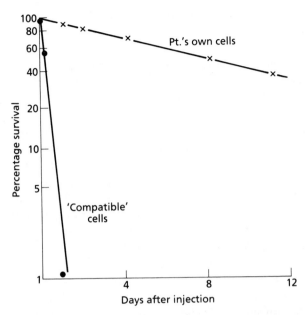

Figure 10.25 Very rapid removal from the circulation of transfused cells, compatible by all the usual serological tests. For comparison, the survival of the patient's own red cells is shown (from Stewart and Mollison, 1959).

The patient was a woman aged 46 years suffering from reticulosarcoma who had been treated with irradiation; during the year in which she had been ill she had received several transfusions. The second had been followed by jaundice, and the fourth and later transfusions by haemoglobinuria. Figure 10.25 shows the survival of red cells which were compatible *in vitro* judged by all tests available including the IAT against enzyme-treated red cells. The figure also shows that the patient's own red cells were removed from the circulation far more slowly, their average life span being about 11 d.

Many similar cases have been reported (see e.g. Heistö *et al.* 1960; Kissmeyer-Nielsen *et al.* 1961; van der Hart *et al.* 1963).

Donor differences. As mentioned above, in one patient investigated by Jandl and Greenberg (1957) the red cells of four donors survived poorly but those of a fifth donor survived normally.

In a patient described by Heistö *et al.* (1962), who developed haemoglobinuria 6 d after the transfusion of 2800 ml blood, tests were subsequently carried out with red cells from eight different donors. The $T_{50}Cr$ varied from 14 d to less than 24 h. Incidentally, the administration of large doses of prednisone did not prevent rapid red cell destruction.

In a patient with sickle cell disease who had had 58 blood transfusions, many different samples of red cells were shown to be rapidly destroyed, although some were completely removed within 24 h whereas others survived normally for 1 week and were then rapidly eliminated. The only cells which survived well were obtained from two siblings (Chaplin and Cassell, 1962). In a case described by Vullo and Tunioli

(1961) red cells from the patient's father survived better than those from another donor.

Cases in which the specificity of an undetectable alloantibody may be inferred

A few cases have been described in which determination of the recipient's red cell phenotype has provided a valuable clue to the specificity of an undetectable alloantibody. For example:

1 In investigating a delayed haemolytic transfusion reaction (DHTR), no evidence of the survival of transfused red cells was found on day 12; the only antigen possessed by all four donors but not by the recipient was c. Tests with ^{51}Cr-labelled red cells showed that c-positive cells underwent rapid destruction (48% survival at 3 h less than 1% at 24 h) whereas c-negative cells had only a slightly reduced survival (93% at 3 h, 80% at 48 h). The patient was then transfused successfully with 8 c-negative units (Davey *et al.* 1980).

2 A patient who had previously received many transfusions received a further transfusion without incident. Two weeks later, another transfusion, this time of 2 units, later shown to be K-positive, caused a haemolytic transfusion reaction characterized by haemoglobinuria and anuria. No alloantibodies could be found. One week later, another transfusion, of 2 units later shown to be K-negative, caused another severe haemolytic transfusion reaction; anti-K was now found but reacting only at room temperature and not at 37°C. Three days later, as the patient's Rh phenotype was found to be ccDEe she was transfused with C-negative units. There was no untoward reaction and the PCV rose by the expected amount; C-negative cells continued to be demonstrable in further samples taken post-transfusion. No antibodies other than anti-K could be detected at any time, using a wide range of sensitive methods (Halima *et al.* 1982b).

3 A woman who had had previous pregnancies and, possibly, a previous transfusion developed a DHTR but did not produce detectable alloantibodies. Following a further transfusion of apparently compatible red cells haemoglobinaemia and haemoglobinuria developed. The patient was found to have the probable Rh genotype *cDE/cDE*. Guessing that the patient might regard e-positive red cells as incompatible, survival tests were done both with e-negative and e-positive cells. Whereas e-negative cells had a normal survival, e-positive red cells were cleared with a $T_{1/2}$ of 4.5–6 h on two separate occasions (Baldwin *et al.* 1983a).

4 A man aged 55 years developed a DHTR after what appeared to be his first transfusion. The second transfusion, given 11 d after the first, produced immediate haemoglobinuria and so did a third transfusion given 2 d later. No red cell alloantibodies could be detected; the patient's probable Rh phenotype was ccDDe. All 6 units which had been transfused to the patient were C-positive. Tests with ^{99m}Tc-labelled red cells showed that cells from two different C-negative donors survived normally (uncorrected survival at 1 h 93.9% and 98.6%) and these units were transfused without reaction. In contrast, cells from one C-positive donor had a survival of 71.1% at 1 h and 28.8% at 4 h (Harrison *et al.* 1986).

Subnormal survival of small amounts of transfused red cells
without demonstrable antibodies

The fact that, when small amounts of ABO-compatible, Rh D-compatible red cells are transfused to a previously untransfused recipient, survival is frequently subnormal, was first recognized by Adner and Sjölin (1957). In estimating the survival of cord red cells transfused to adults they observed that in five of 15 cases, between 6 and 15 d after transfusion there was a sudden increase in the rate of destruction ('collapse') and elimination of the red cells was complete within a month.

A collapse curve had previously been noted in studying a previously untransfused patient with thalassaemia-haemoglobin C disease. When a small volume of red cells was transfused, survival was normal for about 2 weeks but there was then a sudden increase in the rate of destruction and all the cells were eliminated within 30–40 d. Red cells from two other donors survived normally in this patient (Mollison, 1956, p. 354).

The most thorough investigation of the collapse phenomenon yet undertaken was reported by Adner *et al.* (1963). Previously untransfused males were given injections of 3–9 ml red cells, labelled with ^{51}Cr. In 31 cases, donor and recipient were selected as belonging to the same ABO and Rh D group (positive or negative). In ten of the 31 subjects a collapse curve was observed. Nine of these ten subjects received a second injection of red cells from their first donor; in three cases there was rapid destruction but in the remaining six the survival of the red cells of the second injection was normal or only slightly subnormal. Of the three cases showing rapid destruction of the cells of the second injection one had already formed anti-E and another formed anti-Fy^a.

Fourteen additional subjects, all of whom were K-negative, were injected with K-positive blood. Four showed a collapse curve and all of these were given a second injection from their first donor: in two cases the red cells were more rapidly destroyed and one of the two formed anti-E; in the other two recipients the survival of a second injection was normal or only slightly subnormal. Eight of the 14 who showed normal survival of the first lot of red cells were given a second injection; one showed rapid destruction and formed anti-K.

In summary, collapse curves were noted following 14 of 45 first injections of red cells and occurred on average on the 16th day after injection (range 6–33 d). In 13 of these 14 cases a second injection was given; normal or only slightly subnormal survival was found in eight cases and in these no alloantibodies were found. In the remaining five, red cell destruction was observed following a second injection and, in three of these, alloantibodies (two examples of anti-E and one of anti-Fy^a) were detected.

Several other studies in humans have shown an incidence of collapse curves similar to that observed by Adner *et al.* (1963). Brown and Smith (1958) observed 'collapse' of a transfused population of red cells at about 20 d in more than 20% of cases in which red cells which had been through a pump-oxygenator were transfused to other subjects. In most cases no blood group antibodies could be detected in the recipient's serum. In reviewing the total series, G.S. Eadie (personal communication) concluded that 'S-shaped' ('collapse') curves were seen 15 times in 40 survival experiments in 32 recipients. In 38 of the 40 cases the amount of blood injected was 10–20 ml and in the remaining two was 30 and 45 ml respectively. Although at first the phenomenon seemed to be related to the passage of red cells through a pump-oxygenator it was later realized that it occurred irrespective of whether the blood had been through the pump.

In a series studied by E.R. Giblett in 1956, red cells from 1–8 ml of the blood of normal infants were labelled with ^{51}Cr and injected into normal adults. 'Collapse' was

Table 10.3   Incidence of collapse of the red cell survival curve following the transfusion of 1–10 ml red cells to previously untransfused adult recipients

Reference	Donors	Amount of red cells transfused (ml)	Incidence of collapse
Adner and Sjölin (1957)	newborn infants	4–10	5/15
Unpublished observations made by E.R. Giblett	newborn infants	1–8	3/9
Kaplan and Hsu (1961)	newborn infants	2–7	10/41
Adner et al. (1963)*	adults	3–9	14/45
			32/110 (29.1%)
G.S. Eadie (personal communication)†	adults	5–10	15/40

* Following the red cell injections, alloantibodies were detected in three cases in the series of Adner et al. (1963) and in three cases in the series of Brown and Smith (1958), but in no cases in the other series.

† Includes the cases published by Brown and Smith (1958); not included in total above because 40 experiments were carried out in 32 recipients.

observed in three of nine cases and in these no surviving red cells were left in the circulation at 20 d (see Fig. 10.20 for an example).

Kaplan and Hsu (1961) observed that 'collapse' occured in ten of 41 cross-transfusions of small volumes of ^{51}Cr-labelled red cells, '. . . usually [at] about the 14th day after transfusion and in the next week the remainder of the transfused cells are virtually eliminated'.

As Table 10.3 shows, when transfusions of 1–10 ml of Rh D-compatible red cells are given to previously untransfused subjects collapse curves are observed in approximately 30% of cases.

When therapeutic amounts of blood are transfused to previously untransfused subjects premature curtailment of survival is much less common. From a review of more than 100 cases in which the survival of transfused red cells had been followed for not less than 60 d after the transfusion of at least 400 ml blood it was concluded that unexpected shortening of survival was found in only about 5% of cases (Mollison, 1954). A similar incidence was apparent in a series described by Szymanski and Valeri (1971). Forty-four survival studies were carried out by automated differential agglutination in 39 subjects following a transfusion of 450 ml blood; two collapse curves were observed: accelerated destruction set in on about the tenth day after transfusion and all the cells had been eliminated by day 30.

There is some evidence that collapse curves are less common in non-responders to Rh D than in responders, possibly indicating that non-responders to Rh D lack some recognition mechanism for allogeneic red cells (Mollison 1981).

Experiments in animals. Collapse curves were found to be common in cross-transfusion experiments with small volumes of red cells in dogs; collapse occurred at 7–10 d in eight of 30 cases although antibodies were found in only two of the eight (Stohlman and Schneiderman, 1956).

In experiments in rabbits, small volumes of red cells (0.04 ml/kg body-weight) were transfused from Hg-compatible donors. Using a donor of the same inbred strain as that of the recipient, a collapse curve was observed following four of ten first transfusions and survival was subnormal in three more animals. In a second series, using a donor from a different (but still Hg-compatible) strain, a collapse curve following a first injection was observed in six of six animals. In all 16 animals donor red cells with Freund's complete adjuvant were then given but only one of the 16 animals formed a red cell alloantibody (unpublished observations, PLM).

What is the cause of subnormal red cell survival without demonstrable antibodies?
It is tempting to suppose that collapse curves represent primary immunization. In support of this belief, the following observations can be cited: (1) in the series of Adner *et al.* (1963), a collapse curve following a first injection of red cells was sometimes followed by the rapid clearance of a second dose of red cells from the same donor with production of an alloantibody; (2) following a first injection of D-positive red cells to D-negative subjects, collapse curves are commonly observed in responders whereas they are found rarely or not at all in non-responders (Mollison, 1981). Against the belief that collapse curves represent primary immunization, the following can be cited: (1) in the series of Adner *et al.* (1963), in about 50% of cases, a collapse curve following a first injection of red cells was followed by normal survival of a second dose of red cells from the same donor; (2) collapse curves are not found invariably during primary immunization to strong alloantigens, such as D and K. Examples of the normal survival of a first dose of D-positive red cells at 28 d despite the formation of anti-D within the following 6 months were supplied by Samson and Mollison (1975), and an example of the normal survival of a first dose of K-positive red cells for at least 47 d, in a subject who formed anti-K within 10 d of a second injection was described by Adner *et al.* (1963); (3) in rabbits, when Hg (A +) red cells were transfused to Hg (A –) animals, the incidence of collapse curves was 41 of 51 (Smith and Mollison, 1974) but, as stated above, was also high, i.e. 10 of 16, when Hg (A –) red cells were transfused to Hg (A –) rabbits.

The cause of the rapid destruction of red cells in the absence of detectable humoral antibody is unknown.

DESTRUCTION OF RECIPIENT'S RED CELLS BY TRANSFUSED ANTIBODIES

Passively acquired antibodies may destroy either the recipient's own red cells or, when blood from more than one donor is transfused, the red cells of another donor (see pp. 506 and 521). In either case, the mechanism of red cell destruction is similar to that brought about by actively produced antibodies, although the effects tend to be much less severe due to dilution of the transfused antibody by the recipient's plasma and, in the case of anti-A and anti-B, by the inhibiting effect of A and B substances in the plasma and in tissues other than red cells.

In the present chapter, some experimental observations are described; haemolytic reactions arising accidentally are considered in the following chapter.

Destruction of recipient's red cells following the transfusion of plasma containing potent anti-A or anti-B
It was Ottenberg (1911) who first suggested that persons of group O could be used as

'universal donors'. He argued that the anti-A and anti-B agglutinins in the donor's plasma, though theoretically capable of damaging the patient's red cells if the patient belonged to group AB, A or B, would in fact be so diluted in the recipient's plasma as to be harmless. The use of group O blood for transfusion to patients of all groups spread rapidly. At the outset of the Second World War it was accepted that, in practice, the danger of extensive damage to the red cells of recipients of other groups was negligible. Throughout the war, enormous numbers of transfusions of group O blood were given to patients of all groups, without any preliminary matching tests. In the vast majority of cases there was no evidence that undesirable effects were produced. It was well argued that any risks that the procedure carried were small compared with those that would be involved in attempting to group recipients and crossmatch blood under bad conditions.

Nevertheless, the transfusion of group O plasma to group A recipients sometimes causes severe red cell destruction.

Transfusion to human volunteers
The first systematic attempt to assess the effect of transfusions of incompatible plasma was made by Aubert *et al.* (1942b), who transfused plasma containing potent anti-A alloagglutinins to volunteers of group A. By eliminating the complicating factor of the donor's red cells they could be certain that any haemolysis they observed was due to destruction of the patient's own cells. They observed varying degrees of haemoglobinaemia, 'intravascular agglutination' (see below), and hyperbilirubinaemia followed by a progressive reduction in red cell count. The lowest titre of anti-A agglutinin associated with signs of blood destruction was 512. In their hands such anti-A titres were found in the plasma of 40% of group O donors and they therefore concluded that only about 60% of group O individuals could be considered really suitable as universal donors.

Similar findings were reported by Tisdall *et al.* (1946a). In their hands, about 23% of group O persons had anti-A (or anti-B) titres of 640 or higher. The transfusion of 250 ml plasma with an alloagglutinin titre of 600–4000 frequently caused haemoglobinaemia. In one case a volunteer who received plasma with a titre of only 600 developed a sufficient degree of haemoglobinaemia to produce haemoglobinuria. Many patients had rises in serum bilirubin, though none became jaundiced. Tisdall *et al.* also noted the phenomenon described by Aubert *et al.* (1942b) as 'intravascular agglutination'; that is to say, the presence of agglutinates in saline suspensions of blood taken from patients immediately after the transfusions.

In a further series of experiments Tisdall *et al.* (1946b) took blood from a group B volunteer who had been immunized by the injection of group A specific substance, so that his anti-A titre was very high (2500). On one occasion, the injection of as litttle as 25 ml of this plasma into a group A volunteer produced haemoglobinuria. However, after the addition of group-specific substances to the plasma *in vitro*, as much as 250 ml could be injected without producing signs or symptoms. Since the donor of the plasma was group B, the anti-A was probably mainly IgM. In a series of cases, 10 ml of the group-specific substances were added to 250-ml amounts of plasma containing potent agglutinins and transfused to volunteers. No signs of blood destruction were observed in any of the recipients.

One of the difficulties in interpreting these observations is the uncertainty of whether the high-titre agglutinins were IgM or IgG. IgM anti-A and anti-B are far more easily inhibited by soluble blood group substances than are IgG antibodies, so that it would be unsafe to conclude that plasma from group O donors, containing potent anti-A and anti-B, can necessarily be rendered safe by the addition of blood group substances. In fact, at least one case is on record in which a haemolytic transfusion reaction in a group A patient transfused with group O blood occurred despite the addition of AB substance to the plasma before transfusion (Ervin *et al*; 1950).

Observations made by Ervin *et al*. (1950) first called attention to the importance of 'immune' characteristics in causing red cell destruction *in vivo*. They investigated four severe haemolytic reactions in group A patients following the transfusion of group O blood and showed that in all four cases the donor's plasma contained anti-A which was difficult to inhibit and had a higher indirect antiglobulin titre than saline-agglutinin titre. Signs of red cell damage persisted for relatively long periods after transfusion. Thus osmotic fragility was increased for 8–11 d and microspherocytes were seen in films of peripheral blood for approximately 2 weeks after transfusion. The same authors reported the results of giving two transfusions of group O plasma to a group A volunteer. The first transfusion was of plasma with a moderately high saline-agglutinin titre (640) which was readily inhibited by A substance *in vitro* and was presumably wholly or predominantly IgM; no signs of red cell destruction developed. By contrast, when the same volunteer received plasma which had a scarcely higher saline-agglutinin titre (1280) and which probably contained a potent IgG antibody, as judged by the fact that it was not readily inhibited by AB substance, the recipient developed severe intravascular haemolysis and his haematocrit fell from 43% to 24% in 5 d.

Animal experiments

Phenomena very similar to those observed in human beings can be produced in dogs by the transfusion of plasma incompatible with the recipient's red cells (Young *et al*. 1949). Haemoglobinaemia may not be maximal until 5 h after transfusion; some degree of haemoglobinaemia may persist for as long as 72 h. Red cell destruction continues for far longer; for instance in one case the Hb concentration continued to fall for 9 d, whilst spherocytosis and an increase in osmotic fragility persisted for 20 d; as in the human subject, the maximum change in fragility was not seen until 24 h after transfusion.

The above experiments were all performed with plasma capable, *in vitro*, of haemolysing the red cells of the recipient dog. Young *et al*. (1950) performed further transfusion experiments with plasma which, *in vitro*, was not capable of haemolysing red cells and appeared to contain alloagglutinins only. Transfusion of such plasma produced no haemoglobinaemia, bilirubinaemia or increase in osmotic fragility and no increase in bile pigment excretion.

Summary of effects of incompatible plasma (anti-A and anti-B)

The following summary is based partly on the experimental work just described, partly on unpublished observations made with H. Chaplin, H. Crawford (Morton) and M.

Cutbush (Crookston) in 1952, and partly on various transfusion accidents described in the following chapter.

Haemoglobinaemia tends to be slight and haemoglobinuria is unusual.

Jaundice occurring within a few hours of transfusion has been noted occasionally; see, for example, the infants observed by Gasser (1945), referred to in the following chapter.

Progressive anaemia is the most commonly observed sign of red cell destruction; PCV may continue to fall for at least 1 week after transfusion; see Fig. 11.1 for an example.

Spontaneous agglutination of whole blood samples withdrawn from the recipient is an invariable feature. It occurs even when plasma containing relatively weak anti-A is transfused:

In a group A subject transfused in 20 min with 340 ml blood from a donor whose serum had a saline-agglutinin titre of 64 and a haemolysin titre of 4, a sample of blood taken immediately after transfusion showed strong spontaneous agglutination; this was best demonstrated by spreading a drop of blood on an opal tile. Three hours later the sign was still present, but was weaker; the next day it was not present. In patients transfused with potent anti-A, spontaneous agglutination of blood samples *in vitro* may persist for more than 24 h.

The direct antiglobulin test becomes positive in group A subjects transfused with plasma containing even weak immune anti-A. In the subject referred to in the paragraph above the DAT was definitely positive immediately after transfusion, was weakly positive the next day, and was negative thereafter. In patients transfused with potent immune anti-A the DAT may remain positive for as long as 1 week.

The osmotic fragility of the patient's red cells increases when incompatible plasma is transfused. As reported by Ervin *et al.* (1950) the changes are greater 24 h after transfusion than immediately after transfusion; they are almost maximal 3 h after transfusion; osmotic fragility may remain elevated for at least 11 d and during this period films of peripheral blood show microspherocytosis.

Destruction of recipient's red cells by transfused or injected anti-D
Only experimental observations are described in this section; for accidents in clinical practice see the following chapter.

Transfusion of plasma containing anti-D
The effect of transfusing anti-D-containing plasma to D-positive subjects was investigated by Jennings and Hindmarsh (1958): the transfusion of 200 ml plasma containing incomplete anti-D with an indirect antiglobulin titre of 256 produced a direct antiglobulin reaction at 24 h, with spherocytosis, and the recipient's Hb concentration fell by 2.5 g/dl during the following week. In a second case, in which 250 ml plasma with a titre of 128 was transfused, the recipient's bilirubin concentration rose to

2.5 mg/dl at the end of 5 h and the Hb concentration fell by 2.6 g/dl in 1 week. In several recipients transfused with plasma containing antibodies with titres between 8 and 16 there was no definite evidence of red cell destruction.

In a series of cases published by Mohn *et al.* (1961) in which normal volunteers received 250 ml plasma containing moderately potent anti-D (or anti-c or anti-K or anti-M), there were no definite signs of red cell destruction (due partly perhaps to the fact that the red cell volume of the recipients was considerably greater than in the subjects studied by Jennings and Hindmarsh (1958)). In one subject transfused with serum containing an exceptionally potent anti-D (indirect antiglobulin titre of 1000; serum albumin titre of 400 000), the PCV fell from 0.48 to 0.22 in 12 d, and spherocytosis and mild haemoglobinaemia persisted for 2 weeks (Bowman *et al.* 1961).

Injections of anti-D immunoglobulin
In one series of D-positive adults with AITP, injected with 750–4500 µg anti-D i.m. and, or, i.v. over a period of 1–5 d, the red cells became coated with 3.2–7.7 µg IgG/ml cells but only minimal signs of red cell destruction developed (Salama *et al.* 1986). In another series, in which the AITP was related to AIDS, 13 µg IgG anti-D/kg were given daily for 3 d, followed by 6–13 µg/kg weekly. In five of six patients, Hb fell by 6–44 g/l (Cottaneo *et al.* 1989).

CHAPTER 11

HAEMOLYTIC TRANSFUSION REACTIONS

FIGURES

A haemolytic transfusion reaction is one in which signs of increased red cell destruction are produced by transfusion. A distinction is made between an immediate reaction (IHTR), in which destruction begins during transfusion, and a delayed reaction (DHTR), in which destruction begins only after there has been an immune response, provoked by the transfusion. Almost invariably, DHTRs are caused by secondary (anamnestic) immune responses.

The previous chapter was concerned mainly with patterns of removal of incompatible red cells from the circulation rather than with any clinical signs produced. The present chapter deals with the various signs and symptoms produced by the transfusion of incompatible blood and also considers haemolytic reactions due to causes other than incompatibility.

Intravascular and extravascular destruction

Traditionally, following Fairley (1940), red cell destruction is classified as either intravascular, characterized by rupture of red cells within the blood stream and liberation of Hb into the plasma, or as extravascular, characterized by phagocytosis of red cells by macrophages of the mononuclear phagocyte system (MPS), with subsequent liberation of bilirubin into the plasma. Rupture of red cells throughout the circulation (intravascular destruction) is brought about only by those antibodies which activate the whole of the classical complement pathway, the terminal complex C8–9 causing breaches in the red cell membrane. In contrast, antibodies which either fail to activate complement, or activate it only to the C3 stage, can destroy red cells only by mediating a reaction with cells of the MPS. It was initially believed that this reaction consisted simply of phagocytosis but when the interaction of antibody-coated red cells with monocytes was studied *in vitro*, it was found that the red cells could also be lysed outside the monocyte (see Chapter 3). In any case it was known that red cell destruction *in vivo* by a non-complement-activating antibody such as anti-Rh D might be accompanied by haemoglobinaemia. Thus, both Hb and bilirubin may be liberated into the plasma following 'extravascular destruction'. It is clear then that in this context 'extravascular' means 'outside the main blood vessels', i.e. within the liver and spleen, and does not mean 'intracellular'. In describing red cell destruction caused by alloantibodies, terms that are more explicit than intravascular and extravascular are C8–9 mediated and macrophage mediated, but the traditional terms are used as a rule in this chapter.

Intravascular destruction may be produced by antibodies such as anti-A and anti-B which are readily lytic *in vitro*, although it is common for a large proportion of ABO-incompatible red cells to be removed by erythrophagocytosis rather than by lysis in the plasma. Other causes of intravascular lysis are osmotic damage to red cells by preliminary contact with 5% dextrose *in vitro* and the injection of water into the circulation. High levels of plasma Hb may be produced by the injection of red cells which have been lysed *in vitro*, for example by accidental overheating or freezing. Antibodies which are non-lytic *in vitro* bring about destruction which is predominantly extravascular although, as mentioned above, the process may be accompanied by some degree of haemoglobinaemia. The removal of non-viable stored red cells from the circulation is a strictly extravascular process.

INTRAVASCULAR DESTRUCTION

Red cell destruction by rapidly lytic antibodies

The importance of haemolysins as opposed to mere agglutinins was recognized very early in the practice of human transfusion. Indeed, Crile (1909) went so far as to say that in his opinion agglutinins could be disregarded. Similarly, Ottenberg and Thalheimer (1915), as a result of crosstransfusion experiments in cats, some of which developed agglutinins and some lysins, concluded that there was a complete correspondence between lysis *in vitro* and lysis *in vivo*, confirming their opinion that 'similar tests for human transfusion can be relied on completely to prevent haemolytic accidents'.

Overwhelmingly the most important lytic antibodies in human serum are anti-A and anti-B; haemolytic antibodies of other specificities (e.g. anti-PP_1P^k, anti-Vel) have been known to produce similar effects *in vivo*, but are very rare. Lewis antibodies, which are relatively common, produce only slow lysis *in vitro* and only very rarely produce lysis *in vivo*. Kidd antibodies also occasionally lyse untreated red cells but usually, at least, produce predominantly extravascular destruction and are therefore considered in a later section.

Haemolytic transfusion reactions due to antibodies such as anti-A_1 and anti-P_1 which, even when active at 37°C, are usually non-lytic for untreated red cells although they may lyse enzyme-treated red cells, are described in the section on extravascular destruction.

Destruction of transfused ABO-incompatible red cells

As described in the previous chapter up to 90% of the cells may be lysed in the blood stream when a very small volume of incompatible red cells is injected and at least 50% of the cells may be lysed in the blood stream even when a relatively large volume of blood is transfused.

Mrs H. had a serious vaginal haemorrhage after an operation for sterilization and her blood pressure became unrecordable. Her past notes recorded that she belonged to group A and a transfusion of group A blood was begun without any tests. Fifteen minutes later the laboratory reported that a second unit of group A blood that had been matched against the patient's serum, with a view to continuing the transfusion, was incompatible. Forty minutes after the beginning of the transfusion of group A blood the patient started to shiver. Thirty minutes after this a blood sample was obtained and it was found that the patient was group B with no surviving group A cells. The plasma Hb concentration was 10 g/l, corresponding to about 65% of the concentration expected if all the cells had been lysed and none of the Hb had yet disappeared from the plasma. Although the patient passed relatively little urine in the following 24 h the urinary output subsequently rose and thereafter her course was uneventful.

In the following case, a plasmapheresis donor of group O was inadvertently given the red cells of a different donor, who was group A.

Mrs H. was a regular plasmapheresis donor. On the day in question, after she had given blood and before red cells were reinfused into her, she was asked, as usual, to confirm that the signature on the pack was her own. She nodded in agreement but afterwards admitted that she had not seen the signature clearly but felt that, in any case, she could trust the doctor. Within 2 min of the start of the red cell infusion she 'blacked out', felt very frightened and had pain all over, especially over the sternum and lower abdomen. The development of the symptoms was ascribed by the medical attendant to too-rapid infusion and the rate was slowed and infusion completed in about 25 min. After a rest Mrs H. drove home.

One and a half hours later Mrs H. felt very unwell and had diarrhoea and vomiting. She passed a good quantity of urine but did not notice the colour. Three and a half hours after receiving the red cells she was visited by her own doctor who gave her an injection of frusemide. Six hours after receiving the red cells she passed a large volume (about 1 litre) of red urine; the urine Hb concentration was 0.4 g/l and the plasma Hb concentration was 2.6 g/l. The blood contained about 1.7% of group A red cells, the rest being group O. The concentration of fibrin degradation products in the serum was 80 μg/ml, indicating mild disseminated intravascular coagulation (DIC). On the following morning plasma Hb was 0.55 g/l and the urine was now a normal colour. Three weeks after the episode creatinine clearance was normal.

Red cells present as 'contaminants'. When the donor is ABO-incompatible an IHTR may be provoked by red cells present in transfused platelet preparations or in bone marrow cell suspensions, even when the latter have been treated with a sedimenting agent to separate off the bulk of the red cells (Dinsmore *et al.* 1983).

Transplacental haemorrhage (TPH). When the fetus is ABO incompatible, a large TPH may be associated with haemoglobinuria in the mother. One such episode which followed an easy external cephalic version under general anaesthesia was reported by Pollock (1968). The mother (group O) passed fetal Hb in the urine (0.2 g Hb/dl). Four weeks later a group A infant was born; the placenta showed a small area of separation. Of 14 further cases of external version, fetal cells were found in only one and in this case the mother's blood had not been examined before version.

In another case, abruptio placentae followed a car accident following which the mother (group A) gave birth to a stillborn group B infant. The mother exhibited haemoglobinaemia and haemoglobinuria (Glasser *et al.* 1970). In a case described by Samet and Bowman (1961) the group O mother of a B infant developed haemoglobinuria, acute tubular necrosis and DIC.

As described later in this chapter, episodes of intravascular haemolysis following the transfusion of incompatible red cells are sometimes followed by renal failure and by the production of various other untoward signs.

In patients whose serum contains non-lytic or only very weakly lytic anti-A or anti-B, following the transfusion of ABO-incompatible blood the level of plasma Hb may be less than 1 g/l and no Hb is passed in the urine. In fact, it is only when anti-A and anti-B are relatively potent that destruction is predominantly intravascular.

After the transfusion of incompatible blood, erythrophagocytosis may be observed in samples of peripheral blood (Hopkins, 1910; Ottenberg, 1911). Gross leucopenia may be produced, due apparently to the adherence of leucocytes to red cells and to each other. Jandl and Tomlinson (1958) found that after the injection of 10 ml ABO-incompatible red cells, the total leucocyte count sometimes fell from 9000 to 4000 per μl in 5 min. The biggest effect was on the mature granulocytes and monocytes. In further experiments they showed that the injection of as little as 0.05 ml incompatible red cells (5×10^8 cells) caused a significant fall in leucocytes. They calculated that as many as 15 leucocytes were removed for each incompatible red cell injected. Intravenous injection of the stroma of compatible cells produced no effect but the injection of the stroma of incompatible cells produced leucopenia. Incidentally, the injection of A substance into O subjects produced leucopenia in six of seven instances.

Frequency of ABO-incompatible transfusions

From one large series it was estimated that about one in 1000 patients received the 'wrong' blood, usually due to failure to identify the patient correctly (see p. 367). On the other hand, Mayer (1982) recorded only 27 haemolytic reactions due to ABO incompatibility in almost half a million transfusions, a frequency of one in 18 000, suggesting that only about one in 6000 patients received the wrong blood.

The record of the Mayo Clinic is outstanding. In the period 1964–73, in the course of transfusing 268 000 units blood, there was only one occasion on which, as a result of misidentification, ABO-incompatible red cells were transfused (Pineda *et al.* 1978b). This remarkable record must surely be due to the system at the Mayo Clinic whereby blood bank personnel have total control of blood units from the time when they are withdrawn from the donor to the time when they are given to the recipient. Blood bank nurse transfusionists administer almost all blood which is given to patients in their rooms and monitor all transfusions given in operating theatres (Taswell *et al.* 1981, supplemented by personal communication from H.F. Taswell); see also pp. 367–368.

Mortality rate associated with ABO-incompatible transfusions
As already described, the transfusion of ABO-incompatible blood may cause the death of a patient either by initiating DIC or by precipitating renal failure. In one series of 40 patients who received incompatible blood, four died as a direct result of the transfusion. All four patients had been transfused during or immediately after major surgery. Severe and persistent hypotension was the main clinical manifestation. All four patients had DIC; two died within 24 h from irreversible shock and two after about 4 d when manifestations of acute uraemia appeared (Wallace, 1977). The seriousness of DIC as a complication of ABO-incompatible transfusion is emphasized by the experience of Binder *et al.* (1959); of five patients transfused with ABO-incompatible blood who developed a haemorrhagic diathesis, all died. Nevertheless, in the majority of patients who receive ABO-incompatible blood, DIC is mild or undetectable and renal failure does not develop.

In one hospital in the USA 13 cases of ABO-incompatible transfusions came to light in a period of 17 years, during which approximately 300 000 units blood were transfused to 75 000 patients. Of the 13 recipients of ABO-incompatible blood three received 50 ml or less, five received at least 0.5 unit, and five received 1 unit or more. A few of the recipients were transfused during surgery and one developed bleeding associated with DIC; none of the 13 became oliguric and all recovered uneventfully (Mollison, 1979, p. 573).

In another series of 12 patients not one developed abnormal bleeding or any sign of interference with renal function. Three patients received less than 50 ml incompatible blood, transfusion being discontinued because of the development of severe symptoms. Six patients received between 200 and 600 ml blood; of these only one developed immediate symptoms, which were ignored because the subject was a plasmapheresis donor who was believed to be receiving her own red cells (see above); this patient and one of the others developed haemo-globinuria. Of two patients who received 1 litre and one who received 4 litres ABO-incompatible blood only one developed immediate symptoms which were ignored by the doctor in charge because the patient was believed to be 'neurotic'; this patient developed a rigor but the other patient developed only trivial symptoms (Mollison, 1983, p. 649).

In December 1975 it became mandatory in the USA to report immediately to the Food and Drug Administration (FDA) 'when a complication of blood collection and transfusion is confirmed to be fatal'. The information collected between 1976 and 1978 was reviewed by Schmidt (1980a,b) who considered that in only 39 of the 69 cases could transfusion be regarded as the primary cause of death. In 24 of the 39, death was due to an incompatible transfusion; 22 of the 24 were immediate reactions due to transfusion of ABO-incompatible blood and the remaining two were DHTRs associated with anti-c or anti-E. Almost the same series of cases was reviewed by Honig and Bove (1980), but in their paper the emphasis was laid on the errors which had led to the transfusion of incompatible blood. They concluded that of 44 acute haemolytic reactions 38 were due to ABO incompatibility. Both reviews emphasized that the commonest cause of ABO-incompatible transfusion is failure to identify the recipient correctly and that the commonest place where incompatible blood is transfused is the operating theatre.

Deaths reported to the FDA in the 10-year period from 1976 to 1985 (inclusive) were reviewed by Sazama (1990). Of the cases due apparently to red cell incompatibility, 158 were due to acute haemolysis (ABO incompatibility in 131) and 26 to delayed haemolysis (mainly anti-c and anti-Jk^a); recipient deaths from other causes are described in Chapter 15 and donor deaths in Chapter 1.

It seems very likely that the most important factor in determining the outcome of an ABO-incompatible transfusion is the potency of the anti-A (or anti-B) in the patient's plasma. For example, in the case illustrated in Fig. 11.7 (p. 530) in which there were virtually no ill-effects from the transfusion of A blood to an O subject, the anti-A agglutinin titre before transfusion was 32 and the serum was only very faintly lytic. On the other hand, in another case, gross haemoglobinaemia with complete defibrination of the blood, followed by renal failure, developed in a group O patient transfused with a unit of A blood during surgery. Ironically, screening of the patient's plasma before transfusion had revealed that her serum would completely lyse a suspension of group A red cells (Mollison, 1979, p. 650).

Destruction of recipient's own red cells by transfused anti-A or anti-B

Clinical signs of red cell destruction develop occasionally after the transfusion of group O blood or plasma to recipients of other ABO groups. As a rule, destruction is predominantly extravascular but it is convenient to consider all haemolytic reactions due to anti-A or anti-B in the same section.

Transfusion of group O blood to recipients of other ABO groups. In investigating a haemolytic reaction in a group A patient transfused with group O blood, Wiener and Moloney (1943) used the method of differential agglutination to show that the transfused red cells had survived and thus demonstrated that the signs of haemolysis were due to destruction of the patient's own red cells. Experimental work on the transfusion of group O blood containing potent anti-A and anti-B to recipients of other groups has been described in the previous chapter. In the present section a few examples will be given of accidental haemolytic transfusion reactions following the transfusion of ABO-incompatible plasma, either in the form of group O blood or as plasma alone.

The following case illustrates many of the features of a severe haemolytic transfusion reaction in a group A patient after the transfusion of blood from a 'dangerous' group O donor:

The patient was a woman aged 23, who had a postpartum haemorrhage, estimated at 800 ml blood. The placenta was removed manually under anaesthesia. Whilst the patient was recovering from the anaesthetic and during the transfusion of a second unit of group O blood she was found to be having a fit; her blood pressure was 80/40 mm Hg. The transfusion was stopped after 800 ml had been given; the patient was treated conservatively and recovered rapidly. Investigation of a blood sample 12 h after transfusion showed that the patient was group A Rh D-positive with approximately 0.9×10^9 group O red cells per litre. As Fig. 11.1 shows, over the following 9 d there was a scarcely measurable decrease in the concentration of group O cells but

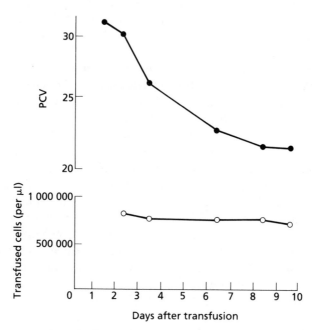

Figure 11.1 Destruction of recipient's own (group A) red cells following the transfusion of group O blood, the plasma of which contained potent anti-A. The transfused cells survived normally and the progressive fall in the recipient's packed cell volume (PCV) was therefore due entirely to the destruction of the patient's own cells.

PCV fell progressively due, evidently, to destruction of the patient's own red cells. The direct antiglobulin test (DAT) was strongly positive for about 48 h after transfusion and more weakly positive for the following week; the test was negative on the tenth day after transfusion. The plasma of the first unit of blood was shown to have an extremely high anti-A titre and to be strongly lytic for group A cells. The donor had received an injection of (horse) anti-tetanus serum 38 d before giving blood (Mollison, 1951, p. 286).

Plasma which has a comparatively low anti-A agglutinin titre (64–256) but contains potent IgG anti-A (indirect antiglobulin titre 1000–5000) may cause serious haemolytic reactions (Grove-Rasmussen *et al.* 1953; Stevens and Finch, 1954).

Ebert and Emerson (1946) noted only about 1% of frank haemolytic reactions in patients of group AB, A or B receiving routine transfusions of group O blood; but they considered that some asymptomatic destruction of recipient's cells was almost invariable after multiple transfusions of group O blood or pooled plasma. They were often able to demonstrate progressive destruction of the patient's red cells for periods up to 1 week after transfusion.

Transfusion of packed red cells from group O blood to recipients of other ABO groups. As described on p. 494, the injection of as little as 25 ml plasma containing potent anti-A may produce haemoglobinuria in a group A subject. It is therefore not surprising that haemoglobinuria has been encountered after the transfusion of a unit of packed O red cells to an A subject. In the case concerned it was estimated that the unit, which had a PCV of 0.70, contained about 95 ml plasma; after 'neutralization' by group A- and

B-specific substances, the plasma had an anti-A indirect antiglobulin titre of 8192. Apart from developing haemoglobinuria, the patient had a rigor and vomited but made an uneventful recovery (Inwood and Zuliani, 1978).

Transfusions of group O plasma from single donors. Gasser (1945) described haemolytic reactions in three group A (or AB) infants, weighing 3.5–4.5 kg, who received 50–90 ml group O plasma; jaundice developed within a few hours. Examination of films of peripheral blood showed striking microspherocytosis; in one case an increase in osmotic fragility was demonstrated. An interesting point in two cases was that plasma from the same donor had been given on the previous day without producing reactions. This suggested that the capacity of the body to inhibit anti-A had been saturated by the first plasma transfusion so that a second transfusion within a short time had a more damaging effect.

Renal failure has been described: a 3-year-old haemophiliac was given a transfusion of 300 ml group O plasma before dental treatment; he vomited before and after the subsequent anaesthetic. By the following morning he was deeply jaundiced and had passed a small amount of almost black urine; his Hb concentration was about 6 g/dl; the DAT was strongly positive. The patient recovered after treatment by peritoneal dialysis. The transfused plasma proved to have a haemolysin titre of 128 and an agglutinin titre of 256 (Keidan *et al.* 1966).

Transfusion of large amounts of low-titre or pooled plasma. Evidence of the damaging effect of the transfusion of large volumes of low-titre ABO plasma was supplied by Topley *et al.* (1963). In some patients with burns, receiving an amount of pooled plasma equivalent to more than three times their plasma volume, haemoglobinuria developed 12–48 h after transfusion and it was calculated that more than 40% of the recipient's red cells were destroyed. The plasma used was prepared from the blood of ten donors of different ABO groups (namely, four group O, four group A and two group B or AB).

In a series of haemophiliacs transfused with large amounts of pooled plasma, haemolytic episodes characterized by a raised serum bilirubin concentration and a positive DAT were common. It was found that the pooled plasma frequently had anti-A titres of 'immune' (non-inhibitable) antibody as high as 64 (Delmas-Marsalet *et al.* 1969).

Anti-A or anti-B in Factor VIII concentrates. A haemolytic reaction due to the administration of large amounts of a Factor VIII concentrate to a group A patient and characterized by a fall in PCV to 0.20, the appearance of microspherocytes in the peripheral blood and a raised plasma Hb level was described by Rosati *et al.* (1970). In a group A patient with a Factor VIII inhibitor who was given approximately 170 000 units Factor VIII, the DAT became positive, Hb fell to 50–60 g/l and the reticulocyte count rose to 54%; batches of the Factor VIII preparation had anti-A indirect antiglobulin test (IAT) titres of 128–512 (Hach-Wunderle *et al.* 1989).

Anti-A and anti-B in immunoglobulin preparations for intravenous use. Episodes of severe intravascular haemolysis were observed in two group B recipients of bone marrow transplants, following the i.v. injection of an immunoglobulin preparation

('Gamimune'), later shown to contain anti-B with a titre of 32, as well as anti-A (Kim *et al.* 1988).

Anti-A or anti-B in platelet concentrates. A severe haemolytic reaction in a group A subject following the transfusion of 4 units platelets from a group O donor, suspended in 200 ml of the donor's plasma, was shown to be due to anti-A in the donor's plasma with an IAT titre of 8192 and the ability to lyse A_1 red cells. The recipient developed haemoglobinuria and the PCV fell from 0.22 before transfusion to 0.16 8 hours later; the DAT became positive (Siber *et al.* 1982).

Incompatibility in a case of parabiosis. Lauer (1941) reported a remarkable case in which the circulation of two sisters, of different ABO groups, became joined for a few days.

In a railway accident a girl sustained severe damage to her foot, involving considerable loss of tissue from the sole. With the object of obtaining tissue to repair this injury, the injured foot was temporarily grafted to the thigh of the patient's sister. The donor of the tissue belonged to group O and the recipient to group A. During the second half of the week following the grafting, both sisters became ill, and it was clear that a connection had been established between their respective circulations. From the point of view of transfusion terminology, each may be regarded as donor and recipient with respect to the other; for the present purpose the terms are here used with respect to giving and receiving of the graft.

The donor (group O), although subjectively well, became jaundiced and febrile and was found to have haemoglobinuria; her red cell count was found to be $3.6 \times 10^9/l$. At the end of the week the recipient (group A) began to vomit and was found to have become very anaemic (red cell count $1.8 \times 10^9/l$); a blood smear showed many normoblasts.

On the eighth day venous samples were taken for examination and the blood of both patients was found to contain only group O red cells, with anti-A and anti-B in the serum. The sisters were promptly separated and both recovered uneventfully.

Further examination of the recipient's blood (originally group A) revealed that no agglutination occurred with anti-A sera, even when abnormally potent sera were used. Four days after the separation, A cells reappeared in the recipient's circulation. After the 14th day anti-A agglutinins were no longer demonstrable in the circulation.

Titration of the recipient's serum on the day of separation showed an anti-A titre of 32 and an anti-B titre of 16. The donor's serum was also titrated on the day of separation. Whereas the anti-B titre was found to be 16, the anti-A titre was 2048. The latter remained at this high level for 3 d and then fell gradually. At the end of 6 months it was found to be only 2.

Destruction of transfused A_1 red cells by passively acquired anti-A
In a case described by Ervin and Young (1950), a patient belonging to subgroup A_2 received a transfusion of 5 units A_1 blood followed by 1 unit group O blood containing immune anti-A. All the transfused A_1 cells were eliminated within approximately 2 d of transfusion and anti-A_1 could be demonstrated in the recipient's plasma. In this case there was no evidence of adverse effects, but in another case in which a patient of subgroup A_2 was transfused with 3 units group A_1 and 1 unit group O blood, jaundice and anuria developed and the patient died (Grove-Rasmussen *et al.* 1951).

Haemoglobinuria following transfusion in patients with haemolytic anaemia

Autoimmune haemolytic anaemia (AIHA). According to Chaplin (1979), haemoglobinuria following transfusion in AIHA is most commonly due simply to increasing the red cell mass subject to autoimmune destruction in patients with a very severe haemolytic process. (The autoantibodies concerned are not necessarily complement-binding but AIHA is included here for convenience.) Haemoglobinuria following transfusion in patients with complement-mediated AIHA may be due to the initial destruction of 'unprotected' red cells, that is, red cells which, unlike the patient's own red cells, have little C3dg on them (see also pp. 453–454). Intravascular lysis due to the supply of complement in the transfused blood seems to be an unusual cause of post-transfusion haemoglobinuria in patients with AIHA; two possible cases, both in patients with cold haemagglutinin disease, were described by Evans *et al.* (1965).

Paroxysmal nocturnal haemoglobinuria (PNH). Patients with PNH react adversely to the transfusion of whole blood with 'discouraging dependability'. The reactions are characterized by shivering and fever with diarrhoea, abdominal pain and headache. During the phase of chill and fever, haemoglobinuria (if present initially) ceases but then there is intense haemoglobinuria which may last for several hours (Crosby and Stefanini, 1952). The mechanism is unknown; it seems likely that some antigen–antibody reaction is involved, leading to the activation of complement, to which PNH red cells are highly sensitive. It has been shown that the interaction of leucocyte antigens and antibodies can cause lysis of PNH red cells *in vitro* (Sirchia *et al.* 1970). Reactions appear to be just as frequent when saline-washed red cells, rather than whole blood or packed red cells, are used for transfusion (Sherman and Taswell, 1977). However, it would seem to be a sound practice to use leucocyte-poor red cells for transfusion.

Symptoms and signs accompanying complement-mediated haemolysis
The activation of complement results in the liberation of C3a and C5a small polypeptides (mol. wt. about 10 000) which act directly on smooth muscle and interact with various cells (e.g. mast cells), to liberate vasoactive substances such as histamine; for further details see p. 142.

Although complement activation is believed to play a key role in producing the various effects including DIC (see below) associated with ABO-incompatibility, there is evidence that the cytokine interleukin-8 (IL-8) may also be involved. IL-8 is liberated when A or B red cells are added to group O serum *in vitro*; it is produced by various cells, including monocytes; it activates neutrophils, leading to the release of thromboplastic substances, and may in this way initiate intravascular coagulation (Davenport *et al.* 1990).

The symptoms and signs produced by complement-mediated lysis associated with the transfusion of ABO-incompatible red cells were vividly described by Oehlecker (1928). As a biological test for compatibility, 5–20 ml blood from a potential donor were injected rapidly and the effects observed. The following is a rough translation of what was noted when the donor was ABO incompatible: 'After one or one and a half minutes the patient becomes restless, breathes deeply and complains of a feeling of oppression, perhaps also of sternal pain. The patient may also have abdominal discomfort and may vomit. The pulse becomes weaker and one often sees a characteristic change in colour; a pale patient may suddenly become strikingly red.' Oehlecker pointed out that usually all the symptoms subside rapidly but that if more blood is injected the same symptoms recur within 1–2 min. Presumably, the constricting pain in the chest is due to a spasm of coronary vessels.

Similar symptoms were noted in some of the early transfusions given to patients from animal donors. For example, the effects of transfusing calf blood to a human subject were reported as follows: after about 200 ml blood had been transfused, the patient 'found himself very hot along his arm and under the armpits'. After a second larger transfusion on the following day (of about 450 ml blood) 'he felt the like heat along his arm and under his armpits which he had felt before . . . and he complained of great pains in his kidneys and that he was not well in his stomach and that he was ready to choke unless they gave him his liberty' (Denis, 1667–8).

Towards the end of the nineteenth century there was a vogue for using lambs as donors and a certain Dr Champneys (1880) reported that he had witnessed more than a dozen transfusions given directly from the carotid vessels of a lamb into the forearm veins of human subjects suffering from phthisis. After a short interval there was difficulty in breathing with a feeling of oppression, then flushing, followed by sweating. On the next day and for a few days subsequently there was 'haematinuria' and, in nearly all cases, urticaria.

Although constricting pain in the chest and pain in the lumbar region has been observed following the injection of 0.7 ml A_1 red cells to a subject whose serum contained potent lytic anti-A (Mollison, 1972a, p. 549), the intravascular lysis of approximately 1 ml ABO-incompatible red cells does not necessarily cause symptoms (personal observations, PLM). Similarly, in a series described by Jandl and Tomlinson (1958) in which 10 ml washed incompatible red cells were injected, only a few subjects developed transient symptoms (lumbar pain, dyspnoea, hyperperistalsis, flushing of the face).

In another series of experiments, Jandl and Kaplan (1960) observed an immediate reaction only when there was intravascular red cell destruction. In this series, ^{51}Cr-labelled group B red cells were injected into a group A patient with hypogammaglobulinaemia whose serum contained no detectable anti-B. The B red cells initially underwent only slow destruction corresponding to a T_{50}Cr of about 5 d. After 5 d various amounts of anti-B were injected, and only when the amount of anti-B was sufficient to produce intravascular lysis were any symptoms noted, namely facial flushing beginning 2 min after injection lasting 4 or 5 min, followed (7 min after injection) by pain in the groins, thighs and lower part of the back, lasting 45 min. Jandl and Kaplan (1960) also found that subjects receiving small injections of red cells of incompatible ABO groups developed a small rise in body temperature but no chills.

Strongly lytic antibodies other than anti-A and anti-B which produce similar effects *in vivo* are very rare. In the first subject in whom anti-PP$_1$P^k (-Tj^a) was identified, a test injection of 25 ml incompatible blood was followed by an immediate severe reaction with haemoglobinaemia (Levine *et al.* 1951a). In a subject with haemolytic anti-Vel transfusion produced a rigor, lumbar pain and anuria (Levine *et al.* 1961b).

The symptoms provoked by the transfusion of incompatible blood are, of course, abolished by anaesthetics (see Young *et al.* 1947) and modified by morphia (Mollison, 1943a, case 3).

In patients who are anaesthetized or are under the influence of drugs during transfusion the only two signs which may call attention to the possibility that incompatible blood has been transfused are, first, hypotension despite apparently adequate replacement of blood, and second, abnormal bleeding.

Disseminated intravascular coagulation associated with intravascular haemolysis

In dogs, the infusion of autologous haemolysed red cells leads to intravascular coagulation (Rabiner and Friedman, 1968). Presumably, thromboplastic substances in stroma (Shinowava, 1951; Quick et al. 1954) are responsible for the initiation of intravascular coagulation. In monkeys, the infusion of sonicated stroma, free of Hb, produces a fall in platelets, fibrinogen and Factors II, V and VIII (Birndorf et al. 1971). Complement activation may also trigger coagulation (Zimmerman and Müller-Eberhard, 1971); see below.

The fully developed syndrome of DIC is characterized by thrombocytopenia, a fall in the levels of Factors V and VIII (particularly the latter), a low level of fibrinogen, and deposition of fibrin thrombi in small vessels. Fibrin degradation products can be demonstrated in the serum.

In experiments in monkeys in which incompatible plasma was transfused, evidence of mild DIC was observed in two animals in which plasma Hb levels reached 6 g/l or more. It was not observed in animals in which the plasma Hb level was below 1 g/l (Lopas et al. 1971). In other experiments in which incompatible allogeneic red cells were transfused, equivalent in amount to 250 ml blood to a human adult, DIC was observed in three of five cases in which there was intravascular haemolysis (average plasma Hb 6.5 g/l) associated with haemolytic antibodies. The main features were a fall in Factors V, VIII and IX and a less consistent fall in fibrinogen concentration and in platelet count. Intravascular coagulation was not observed in two cases in which destruction was predominantly extravascular and associated with predominantly incomplete non-haemolytic antibodies; in these latter cases there was a slow rise of plasma Hb, reaching a peak of about 0.5 g/l in 4 h (Lopas and Birndorf, 1971).

Following the transfusion of ABO-incompatible blood, abnormal bleeding is often observed (Schneider, 1956; Krevans et al. 1957; Moore, 1958; Rock et al. 1969; Sack and Nefa, 1970). In some cases a haemorrhagic state has developed after the transfusion of as little as 100 ml ABO-incompatible blood. If the patient is undergoing operation, uncontrollable bleeding from the wound develops; epistaxis and bleeding from the site of venepuncture have also been observed. A fibrinogen level as low as 15 mg/dl has been reported, with virtually incoagulable blood. Fibrin degradation products (FDP) have been found in the serum, usually in concentrations in the range 250–450 μg/ml but as high as 1900 μg/ml in one case (Sack and Nefa, 1970).

There is some evidence that DIC is more severe for a given level of haemoglobinaemia due to ABO-incompatible transfusion than when due to other causes. For example, in a case described by Slotki et al. (1976) a patient with *Clostridium perfringens* septicaemia developed a plasma Hb level of 40 g/l but with scarcely any evidence of a disturbance of haemostasis. The platelet count remained normal and the level of FDP was only 64 μg/ml. No evidence of DIC was found in a series of glucose-6-phosphate dehydrogenase deficient patients during attacks of favism (Mannucci *et al.* 1969). In rabbits, haemoglobinaemia produced by the i.v. injection of water was not associated with signs of DIC (Slaastad and Eika, 1973). However, plasma Hb reached only about 3.5 g/l.

If it is true that DIC is more severe for any given level of plasma Hb following incompatible transfusion than following intravascular lysis from other causes, some interaction between complement activation and the triggering of coagulation seems to be the most likely cause.

Various interactions have been demonstrated between the complement, kinin, coagulation and fibrinolytic systems (see review by Sundsmo and Fair, 1983); for example, low mol. wt. fragments of Factor XIIa (Hageman factor) may mediate C1 activity (Ghebrehiwet *et al.* 1981). Nevertheless, it is a matter for speculation whether in practice complement activation can, for example, trigger DIC. Although thrombin can cleave complement proteins the concentration required is exceedingly large so that the reaction may not actually taken place in physiological circumstances (Ghebrehiwet *et al.* 1981).

After predominantly extravascular destruction, it is probable that DIC occurs very occasionally. There are two reports in the literature of abnormal bleeding following incompatible transfusion due to antibodies which are not haemolytic *in vitro*: one due to anti-c (Wiener, 1954) and one due to anti-Fy^a (Rock *et al.* 1969).

Renal failure following intravascular haemolysis

The destruction of red cells within the blood stream, resulting in haemoglobinaemia, is sometimes followed by interference with renal function, but it still seems uncertain whether Hb itself is harmful. The infusion of large volumes of stroma-free Hb has been found to have no effect on renal function in dogs and monkeys (Birndorf and Lopas, 1970; Rabiner *et al.* 1970). Nevertheless, there is other evidence indicating that the infusion of even highly purified Hb causes some impairment of renal function (see review of Dzik and Sherburne, 1990). In one study, when 250 ml of a preparation of Hb containing only 1.2% stromal lipid was administered at the rate of 4 ml/min to six well-hydrated healthy men, urinary output fell by 81%, mean creatinine clearance declined and there was transient bradycardia and hypertension (Savitsky *et al.* 1978).

Renal damage associated with intravascular destruction is relatively common when destruction is due to potent lytic antibodies, i.e. anti-A and anti-B, and is rare when destruction is due to non-lytic antibodies; it is also rare when haemoglobinaemia is due to causes other than incompatibility, e.g. the accidental injection of water into the circulation.

The precise way in which renal failure is produced is not known but the initiation of DIC may play a part. In experiments in monkeys, in which haemolytic transfusion reactions were produced, fibrin thrombi were widespread and were found in one case in renal tufts (Lopas *et al.* 1971). Hypotension is doubtless another factor in precipitating renal failure; potent complement activation leads to the release of large amounts of C3a and C5a which in turn release vasoactive peptides from mast cells.

Renal failure following the infusion of stroma
Evidence that the infusion of stroma from incompatible red cells is followed by renal failure was presented by Schmidt and Holland (1967). In one case, in an attempt to depress the titre of a panagglutinin in a patient's plasma, stroma from 4 units red cells was infused. One hour later the patient felt apprehensive, had some fall in blood pressure, a rapid decrease in urinary output and granulocytopenia and thrombocytopenia. Following an infusion of mannitol (25%), urinary flow was rapidly restored.

In a second case, a patient whose serum contained anti-K was given an infusion of stroma from 1 unit K-positive red cells and 3 units K-negative red cells. There was a rigor and severe oliguria lasting 5 d. The authors stated that in 12 other cases in which stroma had been infused, no complications occurred.

These experiments reinforce the conclusion that transfusion of incompatible red cells produces its damaging effect on the kidney not by releasing Hb but by triggering DIC and by activating complement. For a fuller discussion, see Goldfinger (1977).

Effect of incompatible transfusion in an anuric patient. A patient of group O with presumed tubular necrosis following severe injury 1 month earlier was given one-third of a unit of group AB blood in 4 min. The patient felt unwell and temporarily lost consciousness. At 1 h plasma Hb was 4.8 g/l (1.82 g bound to haptoglobin (Hp), the rest free). The plasma was cleared of Hb in about 10 h, during which time the patient excreted 8 ml of faintly orange urine. The episode appeared to delay slightly the onset of diuresis but ultimately renal function was only slightly impaired (Hoffsten and Chaplin, 1969).

Management of suspected immediate haemolytic transfusion reactions
Methods of diagnosing IHTRs and the immediate steps to be taken when an IHTR is suspected are described later in this chapter; the serological investigations to be undertaken are discussed in Chapter 8.

The threats posed by an episode of acute intravascular haemolysis are of renal failure, the management of which is described below, and of DIC, which has no generally accepted treatment (but see Chapter 14).

If DIC is diagnosed and the decision is taken to give heparin, a dosage which has been recommended is 5000 units i.v. immediately, followed by a continuous infusion of 1500 units/h for 6–24 h (Goldfinger, 1977). Heparin treatment carries, of course, the risk of making the situation worse; few reports are available of its effects in dealing with IHTR, although two apparent successes were reported by Rock *et al.* (1969).

Treatment of threatened or established renal failure
Treatment may be divided into three phases: immediate, the period of oliguria, and the period of diuresis.

Immediate treatment. As soon as it is realized that there is intravascular haemolysis, an attempt should be made to promote the flow of urine by: (1) ensuring adequate renal perfusion. Hypovolaemia, if present, should be treated. Dopamine, (infused at 3–5 μg/ kg per min) produces selective renal vasodilatation; (2) administering diuretics. Frusemide may be given in doses of up to 250 mg by infusion over 4 h.

The aim is to achieve a urinary output of at least 0.5 ml/kg per hour and preferably of twice this amount.

The period of oliguric renal failure. Whilst the above measures should be continued, it is extremely important not to administer more water than the patient can excrete. The fluid intake must be rigorously limited to the volume of urinary output plus about 20 ml/h (500 ml/d) to correspond with the patients 'insensible' losses via the lungs, skin and faeces. A patient with renal failure is extremely susceptible to overloading with fluid and can easily develop pulmonary oedema. Electrolytes should be excluded from the patient's fluid intake.

Hyperkalaemia is a frequent cause of cardiac arrest in patients with renal failure. The patient's electrocardiogram (ECG) should be monitored continuously and the serum potassium level measured 4-hourly. If the serum potassium exceeds 6 mol/l, it may be controlled with an infusion of 50% dextrose with added insulin. Calcium chloride (10–20 ml of a 10% solution) can be used in emergency to counteract the effects of hyperkalaemia on the heart. The release of potassium by the catabolism of tissue protein can be retarded by a high calorie intake, which may have to be given i.v.

Metabolic acidosis develops slowly and is, in the early stages at least, compensated by hyperventilation and hypocarbia. Treatment with sodium bicarbonate is deferred for as long as possible because it may exacerbate sodium and water overload and precipitate hypocalcaemia.

The blood urea and creatinine levels should be estimated daily. The dosage of any concurrent drug therapy must be adjusted to take account of the absence of renal excretion. The advice of a nephrologist is essential.

Active intervention (haemofiltration, peritoneal dialysis or haemodialysis) is indicated in the presence of:

1   Uraemic stupor, coma, vomiting, hiccough or fits.
2   Pulmonary oedema. Severe hypoxia may be treated with artificial ventilation (IPPV) until sodium and water have been removed.
3   Hyperkalaemia, i.e. serum potassium concentration 7 mmol/l despite conservative measures.
4   A rapidly rising blood urea, threatening to exceed 30–50 mmol/l, or a serum creatinine threatening to exceed 0.7–1.5 mmol/l. Other biochemical criteria include a plasma bicarbonate of < 12 mmol/l.

The removal of sodium and water makes it possible to give a larger fluid intake and thus facilitates parenteral nutrition and blood transfusion. The invasive measures required to establish filtration or dialysis may cause dangerous bleeding if there is DIC.

The period of diuresis. Urinary output must be matched by an equivalent intake not just of water but also of electrolytes; there is often considerable loss of sodium in the urine. The diet should contain only limited amounts of protein until the blood urea falls below 20 mmol/l.

Lysis from osmotic effects

Damage produced by exposure to 5% dextrose
Haemolytic transfusion reactions have sometimes been observed in patients receiving transfusions of whole blood passed through a bottle containing 5% dextrose and 0.225% saline (Ebaugh *et al.* 1958, cited by DeCesare *et al.* 1964).

Noble and Abbot (1959) noted that if a giving set, of the type in which a filter was inserted into a bottle, was transferred from a bottle of blood to a bottle of dextrose, some red cells were lysed after 12 h. They showed that red cells suspended in excess 5% dextrose or in 4.3% dextrose with 0.18% saline were almost completely lysed after 24 h at room temperature.

Measurements of the amount of lysis observed if blood is mixed with varying proportions of 5% dextrose in water or 0.225% saline, both at room temperature and 37°C, were provided by Ryden and Oberman (1975). No lysis was found even after 15 h at 37°C when blood was mixed with 5% dextrose in normal saline.

Red cells exposed to 5% dextrose in hypotonic saline before transfusion become hypertonic and swollen; when the swelling is equivalent to 160% or more of their original volume, a substantial number are lost following return to the circulation. Red cells with a similar increase in dextrose concentration following exposure to 5% dextrose in normal saline survive normally during the immediate post-transfusion period, suggesting that the increased dextrose concentration *per se* is not damaging (De Cesare *et al.* 1964). On the other hand, delayed damage due to exposure to dextrose has been demonstrated; red cells incubated for only 15 min with 5% dextrose (in water) and returned to the circulation had a normal survival in the first few hours but a survival of only 20–30% at 48 h (Jones *et al.* 1962).

Injection of water into the circulation

The i.v. injection of 100 ml water into an adult produces only trivial haemoglobinaemia (0.1–0.2 g/l) but the injection of 300–900 ml, infused over a period of 1–4 h, produces plasma Hb levels of 2–4 g/l. Water may gain entrance to the circulation if during transurethral prostatectomy the bladder is irrigated with water rather than saline. In patients who already have renal ischaemia the entrance of water into the circulation may apparently precipitate renal failure (all information in this paragraph from Landsteiner and Finch, 1947).

The potential danger of injecting water into the circulation is emphasized by the experience of J. Wallace (personal communication). In two patients seen during the Second World War who were accidentally given 1.5 and 2 litres of distilled water by rapid i.v. injection, rigors, haemoglobinuria and persistent hypotension developed and both patients became oliguric and died.

Despite the evidence that the i.v. injection of large amounts of water is dangerous in humans, very large amounts were given i.v. to rabbits by Bayliss (1920) without producing ill effects.

Insufficiently deglycerolized red cells

The transfusion of red cells which have been stored with glycerol may be followed by haemoglobinuria, due presumably to the osmotic lysis of cells from which glycerol has not been completely enough removed (Bechdolt *et al.* 1986).

Transfusion of lysed blood

If enough free Hb is injected into the circulation the resultant haemoglobinaemia may be misinterpreted as a sign of intravascular haemolysis. Appreciable quantities of free Hb may be injected in any of the following circumstances.

Transfusion of overheated blood

Blood haemolyses if warmed to a temperature of 50°C or more. Accidents occasionally happen when a bottle of blood is placed in a vessel containing hot water with the intention of warming the blood to body temperature.

In a patient observed by J. Wallace (personal communication), the transfusion of 5 units blood which had been accidentally overheated, and thus lysed, was associated with irreversible renal failure and death of the patient.

As discussed in Chapter 15, blood should not be warmed before transfusion except in special circumstances and using methods in which the temperature is carefully monitored.

Landois (1875) showed that red cells were irreversibly damaged by being heated to approximately 50°C. Harris *et al.* (1957) heated ^{51}Cr-labelled red cells to 49.6°C for 15 min and reinjected them into the circulation. Surface counting showed a progressive rise in radioactivity over the spleen reaching a plateau at 60 min. On the following day only 10% of the injected cells were still present in the circulation. The rate of removal from the circulation of red cells previously heated to 50°C is illustrated in Fig. 11.2; although there was no haemoglobinaemia following the injection of the washed, labelled red cells, there would of course be gross haemoglobinaemia following the transfusion of whole lysed blood.

Heating red cells to 46°C for 10 min was found to produce no change in cellular deformability but at 47°C and higher there were progressive changes, and after heating at 50°C the cells became undeformable (Mohandas *et al.* 1978).

Transfusion of blood lysed by accidental freezing

Blood may be accidentally frozen, either by being stored in a refrigerator in which the

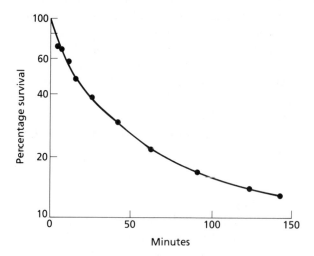

Figure 11.2   Rate of removal from the circulation of red cells damaged by being heated. One millilitre of red cells was taken from a normal subject and labelled with ^{51}Cr. The suspension was then placed in a water-bath at 50°C for 20 min. The red cells were washed three times and the suspension was then reinjected into the donor's circulation. Destruction of the damaged cells appeared to be entirely extravascular (predominantly splenic) and the amount of radioactivity in the plasma never exceeded a level corresponding to 0.5% of the total dose injected (from Mollison, 1961b).

temperature is not properly controlled, or by being placed in a freezer. Oliguria after the transfusion of accidentally frozen blood has been recorded.

Three units of autologous blood, donated 2–4 weeks previously, which had been accidentally frozen at $-20°C$, were transfused during hip surgery. Six hours after surgery, the urine was noticed to be dark red and oliguria developed; there were no signs of shock. The patient required repeated haemodialysis but recovered (Lanore et al. 1989).

Transfusion of infected blood

Blood which is contaminated with certain bacteria becomes grossly haemolysed. The transfusion of such blood may produce haemoglobinuria but this sign is likely to pale into insignificance compared with the very toxic effects of bacteria (see Chapter 16).

Blood haemolysed by being forced through a narrow orifice

It is easy to demonstrate that if blood is pushed with considerable force through a fine needle some of the red cells are lysed. The forcing of blood through narrow openings has been incriminated as the cause of lysis in several different circumstances.

Haemoglobinuria was observed in an infant aged 1 month, 1 h after it had been given a scalp vein transfusion. Fifty-five millilitres of a partially packed suspension of red cells had been injected through a fine needle and it had been noted that considerable pressure was needed to inject the blood. It was shown that, when stored blood was injected through a needle similar to the one which had been used for transfusion, there was very substantial lysis when the rate of injection exceeded about 0.3 ml/s (Macdonald and Berg, 1959).

Haemoglobinuria was noted in a donor who was undergoing thrombapheresis on a continuous flow centrifuge and was believed to be due to the passage of blood through a partially obstructed tube (Howard and Perkins, 1976).

After the unexpected death of several infants following intra-uterine transfusion it was realized that all these cases had occurred since changing to a type of catheter with a much smaller side opening. It was demonstrated that when red cells were injected through the new type of catheter very substantial lysis occurred (Bowman and Pollock, 1980).

Clearance of haemoglobin from the plasma (Fig. 11.3)

Haemoglobin liberated into the plasma dissociates into dimers which bind to Hp. Unbound Hb is partly taken up by the liver and partly excreted (as dimers) in the urine. Free Hb is readily oxidized in the plasma to metHb; after dissociation from globin, haem binds preferentially to haemopexin. The globin split off from Hb is bound by Hp.

Haptoglobin. The plasma normally contains a protein, Hp, which can bind about 1.0 g Hb per litre of plasma. Therefore, when amounts of Hb not exceeding this level are injected or liberated into the blood stream, the Hb circulates as a complex with Hp.

The mol. wt. of Hp varies according to phenotype, being about 100 000 for Hp 1-1 and about 220 000 for Hp 2-1 (Giblett, 1969). Molecules of Hp tend to bind with

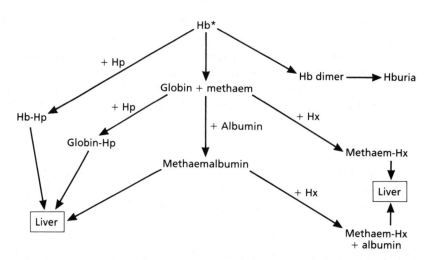

Figure 11.3   Fate of haemoglobin (Hb) liberated into the plasma. OxyHb is rapidly converted to metHb. Hb binds to haptoglobin (Hp) which also binds globin freed by the dissociation of Hb. Hb–Hp and globin–Hp are taken up by the liver. Hb which is not bound to Hp dissociates into half-molecules which pass through the glomerulus and are excreted in the urine. Methaem forms a complex with haemopexin (Hx) which is removed by the liver. When the binding capacity of Hx is exceeded, methaem binds to albumin to form methaemalbumin which is also taken up by the liver.
 * In the absence of free Hp, Hb is taken up directly by the liver.

dimers of Hb rather than with whole molecules (tetramers) of Hb to give a complex of mol. wt. (for Hp 1-1) of 135 000; when whole Hb molecules are bound, the complex has a mol. wt. (for Hp 1-1) of 169 000.

The complex Hb–Hp is taken up by hepatic parenchymal cells (Hershko *et al.* 1972). When the amount of Hb liberated into the plasma corresponds to only a few grams per litre, the Hb (complexed with Hp) is cleared exponentially with a half-time of the order of 20 min (Garby and Noyes, 1959), but at higher Hb levels the clearance system is saturated and a constant amount of approximately 0.13 g Hb per litre plasma is cleared per hour (Laurell and Nyman, 1957; Faulstick *et al.* 1962).

In nephrectomized rabbits, Hb is more rapidly cleared by the liver than are Hb–Hp complexes (Murray *et al.* 1961).

After the injection of radio-iodine-labelled Hp, there is a relatively rapid disappearance for 3 d due to equilibration with an extravascular pool; thereafter, about 10–20% of the i.v. pool is catabolized per day (Böttiger and Molin, 1968). The rate of restoration of Hp in normal subjects was studied by Noyes and Garby (1967): after the injection of amounts of Hb calculated to suppress the Hp level to zero, the level rose to 50% of the pre-injection level in 36 h and to 100% in 7–9 d.

Haemopexin (Hx). Methaem derived from circulating free metHb binds preferentially to Hx. Hx also binds haem from methaemalbumin and may provide the primary clearance route for haem complexed in this way (Müller-Eberhard *et al.* 1969).

The Hp level may be reduced even when the Hx level is normal but reduction in Hx is invariably associated with a reduction in Hp. Assuming that one molecule of Hx binds one molecule of haem, $6\,\mu g$ haem per ml are required to deplete the plasma Hx. Accordingly, depletion of Hx reflects a high concentration of haem in the plasma (Müller-Eberhard *et al.* 1970; Hershko *et al.* 1972).

Hx–haem gives a positive Schumm's test; however, since haem binds preferentially to Hx, the latter is rapidly depleted so that in practice a positive Schumm's test is usually due to methaemalbumin (Rosen and Sears, 1969).

Methaemalbumin. Haem (methaem) which is not bound by Hx binds to albumin to form methaemalbumin, a pigment originally described by Fairley (1940; 1941). Apart from acute haemolytic incidents, methaemalbumin is found in the plasma only when the amount of Hp has been reduced to a negligible level, that is, less than 5 mg/dl (Nynam *et al.* 1959). According to Fairley, the rapid i.v. injection of 14 g Hb into an adult will lead to the formation of sufficient methaemalbumin to give a positive Schumm's test, although about three times this amount of pigment must be present before it can be detected spectroscopically. Methaemalbumin can be detected about 5 h after injecting Hb and then remains detectable for 24 h or more (Fairley, 1940).

Haemoglobinuria

Hb liberated into the plasma dissociates into dimers (see Bunn *et al.* 1969a). When the amount of Hb not bound by Hp reaches about 0.25 g/l, some is excreted in the urine. The clearance of Hb by the kidney is only 5% of that of water; that is, the clearance is equivalent to 6 ml plasma per min per 1.73 m^2 of body surface compared with 100 ml plasma per min for inulin (Lathem, 1959). Reabsorption of Hb by the renal tubules was described by Lathem *et al.* (1960) using the technique of 'stop-flow' analysis. Lowenstein *et al.* (1961) induced plasma Hb levels of approximately 1.8 g/l in normal males and estimated that the amount of Hb reabsorbed by the tubules was of the order of 1.4 mg/min, which was about one-third of the amount being filtered by the glomeruli.

The fact that in most subjects haemoglobinuria occurs only when the plasma level exceeds about 1.5 g/l was of course known long before the role of Hp was appreciated; see Ottenberg and Fox (1938), Gilligan *et al.* (1941) and Yuile *et al.* (1949). These earlier investigators also collected useful information about the time taken to clear the plasma of Hb. For example, when the initial plasma Hb concentration was 0.4–0.6 g/l the plasma was cleared in 5 h; when the initial level was 1.0–2.25 g/l the time was 8 h; and when the initial level was 2.8–3.0 g/l the plasma was not cleared for 12 h (Gilligan *et al.* 1941).

After the injection or liberation of relatively large amounts of Hb into the blood stream up to about one-third may be excreted in the urine. Amberson *et al.* (1949) found that in six persons receiving rapid injections of 12–18 g Hb, the average amount excreted was about 18% of the amount injected. In dogs transfused with incompatible blood, in amounts equivalent to the giving of 200–1000 ml to an adult human, the amount of Hb excreted in the urine varied from 10% to 40% of the amount in the transfused red cells (Yuile *et al.* 1949). (The antibody concerned was readily haemolytic *in vitro*.)

Haemosiderinuria. When free Hb is filtered through the glomeruli, some or all of it is reabsorbed by the renal tubules and the iron released is stored as haemosiderin. If this process continues for a long period, iron-laden cells and free haemosiderin are found in the urine; for references see Bothwell and Finch (1962, p. 413). According to Crosby and Dameshek (1951) haemosiderinuria is invariably found in adults whose plasma Hb concentration exceeds 0.25 g/l. Only microscopical amounts are found when the plasma Hb is below 0.20 g/l, but larger amounts are found when the level exceeds 0.50 g/l.

Bilirubinaemia following injections of haemoglobin
The serum bilirubin concentration may rise by about 0.5 mg/dl (1 mg/dl = 17 μmol/l) after an i.v. injection of 14–21 g Hb, the maximum concentration being reached 3–6 h after injection (Fairley, 1940). A similar rise was noted in a subject injected with 16 g in whom the maximum plasma Hb concentration was 3.8 g/l (Gilligan *et al.* 1941).

According to With (1949) each gram of Hb is converted to 40 mg bilirubin. Therefore the catabolism of 16 g Hb should yield 640 mg bilirubin. If this were liberated into the plasma of an adult who was incapable of excreting bilirubin, the plasma bilirubin concentration would rise by about 10 mg/dl (170 μmol/l), assuming that about half the liberated bilirubin diffused rapidly into the extravascular fluid space (Weech *et al.* 1941). In practice the bilirubin is delivered to the circulation over a period of several hours and excretion almost keeps pace with production.

The catabolism of Hb *in vivo* has been studied in the rat (Ostrow *et al.* 1962). Within 30 min of injecting labelled Hb, labelled bilirubin appeared in the bile; the average time for conversion of the Hb to bilirubin was estimated to be about 3 h. When sensitized red cells rather than Hb were injected, the time taken for conversion of Hb to bilirubin was essentially the same. When large amounts of Hb were injected, a significant fraction of the haem moiety appeared to be degraded to derivatives other than bilirubin. (For further data on the catabolism of Hb, see pp. 390 and 523–524.)

EXTRAVASCULAR DESTRUCTION

Red cell destruction by antibodies which are non-lytic, or only slowly lytic, *in vitro*
Many red cell antibodies, e.g. virtually all examples of anti-D and some examples of anti-K and of anti-Fy^a, do not activate complement at all; others activate complement but mainly to the C3b stage, thus producing negligible lysis of red cells incubated with fresh serum *in vitro*; in all these cases, red cell destruction *in vivo* is due to cells of the MPS. Lewis antibodies lyse red cells *in vitro* but do so only slowly and, with possible rare exceptions, also destroy red cells *in vivo* only with the help of macrophages. As explained above, the destruction by macrophages of red cells coated with IgG, with or without C3b, may be accompanied by haemoglobinaemia.

Antibodies that activate complement only to the C3b stage do not produce symptoms and signs associated with the release of 'anaphylatoxins', i.e. C3a and C5a. Although some C3a must be released in these circumstances, presumably the amount is too small to produce significant effects. C5 is activated only when the number of C3 molecules activated is substantial; see Chapter 3.

Haemoglobinaemia and haemoglobinuria accompanying
macrophage-mediated destruction

Anti-D and anti-C. As discussed in Chapter 3, macrophages can lyse IgG-coated red cells by the action of excreted lysozymes.

In many of the earliest described examples of haemolytic transfusion reactions due to Rh D incompatibility, haemoglobinuria was a feature; most of the patients concerned had been transfused many times with Rh-incompatible blood and had relatively potent antibodies (Wiener and Peters, 1940; Wiener, 1941b; Vogel *et al.* 1943). The transfusion of Rh D-positive blood to subjects whose serum contains only weak or moderately potent anti-D does not, as a rule, cause haemoglobinuria.

Haemoglobinuria is occasionally observed in unimmunized D-negative subjects who have been inadvertently transfused with D-positive blood and then treated with anti-D in the hope of suppressing primary Rh D immunization; see below. Haemoglobinuria has been observed in a case in which anti-C was almost certainly the cause of the incompatibility (see p. 490). Several DHTRs characterized by haemoglobinuria, also due to anti-C, have been observed (see p. 527).

Anti-Jk^a and anti-Jk^b. Incompatible transfusions due to anti-Jk^a and anti-Jk^b are sometimes characterized by haemoglobinuria but it is doubtful whether C8–9-mediated destruction plays a substantial role.

In one case, a woman who had been transfused twice previously (4–5 years earlier) received two transfusions at an interval of 9 d. The first of these two produced no obvious ill effects but 30 min after beginning the second, nausea and shivering developed and the patient passed red urine. A further blood transfusion 3 d later produced a similar clinical picture and this time haemoglobinaemia and methaemalbuminaemia were demonstrated. The patient's serum contained a typical complement-binding anti-Jk^a (Kronenberg *et al.* 1958).

In another case, a woman of 60 years who had never been transfused before but had had five pregnancies was transfused with 300 ml blood and developed a severe febrile reaction with haemoglobinuria. The blood had been passed as compatible but on repeating the tests a very weak anti-Jk^a was found; it was best detected by the indirect antiglobulin method with enzyme-treated red cells and using an anti-IgG serum (Degnan and Rosenfield, 1965). The authors referred to the case mentioned in the preceding paragraph and to two similar cases in the French literature, and emphasized that haemolytic reactions due to anti-Jk^a are characterized by difficulty in detecting the antibody and by the occurrence of haemoglobinuria.

Lewis antibodies. Many examples of anti-Le^a and a few examples of anti-Le^b lyse untreated red cells *in vitro* although lysis occurs only slowly. When small amounts of Le(a +) red cells are injected into the circulation of a patient with potent anti-Le^a the cells are normally cleared by the MPS with the liberation of only traces of Hb in the plasma. Haemoglobinuria has been observed after the transfusion of relatively large amounts of Le(a +) red cells, perhaps simply because the amount of Hb released is then greater, or possibly because, due to slow clearance, the cells have time to undergo lysis in the plasma whilst waiting to be cleared by the 'overloaded' MPS.

In a patient W.B. whose serum contained anti-Le^a, capable of causing slow but appreciable lysis of Le(a +) red cells *in vitro*, 2 ml Le(a +) red cells labelled with ^{51}Cr were injected i.v. and found to be cleared with a half-time of approximately 2 min; the maximum amount of ^{51}Cr found in the plasma during the following 40 min was 2% of the total injected as intact red cells. A few weeks previously this same patient had developed haemoglobinuria following the transfusion of 250 ml Le(a +) blood. It seems possible that the haemoglobinuria was due mainly to the fact that clearance of the large volume of Le(a +) red cells was substantially slower so that there was time for intravascular haemolysis to occur. (A second factor may have been the low Hp level in this patient which would have led to haemoglobinuria at relatively low levels of haemoglobinaemia.)

A similar phenomenon was observed during experiments with stored red cells in rabbits by Hughes-Jones and Mollison (1963). The red cells used for the experiments were rendered non-viable by storage at 37°C in trisodium citrate for 24 or 48 h. *In vitro* these red cells showed relatively rapid spontaneous haemolysis (5% per hour). When small numbers of red cells were injected i.v. they were rapidly cleared by the MPS without liberation of Hb into the plasma; but when very large amounts of the red cells were transfused, so that the MPS was overloaded and complete clearance took more than 24 h, gross haemoglobinaemia and haemoglobinuria developed, presumably because the red cells were lysing within the blood stream while waiting their turn to be phagocytosed by the MPS.

Cold alloantibodies. As described in the previous chapter, cold alloantibodies cause red cell destruction only when they are active at 37°C. Since examples active at 37°C are rare and are very likely to be detected in compatibility testing, particularly when the test is read at a temperature somewhat below 37°C, it is not surprising that the literature contains only a single example of an immediate haemolytic reaction due to anti-P$_1$ (Moureau, 1945) and only five due to anti-M (Broman, 1944; Wiener, 1950; Strahl *et al.* 1955) or anti-N (Yoell, 1966; Delmas-Marselet *et al.* 1967). In fact, in four of the six cases just referred to, no crossmatching at all was carried out before transfusion and in one of the remaining two (Strahl *et al.* 1955) only an agglutination test was carried out although subsequent testing showed that the antibody was readily detectable by IAT.

The thermal range of cold alloantibodies occasionally increases after transfusion and in rare cases these antibodies have been the cause of DHTRs (see below).

Destruction of donor's red cells by passively acquired antibodies

Anti-Rh D. There is now substantial experience of the effect of giving anti-D to D-negative subjects who have been accidentally transfused with D-positive red cells and have then been given an injection of anti-D immunoglobulin (or plasma) in an attempt to suppress primary Rh D immunization. As described earlier, during the rapid destruction of D-positive red cells there is some release of free Hb into the plasma but haemoglobinuria is observed only when the antibody is relatively potent. Two examples are as follows.

Following the inadvertent transfusion of about 200 ml D-positive red cells to a D-negative woman, anti-D was given i.v., resulting in the destruction of almost all the D-positive cells within 30 h; the plasma Hb concentration reached a maximum of 1.5 g/l at about 12 h after the onset of the red cell destruction (Eklund and Nevanlinna, 1971).

In a similar case, although the plasma Hb concentration reached only 1.28 g/l, haemoglobinuria developed and lasted for several hours (Mollison, 1979, p. 576).

The patient was a group B,D-negative woman who was found to have chronic malaria during the last trimester of her first pregnancy. After she had been transfused with 2 units B,D-positive blood it was found that she was D-negative and 2000 μg anti-D (preparation of Hoppe et al. 1973) was administered i.v. over a period of about 1 h. Four hours later the patient passed bright red urine and the plasma Hb concentration was 1.28 g/l. Ten hours after the administration of anti-D, plasma Hb was 1.04 g/l, and 24 h after the infusion was 0.56 g/l; haemoglobinuria persisted for about 24 h. There was no detectable interference with renal function. The occurrence of haemoglobinuria despite the relatively low plasma Hb concentration was probably related to the fact that the plasma Hp concentration before transfusion was low (0.4 g/l), due presumably to the chronic malaria. The anti-D immunoglobulin preparation contained IgG anti-B but in view of the fact that a second infusion of 2000 μg anti-D, 24 h after the first, produced no increase in plasma Hb concentration it was thought to be very unlikely that the anti-B had contributed to the haemolytic episode. (Plasma Hb was 0.42 g/l 12 h after the second infusion and 0.02 g/l 24 h later.)

A healthy D-positive infant with a negative DAT was born 24 h after the administration of the anti-D.

Anti-K. Several cases have been reported in which reactions in K-negative subjects have been due to the transfusion, either simultaneously or at an interval of only a few days, of K-positive red cells from one donor and of K-negative blood containing anti-K from a second donor: (1) a patient was transfused uneventfully with a K-positive unit but, following the transfusion of 1 unit K-negative blood 12–24 h later, a severe febrile reaction developed and the patient was found to have a positive DAT. Serum from the K-negative donor was shown to contain anti-K with an indirect antiglobulin titre of 2048 (Zettner and Bove, 1963); (2) a patient developed anuria after being transfused with 3 units blood, two of which were K-positive and a third of which was K-negative with potent anti-K (titre 2000) in the plasma (Franciosi et al. 1967); (3) a patient who was bleeding was transfused with 10 units blood over a period of 24 h; during the transfusion of the tenth unit chills and fever developed. A few hours later, haemoglobinaemia and signs of DIC were detected but thereafter the patient rapidly improved. One of the 10 units of blood was found to be K-positive and another unit contained anti-K with a titre of more than 1000 (Abbott and Hussain, 1970); and (4) a patient with acute leukaemia developed hypotension, malaise and a severe febrile reaction after the transfusion of a unit of granulocytes suspended in 400 ml plasma with an anti-K titre of 128. Investigations showed that transfusions of granulocytes given during the previous 2 d contained about 30 ml K-positive red cells (Morse, 1978).

Destruction of recipient's red cells by passively acquired antibodies

Very few haemolytic transfusion reactions due to the accidental transfusion of plasma containing anti-D seem to have been described. In one case a patient who received 250 ml fresh frozen plasma following coronary bypass surgery developed a haemorrhagic syndrome 6 h later and was found to have a positive DAT; one of the units of fresh frozen plasma contained anti-D with a titre of 1000. The patient developed renal failure and acute hepatic necrosis but eventually recovered (Goldfinger et al. 1979).

In another case, haemoglobinuria was produced by the accidental transfusion of plasma containing anti-D. The patient was a small boy with hypogammaglobulinaemia who was given a transfusion of plasma with the intention of supplying him with antibodies against cytomegalovirus. Unhappily, he was accidentally transfused with plasma from a hyperimmunized D-negative donor whose plasma contained approximately $100\,\mu g$ anti-D/ml. Haemoglobinuria developed but there were no other untoward signs (Mollison, 1982).

In 12 infants the injection of an IgM concentrate, containing about 10% IgM and 90% IgG and intended to counter Gram-negative bacterial infections, produced mild jaundice and a positive DAT. The preparation was found to have an anti-D titre of 1000 (Ballowitz et al. 1981).

Several cases have been reported in which a dose of anti-D immunoglobulin which should have been given to a D-negative mother was in fact given to her D-positive infant. Details of one case are given in Chapter 12.

Febrile reactions associated with the extravascular destruction
of antibody-coated red cells
The removal of relatively large numbers of non-viable (stored) red cells from the circulation is not associated with the production of symptoms or of fever. Chaplin et al. (1956a) reported that after transfusions of red cells which had been stored at $-79\,°C$ in glycerol and then freed from glycerol by repeated washing, no febrile reactions developed even though in some cases as much as 50 ml red cells was removed from the circulation within about 1 h. Similarly Jandl and Tomlinson (1958) found that the injection of 50 ml red cells rendered non-viable by storage at $37\,°C$ for 48 h did not produce chills, although 90% of the red cells were removed from the circulation within 20 min.

In contrast, in subjects whose serum contained incomplete anti-D the injection of 10 ml washed D-positive red cells produced chills and fever developing after about 1 h in four of four cases (Jandl and Kaplan, 1960). A severe reaction, with shivering, has been observed in a volunteer injected with only 1 ml D-sensitized red cells; the cells were almost all cleared within 1 h and the reaction, accompanied by generalized aching, developed about 2 h after the injection of the cells (Mollison, 1967, p. 576). Similarly, in a D-negative subject, observed by H.H. Gunson (personal communication), whose serum contained approximately $40\,\mu g$ anti-D per ml, following the injection of 0.25 ml red cells of the probable genotype *cDE/cDE*, a feeling of malaise and coldness developed 2–3 h after the injection, with slight shivering, together with pain in the back. The same subject had developed similar symptoms on a previous occasion, when his anti-D concentration was only about $10\,\mu g$/ml, following the injection of 0.5 ml of red cells of the probable genotype *CDe/cde*. On the other hand, many other volunteers with anti-D levels of $40\,\mu g$/ml or more had no reactions following the injection of 0.5 ml D-positive red cells. Similarly, no symptoms have been observed in some 30 subjects (excluding the one mentioned above) injected with 0.5–1.0 ml of red cells heavily coated with anti-D (personal observations, PLM).

In view of the fact that the injection of 10 ml washed A or B red cells to subjects whose serum contains anti-A or anti-B produces only a slight rise in temperature

(0.3°C) and no chills (Jandl and Tomlinson, 1958), it has been suggested that the development of severe febrile reactions following red cell destruction by anti-D may be related to splenic sequestration (Jandl and Kaplan, 1960).

Oliguria associated with extravascular destruction

Oliguria is unusual after Rh-incompatible transfusions. In one series it was observed in none of four cases due to anti-D and in only one of six cases due to anti-c (Pineda *et al.* 1978b), and in another series in only two of ten cases due to anti-D (Vogel *et al.* 1943). This latter series was exceptional in that most subjects can be presumed to have had exceptionally potent anti-D following many transfusions of D-incompatible blood, and that as many as seven of ten had haemoglobinuria, although this finding is relatively uncommon after Rh D-incompatible blood. Anuria was not observed in any of the foregoing cases but it occurred in three of ten cases due to anti-K and in one of nine cases due to anti-Jk^a in a Mayo Clinic series (Pineda *et al.* 1978b).

The cause of the renal damage when incompatibility is due to antibodies other than anti-A and anti-B is a matter for speculation. Some of the antibodies concerned activate complement but they are either non-lytic or only weakly lytic *in vitro*, and bring about extravascular destruction *in vivo*. Since, in these cases, there is almost certainly an association between renal failure and haemoglobinuria, it must be supposed that stroma or its products released into the circulation trigger the events that lead to renal damage. It is, of course, true that the patients concerned are often already seriously ill and may have features such as hypotension which contribute to the development of renal failure.

Possible effects of intravascular agglutinates

Pearce (1904) prepared anti-dog red cell agglutinating serum in rabbits and injected this into dogs. Four minutes after injection, the blood contained large clumps of red cells; at autopsy almost the only lesions were in the liver, where necrosis was found round the portal vessels within 24 h of the injection. Davidsohn *et al.* (1963) also produced hepatic infarcts by injecting heteroimmune sera into mice; there was a very poor correlation between the agglutinin titre of the serum injected and the incidence of infarcts, and it was concluded that the cause of the infarcts was uncertain. On the other hand it should be noted that Stalker (1964), in experiments in animals with high mol. wt. dextran, produced focal necrotic lesions in the liver and myocardium presumably due directly to blocking of small blood vessels by clumped red cells. Agglutinated red cells may possibly block pulmonary capillaries (McKay, 1965, p. 202).

Destruction of red cells rendered non-viable by storage

The removal of non-viable red cells from the blood stream is not associated with the liberation of any detectable amount of Hb into the plasma. This conclusion is based on observations with ^{51}Cr-labelled red cells (Jandl and Tomlinson, 1958; see also Fig. 11.4), and on measurement of plasma Hb using a very sensitive method (Cassell and Chaplin, 1961), and applies to red cells stored in the frozen, as well as in the liquid, state (Valeri, 1965a).

After the transfusion of non-viable stored red cells, the serum bilirubin concentra-

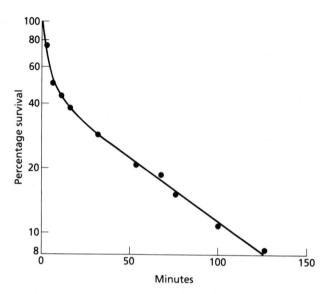

Figure 11.4   Rate of destruction of 'non-viable' stored red cells. A sample of blood was taken from a normal subject and stored at 4°C with trisodium citrate for 2 weeks. The red cells were then washed, labelled with ^{51}Cr, washed again and injected. As the figure shows, the red cells were virtually all removed from the circulation in 2 h. The amount of radioactivity in the plasma never exceeded a level corresponding to 0.2% of the total dose injected.

tion normally reaches a peak about 5 h after transfusion (Mollison and Young, 1942; Vaughan, 1942).

Jaundice is commonly observed in subjects with severe injuries who receive large transfusions of stored blood. In a series of 16 carefully studied cases, hyperbilirubi-naemia reached a maximum about 5 d after the initial transfusion; all the subjects had bilirubin (as well as urobilinogen) in the urine, indicating some interference with liver function. It was suggested that in these circumstances a transfusion of stored blood could be regarded as a test of liver function (Sevitt, 1958; 1959).

Does loading of the mononuclear phagocyte system with non-viable
red cells increase susceptibility to infection?
From experiments in mice, it has been concluded that loading with erythrocytes has some effect on the cells of the MPS which makes them less effective in killing engulfed bacteria (Kaye and Hook, 1963). It is not known whether this finding indicates that the transfusion of large amounts of non-viable red cells is potentially harmful.

DELAYED HAEMOLYTIC TRANSFUSION REACTIONS

When incompatible red cells are transfused, the amount of antibody in the recipient's serum may be too low to bring about rapid red cell destruction or even to be detected, but the transfusion may provoke an anamnestic immune response so that, a few days after transfusion, there is a rapid increase in antibody concentration and rapid destruction of the transfused red cells.

Hédon (1902) was the first to describe a delayed haemolytic transfusion reaction. After finding that whereas rabbit serum agglutinated and lysed red cells from pigs, horses and humans, it had scarcely any effect on dog red cells, he tried the effect of transfusing washed dog red cells to rabbits. After removing 120 ml blood from a rabbit over a period of 1 h he transfused it with 50 ml of a saline suspension of dog red cells. For the next 3 d the rabbit passed urine of a normal colour, but on the fourth day haemoglobinuria developed; on the fifth day the urine was black. On the sixth day the urine was deep yellow and by the eighth day after the transfusion it was once more a normal colour. Hédon noted that on about the fourth day after transfusion the serum of the rabbit became haemolytic and strongly agglutinating for dog red cells. When a second transfusion of dog red cells was given to rabbits there was immediate haemoglobinuria and, if a sufficient amount of red cells was transfused, rapid death.

Virtually all DHTRs are due to secondary responses. Most commonly, the recipient has been immunized by one or more transfusions and, or, pregnancies. Occasional DHTRs are observed following the transfusion of ABO-incompatible blood to a subject who has not been transfused previously, but subjects lacking A or B display typical secondary responses when exposed to these antigens and can be regarded as being always primarily immunized. In theory, a DHTR could be caused by a primary immune response but this event is expected to be extremely rare. The most potent red cell alloantigen (apart from A and B) is D; following the transfusion of D-positive blood to a D-negative recipient, anti-D is seldom detectable before 4 weeks and even then is present in only low concentration. No case of a DHTR due to primary immunization to Rh D has been described but two suggestive cases involving immunization to K:6 and C, respectively, have been reported. In both, the interval between transfusion and the onset of red cell destruction was far longer than in the usual DHTR and, in one case at least, previous immunization was unlikely.

(1) A white woman who had had four pregnancies by her K: – 6 husband, but who had had no earlier transfusions, developed a haemolytic syndrome 23 d after being transfused with 3 units blood, one of which was K:6. (The unit was from a black donor; the frequency of the K:6 phenotype is 19% in Blacks but only 0.1% in Whites). The patient's PCV which, 5 d earlier had been 30%, fell to 25%, her reticulocyte count rose to 16% and her serum bilirubin to 2.1 mg/dl; spherocytosis was present. Her serum was found to contain anti-K6; although the DAT was negative, anti-K6 was eluted from her red cells (Taddie *et al.* 1982).

(2) A woman of probable Rh genotype *cDE/cde* with a husband of probable genotype *CDe/CDe*, who had had no earlier transfusions, was transfused with 12 units blood after her first delivery; 5 d later, her Hb concentration was 10.4 g/dl. Four weeks later she developed haemoglobinuria; her Hb was now 8 g/dl and her DAT was weakly positive, with anti-complement only. After a further 5 d, the Hb was 8.9 g/dl, the reticulocyte count was 17% but the haemoglobinuria had ceased. Eight weeks after delivery, anti-C was detectable in the plasma for the first time (Patten *et al.* 1982). Immunization to C during pregnancy may have played some role in this immune response.

Early descriptions of delayed haemolytic transfusion reactions in humans
The case described by Boorman *et al.* (1946), as a 'delayed blood-transfusion-incompatibility reaction' seems to be the first account of a DHTR in humans. The patient was a young woman with pulmonary tuberculosis and haemolytic anaemia; her group was A_2. She was given a large transfusion of group O blood and between 4 and 7 d after this she received 8 units group A blood, of which at least 7 units were

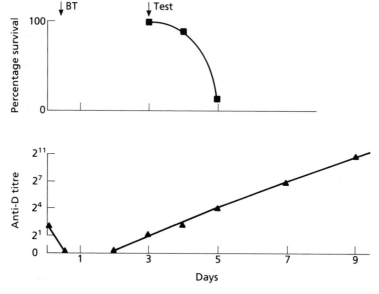

Figure 11.5   Delayed haemolytic reaction due to anti-D. The patient was transfused with 1 unit D-positive blood on day 0 before it was realized that her serum contained a trace of anti-D. There were no signs of red cell destruction and 3 d later when a test dose of 1 ml D-positive red cells was given, only 10% of the cells were destroyed within 24 h. However, between days 4 and 5 almost all the remaining labelled cells and presumably also the transfused red cells were destroyed; the anti-D titre started to increase on day 3 and reached 1000 on day 9 (data from Mollison and Cutbush, 1955).

subsequently shown to be A_1. One week after the last transfusion she became severely jaundiced and anti-A_1, which had not previously been detected in her serum, was now demonstrable (titre 32 at 37°C). It was shown that whereas some 20% of the group O transfused cells were still present in the circulation, there were no surviving A_1 cells.

Other early descriptions of DHTR in humans are as follows: haemoglobinuria developing 8 d after transfusion shown to be due to anti-K (Collins, quoted by Young, 1954); accelerated destruction of Rh D-positive red cells starting on about the fourth day after transfusion (Mollison and Cutbush, 1955; Fig. 11.5); accelerated destruction of group B cells about 5 d after transfusion to a group A subject (R.E. Davies, 1956, quoted by Mollison, 1961b, p. 446); and jaundice and oliguria developing 10 d after the first of a series of transfusions, shown to be due to anti-k (Fudenberg and Allen, 1957).

Clinical features of delayed haemolytic transfusion reaction
The most constant features are fever and a fall in Hb concentration (Pineda *et al.* 1978a). Other features which are often observed are jaundice and haemoglobinuria.

Jaundice
The onset of jaundice is most common on days 5–7 after transfusion (Pinkerton *et al.* 1959; Joseph *et al.* 1964; Stuckey *et al.* 1964; Day *et al.* 1965; Morgan *et al.* 1967; Rauner and Tanaka, 1967). On the other hand, jaundice may occur as late as about

10 d after transfusion (Croucher *et al.* 1967). In nine cases reported by the foregoing authors, where adequate data were given, the mean number of days after transfusion at which jaundice was noted was 6.9.

Haemoglobinuria

It is not uncommon for haemoglobinuria to be observed in patients with DHTRs, and it may occur in association with antibodies with many different specificities, e.g. anti-Jk^a (Rauner and Tanaka, 1967); anti-Jk^b (Kurtides *et al.* 1966; Holland and Wallerstein, 1968); anti-C (or Ce), in five cases described by Pickles *et al.* (1978); anti-c (Roy and Lotto, 1962); anti-c plus anti-M (Croucher *et al.* 1967); anti-U (Meltz *et al.* 1971; Rothman *et al.* 1976); anti-HI, -Jk^b, -S and -Fy^b (Giblett *et al.* 1965); anti-E, -K, -S and -Fy^a (Moncrieff and Thompson, 1975); and anti-c, -E and -Jk^b (Joseph *et al.* 1964). In these 15 cases the mean interval between transfusion and haemoglobinuria was 7.9 d.

The association of anti-C (or -Ce) with haemoglobinuria is very surprising. Apart from the five cases mentioned in the preceding paragraph, in all of which the antibody titre was relatively low, at least three cases have been encountered at the Puget Sound Blood Center, all characterized by intravascular haemolysis associated with anti-C reacting weakly *in vitro* (E.R. Giblett, personal communication, 1981).

Renal failure

DHTRs are only occasionally followed by renal failure. Moreover, when this complication does occur it is usually difficult to know what part, if any, has been played by the transfusion reaction, since the patients concerned often have concomitant failures of other systems. For example, although renal failure occurred in the case reported by Meltz *et al.* (1971), associated with anti-U, no evidence that the renal damage was due to intravascular lysis was presented. In a case reported by Holland and Wallerstein (1968), due to anti-Jk^b, oliguria and uraemia developed about 2 weeks after the transfusion of 3 units Jk (b +) blood; it should be noted that an additional unit of Jk (b +) blood was transfused at about the time of onset of oliguria.

Although renal failure was noted in four of 23 DHTRs reported from the Mayo Clinic by Pineda *et al.* (1978a), all the patients had serious underlying disease; in a later series from the same clinic there was not a single case of renal failure in 37 patients (Moore *et al.* 1980).

Interval between transfusion and the time of maximal red cell destruction

As judged by the day on which jaundice or haemoglobinuria are noted, the maximal rate of red cell destruction seems to occur between about the fourth and 13th day after transfusion, although signs of destruction are commonest on about the seventh day (see above).

In the case illustrated in Fig. 11.5, it was possible to say precisely when the maximum rate of red cell destruction occurred. Following the transfusion of D-positive blood to a subject whose serum was later shown to have contained a trace of Rh D antibody (indirect antiglobulin titre 2) there was no fall in Hb concentration for 3 d, after which time a test dose of 1 ml ^{51}Cr-labelled D-positive red cells was injected; only 10% of the cells were destroyed in the first 24 h, but during the following 24 h, i.e. between 4 and 5 d after the transfusion, virtually all the remainder were destroyed.

An example of destruction occurring even earlier after transfusion is shown in Fig. 11.7. It appears that there was substantial destruction between days 2 and 3 with an increase in the rate of destruction after day 4.

When signs of red cell destruction develop within 24–48 h of transfusion, the explanation seems always to be that the patient has been transfused during the development of a secondary response to a transfusion given some days previously. A case described by Lundberg and McGinniss (1975) of an A_2B patient who developed anti-A_1 is a good example. The patient had been sensitized by an initial transfusion of A_1-positive blood (i.e. A_1 or A_1B) and received a second transfusion of A_1-positive blood 6 weeks later. A third transfusion of A_1-positive blood, given 5 d after the second, was followed within 48 h by signs of red cell destruction, evidently because a secondary response to the second (not the third) transfusion was developing. Anti-A_1, which was not detected in the compatibility test at the time of the second transfusion, was active at 37°C 4 d later.

In one exceptional case signs of red cell destruction developed only about 3 weeks after the transfusion of 6 units given during a splenectomy; anti-Fy^b was detected in the patient's serum. It was suggested that the late onset of red cell destruction might somehow have been associated with the splenectomy (Boyland et al. 1982).

In DHTR, it is usually impossible to find incompatible cells in the recipient's circulation more than about 2 weeks after the transfusion, although in the case illustrated in Fig. 11.6 incompatible cells could still be detected 3 weeks after transfusion.

Occasionally, signs of an IHTR and of a delayed reaction are combined as when the recipient has a relatively low-titre antibody so that there are only very mild signs of red cell destruction at the time of transfusion and further signs of destruction develop a few days later as the antibody reappears in the circulation. An example of such a reaction is shown in Fig. 11.7.

Haematological and serological features
of delayed haemolytic transfusion reactions

Haematological findings
The regular occurrence of anaemia has already been described.

Spherocytosis is often noted in blood films taken from patients during DHTR and may be the first indication that red cell destruction is occurring, as in the following case:

The patient, Mrs N.G., aged 47 years, was group A,D negative; she had never been transfused and because of this and her age, and the fact that it was considered that many units of blood would be needed during arterial surgery, it was decided to transfuse her with D-positive blood. Screening of her serum by IAT and by a test with enzyme-treated red cells failed to reveal the slightest trace of Rh D antibody.

During operation 6 units A,Rh D-positive blood were transfused. Five days after operation she appeared pale and her Hb concentration was found to have fallen slightly; examination of a

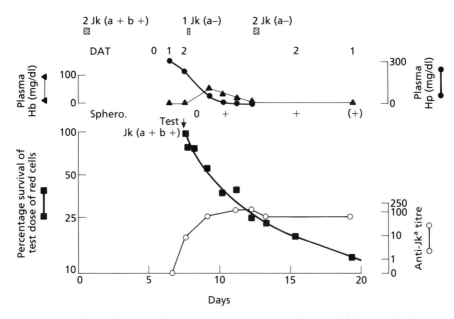

Figure 11.6 Very slow destruction of transfused red cells in a delayed haemolytic transfusion reaction due to anti-Jk^a. The direct antiglobulin test (DAT) became weakly positive 6 d after an uneventful transfusion but no abnormal alloantibodies could be detected in the plasma. In order to investigate this finding a dose of ^{51}Cr-labelled red cells was injected. On the same day anti-Jk^a was detected in the plasma and it became clear that the positive DAT was associated with the fact that Jk (a +) red cells had been transfused. Although the titre of anti-Jk^a rose to 64 on day 9 and to 128 by day 12, the labelled red cells, and presumably the transfused red cells, were eliminated slowly, over a period of 3 weeks after the original transfusion. It may be relevant that the patient's spleen had been removed at the time of the original transfusion and that the antibody was complement-activating. The maximum rate of red cell destruction occurred on about days 8–10 when there was very mild haemoglobinaemia and a fall in plasma haptoglobulin (Hp) (from Mollison and Newlands, 1976). ▨, units of blood transfused; haptoglobulin (Hp) Sphero, spherocytes in blood film.

stained blood film showed the presence of numerous spherocytes intermingled with normal red cells. The DAT was strongly positive and anti-D was found in the serum.

The patient had had two pregnancies, the last of which had occurred 17 years previously; both infants had been regarded as entirely normal.

When large amounts of blood have been transfused, the majority of the red cells in the patient's blood may be involved in a subsequent DHTR, and a picture closely resembling AIHA may result, as in a case described by Croucher *et al.* (1967).

The patient had had two pregnancies and a blood transfusion between 16 and 18 years previously. On the present occasion she had been transfused with 9 units blood in 6 d because of severe bleeding from fibroids. On day 6 she underwent a hysterectomy but, although the bleeding stopped, her Hb concentration continued to fall. From day 7 onwards, and up to about day 20, spherocytes were present in her peripheral blood films. Jaundice was noticed on day 9, beginning to fade on day 13. Her urine contained 'blood' on day 10; on the same day her Hb concentration was found to have fallen to 6.2 g/dl; the reticulocyte count was 13%, the serum bilirubin concentration 4.5 mg/dl and the Hp concentration nil; the DAT was strongly positive. A minor degree of red cell autoagglutination was observed and the serum reacted with

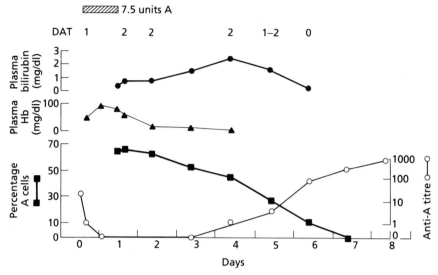

Figure 11.7 Very mild immediate haemolytic reaction combined with a delayed haemolytic reaction following the transfusion of 7.5 units group A blood to a group O subject whose plasma contained a relatively low-titre anti-A (32). The only immediate sign of red cell destruction was transient haemoglobinaemia. During the following 3 d no anti-A could be detected in the plasma although there was appreciable destruction of group A red cells from day 2 onwards and the serum bilirubin concentration reached a peak on day 4. Following the reappearance of anti-A, red cell destruction accelerated and was complete by day 7. Estimates of the survival of group A red cells were made by the differential agglutination/^{51}Cr method described in Appendix 7. As indicated, the direct antiglobulin test (DAT) became negative by day 6. However, the results shown refer to tests with anti-IgG. With anti-C3d the test was still positive on day 11 (Mollison, 1979, p. 579, supplemented by unpublished data).

all 30 samples tested. On the findings, the diagnosis of AIHA seemed possible. However, a sample composed largely of the recipient's own red cells was obtained by differential centrifugation and these cells were found to have a negative DAT and did not react with the patient's own serum; it was now demonstrated that the patient's serum contained the alloantibodies anti-Fy^a, anti-Ce and anti-e.

Serological findings

Positive direct antiglobulin test. Characteristically, the DAT becomes positive a few days after transfusion and remains positive until the incompatible transfused red cells have been eliminated (but see below). By making an eluate from the red cells it may be possible to identify the alloantibody responsible for the reaction at a time when antibody can be detected only with difficulty in the patient's plasma.

Antibody in plasma. It is a typical feature of DHTRs that even when some antibody has been present in the recipient's plasma immediately before transfusion no free antibody is found for a few days after transfusion. Typically, antibody becomes detectable between about 4 and 7 d after transfusion and reaches a peak value between 10 and 15 d after transfusion.

A D-negative patient was transfused with 6 units D-positive blood during arterial surgery because sufficient D-negative blood was not immediately available and because no anti-D had been detected in his serum before transfusion. A routine blood film 5 d after transfusion showed striking microspherocytosis which led to the discovery that the DAT was strongly positive and that there was potent anti-D in the serum. Retesting of the pre-injection sample of serum showed a very low concentration of anti-D, estimated at $0.004\,\mu g/ml$; subsequent estimates were as follows: day 6, $90\,\mu g/ml$; day 9, $500\,\mu g/ml$ and day 12, $460\,\mu g/ml$ (estimates on AutoAnalyzer by W.J. Jenkins; 9 d value checked by ^{125}I-labelled antiglobulin method by N.C. Hughes-Jones). In a case reported by Beard et al. (1971) the anti-D concentration was higher on day 14 ($162\,\mu g/ml$) than on day 8 ($95\,\mu g/ml$).

In some subjects who develop a DHTR it turns out, in retrospect, that the reaction could have been prevented by better pre-transfusion testing. That is to say, detectable alloantibody was present but, either because tests were insufficiently sensitive or were omitted altogether, the presence of the antibody was overlooked. In other subjects, testing of the pre-transfusion sample by all available methods fails to reveal the presence of an antibody.

Examples of the importance of using the most sensitive conditions for antibody detection in preventing DHTR were supplied by Moore et al. (1980). In four cases in which no antibody had been detected pre-transfusion, using two drops of serum to one drop of cell suspension, antibodies (either anti-E or anti-Jk^a) were detected when the ratio of serum to cell suspension was increased to 3 : 1 or 4 : 1.

Similarity of the clinical and serological features of delayed haemolytic transfusion reactions and autoimmune haemolytic anaemia

When a patient abruptly develops signs of increased red cell destruction, such as a falling Hb concentration together with jaundice, and investigation shows a positive DAT together with spherocytosis, a diagnosis of AIHA rather than DHTR may be made (see above). The mistake is serious if it leads to the transfusion of incompatible blood. In a DHTR it may be possible to identify the antibody responsible for the reaction by preparing an eluate from the patient's red cells. In any case, red cells which are compatible with the eluate should be transfused if the patient requires more blood.

Some other serological findings in delayed haemolytic transfusion reactions

Persistent direct antiglobulin reactions following delayed haemolytic transfusion reaction. Some DHTRs are first diagnosed when the recipient requires a further blood transfusion and routine tests show that the DAT is positive, having previously been negative. It is to be expected that, as the amount of the antibody concerned increases in the recipient's plasma, the surviving incompatible red cells will become coated with a sufficient amount of antibody to give a positive DAT and that the test will remain positive until the incompatible cells have been cleared from the circulation. In practice, the situation is more complex than this because the DAT may remain positive after all transfused cells have been cleared from the circulation.

In one series of DHTR, the DAT was found to be positive with anti-C3d 11 d or more after the last transfusion in at least 21 of 26 cases. The DAT often remained positive for at least 3 months. In a minority of cases the red cells reacted with anti-IgG as well as with anti-C3d (Salama and Mueller-Eckhardt, 1984). In another series, mainly of 'DSTR' (see below), the DAT also remained positive for long periods after transfusion, i.e. for at least 25 d in 13 of 15 cases; in this series the red cells reacted with anti-IgG in 12 of 15 cases, with anti-complement as well in five and with anti-complement alone in one (Ness *et al.* 1990). In both the foregoing series, in a minority of cases, alloantibody apparently having the same specificity as that in the serum could be eluted from circulating red cells many weeks after transfusion. These various findings await an explanation.

Development of cold autoagglutinins. As described on pp. 292–293, after repeated transfusions in rabbits, cold autoagglutinins may develop. It seems that, in humans also, potent cold autoagglutinins may sometimes develop in association with allo-immunization.

In a case described by Giblett *et al.* (1965), a boy aged 15 years with thalassaemia major who had received several previous transfusions was again transfused without immediate ill-effect but 7 d later complained of back pain and passed red urine. During the following days the liver enlarged rapidly, his PCV fell precipitously and methaemoglobinaemia was detectable; during a 3-d period his DAT was positive and a potent cold agglutinin of specificity 'pseudo-anti-IH' appeared in his serum. The authors concluded that the episode of red cell destruction was probably not due to this agglutinin but to other antibodies such as anti-S and anti-Fy^b which later became detectable in the patient's plasma.

A rather similar case was encountered by G.N. Smith (personal communication). In a child aged 11 years with thalassaemia major, the transfusion of 2 units blood produced an initially satisfactory response but 6 d after transfusion severe anaemia (Hb 3 g/dl) and jaundice developed. Anti-E, anti-Fy^b and anti-Jk^b were found in the serum together with a potent cold autoagglutinin of a specificity related to H. Although the autoagglutinin was active up to a temperature of about 30°C *in vitro* and was associated with a positive DAT (complement only) it was uncertain whether it contributed to the haemolytic process.

Are the recipient's own red cells destroyed at an accelerated rate in some DHTR?
The finding, referred to above, that following a DHTR the recipient's red cells may develop a positive DAT which persists for at least many weeks does not, of course, imply that the cells are undergoing accelerated destruction. Indeed, it is very difficult to find convincing descriptions of increased destruction of the recipient's red cells during or following a DHTR. Excluding cases in which the recipient had an AIHA preceding transfusion, the only cases in the literature appear to be the following:

In an Rh D-immunized patient who had been transfused on several occasions with D-positive blood, anaemia developed and it was suggested that the patient's own red cells were being destroyed as well as the transfused ones (Wiener, 1941b). The fact that the patient was suffering from a malignant blood disease makes it difficult to draw definite conclusions from this case.

On the other hand, in the case described by Polesky and Bove (1964), there was very good evidence of accelerated destruction of the patient's own red cells following a haemolytic transfusion reaction due to anti-Jk^a. By a fortunate chance the patient's own red cells had been labelled with ^{51}Cr for a red cell survival study and had been shown to be surviving normally for 1 week before the incompatible transfusion was given. After the haemolytic reaction due to anti-Jk^a, there was a very rapid and substantial increase in the rate of destruction of the patient's own red cells. There seems to be a possible analogy here with the syndrome of post-transfusion purpura (Chapter 15).

Frequency of delayed haemolytic transfusion reactions

In three successive series from the Mayo Clinic over the period 1964–80, the frequency with which DHTRs were diagnosed, in relation to the numbers of units of blood transfused, increased as follows: 1964–73, one per 11 650; 1974–7, one per 4000; and 1978–80, one per 1500. The increase was attributed to a number of factors, including the introduction of more sensitive methods of antibody detection and a greater awareness of the syndrome, leading to an increasing tendency to include asymptomatic cases (Taswell *et al.* 1981). This latter point raises the question of the criteria for diagnosis.

The definition of a DHTR is accelerated destruction of transfused red cells after an interval, during which the recipient mounts an immune response to an antigen carried by the transfused cells. The problem is that, whereas it is relatively easy to demonstrate that a 'new' antibody has been produced following transfusion, it may be difficult to diagnose accelerated destruction of transfused red cells. The usual clinical criteria of increased destruction, namely fever and progressive anaemia, sometimes accompanied by jaundice or haemoglobinuria, have been discussed above, but the absence of all of these signs clearly does not exclude relatively minor increases in the rate of destruction. An example of a subclinical DHTR is given in Fig. 11.6.

In one series, 'new' antibodies developed within 30 d of transfusion in one of 151 recipients, but the frequency of signs of a DHTR was one in 854 recipients (Ness *et al.* 1990). These authors suggested that the term 'delayed serological transfusion reaction (DSTR)' should be used for cases in which no signs of increased destruction were found, but this term is not very satisfactory, since the assiduity with which signs of destruction are sought is so variable. The authors themselves relied on retrospective chart reviews. In comparing 127 cases of DHTR with 95 cases of red cell sensitization not associated with overt signs of DHTR, it was found that Kidd and Duffy (but not Rh or Kell) antibodies were significantly more likely to be associated with DHTR than with uncomplicated red cell sensitization (Pineda *et al.* 1987).

In the various series considered so far, the reasons for testing patients after transfusion when they did not exhibit signs suggesting a DHTR were not given, but it seems safe to assume that not every patient who had been transfused was tested for the development of a new antibody in the post-transfusion period. A prospective study in which patients were tested routinely is therefore of substantial interest. The series comprised 530 patients, 183 of whom had been pregnant or had been transfused previously. All were tested 1 week after they had undergone cardiac surgery involving transfusion, most commonly of 2–6 units. Of the 530, 2% developed new antibodies but not one developed a positive DAT or signs of red cell destruction (Hewitt *et al.* 1988). The results of this survey suggest that routine post-transfusion testing would not bring to light many cases which are at present missed. In a series in which no special effort was being made to detect DHTR, the incidence was one per 524 patients transfused (Croucher, 1979).

A high incidence of DHTR was reported in a small series of patients undergoing partial exchange transfusion in sickle cell disease. Of 18 patients, three developed a DHTR (Diamond *et al.* 1980). Similarly, in a series of 107 patients with sickle cell disease who received regular transfusions, 14 developed a DHTR (Vichinsky *et al.* 1990).

Relative frequency with which different alloantibodies are involved

In estimating the relative frequency with which different antibodies are involved, reviews of individual case reports may be misleading since there must be a tendency to report the unusual. Perhaps the best estimates can be obtained by analysing experience from particular centres over a relatively long period. Three such series are available for analysis: (1) Mayo Clinic, 1964–73, 23 cases (Pineda *et al.* 1978a); (2) Mayo Clinic, 1974–7, 37 cases (Moore *et al.* 1980); and (3) Toronto General Hospital, 1974–8, 40 cases (Croucher, 1979).

In each series there were some cases in which more than one alloantibody was found in the patient's serum. In the following analysis the published figures for the number of such cases have been revised slightly as follows: first, when both alloantibodies belonged to the same blood group system, e.g. anti-c and anti-E, the patient has been regarded as having only a single antibody; second, when one of the alloantibodies was known to be a common cause of a DHTR, such as anti-Jk^a, and the second alloantibody was a cold agglutinin such as anti-P_1, which hardly ever causes a DHTR, the case has again been regarded as having only one specificity, i.e. anti-Jk^a in this example. With these minor revisions the figures for the 100 cases were as follows: only one alloantibody found, 90 cases; two alloantibodies found, ten cases; of the cases in which only one antibody was found the specificities of the antibodies were as follows: Rh system, 31 (34.4%); Jk system, 27 (30%); Fy system, 13 (14.4%); Kell system, 12 (13.3%); MNSs system, 4 (4.4%); others, 3 (3.3%). Among the ten cases in which more than one specificity was found, the specificities were as follows: Rh, 8; Kell, 6; Jk, 3; Fy, 2; and S, 1. In Chapter 3 (Table 3.6) these figures are compared with the relative frequencies with which the different red cell alloantibodies are found in random transfusion recipients and in patients who have had haemolytic transfusion reactions.

Further details of the figures given above are as follows: of the 90 cases in which only one antibody was involved, Rh system: anti-D or -D,-E, 3; -c, 5; -c,-E, 6; -E, 12; -C or -C^w, 3; -C,-E, 1; -e, 1; Jk system; 27 (-Jk^a, 24; -Jk^b, 23); Fy system; 13 (all -Fy^a); Kell system; 12 (all anti-K); MNSs system: 4 (-M, 2; -S, 1; -s, 1); anti-A_1, 1; anti-Le^a,-Le^b (see comment below), 1; unidentified, 1.

As expected, anti-D has been involved relatively infrequently, that is when, due to a shortage of D-negative blood, D-positive blood is transfused to a D-negative subject whose plasma lacks detectable anti-D but who has been sensitized in the past either by previous transfusion or previous pregnancy (see pp. 528–529 for an example of the latter).

Antibodies not mentioned in the above list but mentioned earlier in the chapter include anti-A, -B, -k, -Fy^b and -U. Others which have been implicated include anti-ce(f) (O'Reilly *et al.* 1985); anti-N (Ballas *et al.* 1985); anti-Lu^b (see paragraph below); anti-Di^b (Thompson *et al.* 1967); anti-Do^b (Moheng *et al.* 1985) and anti-Co^b (Squires *et al.* 1985).

A DHTR due to anti-Lu^b was described by Greenwalt and Sasaki (1957); jaundice developed 10 d after the transfusion of Lu(b+) blood and the patient's serum was found to contain methaemalbumin. Another case was encountered by M. Metaxas (personal communication). A man who developed severe gastrointestinal bleeding received 19 units blood in 5 d. On day 8 his PCV was 0.47 but 2 d later it started to fall and was 0.22 on day 22. Serum bilirubin concentration reached approximately 20 mg/dl (340 µmol/l) on day 14. On the following day anti-Lu[b] with a titre of 256 was found in his serum. It was uncertain whether a trace of antibody might have been present before this series of transfusions because serological tests had been read only macroscopically. A case in which anti-Lu[b] was present 2 weeks after transfusion (agglutinin titre 2048), but was not detectable before transfusion, was described by Croucher et al. (1962).

Cold alloantibodies have only very rarely been involved, i.e. anti-A$_1$ in five published cases (Boorman et al. 1946; Salmon et al. 1959b; Perkins et al. 1964; Lundberg and McGinniss, 1975; Pineda et al. 1978a); anti-P$_1$ in one (DiNapoli et al. 1977); and anti-M in one (Alperin et al. 1983).

Lewis antibodies were believed to be responsible for a DHTR in the series of Pineda et al. (1978a) but the case was investigated retrospectively 11 d after the last transfusion and there must be some doubt about the diagnosis (see Mollison, 1983, p. 661).

DHTR associated with ABO-incompatible bone marrow transplantation. In the first case to be reported, a patient of group O was prepared for a transplant of bone marrow from a group AB donor by a plasma exchange of 11 litres, which reduced the anti-A and anti-B titres of the plasma to low levels. Four units of group AB cells were then transfused without reaction, followed by the bone marrow. It was estimated that the total volume of AB cells transfused, including those in the transplanted marrow, was 1625 ml. On the sixth day after transplantation the patient became acutely dyspnoeic and was found to have a PCV of 0.18, a positive DAT and hyperbilirubinaemia with extensive agglutination of red cells on a blood smear. Anti-A and anti-B were eluted from circulating red cells. The patient was given group O red cells and corticosteroids and recovered rapidly (Warkentin et al. 1983).

Mortality associated with delayed haemolytic transfusion reactions
When patients die during the period when they are experiencing a DHTR it is usually very difficult to say to what extent the transfusion reaction has contributed to their deaths. For example, in the series of Pineda et al. (1978a) there were three deaths, but the authors commented that there was serious underlying disease in all cases and that the 'haemolytic reaction merely complicated a tempestuous course that was undoubtedly lethal'. On the other hand, cases have been described in which the occurrence of a DHTR appears to have tipped the scale decisively against the patient's recovery. Perhaps the most clear-cut example was a case described by Bove (1968), in which a man aged 32 years was transfused with 10 units during an operation for the repair of a hiatus hernia. His progress was good until the seventh day after operation when chills and fever developed, the PCV fell from about 0.40 to 0.25 and haemoglobinuria was noted. Anti-Fy[b] and anti-Jk[a] were found in the serum and the DAT was strongly positive. The patient became anuric and progressively more anaemic and died 8 d after the onset of the haemolytic syndrome. A rather similar case, though in a man aged 72 years, was described by Hillman (1979). Sudden fever, cyanosis and acute respiratory distress developed on the sixth day after a partial gastrectomy and blood transfusion. There was haemoglobinuria and the DAT was positive. Anti-E and anti-c were found in the serum; the patient developed anuria and died.

Haemolytic syndrome after grafting due to an immune response by lymphocytes in graft

Transplanted organs contain lymphocytes; unless the organ is irradiated before transplantation the lymphocytes may survive in the host, particularly when the host is receiving immunosuppressive treatment, and mount an immune response against host antigens. Haemolytic syndromes have frequently been observed 1–2 weeks after the transplantation of organs from group O donors to recipients of other groups. In the first reported case, 7 d after the transplantation of a lung from a group O donor to a group A recipient, potent anti-A was demonstrated in the recipient's serum. The authors speculated that the agglutinin might have been produced 'by lymphoreticular tissue transplanted with the lung' (Beck et al. 1971). Many examples of haemolytic syndromes developing after grafting, associated with the development of antibodies outside the ABO system, have also been described. The fact that antibodies developing after grafting are alloantibodies (derived from the graft donor) and not autoantibodies has been demonstrated by showing that they are of the same Gm type as the donor (Ahmed et al. 1987; Swanson et al. 1987).

Renal grafts. Many cases have been reported of severe haemolytic syndromes developing following the transplantation of a kidney from a group O donor to a group A or B recipient (e.g. Bird and Wingham, 1980; Contreras et al. 1983b). In reporting three cases, Mangal et al. (1984) stated that a retrospective analysis of their records showed that of four earlier cases in which an unirradiated kidney from a group O donor had been transplanted to a group A or B recipient receiving cyclosporine, three had developed 'pseudo-autoantibodies' (i.e. anti-A or anti-B); no such antibodies had been observed in 21 recipients of irradiated kidneys treated either with azathioprine or cyclosporine. Some detailed studies on two further patients were reported by Bevan et al. (1985).

The production of Rh antibodies by lymphocytes in transplanted kidneys has also been described. In one case, cadaver kidneys from an O,D-negative donor with weak anti-D in the plasma were transplanted to two D-positive subjects; both developed rejection episodes with anti-D in the serum and a positive DAT about 3 weeks later (Ramsey et al. 1986). Similarly, anti-c associated with immune red cell destruction developed in the recipient of a cadaver kidney from a donor whose serum contained anti-c (Herron et al. 1986). In another case of the development of anti-c, the donor was a D-positive subject who had been transfused with 4 units D-positive blood 5–7 d before death and was presumed to have been thereby primarily immunized to c (Hjelle et al. 1988).

In an e-positive patient who developed anti-e following a renal transplant from a living donor (the mother), there was a severe haemolytic anaemia lasting for 4 months (Swanson et al. 1985).

Bone marrow cannot, of course, be irradiated if the graft is to fulfil its desired function, and many haemolytic reactions have been observed in bone marrow-graft recipients due to donor lymphocyte-derived incompatible antibody.

In a series of six cases, five were due to anti-A or anti-B and one to anti-D produced by donor lymphocytes. The maximum rate of red cell destruction was found

9–16 d after grafting. It was noted that although red cell antibody against recipient antigens was frequently produced after giving group O marrow to A or B recipients or D-negative marrow to D-positive recipients, only 10–15% of patients developed clinically significant red cell destruction. In a further retrospective series three of seven D-positive patients receiving D-negative marrow produced donor-derived anti-D. These subjects continued to produce anti-D for periods of up to 1 year after grafting. On the other hand, of 16 patients in whom donor-derived anti-A or anti-B was found, antibody production was only transient (Hows *et al.* 1986). The authors speculated that greater abundance of A and B antigens induced tolerance.

Heart–lung transplants. In nine of 84 cases, the donor was group O and the recipient group A, B or AB; among these nine, six developed anti-A or anti-B or both after transplantation (Hunt *et al.* 1988).

Liver grafts. Following the grafting of ABO-unmatched liver, i.e. donor plasma-ABO-incompatible with the recipient's red cells, anti-A or anti-B (of donor origin) were detected 8–16 d after grafting in eight of 29 (28%) evaluable recipients. IgG was detected on the patient's red cells in most cases and complement in all cases. There was evidence of destruction of the recipient's red cells in five cases, starting 5–8 d after surgery, lasting for 7–19 d and characterized by hyperbilirubinaemia and a substantial fall in PCV (Ramsey *et al.* 1984).

In a larger series the findings were similar: anti-A and anti-B were detected in 22 of 60 cases in which ABO-unmatched liver was transplanted, and a haemolytic syndrome in 13 of 19 evaluable cases (Ramsey *et al.* 1989a).

In one reported case, in which a haemolytic syndrome developed in an A_2 subject following the transplant of a group O liver, red cell destruction was attributed to anti-A_1 (Brecher *et al.* 1989), but a more likely interpretation is that anti-A was responsible and that anti-A_1 was detected because it was not bound strongly by the A_2 red cells (cf. the case reported by Contreras *et al.* 1983b, following a renal transplant).

INVESTIGATION OF HAEMOLYTIC TRANSFUSION REACTIONS

The need to search for signs of blood destruction
Since large amounts of red cells or Hb can be rapidly removed from the circulation without causing either haemoglobinuria or jaundice, the diagnosis of a haemolytic reaction cannot be excluded with certainty without laboratory tests. The following case is a striking example:

The patient was an elderly woman with carcinoma of the stomach who was transfused with a unit of citrated blood (equivalent to 420 ml whole blood). By mistake she was given old blood which was awaiting return to the transfusion centre, instead of the fresh blood which had been selected for her. The unit of blood she received had been stored in a blood bank for 19 d and had then stood at room temperature for a further 4 weeks. The transfusion was completed in less than 3 h. After transfusion the patient developed a temperature of 38.3 °C and a pulse rate of 135/min, and the doctor in charge asked for further investigation. A venous sample taken an hour after transfusion showed the plasma Hb to be 1 g/l. A sample of urine passed an hour after transfusion contained no free Hb. Differential agglutination tests showed that there were no surviving donor cells. Two hours later the degree of haemoglobinaemia had diminished but the serum bilirubin had risen considerably. The patient did not become jaundiced. In summary, this elderly patient eliminated 400 ml blood within 4 h without any overt signs of red cell destruction (Mollison, 1943a, case 10).

Some common difficulties in carrying out the investigation

In maintaining a high standard of safety in blood transfusion, it is of the greatest importance to investigate the cause of every haemolytic transfusion reaction. The difficulties of doing this are two-fold; first, as has just been emphasized, many transfusion reactions which are in fact haemolytic do not produce obvious clinical signs of blood destruction. Sometimes the only hint that a haemolytic reaction has occurred is a small increase in a patient's body temperature. It is a good practice to record the temperature at half-hourly intervals during the transfusion and for 2 h after its end, and to pay attention to any rise observed. This practice is perhaps most helpful when a patient is having a series of transfusions; if it is found that as a rule there is no fever following transfusions, then on any particular occasion when a fever develops, there will be a clear indication to search carefully for a cause.

The second difficulty in investigating haemolytic reactions is the absence of important sources of evidence. For example, by the time it is realized that a haemolytic reaction may have occurred the blood pack may have been discarded. It should be a routine practice to leave a few millilitres of blood in every container after transfusion and to keep the pack in a refrigerator for at least 24 h. It is equally important to take a pre-transfusion sample of blood from every patient. It might appear that a sample of blood could very well be obtained from the patient only when the suspicion of a haemolytic transfusion reaction had been aroused. However, a sample taken before transfusion may help in the investigation in three ways.

First, the patient's full blood groups can be determined. This may be very important in the identification of a blood group antibody present in the serum; e.g. if the patient is found to be Fy (a +), he or she cannot have formed anti-Fy^a. In a sample taken after transfusion there may be large numbers of transfused cells, even though the cells are incompatible, and it may be difficult or impossible to decide the group of the patient's own cells.

Second, the presence of blood group antibodies can be determined with certainty. After the transfusion of incompatible blood, the antibody may all, or almost all, be adsorbed on to the transfused cells. It is true that this implies that, if a further transfusion of incompatible blood is now given, the cells will not be rapidly destroyed, but in a few days' time the amount of antibody in the circulation will usually increase rapidly and all incompatible cells will then be rapidly eliminated.

Third, it may be useful to make comparisons between pre- and post-transfusion values of serum bilirubin, serum Hp, etc.

Methods of investigation

In investigating a haemolytic transfusion reaction the first anxiety is that the wrong blood may have been given; a reasonable first step is therefore to check that the blood given was in fact the blood selected for the patient. If it is found that the wrong blood has been given, it should be remembered that this often implies that the 'right' blood has been given to another patient and this question should be immediately looked into.

Assuming that obviously incompatible blood has not been given, the investigation of a suspected haemolytic transfusion reaction falls conveniently into two parts: (1) obtaining evidence of increased red cell destruction; and (2) identifying the cause of the increased destruction.

Before discussing some of the tests to be applied it may be useful to summarize the more important steps to be taken.

Routine procedure in suspected haemolytic transfusion reactions

As soon as a haemolytic transfusion reaction is suspected the transfusion should be stopped (but the line kept open with saline) and a venous sample taken from the patient. Steps should be taken to secure the residues of all units of blood which have been transfused and any sample of serum or whole blood taken from the patient before transfusion.

Evidence of increased red cell destruction. The post-transfusion blood sample should be centrifuged and the supernatant plasma examined for Hb and for increased bilirubin. When there is sufficient pre-transfusion plasma this may be used as a control. The first sample of urine passed by the patient after transfusion should be obtained and examined for Hb and for urobilinogen.

If the post-transfusion blood sample is taken some hours after transfusion, when the plasma may have been cleared of Hb, it will be worth looking for methaemalbumin (Schumm's test) and estimating plasma Hp.

Identifying the cause. The most important step will be to repeat the crossmatching test. This and other steps to discover a serological cause of a suspected haemolytic transfusion reaction are described in Chapter 8.

When no serological cause can be found, suspicion should fall on the condition of the donor red cells at the time of transfusion (see pp. 513–515).

Some of the tests to be carried out in investigating haemolytic transfusion reactions must now be described more fully.

Visual detection of haemoglobinaemia

In withdrawing blood samples, special precautions must be taken to prevent haemolysis. Probably the commonest cause of haemolysis in blood samples is the drying of small amounts of blood with subsequent liberation of Hb when the dried blood is mixed with the rest of the sample. Therefore, one of the most reliable ways of obtaining an unhaemolysed sample is to take the blood into a syringe which has been rinsed with sterile saline. Other important points are to use a reasonably wide-bored needle and, when the sample has been obtained, to remove the needle from the syringe before ejecting the sample slowly into a suitable container with anticoagulant. The top of the container can be covered with parafilm and the contents mixed gently. It is again important not to allow any blood to dry on the walls of the container. Thus either the container should be filled almost to the top with blood or the container should be centrifuged immediately before any blood can dry on its walls. It is a good practice to examine the part of the container above the level of the blood before centrifugation and to wipe away, with some cotton wool on a stick, any traces of blood. When these precautions are observed, the amount of free Hb in the plasma should not exceed 0.02 or 0.03 g/l.

A sample of plasma which contains about 0.2 g of Hb/l plasma will appear very faintly pink or light brown if examined in a thickness of about 1 cm. Even smaller amounts of Hb can be detected with a small spectroscope. Quantities of Hb of the order of 1 g/l make the plasma appear red.

Estimation of plasma haemoglobin concentration
In the past, methods employing benzidine were widely used, e.g. Crosby and Furth (1956) and Hanks *et al.* (1960), the latter modification being extremely sensitive and giving normal values of less than 0.01 g/l. After it was realized that benzidine is carcinogenic, *o*-tolidine was substituted, but this substance is also carcinogenic. Provided that a high degree of sensitivity is not required, plasma Hb can be satisfactorily estimated by direct spectrophotometry (Cripps, 1968).

Detection of methaemalbuminaemia
When the plasma contains Hb, detectable by naked eye examination, it is usually pointless to look for methaemalbumin. However, if the sample has been obtained 12 h or more after transfusion and the plasma contains only traces of Hb, which might have been produced by careless taking of the sample, it is worth carrying out a spectroscopic examination. The α-band of methaemalbumin lies at 623–624 nm, whilst that of methaemoglobin lies at 630 nm.

When methaemalbumin cannot be detected spectroscopically, Schumm's test, which is much more sensitive, should be used.

Estimation of serum haptoglobin
In theory, estimation of serum Hp concentration should be most useful a day or two after a suspected haemolytic reaction. If any appreciable amount of Hb has been liberated into the plasma it will all have been cleared but the plasma Hp level will be very low.

Hp concentration is most conveniently estimated by the Mancini method, using commercially available plates. If an estimate of the Hb binding capacity of the plasma is wanted, probably the most convenient method is to add an excess of Hb to the sample of plasma concerned and to pass the sample through a Sephadex G-100 column. The Hb and Hb–Hp are eluted in separate peaks so that the Hb-binding capacity of the Hp can be estimated (Lionetti *et al.* 1964; Ratcliffe and Hardwicke, 1964).

In practice the usefulness of Hp estimation is limited by the wide range of normal values, given by Ratcliff and Hardwicke (1964) as 106.8 ± 25.9 for males and 82.7 ± 20.2 for females, expressed as Hb-binding capacity (mg/dl). Because occasional normal individuals have a very low level of plasma Hp, the finding of a low level following a suspected haemolytic episode is of limited value unless by chance the subject's pre-transfusion level has been estimated.

Detection of haemoglobinuria
When relatively low concentrations of oxyhaemoglobin are present in urine the sample

appears red, but when high concentrations are present it may appear black when viewed by ordinary light; the red colour can be seen if the sample is examined against an intense source of light. The presence of Hb can be confirmed by using commercially available chemical tests.

Oxyhaemoglobin in urine may be converted to methaemoglobin; if desired, the two pigments can be distinguished by spectroscopy. The bands of oxyhaemoglobin lie at 578 nm (α) and 540 nm (β) in the yellow and green parts of the spectrum respectively; the α-band of methaemoglobin lies in the red at 630 nm. For the demonstration of this band, the urine must not be alkaline, since the band is not present in alkaline solution.

Detection of hyperbilirubinaemia

Following extravascular destruction, the serum bilirubin concentration increases, reaching a peak not less than 3–6 h after the episode of destruction (see pp. 518 and 524). As mentioned above, when accelerated destruction of transfused red cells is suspected, the patient's plasma should be examined for Hb; if the plasma is not pink, hyperbilirubinaemia should be looked for; it is helpful to compare the colour of the sample with that of one taken before transfusion. If the post-transfusion sample is definitely yellow, the bilirubin concentration should be recorded.

Tests for the survival of transfused red cells

Wiener (1941a,b; 1942a,b) was the first to insist on the importance of tests for red cell survival in demonstrating incompatibility; and he first used the term 'inapparent haemolysis' to describe those cases in which, despite the absence of clinical signs of blood destruction, the red cells leave the circulation at a greatly increased rate.

Differential agglutination. Quantitative estimates can be made if the donor lacks some red cell antigen which is present on the recipient's red cells, e.g. when group O blood has been transfused to a patient of group A, or M – blood has been transfused to a patient who is M +, and when a suitable potent agglutinating serum is available (i.e. anti-A or anti-M in the examples given).

As described in Appendix 7, differential haemolysis after ^{51}Cr-labelling can be used to provide quantitative estimates of the proportion of red cells of different ABO groups in a sample, e.g. A and O. It is thus possible either to estimate the survival of group O cells in an A recipient or of A red cells in a group O recipient; a case in which this method was applied to estimate the survival of a large volume of transfused A blood in an O recipient has been described above (see Fig. 11.7).

Flow cytometry can be used to estimate the survival of transfused red cells when there are antigenic differences between donor and recipient; for examples and brief discussion, see Chapters 9 and 10. Compared with differential agglutination and visual counting of cells, the method is more sensitive and more accurate, but not every laboratory has access to a flow cytometer.

Qualitative or semi-quantitative estimates of survival may be made in three ways: (1) by looking for agglutinates in a sample of blood taken from the recipient; (2) by doing a DAT; or (3) by applying the method of direct differential agglutination (see Appendix 7).

1   Agglutinates may be found in samples of the recipient's blood for a day or two after the transfusion of blood of the wrong ABO group.

Mrs D. was an elderly woman with carcinoma of the lung. Her blood group was O but she was inadvertently given 600 ml group B blood. A sample of urine passed after transfusion was noted to be red but was not tested. The next day, the patient's blood contained a number of group B cells. These were apparent as small clumps visible microscopically in a saline suspension of the patient's blood; the clumps could be increased in size by the addition of anti-B serum. As anticipated, the titre of anti-B in the patient's serum on the day after transfusion was very low (Mollison, 1943, case 4).

2   The DAT on samples taken from the recipient becomes positive when the recipient's serum contains an incomplete blood group antibody and incompatible red cells are present in the circulation. In D-negative patients whose serum contains potent anti-D, circulating D-positive red cells may sometimes be visualized as microspherocytes. Often some of these cells form small clumps — a not unexpected finding since red cells heavily coated with anti-D tend to agglutinate in undiluted serum.

If the circulation contains predominantly donor red cells, virtually all the cells may appear to be agglutinated by an antiglobulin serum and this may suggest that the recipient has developed AIHA (see above). When reticulocytes are present, the recipient's own cells can be separated from transfused cells by centrifugation (see end of Chapter 8).

Occasionally, a positive DAT following transfusion is due to the presence in the donor's plasma of an antibody which is incompatible with the recipient's red cells. For example, the transfusion of potent anti-A plasma to a group A recipient regularly produces a positive DAT (see Chapter 10).

3   Direct differential agglutination has a restricted scope and depends for its success on chance. Thus if the recipient happens to be group N and the transfused red cells happen to be group M, a test with anti-M can be used to discover whether or not any of the transfused cells are still present in the recipient's circulation (see Wiener, 1941a).

Determination of the serological cause of a haemolytic transfusion reaction
See Chapter 8.

Tests when no serological cause can be demonstrated
The supernatant plasma of the unit or units of transfused blood should be inspected for free Hb; if the concentration appears to be higher than expected for the period of storage, an attempt must be made to discover why the blood is haemolysed. The possibility that the blood is infected should be considered and cultures made. In any case, enquiries about the conditions under which the blood was stored and subsequently handled must be made, to determine whether the blood has been frozen or overheated.

CHAPTER 12

HAEMOLYTIC DISEASE OF
THE FETUS AND THE NEWBORN

Definition

Haemolytic disease of the newborn (HDN) is a condition in which the life span of the infant's red cells is shortened by the action of specific antibodies derived from the mother by placental transfer; the disease begins in intra-uterine life and may result in death *in utero*. In liveborn infants, the haemolytic process is maximal at the time of birth and thereafter diminishes as the concentration of maternal antibody in the infant's circulation declines. On the other hand, for reasons explained below, jaundice and anaemia become more severe after birth.

A positive direct antiglobulin test (DAT) in a newborn infant does not establish the diagnosis of haemolytic disease. It is known that D-positive red cells may survive normally in a newborn infant with a positive DAT due to anti-D (Mollison 1951, p. 382) and that many infants with a positive DAT have no signs of increased red cell destruction. In practice it is often difficult to decide whether there is any increased red cell destruction because, in almost all newborn infants, serum bilirubin concentration rises during the first 2–3 d of life (Davidson *et al.* 1941) and there is a progressive fall in Hb concentration, which continues for a period of about 2 months.

Transfer of antibodies from mother to fetus

In humans, the transfer of antibodies from mother to fetus takes place only via the placenta. The only immunoglobulin transferred is IgG, which is bound by an Fc receptor on the plasma membrane of the placenta (van der Meulen *et al.* 1980b). The transfer of IgG is an active process and takes place only from mother to fetus and not in the reverse direction.

In the first 12 weeks of gestation only small amounts of IgG are transferred, although when the mother's serum contains relatively potent anti-D the DAT on the fetal (D-positive) red cells may be positive as early as 6–10 weeks (Mollison, 1951; Chown, 1955). At about the 24th week of pregnancy the mean IgG concentration in the fetus is 1.8 g/l and thereafter rises exponentially until term (Yeung and Hobbs, 1968). At term the IgG level in the infant tends to be higher than in its mother; only slight differences have been found in some series (e.g. Lee *et al.* 1986), but in one the differences in mean values were substantial, viz. infants 15.12 g/l, mothers 12.60 g/l (Kohler and Farr, 1966).

The rate of transfer of IgG from mother to fetus at term is relatively slow (DuPan *et al.* 1959). When labelled IgG was injected into pregnant women at various intervals before delivery, even after 12 d the concentration in the infant's serum was only about 40% of that in the mother's (Gitlin *et al.* 1964). The rate of transfer of anti-Rh D across the placenta may well be the rate-limiting step in the reaction between maternal anti-D and the fetal red cells (Hughes-Jones *et al.* 1971b).

By giving large doses of IgG i.v. to a pregnant woman with hypogammaglobulinaemia throughout the third timester it has proved possible to increase the fetal serum IgG concentration substantially (Hammarström and Smith, 1986). Evidence that large doses of IgG given i.v. to mother or fetus diminish the severity of HDN is discussed later.

IgG subclasses. IgG1 levels begin to rise at an earlier stage of gestation than IgG3 levels (Morell *et al.* 1971; Schur *et al.* 1973). Although fetal to maternal ratios of all four IgG subclasses were found to be similar in cord serum by Morell *et al.*, others have found a relative deficiency of IgG2 (Wang *et al.* 1970; Hay *et al.* 1971). Whereas the relative concentration of IgG1 in fetal serum compared with maternal serum is 1.77, for IgG2 the figure is 0.99 (Einhorn *et al.* 1987). These findings are consistent with the observation that Fc receptors in placental tissue bind IgG1 with higher affinity than IgG2 (McNabb *et al.* 1976).

Persistence of anti-D in the infant after birth. In D-negative infants with passively acquired anti-D, the antibody titre declines with a $t_{1/2}$ of 2–3 weeks; due to the growth of the infant the titre declines a little more rapidly than expected from catabolism alone. As an example, when the titre at the time of birth is 128, the antibody will still be just detectable after 100 d. In D-positive infants not treated by exchange transfusion, the DAT may remain positive for at least 3 months.

IgG red cell alloantibodies causing haemolytic disease

The commonest IgG red cell antibodies in human serum are anti-A and anti-B, although, as described in Chapter 4, relatively high concentrations are found only in group O subjects. Anti-A and anti-B cause a mild haemolytic syndrome in about one in 150 of all births; they seldom cause severe haemolytic disease.

The antibody involved in most cases of moderate or severe haemolytic disease of the fetus is anti-D, and this antibody continues to be the commonest cause of death from haemolytic disease. Nevertheless, its importance relative to that of other alloantibodies has diminished substantially following the introduction of suppressive therapy with anti-D immunoglobulin. For example, the number of deaths registered in England and Wales from haemolytic disease due to anti-D fell from 106 in 1977 to 34 in 1983 (Clarke and Whitfield, 1979; Clarke et al. 1985). The number of deaths from haemolytic disease due to anti-c was the same in each of these 2 years, namely four. Similarly, if one compares the results of antenatal screening tests in periods before and after the introduction of suppressive therapy there has been a substantial change in the frequency with which anti-D is found in relation to anti-c. For example, in one series before the introduction of suppressive therapy the ratio was 74 : 1 (Giblett, 1964) and in one series after the introduction of suppressive therapy it was 10 : 1 (Kornstad, 1983).

Haemolytic disease due to anti-D tends to be more severe than haemolytic disease due to anti-c. Of infants with a positive DAT due to anti-D, about 60% need exchange transfusion, but for anti-c the figure is 30% or less. As a cause of death from haemolytic disease, anti-K is next in importance after anti-c.

The presence of red cell alloantibodies in the serum of pregnant women is often the consequence of a previous transfusion rather than of pregnancy. For example, a history of transfusion is common in pregnant women whose serum contains anti-c, anti-K and anti-Fy^a (Greenwalt et al. 1959; Weinstein and Taylor, 1975; Astrup and Kornstad, 1977; Pepperell et al. 1977).

The list of antibodies which have been claimed to have caused HDN includes virtually every one which can occur as IgG, i.e. in the Rh system: anti-D -c, -C, -C^w, -C^x, -e, -E, -E^w, -ce, -Ce^s, -Rh32, -Go^a, -Be^a, -Evans, -Riv, anti-LW; in the Kell system: anti-K, -k, -Ku, -Kp^a, -Kp^b, -Js^a, -Js^b, -K14 and K24; in the Duffy system: anti-Fy^a and -Fy3; in the Kidd system: anti-Jk^a, -Jk^b and -Jk3; in the MNSs system: anti-M, '-N', -S, -s, -U, -Vw, -Far, -M^v, -Mit, -Mt^a, -Mur, -Hil, -Hut and -En^a; in other systems: -PP$_1$P^k; anti-Lu^a, -Lu^b and -Lu^9; anti-Di^a and -Di^b; anti-Yt^a and -Yt^b; anti-Do^a; anti-Co^a; antibodies to the following low frequency antigens: Wr^a Bi, By, Fr^a, Good, Rd, Re^a Zd; and antibodies to the following high frequency antigens: At^a, Jr^a, Lan and Ge (for references to most of the above see Nossaman, 1981; Vengelen-Tyler, 1984). The only antibodies in the foregoing list which have been associated with moderate or severe haemolytic disease are the following: all the Rh specificities mentioned, anti-K, -Jk^a, -Js^a, -Js^b, -Ku, -Fy^a, -M, -N, -s, -U, -PP$_1$P^k, -Di^b, -Lan, -LW, -Far, -Good, -Wr^a, -Zd (for references see Vengelen-Tyler, 1984).

HAEMOLYTIC DISEASE OF THE FETUS AND NEWBORN DUE TO ANTI-Rh D (Rh D HAEMOLYTIC DISEASE)

In a case described by Levine and Stetson (1939), in which it was first demonstrated that a woman might become immunized to an alloantigen present in the red cells of her fetus, the fetus was stillborn, although the fetal death was not attributed to the antibody (subsequently shown to be anti-Rh D). The role of anti-D in causing HDN was amply documented in the paper of Levine et al. (1941).

Since Rh antigens are present only on red cells, Rh D immunization develops in D-negative subjects only after the i.v. or i.m. injection of D-positive red cells or following transplacental haemorrhage (TPH) from a D-positive fetus.

Rh D immunization due to the deliberate or accidental injection of D-positive red cells into D-negative subjects has been dealt with in Chapter 5. Rh D immunization caused by (TPH) must now be considered.

Immunization by pregnancy; transplacental haemorrhage

TPH from the fetus into the mother's circulation was first clearly demonstrated by Chown (1954) when he investigated a case in which a newborn infant had an Hb concentration of only 7.8 g/dl; 5–10% of the red cells in the mother's circulation were of the infant's blood group. Chown estimated that the fetus had lost 200–300 ml blood, probably over a period of weeks. Within 3 weeks of delivery more than half the D-positive cells had been removed from the mother's circulation and a trace of anti-D was already detectable.

In a similar case described by Gunson (1957) a newborn infant was found to have an Hb concentration of 9.5 g/dl; 3.6% of the red cells in the mother's circulation were of the fetal group. By the end of 2–3 months all the fetal red cells, which were D-positive, had been cleared from the mother's circulation and anti-D was detectable.

Cases such as the two just described, in which very substantial numbers of fetal red cells are present in the mother's circulation, are rare. The fact that small numbers of fetal red cells very frequently cross the placenta was recognized only after the introduction of the 'acid-elution' method of differential staining which permits the detection of very small numbers of fetal red cells in the mother's circulation.

Detection of fetal red cells by the acid-elution method

In this method, blood films are fixed in alcohol and then treated with an acid buffer (pH 3.3). Adult Hb but not fetal Hb is soluble at this pH so that (after counter-staining) fetal red cells stand out as dark cells in a field of ghosts (Kleihauer et al. 1957; Betke and Kleihauer, 1958; Kleihauer and Betke, 1960). Details are given in Appendix 9.

In interpreting results obtained with the acid-elution method the presence of an increased percentage of adult red cells containing fetal Hb (F cells) may cause difficulty. First, amongst the normal population, adults of both sexes may have some form of hereditary persistence of fetal Hb (HPFH), most commonly the so-called Swiss type (heterocellular) HPFH; using the acid-elution method, F cells are found in small numbers in 1–2% of normal adults. Second, in about 25% of pregnant women, the level of maternal Hb F rises above the upper limit of normal (0.9%), starting at about 8 weeks, and may reach 7%; the increase may persist until about the 32nd week. When blood films from adults are examined by the acid-elution method there are some cells which stain so darkly as to be indistinguishable from cells of fetal origin and there are many additional cells which give intermediate staining (Pembrey *et al.* 1973).

Using a very sensitive method employing fluorescein-labelled anti-Hb F, some F cells are found in all normal subjects, with an upper limit of 4.4% (Miyoshi *et al.* 1988; Sampietro *et al.* 1992). In a survey of normal adults in Japan, 11% of males and 20% of females had more than 4.4% of F cells, suggesting that the level of F cells in normal adults may be sex-linked (Miyoshi *et al.* 1988). When the immunofluorescence method is used to examine the blood of pregnant women, an increase in F cells is always found in the second trimester; the increase starts at about 16 weeks and is usually maintained until 24–28 weeks (Popat *et al.* 1977).

Quantitation of fetal red cells by the acid-elution method. Various methods have been used to estimate the amount of fetal red cells present in the maternal circulation. The best one is to express the number of fetal red cells present as a proportion of adult cells in the same sample, although in order to deduce the absolute amount of fetal red cells present, various points must be taken into account:

1 That fetal red cells are larger than adult cells so that the volume present will be greater than that indicated by the number present.
2 That not all fetal red cells stain darkly by the acid-elution method.
3 That an arbitrary figure for maternal red cell volume has to be assumed.

Making the following assumptions: (1) that fetal red cells have a volume about 22% larger than adult red cells; (2) that about 92% of fetal red cells stain darkly; (3) that the average red cell volume of a recently delivered woman is 1800 ml, then if the proportion of fetal to adult cells observed is 1 : 2000, the absolute volume of fetal red cells present is estimated to be:

$$\frac{1800}{2000} \times \frac{122}{100} \times \frac{100}{92} \quad \text{or} \quad \frac{2400}{2000} = 1.2 \text{ ml}$$

Thus the simple rule of thumb is (Mollison, 1972b):

volume of fetal red cells (ml) in the mother's circulation

$$= \frac{2400}{\text{no. of adult : no. of fetal red cells in maternal blood}}$$

This formula turns out to give almost exactly the same answer as the one proposed by Kleihauer (1966): TPH (ml blood) × (ratio fetal to adult cells as a percentage) × 50, i.e. taking the above example = 0.05 × 50 = 2.5 ml blood or 1.25 ml red cells. The formula assumes that the maternal blood volume is 5 litres, that all fetal cells stain darkly and that the MCV of fetal cells is the same as that of adult cells.

The method of estimating the size of TPH from the number of darkly staining cells per low-power field has been quite widely used but is very inaccurate. One important source of error is variability in the thickness of blood films; in one survey, the density of adult cells per mm^2 in different laboratories was found to vary from about 1000 to 16 000 (Mollison, 1972b).

If the number of adult red cells in a given area is determined, and the number of darkly stained cells expressed as a proportion of the total number of cells present, accuracy is improved. The accuracy of fetal cell counts in different laboratories was assessed by distributing samples of adult blood to which known amounts of fetal red cells had been added. Laboratories were asked to determine the ratio of fetal to adult red cells present. When the number of fetal red cells present was very small, e.g. corresponding to a ratio of $1 : 10\,000$ adult cells, there was an almost ten-fold difference between the lowest and highest estimates, but when the amount of red cells present corresponded to about $1 : 1000$ or more, equivalent to a TPH of 2 ml or more, and the estimates were interpreted by the method described above, almost all values fell within 50–200% of the correct ones (Mollison, 1972b). A method of making quantitative estimates of the extent of TPH is described in Appendix 9.

A method which should be suitable for the accurate estimation of TPH of 10 ml red cells or more is as follows: a droplet of exactly $1\,\mu l$ of a $1 : 1000$ dilution of maternal blood is allowed to dry on a slide and then stained; all the darkly staining cells are counted and from the number the size of TPH can readily be estimated. The method proved satisfactory with mixtures containing at least 0.5% of fetal blood though very inaccurate for assessing small TPHs (Corsetti *et al.* 1988).

Serological methods of detecting transplacental haemorrhage

Rosetting tests. In looking for small numbers of fetal D-positive red cells in the circulation of an Rh D-negative mother the method is as follows: anti-D is added to a sample of red cells taken from the mother in order to coat any D-positive cells that may be present; the red cells are washed; D-positive 'detector' red cells (enzyme treated) are now added and form rosettes round any D-positive cells present in the original sample. This method was first used by Jones and Silver (1958) to detect small numbers of red cells in the mother's circulation and was used by Helderweirt (1963) to look for maternal D-positive red cells in D-negative infants; as detector cells, papain-treated D-positive cells were found to be better than untreated D-positive cells. A similar method was used by Sebring (1984) in looking for D-positive fetal cells in D-negative mothers. When 15 ml or more of fetal cells were present in the mother's circulation they were detected by rosetting in 99–100% of cases. On the other hand, when the same maternal sample was incubated with anti-D and then tested by the indirect antiglobulin method (IAT) (a technique sometimes referred to as a D^u test) the D-positive cells were missed in 15% of cases. In one version of the rosetting test available as a kit (from Gamma Biologicals), the method is as follows: a sample of maternal red cells is incubated with chemically modified anti-D; after washing, ficin-treated *ccDEE* red cells are added as detector cells and the result is read immediately. True positives due to the presence of D-positive fetal cells may not be distinguishable from results observed when testing a weak D (D^u) blood sample. The acid-elution (Kleihauer–Betke) test should be done to confirm the presence of fetal red cells and to provide a quantitative estimate.

The observations referred to above indicate that D-positive red cells can be detected with near certainty when the ratio of D-positive to D-negative red cells is one or more per 100. Using the same method (mixed agglutination) others have concluded that as few as one in 1000 foreign cells can be detected (Gemke *et al.* 1986).

Solid-phase indirect immunofluorescence. In this method the red cells are attached to wells of microtitre plates pre-treated with poly-L-lysine, followed by treatment with fetal calf serum and washing. The appropriate antibody (anti-A, anti-D, etc.) is added. To prevent quenching of the fluorescent signal by haemoglobin the red cells are lysed using a hypotonic buffer. Fluorescein-labelled antiglobulin serum is added and the preparations examined. Using several different red cell alloantibodies, foreign red cells could be detected when they were present in a ratio as low as one in 4000 (Gemke *et al.* 1986).

Flow cytometry. The fluorescence-activated cell sorter has been used to make quantitative estimates of small numbers of D-positive red cells present in a predominantly D-negative sample. The sample is first treated with anti-D and then with fluorescein-labelled anti-IgG. Although it has been claimed that, with this method, one in 100 000 D-positive cells can be detected (Medearis *et al.* 1984), others have found that, because purely D-negative samples have occasional positively staining cells, the sensitivity of the method is nearer to one in 1000 (N.C. Hughes-Jones, personal communication; personal observations, CPE).

Detection of α-fetoprotein in maternal serum

Alpha-fetoprotein (α-FP) is a glycoprotein of mol. wt. 69 000 which is an analogue of albumin; in the fetus plasma levels are at a maximum of 3–4 mg/ml at about the 13th to 15th week of pregnancy, falling to about 50 μg/l at term. In most pregnant women the plasma level is about 35 ng/ml in the first trimester, rising to a maximum of about 200 ng/ml at the 8th to 9th lunar month of gestation (Seppala and Ruoslahti, 1972; Caballero *et al.* 1977). Since the level of α-FP is so much higher in the fetus than in the mother, changes in maternal serum concentration are potentially a very sensitive index of TPH. On the other hand, since the concentration of α-FP in the maternal serum increases during pregnancy, small changes are impossible to interpret. In a comparison between the acid-elution method and the estimation of α-FP in detecting and quantitating TPH, a few discrepancies were noted (Lachman *et al.* 1977). Some but not all of these discrepancies were due to the fact that measurement of serum α-FP concentration is the more sensitive of the two tests.

Frequency of transplacental haemorrhage

First two trimesters. The increase in Hb F observed in about 25% of women between about the eighth and 32nd weeks of pregnancy complicates the interpretation of counts of fetal cells made by the acid-elution method during this period. Nevertheless, some deductions can be made, particularly when findings in two different types of cases have been compared by the same observer. For example, Liedholm (1971) found that in women who had had ectopic gestations, blood samples taken 3 h or more after laparotomy contained substantially greater numbers of fetal red cells than samples taken from women with normal gestations at the same stage of pregnancy. Incidentally, in the women with ectopic gestations, blood had been found in the abdominal cavity in almost every case.

Jørgensen (1975) compared findings in women who had spontaneous abortions in the first or second trimester with those in women with normal pregnancies at the same stage. Hb F cells were found in 35% of the aborters but in only 13% of normal women. The amount of red cells in the circulation was never more than about 0.05 ml. In women undergoing induced abortions, comparisons of blood samples before and after the operation showed an increase in the number of Hb F cells in 17%. The extent of the haemorrhage was greater than 0.05 ml red cells in 5% and greater than 0.5 ml in 2%.

Third trimester. Most authors have found that the proportion of women in whom fetal red cells can be detected is greater towards the end of pregnancy than in the earlier stages. For example, Cohen *et al.* (1964) found cells almost twice as frequently in the third trimester as in the second and Krevans *et al.* (1964) found fetal cells only rarely in the first and second trimesters, but commonly in the third.

Quantitative estimates have varied widely. Some figures for the frequency with which fetal cells can be identified in the maternal circulation are as follows: at 28–30 weeks, 0.40% and at 30–39 weeks, 1.84% (Bowman and Pollock, 1987); at 28 weeks, 5.8% and at 34 weeks 7.0% (Huchet *et al.* 1988); and in the last trimester, 3.5% (Woodrow and Finn, 1966). As one might expect, the discrepancies arise from the number of women estimated to have very small TPHs, which are difficult to determine with certainty. For TPHs of 2.5 ml or more of red cells the discrepancies were relatively minor, namely at 30–39 weeks, 0.94% (Bowman and Pollock, 1987) and at 34 weeks, 0.5% (Huchet *et al.* 1988).

Amniocentesis. The use of methods, particularly ultrasonography, for localizing the placenta has greatly reduced but has not abolished the risk of causing TPH during amniocentesis. In one retrospective survey covering the period 1981–1984, of almost 1000 women on whom amniocentesis had been performed at 16–18 weeks' gestation for diagnosing genetic disorders, 2.6% had a TPH > 0.1 ml of fetal red cells due, presumably, to placental trauma. In 1.6% of the women the TPH was estimated to be 1 ml or more. In approximately 1200 women having an amniocentesis between 32 and 38 weeks' gestation to assess Rh D haemolytic disease 2.3% had a TPH of > 0.1 ml and 1.8% of > 1 ml (Bowman and Pollock, 1985).

The risk of Rh D immunization following amniocentesis is greater than these figures imply. In one series of D-negative women with D-positive infants, anti-D developed in three of 58 who were not given anti-D, even though no fetal cells had been detected following amniocentesis; of 59 women who were given anti-D Ig after the amniocentesis, not one became immunized (MRC, 1978). Rapid rises in maternal anti-D concentration following amniocentesis were observed in several cases in another series (Grant *et al.* 1983).

Chorionic villus sampling (CVS). This procedure can be carried out as early as 8–11 weeks of gestation for the diagnosis of genetically determined diseases (Modell, 1985) or for determining fetal blood groups (Kanhai *et al.* 1984).

Using a solid-phase microfluorescence technique, fetal red cell antigens could be detected in all of 11 cases in which they carried an antigen (A, B, c or E) not present on the maternal cells (Gemke *et al.* 1986).

In 161 patients undergoing CVS at 7–14 weeks, no fetal red cells could be detected by the acid-elution method. On the other hand, the maternal α-FP level rose significantly in 49%; the chance of an increase was correlated with the number of attempts at biopsy. It was concluded that as few attempts as possible should be made and that in any case, when the mother was D negative, a dose of anti-D Ig should be given (Warren *et al.* 1985).

During normal delivery, TPH is relatively common. In one series in which fetal red cells were detected in the blood of 59 of 200 women immediately after delivery, it was concluded that in 40 of the cases the TPH had occurred during delivery (Woodrow *et al.* 1965).

If the placental blood is allowed to drain freely, immediately after the cord has been tied and the infant separated, the incidence and magnitude of TPH are substantially reduced (Terry, 1970; Ladipo, 1972).

Following normal delivery. In three series, in each of which the blood of between 2000 and 5000 recently delivered women was examined, estimates of the extent of TPH were similar (Fig. 12.1).

In Fig. 12.1 the magnitude of TPH on a logarithmic scale is plotted against cumulative frequency, also on a logarithmic scale. The fact that the data can be reasonably well fitted by a straight line is convenient since it is easy to read off the expected frequency of interpolated values. As the figure shows, about 1% of women have 3.0 ml or more of fetal red cells in their circulation at the time of delivery and 0.3% have 10 ml or more. The latter estimate agrees closely with that of Bartsch (1972)

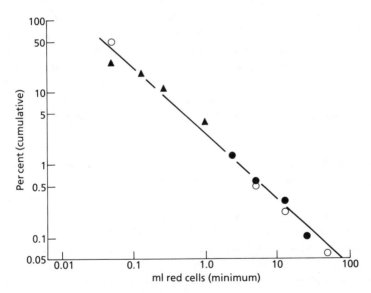

Figure 12.1 Estimates of the extent of transplacental haemorrhage at the time of delivery in three different series: 1 (▲), Woodrow and Donohoe (1968); 2 (○), E. Borst-Eilers (personal communication); 3 (●), Poulain and Huchet (1971).

Only women with ABO-compatible infants were included in the first series; in the other two series, the cases were unselected. Each point indicates the percentage of women found to have *x* ml or more of fetal red cells in their circulation immediately after delivery.

who estimated that 0.2% of recently delivered women had more than about 10 ml fetal red cells in their circulation and it also agrees with data collected by Zipursky (1971), based on about 8000 cases from seven different centres, that about 0.3% of recently delivered women had 15 ml or more of fetal red cells in the circulation.

The data plotted in Fig. 12.1 suggest that the fact that fetal red cells can be detected in the circulation of only about 50% of recently delivered women, using the acid-elution method, is due simply to the relative insensitivity of the method.

Effect of ABO incompatibility. When the fetus is ABO incompatible with the mother, fetal red cells are less frequently detected in her circulation and then only in small numbers.

In two large series, when the fetus was ABO incompatible, fetal red cells were found in 19% and 24.7% of cases, respectively, compared with 50% and 56%, respectively, when the fetus was ABO compatible (Cohen and Zuelzer, 1967; Woodrow and Donohoe, 1968). Moreover, when the fetus was ABO incompatible, the amount of fetal red cells was usually very small, e.g. 0.1 ml or more in only 1.9% of cases when the fetus was ABO incompatible, compared with 18.5% when it was compatible (Woodrow and Donohoe, 1968).

Similarly, in the series of Schneider (1969) 0.05 ml or more of red cells were found in 0.5% of cases when the fetus was ABO incompatible but in 23.1% of cases in which it was ABO compatible.

Caesarean section and manual removal of placenta are associated with a considerable increase in the number of fetal red cells found in the maternal circulation: in one series the incidence of those with fetal cells was 23.5% compared with only 5.2% in mothers who had had a normal labour (Finn *et al.* 1963) and in another series the number of women with more than 0.5 ml fetal blood in the circulation was about 11% after a caesarean section or manual removal of the placenta compared with less than 1% in women with uncomplicated deliveries (Zipursky *et al.* 1963a,b). Similarly, of women who had had a TPH corresponding to 5 ml or more of fetal red cells, 12% had had manual removal of the placenta compared with 1% in controls; incidentally, fetal distress during labour was also significantly more frequent when there was a TPH of 5 ml or more (Li *et al.* 1988).

'Late' entry of fetal red cells into the maternal circulation, via the peritoneal cavity. There seem to be two possible routes by which fetal red cells may reach the mother's peritoneal cavity and thence make their way into her circulation. First, if they are spilled into the uterine cavity, they may pass into the peritoneal cavity by the fallopian tubes. Occasionally this can be observed after vaginal termination of pregnancy, when this is followed immediately by tubal ligation or diathermy. Second, fetal red cells may be spilt into the peritoneal cavity at hysterotomy or caesarean section. In one series of 46 women who underwent caesarean section, fetal cells were not detected in any of the cases at 4 h but were found in six cases at 6 d (Hindemann, 1966).

Massive transplacental haemorrhage

A massive TPH may be arbitrarily defined as one of more than 25 ml red cells (50 ml blood). TPHs of this magnitude occur in approximately one per 1000 pregnancies

(Renaer *et al.* 1976) (see also Fig. 12.1). If the blood volume of an infant at term is taken as 270 ml plus 120 ml in the placental circulation, i.e. 390 ml, a haemorrhage of 50 ml is equivalent to 13% of the circulating blood volume.

The cause of most massive TPHs is unknown, but occasionally the cause can be identified, as when there is maternal trauma, e.g. a fall or a car accident, or when there is a placental chorioangioma (Sims *et al.* 1976) or a uterine choriocarcinoma (Blackburn, 1976). From a review of the literature and from 64 personally observed cases, it was concluded that more than 50% of women with a TPH of 15 ml or more of fetal red cells have no history of any of the risk factors commonly believed to be important, e.g. intrapartum manipulation or placenta praevia. The few risk factors which were associated with large TPHs included premature separation of the placenta, manual removal of the placenta, and fetal death (Sebring and Polesky, 1990).

The fetus may suffer a single haemorrhage, or may be subject to chronic haemorrhage. The two types of haemorrhage may produce different clinical pictures in the infant; in some circumstances the mother may be affected by a massive TPH (see below).

When the fetus is ABO incompatible, a large TPH may be masked. In two cases reported by Cohen and Zuelzer (1967) in which infants were born with Hb concentrations of 3.5 and 6.9 g/dl, respectively, the percentage of fetal red cells demonstrable in the mother's circulation was 0.6% and 1.9%, respectively. Since these infants must have lost amounts of red cells of the order of 100 ml, at least 6% of the cells in the mother's circulation would have been expected to have been of fetal origin if they had survived normally, i.e. had been ABO compatible.

Effect on fetus. Of women who had had a stillbirth, 4.5% were found to have the equivalent of 25 ml or more of fetal red cells in their circulation (Huchet *et al.* 1975). This incidence is far higher than in a random series, leading to the conclusion that some stillbirths are caused by a massive TPH.

When a massive TPH occurs during delivery the infant may be in a condition of oligaemic shock at birth but with a more or less normal Hb concentration since there has been too little time for haemodilution. On the other hand, when there has been chronic severe bleeding the infant may be born with severe anaemia with signs of intense blood regeneration (Huchet *et al.* 1975; Renaer *et al.* 1976; Sims *et al.* 1976); very occasionally, hydrops has been observed (Weisert and Marstrander, 1960; Pai *et al.* 1975; Renaer *et al.* 1976; Debelle *et al.* 1977). Chronic fetal–maternal bleeding may be responsible for iron deficiency anaemia in the fetus (Pearson and Diamond, 1959; Miles *et al.* 1971).

Effect on the mother. When the fetus is ABO incompatible, a large TPH may be associated with haemoglobinuria in the mother. One such episode followed an easy external cephalic version under general anaesthesia. The mother (group O) passed fetal Hb in the urine (0.2 g Hb/dl). Four weeks later a group A infant was born; the placenta showed a small area of separation (Pollock, 1968). In 14 further cases of external version, fetal cells were found in only one, and in this case the mother's blood had not been examined before version. In another case, *abruptio placentae* followed a car accident, following which the mother (group A) gave birth to a stillborn group B infant.

The mother exhibited haemoglobinaemia and haemoglobinuria (Glasser *et al.* 1970). In a case described by Samet and Bowman (1961) the group O mother of a B infant developed haemoglobinuria, acute tubular necrosis and disseminated intravascular coagulation, due presumably to TPH.

The passage of red cells from mother to fetus

The passage of red cells from mother to fetus is far less common than traffic in the reverse direction. Cohen and Zuelzer (1964) used fluorescein-labelled anti-D and anti-B and identified 'a few' maternal cells in the circulation of three of 82 newborn infants. Helderweirt (1963), using the modification of the minor population (rosetting) test described above, detected maternal red cells in 70% of infants, but the total volume of maternal red cells in the infant exceeded 0.01 ml in only two of 92 cases. A very rare case in which a massive materno-fetal haemorrhage was associated with non-immunological hydrops fetalis is described on p. 559.

Frequency of opportunities for Rh D immunization in pregnancy

In about one of every ten pregnancies in Whites, the mother is D negative and the fetus is D positive. The calculation is as follows: 17% of women are D negative; 83% of their partners are D positive and 17% are D negative. Of the 83 D-positive partners, 35 are *DD* and 48 *Dd*. All children born to the homozygous (*DD*) fathers will be D positive but only half those born to the heterozygous (*Dd*) fathers will be D positive. Thus, of every 100 pregnancies, the number in which the fetus is D positive and the mother is D negative will be:

$$17\left(\frac{35}{100} + \frac{0.5 \times 48}{100}\right) = 10$$

An alternative way of calculating this is to say that a D-negative woman can produce a D-positive fetus only if her partner transmits the *D* allele. The frequency of the combination D-negative mother with D-positive fetus is given by: (frequency of the phenotype D negative) × (frequency of the *D* allele), i.e. $0.17 \times 0.59 = 0.10$, or 10%.

When primary Rh D immunization is induced in a first pregnancy, the amount of anti-D produced is almost always too small to produce haemolytic disease in the fetus. In considering the opportunities for producing Rh D haemolytic disease, one must therefore calculate how frequently a D-negative woman gives birth to two D-positive infants. Since family size is often restricted to two children, one may consider how often a D-negative woman has two D-positive infants in succession. When her partner is *DD*, all her infants will be D positive, but when he is *Dd*, the chance that he will pass on *D* twice in succession is only one in four. Thus, of every 100 second pregnancies, the number in which a D-negative woman is carrying her second D-positive infant is given by:

$$17\left(\frac{35}{100} + \frac{0.25 \times 48}{100}\right) = 8$$

In calculating the frequency of opportunities for immunization to Rh D, account must be taken of the fact that primary immunization to Rh D is rare when the fetal red cells are ABO incompatible with the mother's serum, as occurs, in Whites, in about 20% of pregnancies. Thus, the figure of 8 must be multiplied by 0.8 (80%) to give an estimate of the number, i.e. about 6, of second pregnancies in every 100 in which a D-negative mother would be expected to have an infant with Rh D haemolytic disease if: (a) every first pregnancy with an ABO-compatible, D-positive infant induced primary immunization to Rh D; and (b) every subsequent pregnancy with a D-positive infant resulted in haemolytic disease. The frequency of Rh D haemolytic disease in the era before immunoprophylaxis, was about one-sixth of this, i.e. one per 100 second pregnancies. The main reasons why, in five of six cases, in the absence of immunoprophylaxis, the second infant is not affected with haemolytic disease are, first, that the amount of TPH is often too small to induce primary immunization, and, second, that even when the amount is large enough to induce primary immunization in some subjects, in others (non-responders) it is not.

In the preceding paragraph, for convenience, a positive DAT has been regarded as diagnostic of haemolytic disease. As discussed above, some infants with a positive DAT due to maternally derived alloantibody have no signs of increased red cell destruction. However, in practice there is no way of distinguishing in a newborn infant between no increased red cell destruction and a slight increase in red cell destruction and so, in calculating the frequency of the disease, all infants with a positive DAT have to be included.

Primary Rh D immunization caused by pregnancy

Abortion

There is evidence that significant TPH occurs only after curettage and does not occur after either threatened or incomplete spontaneous abortions (Katz, 1969; Matthews and Matthews, 1969; Jørgensen, 1975). In fact, evidence that spontaneous abortion occurring in the first trimester can cause primary Rh D immunization scarcely exists. In one series of women who had not been given anti-D Ig after an abortion occurring in the first 12 weeks of pregnancy and who developed anti-D during the following pregnancy, there were eight in whom the abortion had been spontaneous. In these eight cases, anti-D developed only during the last weeks of the succeeding pregnancy, and immmunization might well have been initiated by TPH occurring during the second pregnancy rather than by the previous abortion (L.A.D. Tovey, personal communication).

Following induced abortion in D-negative primiparae, anti-D was found within the first 3 months of the following pregnancy in 1.5% and by term in 3.1% of the women (Simonovits et al. 1980). A similar frequency was found in another series, in which termination in the second month of pregnancy seemed to carry about the same risk of inducing immunization as termination carried out later (Hočevar and Glonar, 1974). Since 40% of fetuses carried by D-negative women are expected to be D positive, the frequency with which immunization to Rh D occurs following the induced abortion of a D-positive fetus must be higher than 3%. Even after making allowance for the fact that some women must become primarily immunized during the following pregnancy, the overall risk of immunization following the termination of pregnancy in a D-negative woman seems to be at least 4%.

Anti-D present by the end of a first full-term pregnancy

In D-negative women with no history of previous transfusion who are tested at the end of their first pregnancy with a D-positive infant, anti-D is found in approximately 1%, e.g. 0.8%, deduced from the data of Hartmann and Brendemoen (1953); 0.71%, (Eklund, 1973); 0.9%, i.e. 18 in 2000 (Tovey *et al.* 1983). An apparently much higher incidence, namely 62 in 3533, or 1.8%, was reported in a Canadian series (Bowman *et al.* 1978). However, the series included some women who had been pregnant previously and some in whom anti-D was not present at delivery although present 3 d later. If only primiparae are considered and only those in whom anti-D was found by the time of delivery, the figures become 34 in 2767, or 1.2% (excluding one woman in whom anti-D was detected at 11 weeks). The remaining discrepancy between this figure and those (0.7–0.9%) reported by others can be explained by the fact that, in almost one-third of the Canadian cases, the anti-D was detectable only in the AutoAnalyzer or by enzyme methods. If only cases in which the antibody was detectable by IAT are included, the figures become the same as those reported by others.

When anti-D develops during a first pregnancy, it is most commonly first detectable in the last few weeks: in one series, antibody was detected between 36 weeks and term in 50% (Eklund, 1971); in another, antibody was detected in about 40% at 34 weeks, though not at 28 weeks, and in the remaining 60% was found for the first time at delivery, having been undetectable at 34 weeks (Tovey *et al.* 1983). In the Canadian series, among the 34 primiparae (see above), anti-D was first detected by 28 weeks in two, by 34 weeks in three more, between 35 and 40 weeks in 15 more, and immediately after delivery in the remaining 14; antibody was found in a further ten for the first time 3 d after delivery (Bowman *et al.* 1978).

Cases in which anti-D was detected 8 d after delivery, having been undetectable at the time of delivery, were originally reported by Bishop and Krieger (1969) and were also noted by Jørgensen (1975).

The evidence that, in a substantial number of D-negative women, primary immunization to Rh D occurs during pregnancy indicates that anti-D Ig must be given antenatally as well as postnatally if Rh D haemolytic disease is to be prevented in as many cases as possible.

Anti-D first detected 3–6 months after a first pregnancy,
or during or after a subsequent pregnancy

Estimates of the incidence of anti-D in D-negative women 6 months after the birth of a first D-positive, ABO-compatible infant range from 4.3% in 1012 mothers (Eklund and Nevanlinna, 1973) through 7.7% in 337 mothers (Borst-Eilers, 1972) and 8.2% in about 400 mothers (Woodrow, 1970) to 9.0% in 106 mothers (Jørgensen, 1975). When antibody is present at 6 months it can almost always be detected at 3 months (Eklund and Nevanlinna, 1973).

After the birth of a first D-positive infant to a D-negative mother, a relationship can be demonstrated between the number of fetal red cells demonstrable in the mother's circulation at the time of delivery and the chance that anti-D will appear. When no fetal cells are detectable, anti-D is found in only about 3% of cases, whereas when the amount is 0.1 ml or more anti-D is found in about 31% of cases (Woodrow, 1970).

Similar findings were reported by Spensieri *et al.* (1968). In the series of Woodrow (1970) in which 8.2% of D-negative mothers had anti-D in their plasma 6 months after their first pregnancy with a D-positive fetus, by the end of a second pregnancy with a D-positive fetus the frequency of anti-D was 17% (or one in six). The appearance of anti-D in a further 9% of women during the second pregnancy must have been due, in the great majority of cases, to a secondary response during the second pregnancy, so that the conclusion is that, for every woman who develops serologically detectable anti-D following a first pregnancy, there is another who has been primarily immunized but who requires a further stimulus to produce sufficient anti-D to be detectable serologically.

Anti-D developing during or following a second or later pregnancy may of course be due to primary Rh D immunization initiated during that pregnancy. Anti-D detected only during the last few weeks of pregnancy or after the pregnancy is likely to be due to primary immunization occurring during that pregnancy, whereas anti-D detected early in a pregnancy is likely to represent secondary Rh D immunization.

After delivery it is not uncommon for the titre of anti-D to increase, reaching a peak 1–3 weeks postpartum (Boorman *et al.* 1945a).

Fetal factors which may affect Rh D immunization

There is evidence that R_2r infants are more effective in sensitizing their mothers to Rh D than are infants of other phenotypes (Murray, 1957).

There is also evidence which suggests that the D-positive infant which initiates Rh D immunization is more frequently male than female. The sex ratio, M : F, in one series was 1.44 : 1, control 1.05 (Renkonen and Seppälä, 1962), in another was 1.74 (Renkonen and Timonen, 1967), and in another 1.5 (Woodrow, 1970). In one more series, 18 of 21 D-positive infants who initiated Rh D immunization in their mothers were male (Scott, 1976).

Influence of ABO incompatibility on Rh D immunization in pregnancy

The fact that immunization to Rh D during pregnancy is less common when the father is ABO incompatible with the mother was noted by Levine (1943). In a series of matings between D-positive fathers and D-negative mothers who had given birth to infants affected with HDN, 24.7% were ABO incompatible (father's red cells vs. mother's serum) compared with 35% of ABO-incompatible matings expected in the general population. (For a later review, see Levine, 1958.)

It has been estimated that (in Whites) group A incompatibility between infant and mother gave 90% protection and B incompatibility gave 55% protection against Rh D immunization (Murray *et al.* 1965). Evidently, this subject has become far less important since the introduction of immunoprophylaxis. Those interested should consult the papers of Nevanlinna and Vainio (1956) and Nevanlinna (1965). Other references were given by Mollison (1979, p. 338).

Do Rh D-negative infants get immunized by maternal Rh D-positive red cells?

Although it has been claimed that some D-negative infants born to D-positive mothers develop anti-D within the first 6 months of life, the data have never seemed convincing (for references and discussion see Mollison *et al.* 1987, p. 653). Incidentally, tests on the maternal grandmothers of infants with HDN have failed to show any significant excess of D positives amongst them (Booth *et al.* 1953; Owen *et al.* 1954; Ward *et al.* 1957).

Clinical manifestations of Rh D haemolytic disease

Haemolytic disease due to anti-D shows a wide spectrum of severity. In some D-positive infants whose red cells are coated with anti-D, as demonstrated by a positive DAT, there are no signs of red cell destruction. In infants in whom signs of red cell destruction are present, they may be so mild as to be recognized only by the development of mild jaundice on the first day or two of life and a slightly-more-rapid than normal fall in Hb concentration during the first 10 d or so; see Fig. 12.2. (In all newborn infants the Hb concentration falls because red cell production decreases rapidly after birth, and remains depressed until the Hb concentration falls to about 10 g/dl.)

In more severely affected infants, jaundice may develop very rapildy (icterus gravis neonatorum). Unless the infant is treated promptly by exchange transfusion it may develop kernicterus, a syndrome characterized by signs of damage to the brain. Of infants who develop kernicterus, about 70% die between about the second and fifth days of life and are found at autopsy to have yellow staining of the basal ganglia of the brain. Those who survive have permanent cerebral damage, characterized by choreo-athetosis and spasticity; some infants show high-frequency deafness as the only sign.

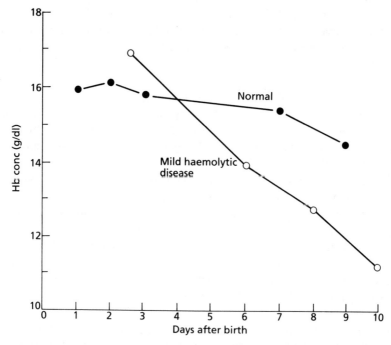

Figure 12.2   Rate of fall of haemoglobin (Hb) concentration in an infant mildly affected with haemolytic disease of the newborn, contrasted with the changes in a normal infant (from Mollison, 1951, p. 385).

There is a close relationship between the peak serum bilirubin concentration and the development of kernicterus. In mature infants, kernicterus seldom, if ever, develops in association with serum bilirubin concentrations of less than 18 mg/dl (306 μmol/l) (Mollison and Cutbush, 1951; 1954), although in premature infants there is some evidence that kernicterus develops at lower bilirubin levels (Ackerman et al. 1970).

In infants with a still more severe haemolytic process, profound anaemia develops and the infants may die in utero at any time from about the 17th week of gestation onwards.

In a series in which blood samples were obtained by fetoscopy at 18–24 weeks from 29 fetuses with severe haemolytic disease there were 14 with Hb values of less than 4 g/dl and ten of these had the syndrome of hydrops fetalis (Nicolaides et al. 1985a). In this syndrome there is ascites and generalized oedema together with gross enlargement of the liver and spleen and, in many cases, of the heart. The oedema has been ascribed to the low serum albumin concentration which is almost always found (Phibbs et al. 1974). The finding of a relatively high concentration of albumin in the ascitic fluid suggests that damage to vascular endothelium, secondary to chronic hypoxia, may be an important feature in lowering the serum albumin concentration (Nicolaides et al. 1985b).

Severe hydrops fetalis is complicated by intravascular coagulation with widespread pulmonary haemorrhage and, in many cases, subarachnoid haemorrhage (Ellis et al. 1979). The outlook for infants with established or threatened hydrops due to haemolytic disease has been dramatically improved by the introduction of intravascular transfusion in utero (see below).

Non-immunological hydrops occurs in about one in 3500 births (Macafee et al. 1970; Hutchinson et al. 1982). The list of causes is very long; among the commonest are cardiac abnormalities, chromosomal abnormalities and the twin-to-twin transfusion syndrome (Holzgreve et al. 1985). A single case has been described of hydrops due to a massive transfer, estimated at 470 ml blood, from the maternal into the fetal circulation (Bowman et al. 1984).

The mortality rate of non-immunological hydrops is over 80% (Holzgreve et al. 1985). The subsequent infant is almost always normal (Macafee et al. 1970).

Before the introduction of immunoprophylaxis with anti-D Ig, more than 80% of cases of fetal hydrops were due to haemolytic disease (Macafee et al. 1970). Now, the percentage is less than 20.

Pattern of haemolytic disease in successive siblings
When anti-D develops during the first pregnancy it can seldom be detected as early as the 28th week and is most commonly first detected during the last few weeks of pregnancy (see above). Moreover, when anti-D does develop during a first pregnancy, the titre of the antibody is usually low. Accordingly, a D-positive infant born following a first pregnancy in a woman who has not previously been immunized to D very seldom shows clinical signs of haemolytic disease, and may simply have a positive DAT. When severe haemolytic disease is observed in a first-born infant it must always be suspected that the mother was immunized before the pregnancy, either by a previous blood transfusion or by a previous abortion.

In the first-affected infant (i.e. in most cases, born to a mother following a second or later pregnancy) haemolytic disease tends to be less severe than in subsequent affected siblings. For example, in first-affected infants the stillbirth rate is 6% (Walker *et al.* 1957) but in second-affected and later infants is about 29% (Mollison, 1979, p. 677). After the second-affected infant there is no tendency for the disease to become progressively more severe (H.R. Nevanlinna, personal communication, 1964; for further details, see previous editions of this book). Accordingly, in women who have had an affected infant the history is very helpful in giving a prognosis for any future infants. For example, the risk of stillbirth in a woman who has previously had a mildly affected infant is of the order of 2%, whereas in a woman who has had one previous stillbirth the risk of a subsequent stillbirth is as high as 70% (Walker *et al.* 1957).

Significance of a previous transfusion to the mother
Although the prognosis for infants of women who have previously been transfused with D-positive blood is not essentially different from that of other affected infants (Nevanlinna, 1953), this generalization does not seem to apply if only first-affected infants are considered (Levine and Walker, 1946; Levine *et al.* 1953; Mollison and Cutbush, 1954). The greater severity of the disease in first-affected infants born to previously transfused mothers is presumably due simply to the fact that a transfusion is a better primary stimulus than a small TPH.

Routine tests to detect Rh D immunization
All so-far-unimmunized women should have their Rh D group determined on at least two occasions: (1) during pregnancy; and (2) at the time of delivery.

Tests for anti-D
The sera of all D-negative women should be tested for anti-D at the time of their first antenatal visit, i.e. at about the 12th week of gestation. In women believed to be pregnant for the first time, anti-D will be found only in occasional subjects, who have either had a previous transfusion of D-positive blood or who have had a previous abortion. In women known to have been pregnant before, the presence of anti-D at 12 weeks will usually be due to failure to administer anti-D immunoglobulin following an earlier pregnancy. In D-negative primiparae, whether or not anti-D is found at 3 months, the serum should be tested again at about 20 weeks. If there is still no detectable anti-D no further tests need be made until 28 weeks when, if there is again no detectable antibody, a dose of anti-D immunoglobulin should be given.

If anti-D is found at 20 weeks but only in low concentration (see below), further tests at monthly intervals will be sufficient. If the antibody concentration increases, tests at shorter intervals will be indicated.

All D-negative women should have their serum tested at the time of delivery so that those who are not already primarily immunized, and whose infants are D positive, may be given an injection of anti-D immunoglobulin. In those women who have become primarily immunized, the infant, if D positive, can be tested for signs of haemolytic disease. The relation between anti-D concentration and the severity of Rh D haemolytic disease is considered below.

Changes in anti-D concentration when the infant is D negative. Significant rises in anti-D titre in women carrying a D-negative fetus were found in four of 239 cases by Hopkins (1970b) and in 13 of 300 by Fraser and Tovey (1976).

Antenatal tests for alloantibodies in D-positive women

When D-positive women form antibodies such as anti-c or anti-E, or alloantibodies outside the Rh system such as anti-K, there may be serious delay in diagnosing haemolytic disease in their infant after birth unless antenatal tests have revealed the presence of the antibody. It is therefore most desirable to screen the serum of all pregnant women for alloantibodies well before term, so that when alloantibody is found there is adequate time for its identification, for testing the father, and for making arrangements for the treatment of the infant, if this should prove to be necessary. Serum should be tested at about 12 weeks and again at 34 weeks. When an antibody is found at 12 weeks, further tests must be made at about monthly intervals, as when anti-D is present.

Even when an antibody is found which reacts only with enzyme-treated red cells, its concentration should be monitored. One example of anti-E which, early in pregnancy, was detectable only with enzyme-treated cells, had an IAT titre of 512 by the end of pregnancy and caused moderately severe HDN (Garner *et al.* 1991).

Antenatal assessment of severity

The severity of haemolytic disease can be assessed most reliably by fetal blood sampling but the procedure carries a small risk to the fetus. Accordingly, various non-invasive methods of assessment are used in the first instance and fetal blood sampling is used only in selected cases.

Estimation of maternal antibody concentration

Estimations of antibody concentration are simple to make and are useful mainly in two ways. First, in distinguishing between mildly affected infants and others. When a very low result is obtained, the infant is very unlikely to be severely affected. Estimations made in the AutoAnalyzer are better correlated with severity than are simple determinations of titre. In one series, in 78 cases in which the anti-D concentration remained below 4 iu/ml (0.8 µg/ml), no infant had a cord Hb below 10 g/dl and only three infants needed an exchange transfusion whereas, of 106 mothers with anti-D levels above 4 iu/ml, 23 infants had cord Hb concentrations below 10 g/dl and 79 infants required exchange transfusion (Bowell *et al.* 1982). The authors suggested that when the mother's anti-D concentration remained below 4 iu/ml, amniocentesis was unnecessary. The other circumstance in which the results of antibody estimates are helpful is when, as a result of testing serial samples, an increase in antibody concentration is observed. In interpreting apparent changes in antibody concentration, it is essential to compare the latest sample with earlier samples by testing the samples together.

Relation between IgG subclass of anti-D and severity

Discrepant results have been reported. In one series in which samples obtained from D-sensitized women at 30–34 weeks of pregnancy were tested, the infant was severely or very severely affected in 24 of 28 cases in which both IgG1 and IgG3 anti-D were present, but in only four of 38 when only IgG1 was present and in only one of six when only IgG3 was present (Zupanska *et al.* 1989). In a second series, severe disease, as judged by the proportion of infants with a cord bilirubin concentration greater than 6 mg/dl (102 μmol/l), was significantly more frequent when the anti-D was IgG1 alone than when it was IgG3 alone or a mixture of IgG1 and IgG3 (Parinaud *et al.* 1985). In the same series, the infant was more likely to have an Hb concentration of < 100 g/l when the anti-D was Gm(1) and Gm(4). In a third series, there was no difference in severity between cases in which IgG1 anti-D alone was present and those in which both IgG1 and IgG3 were found; as in the first series, the disease was always mild in the small number of cases in which only IgG3 anti-D was found (Pollock and Bowman, 1990). It should be noted that when only IgG3 was present the antibody titre never exceeded 4.

Cellular bioassays in the assessment of severity
Bioassays are substantially more cumbersome to perform than estimates of antibody concentration but are expected on theoretical grounds to give better predictions of severity. Monocyte monolayer assays (MMAs), applied to maternal serum, have been found to distinguish between mildly and severely affected infants (Nance *et al.* 1989; Zupanska *et al.* 1989). MMAs were more reliable than amniotic fluid measurements in predicting the need for treatment (Nance *et al.* 1989). In another series, the results of an MMA test were compared with the grade of severity of HDN and the correlations were only fairly good, e.g. 30 cases in which the MMA test gave a low result, 20 infants were moderately affected, and of 11 cases in which a mild result was obtained with the MMA test, five infants were severely or very severely affected; the results of the MMA test gave better predictions than did IAT titres (Zupanska *et al.* 1989).

In a series in which the results of an antibody-dependent, cell-mediated, monocyte-dependent cytotoxicity (ADCC(M)) assay were compared with IAT titres, either at 32 weeks or at term, severe disease was correctly predicted in 75% by ADCC(M) but only in 15% by IAT titre (Engelfriet and Ouwehand, 1990). In a small series in which an ADCC assay with lymphocytes (ADCC(L) assay) was used, of ten women, all of whom had anti-D concentrations of 20 iu/ml or more, three had low assay values and these were the only ones whose infants did not require exchange transfusion (Urbaniak *et al.* 1984).

In a study in which samples were tested 'blind' by several different laboratories, the frequency of correct results with various assays was as follows: ADCC(M), 60%; ADCC(L), 57%; chemiluminescence (CL), 50%; adherence and phagocytosis with peripheral blood monocytes, 41% and with U937 cells or cultured macrophages, 32%. In many cases, maternal samples were taken only some time after delivery which may explain why the frequencies of correct results were not higher (Report from Nine Collaborating Laboratories, 1991). Nevertheless, in the same study, when the infant was too mildly affected to require exchange transfusion, ADCC assays, both with monocytes and with lymphocytes, gave correct predictions in as many as 18 of 20 tests. The frequency of correct predictions was substantially lower when there was moderate or severe disease. In another study, the results of a CL test, an ADCC(M) test, and a test for the number of anti-D molecules bound per cell were all quite well correlated with severity although those of an ADCC(L) test and of a rosetting test with cultured monocytes (U937 cells) were not (Hadley *et al.* 1991).

In one more study, the severity of haemolytic disease *in utero*, as judged by the PCV of a blood sample obtained by cordocentesis, was compared with the results of various tests made on maternal serum. Whereas severity was well correlated with the results of ADCC(M) assays, it was only weakly correlated with anti-D concentration, IgG subclass and the results of a macrophage-binding assay (Garner *et al.* 1992).

False-positive results when the fetus is D negative
A relatively high anti-D concentration and a positive cellular bioassay may be found when the fetus is D negative; for examples, see Urbaniak *et al.* (1984) and Nance *et al.* (1989).

Effect of Fc receptor blocking antibodies on interpretation of antibody assays
In about 4% of second or later pregnancies, the mother forms an antibody which blocks the Fc receptor on fetal monocytes, thus interfering with the binding of IgG-coated red cells to the monocytes and reducing or even preventing the haemolytic process (Ouwehand and Engelfriet, 1990). Fc receptor blocking antibodies were present in seven of 13 cases in which, despite the presence of potent anti-D in the mother's serum (ADCC(M) test giving > 80% lysis), the infant was very mildly affected or unaffected, and were not found in any of 14 infants suffering from severe HDN. In six of seven cases, Fc receptor blocking antibodies had anti-HLA-DR specificity (Dooren *et al.* 1992a).

Amniocentesis in the estimation of severity of haemolytic disease
Estimation of the amount of bile pigment in amniotic fluid is performed by measuring the difference in optical density at 450 nm (OD 450) between the observed density and an extrapolated base line (Fig. 12.3). The optical density of amniotic fluid falls during the last 13 weeks of pregnancy so that the stage of pregnancy has to be taken into account when interpreting the findings. Figure 12.4 shows a chart produced by Liley (1961) to indicate the approximate severity of disease for a particular OD 450 at any stage of pregnancy from 27 weeks onwards.

If the lines in Liley's chart are extrapolated to earlier stages of pregnancy, misleading results are obtained. For example, in one series, if results had been interpreted in this way, ten of 31 severely anaemic fetuses (Hb < 6 g/dl) would not have received an intra-uterine transfusion, whereas many mildly affected fetuses would have been treated unnecessarily (Nicolaides *et al.* 1986).

Examination of the fetus by ultrasonography
Ultrasonography can be used to diagnose hydrops fetalis as indicated by ascites, pleural or pericardial effusions and skin oedema (Bowman, 1983); In fetuses of 18–24 weeks, ascites diagnosed in this way is always associated with Hb levels of less than 4 g/dl (Nicolaides *et al.* 1985a). Repeated examination of the fetus by ultrasonography can detect early signs of cardiac decompensation, i.e. a small pericardial effusion or dilatation of cardiac chambers.

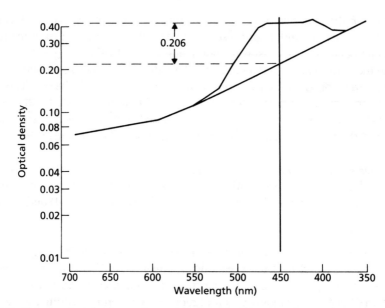

Figure 12.3 Plot of optical density readings of amniotic fluid from an Rh D-immunized woman at the 35th week of pregnancy. The optical density at 450 nm (OD 450) is expressed as the height (in this case 0.206) above the conjectural base line (slightly modified from Bowman and Pollock, 1965).

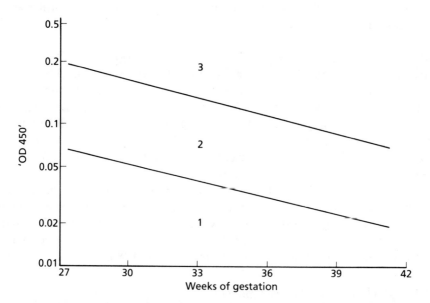

Figure 12.4 Liley's three zones, indicating the approximate severity of haemolytic disease, from readings of the OD 450 of amniotic fluid (see Fig. 12.3) during the last trimester of pregnancy. Zone 1 indicates a mildly affected or unaffected infant, whereas zone 3 indicates a high probability of hydrops and fetal death; the significance of zone 2 is intermediate. In the original paper the chart begins, as here, at 27 weeks 1 day, i.e. at the start of the 28th week of gestation (Liley, 1961). Subsequently, the lines were extrapolated to 20 weeks but then provided a far less reliable guide (see text).

Combined with monitoring of the fetal heart rate, sonographic examination makes conservative management of the fetus possible and helps to avoid unnecessary intervention (Frigoletto *et al.* 1986).

Fetal blood sampling

The preferred method of obtaining blood from the fetus *in utero* is by inserting a needle percutaneously and guiding it by ultrasonographic monitoring into the umbilical vein. In 394 women in whom 606 fetal samplings were carried out by this method before the 24th week, the pregnancy loss rate was 0.8% (Daffos *et al.* 1985).

It is essential to confirm that the sample obtained is of pure fetal blood. A rapid method is to determine the MCV in an automated blood counter; fetal values are 118–135 μ^3. Examination of a blood film stained by the Kleihauer–Betke method (see Appendix 9) is a more accurate method of excluding the presence of maternal red cells but takes substantially longer. Another reliable method is to visualize the streaming of microbubbles in the umbilical vein during the infusion of saline (King and Sacher, 1989).

It is now routine practice to determine the fetal PCV or Hb concentration before intra-uterine transfusion. Figure 12.5 shows the Hb concentration from 17 weeks to term of 106 non-hydropic and 48 hydropic infants with Rh D haemolytic disease. The figure also shows the range of values in 200 normal fetuses and ten cord samples obtained at the time of delivery. As the figure shows, the Hb concentration of normal fetuses was found to increase from 11 g/dl at 17 weeks' gestation to about 13.5 g/dl at 32 weeks and to 15.0 g/dl at term (Nicolaides *et al.* 1988), although this latter value is substantially below the generally accepted value of about 16.5 g/dl for the cord blood of normal mature infants.

A paper giving more details of the 110 fetuses in this series sampled between 15 and 21 weeks gave the following values before 22 weeks: for Hb, between 12.3 and 13.0 Hb g/dl, and for PCV, 0.373–0.393; there was no obvious trend towards higher

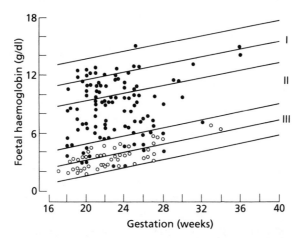

Figure 12.5   Haemoglobin concentrations of 48 hydropic (O) and 106 non-hydropic (●) fetuses with HDN due to anti-D, at the time of taking the first sample from each fetus. Zone I indicates the zone of normal values (the lines mark the mean and limits of ± 2 SD), based on samples from 200 normal fetuses undergoing prenatal tests. Zone III indicates the mean ± 2 SD for hydropic fetuses, and zone II is that of moderate anaemia (from Nicolaides *et al.* 1988).

values during this period although values for six fetuses at 15 weeks were slightly lower (Millar *et al*. 1985). In another series, of 163 fetuses of 18–30 weeks' gestation, Hb increased from 11.47 g/dl at 18–20 weeks to 13.35 g/dl at 26–30 weeks; corresponding figures for PCV were 0.359–0.415 (Forestier *et al*. 1986).

It has been suggested that the severity of haemolytic disease *in utero* should be assessed on the basis of the deviation of the observed Hb from the normal mean for the period of gestation; a deficit of 2 g/dl is diagnosed as mild, of 2–7 g/dl as moderate, and of > 7 g/dl as severe (Nicolaides *et al*. 1988).

Assessment of severity in the newborn infant

Since about 40% of infants born with a positive DAT require no treatment, whereas others need exchange transfusion if they are to be prevented from developing kernicterus, assessment of severity at the earliest possible moment is desirable. As explained below, there is a special advantage in testing cord blood rather than blood obtained from the infant after birth.

The best single criterion of severity of haemolytic disease is the cord Hb concentration, although in practice other criteria are always taken into account. The reason for preferring to test cord blood to blood obtained from the infant after birth is simply that during the few minutes after delivery a variable amount of blood is transferred from the placenta to the infant (Budin, 1875; DeMarsh *et al*. 1942; Yao *et al*. 1969). Accordingly, interpreting Hb values in infants shortly after birth presents just the same difficulties as interpreting the significance of Hb values in any other subject who has recently been transfused with an unknown amount of red cells. The postnatal rise in Hb concentration has the effect of widening the normal range of values. Whereas the normal range (mean ± 2 SD) of Hb values in cord blood is approximately 13.6–19.6 g/dl, the range in samples taken on the first day of life is approximately 14.5–22.5 g/dl (Mollison and Cutbush, 1949a). These figures refer to venous samples. In newborn infants skin prick samples tend to give distinctly higher values (for references see Mollison, 1961b, pp. 579–80). The practical importance of Hb changes in the immediate postnatal period is illustrated in Fig. 12.6. In the case shown, an infant with moderately severe haemolytic disease had a cord Hb concentration of 12.8 g/dl, a value definitely below the lower limit of normal, whereas a sample taken a few hours after birth was within the normal range.

Before the introduction of prophylactic anti-D immunoglobulin to suppress Rh D immunization, almost 50% of affected infants had cord Hb concentrations of 14.5 g/dl or more, 30% had cord Hb values between 10.5 and 14.4 g/dl, and about 20% had Hb values between 3.4 and 10.4 g/dl (Mollison, 1956, p. 464). The probability of survival diminishes as the cord Hb concentration falls (Mollison and Cutbush, 1951; Armitage and Mollison, 1953); there is also a correlation between cord bilirubin concentration and severity, although the relation is less close than that between cord Hb concentration and severity (Mollison and Cutbush, 1949a).

Most infants with a cord Hb concentration within the normal range do not require exchange transfusion; in these infants estimation of cord plasma bilirubin concentration is valuable and a cord level of 4 mg/dl (68 μmol/l) or more (normal range 0.7–3.1 mg/dl (12–53 μmol/l)) may be an indication for exchange transfusion (Walker, 1958).

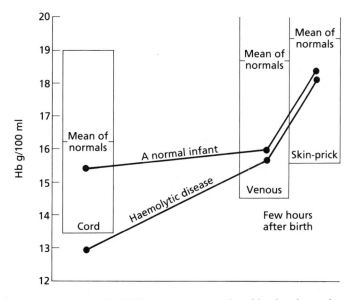

Figure 12.6 Changes in haemoglobin (Hb) concentration produced by the placental transfer of blood tend to mask mild degrees of anaemia in newborn infants. Often the Hb concentration of skin-prick samples is much higher than that of venous samples and this is a second factor which may mask anaemia. In the case illustrated here, an infant with haemolytic disease of the newborn has a cord Hb concentration below the normal range, but after birth its Hb concentration is as high as that of many normal infants (from Mollison and Cutbush, 1949a).

When exchange transfusion is not indicated immediately, serum bilirubin concentration should be estimated every few hours so that if the concentration threatens to rise to a dangerous level exchange transfusion can be carried out in good time.

Estimation of the amount of antibody on red cells of affected infants
In one series, the amount of anti-D on the cord red cells varied from 0.4 to 18.0 μg/ml cells. The amount of antibody on the red cells was not highly correlated with either the infant's cord Hb concentration or the cord serum bilirubin concentration (correlation coefficient about 0.6). All 13 infants with more than 8 μg anti-D per ml red cells required treatment, but even at a level of 2 μg anti-D per ml, six of 14 infants required treatment (Hughes-Jones *et al.* 1967). In cases in which, due to a misunderstanding, a dose of 150–300 μg anti-D has been given to a D-positive infant, instead of to its D-negative mother, only a very mild haemolytic syndrome has as a rule been produced. In one such case the infant's red cells were shown to be coated with approximately 1.5 μg anti-D per ml (Marsh *et al.* 1970; see Fig. 12.7).

Treatment of haemolytic disease of the fetus and newborn

Antenatal

Plasma exchange in the mother. Although at first sight intensive plasma exchange in women immunized to Rh D seems entirely rational and might be expected to lead to a substantial lowering of the concentration of anti-D, to the benefit of the D-positive fetus *in utero*, results of this treatment have in fact been very variable.

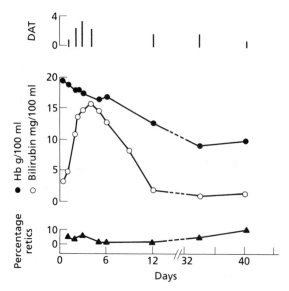

Figure 12.7 Changes in haemoglobin (Hb) concentration (●—●); serum bilirubin concentration
(O—O); reticulocyte count (▲—▲); and direct antiglobulin test (DAT; positive reactions graded from 0
to 4) in a D-positive infant injected, 5 h after birth, with 200 μg anti-D (from Marsh *et al.* 1970).

Some of the best results have been observed following the removal of relatively
small amounts of plasma. For example, the removal of only 250 ml plasma every week
for 20 weeks was shown in eight hyperimmunized male volunteers to decrease
antibody levels to 20% of their initial values in five of the subjects, and it was then
shown that similar results could be obtained in D-immunized pregnant women.
Moreover, among those women in whom antibody levels were reduced to the greatest
extent, most of the infants were liveborn and survived (Rubinstein, 1982).

Favourable results were also observed in a series of D-immunized women, almost
all of whom had had a previous stillbirth. Following weekly plasma exchange of
600 ml, beginning at 10–12 weeks of pregnancy and continuing to term, ten of 18
pregnancies resulted in the birth of an infant, at the 34th week of pregnancy or later,
which survived (experience cited by van't Veer-Korthof *et al.* 1981). Plasma exchange
produced no consistent change in the IgG subclass composition of the anti-D (van't
Veer-Korthof *et al.* 1981).

When larger amounts of plasma are removed, antibody concentrations can sometimes be kept at about 50% of their initial values for periods of at least 3 months
(Robinson and Tovey, 1980), but in other cases antibody levels are reduced only
transiently and then not only rise again but often surpass their initial concentration.

The failure to produce a sustained lowering of antibody levels in humans when large
amounts of plasma are removed is not unexpected in view of the finding that, in rabbits,
exchange transfusion resulting in immediate lowering of antibody concentration by an average of
67% was followed by a 'rebound', resulting in an average doubling of the initial antibody
concentration 8 d after exchange. When the donor plasma contained antibody of the same
specificity as that in the recipient animal, only a small rebound was observed, shown to be due to

redistribution of antibody between the extravascular space and the plasma (Bystryn *et al.* 1970). These results suggest that plasma antibody concentration plays an important part in regulating antibody production.

In some cases in which antibody levels increase following plasma exchange, an antigenic stimulus introduced in the course of treatment can be identified. For example, in the series of Barclay *et al.* (1980), following intensive plasma exchange, titres rose dramatically in two women who were subsequently shown to be carrying D-negative infants. In these cases it seemed that the source of the antigenic stimulus could have been stroma from D-positive red cells present in the fresh-frozen plasma from a D-positive donor used in the plasma exchange. In cases in which the fetus is D positive there is an increased risk that D-positive cells will be introduced into the mother's circulation during diagnostic amniocentesis or therapeutic intra-uterine transfusion.

Although repeated large plasma exchanges cannot be relied upon to maintain antibody concentration at lower-than-initial levels, they do seem to have this effect in some cases. For example, in one series of Rh D-immunized women in whom a mean volume of 3.5 litres plasma was exchanged on average twice a week, the anti-D level was rapidly lowered and maintained at a lower level than previously in 15 of 35 cases. In the remaining 20, the anti-D level remained high despite intensive plasma exchange or was lower only until about the 30th week of pregnancy, after which an uncontrollable rise occurred. The overall survival rate among the 33 D-positive infants was 70% (Robinson, 1984). The difficulty in interpreting these findings lies in the fact that there was no control series, results simply being compared with those obtained in the past before plasma exchange was introduced. Since, in centres where plasma exchange is not practised, the survival rate for severely affected fetuses has improved substantially during the last decade or so, the role played by plasma exchange is very difficult to evaluate. In view of the substantial inconvenience and expense involved, and of the slight risk of fatal overloading of the circulation (Huestis, 1983b), plasma exchange cannot be recommended for routine use. In those few centres with a large experience of intravascular transfusion of the fetus *in utero*, plasma exchange has a very limited application because deaths *in utero* from haemolytic disease are unknown before about 17 weeks, and i.v. transfusion becomes possible as early as the 18th week of gestation (Nicolaides and Rodeck, 1985).

It has been suggested that plasma exchange should be reserved for the woman with a previous history of hydrops developing before 24–26 weeks' gestation, with a homozygous (*DD*) partner. Intensive plasma exchange should then be begun at 10–12 weeks, with fetal blood sampling at 19–22 weeks (Bowman, 1990).

Adsorption of alloantibodies on to red cells. A possible method of removing specific alloantibodies from the mother's serum is to withdraw substantial quantities of plasma, absorb the plasma with appropriate red cells and return the plasma to the mother (see Chapter 1). The method involves the risk of introducing foreign red cells and thus of further increasing the mother's antibody concentration.

Injections of IgG into the mother's circulation, given (i.v.) as a single course totalling 2 g/kg over 5 d, or as repeated weekly injections of 1 g/kg, have been tried in conjunction with plasma exchange or with intravascular transfusion of the fetus in two very small series of cases, with apparent benefit in one series but not in the other (Berlin *et al.* 1990; Chitkara *et al.* 1990). In two much larger series in which i.v. Ig was given, (see following paragraph) there was suggestive evidence that the severity of haemolytic disease in the fetus was reduced. However, because there was great variability in previous obstetric histories, in the stage of pregnancy at which treatment was started and in the number of courses of Ig given, definite conclusions cannot yet be reached.

In the first series, 24 Rh D-immunized women with anti-D levels of more than 5 iu/ml were injected with 0.4 g Ig/kg per day for 4–5 d, sometimes followed by similar courses at intervals of 2–3 weeks, depending on when treatment was started (sometimes before 20 weeks, sometimes after 28 weeks). No other antenatal treatment was given. Twenty-one infants survived. Of 13 cases in which the mother had lost a previous infant with HDN (10 of 13 with hydrops), ten infants survived after one or two postnatal exchange transfusions; in these ten cases, 7 of the mothers had received 1–2 courses of i.v. Ig, the remaining three having received 3–7. The three fetuses which were lost were already hydropic when treatment with i.v. Ig was started. In the series as a whole, after injections of Ig were started, the concentration of maternal anti-D and of bilirubin in amniotic fluid tended to fall (Margulies *et al.* 1991).

In the second series, 50 Rh D-immunized women with anti-D levels exceeding 5 iu/ml, all of whom subsequently gave birth to D-positive infants, were injected with 0.4 g Ig/kg per day for 4 d every 2 weeks. In some cases no other antenatal treatment was given but in an unspecified number, the women were also treated with plasma exchange. Of the 50 women, 18 had lost a previous infant from haemolytic disease. Following the pregnancies in which i.v. Ig was injected, three infants died *in utero* and the remainder survived without intra-uterine transfusion and were born at 37 weeks or later (C. De la Camera and R. Arrieta, personal communication).

Injected IgG (i.v. Ig) might act by blocking Fc receptors on fetal macrophages (cf. p. 458); by interfering in some way with antibody synthesis; or by blocking the placental transfer of antibody to the fetus: in perfusion experiments with a lobule of human placenta, a plasma level of 20 g/l IgG in the maternal circulation, produced by injecting commercial i.v. Ig, inhibited the transfer of the alloantibody anti-Pl^{A1} (HPA-1a) (Morgan *et al.* 1991).

Transfusion of the fetus in utero. Intraperitoneal transfusion was the first method to be used (Liley, 1963). In this method, red cells are injected into the peritoneal cavity of the fetus, whence they are taken up into the blood stream via the subdiaphragmatic lacunae and right lymphatic duct. Uptake is dependent on diaphragmatic movements (Menticoglou *et al.* 1987) and intraperitoneal transfusions are therefore useless in those hydropic fetuses who have no such movements. Although intraperitoneal transfusion has been largely superseded by intravascular transfusion, it still has a place. It is easy to perform and may also be used in combination with intravascular transfusion to increase the total volume of blood given to the fetus, thus prolonging the interval between transfusions (Nicolini and Rodeck, 1988; Rodeck and Letsky, 1989).

Intravascular transfusion was first performed by fetoscopy (Rodeck *et al.* 1984) but is now performed through a needle inserted into the umbilical vein by ultrasonographic guidance (Daffos *et al.* 1984; Grannum *et al.* 1986; Nicolaides *et al.* 1986; Berkowitz *et al.* 1988).

The results of intravascular transfusion have been spectacular. In one early series of 29 fetuses severely affected with Rh D haemolytic disease (ten with hydrops) treated at 18–24 weeks, 25 survived (Rodeck *et al*. 1984). In another series, 16 of 22 hydropic fetuses survived and three of the six deaths were at 19–22 weeks in the fetuses of i.v. drug abusers (Bowman, 1990). In a third series, the survival rate of fetuses developing hydrops before 26 weeks was 61%, and of those developing hydrops later was 100% (Grannum and Copel, 1988).

In ten published series of fetuses with severe haemolytic disease treated by intravascular transfusion *in utero*, of those with hydrops 66 of 96 (69%) survived, compared with 114 of 134 (85%) of those without hydrops. Hydrops was reversed in 60% of cases and in these, the survival rate was 92%, compared with 43% in those cases in which hydrops was not reversed (Tannirandorn and Rodeck, 1990). Even in very experienced hands, a single intravascular transfusion has a mortality rate of 2% (Rodeck and Letsky, 1989).

It is customary to use blood which is less than 72 h old. The red cells should be group O, D negative, K negative and should be crossmatched with the mother's serum; the PCV of the red cell preparation should be 0.70–0.85. To avoid the risk of graft versus host disease, the preparation should be irradiated or the white cells should be removed by filtration. The blood should be screened for HbS and for anti-CMV, as well as being submitted to all the usual tests.

Following intra-uterine sampling or transfusion of the fetus, donor red cells may enter the maternal circulation, either by being shed into the mother's peritoneal cavity or by entering maternal blood vessels in the placenta, and may stimulate the formation of 'new' alloantibodies or increase the concentration of existing ones.

In two series of Rh D-sensitized pregnancies managed differently, when fetal blood sampling was used other alloantibodies were found during pregnancy in three of 63 cases and in a further two of 38 examined after delivery; in contrast, when only amniotic fluid examinations were used, other antibodies were found during pregnancy in one of 52 cases and in one of 22 examined after delivery (Pratt *et al*. 1989). The development of alloantibodies within 2–4 weeks of giving intraperitoneal transfusions to fetuses has been recorded in three cases: anti-Fy^b in a woman who had already formed anti-Ce (Contreras *et al*. 1983c), and anti-Jk^a and a combination of anti-Fy^b, -Jk^b and -S in two other women (Barrie and Quinn, 1985).

Following a series of 68 fetal intravascular transfusions, TPH, as judged by an increase of at least 50% in the level of maternal α-FP, occurred in 27 cases (40%). The frequency was much higher (66%) in women with an anterior placenta than in those in whom the placenta was posterior or fundal (frequency of TPH, 17%). The mean estimated volume of TPH was 2.4 ml (blood). When the volume of TPH following the first intravascular transfusion exceeded 1 ml, the mother's anti-D titre rose by more than 150% within the following 3 weeks (Nicolini *et al*. 1988a).

Premature delivery. At a time when premature delivery was being practised only occasionally, it was found that approximately 50% of all stillbirths due to haemolytic disease occurred after the first 35 weeks of pregnancy (Allen, 1957; Walker *et al*. 1957). Because of the high mortality rate in premature infants at that time, there was reluctance to carry out premature delivery before about the 35th week of pregnancy but, with the steadily increasing success in the care of prematurely delivered infants, delivery is now carried out as early as 30–32 weeks with high survival rates.

Postnatal treatment of the infant

Exchange transfusion (using D-negative blood) greatly increases the survival rate and almost removes the risk of kernicterus (Allen *et al.* 1950; Mollison and Walker, 1952). In the method introduced by Diamond (1947), blood is withdrawn and injected, intermittently, through a plastic catheter passed up the umbilical vein (see Apendix 10). The primary object of exchange transfusion is to remove D-positive red cells which, in a severe case of HDN, may have a survival time as short as 2 or 3 d (Mollison, 1943b). (In contrast, D-negative red cells almost always survive normally (Mollison, 1951, p. 398).) The secondary object of exchange transfusion is to remove bilirubin already present in the plasma. It is possible to predict accurately the volume of D-positive red cells remaining in the infant's circulation if the infant's initial PCV and body-weight are known; a nomogram was published by Veall and Mollison (1950). However, the amount of bilirubin removed is more difficult to calculate since during exchange transfusion bilirubin enters the plasma from the extravascular space. For this reason most clinicians like to exchange relatively large volumes of blood, e.g. 200 ml/ kg, and to spend some time, e.g. 60–90 min, over the exchange transfusion.

Plasma-reduced blood with a PCV of at least 0.60 should be used for exchange transfusion; the blood should be group O, D negative and K negative, and should be crossmatched with the mother's serum; it should be less than 5 d old. The blood should be screened for HbS and for anti-CMV, as well as being submitted to all the usual tests.

Phototherapy to reduce serum bilirubin concentration. On exposure to light, particularly in the region of 420–480 nm, bilirubin is converted to the non-toxic pigment, biliverdin. Exposing jaundiced newborn infants to a suitable fluorescent light lowers serum bilirubin concentration (Cremer *et al.* 1958; Costa Ferreira *et al.* 1960), an effect which was confirmed in a controlled trial (Tabb *et al.* 1972). Evidently, samples of serum for bilirubin estimation must be protected from light.

Phototherapy is used in an attempt to prevent or postpone exchange transfusion but it is not used as the sole method of therapy in any case in which exchange transfusion would otherwise be indicated.

Intravenous IgG to reduce need for exchange transfusion. In a trial, infants were randomly assigned as soon after birth as possible to receive phototherapy alone or phototherapy plus high-dose IgG (500 mg/kg over a 2-h period). Serum bilirubin was monitored 6-hourly. Exchange transfusion was required in 11 of 16 infants receiving only phototherapy but in only two of 16 who also received IgG (Rubo and Wahn, 1991).

Suppression of Rh D immunization which would otherwise follow pregnancy

As pointed out in Chapter 5, Rh D immunization can be prevented by giving 20 µg or more anti-D immunoglobulin for every 1 ml D-positive red cells introduced into the circulation. So far as Rh D immunization by pregnancy is concerned there are two causes of failure to prevent immunization when anti-D immunoglobulin is given: either the dose of anti-D is insufficient or it is given too late, that is to say after primary Rh D immunization has been induced.

When anti-D immunoglobulin was first used to prevent Rh D immunization associated with pregnancy, it was injected immediately following delivery. It was assumed that if given during pregnancy it would harm the fetus and that, in any case, TPH occurred mainly during delivery so that treatment immediately after delivery would be effective. It eventually became clear that in a minority of cases primary Rh D immunization occurs during pregnancy so that when anti-D is injected only postnatally there is a regular, though small, failure rate.

The results of giving anti-D only postnatally will be considered first.

Administration of anti-D only postnatally

Failure rates at 6 months. When 100–300 μg anti-D immunoglobulin are injected immediately after delivery the number of D-negative women who develop anti-D within the following 6 months is 0.1–0.5%. For example, 34 of 33 260 (0.1%) in Finland where women were treated with 250 μg anti-D (Eklund, 1978); 55 of 16 142 (0.34%) in women treated in Scotland with either 100 or 200 μg anti-D (I. Cook, personal communication), and 16 of 3113 (0.51%) in an Australian series. The somewhat higher failure rate in this latter series does not seem to have been due to the inclusion of women already immunized before being treated since anti-D was detected in 0.71% at delivery and these women were excluded (Davey, 1976b).

Failure rates at the end of a second D-positive pregnancy. From what has been said already, the minimum failure rate expected is about 1.5%, i.e. an incidence of 0.7% in each of the two pregnancies due to primary immunization occurring during the pregnancy and an additional 0.2% or so for failures due to a TPH at the time of the first delivery too large to be covered by a dose of 300 μg anti-D or less. In fact, failure rates of the order expected have been observed in many series; e.g. 1.86% (Davey, 1976b, supplemented by personal communication); approximately 1.5% (Eklund, 1978); and approximately 1.5% in women treated with 50, 100 or 200 μg anti-D in a controlled trial (see Table 12.1).

When anti-D is detected for the first time during a second pregnancy in a woman who has been given anti-D Ig after her first pregnancy, there are two possible

Table 12.1   Controlled trials of anti-D dosage in suppressing Rh D immunization (MRC, 1974a)

Dose* (μg)	% of women with anti-D[†]	
	6 months after first pregnancy	At the end of second pregnancy
200	0.2	1.5
100	0.2	1.1
50	0.4	1.5
20	1.4	2.9

All women D-negative with two D-positive infants, the first being ABO compatible.
* Anti-D injected i.m. within 36 h of delivery of first infant.
[†] Detected by indirect antiglobulin test.

explanations: (1) sensitization to D occurred by the time of the first delivery but anti-D was produced in detectable amounts only after the further stimulus of a second pregnancy; (2) primary immunization to D occurred only during the second pregnancy. It seems that the second explanation is usually the right one; the evidence is that in these cases the antibody develops only towards the end of the second pregnancy, e.g. in the last 4 weeks in 50% of the cases in one series (Eklund, 1978).

Effect of different amounts of anti-D given immediately after delivery. In a 'blind' trial conducted by a working party of the Medical Research Council (MRC) and begun in 1967 in the UK, different doses of anti-D were given to four groups of women (about 450 women in each group). Over the dose range 200 to 20 μg there was a significant, though small, trend towards an increase in the failure rate (see Table 12.1). Approximately 200 women in each of the four groups were followed through a second pregnancy with a D-positive infant; the differences in the failure rates in the different groups were not statistically significant although failures were suggestively more frequent with the 20 μg dose than with the larger doses.

Standard doses of anti-D for postpartum injection. Although there is evidence that an i.m. dose of 20 μg anti-D per ml D-positive red cells is completely effective in suppressing Rh D immunization, in order to allow a margin of safety it has been recommended that the standard dose should be 25 μg per ml cells (WHO, 1971). In theory then, when 300 μg anti-D is given routinely, only women with a TPH exceeding about 12 ml red cells, that is to say about 0.2% of all recently delivered women, require extra anti-D. In detecting these exceptional cases the rosetting test described on p. 548 is very suitable since it has been shown to be reliable in detecting 15 ml or more of fetal red cells. When 100 μg anti-D is the standard dose, women with a TPH exceeding 4 ml red cells, that is to say, about 0.7% of all recently delivered women, should receive extra anti-D. To detect these women it has been proposed that a blood film should be taken from all women at risk and stained by the acid-elution method. A simple method of screening based on the examination of five low-power fields of known area and red cell density has been proposed (see Appendix 9). When the number of darkly staining cells exceeds certain limits, a quantitative estimate of the size of the TPH should be made, and extra anti-D given as necessary to bring the total dose to correspond to 25 μg per ml fetal red cells. Although screening for unusually large TPHs does not seem to be done universally there is no evidence that the failure rate of suppressive treatment is higher with the standard dose of 100 μg anti-D than with 300 μg (McMaster Conference, 1977; Tovey *et al.* 1978). Nevertheless, the UK seems to be the only country in which the standard dose is 100 μg; in the USA and elsewhere, 300 μg is the standard dose. Incidentally, the UK is also the only country in which anti-D concentration is expressed as iu/ml (1 μg = 5 iu). Reasons why the present authors consider the use of iu in this context to be pointless are given in Chapter 8.

   In women in whom an unusually large TPH has been detected and who have been given extra anti-D Ig, tests are sometimes done to confirm that an adequate dose has been given. One practice is to look for the presence of anti-D in the maternal plasma but this is unsound in principle since, even when the antigen concentration is low, not all the antibody will be bound, however little is given. Furthermore, the method has been shown to be of no practical value (Ness and Salamon, 1986). The method which seems most likely to be worthwhile is to test for clearance of fetal red cells from the maternal circulation, e.g. by using a rosetting test. Although a relationship between clearance and immunosuppression has yet to be firmly established, the two seem at least to be associated; see pp. 120–121 for further discussion.

In women undergoing termination of pregnancy up to 20 weeks' gestation, a common practice is to give 50 μg anti-D, although few observations have been made on the effectiveness of this procedure. In one series of 3080 women treated with 50 μg anti-D following therapeutic abortion only 13 (0.42%) were found to be immunized during a second pregnancy (I. Simonovits, personal communication), suggesting a very low failure rate of suppression.

From 20 weeks onwards the dose used should be the same as for women at term (e.g. in the USA, 300 μg). As for term deliveries, a screening test should be done to detect women with unusually large TPHs, who require additional anti-D.

Antenatal administration of anti-D

As described above, a single pregnancy with a D-positive, ABO-compatible infant initiates primary Rh D immunization in about one in six (17%) of D-negative women. When anti-D immunoglobulin is given postnatally, the incidence of primary Rh D immunization falls to about 1.5%, as judged by the development of anti-D by the time of delivery of a second D-positive infant. Thus, in some 90% of cases Rh D immunization which would otherwise follow pregnancy can be prevented by giving anti-D postnatally. As described below, it seems likely that most of the remaining 10% of cases can be prevented by antenatal treatment.

Safety of antenatal treatment. Although it was at first believed that injecting anti-D into a D-negative woman pregnant with a D-positive fetus was potentially dangerous, further consideration and practical experience show that the fear is groundless.

In D-positive infants born to mothers who are actively immunized to Rh D, the total amount of anti-D in the infant is only about 10% of that in the mother (Hughes-Jones *et al.* 1971b). Accordingly, when 300 μg anti-D is injected into the mother, even if equilibration across the placenta occurred immediately, not more than about 30 μg would be expected to be in the infant. In fact, as discussed on p. 544, IgG is transferred relatively slowly across the placenta. Accordingly, by the time that equilibrium is reached a considerable amount of the anti-D which has been injected into the mother will have been catabolized and the total amount reaching the infant will be less than 30 μg.

In trials in which 300 μg anti-D were given to D-negative women at the 28th week and again at the 34th week of pregnancy, although as many as 28% of ABO-compatible D-positive infants had a weakly positive DAT the cord serum bilirubin concentration never exceeded 3.4 mg/dl (58 μmol/l) and no infant developed hyper-bilirubinaemia severe enough to require phototherapy (Bowman *et al.* 1978). In a few cases in which D-negative women were given four doses of 300 μg anti-D between about the 12th and 34th weeks of pregnancy in an attempt to turn off the immune response following the discovery of low concentrations of maternal anti-D reacting only with enzyme-treated cells, not all the D-positive infants born subsequently had a positive DAT (J.M. Bowman, personal communication).

Results observed with antenatal treatment. Although no properly controlled randomized trials have been conducted there is highly suggestive evidence that the administration of anti-D immunoglobulin during pregnancy suppresses primary immunization to Rh D in most women in whom it would otherwise occur. In one series in which almost 10 000 D-negative women carrying D-positive fetuses were given an injection of anti-D at 28 weeks (either 300 μg i.m. or 240–300 μg i.v.), less than 0.1% developed anti-D by full term, whereas previous experience indicated that without antenatal anti-D the incidence would have been 1.8% (Bowman, 1984). As explained on p. 556, the figure of 1.8% is substantially greater than that reported by others, but the discrepancy can be explained.

In another series in which, unlike the one just referred to, only primiparae were included, of 1238 D-negative women carrying D-positive fetuses who were injected both at 28 and 34 weeks with 100 μg anti-D, only 0.16% developed anti-D by the time of delivery. In an earlier series from the same centre in which women were given anti-D only after delivery, 0.9% formed anti-D by the end of pregnancy (Tovey *et al.* 1983). The foregoing figures give a slightly too favourable impression of the success of antenatal immunoprophylaxis with anti-D because in both series a few additional women developed anti-D either 6 months after delivery or during a second pregnancy. In the first series, in which most of the women were tested at 6 months, there were two in whom anti-D was detected for the first time, an incidence of very approximately 0.02%; of an unknown number who had a second D-positive pregnancy there were another two who developed anti-D before the 28th week (Bowman, 1984). In the second of the two series quoted above anti-D developed during a second pregnancy with a D-positive infant in two of 325 women, but in neither case did the antibody appear to cause clinically significant haemolytic disease.

Optimal amount of anti-D for antenatal injection. From the data of Bowman *et al.* (1978) it appears that treatment should be given as early as 28 weeks. If it is arbitrarily assumed that there should be at least 25 μg anti-D in the mother just before delivery and if only a single dose of anti-D immunoglobulin is to be given, then 300 μg given at 28 weeks is barely sufficient. Assuming a $t_{1/2}$ of 21 d for passively administered IgG anti-D in a D-negative woman carrying a D-positive fetus (Eklund *et al.* 1982), on the average 19 μg will remain in the mother at term.

The administration of 300 μg anti-D at 28 weeks is convenient in countries where 300 μg or thereabouts is the standard dose to be given postpartum since the same preparation can then be given on the two occasions. On the other hand, in countries where the standard postpartum dose is 100 μg it may prove preferable to give two doses of 100 μg during pregnancy, at 28 weeks and 34 weeks, respectively. This dosage will in fact result in a rather higher concentration of anti-D in the mother's plasma immediately before delivery than when a single dose of 300 μg is given at 28 weeks, will result in a certain saving of anti-D, and will avoid the confusion of having two different-sized doses to be administered antenatally and postnatally. In conclusion, two different dose-schedules can be recommended at the present time: 300 μg to be given at 28 weeks and immediately after delivery, and 100 μg to be given at 28 weeks, 34 weeks and immediately after delivery. (In some countries 250 μg rather than 300 μg is used, and in others 125 μg rather than 100 μg. There is no reason to believe that these differences materially affect the results and, in any case, it must be remembered that the anti-D assays are not very precise so that the amounts actually given are known only approximately.)

Intravenous administration of anti-D. As discussed in Chapter 5, it is possible that when anti-D is given i.v. at the same time as an injection of D-positive red cells, the dose of antibody required for the suppression of primary Rh D immunization may be only half as great as when the anti-D is injected i.m. There is therefore a potential advantage in giving anti-D i.v. rather than i.m. immediately following delivery when it is likely that any D-positive red cells in the circulation have arrived there only recently. In practice, because of the increased risk of transmitting viral infections when Ig is given i.v. (see Chapter 16) and because the methods used for viral inactivation in some preparations are suspect, the i.m. route should be used whenever possible. When giving anti-D antenatally there does not seem to be any potential advantage in i.v. administration since the object is to protect against Rh D immunization over a period of many weeks and since, within 3 d of giving anti-D, plasma levels are the same whether the injection has been given i.v. or i.m. (see Table 10.1 on p. 471).

Occasional reactions have been reported following the i.v. injection of anti-D immunoglobulin prepared by fractionation on DEAE Sephadex (Hoppe *et al.* 1973); at one centre only seven reactions, only two of which were severe enough to require treatment, were noted following injections to 80 000 women (H. Hoppe, personal communication). In another series, transient marked flushing and mild chest discomfort were noted in two of 2792 women. The reactions were thought to be due to aggregated material in vials which had too high a moisture content (Bowman *et al.* 1980). In a third series not a single untoward reaction was reported amongst 120 000 recipients (J.R. O'Riordan, personal communication).

Changes in the incidence and mortality of haemolytic disease

As described in Chapter 3, before the introduction of immunoprophylaxis of Rh D haemolytic disease, the frequency of the disease, both in England and in North America was about one per 170 births. Assuming an average family size of more than two children, this figure is close to expectation: the frequency of the disease in first pregnancies is very low (less than one per 1000 births), in second pregnancies is about one per 100 births, and in subsequent pregnancies is somewhat greater.

Immunoprophylaxis with anti-D became available in 1968–70. In one North American hospital, the frequency with which anti-D was found in pregnant women declined from one in 238 in 1974 (Walker, 1984) to one in 963 in 1988 (Walker and Hartrick, 1991). In this latter series, the frequency of a positive DAT in newborn infants due to anti-D was one in 1190; in the hospital concerned, anti-D had been given to mothers antenatally as a routine since 1985. In a nationwide survey in the USA, the frequency of HDN in 1986 was estimated to be one in 943 births (Chavez *et al.* 1991), although the survey was based on only 18.2% of the total births for that year and some cases, e.g. stillbirths, may have been excluded. In an English region, the decline in a comparable period was substantially less, namely from one in 210 in 1974 to one in 497 in 1988 (G.J. Dovey, personal communication). The difference may have been due to the more widespread use of antenatal immunoprophylaxis in North America.

Even if anti-D Ig had been given to all previously unimmunized D-negative women delivered of a D-positive infant from 1970 onwards, some women immunized before that time would still be giving birth to affected infants until about 1995. From about then onwards, if it could be assumed that anti-D Ig had been given, after delivery, to all previously unimmunized women, the frequency with which anti-D was found in pregnant women would be expected to be about one in 2000, since postnatal immunoprophylaxis is about 90% effective (McMaster Conference, 1977). Antenatal immunoprophylaxis, when widely applied, can be expected to reduce the frequency of anti-D in pregnant women to one in 10 000 or less.

Although the frequency of Rh D haemolytic disease has declined only five- to ten-fold, the death rate from the disease has declined to a far greater extent. Before giving details, it is necessary to explain that figures based on registered deaths have been found to be seriously inaccurate. In England and Wales for each of the years 1953 and 1955, approximately 400 deaths were registered as being due to HDN. When a detailed enquiry was made and the clinical notes of each infant scrutinized, supplemented by correspondence with the clinician in charge as necessary, only about 310 deaths in each year (about one in 2180 births) were found to have been due to HDN (Walker and Mollison, 1957). A similar enquiry was made for deaths registered as due to HDN in England and Wales for the years 1977–90 (Clarke and Mollison, 1989; Hussey and Clarke, 1991; C.A. Clarke, personal communication). At the beginning of the study, registered deaths were greater than deaths actually due to haemolytic disease by about 50%, although 10 years later, the number of deaths falsely certified as due to haemolytic disease had fallen substantially. On the other hand, registered deaths in England and Wales underestimate the true death rate because stillbirths before the 28th week are not registrable. In the past, many deaths *in utero* from HDN must have been unrecorded but the increasingly successful intra-uterine treatment of HDN is making this source of error less important.

By 1989 the registered death rate from Rh D haemolytic disease in England and Wales, based on examination of clinical notes but excluding deaths before the 28th week of pregnancy, had fallen to about one in 65 000 births (Hussey and Clarke, 1991), compared with the figure for 1953, given above, of one in 2180 births.

Figure 12.8 shows the registered deaths from Rh D haemolytic disease for England and Wales for the years 1977–90; those cases in which the mother had become immunized to Rh D despite postnatal treatment with anti-D Ig are plotted separately. In the period 1977–88 there was only a modest fall in the number of such cases, in keeping with the idea that these cases could have been prevented only by antenatal treatment, and as expected from the fact that as late as 1988 very few women in England and Wales were being given anti-D Ig antenatally. The much lower number of these cases in 1989 and 1990 seems likely to have been due mainly to improved treatment of the affected fetus.

Deaths from HDN due to antibodies other than anti-D showed no change between 1977 and 1990, the number being three or four in 12 of the 14 years. Of the total of 49, 32 were associated with anti-c, with or without anti-E, 11 with anti-K alone, four with both anti-K and anti-c or anti-E, one with anti-E alone and one with anti-C alone.

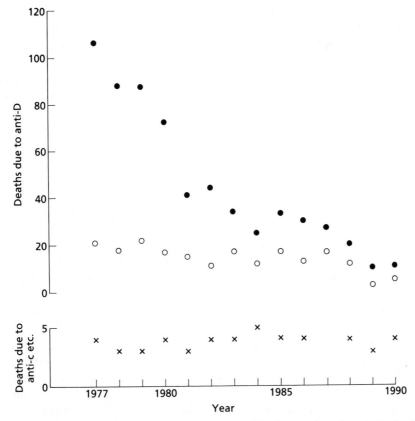

Figure 12.8 Registered deaths due to haemolytic disease of the fetus and newborn in England and Wales, 1977–90 (data for 1977–89, see Clarke and Mollison (1989); for 1989, see Hussey and Clarke (1991); for 1990, C.A. Clarke, personal communication.) ●, Total deaths due to anti-D; ○, deaths due to anti-D in which the mother had been treated with anti-D immunoglobulin following previous deliveries; ×, deaths due to antibodies other than anti-D (mainly anti-c and anti-K); for details see text.

The most important steps in preventing Rh D immunization by pregnancy

First, in order to minimize the risk that, due to a technical or clerical error, a D-negative woman will be reported as D-positive and thus not be given anti-D immunoglobulin after delivery, the D group of all so-far-unimmunized women should be determined (using two different anti-Ds) on at least two separate occasions: (1) during pregnancy; and (2) at the time of delivery. In addition, the following steps are recommended for all so-far-unimmunized D-negative women:

1 Since anti-D immunoglobulin is sometimes withheld because a report on the infant's D group has not yet been received, anti-D immunoglobulin (100 μg or more) should be given to all D-negative women within 72 h of delivery, unless the infant has been shown to be D negative.

2 After delivery, if the infant is D positive, a screening test for fetal red cells should be made on a sample of the mother's blood; if this is positive a quantitative estimate of the number of cells present should be made (see Appendix 9) and extra anti-D given if indicated.

3 All D-negative women should be given a dose of anti-D immunoglobulin after induced abortion. Up to the 20th week a dose of 50 µg anti-D is sufficient; after that, 100 µg or more should be given. The case for giving anti-D after spontaneous abortions in the first trimester is not strong (see p. 555) and practice varies.

4 After obstetric interference, e.g. amniocentesis or version, anti-D immunoglobulin should be given, whether or not fetal red cells can be demonstrated in the mother's blood. In women who are 20 or more weeks pregnant, a test for fetal red cells should be made and extra anti-D immunoglobulin given when indicated. Up to the 20th week of pregnancy, only 50 µg need be given, but if the pregnancy continues further anti-D should be given, e.g. 300 µg at 28 weeks or 100 µg at 28 weeks and again at 34 weeks.

Women with partial D

A woman who is apparently very weak D (D^u) may really be partial D and may then develop anti-D as a result of a pregnancy with a fetus whose red cells carry the D epitopes which she lacks. In two reported cases (Davey, 1976a; Lacey, 1978), the mother's red cells belonged to category VI and, in both, the mother had apparently been immunized by pregnancy alone. In the second of the two cases, the infant was severely affected and died.

In the years 1976–85, 28 pregnant D-positive women with anti-D in their serum were tested at various centres of the National Blood Transfusion Service in the UK; most of the women either belonged to category VI or had red cells which reacted too weakly with anti-D to be categorized. Twenty-six of the 28 infants were normal or only mildly affected; in most of these cases the titre of anti-D in the mother's serum was low although in a few cases it was in the range 20–256; of the remaining two infants, one required an exchange transfusion, and one died *in utero* at 37–38 weeks (maternal anti-D titre in this case was 128).

When a woman is grouped as weak D (D^u) for the first time after delivery it is essential to do a screening test for fetal red cells since she may in fact be D negative with a substantial number of D-positive fetal red cells in her circulation and not only need anti-D immunoglobulin but require more than the standard dose.

D-negative woman with a partial-D infant

In a case described by Revill *et al.* (1979) a D-negative woman, whose infant was typed as D positive, was given 100 µg anti-D immunoglobulin after it had been estimated that her circulation contained approximately 4 ml fetal red cells. Despite a second dose of 100 µg of anti-D 72 h later, the fetal red cells were not cleared from the maternal circulation and it was then shown that the infant's red cells not only reacted weakly with anti-D but failed altogether to react with some anti-D sera, indicating that they were partial D. *In vitro*, the red cells reacted relatively weakly with the anti-D Ig that had been injected (P. Tippett, personal communication).

HAEMOLYTIC DISEASE DUE TO ANTIBODIES OTHER THAN ANTI-D, ANTI-A AND ANTI-B

A list of the various red cell alloantibodies which can cause haemolytic disease is given near the beginning of this chapter; after anti-D, anti-c is easily the most important.

Haemolytic disease due to anti-c

Anti-c (with or without anti-E) is found in about 0.7 per 1000 pregnant women, e.g. 177 of 280 000 (Bowell et al. 1986b); 65 in about 90 000 (Tovey, 1986). The frequency of haemolytic disease due to anti-c is substantially lower than this, for two reasons: first, since 40–50% of pregnant women with anti-c have been immunized by transfusion (Astrup and Kornstad, 1977; Bowell et al. 1986b), the fetus is relatively often c negative; and second; since the antibody is often present in low titre, a substantial number of c-positive infants have a negative DAT. For example, of 42 c-positive infants born to mothers with anti-c, ten had a negative DAT; in three of the ten the antibody was detectable only with enzyme-treated red cells. In 24 of 42 infants, including the ten with a negative DAT, the titre of anti-c was 8 or less (Astrup and Kornstad, 1977). In another series, the titre of anti-c was 8 or less in 129 of 177 (Bowell et al. 1986b). In two series, only about 20% of c-positive infants born to mothers with anti-c required exchange transfusion (Astrup and Kornstad, 1977; Hardy and Napier, 1981). In the several series referred to above no stillbirths and only one neonatal death were recorded. In contrast, in another series, of 62 c-positive infants born to c-immunized women over a 40-year period, 20 required transfusion and eight were either stillborn (with hydrops) or died in the neonatal period (Wenk et al. 1985). In England and Wales in 1977–87, among approximately 7000 000 births, there were 26 infants recorded as dying from HDN due to anti-c (Clarke and Mollison, 1989), that is, approximately one per 250 000 births; even at the end of this period, that is, in 1987, the death rate from HDN due to anti-D was still very much higher, i.e. one per 25 600 births.

Haemolytic disease due to other Rh antibodies

Anti-E alone is the Rh antibody found most commonly after anti-D. In one series, it was present in 97 of about 90 000 pregnancies (Tovey, 1986). The antibody is often naturally occurring and is then sometimes detectable only with enzyme-treated red cells. Anti-E very seldom causes haemolytic disease.

Anti-C was found in 38 of 280 000 pregnancies (0.14 per 1000); it was about five times commoner in ccDEE than in ccDEe women; of infants tested at birth, two of three had a negative DAT and there were no deaths from HDN (Bowell et al. 1988).

Anti-e is a very rare cause of HDN; the disease is usually mild (Moncharmont et al. 1990).

Anti-Rh29 in Rh-null pregnant women has been associated both with mild (Bruce et al. 1985) and severe (Portugal et al. 1990) HDN.

Haemolytic disease due to anti-K or anti-k

Anti-K is found in about one per 1000 pregnant women, e.g. 127 of 127 000 (Caine and Mueller-Heubach, 1986); 27 of 40 000 (Tovey, 1986, estimates for 1982 only); 407 of 350 000 (Mayne et al. 1990). The frequency of HDN due to anti-K is much lower since in most cases the infant is K negative, e.g. in 80% in one series (Caine and Mueller-Heubach, 1986). A history of previous transfusion was elicited from 88% of K-immunized pregnant women in one series (Mayne et al. 1990) and from 80% in another (Pepperell *et al.* 1977). The frequency of severe haemolytic disease due to anti-K was five (all hydropic) of 13 K-positive infants in one series (Caine and Mueller-Heubach, 1986) and two (stillborn) of ten K-positive infants in another (Mayne *et al.* 1990a). In this latter series six of ten K-positive infants had a positive DAT but some infants with K-positive fathers were not tested so that the exact frequency of HDN due to anti-K could not be determined.

Over the period 1977–90 in which, in England and Wales, there were approximately 9000 000 births, there were 15 registered deaths from HDN in which the mother's serum contained anti-K, either alone (11 cases) or together with anti-c or -E (four cases); see above.

In a few cases of HDN due to anti-K it has been noted that the percentage of reticulocytes in the fetal blood is much lower than expected from the Hb level in comparison with cases due to anti-D (J. Bennebroek-Gravenhorst, personal communication). Furthermore, it has been found that hydrops fetalis may develop very rapidly in cases in which amniotic fluid bilirubin measurement has indicated mild to moderate disease. A possible explanation would be that anti-K has a disproportionate effect (compared with anti-D) on red cell precursors, causing relatively more anaemia and less jaundice (F.D. Frigoletto, Jr, personal communication).

Another feature of haemolytic disease due to anti-K, which has been noted occasionally, is a poor correlation between the severity of the disease and the titre of antibody in the mother's serum. In one case, hydrops fetalis occurred despite an anti-K titre of only 2 at the 37th week of pregnancy (L. McDonnell, personal communication). In another, hydrops at 23 weeks, associated with an Hb concentration of 22 g/l, was associated with a maternal anti-K titre of 8 (Bowman *et al.* 1989).

Haemolytic disease due to anti-k is very rare. As in HDN due to anti-K, the disease may be severe despite a low maternal antibody titre. For example, in a case in which the mother's anti-k titre was 16, the infant's Hb concentration at 31 weeks was only 60 g/l and three intravascular transfusions were given to the infant *in utero* (Bowman *et al.* 1989). In another case, despite a maternal anti-k titre of only 8–16, the infant, after being born spontaneously at 33 weeks, had an Hb concentration of 76 g/l (Anderson *et al.* 1990).

Other antibodies of the Kell system (anti-Js^a, -Js^b and -K^u) have been implicated in mild or moderate haemolytic disease (for references see Vengelen-Tyler, 1984).

Haemolytic disease due to Duffy and Kidd antibodies

Anti-Fy^a usually causes mild haemolytic disease, although among 11 cases reviewed by Greenwalt *et al.* (1959) there were two deaths. Mild haemolytic disease due to anti-Fy^3 has been reported (Albrey *et al.* 1971).

Anti-Jk^a can cause severe haemolytic disease (Matson *et al.* 1959). In one unusual case in which anti-Jk^a was present throughout pregnancy in a Jk (a –) mother, and at term had a titre of 64, the infant showed no signs of haemolytic disease even though the antibody could be eluted from its red cells and was present in its serum to a titre of 64. The infant's red cells were agglutinated by anti-C3d but not by anti-IgG (Dorner *et al.* 1974).

Haemolytic disease due to antibodies of the MNSs system

Haemolytic disease due to anti-M. When anti-M develops during pregnancy, it may fail to affect the fetus (see Bowley and Dunsford, 1949). In rare cases haemolytic disease develops and is occasionally responsible for hydrops fetalis (Stone and Marsh, 1959; Matsumoto et al. 1981). In both of these cases the anti-M in the mother's serum was very potent. In cases in which the infant is mildly or moderately affected with haemolytic disease due to anti-M there are two features that resemble ABO haemolytic disease rather than Rh haemolytic disease: first, the DAT is only weakly positive but unwashed red cells agglutinate spontaneously in a colloid medium, and second, the osmotic fragility of the red cells may be greatly increased (Stone and Marsh, 1959; Freiesleben and Jensen, 1961).

Haemolytic disease due to anti-S and anti-s is very occasionally severe or even fatal (Levine et al. 1952; Issitt, 1981, p. 43).

Haemolytic disease due to anti-U may be severe (Issitt, 1985, p. 322) or even fatal (Burki et al. 1964).

Haemolytic disease due to anti-PP$_1$P^k
HDN of varying severity has been reported. In one case the IgG component of the antibody in the mother's serum had a titre of 16 (Hayashida and Watanabe, 1968). In another, in which the infant had an Hb concentration of 8.7 g/dl, the DAT was only weakly positive (Levene et al. 1977).

HAEMOLYTIC DISEASE OF THE NEWBORN DUE TO ANTI-A AND ANTI-B (ABO HAEMOLYTIC DISEASE)

Anti-A and anti-B occurring in group B and A subjects are predominantly IgM, but in O subjects are at least partly IgG. In 15% of all pregnancies in Whites the mother is O and her infant is A or B, but clinically obvious haemolytic disease is comparatively rare. There seem to be two main reasons for this finding: first, the A and B antigens are not fully developed at birth, and second, A and B substances are not confined to the red cells so that only a small fraction of IgG anti-A and anti-B which crosses the placenta combines with the infant's red cells. The protective effect of A and B determinants in fluids and tissues other than red cells was discussed by Tovey (1945), Wiener et al. (1949) and Høstrup (1963b).

Using sensitive methods, small amounts of IgG anti-A or anti-B are commonly found on the red cells of group A and B infants born to group O mothers (Hsu et al. 1974b). Although severe HDN due to anti-A and anti-B is relatively rare, minor degrees of red cell destruction are common, as shown by the incidence of neonatal jaundice and by the slight lowering of the Hb concentration in ABO-incompatible infants compared with ABO-compatible infants.

Incidence
ABO haemolytic disease must be defined before its incidence can be estimated. For

Table 12.2 Effect of ABO incompatibility between infant's red cells and mother's serum on cord blood findings (from Rosenfield and Ohno, 1955)

	No. of cord blood samples*	Mean values		
		Haemoglobin concentration (g/dl)	Reticulocytes (%)	Bilirubin concentration (mg/dl)[†]
A Infant's red cells compatible with mother's serum	2256	16.05	4.34	2.11
B Infant's red cell incompatible with mother's serum; infant's direct antiglobulin test negative	558	15.82	4.53	2.22
C As B, but direct antiglobulin test positive	89	14.85	5.94	2.96

* Haemoglobin estimates were made on all samples, and reticulocyte counts and bilirubin estimates on almost all samples.
[†] 1 mg/dl = 17 μmol/l.

birth, the incidence was estimated to be one in 180 (Halbrecht, 1951); taking the faintest trace of jaundice in the first 24 h as the criterion, the incidence was as high as one in 70 in another series (Valentine, 1958).

In two series in which the Hb concentration and bilirubin concentration of cord blood were measured in ABO-compatible and ABO-incompatible infants born to group O mothers, it was found that values for Hb concentration were slightly lower, and those for bilirubin concentration slightly higher, in ABO-incompatible infants. In the first of these series the DAT was positive in 14% of the ABO-incompatible infants and in these the Hb concentration was distinctly lower and the bilirubin concentration distinctly higher than in the infants with a negative antiglobulin test (Table 12.2). In the second series, a positive DAT was found in as many as 32.8% of the ABO-incompatible infants and anti-A or anti-B could be eluted from the infant's red cells in a further 38%, but clinically significant disease, judged by a peak bilirubin concentration of more than 12 mg/dl (204 μmol/l) together with anaemia and reticulocytosis, was diagnosed in only 27 of the 680 infants, i.e. in one in 125 of all newborn infants or one in 25 ABO-incompatible infants (Desjardins *et al.* 1979).

Cases of HDN due to anti-A or anti-B which are severe enough to need exchange transfusion are relatively rare, e.g. none amongst 1500 newborn infants (Rosenfield, 1955); three of 14 000 consecutive births (Mollison, 1956, p. 505); three of 8000 births (Ames and Lloyd, 1964); and six of 5704 infants born to group O mothers (Voak and Bowley, 1969).

Relative frequency in group A and B infants
If group A and B infants were equally liable to the disease, the ratio A : B in White affected infants should be approximately 2.7 : 1. In the series of Fischer (1961) the ratio was 3.7 : 1, suggesting that, in Whites, group B infants are slightly less liable than

group A infants to develop haemolytic disease. On the other hand, in another study a positive DAT was found to be relatively commoner in group B than in group A infants, both in Whites and in Blacks (Peevy and Wiseman, 1978).

Racial differences

There is apparent disagreement about the relative frequency of ABO haemolytic disease in Blacks and Whites. The disease was found to be commoner in Blacks by Kirkman (1977), but in another series, although a positive DAT was commoner in Black than in White infants, there was no difference in bilirubin levels or in the need for phototherapy (Peevy and Wiseman, 1978).

In assessing the relative frequency of ABO haemolytic disease in Blacks and Whites, a complication is introduced by the fact that in ABO-compatible infants hyperbilirubinaemia is commoner in Whites than in Blacks. Accordingly, if, for example, all ABO-incompatible infants whose serum bilirubin concentration exceeds 170 μmol/l are considered to have ABO haemolytic disease, the disease will appear to be much commoner in Whites than it really is. One way of assessing the effect of ABO incompatibility is to compare various indices, i.e. the DAT, the age at the onset of jaundice, and the maximum recorded serum bilirubin concentration, in ABO-incompatible and ABO-compatible infants. When this was done, in a very careful study in which Black and White infants were being treated in the same nursery, ABO haemolytic disease was found to be clearly commoner in Blacks than in Whites, the relative frequency being between 2 and 6 : 1, depending on the particular criteria chosen for diagnosis (Kirkman, 1977).

In a survey in Nigeria, the serum of about one-third of group O subjects was found to have strong lytic activity for A or B cells, anti-B lytic activity being commoner than anti-A lytic activity; moderate or severe jaundice, defined as a serum bilirubin concentration exceeding 10 mg/dl (170 μmol/l with a positive DAT was found to develop in about one-third of infants whose red cells were lysed *in vitro* by their mother's serum (Worlledge *et al.* 1974). These figures indicate that the frequency of ABO haemolytic disease of the newborn in Nigeria is about 5% of births.

From a survey of almost 3000 newborn Arab infants it was concluded that ABO haemolytic disease was about as common in Arabs as in Blacks and that the disease tended to be more severe in Arabs than in Europeans: exchange transfusion for ABO haemolytic disease was carried out on one in every 500 newborn Arab infants (Al-Jawad *et al.* 1985).

A factor which might be expected to produce relatively severe HDN in Blacks is the relatively strong expression of A and B which they have (see Chapter 4). Although the relative potency of anti-A and anti-B has in the past been suspected of being racially determined, recent work indicates that environmental factors may be more important (see Chapter 4).

Familial incidence

In about 50% of families in which ABO haemolytic disease is diagnosed, the first ABO-incompatible infant in the family is affected (Mollison, 1951, p. 391).

In families in which ABO haemolytic disease is mild, an affected infant may be followed by a clinically unaffected infant. On the other hand, when severe disease occurs it is likely to be followed by similarly severe disease in subsequent infants of the same blood group.

Mrs Bak. First infant born February 1960; rapidly developed jaundice and found to have erythroblastaemia; diagnosed as having haemolytic disease due to anti-A; exchange transfusion given but infant died. Second infant born April 1961; cord Hb 11.6 g/dl, DAT weakly positive; blood film showed numerous normoblasts and microspherocytes; osmotic fragility: 50% lysis in 0.590% NaCl (grossly increased). The infant was given one exchange transfusion and made excellent progress. Third infant born November 1962; cord blood findings almost identical to those of the second infant, e.g. cord Hb 11.8 g/dl; DAT weakly positive, infant was treated by exchange transfusion and recovered uneventfully. As the findings indicate, the degree of severity of the haemolytic process appeared to be almost identical in the second and third infants. The titre of IgG anti-A in the mother's serum, estimated by the method of Polley et al. (1965), was virtually the same at the time of birth of these two infants, namely 4096 and 8192, respectively.

Serological findings in mothers

ABO group
Mothers of infants with ABO haemolytic disease almost invariably belong to group O (Rosenfield, 1955), evidently because IgG anti-A and anti-B occur far more commonly in group O than in group B and A mothers (Rawson and Abelson, 1960b; Kochwa et al. 1961). In one series of 45 cases the mother was group O in 43 instances and subgroup A_2 in the remaining two; A_2 mothers produced much stronger 'incomplete' anti-B than A_1 mothers (Munk-Andersen, 1958).

IgG anti-A and anti-B
The simplest and most satisfactory test is to treat the mother's serum with a reducing agent (e.g. DTT) to inactivate IgM antibodies and then determine the anti-A or anti-B titre by IAT using an anti-IgG serum (Voak and Bowley, 1969). Using this method, a titre of 512 or more was found to be very suggestive of haemolytic disease. An earlier study, using a modification of the partial neutralization test of Witebsky, had shown that in ABO haemolytic disease the indirect antiglobulin titre was almost always in the range 64–16 000, and was 1000 or more in 13 of 18 cases in which an infant needed an exchange transfusion (Polley et al. 1965).

IgG subclasses of anti-A and anti-B. As described in Chapter 4, all anti-A and anti-B from pregnant women have been found to be at least partly IgG_2. Since this subclass is unable to mediate red cell destruction, it is understandable that there is a relatively poor correlation between antibody titre and the severity of ABO haemolytic disease and that severe cases of haemolytic disease are uncommon.

Antibody-dependent cell-mediated cytotoxicity assays with monocytes assays
In a large number of cases in which an ADCC(M) assay gave negative results, i.e. < 10% lysis, the infant never showed signs of red cell destruction; in three cases in which the ADCC assay was strongly positive, i.e. > 45% lysis, the infant was severely affected and needed more than one exchange transfusion. In cases in which there was 10–45% lysis in the assay, the degree of affection could not be predicted. The

discrepancy between the results of the assay and the severity of red cell destruction in the infant appeared to be due to using standard adult red cells in the assay. When the infant's red cells were used, the degree of lysis was strongly affected by the number of A or B sites on the red cells (Brouwers *et al.* 1988b).

Serological findings in infants

The direct antiglobulin test using anti-IgG

In infants with relatively severe ABO haemolytic disease the amount of antibody on the cells was found to be less than 220 molecules per cell (0.6 μg IgG/ml red cells) in ten of 15 cases (Romano *et al.* 1973). Since, when the spin-tube antiglobulin test is used, the minimum number of antibody molecules which can be detected is about 100–150 (see p. 341), it is not surprising that in mildly affected infants the DAT may be negative. When a very sensitive method is used some anti-A or anti-B can be demonstrated on the red cells of virtually all ABO-incompatible infants. When the DAT was carried out in an AutoAnalyzer, using a low-ionic-strength medium with enhancing agents, the red cells of 13 A_1 and eight B infants, all apparently healthy, gave positive results. The authors calculated that there were between eight and 85 molecules of IgG per red cell (Hsu *et al.* 1974b). Incidentally, the DAT was positive in only one of seven A_2 infants.

It is evident that there is an apparent substantial discrepancy between the findings in haemolytic disease due to anti-D, on the one hand, and to anti-A and anti-B, on the other. In Rh D haemolytic disease, infants may have a strongly positive DAT without showing any clinical signs of disease, whereas in ABO haemolytic disease they may be clinically affected but have a negative or only very weakly positive test. It has been suggested that in ABO haemolytic disease the findings in DATs do not indicate correctly the amount of antibody bound to the red cells *in vivo*. Romans *et al.* (1980) showed, for single examples of IgG anti-A and anti-B, that these antibodies must be bound by both combining sites (monogamous bivalency) to be detectable in the antiglobulin test.

The presence of A antigen sites on unbranched chains of glycolipids or glyco-proteins on the surface of the red cells of newborn infants would make it difficult for molecules to bind bivalently because the sites on unbranched chains are not close enough together. Incidentally it would also make it difficult for molecules binding univalently to co-operate in activating C1 (cf. p. 138).

Although the foregoing explanation is intellectually satisfying, it may not be correct. For one thing, the claim that the binding of anti-A to adult group A red cells is predominantly bivalent has been challenged by Romano *et al.* (1983), who found that the binding constants of anti-A and its Fab derivative were similar with both adult and newborn group A red cells. Other observations which appear to be incompatible with the hypothesis of Romans *et al.* (1980) have been discussed previously (Mollison, 1983, p. 695). To take one example, if cord group A_1 red cells are coated with ^{125}I-labelled human IgG anti-A, some 90% of the antibody appears to be firmly bound by the red cells (N.C. Hughes-Jones, personal communication, 1981). It seems that further experimental work is needed to define precisely the extent and nature of the binding of IgG anti-A and anti-B to the red cells of newborn infants.

The direct antiglobulin test using anti-C3d
Even in severe ABO haemolytic disease the infant's red cells do not react with anti-C3d (Mollison, 1983, p. 694). This finding is due partly to the weak expression of A and B antigens on the red cells of newborn infants but also to the relatively low level of complement in the serum of newborn infants (Brouwers *et al.* 1988a).

Elution of antibody from infant's red cells
In ABO haemolytic disease, when the DAT is only weakly positive or even negative, eluates from the infant's red cells may give strong indirect antiglobulin reactions with adult A_1 red cells (Voak and Bowley, 1969). The explanation for the finding seems to be that the elution procedure results in a considerable concentration of antibody (Voak and Williams, 1971; Romano *et al.* 1973).

There is a relation between crossreactivity of eluates, e.g. reaction of an eluate from group A cells with B cells as well as with A cells, and severity, simply because there is a relation between crossreactivity and potency (see Chapter 4).

Spontaneous agglutination of red cells
Red cells from infants with ABO haemolytic disease tend to clump spontaneously when suspended in plasma (Wiener *et al.* 1949). Similarly, in observations on a series of moderately severely affected infants it was noticed that 'blood freshly drawn from the infant formed large clumps which were easily seen when the blood was allowed to flow down the side of a tube or was examined on an opal glass tile'; the authors pointed out that if blood is taken from a patient of group A_1 who has received a transfusion of plasma containing potent anti-A, it behaves in the same way (Crawford *et al.* 1953a).

The tendency of red cells taken from infants with ABO haemolytic disease to clump spontaneously was reinvestigated by Romano and Mollison (1975). Red cells coated with small amounts IgG anti-A and then washed were found to be almost as readily agglutinated by ABO-compatible plasma as by anti-IgG. Plasma was very much more effective than serum in potentiating agglutination. In a series of infants suspected of having ABO haemolytic disease, a test for autoagglutination, performed by mixing red cells with their own plasma on a slide, was positive in 23 of 25 cases, whereas the DAT was positive in only 20 of the cases (Romano *et al.* 1982).

The observation described by Lewi and Clarke (1960) presumably also demonstrates some change in the surface charge of the red cells of affected infants. Washed red cells from infants suspected of having haemolytic disease of the newborn due to ABO incompatibility were suspended in PVP and were found to sediment far more rapidly than similarly treated red cells from normal infants.

Reactivity of infant's red cells with anti-A and anti-B in vitro
As described in Chapter 4, the red cells of newborn infants react relatively weakly with anti-A and anti-B *in vitro*. Haemolytic disease of the newborn due to anti-A is observed only in infants who are genetically A_1 (Zuelzer and Kaplan, 1954). At the time of birth the red cells of such infants may fail to react with anti-A_1, although samples taken when the infant is a few months old do react (Crawford *et al.* 1953a). No case of HDN due to anti-A in an infant unequivocally belonging to subgroup A_2

as shown by tests at least many months after birth, has yet been described.

One puzzling observation is that, whereas the red cells of healthy infants who are genetically A_1 are agglutinated at the time of birth by an extract of *Dolichos biflorus*, red cells from genetically A_1 infants with haemolytic disease due to anti-A may fail to be agglutinated by an extract of *Dolichos* (Gerlini *et al.* 1968). The cause of this finding has never been demonstrated but blocking of antigen sites by bound IgG anti-A seems to be a possibility.

Premature infants seem to be protected from ABO haemolytic disease, presumably because there are fewer A and B sites on the red cells than on the cells of full-term newborn infants (Schellong, 1964).

Secretor status of infant

It seems that the secretor status of the infant plays little or no part in protecting it against ABO haemolytic disease. In fact, the ratio of secretors to non-secretors is slightly higher than expected; see Voak (1969) who also quotes several earlier papers in support. The excess of secretors may be related to the fact that secretor infants are more prone to induce immune responses in their mothers, see Chapter 4.

Haematological findings

Haemoglobin concentration

In moderately severe ABO haemolytic disease, the Hb concentration of cord blood may be below normal limits (Mollison and Cutbush, 1949b; see also the cases described above). After birth, due to the wider range of normal Hb values which then prevails; it is unusual to find infants who are definitely anaemic. Compared with Rh D haemolytic disease, ABO haemolytic disease is a short-lived affair and it is unusual for anaemia to be found after the first 2 weeks or so of life.

Reticulocytosis and erythroblastaemia

A slight increase in reticulocytes is a common feature in HDN due to ABO incompatibility (Rosenfield, 1955). In the series of fairly severe cases collected by Crawford *et al.* (1953a) the reticulocyte count exceeded 15% in six of 11 cases. In five of these cases there were 30 or more nucleated red cells per 100 leucocytes.

Spherocytosis and changes in osmotic fragility

Microspherocytes are frequently prominent in blood films from infants with ABO haemolytic disease (Grumbach and Gasser, 1948). Similarly, red cell osmotic fragility is almost always above normal limits, at least in moderately severe cases, whereas in Rh D haemolytic disease, even in severe cases, only minor increases in osmotic fragility are found and spherocytosis is unusual (Crawford *et al.* 1953a). In ABO haemolytic disease, the changes in osmotic fragility may persist for as long as 2 or 3 weeks after birth.

Changes in bilirubin concentration

Although the rise in serum bilirubin concentration is usually only moderate and can be controlled by phototherapy, occasional cases of kernicterus have been reported

(Grumbach and Gasser, 1948) so that, as mentioned above, early exchange transfusion is occasionally indicated.

Management of ABO haemolytic disease

Routine antenatal tests not indicated

ABO incompatibility seldom causes severe haemolytic disease and routine antenatal tests to assess the potency of anti-A and anti-B are not indicated. In women who have a history suggesting that a previous infant has been affected with ABO haemolytic disease, cord blood should be taken and tested as soon as possible after birth.

The authors have been able to find only two convincing cases of hydrops fetalis due to ABO incompatibility. In both, abnormal swelling of the mother's abdomen at 32–34 weeks prompted an examination of the fetus by ultrasonography and revealed fetal hydrops. In the first case, the infant was born by caesarean section at 32 weeks and found to be group A with a strongly positive DAT; haemoglobinuria was noted. The cord PCV was reported to be 0.43, but 1 h after birth was 0.30. Packed group O red cells were transfused but the infant died at 20 h. Two previous infants had had severe neonatal jaundice. The mother's IgG anti-A titre was 4000 (Gilja and Shah, 1988). In the second case, the infant was born by caesarean section at 34 weeks and found to be group B with a positive DAT. The cord blood PCV was 0.20, identical to that of an umbilical sample taken while the infant was still *in utero*. At the time of the report the infant remained gravely ill. The mother's anti-B titre was reported as 65 536 (Sherer *et al.* 1991).

Exchange transfusion in ABO haemolytic disease

Since severe anaemia is very uncommon, the main indication for exchange transfusion is the threat of serious hyperbilirubinaemia, leading to kernicterus. Moderate hyperbilirubinaemia can be controlled by phototherapy.

When exchange transfusion is judged to be necessary, group O blood should be used. Provided that the donor's plasma has been screened so as to exclude donors with potent anti-A or anti-B, the antibodies in the transfused plasma are unlikely to exacerbate the haemolytic process. A better solution is to use group O red cells suspended in group AB plasma, preferably from an ABH secretor.

Phototherapy

The mode of action of phototherapy in lowering serum bilirubin concentration is described briefly on p. 572. In those full-term infants with ABO haemolytic disease whose serum bilirubin concentrations threaten to rise to dangerous levels, phototherapy is often sufficient to control the situation. Some recommendations about monitoring bilirubin levels and indications for phototherapy were given as follows: if the cord serum bilirubin concentration is known to have been > 4 mg/dl, estimate bilirubin every 4 h; otherwise, estimate bilirubin 6-hourly. Phototherapy should be begun if the bilirubin level reaches 10 mg/dl within 12 h, or 12 mg/dl (68 μmol/l) within 18 h, or 14 mg within 24 h or 15 mg/dl thereafter (Osborn *et al.* 1984). Of 44 infants diagnosed by these authors as having ABO haemolytic disease, only four required phototherapy.

Injection of A or B trisaccharides

In two infants with severe haemolytic disease due to anti-A the i.v. injection of 50 mg

A-specific trisaccharide (Chembiomed) had an apparently beneficial effect (Romano *et al.* 1985).

Haemolytic reactions after transfusing A or B red cells

When red cells from adult group A or group B donors are transfused, the red cells will almost always have more A and B sites than the infant's own red cells and are likely to undergo more rapid destruction.

In one case in which an infant with HDN was given an exchange transfusion with A_1 blood, the infant developed haemoglobinuria and died (Carpentier and Meersseman, 1956). In two other group A infants with haemolytic disease due to anti-A, the use of group A blood, for exchange transfusion in the first case, and for a simple transfusion in the second, led to a substantial increase in jaundice and the development of kernicterus. The authors noted that the DAT became positive only after the transfusion of group A blood and then gave a mixed-field appearance, evidently because only the transfused group A red cells from adult donors were agglutinated (Sender *et al.* 1971).

Danger of transfusing A or B red cells from adult donors to A or B premature infants born to group O mothers. As described above, A and B antigens are particularly weak in premature infants; maternal IgG anti-A or anti-B may therefore be present without causing a haemolytic syndrome. However, a haemolytic transfusion reaction may be produced if group A or B red cells from adult donors are transfused. In three cases described by Falterman and Richardson (1980), haemolytic reactions were observed in infants with birth-weights between 1280 and 1560 g (30–32 weeks' gestation). In all three infants the DAT was negative in the first 2 days of life but, after transfusion of red cells of the infant's ABO group, hyperbilirubinaemia developed in all three cases and haemoglobinuria occurred in two. The authors described the infants as suffering from unrecognized ABO haemolytic disease, but to the present authors that seems to be a misconception.

CHAPTER 13

IMMUNOLOGY OF LEUCOCYTES, PLATELETS AND PLASMA COMPONENTS

FIGURES

TABLES

Leucoagglutinins were first recognized in patients with agranulocytosis and appeared to be autoantibodies (Dausset and Nenna, 1952). However, the fact that the patients concerned had been transfused repeatedly was soon noted and the possibility that the antibodies might be alloimmune was considered (Dausset, 1953). This idea was put forward more confidently by Miescher and Fauconnet (1954) who first clearly demonstrated an alloantibody in a patient who had received many transfusions: leucocytes from only 32% of normal subjects were agglutinated. The inheritance of leucocyte antigens was demonstrated decisively by Dausset and Brécy (1957) in a study on monozygotic twins. The first leucocyte alloantigen to be clearly defined was originally named MAC (Dausset, 1958). It later proved to belong to a very complicated and important polymorphic system of human leucocyte antigens (HLA) and MAC was subsequently termed HLA-A2 (see below). Other important alloantigens are those specific for granulocytes (Lalezari et al. 1960) and platelets (van Loghem et al. 1959).

THE HLA SYSTEM

The HLA antigens are the most important alloantigens in determining the compatibility of tissue and bone marrow grafts. They are also those against which alloantibodies are frequently formed after blood transfusion and in pregnancy. The antigens of the HLA system constitute the major histocompatibility complex (MHC) and have important biological functions. Early work on the definition of HLA antigens was made very difficult by the poor reproducibility of leucoagglutination. This problem was partly overcome by applying computer analysis to the results (van Rood and van Leeuwen, 1963). More rapid progress became possible with the replacement of leucoagglutination by lymphocytotoxicity tests. A further important development was the realization that HLA antibodies are frequently formed in pregnancy (Payne and Rolfs, 1958; van Rood, 1958). Antibodies formed in pregnancy are directed against a limited number of HLA antigens, in contrast to those developed after blood transfusion. The HLA antigens first detected were found to be encoded by three closely linked genes: HLA-A, -B and -C. The observation that lymphocytes from two unrelated individuals could stimulate each other to blast formation when cultured together (mixed lymphocyte culture, MLC test), and that the antigens responsible for this stimulation are inherited together with HLA antigens, led to the discovery of HLA-D (Bach and Hirschhorn, 1964; Bain et al. 1964). In a recombinant family it was shown that the HLA-D gene is different from the HLA-A, -B and -C genes (Eijsvoogel et al. 1972). The definition of the HLA-D antigens was hampered by difficulties in interpreting the results of the MLC test. An important step forward was the development of techniques by which these antigens can be detected serologically on B cells (van Rood et al. 1975; 1976a,b). By using these techniques it was shown that there are several different genes in the D region of the HLA system (see below).

HLA genes and antigens

The very polymorphic genes of the HLA system are localized on the short arm of chromosome 6 (Breuning et al. 1977). The A, B and C genes, named class I genes, are closely linked to each other as are the genes of the D region, the class II genes. In the D region there are three sets of genes, DR, DQ and DP (see below). The linkage between the A, B and C genes and those of the D region is somewhat less close because these two sets of genes are separated by genes which encode the complement factors C2, C4a, C4b and Bf (class III genes) and genes which code for enzymes and cytokines (class IV genes) (Fig. 13.1).

The linkage between the genes of the HLA system is so close that crossing over within the region is rare; therefore alleles of the HLA genes present on one chromosome usually segregate together within a family. The HLA genes follow Mendelian inheritance and the two alleles of each individual gene are expressed co-dominantly (e.g. HLA-A1-A11).

The set of alleles of the various HLA genes present on a single chromosome is known as a haplotype. Two siblings who inherit the same haplotypes from their parents are thus HLA identical, unless crossing over has occurred.

Although crossing over within the HLA region is rare with random assortment, equilibrium is expected to be established over a long period of time, so that particular

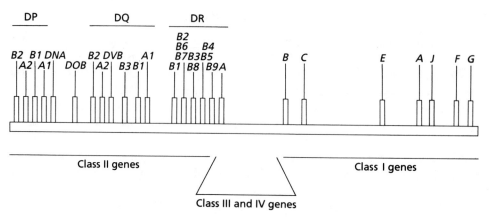

Figure 13.1 DNA of the class I and class II chromosomal regions, analysed by the Southern blot technique. Class I genes: *A*, *B* and *C*, producing corresponding HLA antigens; *E*, *F*, *G* and *J*, producing class I proteins of unknown function. Class II genes: DP subregion *A1*, *A2* = α genes *DPA1*, *DPA2*; *B1*, *B2* = β genes *DPB1*, *DPB2*; between DP and DQ regions, *DNA* and *DOB* = genes of unknown products. DQ subregion *A1*, *A2* = α genes *DQA1*, *DQA2*; *B1*, *B2*, *B3* = β genes *DQB1*, *DQB2* and *DQB3*. *DVB* = gene of unknown product. DR subregion *A* = non-polymorphic α chain gene; *B1* – *B9* = β genes *DRB1* – *DRB9*. For further details, see text.

combinations of alleles at, for example, the *A* and *B* loci or at the loci of the *D* region should not be any commoner than predicted from the product of their relative frequencies in the population. However, in fact, in any given population, certain combinations of alleles or haplotypes are more frequent than expected, a phenomenon described as 'linkage disequilibrium'. Patterns of linkage disequilibrium vary in different populations. For example, the frequency of HLA-A1-B8 in European Caucasians is 8.8% whereas the expected frequency of this haplotype is 1.6% if mating is random.

Molecular biology has provided new possibilities of studying HLA polymorphism directly at the DNA level. In restriction fragment length polymorphism (RFLP) analysis, genomic DNA cleaved by specific bacterial enzymes called restriction endonucleases at polymorphic restriction sites in the DNA is analysed by the Southern blot technique. In this technique, after separation by agar gel electrophoresis, the DNA fragments are hybridized with labelled, cloned single-stranded complementary DNA (cDNA) sequences from the HLA chromosomal region as probes (Wake *et al.* 1982). The length of the fragments depends on the HLA genotype, and it has been shown that specific RFLP patterns are associated with specific serological types (Wake *et al.* 1982; Andersson *et al.* 1984).

A more sophisticated approach is to use synthetic oligonucleotides as probes which correspond to the DNA of a specific allele of a single HLA gene (allele specific oligonucleotides, ASO) in combination with the polymerase chain reaction (PCR) technique. This method makes it possible to study the polymorphism of individual genes (exons) at the DNA level and permits the identification of specific alleles differing from others by only a single nucleotide (Angelini *et al.* 1986; Saiki *et al.* 1986).

Nomenclature
Nomenclature for the HLA genes and antigens is regularly brought up to date by the WHO Nomenclature Committee for factors of the HLA system. The following terms are used: for class I genes HLA-*A*, *-B* etc; for class II genes the prefix *D* followed by a letter (e.g. *R*) for the subregion and by the letters *A* or *B* to indicate whether the gene codes for the α- or β-chain, e.g. *DRA*, *DQB* etc.; numbers of four digits are used to designate the alleles of a particular gene; the first two digits describe the serologically defined antigen with which the allele is (or alleles are) most closely associated, and the last two or three digits complete the number of the allele as defined by molecular techniques (DNA typing, oligonucleotide typing, nucleotide and amino acid sequencing, cloning), e.g. *A0101* for the allele which encodes the A1 antigen and *A0201*, *A0202*, etc. for the alleles associated with the antigen A2; the serologically defined antigens encoded by alleles of each gene are also numbered: A1, A2 etc.; w used to indicate that the specificity was provisional, but in future all serological specificities will be named on the basis of correlation with an identified sequence. The letter 'w' can therefore be dropped with three sets of exceptions: (1) Bw4 and Bw6 to distinguish them as epitopes from those encoded by other alleles of the *HLA-B* gene; (2) the C antigens for which the w is retained throughout to avoid confusion with the nomenclature of the complement system; (3) the Dw specificities which were defined in the MLC test and the DP specificities which were defined by a secondary response of T lymphocytes which had been primed by a first step in the MLC (primed lymphocyte typing) (Bodmer *et al.* 1992).

Class I genes and antigens
Southern blot analysis of the DNA of the class I chromosomal region has shown that in addition to the *A*, *B* and *C* genes, there are several other class I genes (see Fig. 13.1). Three of these genes, *E*, *G* and *F*, have been shown to produce class I proteins (Koller *et al.* 1988; 1989), the function of which is, however, still unknown. Another gene, *HLA-J* is a pseudogene (i.e. a non-functional gene).

The product of the HLA class I genes *A*, *B* and *C* are separate molecules carrying the HLA-*A*, *B* and *C* antigens, respectively. The class I molecules are transmembrane glycoproteins and consist of a transmembrane glycosylated polypeptide chain of mol. wt. 43 000 (the α, or heavy, chain), which carries the polymorphic determinants, linked non-covalently to β_2-microglobulin (β_2m), a non-glycosylated polypeptide of mol. wt. 12 000 (the β, or light, chain), which is encoded by a gene on chromosome 15 (Snary *et al.* 1977a; Barnstable *et al.* 1978). The extracellular part of the heavy chain consists of three domains: α_1, α_2 and α_3 (see Fig. 13.2).

The class I antigens are detected by alloantibodies and, in some cases, also by monoclonal antibodies, using a complement-dependent lymphocytotoxicity test (see later).

The three-dimensional structure of HLA-A2 has been revealed by X-ray crystallographic analysis, (Bjorkman *et al.* 1987a). The α_3 and β_2m domains have tertiary structures similar to domains in the constant region of immunoglobulins (see Chapter 3). The top of the molecule is formed by pairing the α_1 and α_2 domains, which together form the antigen peptide-binding cleft. The majority of the polymorphic determinants

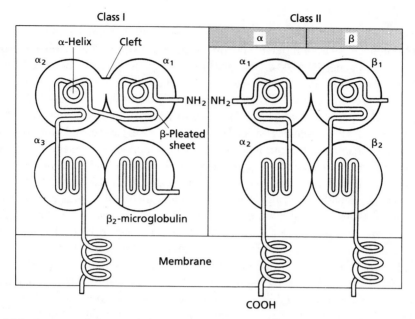

Figure 13.2 Structure of class I and class II HLA molecules, showing domains and transmembrane segments (from Roitt, 1988).

in class I molecules occur on the floor of this cleft, either pointing into it or pointing upwards, which strongly implies that this is the antigen peptide-binding region (Bjorkman *et al.* 1987b) (see Fig. 13.3). Thus, it is now possible to understand the nature of antigen binding to HLA molecules (see below).

The HLA-A, -B and -C antigens are expressed on all nucleated cells except spermatozoa and placental trophoblast; they are also found on platelets but only some class I antigens have been detected on red cells (see Chapter 6). The number of class I antigens on various cells differs and, particularly on platelets, some of the antigens are expressed rather weakly.

The use of a one-dimensional isoelectric focusing technique for the analysis of class I antigens has been shown to be particularly important in recognizing subtypes of HLA-A, -B and -C gene products (Neefjes *et al.* 1986; Frenz *et al.* 1989; Yang, 1989).

The alleles of the class I genes and the class I antigens which have been agreed by the WHO Nomenclature Committee (Bodmer *et al.* 1988; 1991; 1992) are listed in Table 13.1.

Class II genes and antigens
The polymorphism of the class II genes at the DNA level is greater than the polymorphism defined by serological typing and by the MLC test. Molecular genetics has shown that there are at least three series of class II genes: *DR, DQ* and *DP*.

In the DR subregion there is a single α-chain gene (*DRA*) with two alleles whose products have not been recognized. There are nine *DRB* genes, five of which are pseudogenes (*DRB2, DRB6, DRB7, DRB8* and *DRB9*). The presence of seven of the DR

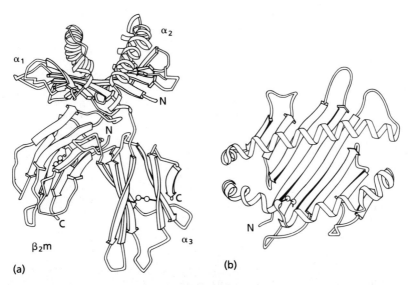

(a)

(b)

Figure 13.3 Schematic representations of the crystallized structure of the HLA-A2 molecule. (a) The four domains, with the α_1 and α_2 domains forming a putative peptide binding region. (b) Top surface of the molecule. The putative antigen binding groove is shown, made up of a β-pleated sheet flanked by two α-helices (from Bjorkman *et al.* 1987a).

genes (except *DRB1* and *DRB9*) is restricted to certain DR haplotypes. The genomic organization of the DR region is shown in Fig. 13.4. The *DRB1*, *DRB3*, *DRB4* and *DRB5* genes encode four separate DR molecules. *DRB1* encodes the major DR antigens detected serologically, whereas the *DRB3* gene codes for DR52, the *DRB4* gene for DR53 and the *DRB5* gene for DR51.

In the DQ subregion there are two α genes *DQA1* and *DQA2* and 3 β genes *DQB1*, *DQB2* and *DQB3*. *DQB3* is a pseudogene. The *DQA1*, *DQB1* and *DQB2* genes are polymorphic but only the products of the *DQB1* gene have been serologically recognized.

In the DP subregion there are also two α and two β genes: *DPA1*, *DPA2*, *DPB1* and *DPB2*. *DPA1* and *DPB1* encode polypeptide chains whereas *DPA2* and *DPB2* are pseudogenes.

In the D region there are three other genes, *DNA*, *DOB* and *DVB*, whose products are as yet unknown.

All class II molecules consist of two transmembrane glycoprotein chains of mol. wt. 33 000 (the heavy or α-chain) and 28 000 (the light or β-chain), respectively (Snary *et al.* 1977b). The extracellular part of both chains consists of two distinct domains: α_1, α_2 and β_1, β_2. The domains distal to the cell surface carry most of the polymorphic determinants. The constant domain near the cell surface is very similar to the constant domain of immunoglobulin heavy chains (Shackleford *et al.* 1980; 1982) (see Fig. 13.2). The class II antigens are detected by alloantibodies and, in some cases, also by monoclonal antibodies, using a complement-dependent cytotoxicity test on isolated B lymphocytes or a two-colour immunofluorescence test on unseparated cells (van Rood *et al.* 1976b).

Table 13.1 Class I alleles and antigens

Allele	Antigen	Allele	Antigen	Allele	Antigen
A*0101	A1	B*0701	B7	Cw*0101	Cw1
A*0201	A2	B*0702	B7	Cw*0102	Cw1
A*0202	A2	B*0703	B703	Cw*0201	Cw2
A*0203	A203	B*0801	B8	Cw*02021	Cw2
A*0204	A2	B*1301	B13	Cw*02022	Cw2
A*0205	A2	B*1302	B13	Cw*0301	Cw3
A*0206	A2	B*1401	B14	Cw*0302	Cw3
A*0207	A2	B*1402	B65(14)	Cw*0401	Cw4
A*0208	A2	B*1501	B62(15)	Cw*0501	Cw5
A*0209	A2	B*1502	B75(15)	Cw*0601	Cw6
A*0210	A210	B*1503	B72(70)	Cw*0701	Cw7
A*0211	A2	B*1504	B62(15)	Cw*0702	Cw7
A*0212	A2	B*1801	B18	Cw*0801	Cw8
A*0301	A3	B*2701	B27	Cw*0802	Cw8
A*0302	A3	B*2702	B27	Cw*1201	—
A*1101	A11	B*2703	B27	Cw*1202	—
A*1102	A11	B*2704	B27	Cw*1301	—
A*2301	A23(9)	B*2705	B27	Cw*1401	—
A*2401	A24(9)	B*2706	B27		
A*2402	A24(9)	B*2707	B27		
A*2403	A2403	B*3501	B35		
A*2501	A25(10)	B*3502	B35		
A*2601	A26(10)	B*3503	B35		
A*2901	A29(19)	B*3504	B35		
A*2902	A29(19)	B*3505	B35		
A*3001	A30(19)	B*3506	B35		
A*3002	A30(19)	B*3701	B37		
A*31011	A31(19)	B*3801	B38(16)		
A*31012	A31(19)	B*3901	B39012		
A*3201	A32(19)	B*3902	B3902		
A*3301	A33(19)	B*4001	B60(40)		
A*3401	A34(10)	B*4002	B40		
A*3402	A34(10)	B*4003	B40		
A*3601	A36	B*4004	B40		
A*4301	A43	B*4005	B4005		
A*6601	A66(10)	B*4101	B41		
A*6602	A66(10)	B*4201	B42		
A*6801	A68(28)	B*4401	B44(12)		
A*6802	A68(28)	B*4402	B44(12)		
A*6901	A69(28)	B*4403	B44(12)		
A*7401	A74(19)	B*4501	B45(12)		
		B*4601	B46		
		B*4701	B47		
		B*4801	B48		
		B*4901	B49(21)		
		B*5001	B50(21)		
		B*5101	B51(5)		
		B*5102	B5102		
		B*5103	B5103		
		B*5201	B52(5)		
		B*5301	B53		
		B*5401	B54(22)		
		B*5501	B55(22)		
		B*5502	B55(22)		
		B*5601	B56(22)		
		B*5602	B56(22)		
		B*5701	B57(17)		
		B*5702	B57(17)		
		B*5801	B58(17)		
		B*7801	B7801		
		B*7901	—		

The numbers in parentheses represent the related public antigens.
* The number which follows represents an allele.
w is used to avoid confusion with the nomenclature of complement.

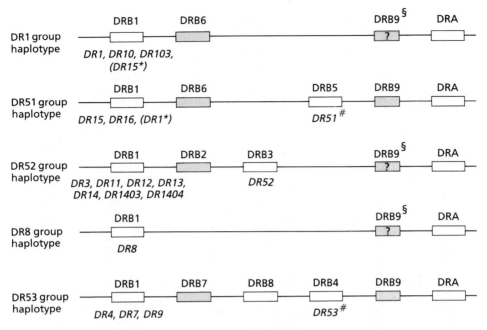

Figure 13.4 Genomic organization of the HLA-DR region and encoded products (specificities) (from Bodmer *et al.* 1992).

Pseudogenes are indicated by shaded boxes, expressed genes by open boxes. The serological specificity encoded by a gene is shown underneath in italics.

* Rarely observed haplotypes.

\# DR51 and DR53 may not be expressed on certain haplotypes.

§ The presence of DRB9 in these haplotypes needs confirmation.

The crystal structure of class II molecules has not yet been established, but a hypothetical model for peptide binding to class II molecules similar to that of class I molecules has been produced (Brown *et al.* 1988). The expression of class II antigens is restricted to B cells and to antigen-presenting cells such as macrophages, dendritic cells and Langerhans, cells. Class II antigens are also present on activated T lymphocytes and some tumour cells (Winchester and Kunkel, 1979).

Two-dimensional gel analysis has shown that class II molecules are more polymorphic than expected from the serological data (Knowles, 1989).

As mentioned above, a polymorphism (Dw) encoded by the *D* region has been defined by using the mixed lymphocyte culture (MLC) and homozygous typing cells. The exact relationship between the Dw factors and the polymorphic determinants encoded by the *DR*, *DQ* and *DP* genes is not known. However, most of the Dw specificities are included in DR specificities and it is therefore probable that the differences in response in the MLC mainly reflect HLA-DR incompatibilities.

The alleles of the class II genes and the class II antigens and determinants which have been agreed by the WHO Nomenclature Committee in 1987 and 1990 (Bodmer *et al.* 1988; 1991) are listed in Table 13.2.

Class III and IV genes
Since the products of these genes are not leucocyte antigens, they will not be discussed

Table 13.2   Class II alleles and antigens or determinants

Allele	Antigen	Allele	Antigen	Allele	Determinant
DRA*0101	—	DQA1*0101	—	DPA1*0101	—
DRA*0102	—	DQA1*0102	—	DPA1*0102	—
DRB1*0101	DR1	DQA1*0103	—	DPA1*0103	—
DRB1*0102	DR1	DQA1*0104	—	DPA1*0201	—
DRB1*0103	DR103	DQA1*0201	—	DPA1*02021	—
DRB1*1501	DR15(2)	DQA1*03011	—	DPA1*02022	—
DRB1*1502	DR15(2)	DQA1*03012	—	DPA1*0301	—
DRB1*1503	DR15(2)	DQA1*0302	—	DPA1*0401	—
DRB1*1601	DR16(2)	DQA1*0401	—	DPB1*0101	DPw1
DRB1*1602	DR16(2)	DQA1*0501	—	DPB1*0201	DPw2
DRB1*0301	DR17(3)	DQA1*05011	—	DPB1*02011	DPw2
DRB1*0302	DR18(3)	DQA1*05012	—	DPB1*02012	DPw2
DRB1*0303	DR18(3)	DQA1*05013	—	DPB1*0202	DPw2
DRB1*0401	DR4	DQA1*0601	—	DPB1*0301	DPw3
DRB1*0402	DR4	DQB1*0501	DQ5(1)	DPB1*0401	DPw4
DRB1*0403	DR4	DQB1*0502	DQ5(1)	DPB1*0402	DPw4
DRB1*0404	DR4	DQB1*05031	DQ5(1)	DPB1*0501	DPw5
DRB1*0405	DR4	DQB1*05032	DQ5(1)	DPB1*0601	DPw6
DRB1*0406	DR4	DQB1*0504		DPB1*0801	—
DRB1*0407	DR4	DQB1*0601	DQ6(1)	DPB1*0901	—
DRB1*0408	DR4	DQB1*0602	DQ6(1)	DPB1*1001	—
DRB1*0409	DR4	DQB1*0603	DQ6(1)	DPB1*1101	—
DRB1*0410	DR4	DQB1*0604	DQ6(1)	DPB1*1301	—
DRB1*0411	DR4	DQB1*0605	DQ6(1)	DPB1*1401	—
DRB1*0412	DR4	DQB1*0606		DPB1*1501	—
DRB1*11011	DR11(5)	DQB1*0201	DQ2(1)	DPB1*1601	—
DRB1*11012	DR11(5)	DQB1*0301	DQ7(3)	DPB1*1701	—
DRB1*1102	DR11(5)	DQB1*0302	DQ8(3)	DPB1*1801	—
DRB1*1103	DR11(5)	DQB1*03031	DQ9(3)	DPB1*1901	—
DRB1*11041	DR11(5)	DQB1*03032	DQ9(3)	DPB1*2001	—
DRB1*11042	DR11(5)	DQB1*0304	DQ7(3)	DPB1*2101	—
DRB1*1105	DR11(5)	DQB1*0401	DQ4	DPB1*2201	—
DRB1*1201	DR12(5)	DQB1*0402	DQ4	DPB1*2301	—
DRB1*1202	DR12(5)			DPB1*2401	—
DRB1*1301	DR13(6)			DPB1*2501	—
DRB1*1302	DR13(6)			DPB1*2601	—
DRB1*1303	DR13(6)			DPB1*2701	—
DRB1*1304	DR13(6)			DPB1*2801	—
DRB1*1305	DR13(6)			DPB1*2901	—
DRB1*1306	DR13(6)			DPB1*3001	—
DRB1*1401	DR14(6)			DPB1*3101	—
DRB1*1402	DR14(6)			DPB1*3201	—
DRB1*1403	DR14(6)			DPB1*3301	—
DRB1*1404	DR14(6)			DPB1*3401	—
DRB1*1405	DR14(6)			DPB1*3501	—
DRB1*1406	DR14(6)			DPB1*3601	—
DRB1*1407	DR14(6)				
DRB1*1408	DR14(6)				
DRB1*1409	DR14(6)				
DRB1*1410	DR14(6)				
DRB1*0701	DR7				
DRB1*0702	DR7				
DRB1*0801	DR8				
DRB1*08021	DR8				
DRB1*08022	DR8				
DRB1*08031	DR8				
DRB1*08032	DR8				
DRB1*0804	DR8				
DRB1*0805	DR8				
DRB1*09011	DR9				
DRB1*09012	DR9				
DRB1*1001	DR10				
DRB3*0101	DR52				
DRB3*0201	DR52				
DRB3*0202	DR52				
DRB3*0301	DR52				
DRB4*0101	DR53				
DRB5*0101	DR51				
DRB5*0102	DR51				
DRB5*0201	DR51				
DRB5*0202	DR51				

The numbers in parentheses represent the related public antigen.

* Means that the number which follows represents an allele of the gene.

w is used because the DP specificities were determined by primed lymphocyte typing.

further. However, it should be mentioned that the Chido and Rodgers blood group antigens are located on the products of the genes which encode the complement factors C4A and C4B (see Chapter 6).

Crossreactions in the HLA system

Sera from subjects alloimmunized against HLA antigens are frequently crossreactive as shown by the following example: a given serum may react with two different serologically defined antigens, e.g. HLA-B51 and HLA-B52, but antibodies recognizing these two specificities individually cannot be separated from that serum. The antibodies in such a serum are in fact directed against a different antigen, HLA-B5 in this example, which occurs together with B51 and B52. Thus the antibodies (anti-B5) crossreact with B51- and B52-positive cells.

The explanation for this kind of crossreactivity is as follows: owing to multiple mutations within the HLA genes, a single allele of a gene may code for different, separate polymorphisms on the single HLA molecule it produces. The frequencies of the epitopes encoded by these different polymorphisms within a single allele differ greatly. Some have a very high frequency, e.g. HLA-B4 and HLA-B6, and are named public or supratypic antigens. At the other end of the scale are antigens with a very low frequency (e.g. 1–2%) which are named private antigens. Thus, epitopes with different frequencies in the population, and against which separate alloantibodies can be made, occur on a single HLA molecule and this is the basis of the crossreactivity: antibodies against public antigens (also called crossreactive antigens) react with cells carrying different private antigens. Public antigens occur together with particular private antigens which form crossreactive groups (CREGs) of (private) antigens. The higher the frequency of the public antigen in the population the more important are antibodies against the antigen for crossreactivity. Thus, anti-HLA-B4 and -B6 are responsible for much of the crossreactivity among the HLA-B antigens.

The occurrence of crossreactive antigens is also responsible for what are called 'splits' of HLA antigens. Frequently a crossreactive antigen, e.g. the antigen B5 as in the above example, was defined before the two private antigens B51 and B52, together with which it occurs. Later, when antibodies recognizing B51 and B52 were found, the B5 antigen was 'split' into B51 and B52 (see Table 13.2).

HLA antigens in plasma

HLA-A2 and HLA-B7 were the first to be demonstrated in plasma (Charlton and Zmijweski, 1970; van Rood et al. 1970). Using monomorphic monoclonal antibodies coated on to immunobeads and one-dimensional isoelectric focusing followed by immunoblotting using specific class I antisera, all serologically defined antigens defined to date have been detected in plasma (Doxiadis and Grosse-Wilde, 1989).

The function of HLA antigens

The main biological function of the HLA molecules is to present antigen to T cells and the HLA antigens therefore play an important role in regulating the immune response. Class I molecules present foreign antigens to cytotoxic T cells (CTL). CTL can only lyse target cells carrying the foreign antigens, provided that, in addition to the foreign antigen for which the CTL carries a specific receptor, the target cell carries class I antigens which are also present on the CTL. The CTL recognizes the antigen accommodated in the groove of the class I molecule on the target cell (see above and Fig. 13.3). This phenomenon, named HLA restriction, was first described in the mouse (Zinkernagel and Doherty, 1974).

The main biological function of class II molecules is also presentation of antigen, particularly to helper T cells, the stimulation of which is required for an effective immune response to most antigens. Class II genes are 'immune response genes' because of this function of their products. Class II antigens thus regulate antigen presentation and the generation of effector T cells (Thorsby, 1984).

Evidently, class II molecules carrying some antigens present certain foreign antigens more efficiently than class II molecules carrying other antigens, and this difference influences the immune response against such foreign antigens. A striking example of this influence in humans is the very strong association of HLA-DR52a with the formation of anti-HPA-1a ($=$ Zw^a, P1^{A1}) in HPA-1(a$-$) subjects (Reznikoff-Etiévant et al. 1981; 1983; Taaning et al. 1983; de Waal et al. 1986; Valentin et al. 1990). Probably, this immune response function of class II antigens is also the basis of the association of these antigens with many diseases in which the immune response is in some way involved.

HLA antibodies

Development of HLA antibodies after transfusion
A very high incidence of HLA antibodies is observed in patients having transfusions from many different donors because such patients are thus exposed to a wide range of HLA antigens. However, even in subjects exposed to the blood of a single donor, the incidence of HLA antibodies is quite high. In a series in which patients awaiting renal grafting were given three transfusions at 2-weekly intervals from a potential donor, who in each case had a haplotype identical with one of the recipient's haplotypes, HLA antibodies developed in some 30% of recipients (Salvatierra et al. 1980).

After massive blood transfusion, which used to be associated with open heart surgery, lymphocytotoxic antibodies and, or, leucoagglutinins may be found in almost all subjects, provided that repeated tests are made, since sometimes the antibodies can be detected only transiently. In a series in which patients were tested at 1 week and usually also at 2, 4 and 12 weeks after open heart surgery, 52 of 54 developed leucocyte antibodies; 12 weeks after transfusion antibodies were present in only 62.5% of the subjects (Gleichmann and Breininger, 1975). The majority of HLA antibodies formed after blood transfusion are directed against class I antigens.

Some patients never become immunized despite repeated transfusions of blood, or of platelets. Such subjects are considered to be non-responders to HLA. HLA antibodies are the most important cause of refractoriness to platelet transfusions (see later) and of febrile transfusion reactions (see Chapter 15).

Development of HLA antibodies in pregnancy
In primiparous women, lymphocytotoxic class I antibodies may be found as early as the 24th week of pregnancy and are present by the last trimester in 10% of women (Overweg and Engelfriet, 1969). Estimates of the incidence of lymphocytotoxic anti-

bodies after a first pregnancy vary widely: 4.3% (Ahrons, 1971), 9.1% (Nymand, 1974), 13% (Overweg and Engelfriet, 1969) and 25% (Goodman and Masaitis, 1967). The discrepancies may well be due to the varying extent of the panels of lymphocytes with which the sera were tested and the sensitivity of the techniques applied. The majority of HLA antibodies developed in pregnancy are directed against class I antigens.

There is a tendency for women to make antibodies against only certain of the HLA antigens to which they are exposed in pregnancy. In multiparous women who had had at least four pregnancies, and were therefore likely to have been exposed to antigens encoded by both of their partner's haplotypes, the frequency of antibodies against only a single paternal antigen was the same as in primiparous women (Tongio et al. 1972).

The specificity of HLA antibodies formed was found to be more commonly anti-HLA-B than anti-HLA-A by Tovey et al. (1973). Similarly, the ratio of B antibodies to A antibodies was found to be 93 : 56 by Minev (1975). Although HLA antibodies are usually immunoglobulin G (IgG), there is no evidence that they damage the fetus.

Monoclonal HLA antibodies
Most murine monoclonal HLA antibodies are directed against non-polymorphic determinants of the HLA molecules (Brodsky et al. 1979; Trucco et al. 1979); some antibodies detect a polymorphism which is different from those detected by allo-antisera (Quaranta et al. 1980). However, many murine monoclonals which recognize HLA antigens as defined by alloantisera have been described, particularly anti-DR and anti-DQ (for a survey of the latter, see Marsh and Bodmer, 1989).

In addition, many human monoclonal HLA antibodies, against both class I and class II antigens, have now been described.

Changes in recipient's lymphocytes after blood transfusion
Following the transfusion of large amounts of fresh or stored blood, changes develop in the recipient's lymphocytes after an interval of about 1 week. Atypical lymphocytes increase by a factor of five or more and, or, there is an increased rate of incorporation of ^{3}H-thymidine in vitro. Values return to the pre-transfusion level by about 3 weeks. Changes are not seen after transfusion of frozen and washed (leucocyte-depleted) red cells (Schechter et al. 1972). Confirmatory observations were published by Hutchinson et al. (1976). The changes are interpreted as a response to donor HLA antigens (presumably of the Dw series) and may be regarded as those of an MLC in vivo.

Some features of HLA antibodies
HLA antibodies formed after blood transfusion or pregnancy are characteristically IgG. They are complement activating and have cytotoxic properties and, like most granulocyte-reactive IgG antibodies, are leucoagglutinins (see below). HLA antibodies may be naturally occurring. Using very sensitive techniques, weak HLA antibodies, particularly anti-B8, have been demonstrated in the serum of about 1% of normal donors who had had no pregnancies or transfusions (Tongio et al. 1985); these antibodies are usually IgM and, in the cytotoxicity test, they react only with B cells, on which class I antigens are more strongly expressed than on T cells.

HLA and tissue grafting

Renal grafts

Significance of HLA antibodies. When HLA antibodies directed against antigens present in the donor are present in the recipient of a renal graft, acute or hyperacute rejection of the graft will occur. It is therefore necessary to do a crossmatch between the patient's serum and the B and T lymphocytes of the donor. Not all antibodies detected in the crossmatch are harmful. IgM B and T cell autoantibodies, which may be present in the serum of dialysis patients and which react better in the cold, are not harmful (see Ting, 1983).

Significance of matching for HLA. In a study for the ninth International Histocompatibility Workshop, of 1973 patients given a first cadaver renal transplant, matching for HLA antigens between donor and recipient was found to be clearly beneficial for graft survival. The best correlation between graft survival and HLA match was observed when the HLA-B and -DR loci were analysed together. Matching for HLA-A gave no further benefit (see Opelz, 1984) a conclusion which was confirmed in a study comprising 4219 patients who received conventional immunosuppressive therapy and 4066 patients who in addition received cyclosporin A (Opelz, 1985).

In the largest and most recent study in which 240 laboratories participated, the results of 30 000 first cadaver kidney transplants were analysed (Opelz, 1988). The influence of HLA matching was investigated separately in cases in which the donor and recipient were typed for all the known 'splits' of the HLA-A and HLA-B antigens and in those in which typing was restricted to the broad antigens. At 3 years there was an 18% difference in survival rates of grafts with zero or four mismatches between donors and recipients typed for A and B antigen splits, but only a 2% difference when typing was restricted to broad antigens. When A, B and DR antigens were considered together, the differences in the rates of survival were 31% and 6%, respectively, in the two groups. It was concluded that typing for antigen splits is important and that the potential benefit of HLA matching in renal transplantation is greater than currently accepted. In another recent study the benefit of matching for HLA-B and HLA-DR was confirmed in 1001 cases (Dyer *et al.* 1989).

It is of interest that the benefit of matching for DR only lasted until approximately 5 months after transplantation, whereas the benefit of matching for HLA-B lasted over the whole 3-year period studied (Thorogood *et al.* 1990). In this study no effect of matching for HLA-A was seen.

For a discussion of the possible effects of Lewis groups on renal transplants see p. 184.

Liver grafts and heart–lung grafts
In some animal models the liver has been found to be 'immunologically privileged' because it is less liable to immunological rejection than, for example, the kidney (Calne *et al.* 1969; Kamada *et al.* 1981). Clinical experience, however, has not demonstrated such privilege in humans (Pichlmayer *et al.* 1987). Thus matching for HLA is probably as important in liver as in kidney transplantation, but is much more difficult in practice, as it also is in heart–lung grafts (Cabrol *et al.* 1987).

Effect of previous transfusion on success of renal graft

As mentioned above, in patients who have antibodies against HLA antigens of the donor, renal grafts undergo acute rejection. On the other hand, blood transfusion has been shown to have a striking effect in improving the survival of subsequent renal grafts in subjects who have not developed cytotoxic antibodies, or who have done so and have received renal grafts from HLA-compatible donors (Opelz *et al.* 1973; van Hooff *et al.* 1976). Leucocytes in the donor blood have been found to be essential for the beneficial effect (Persijn *et al.* 1984).

After the introduction of cyclosporin, the giving of transfusions before grafting was found to confer little additional benefit (Kaban *et al.* 1983; Lundgren *et al.* 1986; Opelz, 1987). However, in a recent survey, transfusions improved the 1-year graft survival rate by 8% ($P < 0.01$) in recipients of a one-DR mismatched graft and by 10% ($P < 0.01$) in recipients of a two-DR mismatched graft (Iwaki *et al.* 1990). Two to four transfusions from random donors were sufficient to obtain this effect. It was concluded that in spite of the use of cyclosporin, the practice of giving deliberate transfusions before grafting should not be abandoned.

When a kidney of a live donor is used, it is possible to give both transfusion and graft from the same donor. Donor-specific blood transfusions (DST) lead to increased graft survival rates (e.g. see Salvatierra *et al.* 1981b; 1986; Kaplan *et al.* 1984). A disadvantage of DST is that the patient may become immunized against HLA antigens of the donor. In animal models it was found that heat treatment of the donor blood (Martinelli *et al.* 1987), or pre-treatment of the recipient with donor leucocytes coated with antilymphocyte antibody, diminished the chance of immunization (Susal *et al.* 1990). Treatment of the patient with azathioprine also had this effect (Anderson *et al.* 1982).

It was also found that immunization occurred significantly less frequently in recipients of transfusions who shared one HLA-DR antigen with the donor than in recipients who were mismatched for two DR antigens (Lagaaij *et al.* 1989). The survival of cadaver kidney grafts in recipients who were given transfusions, and who shared one HLA-DR antigen with the blood donors, was significantly better (81% at 5 years) than in recipients who were given transfusions from donors who were mismatched for both DR antigens (57% at 5 years), or in recipients who were not transfused (45%).

The mechanism responsible for the blood transfusion effect is not known. Several mechanisms have been suggested: (1) the induction of increased suppressor cell activity (Marquet and Heystek, 1981; Quigley *et al.* 1989); (2) decreased natural killer cell activity (Gascon *et al.* 1984); (3) specific unresponsiveness due to idiotype antibodies, which inactivate T cell clones (Woodruff and van Rood, 1983; Kawamura *et al.* 1989); (4) impairment of the function of the mononuclear phagocyte system (MPS) by iron overload (de Sousa, 1983); (5) deletion of clones of cells which are first activated by blood transfusion and then killed or inactivated by high-dose immunosuppressive therapy during the anamnestic response after transplantation (Terasaki, 1984); (6) the production of non-cytotoxic, Fc-receptor-blocking antibodies (McLeod *et al.* 1985; Petranyi *et al.* 1988); and (7) a specific functional clonal deletion of precursors of cytotoxic T lymphocytes, which are 'vetoed' either by donor T cells when there is a class I incompatibility, or by radiation-resistant non-T cells in the case of a class II incompatibility (van Twuyver *et al.* 1989; 1990). Transfusion of blood from a donor who shares one HLA haplotype with the patient, or one HLA-B and one HLA-DR antigen, induces tolerance to donor antigens, probably because low-grade partial chimerism is induced (van Twuyver *et al.* 1991).

Effect of previous transfusion on success of bone marrow grafting

Previous transfusion, particularly from close relatives, prejudices the success of subsequent bone marrow grafting. The chance of rejection of the graft increases with the number of transfusions. If future recipients of a bone marrow graft need to be transfused, they should be given leucocyte-depleted blood, or blood components, from random donors and not from relatives. The discrepancy between the effect of transfusion on grafted bone marrow and the effect on renal grafts has not been explained. The development of graft versus host disease after the transfusion of allogeneic leucocytes is described in Chapter 15.

Effect of transfusion on tumour growth and recurrence of cancer

A retrospective analysis of the recurrence rate of carcinoma of the colon after surgical resection suggested that the 5-year disease-free survival rate was reduced by blood transfusion given at the time of surgery (Burrows and Tartter, 1982). However, the results of numerous subsequent reports are contradictory.

In several studies the effect of blood transfusions was found to be unfavourable, but in several others no difference in the prognosis of transfused and non-transfused patients was observed, e.g. in a prospective study on 58 patients, only 35 of whom received a transfusion (Quintiliani *et al.* 1991).

Experimental models in rats have also yielded conflicting results: allogeneic blood transfusions have been found to inhibit the growth of transplanted tumour cells, to produce mixed results, or to be without effect (Oikawa *et al.* 1977; Marquet *et al.* 1986; Zeller *et al.* 1986). For a survey of the subject, see van Aken (1989). It seems that the important question whether cancer is more likely to recur in patients who have received a blood transfusion needs further evaluation.

Effect of transfusion on infections

In ten of 12 studies in which the association between infection and previous blood transfusions was investigated, it was found that transfusion was significantly associated with an increased risk of bacterial infection (for a survey see Blumberg *et al.* 1990). These studies consistently showed a post-operative infection rate of about 20–30% in patients who received allogeneic transfusions and a rate of 0–10% in patients who were not transfused or who received autologous blood. However, no effect of blood transfusion was seen on bacterial peritonitis in a mouse model (Goldman *et al.* 1991).

Possible role of HLA in habitual abortion

It has been suggested that parental sharing of HLA antigens might be an important immunological factor as a cause of habitual abortion. It is thought that 'blocking antibodies', normally produced by the maternal immune system and which protect the fetus, are absent in such cases (for reviews, see Adinolfi, 1986; Scott *et al.* 1987b). It has been found that non-cytotoxic antibodies, directed against paternal antigens expressed on activated T cells, are detectable in the serum of pregnant women. A strong correlation was found between absence of such antibodies and habitual abortion (B. Genetet, unpublished observations).

Immunization of women with leucocytes has been employed with the object of correcting the immunological unresponsiveness (Taylor and Falk, 1981; Beer et al. 1985). A problem of assessing the benefit of such immunization is that the chance of a successful pregnancy after three abortions is about 60% (Regan, 1991). Only one prospective randomized trial (Mowbray et al. 1987) has shown an apparent benefit; in another trial, no clear advantage of leucocyte injection was observed and the authors expressed their concern about severe growth retardation seen in some fetuses (Beer et al. 1985).

The opinion has been expressed that immune therapy in women with habitual abortion should be restricted to scientific trials until its efficacy has been formally established (Moloney et al. 1989).

OTHER ANTIGENS FOUND ON LEUCOCYTES

Some red cell antigens are also found on leucocytes; see Chapters 4 and 6.

Group 5 system

This system, which is independent of HLA, has two antigens, 5a and 5b, which are present on lymphocytes, granulocytes and platelets (van Rood and Eernisse, 1968) and detectable on red cells in the AutoAnalyzer (Rosenfield et al. 1967a). Anti-5b is the commonest specificity found when the sera of pregnant women are tested for leucoagglutinins (Lawler and Shatwell, 1967). Potent anti-5b agglutinins in transfused plasma can cause transfusion-related acute lung injury (TRALI) (Nordhagen et al. 1986). The gene encoding the antigens of the group 5 system is located on chromosome 4 (van Kessel et al. 1983).

Antigens on granulocytes, monocytes and lymphocytes

Two such antigens have been described: Mart, with a frequency of 99.1% (Kline et al. 1982) and OND, with a frequency of 95%. The Mart antigen is located on the α-chain of the receptor (CR3) for iC3b and OND is located on the α-chain of the LFA-1 molecule (van der Schoot et al. 1992).

Antigens on granulocytes and monocytes

The following antigens have been shown to be present on granulocytes and monocytes: HGA-1 (Thompson et al. 1980a) and the HMA-1 and HMA-2 antigens, products of a bi-allelic gene (Jager et al. 1986). The AYD antigen is shared by granulocytes, monocytes and endothelial cells (Thompson and Severson, 1980). The 9[a] antigen, which was first thought to be granulocyte specific, is also expressed on monocytes (Jager et al. 1986).

Antigens found only on granulocytes (see Table 13.3)

The neutrophil-specific antigens NA1 and NA2 are products of alleles which form a bi-allelic system (Lalezari et al. 1960; Lalezari and Radel, 1974). Exceptions to the

Table 13.3   Antigens found only on granulocytes

Gene (locus)	Antigens	Phenotype frequency (%)	Genotype frequency
NA	NA1	61.2	0.32
	NA2	89.6	0.68
NB	NB1	90.8	0.72
NC	NC1	94.5	0.80
ND	ND1	98.5	0.88
NE	NE1	22.9	0.12
HGA-3	HGA-3a	21.5	0.11
	HGA-3b	23.9	0.13
	HGA-3c	16.1	0.08
	HGA-3d	52.6	0.31
	HGA-3e	17.2	0.09
GA	A,1,2,3,4,5		
GB	B,20,21,22,23,24		
GC	C,40,41,42,43		
GR	GR1		0.18
	GR2		0.35

inheritance of the NA antigens first suggested the possibility of a silent allele at the NA locus (Lalezari *et al.* 1975b; Clay and Kline, 1985). The NA antigens are located on the FcR III of neutrophils (Huizinga *et al.* 1990). The antigens are therefore encoded by the neutrophil FcR III gene. A deletion of this gene has now been convincingly demonstrated (Huizinga *et al.* 1991). The FcR III on neutrophils is a phosphatidylinositol-linked molecule (Huizinga *et al.* 1989).

Other granulocyte-specific antigens which may be specific for neutrophils, are as follows: NB1, NC1, ND1, NE1 and HGA-3a,b,c,d,e (Lalezari *et al.* 1971; Verheugt *et al.* 1978; Claas *et al.* 1979; Thompson *et al.* 1980a) and the less well defined GA, GB, GC antigens and GR1, GR2 antigens (Hasegawa *et al.* 1975; Caplan *et al.* 1977). Most granulocyte-specific antigens have been defined by alloantibodies, but ND1 and NE1 have been defined by autoantibodies. These granulocyte-specific antigens appear to be true differentiation antigens since they appear at the myelocyte or metamyelocyte stage, or even later (Lalezari, 1977; Evans and Mage, 1978; Thompson *et al.* 1980a).

The NB1 antigen is present on a 58–64 kD surface glycoprotein which is also present in secondary granules (Stroncek *et al.* 1990). The NB1 antigen is expressed on only a subpopulation of granulocytes. The percentage of NB1-positive granulocytes varies greatly among healthy subjects (Goldschmeding *et al.* 1992b).

Granulocyte-specific antibodies may be responsible for four different clinical syndromes: (1) neonatal alloimmune neutropenia; (2) febrile reactions following trans-fusion; (3) pulmonary infiltrates following transfusion, often referred to nowadays as acute transfusion-related lung injury (TRALI); and (4) autoimmune neutropenia.

Neonatal alloimmune neutropenia
This syndrome, analogous to haemolytic disease of the newborn, is usually recognized because of infection in a newborn infant. The degree of neutropenia is very severe and

the mother's serum contains potent IgG antibodies against granulocyte-specific antigens (Lalezari and Bernard, 1966).

In reviewing the syndrome, Lalezari and Radel (1974) described results in 19 infants in ten families. The specificity of the antibody in three families was anti-NA1; in one, anti-NA2; in four, anti-NB1; in one, anti-NC1; and in one, not determined. In four of the families the first-born infant was affected.

A prospective survey of some 200 pregnant women, either primiparae at term or multiparae, in which the woman's serum was tested against her partner's granulocytes and lymphocytes, indicated that the incidence of granulocyte-specific antibodies was about 3% (Verheugt et al. 1979). The incidence of diagnosed cases of neonatal alloimmune neutropenia is much lower.

Febrile reactions following transfusion are described in Chapter 15.

Acute transfusion-related lung injury due to transfused leucoagglutinins is described in Chapter 15.

Autoantibodies to granulocytes

In the first case in which it was shown convincingly that autoantibodies may be responsible for neutropenia, a female infant who had had severe infections was found, at the age of 7 months, to have a neutrophil count of $1.0 \times 10^9/l$. It was shown subsequently that the peripheral blood contained less than 3% of mature neutrophils and that the bone marrow contained virtually no mature granulocytes, although it did contain normal granulocyte precursors. The serum contained the neutrophil-specific autoantibody anti-NA2 with a titre of 16–256; the antibody was mainly IgG and the patient was NA(2 +). On steroid therapy the granulocyte count rose to $310 \times 10^9/l$ and the leucoagglutinin titre fell to 2, but on stopping steroids there was a relapse (Lalezari et al. 1975b). Several further cases with autoantibodies to neutrophil-specific alloantigens have been described in which there was a good inverse correlation between the granulocyte count and the potency of the autoantibody; see, for example, McCullough et al. (1988a).

Results in cases of chronic neutropenia or neutropenia accompanying another disease (secondary neutropenia) and in which no specificity of the neutrophil reactive Ig could be found, are difficult to interpret.

Clinically important autoantibodies which react with neutrophil cytoplasmic antigens, but which are not associated with neutropenia, have been described: (1) cANCA (classic antineutrophil cytoplasmic antibody), found mainly in the serum of patients with Wegener's granulomatosis (van der Woude et al. 1985). This autoantibody is directed against a 29-kD serine protease (Goldschmeding et al. 1989); (2) antimyeloperoxidase, found in patients with idiopathic necrotizing and crescentic nephritis or septicaemic arteritis, Wegener's granulomatosis or Churg Strauss syndrome (Falk and Jeunette, 1988; Goldschmeding et al. 1992a).

Treatment of autoimmune neutropenia

Patients with autoimmune neutropenia usually respond to treatment with steroids, but often relapse when the dose of steroids is diminished. Treatment with high-dose intravenous Ig (e.g. 19 mg/kg per day) has been successful in many cases (Pollack *et al.* 1982; Bussel *et al.* 1983).

Drug-induced immune granulocytopenia

Mechanisms responsible for drug-induced immune neutropenia are similar to those involving red cells (see Chapter 7). The classic case of pyramidon-induced granulocytopenia described by Moeschlin and Wagner (1952) is an example of the mechanism in which the drug does not bind firmly to the cells, but in which drug–antibody complexes attach to the cell. Drug-induced neutrophil antibodies may be directed against a metabolite of the drug (Salama *et al.* 1989).

Levamisole may induce the formation of true granulocyte autoantibodies in a way comparable to that in which α-methyldopa induces the formation of red cell autoantibodies (Pegels *et al.* 1980; Thompson *et al.* 1980b).

In many cases, both drug-dependent and true granulocyte autoantibodies are found (Salama *et al.* 1989).

Antigens found only on lymphocytes

In addition to HLA antigens (see above), to some red cell antigens (see Chapter 5), 5a and 5b antigens, and antigens also present on granulocytes and monocytes, lymphocytes carry antigens which do not occur on other cells.

Alloantigens on T_γ and, or, T_μ lymphocytes, encoded by genes outside the HLA system, have been described (Ferrara *et al.* 1979; van Leeuwen, 1979; van Leeuwen *et al.* 1980). Two bi-allelic systems, one on T_γ cells with the antigens TCA1 and TCA2, and one on T_μ cells with the antigens TCB1 and TCB2, were described by van Leeuwen *et al.* (1982a). Non-HLA antigens detectable only on activated T lymphocytes were described by Gerbase de Lima *et al.* (1981) and Wollman *et al.* (1984). The clinical significance of these lymphocyte-specific alloantigens is still uncertain. However, a case of alloimmune lymphocytopenia of the newborn, due to maternal lymphocyte-specific antibodies, resulting in severe combined immune deficiency was reported by Bastian *et al.* (1984).

Cold autoantibodies to lymphocytes

Anti-I and anti-i, see Chapter 4.

Other cold autoantibodies. In patients with various diseases, including systemic lupus erythematosus (SLE), and in some normal subjects, cold autolymphocytotoxins unreactive with red cells are found; their specificity has not been determined, but some of them were found to be reactive only with T cells (Michlmayr *et al.* 1976), T_μ and B cells (Meyer *et al.* 1982) or subpopulations of T cells (Abe *et al.* 1983; Yamada *et al.* 1985). The cell specificity of these cold cytotoxins correlates with a deficiency of the corresponding cell population in the circulation. One report suggested that cold autolymphocytotoxins may be responsible for acute tubular necrosis in transplanted cadaver kidneys and that this damage can be mitigated by warming the kidney before transplantation (Lobo *et al.* 1980). More work has to be done before the clinical significance of these antibodies can be properly evaluated.

Lymphocyte autoantibodies reactive at 37°C in vitro
An investigation of lymphocytotoxic activity in the serum of 59 patients with hypogammaglobulinaemia showed that this condition is only rarely caused by autoantibodies (MacDonald *et al.* 1982). Two exceptions have been described: a patient with
hypogammaglobulinaemia associated with ulcerative colitis and with cytotoxic autoantibodies reacting with B lymphocytes at 37°C (Tursz *et al.* 1977), and a patient with
acquired hypogammaglobulinaemia with autoantibodies specific for T helper cells,
leading to increased activity of T suppressor cells (Rubinstein *et al.* 1981).

Antilymphocyte antibodies have also been found in patients with AIDS or AIDS-
related complex (Klosters *et al.* 1984). Antibodies reactive with both T and B cells, with
T cells only, and with HLA class II antigens have been described (Kiprov *et al.* 1984;
Tomar *et al.* 1985; de la Barrera *et al.* 1987). These antibodies are thought to
contribute to the development of immunodeficiency.

Antigens found only on monocytes
In addition to HLA class I and class II antigens, and the antigens shared by monocytes
and granulocytes mentioned above, monocytes carry alloantigens which do not occur
on other blood cells. Some of these antigens (EM antigens) are also present on
endothelial cells (Moraes and Stastny, 1977; Claas *et al.* 1980; Cerilli *et al.* 1981;
Stastny and Nunez, 1981); others are monocyte specific (Baldwin *et al.* 1983b; Paul
et al. 1984; Cerilli *et al.* 1985). Antibodies against EM antigens are detrimental to
transplanted kidneys and may be involved in graft versus host disease. Anti-EM
antibodies and antibodies reacting with monocytes, tubular endothelium and kidney
cells in the cortex can be eluted from rejected kidneys (Joyce *et al.* 1988). The
significance of monocyte-specific alloantibodies needs further evaluation.

TESTS FOR LEUCOCYTE ANTIBODIES AND ANTIGENS

HLA antibodies
In detecting antibodies against class I determinants, the lymphocytotoxicity test is most
commonly used. For the detection of DQ and DR antibodies, the two-colour fluorescence test as described by van Rood *et al.* (1976b) is often used. Alternatively,
separated B lymphocytes can be used in the lymphocytotoxicity test to detect anti-DR
and anti-DQ. Lymphocytes which have been frozen have proved to be entirely satisfactory for this purpose. Dw determinants are detected using MLC and homozygous typing
cells (see below).

HLA antigens
In serological typing for HLA antigens the same techniques are used as for detecting
antibodies. There is a great deal of crossreactivity between molecules carrying
particular HLA antigens encoded by alleles of each gene, e.g. between molecules
carrying A1, A3 or A11 (see p. 601). Crossreactivity and the lack of antisera with a
single specificity lead to difficulties in HLA typing; therefore several antisera must
be used in typing for any particular antigen. As mentioned above, another technique
for detecting HLA determinants is one-dimensional isoelectric focusing; for a

description of this technique, see Neefjes *et al.* (1986). Dw and DP determinants are detected using MLC reaction and homozygous typing cells. For DP this technique is being replaced by DNA typing and by typing with monoclonal antibodies (Bodmer *et al.* 1987).

HLA genes and alleles

As described above, techniques are now available for studying HLA genes and even particular alleles at the DNA level. These techniques are particularly important for determining class II genes since reliable sera recognizing their products are very scarce or are not available.

Lymphocytotoxicity test

This is the standard test for determining HLA class I antigens. Lymphocytes are incubated with antibody and rabbit complement, and a dye (trypan blue or eosin) is then added; if the lymphocytes carry an antigen corresponding to the antibody, complement is fixed, the cell membrane is damaged, and dye enters the cell and stains it (blue or red). The percentage of stained cells is counted. Live cells are unstained, smaller and refractile. It is essential to use a pure lymphocyte suspension since platelets carry A, B and C antigens and granulocytes are always killed in the cytotoxic assay and stain aspecifically. Details of the NIH-recommended lymphocytotoxicity test, using microdroplets, were given by Terasaki *et al.* (1973).

For the determination of DR and DQ antigens by lymphocytotoxicity, B lymphocytes can be isolated: (1) by removing the T lymphocytes from a lymphocyte suspension by rosetting with 2-aminoethylisothiouronium bromide-treated sheep red cells, the T cell rosettes being removed by centrifugation on ficoll-hypaque (density 1.077) (see Pellegrino *et al.* 1976); (2) by the use of nylon fibre columns (see Wernet *et al.* 1977); or (3), best of all, by the use of magnetic beads coated with monoclonal antibodies specific for class II epitopes (Vartdal *et al.* 1986). For DR and DQ typing the antisera must first be absorbed with pooled platelets to remove class I antibodies.

Monoclonal anti-HLA reagents, if available, have the great advantage of being monospecific.

The mixed lymphocyte culture

This test was described by Bain *et al.* (1964). The principle is to irradiate, or add a substance such as mitomycin C to, one sample, e.g. the donor's, and to mix these lymphocytes with those from another subject, e.g. a potential recipient. Irradiation, or treatment with mitomycin C, prevents lymphocytes from transforming to blast cells but does not destroy their ability to stimulate other lymphocytes, i.e. their antigens are left intact. Blast transformation of the untreated lymphocytes indicates that they have recognized a foreign antigen on the treated lymphocytes (see Bach and Voynow, 1966), and this transformation can be assessed by measuring the incorporation of tritiated thymidine (one-way MLC).

In the MLC the lymphocytes which stimulate are B cells and monocytes carrying Dw determinants and class II antigens. Those that respond are T cells (Potter and Moore, 1977).

If irradiated or mitomycin C-treated stimulator cells, homozygous for a Dw determinant (homozygous typing cells, or HTC), are used they can only stimulate untreated lymphocytes which do not carry the Dw determinant for which they are homozygous. Thus, panels of HTC are used to identify Dw determinants (Bradley *et al.* 1972).

The two-way MLC, in which the lymphocytes in both samples are able to respond by blast formation, is used as a final test for HLA identity of donors and recipients of bone marrow who are serologically identical.

Granulocyte antibodies

In detecting granulocyte-specific antibodies, (1) granulocyte agglutination and (2) immunofluorescence with paraformaldehyde-fixed granulocytes and fluorescein-labelled F(ab')$_2$ fragments of anti-Ig are widely used. A granulocyte cytotoxicity test has also been used but its value now seems doubtful since no correlation has been found between the results of this test and *in vivo* survival of granulocytes (McCullough *et al.* 1981; 1982). Antigen capture assays, which have been described for the detection of platelet antibodies, can also be applied with granulocytes. For a description of these techniques, see pp. 628–629.

The granulocyte agglutination technique

Pure granulocyte suspensions are prepared by dextran sedimentation of EDTA-anticoagulated blood followed by centrifugation of the supernatant on ficoll-hypaque (density 1.077), and the contaminating red cells in the cell pellet are lysed with ammonium chloride or distilled water. Agglutination is carried out in microplates.

Granulocytes, in contrast to red cells and platelets, are agglutinated by two different mechanisms: (1) like red cells and platelets they are agglutinated by crosslinking of cells by IgM antibodies; (2) an entirely different mechanism is responsible for agglutination of granulocytes by IgG antibodies. In this case agglutination results from a response to sensitization by antibodies, which requires active cell participation. Sensitization does not lead to immediate agglutination but to the formation of pseudopods. The granulocytes slowly move towards each other until membrane contact is established (Lalezari and Radel, 1974). This process is time and temperature (37°C) dependent. It is not clear whether agglutination is due to changes in membrane-bound molecules which cause granulocytes to adhere to each other, or whether IgG antibodies on one granulocyte adhere to Fc receptors on other granulocytes. In any case, both IgM and IgG antibodies can be detected in the granulocyte agglutination test. Both granulocyte-specific and HLA-A, -B and -C antibodies are detected, but HLA antibodies are better detected by the lymphocytotoxicity test.

Granulocyte immunofluorescence technique (GIFT)

Purified suspensions of granulocytes are prepared as described above. The granulocytes are fixed with paraformaldehyde, incubated with the serum to be tested, then washed and finally incubated with fluorescein-isothiocyanate-labelled anti-Ig serum. In fact, the Fab or F(ab')$_2$ fragments of the IgG fraction of anti-human Ig are used because whole IgG anti-Ig tends to bind to the Fc receptor on granulocytes. With the above modifications, the fluorescein-labelled antiglobulin test is more sensitive than granulocyte agglutination for the detection of IgG antibodies (Verheugt *et al.* 1977).

Again, both granulocyte-specific and HLA-A, -B, -C antibodies are detected, but HLA antibodies are better detected by the lymphocytotoxicity test.

Unfortunately, with the GIFT, not only antibodies but also preformed immune complexes cause positive reactions, due to adherence to Fc and complement receptors (Camussi *et al.* 1979; Engelfriet *et al.* 1984a). There are three possible ways of distinguishing between antibodies and fixed immune complexes: (1) preparation of an eluate from positively reacting granulocytes. Eluted antibodies will again react with granulocytes while immune complexes are usually dissociated by the elution procedure (Helmerhorst *et al.* 1982); (2) testing the serum under investigation in an ADCC assay on granulocytes; or (3) blocking Fc receptors on target granulocytes with monoclonal antibodies (Engelfriet *et al.* 1984). In practice, it is very difficult to distinguish between autoantibodies and bound immune complexes, because there are seldom enough cells to prepare an eluate and because the results of the ADCC assay on patient's granulocytes are difficult to interpret.

ANTIGENS ON PLATELETS

Antigens shared with other cells

HLA antigens. There is evidence that the presence of HLA-A, -B, -C antigens on platelets is due primarily to adsorption of HLA antigens from plasma (Lalezari and Driscoll, 1982). The number of some of the class I antigens on platelets (e.g. B8, B44) varies greatly in different subjects. D-region antigens are not detectable on platelets.

Red cell antigens found also on platelets. ABH, Lewis, I, i and P antigens on platelets are described in Chapter 4. Using a sensitive two-stage radioimmunoassay the major antigens of the Rh, Duffy, Kell, Kidd and Lutheran systems have been shown to be absent from platelets (Dunstan *et al.* 1984).

Antigens found on platelets and not on other blood cells (see Table 13.4)
Several systems have been defined whose antigens in the peripheral blood occur only on platelets. Some of these antigens are also found on other cells such as endothelial cells. A new nomenclature for these antigens has recently been accepted by the International Society of Blood Transfusion and the International Committee for Standardisation in Hematology (von dem Borne and Décary, 1990). These platelet-specific antigen systems are named human platelet antigen (HPA) systems; the systems are numbered in the order of the date of publication and the antigens are designated alphabetically in the order of their frequency in the population.

HPA-1 system (Zw, Pl^A)
The first system to be described was recognized by van Loghem *et al.* (1959) when a serum was found which would agglutinate some samples of platelets but not others; the antigen was named Zw^a when an antithetical antigen (Zw^b) was recognized (van der Weerdt *et al.* 1963). The system is now named HPA-1 and the antigens, HPA-1a and HPA-1b. Ninety-eight per cent of Caucasian subjects are HPA-1(a +) and 27%, HPA-1 (b +).

Table 13.4 Alloantigens found on platelets and not on other blood cells

Gene (locus)	Antigens	Phenotype frequency in Caucasians (%)	Gene frequency in Caucasians (%)
HPA-1 (Zw, P1^A)	HPA-1a (Zw^a, P1^{A1})	97.6	0.855
	HPA-1b (Zw^b, P1^{A2})	26.8	0.155
HPA-2 (Ko, Sib)	HPA-2a (Ko^b)	99.4	0.923
	HPA-2b (Ko^a, Sib^a)	14.3	0.074
HPA-3 (Bak, Lek)	HPA-3a (Bak^a, Lek^a)	87.7	0.63
	HPA-3b (Bak^b)	60.3	0.37
HPA-4 (Pen, Yuk)	HPA-4a (Pen^a, Yuk^b)	99.9*	0.99*
	HPA-4b (Pen^b, Yuk^a)	1.7	0.01
HPA-5 (Br, Hc, Zav)	HPA-5a (Br^b, Zav^b)	99.2	0.89
	HPA-5b (Br^a, Zav^a, Hc^a)	20.6	0.10
DUZO	DUZO	18.0	0.094
Pl^E	Pl^{E1}	99.9	0.968
	Pl^{E2}	5.0	0.025
Pl^T	P1^{T1}	98	> 0.98
Gov	Gov^a	81	0.532
	Gov^b	74	0.468
Sr	Sr^a	0.01	

* Frequency in Japanese people.

A complement-fixing antibody described by Shulman et al. (1961) reacting with an antigen Pl^{A1} was subsequently shown to have the same specificity as anti-Zw^a. HPA-1a and HPA-1b are alleles. Anti-HPA-1a is associated with most cases of post-transfusion purpura and alloimmune neonatal thrombocytopenia (NATP).

HPA-1a and -1b antigen sites are situated on the membrane glycoprotein IIIa (Kunicki and Aster, 1979; van der Schoot et al. 1986). The HPA-1 polymorphism is due to the substitution of a single base pair in the coding DNA at position 33, coding for leucine in HPA-1a and for proline in HPA-1b (Newman et al. 1989). Patients with Glanzmann's thrombocytopenia type I have no detectable membrane glycoprotein IIIa (or IIb) on their platelets and are therefore unable to express the HPA-1 antigens (Kunicki et al. 1981a; van Leeuwen et al. 1981). Glanzmann's disease may therefore also be called 'Zw (HPA-1)-null disease' (van Leeuwen et al. 1981; Devine and Rosse, 1984).

The HPA-1 polymorphism seems to be absent in Japanese people (Shibata et al. 1986a).

HPA-2 system (Ko)
A second bi-allelic system, Ko (HPA-2), was described by van der Weerdt et al. (1962).

Sixteen per cent of subjects were found to be HPA-2 (b +) (Ko (a +)) and 99% were HPA-2 (a +) (Ko (b +)). Like anti-HPA-1a, anti-HPA-2a and -2b were detected by platelet agglutination. The HPA-2 antigens are situated on GPIb/IX (Kuijpers *et al.* 1989). The polymorphism is due to the substitution of a single nucleotide in the DNA at position 434 which codes for the β-chain of GPIb, to give methionine in HPA-2b and threonine in HPA-2a at position 145 (Kuijpers *et al.* 1992a).

A platelet antigen Sib[a], described by Saji *et al.* (1989), was shown to be identical to Ko[a] (Kuijpers *et al.* 1989).

HPA-3 system (Bak, Lek)

The platelet antigen, Bak[a] (HPA-3a) is present in about 90% of the Dutch population (von dem Borne *et al.* 1980). The first example of anti-HPA-3a was responsible for NATP.

An antigen, Lek[a], at first found to be closely associated serologically with Bak[a] (Boizard and Wautier, 1984) was subsequently shown to be identical with it (von dem Borne and van der Plas-van Dalen, 1986).

HPA-3a is present on glycoprotein IIb (Kieffer *et al.* 1984; van der Schoot *et al.* 1986). The antigen HPA-3b, antithetical to HPA-3a, was described independently by Kickler *et al.* (1988a) and Kiefel *et al.* (1989a). In both cases anti-HPA-3b was responsible for post-transfusion purpura. The HPA-3 polymorphism is also due to the substitution of a single base pair in the coding DNA, to give isoleucine at amino acid residue 843 in HPA-3a and serine in HPA-3b (Lyman *et al.* 1990).

HPA-4 system (Pen, Yuk)

Another bi-allelic system, Yuk (HPA-4) was described by Shibata *et al.* (1986a,b). Both the low frequency antigen Yuk[a] (HPA-4b) and the high frequency antigen Yuk[b] (HPA-4a) were detected with antibodies which were responsible for NATP.

The antigen, Pen[a], which had been described by Friedman and Aster (1985), proved to be identical with Yuk[b] (R.H. Aster and Y. Shibata, unpublished observation). HPA-4a is present on GPIIIa (Furihata *et al.* 1987; Santoso *et al.* 1987). The HPA-4 polymorphism may be absent in the Caucasian population (Friedman and Aster, 1985; Kiefel *et al.* 1988). The Yuk polymorphism is due to the substitution of a single nucleotide in the DNA which encodes the GPIIIa protein, coding for arginine at position 526 in HPA-4a and for glutamine in HPA-4b (Wang *et al.* 1991).

HPA-5 system (Br, Hc, Zav)

The antigens Br[a](HPA-5b) and Br[b](HPA-5a) were described by Kiefel *et al.* (1988; 1989b). The HPA-5 antigens are present on glycoprotein Ia (Kiefel *et al.* 1989b; Santoso *et al.* 1989). Anti-HPA-5a and -5b have been responsible for NATP. Most HPA-5 antibodies are unreactive in the immunofluorescence test and can best be detected by a glycoprotein-specific assay (see below). The lack of reactivity is probably due to the low number of antigenic sites (Kiefel *et al.* 1989b). The bi-allelic Zav system described by Smith *et al.* (1989) is identical with HPA-5, and the antigen Hc[a] (Woods *et al.* 1989) is the same as HPA-5b.

Obsolete systems and systems not yet included in the HPA nomenclature

DUZO. Moulinier (1957), using the antiglobulin consumption technique, demonstrated a platelet antibody in the serum of a woman whose four children had died from neonatal purpura. The corresponding antigen was termed 'DUZO'. However, no second example of anti-DUZO has been found and this antigen has therefore become obsolete.

Pl^E system. The two alleles of this system (Pl^{E1} and Pl^{E2}) were defined by Shulman *et al.* (1962; 1964). This system has not been included in the HPA nomenclature because anti-Pl^{E1} was probably an isoantibody from a patient with Bernard–Soulier syndrome and anti-Pl^{E2} is no longer available (Shulman and Jordan, 1987).

Pl^T antigen. An antigen, Pl^T, with a very high frequency was described by Beardsley *et al.* (1987). It is present on glycoprotein V.

Gov system. A bi-allelic system with the alleles Gov^a and Gov^b was reported by Kelton *et al.* (1990). Anti-Gov^a was found in a patient with post-transfusion purpura.

Sr antigen. An antigen, Sr^a, which has been detected in only a single family, has been described (Kroll *et al.* 1990). The Sr^a antibodies by which it was defined were responsible for NATP. The antigen is located on GP IIIa.

Nak. The antigen Nak^a is absent in 3–11% of Japanese people and is present on GPIV (Ikeda *et al.* 1989). However, the Nak antigen appears to be a non-polymorphic determinant of GPIV, Nak (a –) subjects being deficient for GPIV. Anti-Nak therefore is not an alloantibody, but an isoantibody (Yamamoto *et al.* 1990c).

Presence of platelet-'specific' antigens on other cells
The antigens of the HPA-1 system are present on endothelial cells (Leeksma *et al.* 1987; Giltay *et al.* 1988a). HPA-1a has also been detected on vascular smooth muscle cells and fibroblasts (Giltay, 1988b).

As mentioned above, the HPA-5 antigens are present on the glycoprotein Ia–IIa complex which is also known as VLA2 (very late activation antigen 2) (Pischel *et al.* 1988), e.g. the VLA2 molecule of activated T cells (Santoso *et al.* 1989). The HPA-5 antigens are probably also present on endothelial cells, which also express VLA2. The antigen Hc^a (Woods *et al.* 1989), which is identical with HPA-5b, is also present on the VLA2 molecule.

Alloimmunization to platelet antigens

Diminished platelet survival following repeated transfusion
In patients who receive repeated transfusions, platelet survival may become progressively shorter, presumably due to the formation of antibodies reactive with platelets (Sprague *et al.* 1952; Stefanini *et al.* 1952).

In two subjects studied by Aster and Jandl (1964), following repeated transfusions the survival of the transfused platelets was reduced even though no platelet antibodies could be detected. In one recipient three successive platelet transfusions were given from the same donor; platelet survival was normal after the first two transfusions but after the third the disappearance half-time was 19 h and surface counting indicated clearance in the spleen. In the second recipient, after a sixth platelet transfusion the platelets were removed with a half-time of less than 30 min, with clearance in the liver and spleen. Although platelet antibodies were not detected in these two cases the only tests used were agglutination and complement binding and it is known that these tests fail to detect most alloantibodies reactive with platelets (see below).

In determining the success of platelet transfusion, estimation of the increase in the platelet count 1 h after transfusion is valuable. A method of standardizing results, to give a 'corrected count increment' is described on p. 648.

Role of HLA class I antibodies in refractoriness to platelet transfusions

According to Shulman (1966), platelet antibodies can be detected in 5% of subjects who have received one to ten transfusions, in 24% of those who have received 25 to 50 transfusions, and in 80% of those who have received more than 100 transfusions. It has since been observed that whereas only 40–70% of patients with leukaemia become immunized by transfusion (Dutcher *et al.* 1981b; Holohan *et al.* 1981), the number is much higher (88–100%) in patients with aplastic anaemia (Dutcher *et al.* 1980; Holohan *et al.* 1981), probably because these patients do not receive immuno-suppressive therapy.

The great majority of patients who become alloimmunized after receiving multiple transfusions of platelets from random donors have antibodies directed against HLA class I antigens (Schiffer *et al.* 1976).

In some patients the titre of HLA antibodies decreases or the antibodies may even become undetectable despite continued transfusion of platelets from random donors. In most cases, after becoming undetectable, the antibodies do not reappear and the increment after transfusion of platelets from random donors then remains satisfactory (Lee and Schiffer, 1987; see also McGrath *et al.* 1988).

Role of platelet-specific antibodies

Even when HLA-matched platelets, either from close relatives or from random donors, are given, 19% of recipients become refractory, suggesting that platelet-specific alloantibodies may also be responsible for refractoriness (Schiffer, 1987). However, cases in which platelet-specific antibodies responsible for refractoriness have been identified have only recently been described, i.e. anti-HPA-2b (Saji *et al.* 1989) and anti-Nak^a (Ikeda *et al.* 1989). In both cases, the response to antigen-negative platelets was good. In some patients, the formation of platelet-specific antibodies is transient (McGrath *et al.* 1988). The management of alloimmunized patients is described below.

Prevention of alloimmunization against HLA class I antigens

There is strong evidence that it is the leucocytes in the platelet concentrate rather than the platelets themselves which induce the formation of HLA antibodies. In rats and mice purified platelets do not induce the formation of antibodies against histocompatibility antigens (Welsh *et al.* 1977; Claas *et al.* 1981). Formation of such antibodies occurs if the platelet suspension is contaminated with leucocytes, but platelets alone are capable of inducing an anamnestic immune response.

In the first study in humans, admittedly unrandomized, of patients transfused with platelet concentrates containing 10–20% of the leucocytes present in whole blood, 26 of 28 (93%) became refractory to transfusion of platelets from random donors. In a subsequent period 68 patients were transfused with red cells filtered through cotton wool, which removed 97% of the leucocytes, or with leucocyte-poor platelet concentrates obtained by an additional centrifugation step (residual leucocytes 5×10^6 per unit). Of these 68 patients, only 16 (24%) became refractory (Eernisse and Brand, 1981).

Similar results have been obtained by many others, notably in randomized studies (Murphy *et al.* 1986; Andreu *et al.* 1988; Sniecinski *et al.* 1988; Saarinen *et al.* 1990; van Marwijk Kooy *et al.* 1991).

In a large prospective study, 21% of patients (69 of 335) who had not been previously transfused developed lymphocytotoxic antibodies after transfusion of filtered red cell concentrates and leucocyte-poor platelet concentrates obtained by an additional centrifugation step. However, only 31 of the 69 developed antibodies of multiple specificities, necessitating transfusion of HLA-matched platelets. More female patients who had been pregnant (21%) became refractory than female patients who had not, or male patients, or children (9%), which illustrates the importance of pre-sensitization (Brand *et al.* 1988).

Although foreign antigen is presented to helper T cells by the subject's own HLA class II-positive antigen presenting cells (APCs), it seems that for the presentation of foreign class I antigens, class II-positive APCs of the donor are essential (Lechler and Batchelor, 1982; Sherwood *et al.* 1986).

Dendritic cells of donor origin are probably the class II-positive donor cells responsible for antigen presentation (Deeg *et al.* 1988). Thus, alloimmunization against class I antigens should be prevented when class-II positive cells have been either removed from red cell or platelet concentrates, or have been inactivated.

Removal of leucocytes
In deciding which is the best method for preparing leucocyte-poor platelet concentrates, and red cell concentrates, the minimum number of leucocytes capable of inducing alloimmunization against class I antigens should be the decisive factor. Unfortunately this number is not exactly known. However, the results of Sirchia *et al.* (1982) suggested that HLA immunization does not occur when red cell concentrates with fewer than 10^6 leucocytes are transfused. Similarly, no HLA immunization was seen in patients receiving platelet concentrates containing fewer than 5×10^6 leucocytes, whereas five of 12 patients receiving 15×10^6 leucocytes developed HLA antibodies (Fisher *et al.* 1985). No immunization occurred in 47 patients (21 in one series and 26 in another) transfused with platelet concentrates containing fewer than 10^6 leucocytes per unit (Saarinen *et al.* 1990).

Considering these figures, it is assumed that to avoid primary immunization against HLA class I antigens the total number of leucocytes transfused in a red cell or platelet concentrate must be less than 10^7. The only available method of achieving this figure is filtration through cotton wool, cellulose acetate or polyester.

Many different filters are available, but not all of them are satisfactory. Fewer than 10^7 leucocytes were counted in red cell concentrates from single units filtered through the following filters: Sepacell R-500 (Pikul *et al.* 1989; Bodensteiner, 1990; Reverberi and Menini, 1990); Erypur (Pikul *et al.* 1989; Reverberi and Menini, 1990); Cell Select (Pietersz *et al.* 1989a); Cell Select A (Pietersz *et al.* 1989a); Pall RC 50 (Bodensteiner, 1990); Leucostop and Leucoseize (Reverberi and Menini, 1990); and Erypur Prestomat (Pikul *et al.* 1989).

Using the Pall 100 and the Imugard IG 500 filters, many filtered red cell concentrates contained more than 10^7 leucocytes (Freedman *et al.* 1991). After a second filtration the number of residual leucocytes was always $< 5 \times 10^6$. Of filtered six-unit platelet concentrates 25% contained $> 5 \times 10^6$ leucocytes, but after a second filtration all concentrates had fewer than 10^6 leucocytes (see further below). The effectiveness of leucocyte depletion depended on the pre-filtration white cell count. The residual white cells contained more HLA class II-positive cells after filtration through the polyester filter (Pall 100) than through the cotton wool (Imugard 500) filter.

The very low numbers of leucocytes in filtered concentrates can be determined accurately only by using special methods: red cells can be lysed using ammonium chloride and platelets can be removed using bovine collagen (Vakkila and Myllyla, 1987). Using propidium iodide (PI) to stain the nuclei of leucocytes, one cell per microlitre of platelet concentrate or 11 cells per microlitre of red cell concentrate can be detected (Kao and Scornik, 1989). With PI staining and a flow cytometric technique, counts as low as one leucocyte per microlitre could be reproducibly determined (Bodensteiner, 1989).

To obtain sufficiently low numbers of residual leucocytes, the buffy coat should be removed from red cell concentrates before filtration (Sirchia *et al.* 1982).

For the removal of leucocytes from platelet concentrates the cotton wool filter Imugard IG 500 has been found to be satisfactory using a pool of platelets from eight, five or four units of blood (Sirchia *et al.* 1983; Brubaker and Romnie, 1988; Saarninen *et al.* 1990). The polyester filter Sepacell R-500 removes more than 90% of the platelets (Snyder *et al.* 1988). Platelet recovery is, however, satisfactory if the polyester is coated with the polymer HE X as in the Sepacell-PL filter. Using this filter, the number of residual leucocytes after filtration of a pool of the platelets from ten donors was $0.1–0.2 \times 10^7$ (Miyamoto *et al.* 1989). With another polyester filter, the PL-100, platelet recovery was satisfactory, as was the number of residual leucocytes (Kickler *et al.* 1989; Patten, 1989). Platelet recovery is poor after filtration through cellulose acetate filters, such as the Erypur filter (Brubaker and Romnie, 1988). This problem is overcome if Iloprost, a stable prostacycline 12 analogue, is added to the concentrate (van Marwijk Kooy *et al.* 1989).

In filtering platelet concentrates, the number of units in the pool is important. Using the PL-100 filter, the filtered concentrate contained too many leucocytes when ten units were pooled (Patten and Patel, 1989), but not when six units were pooled (Kickler *et al.* 1989).

A concern regarding the use of leucocyte-depleted concentrates in leukaemic patients is that the duration of the remission of leukaemia has been found to be significantly better in patients receiving standard concentrates than in patients receiving leucocyte-depleted concentrates (Tucker *et al.* 1989). A possible explanation is that graft versus host disease, which is prevented by the removal of leucocytes, has an antileukaemic effect (Weiden *et al.* 1979). An important question is whether all red cell and platelet concentrates should be filtered to prevent immunization against HLA class I antigens. The use of 'bedside' filters appears to be convenient but these filters are as expensive as filters designed for laboratory use and they tend to clog, so that filtration of units in the laboratory is preferable. In any case, it has yet to be established decisively that, in the long term, leucocyte-depleted concentrates fail to induce HLA class I alloimmunization. Furthermore, some patients have already been immunized by previous transfusions or pregnancies. Leucocyte depletion is unnecessary for non-responders, although these subjects cannot at present be identified. Finally, leucocyte depletion is also unnecessary in patients who receive platelet transfusion during a single short episode (not more than a few days). Because of these considerations there is at present no consensus of opinion on the routine application of filtration.

The methods described above aim to remove all but 10^6 or fewer of the leucocytes from each unit of red cells or platelet concentrate, with the object of completely preventing primary immunization to HLA antigens. A routine method has been described in which platelet-rich plasma is prepared by differential centrifugation of the buffy coat from a unit of blood and which results in contamination of platelet concentrates with fewer than about 10^7 leucocytes per concentrate (Pietersz *et al.* 1987). Using a similar method, evidence was obtained that alloimmunization occurred much less frequently than with platelet concentrates from which leucocytes had not been removed (Brand *et al.* 1988).

Inactivation of HLA class II-positive cells
Ultraviolet (UV-B, 280–320 nm) light-irradiated white cells are incapable of stimulating allogeneic responder cells in MLC (Lindahl-Kiessling and Safwenberg, 1971). Because such stimulation is induced by metabolically active HLA class II-positive cells, this finding indicates that such cells are inactivated by UV irradiation. As mentioned above, these cells, and notably dendritic cells, are essential for the induction of primary alloimmunization against HLA class I antigens. To discover whether UV irradiation of class II-positive cells would prevent such alloimmunization, experiments were carried out in dogs. Animals which had received three transfusions of blood from a bone marrow donor before transplantation invariably rejected the marrow graft, but marrow grafts were not rejected by dogs which had received irradiated donor blood (Deeg *et al.* 1986). Furthermore, of 12 dogs which received eight weekly transfusions of UV-irradiated platelets from random donors, only one became refractory, whereas 18 of 21 dogs which received non-irradiated platelets became refractory (Slichter *et al.* 1987).

It is assumed that the inability of UV-irradiated cells to induce alloimmunization against class I antigens is due to inactivation of class II-positive antigen-presenting cells, notably dendritic cells (Deeg *et al.* 1988). Indeed, addition of 12.5×10^3 non-irradiated dendritic cells to UV-irradiated blood restored the ability to immunize canine recipients. UV-irradiated dendritic cells had no such effect (Deeg, 1989).

It has been shown that platelet function is not affected by UV irradiation in the doses applied (Kahn *et al.* 1985; Pamphilon *et al.* 1989; van Prooyen *et al.* 1990). Unfortunately, UV light is not transmitted through standard plastics used for the manufacture of blood bags. However, the Du Pont stericell container, designed for the *in vitro* production of interleukin 2 (IL-2)-activated lymphocytes, is UV light-permeable. Platelet concentrates collected in these bags and irradiated with UV-B in a specially built cabinet had normal *in vitro* function and *in vivo* survival, even after 5 days storage (Pamphilon *et al.* 1990). In this investigation, tests were not made to discover whether irradiation had sufficiently inactivated the class II-positive cells. However, in another investigation in which the same bag and a UV-B irradiator were used it was shown that the ability of irradiated white cells to stimulate allogeneic lymphocytes was completely abolished. Although the stericell bag needs to be modified to allow the use of traditional connecting devices for other bags and transfusion tubing sets, and the UV-B irradiator must also be modified to minimize the rise of temperature during irradiation, the possibility of routinely using UV-B irradition of concentrates is envisaged (Andreu *et al.* 1990).

Using a specially prepared bag made of transparent fluoroseal Teflon, platelet concentrates were UV-B irradiated, resulting in dose-dependent inactivation of lymphocyte responder and stimulator functions with preservation of platelet aggregation responses (Capon *et al.* 1990). Irradiated platelet concentrates were given to four recipients of bone marrow grafts. The transfusions were clinically effective and none of the patients developed HLA antibodies.

UV-B irradiation was found to induce aggregation and degranulation of platelets but only in a dose six times greater than that necessary to inhibit lymphocyte function (van Prooyen *et al.* 1990). A new narrow band UV-B light source tried by these authors had no advantage over the conventional source.

Use of single donors

It has not been clearly established whether alloimmunization can be delayed by the use of platelets from single donors, obtained by thrombapheresis, rather than by using platelets from random donors. In two studies, alloimmunization occurred less frequently (Sintnicolaas *et al.* 1981; Gmür *et al.* 1983). Correspondingly, in dogs given weekly transfusions of platelet pools derived from six animals, refractoriness occurred earlier than in dogs which received platelets from each of the six animals separately (Slichter *et al.* 1986). On the other hand, in another study in patients no advantage of the use of platelets from single donors was observed (Vicariot *et al.* 1984).

Management of alloimmunized patients

As mentioned above, alloantibodies are frequently lost in the course of time, and tests for antibodies should therefore be repeated periodically. If the antibodies disappear, the patient may again respond to platelets from random donors (see above).

Effect of ABO-incompatibility on the survival of transfused platelets. Aster (1965) found that when ABO-compatible platelets were transfused, recovery was 58–75% (average 67%); whereas when ABO-incompatible platelets were transfused it was only 7–48% (average 19%); the subsequent survival of the incompatible platelets was somewhat shorter than that of ABO-compatible platelets.

In a study of 91 thrombocytopenic patients who had become refractory to platelet transfusion, it was found that ABO incompatibility significantly reduced the effectiveness of platelet transfusion. For example, in cases in which ABO-compatible platelets were transfused, the survival rate at 24 h was 37.4% but was only 28.9% when ABO-incompatible platelets were transfused. The authors pointed out that effects of ABO incompatibility are expected to vary considerably in individual cases, depending on such factors as the recipient's titre of anti-A or anti-B and the amount of A or B on the platelets (Duquesnoy et al. 1979).

In a similar study in patients refractory to pooled platelets from random donors, the increment in platelet count at 1 h produced by HLA-selected ABO-compatible platelets was nearly twice that produced by ABO-incompatible platelets: 10×10^9 compared with 5.9×10^9 ($P < 0.01$) (Heal et al. 1987a). When the donor's plasma contained anti-A or anti-B, or both, incompatible with the recipient's platelets, the increment was also clearly smaller. Thus, in dealing with refractoriness, the first step is to use ABO-compatible platelets (Lee and Schiffer, 1989). The expression of the A antigen on platelets from group A_2 donors is very low and in two group O recipients, platelets from group A_2 donors were compatible in vivo (Skogen et al. 1988). Although all the above observations showed the effect of ABO incompatibility on platelet increment rather than on survival, rapid destruction of ABO-incompatible platelets was observed in two group O patients with IgG anti-A or anti-B of high titre (Brand et al. 1986).

Use of HLA-matched platelets
Because the alloantibodies responsible for refractoriness in immunized patients have HLA specificity in the majority of cases, the use of HLA-compatible platelets should improve the results of transfusion in most patients. Only compatibility or matching for HLA-A and HLA-B antigens is indicated since, because of the weak expression of HLA-C antigens on platelets, compatibility or matching for HLA-C antigens does not further improve the increment (Duquesnoy et al. 1977). If the specificity of the HLA-A or HLA-B antibodies (or both) in the patient can be determined, avoidance of the incompatible antigens would be sufficient. Unfortunately it is usually impossible to define the specificity, which leaves the use of HLA-matched platelets as the only alternative. In three patients who did not respond to transfusion of platelets from random donors, far better results were obtained when donors who were unrelated but matched for HLA were used (Yankee et al. 1973).

In a study in which the transfusion of 2–4 units of platelets obtained by thrombapheresis from single donors (usually related to the patient) was compared with the transfusion of four single units obtained from different donors, survival diminished as the number of HLA incompatibilities increased. Moreover, the survival of transfused platelets from HLA-matched single donors was consistently better than that of mismatched donors (Mittal et al. 1976). These observations show that HLA matching will indeed improve transfusion results in many immunized patients. However, the enormous polymorphism of the HLA-A and HLA-B antigens makes it unlikely that HLA-matched platelets will be available for most patients unless the pool of HLA-typed donors is very large, although the availability of donors homozygous for HLA-A and HLA-B is helpful. Therefore the effectiveness of platelets from donors selectively mismatched for crossreactive HLA antigens was evaluated (Duquesnoy et al. 1977).

Transfusions of platelets mismatched for one or two crossreactive antigens were as successful as transfusions of fully matched platelets. However, antibodies against crossreactive antigens occur and their frequency has not been established.

Even if a panel of HLA-typed donors, large enough to ensure HLA-compatible or HLA-matched platelets for most patients, is available, some immunized patients will not respond to HLA-matched platelets. Non-responsiveness is due, presumably, to the fact that these patients have made antibodies against platelet-specific antigens for which matching is very difficult or impossible. Another approach to the provision of compatible platelets must therefore also be considered.

Selection of compatible donors by crossmatching
Of the numerous techniques which have been described for the detection of platelet-reactive alloantibodies, only a few are suitable for use in cross-matching, because most techniques are too laborious for this purpose. In 14 patients who did not respond to transfusions of random platelets, satisfactory increments were produced by 95% of transfusions of platelets compatible by enzyme-linked immunosorbent assay (ELISA) (see below) and by 91% of platelets compatible by the platelet immunofluorescence test (PIFT). The increment was unsatisfactory after seven of ten transfusions of ELISA-positive and after two of four transfusions of PIFT-positive platelets (Sintnicolaas *et al.* 1987).

In another investigation, in 11 patients with broadly reacting HLA antibodies, compatible platelets were selected by a radiolabelled antiglobulin test. There was a great difference between the increment after transfusions of crossmatch-negative platelets: mean after 22 transfusions: $18\,379 \pm 4670$ at 1 h and 7318 ± 3317 at 18–24 h; and after transfusion of crossmatch-positive platelets: mean after 16 transfusions: 2536 ± 3057 at 1 h and 227 ± 657 at 18–24 h (all values $\times 10^9$/l). Two crossmatches were 'false-negative' and one was 'false-positive' (Kickler *et al.* 1988b).

Another crossmatching technique which can be used is a solid phase technique (the mixed red cell adherence assay) in which antibodies are detected on platelets fixed to the wells of microtitre plates, either chemically or by rabbit platelet antibodies, and by using anti-IgG-coated red cells as indicator cells. With this technique it was found that none of 11 transfusions of crossmatch-positive platelets given to immunized patients without clinical conditions which could directly influence the outcome produced a significant increment. In contrast, the increment was satisfactory after 20 of 21 transfusions of crossmatch-negative platelets (Rachel *et al.* 1988). Using the same technique, eight of 14 transfusions of compatible platelets were found to be satisfactory (O'Connel and Schiffer, 1990).

It has been found to be important to determine the increment in platelet count after 24 h (Kickler *et al.* 1988b). In most patients in whom the increment after a transfusion of crossmatch-positive platelets was satisfactory after 1 h, it was low after 24 h. A possible explanation is that the antibodies did not induce immediate destruction of platelets, for example because they were non-complement binding. A possible explanation for false negative crossmatch results is that in the above studies only anti-IgG was used. Both HLA and platelet-specific alloantibodies may be IgM. Such antibodies would not have been detected.

In conclusion, compatible platelets which produce a satisfactory increment can be found for immunized patients even if their antibodies are broadly reacting. If cross-matching is to be applied, the most practical solution is to establish a large panel of thrombapheresis donors whose platelet samples can be stored and crossmatched with the serum of immunized patients in need of platelet transfusions.

The choice of HLA-matched or compatible donors, platelet crossmatching or both for the management of alloimmunized patients will depend on the circumstances in the laboratory concerned.

Use of acid-treated platelets

Platelets were treated with citric acid according to Sugawan et al. (1987) to remove HLA class I antigens. *In vivo* recovery of acid-treated platelets in two healthy subjects was excellent and the survival time was 6.25 d compared with 7.95 d for non-treated platelets. In alloimmunized patients the post-transfusion increment was comparable to that of HLA-compatible platelets (Shanwell et al. 1991).

Neonatal alloimmune thrombocytopenia

This syndrome, first described by Moulinier (1957), is due to destruction of platelets of the fetus or the newborn by IgG alloantibodies made by the mother against platelet-specific antigens present on the fetal platelets but lacking in her. The syndrome has an incidence of about one in 2000–4000 births (Shulman 1991). It often occurs in first-born infants. The typical picture is of a generalized petechial rash developing minutes to hours after birth. Haematomas often occur and there may be bleeding from the gastrointestinal, upper respiratory or urinary tracts. Intracranial haemorrhage occurs in 35–40% of cases and may result in death (10%) or persistent neurological damage (25%) which may become apparent only after a period of time (McIntosh et al. 1973; Naidu, 1983). The severity of the thrombocytopenia often increases in the first 48 h of life and may be due to a rapid postnatal maturation of the monocyte–macrophage system (Shulman et al. 1964). Nevertheless, severe thrombocytopenia may occur early during gestation and intra-uterine intracranial haemorrhage may occur. The thrombocytopenia usually lasts for a few weeks after birth.

In principle, demonstration of platelet-specific (IgG) alloantibodies in the maternal serum is essential in diagnosis. However, the antibodies may not be detectable at the time of delivery and, in any case, because of the insensitivity of available tests, negative results do not exclude their presence. When no antibodies can be detected, tests for relevant platelet-specific antigens in the father and mother and, if possible, in the child may help to make the diagnosis. In some cases, in which no antibodies are detected in the maternal serum at delivery, they may become detectable after 3–6 months.

It is important to ascertain that the mother is not thrombocytopenic, since maternal platelet autoantibodies may also cause neonatal thrombocytopenia. Most cases of NATP are caused by anti-HPA-1a (anti-Zw[a], -Pl[A1]) (Shulman et al. 1964; von dem Borne et al. 1981). In one series this antibody was detected in the serum of 147 (73.9%) of 199 HPA-1(a –) mothers who gave birth to an infant suspected of having NATP. In contrast, platelet-specific alloantibodies were detected in only 19 (5.5%) of 348 HPA-1(a +) mothers whose children were thrombocytopenic at the time of birth.

In 15 of the 19, anti-HPA-5b (anti-Br^a) was detected. This antibody is therefore the second most frequently responsible for NATP (Mueller-Eckhardt, 1991). Thirty-nine cases of NATP due to anti-HPA-5b have recently been described (Kaplan *et al.* 1991). Occasionally other antigens were involved: Pl^{E1} (Shulman *et al.* 1964); HPA-3a (von dem Borne *et al.* 1981); HPA-3b (McGrath *et al.* 1989); HPA-4a and HPA-4b (Friedman and Aster, 1985; Shibata *et al.* 1986a,b); HPA-5b (Kiefel *et al.* 1988); Pl^T (Beardsley *et al.* 1987); and HPA-5a (Bettaieb *et al.* 1991; Kiefel *et al.* 1991).

HLA class I antibodies are often detected in the serum of mothers of infants with NATP but it seems unlikely that HLA antibodies cause NATP. Most class I antibodies are adsorbed on to fetal cells in the placenta and, if they reach the fetal circulation at all, they react not only with platelets but with all nucleated cells.

There is some evidence that potent IgG anti-A or anti-B may cause NATP (Mueller-Eckhardt, 1991).

As mentioned above, a strong association has been observed between the HLA class II antigen DR3 and alloimmunization against HPA-1a (Reznikoff-Etiévant *et al.* 1983; Taaning *et al.* 1983; Mueller-Eckhardt *et al.* 1985b). Association with DR52 appeared to be even stronger (de Waal *et al.* 1986), and the primary association has now been found to be with DR52a, with which DR3 is in linkage disequilibrium (Valentin *et al.* 1990; Décary *et al.* 1991). All 49 women who had made anti-HPA-1a were found to be DR52a positive. Interestingly, no association with HLA was observed in women who had made anti-HPA-1b. The explanation is probably as follows: the affinity of the DR52a-positive class II molecule for the HPA-1 antigenic polypeptide is far greater if leucine is present as in HPA-1a than if proline is present in the same position as in HPA-1b, thus facilitating presentation of the antigen to T helper cells in DRw52a subjects (Kuijpers *et al.* 1992b). DR52a-negative, HPA-1(a –) women are at very low risk of becoming immunized against HPA-1a. A strong association has also been observed between alloimmunization against HPA-5b (Br^a) and DR6 (Mueller-Eckhardt *et al.* 1989b).

Treatment of neonatal alloimmune thrombocytopenia

Pre-natal treatment. In NATP, intracranial haemorrhage may occur *in utero* (Reznikoff-Etiévant, 1988; de Vries *et al.* 1988). Fetal blood sampling by cordocentesis has made it possible to assess the severity of NATP as early as the 20th week of gestation. This technique can also be used to transfuse compatible platelets to reduce the risk of intracranial haemorrhage.

Thrombocytopenia usually does not become severe before the 20th week of gestation (Daffos *et al.* 1988). There are only two documented cases of intracranial haemorrhage before the 30th week (Herman *et al.* 1986; Reznikoff-Etiévant, 1988). Pre-natal treatment is advised in cases in which a previous child was seriously affected and when the fetal platelet count is very low. Weekly transfusions should be begun between weeks 26 and 28, and continued until the fetus is sufficiently mature, when a caesarean section must be performed (Waters *et al.* 1987; Kaplan *et al.* 1988; Nicolini *et al.* 1988b). It may be difficult to obtain compatible donors, who in addition to having negative routine microbiological test results must also be negative for cytomegalovirus antibodies and matched for ABO and Rh D. In cases of emergency the mother's platelets can be used, after being washed to remove the causative antibodies. The platelet concentrates must be γ-irradiated to prevent graft versus host disease. It is particularly important to irradiate concentrates of maternal platelets because they share one HLA haplotype with the fetus or infant (see Chapter 15).

An alternative treatment is to administer high-dose Ig i.v. (1 g/kg per week) to the mother, but results with this treatment are controversial. An increase of the platelet count (mean $\pm$ SD, $72.5 \pm 62 \times 10^9/l$) was seen in six of seven fetuses whose mothers were treated, and all seven infants had platelet counts above $30 \times 10^9/l$ at birth (Bussel et al. 1988). In two cases no effect was seen, but only one course of treatment was given to each (Waters et al. 1987; Kaplan et al. 1988). In another case report, in which the treatment was similar to that used by Bussel et al. (1988), there was no effect on the platelet count (Mir et al. 1988). In a case in which i.v. Ig was given in the last 3 weeks of pregnancy, the platelet count at birth was $161 \times 10^9/l$ (Shwe et al. 1991). Using an isolated perfused lobule of human placenta, i.v. Ig has been shown to inhibit the transfer of anti-HPA-1a (Morgan et al. 1991).

Postnatal treatment. Transfusion of compatible platelets is the treatment of choice (Adner et al. 1969). If no compatible donors are available, washed maternal platelets can be used. An alternative therapy is high-dose i.v. Ig. This treatment was first used successfully in a single case by Sideropoulos and Straume (1984) and subsequently in other cases (Massey et al. 1987; Suarez and Anderson, 1987). Of 12 infants with NATP due to anti-HPA-1a, who were treated with i.v. Ig (doses between 1 and 9 g), ten responded, often with an immediate and sustained increase in the platelet count (Mueller-Eckhardt et al. 1989a).

Neonatal thrombocytopenia due to maternal autoantibodies

Fetuses and newborn infants from mothers with autoimmune thrombocytopenia (AITP) may be thrombocytopenic. Maternal indices do not reliably correlate with the fetal platelet count (Cines et al. 1982; Kelton et al. 1982; Scott et al. 1983; Kaplan et al. 1990). There is a greater risk of thrombocytopenia in the offspring in cases of established AITP than in cases of asymptomatic thrombocytopenia detected during pregnancy (Kaplan et al. 1990). Cordocentesis to determine the fetal platelet count before delivery has been advised in cases in which the mother has AITP or thrombocytopenia of unknown origin with a count $< 100 \times 10^9/l$ (Kaplan et al. 1990). However, because cordocentesis is not without hazard, it has been suggested that it should be avoided until better predictive tests have been devised (Copplestone, 1990). The postnatal treatment of choice of thrombocytopenia due to maternal autoantibodies is high-dose i.v. Ig (Blanchette et al. 1989).

Tests for platelet alloantibodies

Techniques for the detection of platelet antibodies are based on the following principles: a secondary effect of the platelet–antibody interaction, i.e. agglutination, the activation of complement, a disturbance of platelet function or the detection of platelet-bound Ig.

Techniques based on the effect on platelet function have been abandoned because non-immunological factors may affect platelet function *in vitro*.

Techniques based on complement activation have also become obsolete because they are insensitive and most platelet antibodies are non-complement binding. Only IgM antibodies are detected in an agglutination test and, because it is less sensitive than other methods, it is no longer used.

The classical antiglobulin test cannot be applied to platelets because of their tendency to aggregate spontaneously, particularly after having been washed. However, all of the more successful techniques for the detection of platelet antibodies are based on the antiglobulin principle in various ways, e.g. the immunofluorescence test, ELISA and the mixed red cell adherence assay (solid phase). A general problem in these techniques is the presence on platelets of FcRII receptors for IgG which causes binding of inert IgG.

More recently, methods have been developed to detect antibody binding to particular platelet membrane glycoproteins: radioimmunoprecipitation, the immuno-blotting and antigen capture assays, using solubilized glycoproteins in platelet lysates which are captured by monoclonal antibodies.

Of the numerous techniques which have been described, the following are advised for the detection of platelet alloantibodies.

Platelet immunofluorescence test. The improved method described by von dem Borne *et al.* (1978) depends on pre-treatment of platelets with paraformaldehyde (PFA). The advantages of this treatment are a diminished uptake of aggregated IgG and immune complexes together with swelling of the platelets with expulsion of platelet-associated Ig, which overcomes the problem of non-specific fluorescence (Helmerhorst *et al.* 1983; Vos *et al.* 1987). PFA-treated platelets are incubated with serum, then washed, incubated with antiglobulin serum labelled with fluorescein–isothiocyanate, then washed again and examined under a fluorescence microscope. Advantages of this test are: (1) because the fluorescence of single platelets is assessed, aspecific reactions due to cell fragments (see below) are avoided (Shulman *et al.* 1982); (2) a polyspecific anti-Ig reagent for the recognition of IgG, IgM and IgA antibodies can be used.

A disadvantage of the test is its relative insensitivity. It has been shown that at least 1000 molecules of IgG must be bound to a platelet to produce a positive reaction (Tijhuis *et al.* 1991).

The immunofluorescence test described by von dem Borne *et al.* (1978) has been chosen as the standard technique by the ISBT/ICSII working party on platelet serology. An efficient modification of this technique in microplates has been described by Andersen *et al.* (1981).

The enzyme-linked immunosorbent assay. The use of enzyme (peroxidase-labelled) anti-globulin for detecting platelet antibodies was first described by Tate *et al.* (1977). After incubation of sensitized platelets with enzyme-linked antiglobulin serum, substrate is added and the coloured reaction product quantitated spectrophotometrically. The platelets can be coated on to slides or the wells of microplates, and various other enzyme conjugates can be used. A drawback of solid-phase ELISAs is that with some sera IgG is bound quite strongly, and non-specifically, to plastic.

Mixed red cell adherence assay (solid-phase technique). In this assay platelets are fixed to the wells of a microplate coated with antiplatelet antibody, incubated with the serum under investigation and washed. Anti-IgG-coated red cells are then added. If the platelets have been sensitized by antibody, the red cells will cover the platelet monolayers; otherwise the indicator cells will collect in a tight button in the centre of the well. A modification of this technique, in which low-ionic-strength medium is used in sensitizing the platelets, has been described (Rachel *et al.* 1985b).

Monoclonal antibody-specific immobilization of platelet antigens assay (MAIPA). In this assay, target platelets are incubated with a serum under investigation, then washed once and incubated with monoclonal antibodies against a particular platelet glyco-protein (Kiefel *et al.* 1987). The platelets are then solubilized and the lysate is incubated in the wells of microtitre plates coated with polyclonal anti-mouse Ig. Human antibodies in the complex of antigen (i.e. glycoprotein), human antibody and murine monoclonal antibody are then detected with alkaline phosphatase-labelled anti-human Ig and substrate. This assay has the following advantages: the technique is sensitive (e.g. more sensitive than the immunofluorescence test); the glycoprotein against which the platelet antibodies are directed is automatically defined; and contaminating antibodies which may be present in the serum, e.g. anti-HLA class I, do not interfere. Disadvantages of the assay are that, in the detection of unknown antibodies, a panel of monoclonal antibodies must be used and monoclonals to all glycoproteins may not yet be available. Furthermore, if a human antibody is directed against the same epitope as the monoclonal antibody (or an adjacent epitope), false-negative results may be obtained.

Distinction between platelet-specific and HLA antibodies

In the diagnosis of NATP and post-transfusion purpura (see Chapter 15), it is essential to detect platelet-specific alloantibodies and, if they are detectable, to define their specificity. Definition of specificity is often hampered by the presence of strong HLA class I antibodies present in many of the sera under investigation. The problem can be overcome by treating platelets with chloroquine which removes HLA-A and HLA-B antigens (Blumberg *et al.* 1984a). Chloroquine-treated platelets were shown not to react with HLA antisera in the platelet immunofluorescence test, although they reacted with anti-HPA-1a and anti-HPA-3a. After 20 min incubation with chloro-quine, 80% of HLA antigens had been removed whereas there was no effect on GPIIb/IIIa or GPIb/IX. However, after 1 h incubation, approximately 50% of these glycoproteins had been removed (Langescheidt *et al.* 1989). An alternative method of removing HLA class I antigens from platelets is treatment with a citric acid–phosphate buffer (Kurata *et al.* 1989). As mentioned above, if the MAIPA is used to detect platelet-specific alloantibodies, HLA antibodies do not interfere.

Detection of alloantibodies in neonatal alloimmune thrombocytopenia

It is convenient to test the maternal serum first with paternal platelets using the PIFT or, if paternal platelets are not available, with platelets from typed donors. If the result is positive a distinction must be made between HLA class I and platelet-specific antibodies, using chloroquine-treated platelets. If platelet-specific antibodies are de-tected, their specificity must be determined using a panel of phenotyped platelets. If the mother is thrombocytopenic the presence of platelet autoantibodies must be excluded (see below).

If the immunofluorescence test (IFT) with the maternal serum is negative, the presence of platelet-specific antibodies has not been excluded because of the relative insensitivity of the test. A more sensitive test, e.g. the MAIPA (see above), must then be applied. Most anti-HPA-5[a] and -5[b] antibodies are not detected by the IFT but are readily detected by the MAIPA (Kiefel et al. 1987). The specificity of maternal platelet-specific antibodies can be confirmed by phenotyping the maternal and paternal platelets.

Detection of alloantibodies in post-transfusion purpura

In the diagnosis of this syndrome, which occurs 5–7 d after transfusion (see Chapter 15), the detection of platelet-specific alloantibodies in the patient's serum is essential. It is convenient to test the serum first with a panel of phenotyped platelets using the IFT and, if positive results are obtained, to repeat the test with chloroquine-treated platelets. If platelet-specific antibodies are detected, their specificity must be determined. If all reactions in the IFT are negative, it is advisable to test the serum using the MAIPA.

If thrombocytopenia has developed during or immediately after a transfusion, the serum of the donor must be investigated (see Chapter 15).

Crossmatching tests for platelets

As mentioned above, the techniques most widely used for a crossmatch with platelets are the ELISA, PIFT and the mixed red cell adherence assay.

Autoimmune thrombocytopenia

The presence of an antiplatelet factor in the plasma of patients with idiopathic thrombocytopenic purpura (ITP) was first demonstrated by Harrington et al. (1951): plasma from a patient transfused to a normal subject produced an immediate and profound fall in the recipient's platelet count. Autoantibodies can be demonstrated on the platelets of most patients with ITP, and hence the term AITP is now preferred. In AITP, the platelet life span is shortened due to random destruction, by cells of the MPS, of platelets sensitized with autoantibodies. In some patients platelet production is also decreased. The decrease is not due to depressed megakaryocytopoiesis, but to inhibition of the formation or release of platelets, or both (Ballem et al. 1987b); it may also be due to binding of platelet autoantibodies to megakaryocytes, which carry the same antigens as platelets (Vinci et al. 1984; Dunstan, 1986b; Hyde and Zucker-Franklin, 1987).

Using the platelet immunofluorescence test, autoantibodies were detected on the platelets of 69 of 75 (92%) patients with ITP. In 92% of these 69 cases antibodies were also detected in an eluate from the patient's platelets. The platelet-bound autoantibodies were IgG in 92%, IgM in 42% and IgA in 9% of cases. IgG_1 was detected in 82%, IgG_2 in 11%, IgG_3 in 50% and IgG_4 in 20% of the patients with IgG autoantibodies. Complement was never detected on the platelets of these patients (von dem Borne et al. 1986c). Patients with complement-binding autoantibodies have been described but such autoantibodies seem to be very rare (see, for example, Tsubakio et al. 1986; Lehman et al. 1987).

Specificity of platelet autoantibodies
It has been shown that platelet autoantibodies are often directed against non-polymorphic epitopes on GPIIb/IIIa (van Leeuwen *et al.* 1982b; Beardsley *et al.* 1984; Woods *et al.* 1984a; McMillan *et al.* 1987).

Autoantibodies may also react with non-polymorphic epitopes on GPIb (Woods *et al.* 1984b; McMillan *et al.* 1987; Szatkowski *et al.* 1986), on GPIa/IIa and IV (Kiefel *et al.* 1989c) or on GPV (Beardsley, 1989).

Pseudothrombocytopenia and autoantibodies against cryptantigens
In pseudothrombocytopenia the platelet count is spuriously low in EDTA-anti-coagulated blood, due to EDTA-induced platelet agglutination. This phenomenon is caused by platelet autoantibodies which bind to platelets after removal of Ca^{2+} (Pegels *et al.* 1982; von dem Borne *et al.* 1986b).

The antibodies are directed against non-polymorphic cryptantigens on the GPIIb/IIIa complex which are exposed by conformational changes induced by the absence of Ca^{2+}.

Autoantibodies against cryptantigens exposed by fixation with PFA also occur (Magee, 1985; von dem Borne *et al.* 1986b). Neither of these two kinds of autoantibodies causes thrombocytopenia *in vivo*, but they cause misleading positive reactions in techniques in which EDTA- and, or, PFA-fixed platelets are used.

Tests for platelet autoantibodies
A simple technique for detecting these antibodies is the direct immunofluorescence test on the patient's platelets; if the result is positive and sufficient platelets are available, an eluate can be made (see below) to confirm the presence of autoantibodies. As mentioned above, however, the immunofluorescence test is relatively insensitive. Therefore, if the direct immunofluorescence test is negative, a more sensitive test should be applied, e.g. a radio-immunoassay (RIA) to measure platelet-bound Ig (PBIg). Many different versions of this assay have been described. The amount of PBIg found with these techniques is often remarkably high and probably reflects non-specific binding of plasma proteins. An important source of aspecific binding is the presence of platelet fragments in the platelet suspension (Shulman *et al.* 1982). A more specific assay in which monoclonal anti-IgG is used has been described (Lo Buglio *et al.* 1983). The improvement was considered to be due to the restricted specificity and the single binding affinity of the monoclonal reagent, as well as to removal of platelet fragments by centrifugation of the platelet suspension over a discontinuous Percoll gradient.

A slightly modified assay (MARIA), in which a sucrose gradient is used to separate platelets from fragments, has been adapted for the use of monoclonal anti-IgM and anti-IgG subclass reagents (Tijhuis *et al.* 1991). In this assay a platelet suspension containing 10×10^6 platelets is incubated with ^{125}I-labelled monoclonal anti-immunoglobulin in a plastic tube. After incubation, the platelet suspension is centrifuged through a sucrose gradient and, after removal of the sucrose, the tip of the tube is cut off and the radioactivity counted. The non-specific binding of the labelled monoclonal anti-Ig is measured by incubating the same number of platelets with the ^{125}I-labelled monoclonal anti-Ig and a 100-fold excess of non-labelled monoclonal reagent. A positive reaction in the MARIA was found in 21% of 55 patients with AITP in whom the direct fluorescence test was negative (Tijhuis *et al.* 1991).

Elution of antibodies from platelets

Ether-elution method. This is a modification of the method described for red cells by
Rubin (1963). Platelets from EDTA blood are washed and suspended in phosphate-
buffered saline with 2% bovine serum albumin (PBS–BSA) to a final concentration of
0.5×10^9 cells/μl; one volume of this suspension is mixed with two volumes of ether
and shaken vigorously for 2 min. The mixture is incubated for 30 min at 37°C in a
waterbath and shaken frequently. After centrifugation of the mixture, three layers can
be distinguished: the stroma, ether and the eluate, which is removed with a pipette
(von dem Borne *et al.* 1980).

Acid-elution technique. A volume of platelets from EDTA blood is washed three times in
PBS–BSA and the supernatant discarded. A volume of citric acid pH 2.8, equal to that
of the cell pellet, is added. The mixture is incubated for 7 min at room temperature
and then centrifuged at 1000 *g* for 5 min. A volume of NaOH is added to adjust the
final pH to 7.2 (technique used in the laboratory of CPE).

Drug-induced immune thrombocytopenia

Mechanisms responsible for drug-induced immune thrombocytopenia are similar to
those involving red cells (see Chapter 7) and granulocytes (see p. 610). In the classical
example of sedormid-induced thrombocytopenia, the drug does not bind firmly to the
cell, the antibodies being demonstrable only when tested against a mixture of the drug
and platelets (Ackroyd, 1954). In quinine- or quinidine-induced thrombocytopenia the
mechanism is similar. The interaction between the quinine- (or quinidine-) dependent
antibody and platelets probably involves glycoprotein IX or the β-subunit of glycoprotein Ib or both (Berndt *et al.* 1985). In gold-induced thrombocytopenia, true
autoantibodies, reacting independently of the drug, are formed (von dem Borne *et al.*
1986a); the mechanism is thus comparable to that in Aldomet-induced autoimmune
haemolytic anaemia and levamisole-induced granulocytopenia.

SERUM PROTEIN ANTIGENS AND ANTIBODIES

There are a few antibodies to serum proteins which are relevant to blood transfusion.
Antibodies to Factor VIII may seriously impair the response to transfused Factor VIII
but are of IgG$_4$ subclass (Andersen and Terry, 1968) and do not bind complement, and
perhaps for this reason, do not provoke transfusion reactions. Antibodies to determinants on immunoglobulin molecules may interfere with the interpretation of serological tests. Although antibodies to serum lipoproteins are also recognized, they have no
known clinical significance.

IgG

Antibodies with several different specificities are found, reacting respectively with
determinants on native IgG molecules (anti-Gm), with determinants exposed following
the combination of antigen with antibody ('anti-antibodies') and with determinants
exposed by pepsin digestion.

IgG allotypes

These are defined by polymorphic antigenic determinants carried on γ-chains, i.e. the heavy chains of IgG. The existence of Gm groups was first demonstrated by showing that Rh D-positive red cells coated with selected examples of 'incomplete' anti-D were agglutinated by the serum of some patients with rheumatoid arthritis and that the reactions could be inhibited by selected normal sera (Grubb, 1956). Four different determinants are recognized on the heavy chains of IgG_1 and 13 on IgG_3; only one determinant has been recognized so far on IgG_2 and none on IgG_4.

In Gm typing, red cells coated with selected Rh antibodies can be used to identify IgG_1 and IgG_3 markers, e.g. Gm(f) and Gm(5); however, in identifying other markers, such as G2m(n), which are not found (or at least not commonly) on red cell alloantibodies, selected myeloma proteins bound to red cells must be used.

Nomenclature (WHO, 1976). The subclass designation, e.g. (Ig) G1, is followed by m for marker and then (in brackets) a number or a letter since, unfortunately, both numeric and 'alphameric' terminologies are still allowed. Here, the alphameric notation is used, e.g. G1m(a) rather than G1m(1). Some symbols in the alphameric notation consist of letters and numbers, e.g. G3m(b1). The phenotype is written in the numerical order of subclasses, e.g. for a person with G1m(a), G1m(f), G2m(n), G3m(b1) and G3m(g), the phenotype is Gm(af; n; b1g).

Some Gm allotypes are associated with replacement of one amino acid residue by another in the same position of an otherwise identical polypeptide chain, e.g. G1m(z) and G1m(f). The alternative to some Gm allotypes is an antigenic determinant that is not limited to molecules of the subclass concerned but occurs also on other subclasses. Such determinants are described as isoallotypes since they are allotypic in one subclass and isotypic in one or more of the other subclasses.

Anti-Gm may be found in the following circumstances:

1   In patients with rheumatoid arthritis; these sera, known as 'Raggs' (Rheumatoid agglutinators), are autoantibodies, usually have multiple specificities, and exhibit prozones so that few are useful as typing reagents.

2   In normal subjects, some of whom have been transfused or have been pregnant; these sera, known as 'SNaggs' (Serum Normal agglutinators), are usually less potent than Raggs but are usually monospecific and do not exhibit prozones. Moreover, their titre usually remains the same for years. These are the reagents normally used in Gm typing.

3   In normal subjects, usually children, in whom the stimulus for anti-Gm formation can often be shown to have been maternal IgG transferred across the placenta.

4   Polyclonal and monoclonal anti-Gm reagents of animal origin are now available.

Serum from patients with rheumatoid arthritis usually contains a whole family of autoantibodies reacting with many epitopes on the IgG molecule, some of which are revealed only when the IgG is altered in some way, either by being denatured or by reacting with an antigenic site.

Formation of anti-Gm following transfusion

Antibodies, often of recognizable specificities, have been found in patients who have received multiple blood transfusion, particularly children (Allen and Kunkel, 1963; 1966; Stiehm and Fudenberg, 1965).

It seems that, in adults at least, prolonged stimulation is usually required for the production of anti-Gm. A single injection of immunoglobulin produces a scarcely significant increase in the incidence of antibodies against immunoglobulins in parous women (Sturgeon and Jennings, 1968). Similarly, no anti-Gm was detected after a single transfusion followed by an injection of immunoglobulin (Auerswald *et al.* 1967).

Anti-Gm has also been produced by deliberate immunization of volunteer recipients with plasma of incompatible types. Following an initial i.v. transfusion of 125 ml Gm-incompatible plasma, weekly subcutaneous injections of 0.1 ml of the same plasma were given. By about 2 months after the first transfusion three of three recipients had formed anti-Gm (Fudenberg *et al.* 1964).

In one large study in which sera from patients who had been transfused repeatedly were tested against various monoclonal IgGs, evidence was obtained that anti-Gm was frequently not allotype specific but rather resembled rheumatoid factor (Salmon *et al.* 1973).

Formation of anti-Gm after pregnancy
Fudenberg and Fudenberg (1964) reported the finding of anti-G1m(a) in the serum of a pregnant woman whose infant was subsequently shown to be G1m(a); they pointed out that cord serum contains a small amount (1% or less) of endogenous IgG so that there is no theoretical reason why the mother should not be stimulated when the infant's IgG carries determinants which are foreign to the mother.

Response of newborn infant to maternal IgG allotypes
Speiser (1963; see Speiser, 1964) postulated that, during the first few months of life, infants regularly became immunized to maternal Gm allotypes; he demonstrated the presence of anti-G1m(a) in G1m(a –) infants born to G1m(a +) mothers. Similarly, Steinberg and Wilson (1963) showed that the specificity of anti-Gm antibodies in children corresponded to that of the mother's Gm antigens.

IgA
In approximately 50% of IgA-deficient patients anti-IgA antibodies of various specificites are found, i.e. class-specific (anti-α), subclass-specific (anti-α_1 or anti-α_2) or allotype-specific (anti-A2m(1) or anti-A2m(2)). In patients who are not IgA deficient, antibodies of limited specificity may be found, including antibodies reacting with the recognized allotype markers just mentioned.

Class-specific anti-IgA
The prevalence of subjects who are apparently lacking in serum IgA varies according to the sensitivity of the test used. For example, in tests on healthy Finnish blood donors, using a gel diffusion method which could not detect less than 10 μg IgA per ml, one of 396 subjects appeared to lack IgA, but with a radio-immunoassay capable of detecting 0.015 μg/ml only one of 800 lacked IgA (Koistinen, 1975). Similarly, Vyas *et al.* (1975) found that the incidence of IgA deficiency was one in 650 using gel diffusion, which in their hands did not detect less than 100 μg IgA per ml, but was only one in 886 using haemagglutination inhibition, with a sensitivity of 0.5 μg IgA per

ml. The findings of Holt *et al.* (1977) were broadly similar: one in 522 subjects had less than 40 μg IgA per ml and one in 875 had less than 0.5 μg IgA per ml.

Class-specific anti-IgA is found only in IgA-deficient subjects and is then found quite often, even in patients without a history of pregnancy or blood transfusion or injections of blood products. In the series of Vyas *et al.* (1975), 20 of 83 IgA-deficient subjects had anti-IgA, and 13 of these had an anti-IgA titre of more than 256. Only two subjects had a history of injections of blood products. Of seven subjects with anti-IgA interviewed by Koistinen and Sarna (1975) only one had received a transfusion. Again, of 15 totally IgA-deficient subjects reported by van Loghem (1974), eight had anti-IgA but several of these had not been pregnant or received IgA-containing preparations. Anti-IgA was found in one 5-year-old child lacking IgA; the child had not been transfused but evidently might have been immunized by maternal IgA during intra-uterine life (Vyas *et al.* 1970).

In the series of Holt *et al.* (1977) ten of 34 IgA-deficient subjects had antibodies for IgA. Six antibodies were class specific, three were subclass specific (anti-α2), and one had allotypic specificity for A2m(2) (see below).

The role of class-specific anti-IgA in causing transfusion reactions, and the use of IgA-deficient donors for the transfusion of subjects whose serum contains anti-IgA, is discussed in Chapter 15.

Subclass-specific anti-IgA
Anti-α1 and anti-α2 antibodies may be present in addition to class-specific anti-α in the serum of IgA-deficient subjects (van Loghem, 1974). Selective deficiency for IgA$_2$ was described in a patient who developed a severe reaction following transfusion and who was found to have IgG anti-α_2 in her serum (van Loghem *et al.* 1983). Selective absence of IgA$_1$ was detected in six and selective absence of IgA $_2$ in 15 of 93 020 normal donors investigated by Ozawa *et al.* (1985). No anti-α_1 or anti-α_2 was detected in the serum of any of these subjects, none of whom had been transfused or had been pregnant.

Anti-IgA of limited specificity
The term anti-IgA of limited specificity is used for antibodies which react with some, but not all, IgA myeloma proteins. Some examples of anti-IgA of limited specificity may have been anti-α1 or anti-α2 and some have been identified as anti-A2m(2) or anti-A2m(1), reacting with one or other of the two allotypes of IgA$_2$. No allotypes of IgA$_1$ have yet been recognized.

Anti-IgA of limited specificity is found mainly in patients who have been transfused or have received an injection of immunoglobulin, or in women who have had one or more pregnancies.

Of a series of examples of anti-IgA of limited specificity, 19 reacted with one particular myeloma protein, indicating the importance of this particular specificity in alloimmunization and in transfusion reactions (Vyas *et al.* 1969). The possible role of anti-IgA of limited specificity in causing transfusion reactions is discussed in Chapter 15.

IgM
Anti-IgM of limited specificity was first demonstrated by testing sera against CrCl$_3$-treated red cells coated with IgM from patients with Waldenström's macroglobuli-

naemia. Low-titre antibodies were found in the serum of about 2% of normal donors (MacKenzie *et al.* 1967). In a later study the incidence was found to be 4.2% in patients who had had multiple pregnancies and 7.2% in patients who had been transfused repeatedly. Whereas anti-Ig found in normal sera were IgM and almost always had titres of only 1 or 2, those in sera from patients immunized by transfusion or pregnancy were IgG and always had titres of 8 or more (Leikola *et al.* 1971). In another study the incidence of anti-IgM of limited specificity was found to be as high as 21.3% in patients who had had five or more transfusions. It was noted that many of the sera reacted with the same IgM coats and it was also found that the sera would agglutinate Le^a-sensitized cells although the titres were seldom more than 4 (Ropars *et al.* 1973). Low-titre anti-IgM of restricted specificity has been found in many subjects with immunodeficiency (Wells *et al.* 1973).

Determinants on light chains

Antibodies analogous to anti-Gm but directed to determinants on κ-chains are termed anti-Km (previously Inv). Three markers, Km(1), Km(2) and Km(3) are recognized. No allotype markers are recognized on λ-chains.

Tests for immunoglobulin allotypes

Agglutination-inhibition method

A volume of 25 μl test serum, diluted appropriately, is mixed in a well of a microtitre plate with an equal volume of anti-Gm, -Am or -Km serum in optimal dilution. An equal volume of a 0.2% suspension of red cells sensitized with incomplete anti-D carrying the corresponding allotype is added. After careful mixing the plate is incubated overnight at 4°C or for 1 h at room temperature and centrifuged. The plates are tilted at an angle of about 60° and reactions are read. If the allotype is present in the serum, agglutination of the sensitized red cells by the anti-allotype serum is inhibited.

Method of passive haemagglutination

The term 'passive agglutination' is used for a reaction in which antigen is attached to a carrier particle (e.g. red cells) which plays a passive role in that it does not itself react with the antibody. Red cells treated with various agents will adsorb protein antigens 'non-specifically'.

Methods employing several different agents have been used to couple proteins to red cells.

Tannic acid. 20 mg tannic acid powder is dissolved in 20 ml PBS to give a 1 mg/ml solution. One millilitre of this solution is diluted 1 : 200 to give a final concentration of 0.02 mg/ml. Pooled group O red cells are washed three times in phosphate-buffered saline (PBS). Ten millilitres of a 0.02 mg/ml solution of tannic acid in PBS is warmed at 37°C for 5 min. 0.6 ml washed packed cells are then added to the tannic acid in 0.2 ml aliquots, mixed after each addition, and the mixture is incubated for 15 min at 37°C. The cells are then washed twice in PBS and are ready to be coated with protein (method used at the North London Blood Transfusion Centre).

Chromic chloride. To one volume of 0.1% $CrCl_3$ in 0.9% NaCl add one volume of protein antigen and then immediately add one volume of three-times washed red cells. After 4 min continuous shaking (very important) at 20°C, wash the red cells three times in 20–40% bovine serum albumin. Coated cells suspended in red cell preservation fluid can be kept for 4–6 weeks without loss of activity. The coated cells are mixed on slides or in the wells of microplates with the antisera to be tested (Gold and Fudenberg, 1967).

The coating proteins, as well as the saline solution, should be phosphate-free (Schanfield and van Loghem, 1986).

Gluteraldehyde. To 3.2 ml protein solution (10 mg in 0.15 mol/l-phosphate buffer, pH 7.3) are added 0.1 ml of a 50% suspension of red cells in saline and 0.1 ml 0.25 mol/l glutaraldehyde solution (prepared from a 25% solution purified with charcoal).

After 1 h at room temperature the mixtures are spun and the cells washed in 3.5 ml diluent (1 ml inactivated normal rabbit serum in 100 ml isotonic saline) and resuspended in 2.5 ml diluent to give a cell concentration of 2%. At 4°C the cells are stable for several weeks (Onkelinx *et al.* 1969).

CHAPTER 14

THE TRANSFUSION OF PLATELETS, LEUCOCYTES AND PLASMA COMPONENTS

TRANSFUSION OF PLATELETS

The therapeutic value of transfused platelets was first demonstrated by Duke (1911). In three thrombocytopenic patients, two of whom were children, bleeding stopped after the direct transfusion of fresh blood; in all cases the bleeding time diminished and in the two cases in which platelet counts were done an increase was observed, lasting for about 3 d.

The survival of platelets *in vivo*

^{51}Cr and ^{111}In as labels
The introduction of ^{51}Cr as a label for platelets (Aas and Gardner, 1958) was a great step forward in providing a means of defining optimal conditions for platelet transfusion, although uptake of ^{51}Cr by platelets is poor compared to that by red cells. ^{51}Cr has now been replaced by ^{111}In ($T_{1/2}$ 2.8 d) or ^{113m}In ($T_{1/2}$ 100 min), complexed with a suitable chelating agent. Although oxine (8-hydroxyquinoline) was used originally (Thakur *et al.* 1976), tropolone is superior because indium tropolonate, unlike indium oxinate, labels cells effectively in the presence of plasma. Optimal labelling with ^{111}In is achieved using a tropolone concentration of 2×10^{-4} mol/l and a plasma concentration of 50% (Danpure *et al.* 1990). Under these conditions, autologous platelets can be

638

used in patients with platelet counts as low as $4 \times 10^9/l$. It may be necessary to alter the conditions when labelling platelets stored in plasma-free synthetic media (see below). Compared with ^{51}Cr, ^{111}In is less radiotoxic and far more suitable for quantitative scintillation camera imaging.

In a population of stored platelets, there does not seem to be any relation between damage due to storage and the uptake of ^{51}Cr or ^{111}In. This finding indicates that survival studies can be used to define optimal conditions for platelet storage (Holme and Murphy, 1983; Snyder et al. 1986a). However, the $T_{1/2}$ and mean life span of stored platelets were found to be significantly longer when ^{51}Cr was used than when ^{111}In was used, which indicates that the estimates of viability of stored platelets may be influenced by the choice of label (Wadenvik and Kutti, 1991). Detailed methods for conducting survival studies with radiolabelled platelets were described by Snyder et al. (1986b). Using their method with ^{51}Cr as the label, Rock and Titley (1990) found that the survival of random donor platelets was significantly longer than when measured with the ^{51}Cr method which they had used previously. This finding confirmed the importance of using identical methods when comparing results between different laboratories. Other factors which make comparisons difficult are differences in sampling and curve-fitting which substantially affect estimates of mean life span (Wadenvik and Kutti, 1991).

Normal survival of platelets in vivo

Although much knowledge about platelet survival in vivo was derived from measurements made with ^{51}Cr, recent studies have been done mainly with ^{111}In. Using the γ scintillation camera, and particularly scintillation camera computer systems capable of dynamic imaging, new information has been obtained about the distribution of platelets in vivo.

Initial survival ('recovery'). If the platelets of a normal subject are labelled with ^{111}In, the initial rapid fall in the plasma concentration of platelets, which is also seen with ^{51}Cr-labelled platelets (Kotilainen, 1969), is complete in 20 min; at 10 min the value is about 5% above the 20-min value (Peters et al. 1980). The term 'recovery' is used for the number remaining in the circulation after this phase of rapid disappearance, expressed as a percentage of the number expected if all the transfused platelets were in the circulation.

Estimates of recovery have been as follows: with ^{111}In, 71% (Heaton et al. 1979) and 72 ± 16% (Heyns et al. 1980); with ^{51}Cr, 67% (Aster, 1965) and 64.6% (Harker and Finch, 1969).

In splenectomized subjects recovery was found to average 90.2% by Harker and Finch (1969), and a similar figure was found by Kotilainen (1969). Conversely, in splenomegaly low values have been found, e.g. between 7% and 27% in congestive splenomegaly (Harker and Finch, 1969). Similarly, Penny et al. (1966) estimated that in gross splenomegaly there might be seven times as many platelets in the spleen as in the circulating blood.

Although it is generally accepted that a fraction of the total circulating platelets is pooled in the spleen (see below), the fact that in splenectomized subjects recovery of labelled platelets is only about 90% (see above) suggests that the rapid disappearance of a proportion of labelled platelets from the blood stream soon after injection may be due partly to damage during labelling.

The disappearance curve may be obtained by plotting the number of circulating labelled platelets against the time since injection. In normal subjects the number falls relatively rapidly in the first 10–20 min but thereafter falls much more slowly. The survival time is taken simply as the time after injection at which survival falls to zero. Estimates of survival time using ^{111}In-labelled platelets are as follows: 9.0 ± 0.7 d (Heyns *et al.* 1980) and 8.10–10.36 d (Bautista *et al.* 1984), findings which are not essentially different from those established with ^{51}Cr-labelled platelets (Kotilainen, 1969; Abrahamsen, 1970). Platelet survival values obtained with ^{111}In fit a linear curve best (Heyns *et al.* 1980; Bautista *et al.* 1984) and it was concluded that ageing determines platelet life span in normal subjects. Two pieces of evidence support this latter view: after an episode of rapid platelet destruction due to quinidine, and after the quinidine had been cleared from the circulation, it is possible to label the population of newly formed platelets and to follow their survival with ^{51}Cr; a plateau-type of disappearance curve was observed with 50% survival at 7 d followed by almost complete disappearance of the labelled population by 9 d (Harker, 1977). In a study described by Corash (1978) platelets were separated by centrifugation into 'heavy', with a mean survival time of about 314 h, and 'light', with a mean survival time of 75 h, the total population having a life span of 190 h. Cohort experiments confirmed that the heavy platelets were the young ones. Incidentally, in the same study it was found that platelets from platelet-rich plasma had a survival time of 155 h, presumably because a certain number of young platelets are spun down with the red cells and leucocytes and excluded from the platelet-rich plasma. Examples of platelet survival curves obtained with ^{111}In are given in Fig. 14.1.

As stated above, the exact survival time of platelets depends on factors such as the choice of label, the labelling procedure, and techniques of sampling and curve-fitting (Rock and Titley, 1990; Wadenvik and Kutti, 1991).

Using ^{51}Cr as a label, it was estimated that about one-third of the total circulating platelets are concentrated in the spleen, exchanging freely with circulating platelets (Aster, 1966; Harker and Finch, 1969). Using ^{111}In-labelled platelets, a scintillation camera and computer-assisted imaging, the splenic pool was estimated to be 29.6% of the total circulating platelets (Heyns *et al.* 1980). A similar figure was arrived at by measuring intrasplenic platelet transit time (Peters *et al.* 1984). There may also be some pooling of platelets in the liver (Heyns *et al.* 1980). The latter authors also measured sites of the destruction of normal platelets and found that the liver and spleen are responsible for the clearance of 72.3% of the total radioactivity, a figure which corresponds closely to values obtained, using ^{51}Cr, by Aster (1966). Most of the activity not in the liver or spleen remains in the thorax and lower abdomen indicating that these regions contain sites of sequestration of senescent platelets.

Relation between platelet count and bleeding time
In patients with thrombocytopenia due to underproduction, the bleeding time is prolonged when the platelet count falls below about 85 × 10^9/l. Below this level the relation between the bleeding time, as determined by the template method of Mielke

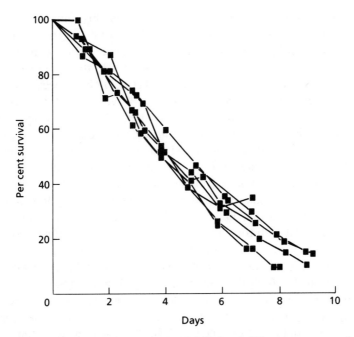

Figure 14.1 Survival curves of autologous platelets labelled with ^{111}In in seven normal subjects. The values at equilibrium after injection were taken as 100% and corresponded to a mean value of 72% (SD 16%) of that expected if all the labelled platelets had been in the circulation. The slopes were best fitted by a linear function and mean survival was found to be 9.0 d (SD 0.71 d). From other data it was concluded that elution of label from the platelets was negligible (slightly modified from Heyns *et al.* (1980)).

et al. (1969), and the platelet count was found to be as follows (Harker and Slichter, 1972):

$$\text{bleeding time (min)} = 30.5 - \frac{\text{platelet count}/\mu l}{3850}$$

e.g. platelet count 10 000/μl

$$\text{bleeding time} = 30.5 - \frac{10\,000}{3850} = 28\,\text{min}$$

In patients with autoimmune thrombocytopenic purpura (AITP) the bleeding time is shorter than that predicted from the platelet count, whereas in conditions in which platelet function is disturbed, as in uraemia or in von Willebrand's disease, bleeding time is prolonged even when the platelet count is normal (Harker and Slichter, 1972).

Storage of platelets in the liquid state

Platelets are usually stored as concentrates. Most commonly, platelets are harvested from single units of blood, either from platelet-rich plasma or from the buffy coat, and resuspended in approximately 50 ml autologous plasma. Storage of platelets under these conditions for more than 3 d results in a decline of platelet function and integrity. The nature of the responsible lesion is not exactly known, but platelet activation may be largely responsible (Fijnheer *et al.* 1990a). Addition to the anticoagulant of inhibitors of platelet activation and an inhibitor of thrombin improved the condition of platelets after 5 d storage (Bode and Miller 1988; 1989). A substantially improved post-storage viability of platelets was seen after storage in a plasma-free electrolyte medium containing glucose, with bicarbonate as a buffer, than after storage in plasma (survival after 7 d storage 144.1 ± 15.9 h and 100 ± 32 h, respectively) (Holme et al. 1987). When platelets were stored in plasma a 50% reduction of the mean population life span occurred after 7.2 d, whereas it occurred after 8.8 d when platelets were stored in a plasma-free medium (Holme et al. 1990). The presence of glucose in the medium leads to the formation of lactic acid and it is for this reason that bicarbonate is added as a buffer. Unfortunately the bicarbonate has to be sterilized and stored at an alkaline pH in a separate container (Holme et al. 1987). It may be possible to avoid the use of glucose and bicarbonate by using a medium containing inhibitors of platelet activation (Holme et al. 1989; Bode et al. 1991). Meanwhile, excellent results have recently been obtained with the commercially available medium plasmolyte A, which contains sodium chloride, sodium gluconate, sodium acetate, magnesium chloride and potassium chloride (Bertolini et al. 1989; Rock et al. 1991a). Recovery after 5 d storage was considerably better (63%) than after 3 d storage in plasma (46%, see below); mean survival was similar. With a medium containing gluconate, acetate and citrate, and platelets prepared by the buffy coat method, results were also good (Fijnheer et al. 1991). The removal of plasma may be beneficial because enzyme systems which affect the biochemical alterations or activation of platelets which occur during storage are removed (Bode and Miller, 1985; Rock et al. 1991).

Although storage of platelets for 7 d is now possible, it is not recommended because there is a significant risk of bacterial contamination of platelet concentrates after 5 d storage (FDA, 1986).

Storage temperature

A temperature of 4°C was used originally, but it was then found that at that temperature platelets lose their discoid shape and their viability and, although their immediate post-transfusion recovery is good and they retain some haemostatic function, their subsequent survival is poor. Storage at 4°C has become obsolete.

Storage at 22°C. Autologous platelets stored in CPD at 22 ± 2°C for 72 h were found to have a mean recovery of 46% and a mean survival time of 7.9 d. Storage in ACD gave similar results (Slichter and Harker, 1976b). Results from another laboratory were almost identical, namely recovery 44%, $T_{1/2}$ 3.8 d (Holme et al. 1978). No differences in recovery or survival of platelets preserved in CPD or CPDA-2, even after 8 h storage of whole blood at room temperature, were found by Bolin et al. (1982). In thrombocytopenic recipients, platelets stored for 72 h had a recovery of 42% and a mean survival of 4.1 d (Slichter and Harker, 1976b).

Storage in CPDA-1 gave very similar results, i.e. for autologous platelets stored for 72 h recovery was 50% and survival 7.3 d; in thrombocytopenic subjects recovery averaged 44% and survival was 3.3 d (Scott and Slichter, 1980).

At 22°C, platelets lose their ability to aggregate in tests using a single activating agent but when two activating agents are used, probably mimicking more closely conditions *in vivo*, synergistic aggregation is observed and platelets stored at 22°C have adequate haemostatic activity (Moroff, 1981; DiMinno *et al.* 1982).

A major limiting factor in storage at 22°C is the fall in pH (Murphy *et al.* 1970) due to lactate production from platelet glycolysis. When pH reaches 6.8 platelet morphology begins to change and it changes dramatically when pH reaches 6.0, and viability is lost. The rate of fall of pH is affected by the number of platelets, the volume of plasma in which they are stored and the availability of oxygen, since deprivation of oxygen leads to increased lactate production (Murphy, 1985). When the pH is above 7.3, platelet morphology also deteriorates and at a pH above 7.5 (at 22°C), post-transfusion viability was very poor (Murphy, 1985).

The effect of different plastics
The use of new, 'second generation', plastics with an increased permeability to oxygen has made it possible to lengthen the period for which the platelets may successfully be stored in plastic containers. With previously used plastic, pH fell below 6.0 after 3 d in platelet concentrates containing more than 8×10^{10} platelets in 50 ml. In containers of the new kind of plastic, there is a continuous linear production of lactate in spite of an adequate oxygen supply. The lactate is buffered by bicarbonate and there is an adequate supply of bicarbonate in 50 ml normal plasma to keep the pH above 6.0 for 7 d (Murphy, 1986).

The following plastics of the new kind have been used:
1 *PL-732* (Fenwal), a polyolefin plastic. Autologous platelets stored for 5 d in a container made of PL-732 had a mean recovery of 51% and a survival $T_{1/2}$ of 3.1. d. In paired studies in the same patient platelet concentrates stored for 5 d in PL-732 were consistently superior to concentrates stored for 3 d in the conventional PL-146 bags (Murphy *et al.* 1984a). In PL-732 bags platelet preservation is reasonably good even after 7 d storage, viz recovery 40.3 ± 7.2% with a survival time of 6.3 ± 1.4 d (Rzad *et al.* 1982). Platelets stored for 5 d in PL-732 have a satisfactory effect in mitigating the haemorrhagic tendency in severely thrombocytopenic subjects (Gunson *et al.* 1983).

Platelets stored for 5 d in PL-732 bags survive satisfactorily, even if whole blood is held for 8 h at 20–24°C before preparation of platelet concentrates (Moroff *et al.* 1984).
2 *CLX* (Cutter), a polyvinylchloride (PVC), plasticized with tri-(2-ethylhexyl) trimellate (TOTM) instead of the conventional di-(2-ethylhexyl) phthalate (DEHP). Mean *in vivo* recovery and $T_{1/2}$ of platelets stored for 5 d in CLX bags were satisfactory (greater than 31% and 3.3 d, respectively), and following storage for 7 d the mean recovery rate was 41% and half-life was 2.8 d (Simon *et al.* 1983). The authors concluded that this new kind of plastic container was promising for storage of platelet concentrates for up to 7 d. Similar results were obtained by Rock *et al.* (1984a); survival of platelets stored for 5 d was 5.1 d with a recovery of 44%.
3 *Teruflexa* (Terumo), a bag made of PVC with a reduced thickness and a larger surface area (400 ml capacity). Survival after 5 d storage was equal to that after storage in PL-732 bags (Holme *et al.* 1989b). A correlation was again found between the number of platelets stored in the bag and the pH after 5 d storage; the lower the number, the higher the pH. In a study in which several second-generation bags were compared, the maximum and minimum number of platelets which could be stored to

keep the pH between 6.9 and 7.4 for 5 d was established. These numbers depended on the oxygen diffusion capacity of the bags (Wallvik and Åkerblom, 1990).

4   F720 (Biotrans), a PVC, with the phthalate ester analogue tri-(2-ethylhexyl)-1,2,4, benzene tricarboxylate as plasticizer. In bags made from this plastic, pH does not decrease in platelet concentrates during storage for 7 d (Koerner, 1984). From all these results it is clear that in bags of the new materials, because the pH remains above 6.0, the storage of platelet concentrates can be extended to 5 d. This conclusion also applies to platelets obtained by a blood cell separator, using a closed system (Buchholz *et al.* 1985).

5   PL-2209 (Fenwal), PVC multiple packs plasticized with butyryl-*n*-trihexyl citrate (BTHC) are suitable for the storage of red cells for 42 d in SAGM and of platelets for 5 d. Apart from being able to use the same plastic for platelets and red cells, there is the advantage that BTHC does not leach into blood components during storage (Gullikson *et al.* 1991; Högman *et al.* 1991c). Although the phthalate ester DEHP has a beneficial effect on stored red cells (see Chapter 9), it is potentially toxic (see Chapter 15).

The effect of some other variables

Effect of contamination of platelet concentrates with leucocytes. In platelet concentrates stored in conventional PL-146 packs, the pH remains significantly higher in leucocyte-poor concentrates (Gottschall *et al.* 1984). However, when the more oxygen-permeable containers are used, a marked decrease of the pH is rarely seen, regardless of the leucocyte content of the platelet concentrate (Moroff and Holme, 1991). Nevertheless, one of the neutrophil proteolytic enzymes which is freed during storage has been shown to decrease the amount of glycoprotein Ib (GPIb) on the platelet surface. The loss of GPIb is accompanied by a loss of platelet responsiveness to ristocetin and thrombin and a decline in the number of high-affinity platelet thrombin receptors (Sloand and Klein, 1990). In general, the level of white cell contamination mirrors the contamination with red cells in platelet concentrates; hence pink or red platelet concentrates should be discarded.

Failure to agitate the platelets leads to a more rapid fall in pH and to reduction in viability by an unknown mechanism, independent of pH (Murphy and Gardner, 1976). In one comparison of agitation versus non-agitation during a 24-h storage period at 22°C, recovery *in vivo* was 51% with agitation but only 23% without (Slichter and Harker, 1976b). The method of agitation has been shown to be important; e.g. the good results reported above with the new plastic PL-732 were achieved by agitating platelet concentrates on a flat-bed agitator at 70 cycles per min; inconsistent results were observed with rotary agitation (Murphy *et al.* 1982). It seems to make no difference whether vertical or horizontal agitation is used (Gunson *et al.* 1983). Comparison of flat-bed agitators with 1.5-inch and 1.0-inch lateral movements revealed no differences with platelets stored in PL-732 and CLX bags as judged by changes *in vitro*. The 1.5-inch shaker is preferable because, due to a more rapid acceleration and deceleration, platelet buttons formed after centrifugation are resuspended more efficiently (Snyder *et al.* 1985). Before agitation is begun, the platelets should remain undisturbed for 1 h. At least when platelets are stored in polyolefin bags, discontinuation of agitation, even for 24 h, has hardly any effect on pH (Moroff and George, 1990). Altogether, the effect of agitation is less important when aerobic metabolism of platelets is maintained (Wallvik *et al.* 1990).

In conclusion, platelets should be stored at 22°C in plasma under conditions in which the pH is maintained at values above 6.8. These conditions can be achieved in first-generation bags by keeping the concentration of platelets below 1.5×10^9 per ml and the concentration of leucocytes below 0.4×10^6 per ml, and by ensuring that the surface for gas exchange is more than 400 cm^2 using normal 600-ml plastic bags, or by using bags made of one of the new kinds of plastic which allow increased gas exchange. Evidently, packs containing platelet concentrates should not be stored on top of each other.

Beneficial effect of brief incubation at 37°C. Platelet morphology and the corrected platelet count increment have been found to improve significantly when platelets stored at 22°C are warmed before transfusion at 37°C for 1 h (Hutchinson *et al.* 1989). The effect on platelet increment is already present 10 min after transfusion, which suggests that the immediate clearance of platelets is reduced by incubation at 37°C (Fijnheer *et al.* 1990b).

Relation between tests on platelets in vitro *and recovery and survival* in vivo
Morphological changes in platelets stored at 20°C are well correlated with post-transfusion viability, concentrates with the highest proportion of discoid platelets having the best survival (Kunicki *et al.* 1975). Similarly, the shape of platelets or their change in shape, and lactate production, were found to be significantly correlated with viability (Holme *et al.* 1990). The shape change is also correlated with a decrease in the amount of ATP and ADP in platelets (de Korte *et al.* 1990).

The percentage of discoid platelets can be assessed by light-scattering measurements (Fratantoni *et al.* 1984) and a method has been devised for assessing platelet viability by visual inspection. If a bag containing platelet concentrate is held near a light source and given a twist, an appearance of swirling, caused by light scattering indicates that the platelets have retained their discoid shape. The swirling is known not to occur when platelets have been stored at 4°C and the pH has fallen to 6.2. A scoring system to assess the magnitude of the swirling phenomenon has been divised (Fijnheer *et al.* 1989; George *et al.* 1989). Visual inspection also helps to detect platelet aggregates; if these are present after storage and gentle agitation, the concentrate should be discarded.

The changes in platelet shape and in mean platelet volume (MPV) in response to EDTA (δ MPV) have been found to be good reflectors of platelet function and can be measured automatically by the use of counters such as the Technicon H1, the Coulter counter, or the Sysmex 2000. The greater the residual function of platelets after storage, the greater the change in size in response to EDTA, measured as δ MPV (Seghatchian *et al.* 1990; Brozović and McShine, 1991).

Storage of platelets in the frozen state

The best results have been found using dimethyl sulphoxide (DMSO) as the cryoprotective agent, and using relatively slow rates of freezing. Murphy *et al.* (1974) found that there was progressively greater damage to platelets at freezing rates exceeding 5°C per min. A final concentration of 5% DMSO was optimal; when the final concentration was 10% rather than 5% initial recovery *in vivo* was about 10% worse; the subsequent viability of the platelets was only slightly less good with a final concentration of 10% rather than 5%.

Conditions for the satisfactory storage of platelets in liquid nitrogen were defined by Kim *et al.* (1976) as follows: suspension of the platelet concentrates in plasma; slow addition of DMSO to a final concentration of 5%; cooling at −1°C per min in a polyolefin plastic bag; rapid thawing (1 min); slow removal of DMSO with final resuspension in a medium of 50% plasma in Hanks' buffered saline solution. Using these conditions, initial post-transfusion recoveries in the recipient were nearly as good as those observed with fresh platelets and viability was low–normal or only slightly subnormal. In 11 thrombocytopenic recipients the transfusion of frozen platelets was followed within 3 h by a shortening of the bleeding time. However, adhesion of frozen-thawed platelets to endothelium has been shown to be significantly reduced (Owens *et al.* 1991), as measured in an apparatus in which adhesion to endothelium was directly measured in a flowing system.

Quite good results with platelets frozen at an uncontrolled rate were reported by Schiffer *et al.* (1982), but poor results with such platelets were obtained by Lazarus *et al.* (1981). Storage in a mechanical refrigerator at −80°C appears to give reasonably satisfactory results (Zaroulis *et al.* 1979). Previously frozen platelets have been shown to deteriorate rapidly after more than 6 h at room temperature (Kim *et al.* 1974).

In nine normal subjects, autologous platelets mixed with glycerol and stored at −80°C for 2 weeks had a mean recovery of 18.3% compared with 47.3% for fresh platelets; survival times were 8.2 d and 9.6 d, respectively (Coates *et al.* 1992).

Indications for platelet transfusions

Thrombocytopenia

Platelets are given to patients with severe thrombocytopenia associated with failure of platelet production to stop or to prevent bleeding. In general, spontaneous bleeding only occurs when the platelet count is below $20 \times 10^9/l$. However, many other factors may influence bleeding in patients with thrombocytopenia, such as conditions causing increased platelet consumption (sepsis, fever, disseminated intravascular coagulation — DIC), conditions causing a decreased response to platelet transfusions (fever, splenomegaly) and conditions causing abnormal platelet function (drugs, renal failure, coagulopathy) (Slichter 1980; McCullough *et al.* 1988b). Thus, although prophylactic platelet transfusions are usually given only to patients with a platelet count below $20 \times 10^9/l$, they are sometimes given to patients with higher counts with one of the conditions listed above.

There is substantial evidence that in patients with platelet counts below about $25 \times 10^9/l$ due to failure of platelet production, platelet transfusions are valuable in preventing haemorrhagic episodes. In a trial in which two different doses of platelets were transfused to children with acute leukaemia with platelet counts of $25 \times 10^9/l$ or less, with no active bleeding within the previous 5 d, comparison with a retrospective 'control' series suggested that platelet transfusions were highly effective in preventing bleeding (Roy et al. 1973). Similarly, in a trial in which patients with acute myeloid leukaemia with platelet counts below $30 \times 10^9/l$ were treated with platelets or with plasma, serious bleeding occurred in six of nine patients receiving plasma but in only three of 12 patients receiving platelets, even though the platelet counts after treatment in the two series were similar (Higby et al. 1974).

Platelet concentrates are commonly given prophylactically to patients with thrombocytopenia secondary either to neoplastic conditions involving the bone marrow or to chemotherapy. If the platelet count is to be kept above $20 \times 10^9/l$, a dose of one concentrate (i.e. platelets harvested from one unit of blood) must be given for each 10 kg body-weight. As soon as the platelet count drops to near $20 \times 10^9/l$, the treatment must be repeated.

Although it has been widely accepted that the platelet count should be kept above $20 \times 10^9/l$ to prevent bleeding, the results of a recent trial in patients with acute myeloid leukaemia indicate that this level is often unnecessarily high. In patients without fever or bleeding, a platelet count of $5 \times 10^9/l$ was found to be adequate, although in patients with these signs the count was kept above $10 \times 10^9/l$ and in those with coagulation disorders, or with anatomical lesions or on heparin, the count was kept above $20 \times 10^9/l$. The maintenance of lower platelet counts in many patients resulted in a large saving in money and reduced the numbers of donors to whom patients were exposed (Gmür et al. 1991).

It has been suggested that in treating patients with epistaxis the platelet count should be raised to $40-45 \times 10^9/l$, and in patients undergoing major surgery to at least $70-80 \times 10^9/l$; for continuing therapy the interval between doses can be increased by raising these levels by 20–30%. It should be noted that there are several reports of patients with platelet counts in the range $40-60 \times 10^9/l$ undergoing major surgery without undue bleeding. Although the bleeding time of the average individual increases when the platelet count falls below about $70-80 \times 10^9/l$, the hazard of post-operative oozing varies with the site of surgery (L.A. Sherman, personal communication).

Patients with aplastic anaemia, dyshaematopoiesis, congenital hypoplastic megakaryocytopenia and Fanconi's anaemia will need supportive platelet transfusion therapy for long periods of time. Since bone marrow transplantation will be considered in the treatment of these diseases (particularly in aplastic anaemia), the only indication for platelet transfusions in these conditions should be serious bleeding. If the platelet count drops below $5 \times 10^9/l$, serious bleeding will always occur and platelet transfusions must be given as soon as possible.

Inherited qualitative defects in platelets

Patients with an inherited defect of platelet function (Bernard–Soulier syndrome, Glanzmann's disease, Wiskott–Aldrich syndrome) must be treated with platelet concentrates when serious bleeding occurs, or before surgery.

Acquired qualitative defects in platelets

An acquired defect of platelet function, due apparently to damage by passage through a pump oxygenator, is sometimes observed in patients following cardiac bypass. Troublesome bleeding may be observed even though the platelet count is above $50 \times 10^9/l$. In these circumstances the transfusion of normal platelets is beneficial (Moriau *et al.* 1977).

Thrombocytopenia due to immune destruction of platelets
Platelet transfusion in neonatal alloimmune thrombocytopenia is discussed in Chapter 13, and in post-transfusion purpura in Chapter 15. Platelet transfusions are seldom indicated in autoimmune thrombocytopenia.

Thrombocytopenia due to consumption of platelets
In thrombotic thrombocytopenic purpura and in the haemolytic uraemic syndrome, the transfusion of platelets tends to aggravate the condition. The effects of platelet transfusion in DIC are less predictable but platelet transfusions are often given when there is serious bleeding associated with thrombocytopenia.

Some other aspects of platelet transfusions

Rise in platelet count to be expected from transfusion
According to Schiffer (1981), the transfusion to an adult weighing 70 kg of one unit of fresh platelets (containing approximately 0.7×10^{11} platelets) produces an immediate post-transfusion increment of approximately $11 \times 10^9/l$. In order to make proper comparisons between different recipients, the number of platelets transfused and the approximate blood volume of the recipient must be taken into account. One formula gives the corrected increment as the rise in platelet count observed multiplied by the surface area (in m^2) divided by (the number of platelets transfused $\div 10^{11}$). For example, taking a 70-kg adult having a surface area of $1.7\,m^2$ and taking the other figures given by Schiffer (see above), the corrected increment would be $11 \times 10^9/l \times 1.7/0.7$ = approximately $27 \times 10^9/l$ (Daly *et al.* 1980). Calculation of the corrected increment at 1 h after transfusion is valuable in three circumstances: (1) when stored platelets are being used, as a check on their efficacy; (2) when platelet transfusions are being given to patients who may have formed alloantibodies; and (3) to check whether HLA-matched or crossmatch-compatible platelets are effective.

Effect of microaggregate filters. When fresh blood is passed through ordinary blood administration sets, not more than 3% of the platelets are trapped on the filter and the post-transfusion survival of the platelets is unimpaired (Morrison, 1966). On the other hand, appreciable numbers of platelets are removed by filters designed to remove microaggregates. For example, in one study the percentage of platelets removed from fresh blood with different filters was as follows: Pall, 16%; Bentley, 9%: Fenwall microaggregate, 24%; Swank, 36% (Dunbar *et al.* 1974).

Stored platelets are apparently not trapped by microfilters. When platelet concentrates from CPD blood were kept at 22°C for 8, 36 or 72 h and passed through the Pall (40 μm) or Fenwall (20 μm) filters, no significant differences were found in the platelet count, in ADP aggregation or in levels of β-thromboglobulin (a marker for the platelet release reaction). Apparently, then, storage even for 8 h seems to render platelets insensitive to activation by filters (Snyder *et al.* 1979).

Repeated transfusions of platelets
Patients who receive repeated transfusions of platelets may develop alloantibodies and the therapeutic effect then becomes progressively less satisfactory. The advantages of using HLA-compatible platelets in these circumstances, and other problems concerning alloimmunization to platelet antigens, are discussed in Chapter 13.

Risks from red cell contamination
Platelet concentrates contain variable numbers of red cells and may induce Rh D sensitization in a D-negative subject (see Chapter 5). When platelet concentrates from D-positive donors are transfused to a D-negative woman who has not yet reached the menopause, provided that the recipient is not already immunized, a dose of anti-D immunoglobulin should be given to suppress primary Rh D immunization.

In thrombocytopenic recipients, i.m. injections are very undesirable and therefore anti-D immunoglobulin should be given i.v. whenever a suitable preparation is available.

Platelet concentrates from cytomegalovirus (CMV) antibody-negative donors
The consequences of primary infection with CMV can be very serious in immunosuppressed patients. For those patients who are anti-CMV negative, platelet concentrates from CMV antibody-negative donors (see Chapter 16) should be made available; alternatively, the platelet concentrate should be depleted of white cells to make it non-infectious for CMV (Gilbert *et al.* 1989).

Use of fresh blood in the treatment of haemorrhagic states
Many clinicians, mainly surgeons, have a strong belief that the transfusion of fresh whole blood can arrest haemorrhage when nothing else will. It is difficult to be sure that this view is incorrect, although if it is correct its scientific basis is unknown. What is certain is that it is highly inconvenient to obtain fresh compatible blood in adequate amounts as the occasion demands, and that when fresh blood is used there is usually no time for testing it properly; omission of tests for HBsAg and anti-HIV is unacceptable. Since virtually all the elements in blood can now be stored satisfactorily and since various concentrates (e.g. Factor VIII and platelets) are available which are more effective than fresh whole blood in treating particular deficiencies, it is doubtful whether there are any circumstances in which fresh whole blood is essential.

THE TRANSFUSION OF LEUCOCYTES

The only white blood cells used for transfusion are granulocytes. When transfused to a patient with severe neutropenia and infection, granulocytes can help to combat the infection.

Labelling of granulocytes; distribution in the circulation
When labelled granulocytes are injected into the blood stream they equilibrate with the total blood granulocyte pool, consisting of cells which 'marginate' along, or adhere to, the walls of venules, and others which circulate freely. Following the i.v. injection of $DF^{32}P$-labelled granulocytes, the concentration in the blood stream is only 45% of that expected if all the granulocytes circulated freely (Cartwright *et al.* 1964). This figure

may slightly underestimate the true percentage of neutrophils which circulate freely, because there is evidence that some DF^{32}P elutes rapidly from labelled granulocytes (Dancey *et al.* 1976). Moreover, when granulocytes were labelled *in vivo* with ^{3}H-thymidine and then transfused to another normal subject, the maximum recovery was 57%, suggesting that only 43% of the granulocytes (rather than 55%) were marginal (Dancey *et al.* 1976). However, using ^{111}In-labelled granulocytes, the marginating granulocyte pool was calculated to be 60% of the total blood granulocyte pool (Peters *et al.* 1985). Granulocytes labelled with ^{3}H-thymidine were found to disappear from the blood stream with a $T_{1/2}$ of 7.6 h. Based on this finding and other data, daily production of granulocytes was estimated to be 0.85×10^9/kg, a figure which is only about half that obtained previously with DF^{32}P; the total marrow metamyelocyte–granulocyte pool was estimated to be 6×10^9/kg (Dancey *et al.* 1976). In a 70-kg man the total pool of marrow granulocytes is thus about 4.2×10^{11}. Taking the granulocyte count in circulating blood at 4.0×10^9/l and assuming a blood volume of 5 litres in a 70-kg man, total circulating granulocytes are estimated to be 2×10^{10} or about one-twentieth of the total marrow granulocyte pool. This estimate agrees well with that of Bierman *et al.* (1962) who, from data obtained following leucapheresis, concluded that the 'extracirculatory' reservoir of granulocytes was on average about 18 times that of the total number of granulocytes in the circulation.

^{111}In combined with a suitable chelating agent is the best label for granulocytes; there is very little elution of the label *in vivo* and labelled granulocytes can be readily detected by surface scanning. Following the injection of ^{111}In-labelled granulocytes there is an immediate accumulation in the lungs but the granulocytes are then redistributed between the liver and spleen. Granulocytes labelled with ^{111}In were cleared from the circulating blood with a $T_{1/2}$ of 7.5 h, confirming results obtained with ^{3}H-thymidine (Thakur *et al.* 1977a). ^{111}In-labelled granulocytes have been used successfully for the localization of abscesses (Thakur *et al.* 1977b; Dutcher *et al.* 1981a) and, combined with imaging, have been used to study the distribution and sites of destruction of granulocytes in normal subjects (Saverymuttu *et al.* 1985).

As determined experimentally in rats by Hollingsworth *et al.* (1957), the large extracirculatory reserve of leucocytes prevents the development of leucopenia following exchange transfusion; after an exchange transfusion carried out with leucopenic rat blood, the recipient mobilized leucocytes so rapidly that severe leucopenia did not develop during the exchange transfusion and 30 min after the transfusion the leucocyte count was back to normal.

Storage of granulocytes

Storage in the liquid state
The effect of storage on granulocyte function is either studied *in vitro* by measuring granulocyte chemotaxis or *in vivo* using ^{111}In-labelled granulocytes.

Anticoagulant
Chemotaxis of granulocytes is maintained satisfactorily for 24 h in ACD and CPD blood (McCullough *et al.* 1974; Strauss and Crouch, 1981). Addition of buffer to the unit may be beneficial if the granulocyte count exceeds 5×10^7/ml (Lane and Lamkin, 1984).

Granulocytes stored in the absence of protein deteriorate rapidly, but chemotaxis is maintained just as well in a synthetic medium supplemented with albumin as it is in autologous plasma (Glasser *et al.* 1985).

Temperature
In vivo studies in humans have shown that post-transfusion kinetics and localization of granulocytes are much better after storage at room temperature than after storage at 4°C (McCullough *et al.* 1978). Post-transfusion recovery, circulation and migration into inflammatory loci remain intact after storage for at least 8 h at room temperature, but a decrease in both recovery and migration into inflammatory loci is seen after storage for 24 h (McCullough *et al.* 1983). Chemotaxis is also maintained much better during storage at room temperature than at 4°C (Lane and Windle, 1979).

Agitation
Agitation of granulocytes during storage leads to a rapid increase in the rate at which their function deteriorates and to extensive lysis of contaminating red cells (McCullough *et al.* 1978). When horizontal agitation is used, maintenance of chemotaxis of granulocytes is strikingly better than without agitation, although, again, lysis of red cells is severe (Miyamoto and Sasakwa, 1987). In conclusion, granulocytes should be stored in plastic bags, with citrate and autologous plasma or with a synthetic medium supplemented with albumin, without agitation and at room temperature. Granulocytes should preferably be used within 8 h of collection. For a survey, see Lane (1990).

Storage in the frozen state
Critical granulocyte functions were found to be severely decreased after freezing and subsequent thawing (Frim and Mazur, 1980). Since no substantial improvements have been reported subsequently, cryopreservation of granulocytes remains a subject of laboratory investigation.

Indications for granulocyte transfusions
Granulocyte substitution therapy is difficult because neutrophils represent only a very small fraction of the formed elements of the blood, whilst because of the very short survival time of these cells almost two and a half times the number of neutrophils present in the circulation at any given time are consumed each day. Thus, for granulocyte transfusions to be effective, very large numbers of granulocytes must be transfused and it is difficult to collect large numbers of these cells.

Therapeutic granulocyte transfusion in infected neutropenic patients

In adults. Several prospective, randomized, controlled clinical trials have shown an increased survival in neutropenic patients given leucocyte transfusions in addition to antibiotics (Higby *et al.* 1975; Alevi *et al.* 1977; Herzig *et al.* 1977; Vogler and Winton, 1977). Most of the patients studied had Gram-negative septicaemia. Significant benefit from the transfusions was seen only when bone marrow recovery was delayed for more than 1 week, but did occur within 2 or 3 weeks and when leucocyte transfusions were given daily for at least 4–7 d in patients with proven infections. However, the number of patients studied in these trials was rather small, the infections in the patients were heterogeneous, and the duration of granulocytopenia differed. In a more recent trial, no benefit was conferred by transfusion of granulocytes, survival being as good in patients treated with antibiotics alone (Winston *et al.* 1982), although the number of granulocytes transfused (approximately 5×10^9 per transfusion) was totally inadequate (Schiffer, 1990).

It has been suggested that granulocyte transfusions should be considered only when the absolute neutrophil count falls to $0.5 \times 10^9/l$ and that, provided that the patient is clinically stable, broad-spectrum antibiotics should be tried for 1–2 d before beginning granulocyte transfusions (Higby and Burnett, 1980).

Granulocyte transfusions have been reported to produce favourable results in patients with chronic granulomatous disease with pyogenic infections (Yomtovian *et al.* 1981).

When therapeutic granulocyte transfusions are given, at least 1×10^{10} functioning granulocytes should be transfused twice a day bearing in mind that normal production in an adult is about 1×10^{11} per day and that only 5–10% of the granulocyte pool is in the circulation. Once granulocyte therapy has been started it should be continued for 4–7 d before reassessing the position. Newborn infants are more likely than adults to benefit from granulocyte transfusions because they have only a small reservoir of neutrophils (Christensen and Rothstein, 1980) with an impaired response to infection (Strauss, 1986).

In alloimmunized patients it is inadvisable to administer transfusions of granulocytes from random donors because the effect of the transfusion will then often be negligible and there is a danger of transfusion reactions (see Chapter 15). For alloimmunized patients compatible donors can be selected by crossmatching (see Chapter 15).

In newborn infants, granulocytes appear to play a critical role in determining survival in the face of bacterial infection. In a trial in which infants were to be transfused with $0.2–1.0 \times 10^9$ granulocytes every 12 h until the neutrophil count was within normal limits, all of seven who needed only a single transfusion recovered, whereas eight of 16 who needed repeated transfusions died, indicating severe depletion of the granulocyte storage pool (Christensen *et al.* 1982).

In a large prospective, randomized study of infants who received granulocyte transfusions, 20 of 21 survived whereas of infants who received only supportive care, only nine of 14 survived (Cairo *et al.* 1987). In a further trial, in infected infants with neutrophil counts below $2.5 \times 10^9/l$, in which treatment was randomized, some infants receiving daily granulocyte transfusions for 3 d and the others receiving i.v. Ig, 1000 mg/kg per day for 3 d, all ten who received granulocyte transfusions survived but only two who received Ig. Taking the two trials together, 30 of 31 infants treated with granulocytes, but only 11 of 21 who received other treatment, survived ($P < 0.004$) (Cairo, 1989).

Granulocyte concentrates given to newborn infants must be irradiated to prevent graft versus host (GvH) disease.

The use of donors with chronic granulocytic leukaemia (CGL) does not seem to have become established, although several studies have shown that there is normally no risk of inducing leukaemia, only temporary engraftment of leukaemic cells having been seen (Brittingham and Chaplin, 1961; Eschbach et al. 1965; Morse et al. 1966; Buckner et al. 1969). The only exception was in a child who had been treated with total body irradiation and methrotrexate in whom there was evidence of engraftment of transfused leukaemic cells (Graw et al. 1970). For other hazards of leucocyte transfusions, see Chapters 15 and 16.

Prophylactic leucocyte transfusions in neutropenic patients
There have been several prospective randomized trials of prophylactic leucocyte transfusions (e.g. Strauss et al. 1981). The results of most of these trials have indicated that leucocyte transfusions had temporary beneficial effects but in none of them was the final outcome improved. One reason for this disappointing result may have been the occurrence of transfusion-related disease (e.g. CMV infections and pulmonary infiltrates). The numbers of leucocytes transfused to these patients were small, but it must be realized that it would be difficult to provide much larger numbers. Thus, particularly with improving antibiotic treatment, the value of prophylactic granulocyte transfusion is very doubtful.

TRANSFUSION OF HAEMOPOIETIC CELLS

The object of transfusing haemopoietic cells is to establish a permanent graft of donor stem cells in the recipient. The fate of a bone marrow graft depends largely on two immunological phenomena: (1) the rejection of transplanted marrow due to an immunological response by the recipient; and (2) an immunological reaction of the grafted immunologically competent cells against the host: GvH disease. Both these reactions depend on histo-incompatibility between donor and recipient and (1) also depends on the immunological competence of the recipient.

Complete identity of histocompatibility antigens is assured only when donor and recipient are identical twins or when autologous marrow is used. Until recently the only allogeneic donors used for bone marrow transplantation were HLA-identical siblings or other relatives, because lethal GvH disease could be expected in all other cases, even if rejection of the graft could be prevented by improved immunosuppressive treatment of the recipient. The removal of T cells from the donor marrow diminishes the risk of GvH disease and makes it possible to use phenotypically HLA-identical donors and even partially HLA-non-identical relatives. For example, successful transplantation of T cell-depleted bone marrow from mismatched fathers has recently been reported in patients with severe combined immunodeficiency syndrome (Fischer et al. 1986; Morgan et al. 1986). Even transplantation of bone marrow not depleted of T cells, from HLA-non-identical relatives, has been successful if the recipients were treated with methotrexate to prevent GvH disease (Beatty et al. 1985). For recent reviews, see Ash et al. (1990) and Hows (1990).

Over the past 10 years, transfusions of autologous blood-derived stem cells instead of, or combined with, autologous bone marrow transplants have been used increasingly. For a satisfactory effect, however, the stem cells must be collected while their

circulating numbers are deliberately expanded either by chemotherapy or by treatment with recombinant granulocyte–macrophage-colony stimulating factor (GM-CSF).
Although the use of blood-derived stem cells seems promising, there are still many
problems which need to be solved. For recent reviews see Kessinger and Armitage
(1991) and Henon *et al.* (1991). Freezing of bone marrow and the evaluation of the
quality of frozen bone marrow is carried out in specialized laboratories and will not be
discussed here.

Effect of incompatibility of grafted cells

ABO incompatibility between donor marrow cells and the recipient's plasma is not a
barrier to successful transplantation (Storb *et al.* 1976; Buckner *et al.* 1978). In a series
of 12 subjects who received ABO-incompatible marrow, not one rejected the graft and
the incidence of GvH disease was no higher than in subjects who received ABO-
compatible marrow (Hershko *et al.* 1980).

When ABO-incompatible bone marrow is injected, steps must be taken to prevent
an immediate haemolytic reaction due to lysis of red cells mixed with the marrow cells.
Originally, plasma exchange was used to diminish the concentration of anti-A and
anti-B in the recipient. This method has been supplanted by a technique in which the
marrow cells are purged almost completely of red cells. In one very satisfactory version
of this method, the harvested marrow is adjusted to a PCV of 0.25 and one volume of
6% hydroxyethyl starch is added to seven volumes of marrow in a plastic bag, which is
then inverted. During sedimentation, the red cells fall to the bottom of the bag and are
removed. After two successive sedimentations only about 2% of the red cells remain,
corresponding to a total of about 4 ml of cells. In 23 patients infused with marrow
treated in this way there were no serious immediate reactions; compared with patients
receiving ABO-compatible marrow, donor-type red cells developed somewhat later and
slightly more red cell transfusion support was needed, but there was no difference in
patient survival (Warkentin *et al.* 1985). An alternative method of removing red cells
from marrow is to use a cell separator (Blacklock *et al.* 1982).

After transplants of ABO-incompatible bone marrow the direct antiglobulin test
(DAT) may become positive after about 3 weeks if substantial numbers of donor red
cells enter the circulation. Anti-A and anti-B may remain demonstrable in the plasma
for some months and the DAT may remain positive during this time. In patients in
whom the alloagglutinins persist, transient haemolysis may develop between 35 and
105 days after transplantation due to lysis of ABO-incompatible donor cells (Sniecinski
et al. 1987). This type of haemolysis has been seen only in patients receiving
cyclosporine and prednisone to prevent GvH disease, and not in patients receiving
methotrexate. Some of the patients need transfusions of group O red cells until
haemolysis subsides (Sniecinski *et al.* 1987). In recipients in whom anti-A or anti-B
persists in high titre, erythropoiesis may be delayed (see, for example, Hows *et al.*
1983). Once the titre of anti-A or anti-B has fallen to 4 or less, erythropoiesis is no longer
suppressed but there may still be accelerated destruction of incompatible red cells
produced by the newly engrafted marrow (Petz, 1991). In some patients thrombopoiesis
may also be delayed (Sniecinski *et al.* 1988).

Lymphocytes in transplanted bone marrow may mount an immune response against host red cell antigens, leading to the development of a haemolytic syndrome 1–2 weeks after grafting; such reactions are commonest when the donor is group O and the recipient A, B or AB, but have also been observed when the donor lymphocytes develop anti-D, etc. (see Chapter 11).

There is evidence that in some of the patients in whom haemolysis is caused by anti-A or anti-B (or both), transfused group O cells are also destroyed due, probably, to the fixation of activated complement factors on to the group O cells ('bystander haemolysis') (see Petz, 1991).

Indications for bone marrow transplantation
In the opinion of the authors this subject is now one for specialists in clinical haematology and it has therefore been omitted from this edition.

HAEMOPOIETIC GROWTH FACTORS

Haemopoietic growth factors are now produced by recombinant technology and have become important in clinical medicine, Since their effect *in vivo* influences the transfusion requirements of the patients treated with them, the subject is briefly described in this chapter.

Erythropoietin

Treatment of patients with renal failure
The major cause of anaemia in patients with end-stage renal disease is a lack of production of erythropoietin, and recombinant human erythropoietin (rHuEPO) is now used successfully to treat the anaemia in these patients (Winearls *et al.* 1986; Eschbach *et al.* 1987; 1989a,b; Lim *et al.* 1989).

Based on many reports, the recommended starting dose of rHuEPO is now generally considered to be 50–100 units/kg three times a week until a PCV of 0.30 is reached. Most patients then require a maintenance dose of about 75 units/kg three times a week but this may vary from 12.5–500 units.

Side-effects of treatment with rHuEPO are hypertension and thrombotic episodes, and iron deficiency which must be treated with iron supplementation. For a survey see Klingemann *et al.* (1991).

Treatment of patients without renal disease
It has been shown that those patients with AIDS and anaemia whose levels of erythropoietin are decreased respond to treatment with rHuEPO, whether the anaemia is due to AIDS itself or to treatment with zidovudine (Rudnick, 1989). Good results have also been obtained in patients with anaemia due to inflammatory diseases (Means *et al.* 1989). Finally, patients who receive rHuEPO can donate more units of blood for autologous blood transfusion than patients who receive a placebo (Goodnough *et al.* 1989). The administration of rHuEPO to autologous blood donors is discussed briefly in Chapter 1.

Colony stimulating factors

Granulocyte-colony stimulating factor (G-CSF) and granulocyte–macrophage-colony stimulating factor (GM-CSF) affect the differentiation of cells of the myeloid series. *In vivo*, GM-CSF has been found to lead to a dose-dependent and sustained increase in the peripheral neutrophil, monocyte and eosinophil counts, whereas the effect of G-CSF is restricted to neutrophils. The factors are now used in the following conditions.

Myeloplastic syndromes

GM-CSF and G-CSF have been found to increase the number of neutrophils in this group of diseases (Vadhan-Raj *et al.* 1987; Antin *et al.* 1988; Ganser *et al.* 1989; Negrin *et al.* 1990). These factors also stimulate the proliferation of leukaemic blasts, although less strongly. In patients with a low blast count, a medium dose of GM-CSF has been shown to improve the neutrophil count without increasing the number of blasts.

Treatment of patients after chemotherapy

Both G-CSF and GM-CSF have been shown to reduce the severity of neutropenia after chemotherapy and to shorten the neutropenic phase significantly (Antman *et al.* 1988; Bronchud *et al.* 1988; Gabrilove *et al.* 1988). Treatment with G-CSF or GM-CSF makes it possible to complete chemotherapy in patients in whom this would otherwise have been impossible.

Bone marrow transplantation

Before the peripheral count begins to recover after bone marrow transplantation, patients are usually severely pancytopenic for 2–3 weeks and are then highly susceptible to bacterial and fungal infections. GM-CSF and G-CSF have been shown to accelerate bone marrow reconstitution and to shorten the pancytopenic phase by 5–7 days (Brandt *et al.* 1988; Nemunaitis *et al.* 1988; Blazar *et al.* 1989; Devereaux *et al.* 1989; Sheridan *et al.* 1989). Because there is a potential risk that the CSFs stimulate the formation of leukaemic blasts, most of the trials have been done in patients with non-myeloid malignancies and mostly in recipients of autologous bone marrow.

Because GM-CSF activates the release of cytokines from monocytes, which are probably involved in the pathogenesis of GvH disease, there is a potential danger that treatment with this factor would increase the risk for GvH disease after transplantation of allogeneic bone marrow. However, in preliminary studies in patients receiving non-T cell-depleted marrow, no increased incidence of GvH disease or aggravation of the disease has been observed (Nemunaitis *et al.* 1988).

Aplastic anaemia

In several trials patients with aplastic anaemia have been treated with GM-CSF, with variable results (Antin *et al.* 1988; Nissen *et al.* 1988; Vadhan-Raj *et al.* 1988; Champlin *et al.* 1989). It has appeared that if there are no detectable progenitor cells in the bone marrow, treatment with GM-CSF has no effect. In patients in whom there is some response, discontinuation of GM-CSF usually results in a decrease of the neutrophil count to pre-treatment levels. Although GM-CSF alone does not affect the platelet count, it has been shown in studies in primates that the combination of

GM-CSF and interleukin 3 (IL-3) leads to an increase in the platelet count (Donahue *et al.* 1988).

Treatment with GM-CSF of patients with aplastic anaemia may be useful until a bone marrow donor has been found.

Other diseases

GM-CSF increases the number of neutrophils in patients with AIDS who develop neutropenia (Groopman *et al.* 1987). Possibly, it may also facilitate HIV infection by increasing the pool of cells which can be infected. At present therefore, treatment with GM-CSF is advised only in patients who are being treated with zidovudine.

In a patient with idiopathic neutropenia, the neutrophil count became normal during treatment with G-CSF (Bonilla *et al.* 1989). The same effect was observed in five patients with congenital agranulocytosis (Jakubowski *et al.* 1989). In cyclic neutropenia, G-CSF reduced the length of the cycle (Hammond *et al.* 1989). Good results have also been obtained in patients with hairy cell leukaemia in whom neutropenia was a problem (Glaspy *et al.* 1988).

Side-effects of colony stimulating factors

The following side-effects have been observed during treatment with GM-CSF: bone pain, low-grade fever, flu-like symptoms such as myalgia, arthralgia, headache, nausea and vomiting. Doses above $500\,\mu g/m^2$ (or $16\,\mu g/kg$) can produce more serious effects, i.e. massive fluid retention and hypotension, and various forms of polyserositis, of which pericarditis may be life threatening. For a survey, see Klingemann *et al.* (1991).

THE TRANSFUSION OF PLASMA COMPONENTS

Plasma fractionation

The transfusion of whole plasma is wasteful in so far as most recipients require only a single protein, e.g. albumin or Factor VIII. Moreover, whereas no practicable method is known of treating whole plasma so as to kill any viruses which may be present in it, albumin or 'plasma protein fraction' (see below), and even freeze-dried cryoprecipitates and Factor VIII concentrates, can be heated to inactivate hepatitis viruses and HIV. Furthermore, immunoglobulin (Ig) separated by alcohol fractionation from whole plasma is virtually free from the risk of transmitting viral hepatitis and probably also HIV (see Spire *et al.* 1984). The Ig fraction contains predominantly IgG.

The incidence of haemophilia A is of the order of 60 cases per million and of haemophilia B of about ten cases per million of the population. The WHO estimates that a minimum of 10 000 iu of Factor VIII are required annually per patient to prevent serious consequences of haemophilia A. However, the International Society of Blood Transfusion (ISBT) estimates that 20 000 iu are required; if 1 litre fresh-frozen plasma (FFP) yields an average of 300 iu when a combination of cryoprecipitate and Factor VIII is used for treatment, then 70 litres FFP are needed annually to supply the needs of each patient. If the high demand for Factor VIII can be met nationally, the available amount of plasma should also cover the need for other plasma proteins,

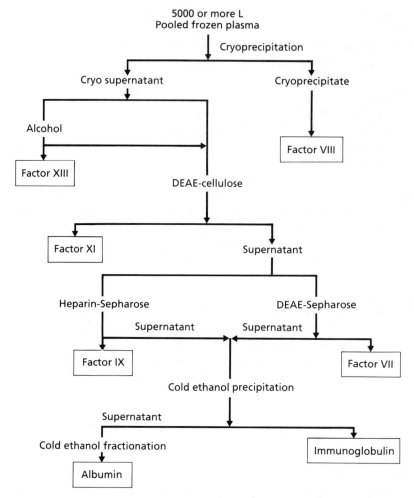

Figure 14.2   Schematic representation of the various blood products (in squares) obtained by step-wise fractionation of large pools of fresh frozen plasma using different cryoprecipitation, ethanol precipitation and adsorption procedures.

including albumin. About 23 g albumin can be prepared from 1 litre plasma. From the 75 million units of whole blood collected annually in the world, 6 million litres of plasma are obtained. An additional 8 million litres are collected by plasmapheresis, making 14 million litres of plasma available for fractionation (see Leikola, 1989; 1990). The most widely used method of fractionating plasma is still that devised by Cohn and his colleagues (1944) or modifications thereof (e.g. see, Kistler and Nitschmann, 1962). An example of a fractionation scheme is shown in Fig. 14.2.

Fresh-frozen plasma
FFP is plasma obtained from a single donor either by normal donation or by plasmapheresis and frozen within 6 h of being collected. It contains all coagulation

factors and great care must be taken during freezing and thawing to preserve their activity.

The thawed material must be stored at $4 \pm 2°C$ for no longer than 24 h before infusion. It must not be refrozen, but it can be used as single donor plasma, i.e. not to replace coagulation factors, for a long period (5 weeks).

Risks of fresh-frozen plasma

The main risk of treatment with FFP is the transmission of viruses, e.g. hepatitis B and C virus, HIV, parvovirus, etc. Allergic reactions may occur after transfusion of FFP, of which the most serious is severe anaphylaxis which may develop in IgA-deficient patients with anti-IgA. Transfusion-related acute lung injury (TRALI) may occur if the FFP contains strong granulocyte-specific or HLA antibodies (see Chapter 15). Because of these risks, FFP should be used only when there is no safer alternative. Ideally, FFP and cryoprecipitate should be prepared from donors who have never been transfused.

Precautions to be taken before injection

FFP containing potent anti-A or anti-B, or FFP which has not been tested for their presence, should not be given to recipients with corresponding red cell antigens. In order to avoid any risk of Rh D immunization, plasma from D-negative donors must be used for D-negative recipients, particularly when they are girls or women of child-bearing age.

Indications for fresh-frozen plasma

There is no justification for the use of FFP as a volume expander because there are safer alternatives (albumin, plasma substitutes) that do not carry the risk of the transmission of viral diseases.

Familial Factor V deficiency. No concentrate of Factor V is available and FFP can be used as a source of Factor V. However, because cryoprecipitate-poor plasma contains 80% of the amount of Factor V in FFP, it can be used as an alternative for FFP (Hellings, 1981).

Severe liver disease. In patients with severe liver disease, there is a deficiency of all coagulation factors. If there is severe bleeding, or the prothrombin time is increased by at least 50% or the concentration of coagulation factors is < 50%, treatment with FFP is indicated. There is no consensus of opinion as to whether FFP should be given routinely to patients with severe liver disease if surgery is required (Oberman, 1990).

Treatment of acquired deficiencies of Factors II, VII, IX and X due to treatment with anticoagulants. In patients receiving anticoagulants in whom it is desired to reverse the anticoagulant effect as soon as possible, e.g. because of bleeding or because surgery is required, in addition to injecting vitamin K, 1–2 units FFP should be transfused. If however, prothrombin complex, which contains factors II, XII, IX and X, is available, it is to be preferred. In the past, there was a risk of transmitting non-A, non-B hepatitis with this product, but prothrombin complex treated with a mixture of an organic solvent and a detergent is safe and therefore safer than FFP (H. Hiemstra, unpublished observations).

Cryoprecipitate-depleted fresh plasma (cryosupernatant)

This is plasma from which about half the fibrinogen, Factor VIII and fibronectin has been removed as cryoprecipitate. The product is also depleted of the largest multimers of von Willebrand factor (vWF) which sediment in the cryoprecipitate fraction and which may be partly responsible for platelet aggregation in thrombotic thrombocytopenic purpura (TTP). Cryosupernatant may be more effective than FFP in the treatment of TTP because it contains the activity that converts endothelial cell-derived, unusually large, vWF multimers to the smaller vWF forms normally found in the circulation. Seven patients with TTP who failed to respond to intensive plasma exchange with whole plasma responded to plasma exchange with cryosupernatant (Byrnes *et al.* 1990).

Transfusion of albumin

If radio-iodine-labelled albumin is injected i.v., its disappearance curve can, as a first approximation, be described by a two-component curve. The initial rapid component represents the mixing of injected albumin with the total exchangeable albumin pool of the body, and the slow component represents normal catabolism (Sterling, 1951).

From a review of published work, and excluding data obtained with unsuitably labelled material, Schultze and Heremans (1966) reached the following conclusions: in a normal adult weighing 70 kg, there is about 125 g albumin in the plasma and 190 g in the interstitial space, so that about 40% of the total body albumin is intravascular. The whole plasma mass exchanges with the tissues more than once a day. The daily turnover of albumin is 10–16 g; since most, if not all, this catabolism takes place in close association with the plasma compartment, the fractional catabolic rate of the plasma albumin is about 10% per day. The fractional rate of catabolism varies in direct proportion to the plasma concentration.

Albumin is available for clinical use either as human albumin in saline containing 4, 4.5, 5, 20 or 25% protein, of which not less than 95% is albumin, or as plasma protein fraction (PPF), available only as a 5% solution, of which at least 83% is albumin. Compared with albumin, therefore, most preparations of PPF contain larger amounts of contaminating proteins. Furthermore, hypotensive reactions attributed to pre-kallikrein activator and acetate have been observed with PPF (Kuwahara, 1980; Ng *et al.* 1981) but not, apparently, with albumin. For these reasons, many clinicians prefer albumin to PPF.

Albumin preparations (including PPF) are heated to 60°C for 10 h with the object of inactivating any viruses, such as hepatitis viruses and HIV, that may be present.

Although albumin contributes 75–80% of the colloid osmotic pressure of the plasma, it is worth recalling that subjects with a genetically determined total absence of plasma albumin in whom the colloid osmotic pressure of plasma is between one-third and one-half normal, may be completely asymptomatic (Bearn and Litwin, 1978). Such subjects show an increase in various plasma globulins and a slight decrease in blood pressure, changes that are regarded as compensatory (Bearn and Litwin, 1978). The indications for infusions of albumin in hypovolaemic patients are discussed in Chapter 2.

Some indications, all infrequent, for the infusion of albumin in normovolaemic subjects are as follows: hypoalbuminaemia secondary to paracentesis for ascites;

pancreatitis; acute nephritis at the outset of steroid therapy; exfoliative dermatitis (Wagstaff, 1984). The commonest indication for the use of albumin is in plasma exchange (see Chapter 1).

Albumin synthesized in vitro. In a large-scale process which is at present being developed, human albumin produced by recombinant DNA technology is synthesized in the yeast *Saccharomyces cerevisiae*. The albumin produced is correctly folded with an authentic N-terminal. Clinical trials have not yet begun (Middleton *et al.* 1991).

Transfusion of fibrinogen

The rate of disappearance of injected fibrinogen has been studied by giving injections to patients with the very rare condition, hereditary afibrinogenaemia: in two cases half the injected fibrinogen disappeared during the first 24 h, presumably due to mixing with the protein 'pool': thereafter the fibrinogen disappeared with $t_{1/2}$ of 4 d (Gitlin and Borges, 1953).

In clinical practice hypofibrinogenaemia is most often encountered as one feature of the syndrome of DIC; in this condition the transfusion of fibrinogen is seldom indicated. Purified fibrinogen prepared by fractionation of pooled plasma carries a high risk of the transmission of viral diseases such as hepatitis and is no longer available. Cryoprecipitate, containing approximately 200–250 mg fibrinogen, prepared from a single donor, is used as a source of fibrinogen.

Disseminated intravascular coagulation

DIC is a condition in which the clotting cascade is activated intravascularly. Liberated thrombin and proteolytic enzymes lead to the intravascular production of fibrin and deposition of platelets, with activation of the fibrinolytic system and an increased level of fibrin degradation products (FDP). In mild DIC the platelet count and the levels of clotting factors may be normal due to compensatory increases in production. As DIC becomes more severe, the levels of clotting factors and platelets fall, a state which may be described as decompensated DIC.

DIC may be precipitated by a wide variety of injuries. Many cases are due to the entry of tissue thromboplastin into the circulation, e.g. after premature separation of the placenta. Other conditions associated with DIC include infections, malignancies, amniotic fluid embolism and intravascular lysis of incompatible red cells.

The cardinal principle of treatment of DIC is to remove the underlying cause since, once this has been done, there is usually a return to normal haemostasis. When the cause cannot be dealt with there may be uncontrollable bleeding. The transfusion of blood may be essential and the replacement of clotting factors has to be considered. This replacement should be guided by coagulation assays and fibrinogen levels. If levels of clotting factors are severely reduced, FFP should be given and, if there is severe thrombocytopenia, platelets are indicated. If the fibrinogen level is very low, cryoprecipitate should be infused. An initial dose of ten bags, to provide 4–6 g, has been suggested (Prentice, 1985). Despite the theoretical objection of adding fuel to the fire, the administration of fibrinogen does not seem to be dangerous.

Since, while DIC continues, fibrinogen, clotting factors and platelets are rapidly consumed, the administration of heparin has been advocated to interfere with coagulation. Administration of an anticoagulant seems particularly indicated in patients who have an underlying disease which it is difficult to treat.

Although there have been no convincing clinical trials to demonstrate that heparin is effective, it is believed to reduce haemorrhage and to increase levels of coagulation factors in particular circumstances, e.g. in the induction treatment of promyelocytic leukaemia, in which the administration of EACA as well as heparin has been advocated (Schwartz et al. 1986). Since, in the presence of thrombocytopenia and hypofibrinogenaemia, full-dose heparinization is believed to be extremely dangerous, an initial dose of 7.5 units/kg per hour has been suggested, to be given immediately before the infusion of platelets and cryoprecipitate (Feinstein, 1988). In treating DIC associated with a haemolytic transfusion reaction, a much larger dose has been recommended; see p. 511.

The transfusion of Factor VIII (anti-haemophilic factor)

Factor VIII levels in haemophiliacs
Severely affected haemophiliacs have no detectable Factor VIII activity in their plasma and suffer from repeated episodes of spontaneous bleeding. Patients whose Factor VIII activity is 1–5% of normal are moderately affected and have infrequent attacks of bleeding. Those with levels exceeding 5% are mildly affected and very seldom have spontaneous bleeding.

Treatment with Factor VIII
Widely varying doses of Factor VIII are used in different haemophilia centres to treat haemorrhages. A common dosage schedule is as follows: 10 iu Factor VIII/kg for minor haemorrhages and 20 iu/kg for major haemorrhages (Kasper et al. 1989). The dose given for a haemorrhage should be the one which the clinician and the patient have found to be promptly effective on previous occasions. Adequate doses may vary from patient to patient and according to the conditions of the individual joint in which the haemorrhage occurs and the severity of the haemorrhage.

Prophylactic administration of Factor VIII
Although the incidence of bleeding can be reduced or even abolished in severe haemophiliacs by prophylactic treatment (Hirschman et al. 1970), the amounts of Factor VIII needed for the general application of such treatment are impracticably large (Aronstam et al. 1976). Nevertheless, prophylactic (maintenance) therapy is sometimes used to prevent haemorrhages. The standard treatment in some centres is routine prophylaxis at a dose sufficient to prevent nearly all haemorrhages, especially in childhood and adolescence. Short-term prophylactic therapy should be considered in patients with frequent haemorrhages, especially if they occur repeatedly in the same joint, or in the presence of chronic synovitis, or if active rehabilitation is planned (Kasper et al. 1989).

Factor VIII levels of healthy donors
The Factor VIII activity in group A donors is on average 8% higher than in group O donors, and the level in males is about 6% higher than in females (Preston and Barr,

1964). Strenuous exercise produces an almost immediate increase in Factor VIII levels, lasting for at least 6 h (Rizza, 1961).

Factor VIII levels can also be increased by injecting DDAVP (1-deamino-8-D-arginine vasopressin). DDAVP is a synthetic derivative of vasopressin which, following i.v. injection, produces a marked, transient, increase in plasma Factor VIII coagulant activity, in Factor VIII-related antigen and in Factor VIII ristocetin co-factor activity in patients with mild or moderate haemophilia A, as well as in patients with von Willebrand's disease. If DDAVP (0.2 μg/kg) is injected into donors 15 min before venesection, the yield of Factor VIII in fractions prepared from the resulting plasma is increased two-fold (Nilsson *et al.* 1979; Mannucci, 1986). However, DDAVP is probably best administered by the intranasal route 1 h before donation to minimize side-effects (Mikaelson *et al.* 1982).

Disappearance of injected Factor VIII from the circulation
When plasma is transfused about 82% of the expected Factor VIII activity is found in the recipient's plasma immediately after infusion; with cryoprecipitates the figure is 70% and with human Factor VIII concentrates 60% (Rizza and Biggs, 1969). Since Factor VIII is removed from the plasma with a half-time of 9–14 h, if infusions are given only every 24 h the level must be expected to have fallen to one-quarter of the maximum post-infusion level by the time that the next infusion is given. When it is important to maintain a relatively high Factor VIII level, e.g. after surgery, it is best to give doses every 12 h.

Choice of Factor VIII-containing material for therapy
Factor VIII can be administered as cryoprecipitate or as Factor VIII concentrate. Only when these are not available should FFP be considered. In FFP, Factor VIII activity is well maintained on storage at −30°C to −40°C. The Factor VIII activity of FFP must not be less than 0.7 iu/ml.

The main risk of treatment with Factor VIII is the transmission of viruses, particularly HIV and hepatitis viruses. The choice of product to use for treatment is largely determined by this risk (see Chapter 16).

Cryoprecipitates
When plasma is fast-frozen and then thawed slowly at 4–6°C, the small amount of protein precipitated is rich in Factor VIII. After decanting almost all the supernatant plasma the protein can be redissolved by warming to give a small volume of solution. The introduction of cryoprecipitate revolutionized the treatment of haemophiliacs by making a highly effective and convenient source of Factor VIII readily available. Cryoprecipitates are available as several different products.

Small-pool freeze-dried cryoprecipitate is prepared from a pool of eight to 12 plasma donations, and the recipient is thus exposed to a much smaller number of donors than when large-pool freeze-dried cryoprecipitate or Factor VIII concentrate is used. Exposure to a smaller number of donors is not important when considering the transmission of HIV since these viruses are inactivated when freeze-dried cryoprecipitate is heated suitably, but is important when considering the risk of transmitting viral hepatitis, particularly non-A, non-B hepatitis, the agents of which are not all inactivated by heating (see Chapter 16). Some 300 iu Factor VIII should be recovered for every kilogram of starting plasma (Hässig and Lundsgaard-Hansen, 1978). The product is relatively stable on storage and easy to transport.

Large-pool freeze-dried cryoprecipitate prepared from approximately 1000 individual cryo-precipitates. Although this product can be heated, or treated with solvent detergent, to inactivate viruses, the chance of transmitting infection, is greater than when small-pool material is used.

'Contaminants' in cryoprecipitates. Cryoprecipitates contain about 30–50% of the original fibrinogen and have about the same titre of anti-A and anti-B as that of the original unit (Rizza and Biggs, 1969; Pool, 1970). Cryoprecipitates may contain enough Rh D-positive red cell debris to sensitize a D-negative patient (see Chapter 5).

Factors which help to maximize the concentration of Factor VIII in the cryoprecipitate are as follows: in addition to the use of DDAVP (see above) obtaining the blood by means of a clean venepuncture, mixing the blood adequately during collection, separating the plasma promptly, minimizing cellular contamination of the plasma, freezing the plasma to lower than $-30°C$ within 2 h of collection, and rapid thawing to recover the cryoprecipitate (Wensley and Snape, 1980). Rapid and controlled thawing of frozen plasma packs, using a microwave oven, has been found to give higher yields of Factor VIII than are obtained by slow thawing overnight (Bass *et al.* 1985). Other important factors which increase Factor VIII yields are agitation (Margolis, 1976) and removal of residual plasma from the cryoprecipitate by siphoning (Mason, 1978). Although the use of heparinized plasma as starting material has been shown to increase the yield of Factor VIII (Rock *et al.* 1979; Smit Sibinga *et al.* 1981; Krackmalnicoff and Thomas, 1983), the resulting cryoprecipitate has poor solubility. Only donations obtained in less than 10 min should be used for the preparation of cryoprecipitates or of FFP. Cryoprecipitate prepared from 1 unit of blood should contain at least 70 iu Factor VIII.

Purified Factor VIII concentrates

Intermediate-purity concentrate. Most fractionation centres use large pools of plasma (500–5000 donations) to prepare this product. The primary procedure is cryoprecipitation, but additional fractionation steps are undertaken to give a higher potency (15–20 iu/ml), stability and solubility than are obtained with the freeze-dried cryoprecipitate. These steps lead to a loss of yield but a method for producing a preparation of intermediate purity with excellent yield has been described (Rock and Palmer, 1980).

High-purity concentrate. Concentrates purified by using affinity chromatography with monoclonal antibodies against Factor VIII have a specific activity of Factor VIIIC of about 3000 iu/mg protein. Even after albumin is added as a stabilizer, the purity is still significantly higher than that of all previously available products. In a group of patients treated with this product for more than 24 months, clinical efficacy, $t_{1/2}$ and recovery were excellent (Brettler *et al.* 1989). The main advantage of purified high potency concentrates was thought to be a less pronounced effect on the immune system of the patients. However, purified concentrate is far more expensive and, despite intensive research in many countries, incontrovertible evidence of its advantages is still lacking (Cash, 1991). Moreover, there is evidence that, particularly in children, some high-potency products more easily induce the formation of Factor VIII inhibitors (Bell *et al.* 1990; Kessler and Sachse, 1990; Montoro *et al.* 1991). Various virus-inactivating procedures have been developed to prevent transmission of viruses by Factor VIII concentrates. These procedures (described in Chapter 16) are particularly important because Factor VIII concentrates prepared from large pools of donor plasma carry a high risk of transmitting viruses.

Synthesis of Factor VIII in vitro. A development of great potential importance is the production of human Factor VIII by recombinant-DNA clones. Clones encoding the complete 2351 amino acid sequence for human Factor VIII have been isolated and used to produce Factor VIII in cultured mammalian cells. The recombinant protein corrects the clotting time of plasma from haemophiliacs and has many of the biochemical and immunological characteristics of plasma-derived Factor VIII. It is hoped that this new technique will make plentiful supplies of Factor VIII available and that the material, being free from viruses, will be safer than plasma-derived Factor VIII (Wood *et al.* 1984).

Clinical trials have shown that *in vivo* recovery and $t_{1/2}$ of recombinant Factor VIII (rFactor VIII) are not significantly different from those of plasma-derived Factor VIII. The rFactor VIII Recombinate (Baxter Highland Division) has been used for the treatment of 55 patients with haemophilia A and found to be effective in acute bleeding episodes, in securing haemostasis during surgery and postoperatively, and for prophylaxis. Only two of 5127 infusions were followed by a mild adverse reaction and inhibitors developed in none of the patients (White *et al.* 1991).

A total of 127 patients with haemophilia A have now been treated with the rFactor VIII Kogenate (Cutter Biological/Miles Inc.). Kogenate has been found to be efficacious for treatment of bleeding episodes and for prophylaxis. The effect of the recombinant product was comparable to that of plasma-derived Factor VIII (Brackmann *et al.* 1991). Of the above 127 patients, 37 had not been treated before with plasma-derived Factor VIII. No immediate or long-term adverse effects were seen but seven of the 37 patients developed inhibitors (Lusher *et al.* 1991).

Animal Factor VIII concentrates. Concentrates prepared from bovine or porcine plasma have 100 times more Factor VIII activity per milligram of protein than normal human plasma. The original preparations were immunogenic and could as a rule be used effectively for only 7–10 d, following which antibodies against the animal protein developed. Polyelectrolyte-fractionated porcine Factor VIII concentrate (PE porcine VIII) appears to be considerably less antigenic and contains negligible amounts of platelet-aggregating factor (Kernoff *et al.* 1981).

Factor VIII inhibitors (antibodies)
Factor VIII inhibitors are found either as alloantibodies in a proportion of haemophiliacs following treatment with Factor VIII-containing materials or, more rarely,

as autoantibodies in non-haemophiliacs. The frequency of Factor VIII antibodies in haemophiliacs was reported to be 6% by Biggs (1974) and to be as high as 15% in selected haemophiliacs with Factor VIII levels of 10% or less by Lusher *et al.* (1980, supplemented by personal communication from P.M. Blatt). As mentioned above, the percentage may be higher in patients treated with monoclonal antibody-purified Factor VIII concentrate.

Patients with Factor VIII inhibitors are relatively refractory to treatment with Factor VIII and must be given very high doses of Factor VIII to secure a response. Concentrates of Factor VIII are effective if the inhibitor titre is less than 20 Bethesda units (B.u.)/ml; with higher titres, Factor VIII concentrates alone are ineffective. Haemophiliacs with Factor VIII inhibitors may show a rise in inhibitor titre following the infusion of Factor VIII; in such patients Factor VIII concentrates are not effective for more than 5–7 d (Blatt *et al.* 1982).

In treating major haemorrhage in haemophiliacs with inhibitors, provided that the inhibitor titre does not exceed 20 B.u./ml, human Factor VIII concentrate should be used initially. In average-sized adults (70 kg) 5000 units of Factor VIII are given initially, followed by 500–1000 units per hour. Thereafter, the dose is adjusted according to the Factor VIII level (Blatt *et al.* 1982). In patients with inhibitor titres exceeding 20 B.u./ml, activated prothrombin–complex concentrates (e.g. Autoplex) appear to be very effective but are very expensive (P.M. Blatt, personal communication). These concentrates bypass the need for Factor VIII in some unknown way.

In patients who require very large amounts of Factor VIII, animal factor concentrates may be very useful. Kernoff *et al.* (1981) reported the results of giving the improved preparation, PE porcine VIII, described above, to four haemophiliacs with Factor VIII inhibitors; repeated infusions were given for periods up to 27 d with very satisfactory results. An antibody response was detected in only one of the four patients. It was concluded that PE porcine VIII was a rational and effective therapeutic alternative to human Factor VIII concentrate in haemophiliacs with inhibitors. Equally good results were obtained in a recent trial (Hay *et al.* 1990). The authors concluded that administration of porcine Factor VIIIC was the treatment of choice in patients with inhibitors which did not crossreact with the porcine product.

In minor bleeding episodes, e.g. haemarthroses, prothrombin–complex concentrates may be tried. In a double-blind, randomized study they were shown to produce significantly better results than a placebo, even though they were only partially effective (Lusher *et al.* 1980).

Increasing numbers of patients with inhibitors have been made immunotolerant to Factor VIII after treatment for several weeks or months with daily or frequent infusions of Factor VIII, sometimes combined with short courses of immunosuppressive agents such as corticosteroids, cyclophosphamide and i.v. Ig (see Kasper *et al.* 1989).

Activated Factor VIII has been found to be beneficial in patients with antibodies against Factor VIII (see below).

Therapy that reduces the amount of Factor VIII required for treatment
In some circumstances, the need for Factor VIII can be reduced by the administration of EACA (ε-aminocaproic acid) (Reid *et al.* 1964).

In a double-blind trial, patients undergoing dental extraction received either EACA (6 g four times daily for 10 d) or a placebo, in conjunction with a single pre-operative dose of Factor VIII concentrate designed to raise the Factor VIII level to 50% of normal. Of ten patients who received the full course of EACA therapy, not one required Factor VIII transfusion, whereas of 12 patients receiving the placebo, seven required Factor VIII transfusion (Walsh et al. 1971).

Tranexamic acid, an isomer of EACA, is more potent and has fewer side-effects than EACA. Given as an initial i.v. dose followed by oral administration four times daily for 5–7 d, it is useful in controlling any form of external bleeding in haemophiliacs such as epistaxis or following dental extraction, but is contraindicated in haematuria.

As mentioned above, DDVAP (0.3 μg/kg) produces substantial increases in Factor VIII levels in patients with mild or moderate haemophilia.

Transfusion of cryoprecipitate in uraemia
In five of six patients with uraemia, bleeding times, which were all more than 15 min before treatment, became normal after the infusion of cryoprecipitate. In four of six patients, major bleeding episodes were controlled (Janson et al. 1980).

Transfusion in patients with von Willebrand's disease
This disorder is a condition with a prolonged bleeding time and decreased levels of Factor VIII (both the coagulant activity and the Factor VIII-related antigen) and of vWr (ristocetin) co-factor. In the majority of patients with von Willebrand's disease, both the Factor VIII defect and the bleeding time can be corrected by giving DDAVP (0.3 mg/kg), which is clinically efficacious in preventing or stopping haemorrhages. However, 10–20% of patients with von Willebrand's disease do not respond to DDAVP and some patients become refractory when repeated transfusions are given over a long period of time (Rodeghiero et al. 1992). Patients who require treatment with plasma products should be given heat-treated cryoprecipitate or Factor VIII concentrate. The latter is now preferred to cryoprecipitate for most patients with von Willebrand's disease (Cohen and Kernoff, 1990).

All the commercially available Factor VIII concentrates of low or intermediate purity appear to be equally effective. More experience is needed to establish the therapeutic effect of high-purity concentrates and of the newly developed von Willebrand Factor concentrates. For planned surgery the products should be given a few hours before operation and the Factor VIII level measured immediately before the operation is begun; if the level is not high enough, more of the product should be given.

Treatment of Factor IX deficiency (Christmas disease or haemophilia B)
Patients with haemophilia B are usually treated with PCC which contains Factors II, VII, IX and X (see below) as well as many other proteins such as other vitamin K-dependent proteins, protein C and protein S, an inter-α-trypsin inhibitor, high-molecular-weight (HMW) kininogen, C4, C5 and C9 (Pejandier et al. 1987). Treatment with PCC may lead to thrombotic disorders and DIC, induced by these contaminating proteins (Aronson & Menache, 1987; Chavin et al. 1988).

Procedures have been developed to produce a highly purified Factor IX concentrate, based either on a combination of three conventional chromatographic steps (Burnouf *et al.* 1989) or on immune-affinity chromatography with monoclonal antibodies against Factor IX (Kim *et al.* 1990; Tharakan *et al.* 1990). Treatment with a purified product has been shown to avoid the side-effects mentioned above (Kim *et al.* 1990).

A wide variety of doses of Factor IX are used in different haemophilia centres to treat or prevent haemorrhages. A common dosage schedule is 20 units Factor IX per kilogram for minor haemorrhages and 40 units for major ones. The dose chosen for a given haemorrhage should be the one which has been found to be promptly effective on previous occasions in the patient concerned (Kasper *et al.* 1989).

The need for Factor IX administration after the extraction of teeth can be considerably reduced by administering DDAVP (Rodeghiero *et al.* 1992).

Concentrates containing Factors II, VII, IX and X (prothrombin–complex concentrates)

Concentrates containing these vitamin K-dependent factors were originally produced for the treatment of inherited Factor IX deficiency but are also used for acquired deficiencies of Factors II, VII, IX and X, e.g. in patients with liver disease or due to coumarin. As described above, these concentrates have also been used for treating minor bleeding episodes in haemophiliacs with inhibitors. The concentrates should be administered rapidly, and immediately after reconstitution.

As mentioned above, prothrombin–complex concentrates are thrombogenic and their use remains controversial except in the treatment of haemophilia B, although, even here, purified Factor IX concentrate will probably replace prothrombin–complex concentrate (see above).

Use of some other coagulation factors

Factor VII
Plasma-derived Factor VII concentrate has been used to treat congenital Factor VII deficiency for several years (Dike *et al.* 1980). Because of the short half-life (3–4 h), frequent infusions are necessary, especially to cover surgery. Activated Factor VII (Factor VIIa) has been found to be effective in haemophiliacs with antibodies to Factor VIII (Hedner and Kisiel, 1983). Factor VIIa is believed to have a Factor VIII bypassing activity. Recombinant Factor VII, which is activated spontaneously during purification, has been successful in covering knee surgery in a patient with haemophilia A and antibodies to Factor VIII (Hedner *et al.* 1988).

Factor XIII
Pasteurized Factor XIII concentrates prepared from either plasma or placenta are used to treat patients with Factor XIII deficiency, a condition which is just as dangerous as haemophilia A or B (Smith, 1990).

Protein C
Protein C is a serine protease zymogen, which is activated by thrombin. Activated protein C attacks the activated forms of Factors V and VIII; it requires a co-factor, protein S. Activated protein C also stimulates fibrinolysis by neutralizing the inhibitor

of tissue plasminogen acivator. Protein C deficiency, whether hereditary or acquired as, for example, in severe liver disease, leads to venous thrombosis. Factor IX concentrate, which contains protein C, has been variably successful in severe protein C deficiency (Tuddenham *et al.* 1989). A human vapour-treated protein C concentrate is now available (Immuno, Vienna). An infant with severe protein C deficiency and purpura fulminans was treated successfully with this concentrate. Long-term therapy was well tolerated (Dreyfus *et al.* 1991).

Fibrin glue

The action of fibrin glue resembles that of the last phase of blood clotting, i.e. the conversion of fibrinogen into fibrin. There are two components of fibrin glue, one consists of fibrinogen with Factor XIII, fibronectin and plasminogen, and the other is a combination of bovine thrombin and calcium chloride. When the two solutions are mixed, thrombin converts fibrinogen into fibrin monomers. Activation of Factor XIII by thrombin in the presence of ionized calcium stabilizes cross-linkage of fibrin monomers, thereby increasing the tensile strength of the clot. The glue has adhesive and haemostatic properties and has been found to enhance wound healing, possibly due to fibronectin. The clot is lysed by the fibrinolytic activity in the wound area. An antifibrinolytic agent, such as aprotinin, can be added to either of the two components to delay clot lysis in areas with a high local fibrinolytic activity, e.g. the lung, the prostate, the uterus and highly vascularized tissues. Fibrin glue is currently used in various kinds of surgery and is commercially available (Immuno, Vienna; Behringwerhe, Germany). For a review of the subject see Brennan (1991).

C1 esterase inhibitor (C1 inh.)

Hereditary functional deficiency of C1 inh. is due to either a deficiency or a dysfunction of the protein. Acquired deficiencies of C1 inh. also occur. This protease inhibitor is involved in the regulation of several proteolytic systems in plasma, including the complement system, the contact system of intrinsic coagulation and kinine release, and the fibrinolytic system (see Cugno *et al.* 1990). Functional deficiency of C1 inh. causes angioneurotic oedema, a serious, potentially fatal, syndrome characterized by attacks of swelling of the subcutaneous tissues and mucous membranes. The pathogenesis of angioneurotic oedema is not completely understood (see Baldwin *et al.* 1991).

Pasteurized C1 inh. concentrates are now available and acute attacks of angioneurotic oedema can be successfully treated with them (Brummelhuis, 1980; Gadek *et al.* 1980). Long-term prophylaxis with C1 inh. concentrate in hereditary as well as acquired C1 inh. deficiency has also been successful (Bork and Witzke, 1989). Activation of the complement and contact systems occurs in septic shock, together with a decrease of plasma C1 inh. levels. Preliminary results show that complement and contact activation can be diminished by treatment with high-dose C1 inh. concentrate (Hack *et al.* 1992).

Injections of immunoglobulin

Survival of injected immunoglobulins

IgG. Of the total IgG, 42–44% is intravascular (Cohen and Freeman, 1960; Solomon *et al.* 1963); accordingly, when IgG is injected, it is distributed in a space rather more than twice as large as that of the plasma volume.

Following i.v. injection, there is a phase of relatively rapid loss due to exchange of IgG between the intravascular and extravascular compartments; equilibrium is reached in about 5 d (Cohen and Freeman, 1960). The daily movement of IgG from the intravascular to the extravascular compartment is equivalent to about 25–30% of the plasma IgG and is of course balanced by a similar transfer in the opposite direction.

When equilibrium has been attained, the plasma level declines with a $t_{1/2}$ of 21 d. The fractional turnover rate of IgG1, IgG2 and IgG4 subclasses is much the same, namely 7–8% per day, but that of IgG3 is much higher, namely 16.8% per day, corresponding to a $t_{1/2}$ of 7 d (Wells, 1980). These estimates are derived from studies with myeloma proteins; estimates made with monoclonal antibodies derived from hybridomas should soon be available. The fractional rate of catabolism is largely independent of plasma IgG concentration so that the total IgG turnover varies directly with the plasma IgG level. The rate of IgG synthesis is thus the primary factor determining the serum IgG level (see Schultze and Heremans, 1966, p. 485). The catabolism of IgG has also been studied by injecting HBs antibodies in high titre, the disappearance of the antibodies being followed with a very sensitive radio-immunoassay. The $t_{1/2}$ of these IgG antibodies was calculated to be 19.7 d (Shibata *et al.* 1983). For other estimates, see pp. 92 and 576.

The i.v. injection of 'standard' Ig preparations, i.e. 16% Ig for i.m. injection (containing predominantly IgG), may produce severe reactions (see Chapter 15). These reactions are particularly troublesome in patients with agammaglobulinaemia or hypogammaglobulinaemia, who may need (over a long period) regular injections of large amounts of Ig, which are difficult to give i.m.

Early Ig preparations suitable for i.v. use resulted in damage to the Fc fragment of IgG and thus to its biological functions. However, several different procedures have now been developed which produce fully functional, well-tolerated preparations of immunoglobulins for i.v. use. One of these procedures is DEAE fractionation and treatment at pH 4 with only traces of pepsin, which does not cleave the IgG molecule, but only breaks up aggregates (Jungi and Barandun, 1985). If i.v. Ig is available in the liquid state, its pH must be low for the sake of purity and stability. A low pH of the product may be associated with pain, erythema and even phlebitis at the injection site. Freeze-dried preparations can be reconstituted immediately before use at a pH of 6.6, thus avoiding the above side-effects. Stable i.v. preparations have a $t_{1/2}$ of 22 d *in vivo*.

Following i.m. injection of IgG the material passes via the lymphatics into the blood stream. Analysis of plasma concentration curves is relatively complex since the influx into the plasma from the site of injection is offset by efflux from the plasma into the extravascular space and also by catabolism. In a study in which ^{125}I-labelled IgG was used, the average fraction of the dose cleared per day from the site of i.m. injection, after injecting 2 ml solution into the deltoid muscle, was estimated to be about 0.37. Plasma levels were almost maximal at 2 d, and corresponded to about 40% of the values which would have been attained immediately after i.v. injection of the same doses (Smith *et al.* 1972); see also Table 10.1 on p. 471. In a single case studied by

Jouvenceaux (1971), surface counting over the site of injection showed that approximately 45% of the total injected dose was cleared per day. In two normal subjects studied by Morell et al. (1980), following the injection of 10 ml 16% Ig into the gluteal region, plasma levels corresponded to 32% of the injected dose on day 5 in one case and 20% on day 7 in the other. In retrospect it seems very likely that uptake was poor because the injections were made into fatty tissue rather than into muscle. One survey indicated that when injections are given into the gluteal region few female patients and fewer than 15% of male patients receive an i.m. injection (Cockshott et al. 1982).

In a study in rabbits the animals were injected simultaneously with ^{125}I-labelled IgG i.v. and ^{131}I-labelled IgG i.m. From a comparison of the levels of the two isotopes in the plasma, the uptake from the i.m. injection sites was deduced without making any compartmental assumptions. The rate of loss of IgG from the injection site was not constant, being faster initially and continuing to decrease at least over the first 7 d; although 70% of the injected IgG had left the injection site by 1–2 d, 10–15% had still not been accounted for in the plasma by 7 d. A similar analysis was attempted for the return from the extravascular space to the plasma. The tentative conclusion was that 80–90% of the IgG returned to the plasma within 6 h but that the other 10–20% had a half-life in the extravascular space of 1–2 d (Smith and Mollison, 1977).

Following subcutaneous injection of IgG into the buttock, the rate of uptake is distinctly slower than after i.m. injection and maximum plasma levels have still not been attained 5 d after injection (Smith et al. 1972).

IgM and IgA
Human Ig preparations contain very little IgM but may contain between 0.2% and 11.8% IgA (Koistinen and Leikola, 1975). About 80% of the total IgM is intravascular; 15–18% is catabolized per day (Brown and Cooper, 1970). About 40% of IgA is intravascular; after equilibration, the level of labelled IgA in the plasma declines with a $t_{1/2}$ of 6 d (Tomasi et al. 1965). For further information, see Schultze and Heremans (1966). Reactions due to anti-IgA are considered in Chapter 15.

Changes in immunoglobulin preparations on storage
In immunoglobulin preparations the IgG sometimes undergoes breakdown to Fab and Fc-like fragments on storage due, it is believed, to traces of plasmin in the preparation (Connell and Painter, 1966). Preparations in which this breakdown has occurred are unsatisfactory since the half-life of the antibody after injection is reduced. Stable IgG preparations can be obtained by careful control of pH during fractionation (Painter and Minta, 1969). The fragmentation of IgG occurs only after isolation of the Ig since, in whole plasma, plasmin is rapidly inactivated by naturally occurring inhibitors (R.H. Painter, personal communication).

Although most IgG antibodies show no obvious change in potency over a period of several years in Ig preparations kept at 4°C, the concentration of anti-D was found to diminish at the rate of about 8% a year over a period of 2–4.5 years in 28 preparations tested by Hughes-Jones et al. (1978). There was no evidence of any appreciable breakdown of IgG molecules in the preparations in the same period.

Use of human immunoglobulin

Prophylaxis of infectious disease. Standard human Ig, prepared for i.m. injection from unselected plasma, is used in protection against hepatitis A, rubella and measles. The immunity conferred by an injection of Ig is, of course, temporary and depends upon the amount of antibody injected. Ordman *et al.* (1944) found that a dose of Ig which would protect children from measles for periods up to 14 d would not protect them for as long as 7–10 weeks. A relatively large dose (450 mg) of Ig provides some protection for periods up to 6 weeks (see Kekwick and Mackay, 1954, p. 58).

In the prophylaxis of hepatitis A the study of Pollock and Reid (1969) suggested that a single dose of Ig (750 mg) may protect for about 5 months.

Hyperimmune Igs prepared from selected donors with high titres of the relevant antibodies are used in the prophylaxis of hepatitis B (see Chapter 16), diphtheria, tetanus, rubella, herpes zoster, rabies, measles and infection with CMV, *Pseudomonas*, etc. Anti-D Ig is used in the prevention of primary Rh D immunization (see Chapter 10).

Anti-HBsAg Ig in very high doses is used for liver transplantation in HBsAg-positive recipients. Specific anti-pertussis toxoid Ig has been shown to reduce significantly the number of whoops in patients with whooping cough (Granström *et al.* 1991).

A decreased incidence of bacterial infections and sepsis and an improved survival rate has been observed in infants with congenital AIDS receiving i.v. Ig (Calvelli and Rubinstein, 1986).

Treatment of hypogammaglobulinaemia. Patients with either congenital or acquired hypogammaglobulinaemia with IgG levels of less than 2 g/l may be regarded as candidates for treatment. Intravenous injection is usually preferred, because of the large amounts of Ig which have to be given. Subcutaneous injection of Ig preparations for i.m. use has also been satisfactory (Roord *et al.* 1982). The recommended dose is 0.2 g/kg body-weight once a month. If the response is unsatisfactory, the dose can be increased or the injections given more frequently. When i.v. Ig is given for the first time or when more than 2 months have elapsed since the previous injection, the Ig should be administered slowly to avoid side-effects such as fever, chills, nausea and vomiting. Anaphylactic reactions are relatively frequent in patients with hypogammaglobulinaemia (see Chapter 15).

Neonatal sepsis. Good results in the treatment of neonatal sepsis, particularly in premature infants, were described by Sidiropoulos *et al.* (1981), who advised routine prophylactic treatment of prematurely born infants weighing less than 1500 g (0.5 g daily for 6 d). In another study, 133 newborn infants were divided into two groups based on whether the duration of gestation was shorter or longer than 34 weeks. The infants were randomly assigned to receive either 500 mg/kg i.v. Ig weekly for 4 weeks or no therapy. Septicaemia and infection-related deaths were significantly less frequent in the group of infants born before 34 weeks who had received i.v. Ig (Chirico *et al.* 1987).

Bacterial infections in adults. In a double-blind study in patients with multiple injuries the prophylactic use of i.v. Ig decreased the incidence of pneumonia by one-third (Glinz *et al.* 1985). It is thought that the best results in bacterial infection will be seen with selected preparations containing antibodies in high titre. Trials with anti-*pseudomonas* Ig prepared from plasma from vaccinated volunteers showed that treatment with the preparation may be life-saving in patients with severe burns (Jones *et al.* 1980). The protective effect of human i.v. Ig preparations in bacterial infection has been shown very clearly in mice (Imaizumi *et al.* 1985). However, results of other trials in patients with severe burns of multiple injuries were not convincing (for a survey see Berkman *et al.* 1990).

Chronic lymphocytic leukaemia (CLL). Hypogammaglobulinaemia is common in patients with CLL, and response to immunization is impaired. The incidence of infections was reduced by 50% in 42 patients with CLL receiving i.v. Ig (400 mg/kg every 3 weeks) compared to the incidence in 42 patients receiving a placebo (Cooperative Group for the Study of Immunoglobulins in CLL, 1988). The beneficial effect of i.v. Ig in CLL has been confirmed in another study (Griffiths *et al.* 1989).

Multiple myeloma. Antibody responses are markedly impaired in patients with multiple myeloma, and infections are common. In a prospective study there was a substantial reduction in bacterial infections in 94 patients treated with i.v. Ig (Schedel, 1986).

Treatment of viral infections. Treatment with i.v. Ig in children with Kawasaki disease, which is probably caused by a retrovirus, has been shown to be effective in several trials (Nagashima *et al.* 1987). Favourable results have been obtained in the treatment of several other viral infections (see Berkman *et al.* 1990).

Autoimmune thrombocytopenic purpura. The potential value of Ig in the treatment of AITP was first demonstrated in a child who was refractory to all conventional therapy. Following a large dose (0.4 g/kg body-weight) of i.v. Ig an immediate rise in the platelet count and a concomitant arrest of the bleeding tendency were observed. In a subsequent study, in all of 13 children, six with acute and seven with chronic AITP treated with i.v. Ig, the platelet count began to rise within 24–48 h. In four of the six patients with acute AITP and in two of the patients with chronic AITP, the platelet count remained normal. In the other children the treatment had to be repeated and one child became resistant to treatment with i.v. Ig (Imbach *et al.* 1981).

Because children with acute thrombocytopenic purpura are at risk for life-threatening haemorrhage early in the disease, treatment with i.v. Ig (1 g/kg per day for 3 d) has been tried in 29 patients by Bussel *et al.* (1985). In all children there was a considerable increase in the platelet count within 24 h. In another study of 94 children with acute thrombocytopenic purpura, 47 were treated with i.v. Ig (0.4 g/kg per day for 5 d) and 47 with corticosteroids. The percentages of children responding to the initial treatment were similar in the two groups (83% and 77%, respectively), but in the cases in which treatment had to be continued, the platelet count rose more rapidly and to higher values in patients treated with i.v. Ig (Imbach *et al.* 1985). In children with acute thrombocytopenic purpura, treatment with i.v. Ig has been advised when the platelet count falls below $10 \times 10^9/l$ (Blanchette and Turner, 1986).

In 15 adults platelet counts rose from a mean of $19 \times 10^9/l$ to a mean of

$122 \times 10^9/l$ after therapy with i.v. Ig for 4 d (Newland *et al.* 1983). However, the increase in the platelet count was maintained in only one of the 15 patients. Despite discouraging long-term results in adults, i.v. Ig has been recommended for patients who are bleeding or who have to undergo surgery, because it induces a significant, albeit short-term, rise in the platelet count in most patients (Oral *et al.* 1984). The mechanism responsible for the effect is unknown, but may be the blocking of the Fc receptor on macrophages or the neutralization of autoantibodies by idiotype antibodies.

The injection of relatively small amounts of anti-Rh D Ig has also been successful in inducing remissions in AITP. In D-positive adults, 750–4500 μg anti-D was given in one series (Salama *et al.* 1986); in another, all of 13 D-positive patients given 2500 μg responded, and a single D-negative patient failed to respond (Boughton *et al.* 1988). Success has also been achieved by giving a single dose of 4 ml D-positive red cells coated *in vitro* with 100 μg anti-D (Ambriz *et al.* 1987). These observations suggest that anti-D produces its beneficial effects by causing D-positive red cells to bind to, and thus block, Fc receptors on macrophages. Nevertheless, this may not be the mechanism. Remission has been reported in one D-negative pregnant woman who had failed to respond to steroids and who was given 120 μg anti-D i.v. (Moise *et al.* 1990). The effective agent in anti-D Ig may be HMW IgG polymers rather than anti-D. Preparations of anti-D Ig contain a substantially higher proportion of HMW IgG polymers than non-specific Ig preparations and these polymers are more effective in blocking Fc receptors (Boughton *et al.* 1990).

Other autoimmune diseases. Intravenous Ig has been used successfully in treating patients with autoimmune neutropenia (Pollack *et al.* 1982; Bussel *et al.* 1983). For the effect of i.v. Ig in autoimmune haemolytic anaemia, see Chapter 7.

Intravenous Ig has also been used in treating patients with other immune disorders: diabetes, systemic lupus erythematosus, chronic inflammatory polyneuropathy, the Guillain–Barré syndrome, myasthenia gravis, pure red cell aplasia, rheumatoid arthritis and amyotropic lateral sclerosis (for references see Berkman *et al.* 1990). Finally, in patients with Factor VIII inhibitors the autoantibody titre was decreased following i.v. Ig administration; this effect was thought to be due to IgG antibodies against idiotypes of the anti-Factor VIII autoantibodies (Sultan *et al.* 1984).

Alloimmune diseases. High-dose i.v. Ig has been used in Rh D haemolytic disease (see Chapter 12), in neonatal alloimmune thrombocytopenia (see Chapter 13) and in post-transfusion purpura (see Chapter 15).

Bone marrow transplantation. Intravenous Ig has been used to modify GvH disease and has been found to decrease CMV-related interstitial pneumonia (Gale and Winston, 1991).

Novel intravenous immunoglobulins
By hybridoma technology, genetic engineering and chemical methods, novel specific monoclonal antibody preparations have been or are being prepared, and may replace polyclonal i.v. Ig for several indications in the future. Both human and murine monoclonals are produced, e.g. against bacterial antigens. To reduce the antigenicity

of murine Igs, antibodies are modified by genetic engineering and drugs, toxins, lymphokines, radionuclides or enzymes are conjugated to monoclonal antibodies by chemical methods (for a survey, see Yap and Williams, 1990). The application of these antibodies is still experimental. However, one murine monoclonal, Orthoclone OKT3, directed against a T lymphocyte-specific antigen, is now licensed and used in the treatment of transplant rejections.

Antithrombin III (AT-III)

There are at lest two types of hereditary AT-III deficiency: the level of AT-III may be low (about 50% of normal) or AT-III may be functionally deficient. In both cases the deficiency is characterized by early manifestations of venous thromboembolism. AT-III inactivates five of the activated coagulation factors. It is probably this function of AT-III at several levels of the coagulation pathway which explains why an apparently modest decrease in AT activity, as in patients with familial low AT-III levels, leads to a thrombotic tendency (Abilgaard, 1984).

AT-III is stable in stored blood (Lundsgaard-Hansen et al. 1983; Inkster et al. 1984) and it is therefore not necessary to use FFP as a source of AT-III. Several methods for the isolation of AT-III have been described (see Wickenhauser and Williams, 1984). Heat-treated AT-III concentrates are now available commercially and are indicated for the prevention or treatment of thromboembolic disorders in patients with hereditary AT-III deficiency (Lechner et al. 1983; Menache et al. 1990).

There are also several causes of acquired AT-III deficiency, but the only circumstances in which AT-III concentrates are definitely indicated are when patients with hepatic cirrhosis are to undergo surgery and when patients are in hepatic coma or pre-coma (Lechner et al. 1983). To ensure careful control the use of AT-III should at present be limited to institutions with special expertise and facilities (Council of Europe, 1984).

Fibronectin

Fibronectin is a glycoprotein widely distributed throughout the body, being found in a soluble form in plasma and in an insoluble form in connective tissue matrices. Several functions of fibronectin have been described; an adhesive function in intracellular attachment and thus probably in wound healing (Yamada and Olden, 1978); a haemostatic function, through its binding to fibrin (Mosher, 1975) and presence in platelets (Plow et al. 1979); and an opsonic function (Saba and Jaffe, 1980). Thus it seems possible that acquired deficiency of fibronectin might adversely affect wound healing, haemostasis and phagocytosis. It has been suggested that impairment of mononuclear phagocyte function in patients following major surgery, trauma, burns or sepsis is associated with diminished plasma fibronectin (Saba et al. 1978; Grossman et al. 1980), and that administration of cryoprecipitate to such patients restores plasma fibronectin levels and results in clinical improvement (Saba et al. 1978).

In a further trial, six patients either undergoing surgery or with severe trauma, with low levels of fibronectin, were treated with purified fibronectin solution (Saba et al. 1986) which produced a significant increase in immunoreactive and functional fibronectin levels; the long-term clinical effects of the treatment were not reported. The results of a controlled trial in patients with severe abdominal infections led to the conclusion that survival or death of the patients was independent of treatment with fibronectin (Lundsgaard-Hansen *et al.* 1985). Furthermore, no correlation was found between fibronectin levels, either at the beginning of, or during, treatment, and the type or number of organs whose function failed. These results are supported by other studies (Rubli *et al.* 1983; Hesselvik *et al.* 1987; Mansberger *et al.* 1989). In all these trials no improvement in organ function was observed after treatment with fibronectin.

Initial, uncontrolled clinical studies have shown a possible beneficial effect of fibronectin in wound healing, e.g. in patients with persistent corneal wounds (Nishida *et al.* 1983; Phan *et al.* 1987). Further placebo-controlled double-blind studies of treatment with fibronectin in patients with corneal lesions or cutaneous wounds are needed to establish the value of this treatment. For a survey, see Powell and Doran (1991).

α_1-antitrypsin (α_1-AT)

α_1-AT is a major serine endopeptidase inhibitor in human plasma and inhibits neutrophil elastase, an enzyme involved in the proteolysis of connective tissue, especially in the lung. Hereditary deficiency for α_1-AT may lead to progressive emphysema. Clinical trials have suggested that replacement therapy in deficient patients may restore the concentration of α_1-AT in plasma and thereby limit the development of emphysema (Gadek *et al.* 1981). A method for the preparation of an α_1-AT concentrate, which can be treated at 60°C for 10 h whilst maintaining excellent inhibitory activity against trypsin and elastase, has been described (Burnouf *et al.* 1987). Another α_1-AT concentrate derived from Cohn fraction IV-1, also treated at 60°C for 10 h (Cutter Biological), has been given to 21 patients homozygous for the deficiency allele (P_1Z) as weekly injections of approximately 4 g for 6 months (Wewers *et al.* 1987). Peak levels in plasma were above the normal upper range. After a rapid decline during the first 2 days after infusion, corresponding to redistribution of α_1-AT into the intravascular space, there was a slower rate of decline consistent with the normal 4–5-day half-life of plasma α_1-AT. The lowest levels before the next injection were always above the threshold level. Diffusion of the infused material across the alveolus and a significant increase in elastase activity in epithelial lining fluid could be demonstrated. Similar results were obtained in another study (Konietzko *et al.* 1988). There are, however, still unanswered questions with regard to replacement therapy with α_1-AT. It has not been established whether such therapy actually prevents the development or the further progress of emphysema. The question as to which deficient patients should be treated has not been answered. Considering the number of deficient patients (e.g. 70 000 in the USA) it is clear that a long-term demand cannot be met by α_1-AT produced from plasma. Recombinant α_1-AT will be needed (for a survey of the subject see Eriksson, 1989).

CHAPTER 15

SOME UNFAVOURABLE EFFECTS
OF TRANSFUSION

FIGURES

Adverse effects due to overloading the circulation have been discussed in Chapter 2 and 9 and haemolytic transfusion reactions in Chapter 11. The present chapter is concerned with some other unfavourable effects which may be produced by transfusion. The transmission of infection from donor to recipient is considered separately in the following chapter.

Immunological reactions involving leucocytes, platelets or plasma proteins

Adverse reactions may be caused by an interaction between leucocytes, platelets or plasma proteins and antibodies directed against them. Complement may be activated as a result of this interaction, leading to the liberation of vasoactive substances. In addition, the destruction of transfused leucocytes may be associated with fever, presumably because of the release of endogenous pyrogen from phagocytic cells (see p. 698).

In practice, when a patient develops signs such as flushing of the face, indicating the release of vasoactive substances, and suggesting that complement activation has occurred, it is often impossible to establish the cause of the reaction.

Diagnosis of the cause is difficult, either because no alloantibodies can be detected, or because the patient has more than one type of alloantibody (e.g. HLA and Am antibodies) in their plasma, when it is usually impossible to decide which, if either, has caused the reaction. On the other hand when fever develops, and potent leucocyte reactive antibodies are found, it is highly probable that these antibodies have caused the reaction. Although the cause of transfusion reactions cannot at present always be determined, it seems likely that most have an immunological basis.

REACTIONS DUE TO LEUCOCYTE ANTIBODIES

Febrile reactions due to antibodies in the recipient

The possibility that leucocyte antibodies might cause transfusion reactions was mentioned by Goudsmit and van Loghem (1953) and by Dausset (1954). The first evidence in support of this hypothesis was produced by van Loghem *et al.* (1956) and was based on a single case in which a patient with leucoagglutinins tolerated leucocyte-poor blood better than whole blood. Very soon after this, abundant evidence in support of the hypothesis was published (Payne, 1957; van Loghem *et al.* 1958).

The role of leucocytes in causing transfusion reactions in patients with leucocyte antibodies was shown very clearly by Brittingham and Chaplin (1957). In five patients who had a history of severe febrile reactions following blood transfusion and whose serum contained leucoagglutinins, the transfusion of a fraction of blood containing more than 90% of the buffy coat produced a severe febrile reaction, but the transfusion, from the same bottle of blood, of red cells and plasma with less than 10% of the buffy coat caused no reaction (Fig. 15.1). The severe reactions were

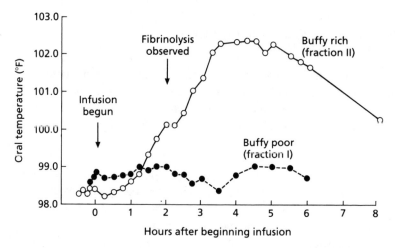

Figure 15.1 Effect of transfusing the 'buffy' coat to a patient whose serum contained leucoagglutinins. Two fractions were prepared from fresh blood, fraction I containing many red cells with very few white cells and platelets, fraction II containing a few red cells and most of the plasma, platelets and white cells. As the figure shows, transfusion of this second fraction produced a very severe febrile reaction whereas transfusion of the first 'buffy-poor' fraction produced no fever (from Brittingham and Chaplin, 1957).

characterized by flushing within 5 min of the start of transfusion, with a feeling of warmth. The patient then felt well for 45 min; about 60 min after the start of the transfusion a severe febrile reaction began.

Complementary observations were made by Payne (1957). Leucoagglutinins were found in 32 of 49 patients with a history of febrile transfusion reactions. Moreover in 13 of 15 patients receiving repeated transfusions, leucoagglutinins were first detected about the time when the patient first started developing transfusion reactions. Blood containing fewer than 0.2×10^9 leucocytes per litre provoked no reaction in these patients.

Brittingham and Chaplin (1961) in a detailed study of a single subject found that 0.4×10^9 leucocytes (the number present in 50 ml normal blood) would not produce a reaction, whereas the injection of 1.5×10^9 or more would regularly do so. The reactions produced by 1.5×10^9 leucocytes were very mild when the titre of the leucoagglutinin was low but severe at a time when the titre was higher. Perkins et al. (1966) studied eight patients and concluded that the least number of leucocytes which would produce a reaction varied from 0.25×10^9 to more than 25×10^9. The degree of temperature elevation was related to the number of incompatible leucocytes transfused (Perkins et al. 1966).

The conclusion is that in preparing leucocyte-poor blood for transfusion to patients who have had febrile reactions due to leucoagglutinins the aim should be to remove at least 90% of the leucocytes.

Features of febrile reactions
When patients develop febrile reactions following transfusion they do not start to feel cold for at least 30 min after the transfusion has started and, often, signs do not develop for 60–80 min (see Fig. 15.2). On the other hand, as mentioned above, when the patient's plasma contains potent leucocyte antibodies, flushing may develop within 5 min of the start of the transfusion, due presumably to complement activation.

Febrile reactions have been produced experimentally in human volunteers by injecting pyrogenic inulin. No symptoms developed for the first hour or so; then the blood pressure started to rise and the subject complained of chilliness. Soon there was a more or less severe chill and the onset of fever. At the peak of the reaction the subject might develop nausea, headache and back pain. At about the time of the chill there was a considerable increase in renal blood flow which lasted several hours. All these manifestations, with the exception of the effect on renal blood flow, could be abolished by giving the subject aminophenazone (amidopyrin) 0.6 g, every 4 h, starting 18 h before the injection of the pyrogen (Smith, 1940).

Fibrinolysis has been observed in association with severe febrile reactions due to leucocyte antibodies (Fig. 15.1). Febrile reactions can also be caused by red cell incompatibility (see Chapter 11) and by platelet incompatibility (see later).

High fever regularly following transfusion in parous women, or in patients who have previously received many transfusions, is very likely to be due to leucocyte antibodies, but mild febrile reactions, observed after only one of a series of transfusions, were found not to be associated with leucoagglutinins by Kevy et al. (1962). Unless leucocyte-poor red cells are readily available they should not be used except in patients who have had at least two severe febrile non-haemolytic reactions.

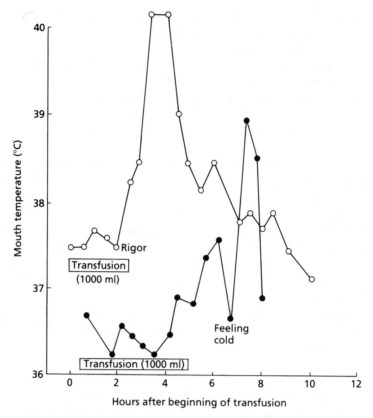

Figure 15.2 Severe febrile reactions following transfusion. ○—○, Transfusion completed in 2 h; rigor (chill) began before the transfusion was finished. ●—●, Transfusion of the same amount of blood in 5.5 h. The temperature started to rise at the end of about 5 h. About 1 h later the patient felt cold, but did not shiver, the temperature then rose and reached its maximum about 2 h after the end of the transfusion.

Febrile reactions in infants

Infants seem incapable of shivering. Perhaps this explains why so little interest is usually taken in an infant's reaction to transfusion. If an infant's temperature is recorded at intervals after transfusion it is not unusual to observe rises in temperature up to 38.5°C or thereabouts. Sometimes the rise in temperature is accompanied by a temporary refusal to feed and by diarrhoea.

Although the infant does not shiver in the early phase of the febrile reaction, it does exhibit pallor and its skin feels cold. The following is an example:

Baby R, aged 5 weeks, was recovering from haemolytic disease of the newborn. Its Hb concentration was 10 g/dl, but it was decided to give a transfusion as the infant was shortly going on a journey by air and would not be under supervision for a long period thereafter.

Seventy-five millilitres of fresh Rh D-negative blood were injected into a scalp vein in 20 min. The infant appeared to have stood the transfusion well, but 75 min later it was pale and refused to feed. During the next 2 h it was restless, and 3 h after the transfusion its pulse rate was 200 per min. Four hours after transfusion the temperature was 39.1°C and the pulse rate 180.

The temperature remained above 39°C for a further 3 h and then fell gradually. Next day the baby appeared perfectly well.

Relative importance of granulocytes and lymphocytes in causing febrile reactions
When blood is passed through a suitable nylon filter, most of the granulocytes and monocytes, but not the lymphocytes, are removed. In patients who had previously developed febrile reactions following the transfusion of whole blood, no fever developed in 75 of 83 cases in which nylon-filtered blood was used, indicating that granulocytes and perhaps also monocytes must play a major role in causing febrile transfusion reactions (Greenwalt et al. 1962).

Role of anti-HLA compared with that of granulocyte-specific antibodies
Granulocytes react with anti-HLA-A, -B and -C, as well as with granulocyte-specific antibodies. Monocytes react with the same HLA antibodies and with antibodies against class II antigens, as well as with monocyte-specific antibodies.

Two studies support the conclusion that HLA antibodies play a predominant role in causing febrile transfusion reactions. In the first, in which sera from 101 patients with a history of non-haemolytic transfusion reactions were tested against granulocytes and lymphocytes by several different methods, the highest percentage of positives was obtained with a modified cytotoxicity test against B lymphocytes; 32% of these positive reactions, probably due to weak HLA-A, -B or -C antibodies, were missed by the standard cytotoxicity test (Décary et al. 1984).

In the second study, in which leucocyte agglutination, lymphocytotoxicity, and immunofluorescence tests using granulocytes, lymphocytes and platelets were applied, HLA alloantibodies were found far more frequently than granulocyte-specific antibodies; alloantibodies of one kind or another were found in every single case; in 36 of 40 patients leucocyte antibodies were found but in the remaining four the antibodies detected were directed against platelet-specific antigens (de Rie et al. 1985). From both studies it was concluded that a large cell panel must be used in looking for alloantibodies in patients who have had febrile reactions following transfusions.

Transfusion-related acute lung injury (TRALI)
A severe, potentially fatal, transfusion reaction caused by leucocyte antibodies is characterized by chills, fever, a non-productive cough, dyspnoea and hypotension. On radiography, numerous nodules, predominantly perihilar, and infiltration of the lower lung fields without cardiac enlargement or engagement of the vessels are found (see Ward, 1970). This reaction, and the fact that it may be caused by injecting leucoagglutinins into a recipient, was first described by Brittingham and Chaplin (1957). Fifty millilitres of blood containing leucoagglutinins with a titre of 256 were transfused to one of the two authors, who developed all of the above-mentioned symptoms.

Several cases of this reaction which is now named transfusion-related acute lung injury (TRALI) have been reported since then. In most cases the responsible antibodies were present in the donor (Ward, 1970; Kernoff et al. 1972; Popovski et al. 1983; Yomtovian et al. 1984; Levy et al. 1986; Gans et al. 1988). However, TRALI may also occur when the antibodies are present in the recipient and granulocytes are transfused (Ward, 1970; Wolf and Canale, 1976; Gans et al. 1988).

The following antibodies have been responsible for TRALI; HLA antibodies (Andrews *et al.* 1976; Campbell *et al.* 1982; Popovski *et al.* 1983; Popovski and Moore, 1985; Gans *et al.* 1988; Eastlund *et al.* 1989); granulocyte-specific antibodies (anti-NA2, Yomtovian *et al.* 1984; anti-NB2, van Buren *et al.* 1990) and anti-5b (Nordhagen *et al.* 1986).

In one study 36 cases of TRALI were diagnosed in a single medical centre (Mayo Clinic) in a period of 2 years (Popovski and Moore, 1985). The authors suggest that TRALI occurs much more frequently than appears from the literature and that the diagnosis is often missed. In this series of cases granulocyte-reactive antibodies were detected in only two of the patients, but were detected in at least one of the donors whose blood was transfused to 32 of the 36 patients, which confirms that TRALI is caused by donor antibodies in the vast majority of cases. In 26 of the cases there was evidence of the presence of HLA antibodies in the donors and in 11 cases the specificity of the, presumably class I, antibodies, could be established. In all these cases the recipient was positive for at least one of the corresponding HLA antigens. In two cases no antibodies could be found in either the donor or the patient.

The exact mechanism and therefore the essential characteristics of the antibodies responsible for TRALI are not clear. However, in an *in vitro* model in which isolated rabbit lungs and 5^b antibodies were used, severe vascular leakage could be induced, but only in the presence of rabbit complement (Seeger *et al.* 1990). This finding implies that activation of complement is essential for inducing TRALI. Fragments of activated C5 injected into rabbits have been shown to produce inflammation of the lungs, characterized by accumulation of neutrophils and oedema (Larsen *et al.* 1980; Henson *et al.* 1982). Thus it seems likely that an essential characteristic of the responsible antibodies is that they bind complement.

It has been suggested that the patient's pre-existing condition plays a significant role in the occurrence of TRALI (Popovski and Moore 1985; van Buren *et al.* 1990). However, severe TRALI occurred in a healthy young male volunteer after the injection of an i.v. Ig preparation containing HLA class I and class II antibodies (Dooren *et al.* 1992b).

In conclusion, TRALI, the most severe transfusion reaction caused by leucocyte antibodies, probably occurs much more frequently than appears from the literature. It is caused by granulocyte-reactive antibodies in the donor in the vast majority of cases; HLA, granulocyte-specific and 5^b antibodies have been responsible for the reaction which may occur in previously healthy subjects.

Leucoagglutinins complicating haemodialysis
Pasternack and Furuhjelm (1964) observed that in a patient who had had a series of dialyses, using the Kolff twin-coil unit, the filter of the unit became blocked during dialysis and that this was due mainly to clumping of leucocytes; the patient's serum contained a leucoagglutinin with a titre 32; the problem was overcome by using leucocyte-poor blood.

Crossmatching of leucocytes
When granulocytes are transfused to subjects who have already formed antibodies it may be possible to secure good survival and avoid reactions by using suitable compatibility tests.

When blood transfusions are given with the sole object of supplying red cells, it is possible to remove the leucocytes by differential sedimentation, filtration, washing, or freezing and thawing.

In patients with acute leukaemia transfused with an average of 0.2×10^{11} granulocytes from a single donor with chronic myeloid leukaemia, reactions occurred after 19 of 21 transfusions in subjects with preformed antibodies but after only six of 57 transfusions in subjects without antibodies. It was recommended that in giving leucocyte transfusions the donor leucocytes should be crossmatched against the recipient's serum partly to avoid reactions and partly because incompatible antibodies inhibit the bactericidal power of granulocytes (Goldstein et al. 1971).

In crossmatching, it seems advisable to use a combination of the granulocyte immunofluorescence test, which is the most sensitive technique for the detection of granulocyte-specific antibodies (Verheugt et al. 1971), and the lymphocytotoxicity test, which is best for the detection of HLA antibodies.

Hazards of leucocyte transfusions
Apart from the immediate immunological reactions which may occur, leucocyte transfusions are quite often followed by a toxic reaction characterized by fever and occasional transient episodes of hypotension. These reactions are probably due to the effect of neutrophils damaged during collection (Goldman et al. 1979). The greatest hazard of using leucocyte concentrates is the possibility of transmitting infectious agents, particularly cytomegalovirus (CMV). The risk is greatest in children (for further details see Chapter 16). Another risk is graft versus host (GvH) disease (see below).

Removal of leucocytes from red cell concentrates

Use of centrifugation to prepare leucocyte-poor blood
The majority of non-haemolytic febrile transfusion reactions in multitransfused patients can be prevented or attenuated by the transfusion of units of blood containing fewer than 0.5×10^9 leucocytes, i.e. less than 20% of the original number (Perkins et al. 1966), prepared simply by centrifugation and removal of the buffy coat.

Use of filters to remove granulocytes
The use of a nylon-mesh column to remove leucocytes was described by Greenwalt et al. (1962). Fresh heparinized blood had to be used and only granulocytes (and monocytes) but not lymphocytes were removed. The most effective method of removing not only granulocytes and monocytes, but also lymphocytes, is to pass the blood through cotton wool. Blood is centrifuged to sediment the red cells but not the platelets. The red cells are resuspended in saline and then filtered. The method results in the removal of 98% or more of the leucocytes and 90–95% of the platelets (Diepenhorst et al. 1972; Diepenhorst and Engelfriet, 1975; Sirchia et al. 1980; Mijovic et al. 1983). The first cotton-wool filters to be described were very effective in removing leucocytes from blood but they were designed for use in the blood bank and some needed water pumps to provide the necessary pressure (Diepenhorst and Engelfriet, 1975). White-cell depletion filters now available remove more than 99% of leucocytes. For further discussion, see Chapter 13.

Other methods of preparing leucocyte-poor red cells

Removal of leucocytes by freezing and thawing. Suspensions of red cells which have been frozen in glycerol, thawed and washed thoroughly appear to be free from the risk of causing febrile transfusion reactions (Chaplin *et al.* 1956a; Haynes *et al.* 1960). Ninety-eight per cent or more of the leucocytes and 100% of the platelets and plasma are removed from each unit of blood; the red cell loss is, on average, 10%.

Removal of leucocytes by washing. Washing of red cells in the Dideco Progress 90 and IBM machines removes 82% and 89% of leucocytes respectively but also removes 3–30% of the red cells. If one attempts to remove 90% of the leucocytes, the loss of red cells is even greater (Hughes and Brozović, 1982).

In summary, in patients who have had previous transfusion reactions and in whom leucocyte-poor red cells are indicated (see above), blood depleted of white cells by centrifugation should be provided initially, since this will be effective in most patients. If the patient still experiences febrile reactions, blood passed through a white-cell depletion filter should be used.

The effect of drugs in suppressing febrile reactions

Smith (1940) and Altschule and Freidberg (1945) showed that pyrogenic reactions could be modified by the previous administration of antipyretic drugs. Dare and Mogey (1954) gave i.v. pyrogens to volunteers and found that if 1 g aspirin was administered at the onset of shivering, all symptoms were suppressed within 20 min in all except the most severe cases; moreover, there was no subsequent rise in temperature. In a single case investigated by Jandl and Tomlinson (1958), 1 g aspirin given to the subject 1 h before the injection of 10 ml Rh D-sensitized cells, followed by three doses of 1 g at 2-h intervals, starting 2 h after the injection, appeared to suppress a febrile reaction. In children, paracetamol rather than aspirin should be used in the prophylaxis of febrile reactions.

There is no good evidence that antihistamines prevent febrile reactions. Wilhelm *et al.* (1955) added 5 mg diphenhydramine hydrochloride to 500 ml blood at the time of collection and found that the patients receiving such blood were as likely to develop febrile reactions as those receiving untreated blood. Hobsley (1958) found that the same was true when the drug used was Piriton (chlorpheniramine maleate), 10 mg being added to 500 ml blood. Wilhelm *et al.* also found that in rabbits the subcutaneous injection of antihistamine drugs 15 min before the i.v. injection of purified pyrogen did not prevent a febrile reaction; the drugs they tested were the two mentioned above and pyribenzamine (tripelennamine hydrochloride).

Effect of rate of infusion

It seems evident that when pyrogenic substances are being infused the rate of infusion will affect the severity of the reactions. This is one reason for using a moderate rate of transfusion, e.g. 500 ml in 1 h in non-urgent cases. Many clinical impressions have been recorded to the effect that febrile reactions are more severe when transfusions are given rapidly (see Grant and Reeve, 1951).

Graft versus host disease

This syndrome is produced when, following successful engraftment of allogeneic T lymphocytes or their precursors, the foreign cells, if they are HLA incompatible, mount an attack against the host tissues.

The main features of GvH disease are: fever and skin rash, which usually begins as a central erythematous, maculopapular eruption which spreads to the extremities and which may progress to generalized erythroderma and the formation of bullae, nausea, vomiting and watery or bloody diarrhoea, lymphodenopathy and pancytopenia due to bone marrow aplasia. There are typical changes in the lymph nodes and the spleen.

GvH disease frequently occurs after bone marrow transplantation and in the last two decades there has been an increasing incidence of GvH disease following blood transfusion: transfusion-associated GvH disease (TA-GvH disease). TA-GvH disease occurs between 4 and 30 d after transfusion and is severe with a mortality rate as high as 90% (see von Fliedner et al. 1982). TA-GvH disease has been observed after transfusion of whole blood, packed red cells, platelet concentrates, granulocyte concentrates and fresh plasma (for a survey see Anderson and Weinstein, 1990).

TA-GvH disease has been reported in four types of recipients.

1   In subjects with immature immunological systems, i.e. in fetuses following intra-uterine transfusion and premature infants after exchange transfusion. Two cases of fatal GvH disease in immunologically normal infants who had been given intra-uterine transfusions at 30 and 32 weeks, with blood which had been kept for not more than 48 h before transfusion, were reported by Parkman et al. (1974). Both infants, born at 36 weeks, were treated by exchange transfusion and died 2–3 weeks after birth. The cells causing the GvH reaction came from the donors used for the exchange transfusion and it was therefore concluded that the role of the intra-uterine transfusion had been to induce tolerance. GvH disease following exchange transfusion in premature infants has been demonstrated by Seemayer and Bolande (1980).

2   In subjects with an impaired immunological system, e.g. thymic alymphoplasia and combined immunodeficiency disease (Hathway et al. 1967; Park et al. 1974). In these cases GvH disease, which may occur following a single transfusion, is often fatal. However, no cases of TA-GvH disease have been reported in patients with AIDS, despite in vitro evidence of profound immunodeficiency (Kaslow et al. 1987).

3   In patients with an immunological system impaired by cytotoxic drugs, e.g. patients with acute leukaemia (Ford et al. 1976) or Hodgkin's disease (Burns et al. 1984).

4   In non-immunocompromised patients TA-GvH disease may occur when the donor is homozygous for one of the patient's HLA haplotypes. In this situation the patient is incapable of rejecting the donor's T lymphocytes, which can react against the HLA antigens encoded by the patient's other haplotype (Sakatibara and Juji, 1986; Ito et al. 1988; Otsuka et al. 1989; 1991; Thaler et al. 1989). The chance that a donor is homozygous for one of the patient's haplotypes is very small in the general population, but greater among first-degree relatives and in populations in which homozygosity for HLA haplotypes is much more frequent as, for example, in Japanese people and the Israelian population.

TA-GvH disease is underdiagnosed because the syndrome usually affects patients who are already severely ill and the combination of symptoms may be wrongly attributed to the underlying disease, intercurrent infection or a severe reaction to a drug. Consequently the frequency of TA-GvH disease is unknown. GvH disease occurred in one of 659 immunocompetent patients following cardiac surgery with transfusion of fresh blood in Japan (Juji *et al.* 1989). However, because homozygosity for HLA haplotypes is relatively frequent in the Japanese population, no conclusions can be drawn concerning the general frequency of TA-GvH disease.

Prevention of transfusion-associated graft versus host disease
In order to avoid the risk of GvH disease from the transfusion of random blood components to patients with immunological deficiency, the transfused materials should be treated with 1500 rad (15 Gy) before being transfused (Graw *et al.* 1970). This dose abolishes the response of lymphocytes in mixed lymphocyte cultures. Incidentally, the dose of radiation required to impair red cell survival is far greater than this: 35 000 rad (350 Gy) or more, according to Schiffer *et al.* (1966).

When first-degree relatives are used as donors, irradiation of the blood has been advised, even in recipients who are not immunocompromised (AABB, 1989; Vogelsang, 1990), although not everyone supports this view (Avoy, 1990).

Whether platelet or red cell concentrates from which the leucocytes have been removed, by filtration, washing, or freezing and thawing, can safely be used is uncertain (Anderson and Weinstein, 1990). It has been shown that frozen and thawed red cell concentrates contain some 2% of residual leucocytes with the capacity to proliferate (Crowley *et al.* 1974). Thus, immunocompetent T cells are present, suggesting that current leucocyte-depletion techniques may not be effective in preventing TA-GvH disease (Anderson and Weinstein, 1990).

REACTIONS DUE TO PLATELET ANTIBODIES

Febrile reactions
The role of platelet antibodies in causing transfusion reactions is rather difficult to assess, first because suspensions of platelets are always contaminated to some extent with leucocytes, and second because platelet alloantibodies are usually associated with leucocyte antibodies. Nevertheless, there is no doubt that the destruction of platelets by alloantibodies may cause adverse reactions. The association was shown convincingly by Aster and Jandl (1964b). HLA-A2-negative recipients were transfused with HLA-A2-positive platelets and, a day or two later, with serum containing anti-HLA-A2. In three of the four recipients, frontal headache developed at 30 min, and at 45–50 min rigors lasting 15–30 min, followed by fever.

Cases in which severe febrile reactions were almost certainly due to incompatible platelets but may have been due partly to contamination with transfused leucocytes were described by Marchal *et al.* (1960) and Cooper *et al.* (1975).

As mentioned above, only platelet-specific antibodies were detectable in the serum of four of 40 patients who developed a typical febrile reaction after transfusion (de Rie *et al.* 1985).

Post-transfusion purpura (PTP)
In this syndrome, profound thrombocytopenia develops approximately 1 week after a transfusion, in association with the presence of platelet alloantibodies.

The first example was recorded by van Loghem *et al.* (1959) in a patient in whom the platelet antibody, anti-Zw[a], was first identified, but it was Shulman *et al.* (1961) who pointed out that there must be a connection between immunization to the platelet antigen and the onset of thrombocytopenia. These latter authors described two further patients with the syndrome, in both of whom anti-Zw[a] (which they renamed anti-Pl[A]) was present. Both patients developed severe generalized purpura with thrombocyto-penia 6–7 d after a blood transfusion. It was postulated that these two patients had been primarily immunized to Pl[A1] previously during pregnancy, and that the subse-quent transfusion of Pl[A1] platelets had stimulated an anamnestic response. It was suggested that for at least 1 week after transfusion sufficient Pl[A1] antigen from transfused platelets had remained to interact with anti-Pl[A1] and had somehow caused the non-specific destruction of the patient's own Pl[A1]-negative platelets (see below). However, the authors did not succeed in demonstrating residual Pl[A1] antigen in their patients. Pl[A1] (Zw[a]) has now been renamed HPA-la; see Chapter 13.

Some of the features of PTP are as follows: almost all the patients are women, most of whom appear to have been immunized by previous pregnancies. In a few cases, women who have either not been pregnant or who have had only HPA-1(a –) children have been immunized by a previous transfusion; one case has been described in a woman who had not been pregnant and had not previously been transfused (Nicholls *et al.* 1970). Among over 200 recognized cases, only five were in men, four of whom had been transfused many years before the transfusion, which was followed by PTP (Shulman, 1991).

Almost all patients have been shown to be HPA-1(a –) with anti-HPA-1a in their plasma during the period of thrombocytopenia. In three of the early cases the patient was HPA-1(a +) (Vaughan-Neil *et al.* 1975; Zeigler *et al.* 1975; Hoak *et al.* 1979); in these cases the possibility that the antibody had another specificity, e.g. anti-HPA-1b, was not investigated. Cases have been described in which anti-HPA-1b was, in fact, demonstrable in the serum of HPA-1(a +) patients who developed PTP (Taaning *et al.* 1985; Ludorf *et al.* 1988). Apart from antibodies to HPA-1 antigens, anti-HPA-3a (anti-Bak[a]) anti-HPA-3b (anti-Bak[b]), anti-HPA-4b (anti-Pen[a], Yuk[a]) and anti-HPA-5b can also be responsible for PTP (Boizard and Wautier, 1984; Simon *et al.* 1988; Kiefel *et al.* 1989; Christie *et al.* 1991).

Anti-HPA-1a has usually been found in its highest concentration on about the seventh day after transfusion and in many cases has disappeared completely within the following month. However, in a case described by Lau *et al.* (1980) the antibody level had fallen to only 50% of its peak after 12 months, and in a case described by Slichter (1982) the antibody remained detectable for 18 months. Of eight cases investigated by Pegels *et al.* (1981), the antibody was wholly IgG in six cases and partly IgG and partly IgM in two. The IgG antibody was wholly IgG1 in five cases and also partly IgG3 in three; in most cases the antibody was capable of activating complement.

Thrombocytopenia has most commonly been first diagnosed on the seventh day after transfusion, the limits being 5–12 d in all but one case (Le Roux *et al.* 1981) and, if untreated, has often persisted for more than 1 month.

Treatment of post-transfusion purpura
Many patients have been treated with steroids, usually without beneficial effect,

although in five cases the administration of prednisone in doses of approximately 1–2 mg/kg per day has produced a prompt rise in platelet count (Vaughan-Neil *et al.* 1975; Seidenfeld *et al.* 1978; Moffat *et al.* 1982; Slichter, 1982; Weisberg and Linker, 1984).

Plasma exchange has proved to be a very effective treatment. Shulman *et al.* (1961) reported a very good response in one case to the exchange of approximately 6 litres of fresh whole blood, and a similarly good response to whole blood exchange was reported by Cimo and Aster (1972), i.e. the platelet count rose from virtually nil to $45 \times 10^9/l$ within 24 h. Subsequently, rapid responses to plasma exchange have been reported by many others, e.g. Lau *et al.* (1980). One case in which plasma exchange (5 litres in 3 d) failed to produce any obvious improvement was described by Erichson *et al.* (1978).

The transfusion of HPA-1(a –) platelets to patients with PTP due to anti-HPA-1a has been thought to be an ineffective form of therapy (Vogelsang *et al.* 1986; Mueller-Eckhardt and Kiefel, 1988). However, a case of PTP has been described in which transient increases in the patient's platelet count and clinical haemostasis have been achieved by multiple transfusions of HPA-1(a –) platelets (Brecher *et al.* 1990).

More recently, treatment with high-dose i.v. Ig has been introduced and has been reported to be successful by Glud *et al.* (1983), Hamblin *et al.* (1985), Becker *et al.* (1985) and Walker *et al.* (1988). A good or excellent response was observed in 16 of 17 patients with PTP, normal platelet counts being reached within a few days. Relapse occurred in five patients, but in these platelet counts became normal after a second dose of i.v. Ig (Mueller-Eckhardt and Kiefel, 1988). In a patient with massive bleeding, who was refractory to corticosteroids, i.v. Ig and plasma exchange, an immediate and sustained rise in the platelet count followed splenectomy (Cunningham and Lind, 1989).

Pathogenesis of post-transfusion purpura

The mechanism of destruction of the patient's own platelets in PTP remains unknown. Shulman *et al.* (1961) suggested that persisting HPA-1a antigens formed complexes with anti-HPA-1a, and that these immune complexes attached themselves to HPA-1(a –) platelets, so-called 'innocent bystanders', which were then phagocytosed. In fact, an increased amount of IgG has been demonstrated on the recipient's platelets in several cases of PTP, viz. ten times the normal amount in one case on the fourth day after the onset of thrombocytopenia (Cines and Schreiber, 1976b); demonstrable by immunofluorescence in two cases during the acute phase of the illness (Pegels *et al.* 1981) and, together with IgA and IgM in five cases, in three of which anti-HPA-1a could be eluted from the patient's HPA-1(a –) platelets (von dem Borne and van der Plas van Dalen, 1985). In two cases anti-HPA-1a could be eluted from the patient's platelets even after the platelet count had returned to normal (Taaning and Skov, 1991).

A possible explanation for the adherence of immune complexes to platelets in PTP is as follows: in all cases of PTP but one (see below), the platelet antigens involved are either on glycoprotein (GP) IIb (HPA-3a, HPA-3b) or on GPIIIa (HPA-1a, HPA-1b; HPA-4a). Although in one case anti-HPA-5b was detectable, anti-HPA-1b was also present (Walker *et al.* 1988). The GPIIb and GPIIIa very easily associate to form the complex GPIIb/IIIa; in fact, under experimental conditions, these proteins can be kept apart only in the absence of Ca^{2+} (Kunicki et al. 1981b; Hagen et al. 1982; Howard et al. 1982b). It seems possible that fragments of HPA-1(a +) platelets, if they contain GPIIb/IIIa, adhere to GPIIb/IIIa on intact HPA-1(a –) platelets. When the platelet fragments are bound to IgG (i.e. anti-HPA-1a) the intact HPA-1 (a –) platelets with the immune complexes on them undergo destruction by the mononuclear phagocyte system (MPS). It is of interest that in patients with Glanzmann's disease on whose platelets there is no GPIIb/IIIa, who have antibodies against determinants on GPIIb/IIIa, PTP has not been observed. Recently a case of PTP due to anti-HPA-5b has been described (Christie et al. 1991). HPA-5b is located on GPIa, which forms a complex with GPIIa. Thus, the above mechanism may also be applicable in this case. An alternative explanation for PTP is as follows: in vitro HPA-1a antigen is bound by HPA-1(a –) platelets from plasma from HPA-1(a +) subjects (Kickler et al. 1986). If plasma containing HPA-1a antigen is transfused to HPA-1(a –) subjects, the antigen may bind to the HPA-1(a –) platelets and thus render them susceptible to destruction by anti-HPA-1a.

Another possible explanation for PTP would be the formation of autoantibodies as a result of the secondary immune response to the alloantigen. In animals, alloimmunization against platelets may induce the formation of autoantibodies and thrombocytopenia (Gengozian and McLaughlin, 1978). In one case of PTP there was evidence of autoantibodies (Stricker et al. 1987), but these could have been present before the platelet transfusion. In any case, because anti-HPA-1a could also be eluted from the patient's HPA-1(a –) platelets, the role of the autoantibodies in inducing thrombocytopenia was, at the most, only partial.

One of the many puzzling features about the syndrome is that in two cases in which HPA-1(a +) blood has been transfused to patients who have previously suffered from PTP, there has been no untoward episode or recall of the antibody (Shulman et al. 1961; Lau et al. 1980). However, PTP may recur. An HPA-1(a –) patient who had had two relatively mild episodes of thrombocytopenia, separated by an interval of 3 years, both occurring a week or two after transfusion was found to have potent anti-HPA-1a in her plasma (Soulier et al. 1979). Another patient had had three episodes of PTP due to anti-HPA-1a (Budd et al. 1985).

Effect of transfusing platelet alloantibodies

Experimental studies

The effect of transfusing plasma containing platelet alloantibodies to a normal subject was described by Harrington (1954). The donor was a person who had himself previously received many transfusions; potent platelet agglutinins were found in his plasma and an injection of 10 ml into a normal subject produced profound thrombocytopenia.

Similarly, Shulman et al. (1961) showed that a transfusion of as little as 5–10 ml plasma containing potent complement-fixing anti-HPA-1a would produce thrombocytopenia in normal HPA-1(a +) subjects. In a subsequent review, Shulman et al. (1964) concluded that the concentration of alloantibody capable of producing effects in vivo was about ten times less than the minimum concentration detectable by the most sensitive tests in vitro.

Further studies were made by Aster and Jandl (1964). ^{51}Cr-labelled HLA-A2 platelets were transfused to four recipients whose own platelets lacked the antigen; 1–2 d later various amounts of serum containing anti-HLA-A2 were injected. This serum, in the presence of positive platelets, fixed complement *in vitro* at a dilution of 1 in 300. In the first recipient the injection of 0.25 ml serum produced clearance of the labelled platelets with a $T_{1/2}$ of 160 min and sequestration only in the spleen. In the second recipient the injection of 0.5 ml serum produced clearance with a $T_{1/2}$ of 80 min with sequestration in both liver and spleen, and the injection of 2.0 ml serum brought about clearance with a $T_{1/2}$ of 15 min and sequestration in the liver. Three of the four subjects developed febrile reactions.

Clinical reactions
Following the transfusion of 80 ml blood, a patient developed a severe reaction characterized by dyspnoea, a rash and fever; there was marked oozing of blood and the platelet count fell from $193 \times 10^9/l$ to $11 \times 10^9/l$. The donor plasma was found to contain anti-HPA-1a with a titre of 1000; the patient was HPA-1(a +). Interestingly, three previous recipients of blood from the same donor had developed unexplained thrombocytopenia (Scott *et al.* 1988). A similar case, in which a patient developed severe thrombocytopenia immediately after receiving a unit of packed red blood cells which contained strong anti-HPA-1a, was described by Ballem *et al.* (1987a).

Granulocytopenia following transfusion of incompatible platelets
In two patients with aplastic anaemia the transfusion of HLA-incompatible platelets was followed by a prolonged decrease in the number of circulating granulocytes. At 20 h the count was still only 30% of the pre-transfusion value and it was still depressed at 48 h. No rebound granulocytosis, as noted after the transfusion of incompatible red cells, was found. HLA-matched platelets did not cause granulocytopenia (Herzig *et al.* 1974). The authors discussed the possibility that the transfusion of incompatible platelets may increase the risk of infection.

REACTIONS DUE TO TRANSFUSED PROTEINS

Immediate-type hypersensitivity reactions following plasma transfusion
Following the transfusion of whole blood or plasma, the recipient may develop an anaphylactic-type reaction; the severest form (anaphylactic shock) is characterized by flushing of the skin, hypotension, substernal pain and dyspnoea, and the mildest simply by urticaria (hives). Intermediate forms are sometimes described as anaphylactoid. Some severe cases of anaphylactic shock are due to an interaction between transfused IgA and class-specific anti-IgA in the recipient's plasma but in many cases the cause of the reaction is unknown. The frequency of severe reactions following the transfusion of blood or plasma is very low; in one series it was one per 20 000 transfusions (Bjerrum and Jersild, 1971). The development of urticaria is relatively common. In one series the incidence was 1.1% (Kevy *et al.* 1962); in another series in which even a few weals were counted the incidence was approximately 3% (Stephen *et al.* 1955).

Hypersensitivity reactions appear to be commoner in patients undergoing plasma exchange on cell separators when plasma is used as the replacement fluid (see Chapter 1). Moreover, there is a tendency for the reactions to get worse when repeated infusions of plasma are given. For example, there may be itching on the first occasion followed by the appearance of a mild rash on the second occasion and by anaphylactoid reactions following further infusions. Occasionally, true anaphylactic reactions are seen with dyspnoea and hypotension (W. Wagstaff, personal communication). Severe hypotension and bronchospasm have been observed in two patients following a first plasma exchange; neither patient had IgA deficiency (K. Shumak, personal communication).

Until recently, it was believed that most if not all of the acute symptoms and signs of immediate-type hypersensitivity reactions were due to the release of fragments of complement components, C3a and C5a. It is now believed that leukotrienes may also play important roles as mediators of these reactions; the substances are outstandingly potent as bronchoconstrictors in humans and are at least as potent vasoconstrictors as angiotensin and more than 1000 times as active as histamine in promoting plasma leakage (Dahlén et al. 1981).

Reactions due to class-specific anti-IgA

Several cases have been described in which the transfusion of only a few millilitres of blood has caused such symptoms as dyspnoea, substernal pain, laryngeal oedema and collapse.

In a case described by Schmidt et al. (1969), in a woman aged 60 years who denied previous pregnancies and had no previous history of exposure to blood antigens, the transfusion of as little as 10 ml blood was followed by severe hypotension and cyanosis. The reaction was at first ascribed to a coincidental pulmonary embolism and a second transfusion, of packed red cells, was begun a few days later. Almost immediately the patient developed light-headedness, sternal pain, nausea, and flushing of the face and upper part of the chest, with hypotension. The symptoms lasted 10 min and were followed by chills and fever. No cause for the reaction could be found and further test transfusions were given to exclude such possibilities as red cell incompatibility. On each occasion, the transfusion of a few millilitres of blood produced very severe anaphylactic reactions. The patient was eventually found to lack IgA and to have a potent IgG, complement-fixing, anti-IgA; the titre of a sample taken before the first transfusion was 1750; after the second transfusion it rose to 17 500.

In a case described by Vyas (1970), an adult male with malabsorption syndrome who had received a transfusion of plasma some years previously was given a further transfusion of plasma. After 10–15 ml had been injected the patient developed redness of the skin, watering of the eyes, shortness of breath and crushing substernal pain. The symptoms disappeared rapidly after stopping the transfusion and giving hydrocortisone. The patient's serum contained class-specific anti-IgA.

In a similar case reported by Ropars et al. (1971), intense malaise, laryngeal oedema, sweating and collapse followed the transfusion of only a few millilitres of whole blood. The patient gave a history of a similar reaction after receiving an injection of Ig i.m. a year previously. The very slow transfusion of washed red cells produced only slight malaise. The patient's serum contained a potent anti-IgA (titre varying from 64 to 1000).

In a case described by Miller *et al.* (1970), red cells which had been frozen and deglycerolized could be transfused without incident provided the rate was slow enough; more rapid infusion produced a mild reaction. The transfusion of washed red cells, cell-free plasma or plasma protein fraction (PPF) all produced a reaction. The patient's own stored blood and blood from donors known to lack IgA was well tolerated.

Vyas and Perkins (1976) suggested that subjects found to have potent, class-specific anti-IgA should be given a card with the information on it.

In one of the patients described by Leikola *et al.* (1973) twice-washed red cells gave only a mild reaction and five-times washed red cells no reaction. In this patient, and in three others whom they described, anaphylactic reactions developed after giving a small amount of whole blood. In one case symptoms developed within a few seconds. All four patients in their series had anti-IgA titres in the range 500–16 000.

Reaction to IgA following injected immunoglobulin
Although Ig preparations usually contain about 95% IgG they also contain some IgA. One serious reaction following the i.m. administration of Ig was shown to be associated with the presence in the recipient's serum of potent anti-IgA; other patients with weaker anti-IgA suffered no reactions (Vyas *et al.* 1968). Anaphylactic reactions due to anti-IgA occur more frequently after i.v. administration of Ig. Reactions have been shown to be particularly severe in patients with IgE anti-IgA (Burks *et al.* 1986; Ferreira *et al.* 1988). The routine screening for anti-IgA in patients to be treated with i.v. Ig has been advocated (McClusky *et al.* 1990). A simple method for screening for anti-IgA has been described (Hunt and Reed, 1990).

Availability of donors who completely lack IgA
It has been recommended that blood donor services should establish a register of IgA-deficient donors (Vyas and Perkins, 1976). Although patients with proven suscep-tibility to donor IgA can be transfused with four to six times washed red cells from ordinary donors, they can only receive platelet or granulocyte concentrates and plasma products prepared from the blood of donors who completely lack IgA. Many transfusion centres now stock fresh-frozen plasma (FFP) made from such donors.

Reactions due to anti-IgA of limited specificity
The term limited specificity applies to antibodies against Am factors and subclass antibodies (i.e. anti-α1 and anti-α2).

The suggestion that anti-IgA of limited specificity might be the cause of anaphy-lactic or urticarial reactions following transfusion was first made by Vyas *et al.* (1969). Most of the cases described below were observed at a time when the specificity of the anti-IgA of limited specificity could not always be established.

In investigating 29 subjects who had had anaphylactic or urticarial reactions following the transfusion of plasma or cryoprecipitates, class-specific anti-IgA was found in three subjects and anti-IgA of limited specificity in 22 (Vyas *et al.* 1969). Although this finding seemed at first to establish the role of anti-IgA of limited specificity in causing anaphylactoid reactions, it now seems that the finding of anti-IgA of limited specificity in these cases may have been, at least to some extent, coincidental. For example, in one other series of six patients whose plasma contained anti-IgA of limited specificity (titre seldom more than 32) not one had had a reaction (Ropars *et al.* 1974).

In another series of 158 patients who had had transfusion reactions characterized by urticaria or mild anaphylactoid symptoms and a slight rise in temperature, only 14 had anti-IgA in their plasma and none of the antibodies had a titre greater than 8. No anti-IgA was found in the plasma of 100 normal donors when fresh IgA proteins were used, although when the IgA was digested or stored at 4°C for 6–8 months, antibodies against this altered IgA could be detected in almost all the sera. The authors emphasized the need for testing antisera against fresh IgA proteins and added that, even then, they doubted whether titres of from 4 to 8 could be considered significant in view of the high sensitivity of agglutination tests with chromic chloride-treated red cells (Koistinen and Leikola, 1977). In a survey using an immunoradiometric assay, the incidence of anti-IgA in patients who had had urticarial transfusion reactions was also about 8% (Homburger *et al.* 1981).

A few cases have been described in which anti-IgA of limited specificity does seem to have been responsible for reactions.

In a case described by Vyas *et al.* (1968), the patient, who had a severe erythematous rash, abdominal pain and difficulty in breathing following the transfusion of 100 ml packed red cells from one donor, showed a rise in anti-IgA titre from 8 to 32. Subsequently she was given 60 ml plasma from the same donor and developed a severe hypersensitivity reaction and lost consciousness. Previously she had been transfused with IgA-deficient plasma without reaction.

Two cases were described by Pineda and Taswell (1975). The first patient was a woman whose second transfusion, given 2 years after the first, was followed by severe urticaria, hypotension and oliguria. A third transfusion given 2 years later produced a similar clinical picture accompanied by apprehension and respiratory distress. The patient's serum contained anti-IgA of limited specificity with a titre of 256. In the second case a man, who may have been transfused previously, was given 2 units blood during operation and a third unit on the following day. After 25–30 ml had been transfused he developed apprehension and restlessness and died 45 min later. The only abnormal finding in his serum was anti-IgA of limited specificity with a titre of 64 before transfusion and of 16 immediately afterwards. Vyas and Perkins (1976) reported four patients of the phenotype A2m(– 1), with normal levels of IgM in their serum, in whom anaphylactoid reactions following transfusion were due to anti-A2m(1) in the recipient's plasma and could be avoided by transfusion of A2m(– 1) or aIgA plasma. In one of these patients the antibody had a titre of 256 and the patient twice had a serious anaphylactic reaction following transfusion of only small amounts of A2m(1) blood (Vyas and Fundenberg, 1970).

Finally, in a patient who developed a life-threatening reaction with shortness of breath, itching, hot flushes substernal pain, marked hypotension and cardiorespiratory arrest after the transfusion of 50 ml pooled platelet concentrate, the serum contained an antibody reactive only with red cells coated with one single A2m(1) protein; the patient subsequently received platelet concentrates from an A2m(1)-negative relative without incident (Strauss *et al.* 1983a).

Other immunoglobulins

IgG

Immediate reactions. When preparations of Ig containing predominantly IgG are injected, adverse reactions may be brought about by at least two mechanisms. First, if the preparation is given i.v. and if it contains a substantial amount of aggregates, complement may be activated with the liberation of vasoactive substances. Second, the preparation may contain prekallikrein activator (PKA), although this now seems to be rare (see below). In most published accounts of reactions, no attempt has been made to determine which of these two mechanisms has been responsible.

In a series reported by Barandun *et al.* (1962) 10 ml of a 160 g/l solution of Ig diluted with 100 ml saline were infused over a period of 90–120 min. Of 70 subjects 20 developed reactions characterized by uneasiness, a rapid pulse and dyspnoea; there was flushing of the face, a feeling of oppression in the chest, and lumbar pain; in a few cases the picture was severe enough to resemble anaphylactic shock. The 70 subjects included 15 with hypogammaglobulinaemia.

Two similar reactions were reported in *Notes on Epidemiology* (1977). In the first case, within 5 min of an i.v. injection there was a tight feeling across the upper chest and neck with nausea and sweating although no hypotension. There was also slight shivering but no fever. The patient was better after 1 h. In the second case 375 mg human Ig diluted 1 in 3 in saline was injected i.v. in 10 min as a test dose. Infusion was followed by tachycardia and flushing of the face, with pain and a feeling of tightness in the neck. The symptoms disappeared in 15 min.

Patients with hypogammaglobulinaemia are especially prone to anaphylactic reactions following the administration of IgG, even when given i.m. (e.g. MRC, 1969). This hypersensitivity may be related to the paucity of tissue-bound Ig in these patients (see review by Barandun and Isliker, 1986).

The i.v. injection of relatively small amounts of IgG, as in vials containing anti-Rh D Ig prepared by fractionation on DEAE Sephadex, seldom causes reactions; see Chapter 12. Similarly, the commercial preparation of anti-D Ig 'Rho-GAM', which contains 300 μg anti-D and, presumably, about 300 mg IgG per 2 ml vial, although intended for i.m. use, has been given i.v. on many occasions without producing any obvious untoward effects (W. Pollack, personal communication).

Reactions associated with repeated i.m. injections of immunoglobulin. Amongst 43 normal adults (the staff of a dialysis unit) receiving 5 ml of a 165 g/l solution of Ig as a source of anti-HBs every 8 weeks, four developed either chills or local oedema or generalized urticaria. Of the 43 subjects, about 80% developed IgE antibodies against other Ig classes and about 60% showed a decrease in IgE levels, lasting for several months (Ropars *et al.* 1979).

Possible role of anti-Gm. Two cases in which anti-G1m(a) appeared to be responsible for a transfusion reaction have been described (Fischer, 1964; Fudenberg *et al.* 1964) but these cases were reported before the role of anti-IgA was appreciated and no investigations were made to exclude anti-IgA as a possible cause. One more recent case, in which the role of anti-IgA was excluded, was described by van Loghem and De Lange (1975). Following a febrile reaction the only anti-protein antibody demonstrable in the patient's serum was anti-G1m(z). The antibody was remarkable in that it was IgG (unlike most Gm antibodies which are IgM) and that it had a titre of 10 000. Tests were not made to determine the subclass of the antibody or whether it bound complement.

Serum sickness-like syndromes due to anti-IgG seem to be very rare. One case followed an i.m. injection of IgG (Mollison, 1979a, p. 631).

The subject was a male volunteer who was given an i.m. injection of a standard preparation of anti-Rh D Ig (100 µg). Three days later he developed polyarthritis affecting particularly the hands. Two days after this he was a little worse but after a further 2 d he had started to improve and within 2–3 weeks of the injection he was completely free of symptoms. He never developed a rash or fever. Ten days after the injection the level of haemolytic complement in his serum was reduced (6 units compared with the normal level of 22–27) and, in the polyethylene–glycol (PEG) test of Johnson *et al.* (1975), significant amounts of C1q and IgG were precipitated. Results on a further sample taken on the following day were similar but 16 d after the injection the level of haemolytic complement was almost normal (20 units) and only trace amounts of C1q and IgG were precipitated in the PEG test. The results were interpreted as typical of the development of immune complexes and their subsequent removal from the circulation within a few days (J.F. Mowbray, personal communication). The subject had had one previous injection of Ig 18 months earlier and it may be significant that the preparation given (which was an experimental one) was known to have contained 15% of denatured material.

A case in which serum sickness-like reactions developed 2 d or more after transfusions of materials containing plasma (e.g. packed red cells) was described by Avoy (1981); the patient's plasma was found to contain 'autoantibodies directed against IgG'.

Effects of immunoglobulin preparations on lymphocyte function. There is evidence that the injection of commercially available Ig preparations may induce dysfunction in the recipient's lymphocytes, including direct inhibition of B cell maturation and activation of suppressor T cells (Durandy *et al.* 1981).

IgM

Anti-IgM of limited specificity was found in 21.3% of 197 subjects who had had five or more blood transfusions, who lacked antibodies against leucocytes or platelets, and about one-third of whom had had a transfusion reaction (shivering, fever or urticaria). There was no reason to believe that the anti-IgM was involved in the febrile reactions (Ropars *et al.* 1973).

Atopens

In a series of atopic subjects, i.e. those known to be sensitive to such common atopens as pollen, dust, milk and egg, the transfusion of pooled serum was almost always followed by moderate of severe urticaria, whereas in normal subjects no more than an occasional weal developed (Maunsell, 1944). Presumably, these reactions were due to IgE anti-atopens.

Histamine and other pharmacological mediators are responsible for the acute inflammatory symptoms and signs of the urticarial response. Fc receptors on mast cells and basophils bind IgE molecules which, on contact with antigen (atopen), are cross-linked, triggering degranulation of the cells and release of mediators. The Fc receptor can also be cross-linked by IgG anti-IgE, by antibodies to idiotypes of IgE, by lectins, by antibodies to the Fc receptor, etc. (Roitt *et al.* 1989).

Hypersensitivity reactions due to passively acquired antibodies. In a classical case described by Ramirez (1919) a patient, who had received a transfusion 2 weeks previously, went for a carriage drive and promptly developed a severe attack of asthma, a thing that had never happened to him before. It was then discovered that the donor of the transfusion had long known that exposure to horses brought on attacks of asthma in him and his skin tests to horse dandruff were strongly positive. The conclusion seems to be that those occasional donors who give a really striking history of hypersensitivity should be rejected.

Reactions due to passively acquired penicillin antibody. In a patient who developed a generalized maculo-papular rash 1 h after receiving 4 units of blood, highly suggestive evidence was obtained that the reaction was due to the presence of penicillin antibody in the plasma of one of the transfused units. The recipient had been receiving ampicillin until the day before transfusion and red cells in a pre-transfusion sample were found to be coated with penicillin; another similar case has been mentioned (McGinniss and Goldfinger, 1971).

Reaction due to passively acquired penicillin. In a patient known to be allergic to penicillin, transfusion was followed by the development of a maculo-papular eruption with pruritus and fever; the donor unit was shown to contain penicillin (Michel and Sharon, 1980).

Sensitivity to nickel
Stoddart (1960) reported two patients who, within 24 h of receiving transfusions of blood or plasma, developed an urticarial rash (generalized in one case, round the site of infusion in the other) apparently due to sensitivity to nickel. Both patients on questioning gave a history of sensitivity to nickel and it was presumed that the nickel–steel shafts of the needles through which the transfusions were given were responsible.

A post-transfusion syndrome in newborn infants
In six of 17 infants who had received multiple exchange transfusions, and in 21 of 35 infants who had received both an intra-uterine transfusion and an exchange transfusion, a benign syndrome characterized by a transient maculo-papular rash associated with eosinophilia and thrombocytopenia developed. The syndrome was thought to represent a host reaction to some constituent of the donor blood rather than some form of GvH reaction since in many cases the donor blood had been irradiated (Chudwin *et al.* 1982). No similar cases have been described.

Prophylaxis and treatment of allergic reactions

Antihistamines

Although antihistamines have been shown to be effective when added to donated blood, two points must be made. First, antihistamines should be given only to those recipients with a history of previous allergic manifestations. Second, when antihistamines are indicated they should not be added to the blood to be transfused but should be given by mouth or, if necessary, by injection. For example, 50 mg diphenhydramine may be given by mouth 1 h before transfusion and a further 50 mg after the start of the transfusion. If antihistamines have not been given and an allergic reaction develops, 25 mg diphenhydramine or 10 mg chlorpheniramine may be given i.v.

The above discussion refers predominantly to the suppression of urticarial reactions. If a severe allergic reaction occurs, adrenaline should be given i.m. or, slowly, i.v.

Use of washed cells in prophylaxis of anaphylactoid reactions

In three patients described by Silvergleid et al. (1977), in whom severe urticaria was associated with the transfusion of suspensions of red cells or platelets, no reactions occurred when washed red cells or platelets were transfused.

SOME NON-IMMUNOLOGICAL REACTIONS

Effects of vasoactive substances

Prekallikrein activator

Hypotension, vasodilatation, nausea, sweating and chest pain have been noted after the rapid administration of certain batches of PPF (Bland et al. 1972; Alving et al. 1978; Culliver and Penington, 1979). The most important substance producing these effects seems to be a degradation product of Hageman factor (Factor XII) known as PKA (Alving et al. 1978), although the effects may also be due to the persistence of appreciable amounts of a peptide with bradykinin-like properties (Horowitz and Mashford, 1980a,b). PKA presumably produces its effects by triggering the generation of bradykinin in recipients (Alving et al. 1978).

In testing batches of human PPF in rats, a good correlation was found between the PKA content of the rapidly infused PPF on the one hand and the generation of kallikrein in the rat's plasma and the fall in its arterial blood pressure on the other (Bleeker et al. 1982).

The temperature to which plasma protein solution is heated appears to be critical in determining the amount of PKA in the final product; heating to 60.5°C can lead to a two- or three-fold diminution in PKA concentration compared with heating to 59.5°C, and can make the difference between the product being potentially reactive on the one hand or innocuous on the other (Marley and Gilbo, 1981). Batches of albumin, as opposed to PPF seldom contain PKA (Alving et al. 1978).

Factor VIII concentrates may also contain PKA (Kuwahara, 1980), as may preparations of Ig.

Now that tests for PKA are part of the quality control of plasma fractions, adverse reactions due to PKA are believed to be rare.

Angiotensin may be generated in plasma pools kept at room temperature. The amounts present are sufficient to affect blood pressure and the aldosterone secretion of human recipients when infused rapidly. In nine different pools the mean level was found to vary between 320 and 830 ng/ml (Vandongen and Gordon, 1969).

Poor plasma volume expansion after plasma transfusion

Several papers have been published suggesting that transfusions of allogeneic plasma are less effective than transfusions of autologous plasma in producing expansion of plasma volume both in dogs (Remington and Baker, 1959) and in humans (Hutchison *et al.* 1960; Hutchison and Burgen, 1963). In reviewing this work, Hillman (1964) pointed out that in all cases fresh plasma or FFP had been used and he suggested that vasoactive substances in such plasma were probably responsible for leakage of plasma from the circulation and for the urticaria which had been observed. Pooled plasma stored at 30–32°C for 6 months was found to produce very satisfactory expansion of plasma volume; in normal subjects transfused with half a litre of plasma there was 74% retention at 1 h and 63% retention at 2 h. No allergic reactions were produced. In subjects venesected before transfusion virtually all the transfused plasma was retained in the circulation for at least 3 h. Evidence that fresh plasma is less effective than stored plasma in restoring blood volume was published by Pareira *et al.* (1964).

Bacterial pyrogens

Lipopolysaccharides of bacterial origin are the most potent pyrogens known; as little as 0.001 μg/kg *Escherichia coli* 08 lipopolysaccharide will produce a rise in body temperature when injected i.v. into rabbits; doses of 1 μg/kg regularly produce leucopenia, and doses of 20–30 μg/kg are fatal. In an adult human 0.1 μg of the same pyrogen may produce slight fever with leucopenia, followed by leucocytosis (Westphal, 1957).

Many bacteria produce pyrogens (Tui and Schrift, 1942) but their presence in solutions for parenteral use is tested for as a routine; solutions which, following infusion into rabbits, cause a rise in temperature are rejected.

Endogenous pyrogens

Endogenous pyrogens are low mol. wt. proteins which are liberated by various leucocytes, particularly blood monocytes, granulocytes and tissue macrophages. Three endogenous pyrogens have been recognized, interleukin-1 (IL-1), interferon and tumour necrosis factor (Dinarello *et al.* 1986). All three factors directly stimulate the synthesis of prostaglandin (PGE$_2$) in the hypothalamus; the effect is to raise the level at which body temperature is set. Presumably, in febrile reactions due to leucocyte antibodies in the recipient, IL-1 is released from donor leucocytes and provokes fever. Febrile reactions following the destruction of red cells by anti-Rh D may be due to the release of endogenous pyrogen from the recipients's tissue macrophages.

Effects of transfusing ice-cold blood

In patients transfused with large amounts of cold (stored) blood, oesophageal temperatures as low as 27.5–29°C have been recorded (MacLean and van Tyn, 1961; Boyan and Howland, 1963).

Boyan (1964) reported observations which appeared to show that massive transfusions of ice-cold blood were very dangerous. Results in patients transfused with cold and warm blood were compared; in both series 3000 ml or more citrated blood were transfused at 50 ml or more per minute. In 25 patients transfused with cold blood at 50–100 ml/min there were 12 episodes of cardiac arrest and in 11 further patients transfused with more than 6000 ml cold blood at more than 100 ml/min there were nine episodes of arrest. By contrast, in 105 patients transfused with warm blood at 50–110 ml/min there were only three episodes of cardiac arrest although in 13 further patients transfused with warm blood at the rate of more than 100 ml/min there were five episodes. The patients in this series were undergoing very extensive operations for terminal cancer and the high incidence of cardiac arrest may not indicate what would be expected in reasonably fit subjects.

Dybkjaer and Elkjaer (1964) reported that during the period 1957–62 they had observed several episodes of ventricular arrhythmia during neurological operations in which a large amount of blood had been transfused. There had been 13 cases of cardiac arrest with 11 deaths. It seemed improbable that the deaths were due either to citrate or potassium toxicity because calcium had been given, and blood less than 1 week old had been used. It was concluded that the administration of cold blood might be responsible and for a further 2-year period warmed blood was used and no deaths occurred. The same authors showed that when warm blood was given body temperature fell only very slightly during operations lasting 3–4 h, whereas with cold blood body temperature sometimes fell by 3°C or more. In one patient whose temperature fell from 37 to 34.8°C and in whom extrasystoles occurred, the administration of calcium was without effect, but the transfusion of warmed blood reversed the signs.

The experimental work of Taylor et al. (1961) suggested that in some circumstances the rapid transfusion of ice-cold blood may be relatively safe. In exchange transfusions in rabbits, blood at 1°C was injected rapidly (10 ml amounts in about 30 s) into a catheter whose tip lay in the external jugular vein near to the right atrium. In a series of experiments designed to test the toxicity of citrate and potassium, blood transfused at 1°C seemed to be no more dangerous than blood injected at 21°C. Indeed there was some evidence that the animal could tolerate larger amounts of citrated, high-potassium blood when this was injected at 1°C (Taylor et al. 1961).

Methods of warming blood

The simplest method is to pass the blood (on its way from the container to the patient) through a coil of tubing in a water-bath at approximately 40°C (e.g. Dybkjaer and Elkjaer, 1964). This method is not ideal mainly because a relatively long piece of tubing is required to achieve the necessary warming and this means that the blood may be exposed to water-bath temperatures for relatively long periods and that considerable pressure may be required to force blood through the tubing. A better method is to use a disposable heat exchanger in which the coils of tubing are warmed by electric heating plates. The use of radio-frequency induction should be avoided because accidents have occurred due to faulty use of the equipment. In any case, blood should be warmed for transfusion only in a few special circumstances such as when massive amounts are being transfused (see above), or in occasional patients who complain of pain at the site of transfusion due to venous spasm.

For a recent review, see Iserson and Huestis (1991).

Citrate toxicity

Plasma normally contains approximately 1 mg citrate/dl expressed as citric acid (Howland *et al.* 1957). During the infusion of citrate the plasma level rises and may reach approximately 100 mg/dl (see below). At such levels serious toxic effects may be observed due to a fall in ionized calcium. In humans these levels have been reached either during exchange transfusion to newborn infants or during rapid transfusions to adults with impaired liver function (see below).

Newborn infants treated by exchange transfusion may receive as much as 600 mg citrate per kg in 1 h and their plasma citrate level may reach 100 mg/dl (Wexler *et al.* 1949). There is no doubt that signs of citrate toxicity may develop during exchange transfusion. In one series of infants receiving 500 ml citrated blood in 100 min, muscle tremors and changes in the electrocardiogram, namely a marked prolongation of the ST segment, were observed. The changes were rapidly reversed by the administration of 4–8 ml 10% calcium gluconate (Furman *et al.* 1951).

Similarly, Gustafson (1951) exchanged 500 ml in 75 min and found gross skeletal muscle tremors after the transfusion of 100–150 ml blood; these could be rapidly abolished by the injection of 2 ml calcium gluconate. The corresponding rate of administration of citrate can be calculated to be approximately 0.03 mmol/kg per min (assuming that approximately 2 g disodium citrate were injected in 80 min into an infant weighing 3 kg). Experiments in animals suggest that such a rate is only just safe. According to Adams *et al.* (1944) the administration of 0.06 mmol/kg per min for 20 min is lethal, although 0.04 mmol/kg per min is safe. Cumulative effects must be considered as well as rate, for Nakasone *et al.* (1954) concluded that there was '. . . an inverse ratio between the rate of i.v. infusion of ACD solution and the cumulative amount of citrate required to produce equivalent ECG changes'. Nevertheless, by keeping the rate of administration at 0.02 mmol/kg per min they were able to inject a total dose of approximately 1.8 mmol citrate per kg (in 90 min). This corresponds to the administration of almost 7 litres of citrated blood to an adult man.

Observations in adults are in general agreement with those in infants and in experimental animals. For example, Howland *et al.* (1957) gave infusions of 40 ml ACD per min for 20–30 min to three anaesthetized patients, a rate corresponding to 6–8 mg citric acid per kg per min, i.e. almost 0.04 mmol/kg per min. The plasma citrate level rose to about 80 mg/dl and there was a prolongation in the QT segment of the electrocardiogram.

In a further paper two series were compared retrospectively: among 152 patients transfused without additional calcium there were three deaths and among 114 patients who had been given calcium there were 13 deaths (Howland *et al.* 1960). However, valid comparison between the two series is impossible since, of patients receiving 20 or more units of blood, 13 of 14 were in the series treated with calcium and there were eight deaths among these. As the authors pointed out, the apparent association of death with the administration of calcium may simply have been due to the fact that calcium was given as a last resort.

Rather surprisingly, the papers just referred to (Howland *et al.* 1957; 1960) are sometimes quoted in support of the idea that citrate intoxication is not a significant problem (e.g. AMA, 1973). As mentioned above, a rate of 0.04 mmol citrate per kg per min (the maximum rate used by Howland *et al.* 1957) is just safe, provided it is not maintained for too long.

Nakasone *et al.* (1954) found that in dogs the toxic changes observed were: a prolongation of QT, *pulsus alternans*, depression of P and T waves and development of muscle tremor. With higher doses the arterial pressure declined to zero and the animal died unless calcium was injected promptly.

In another study in dogs, arrhythmias developed when the blood citrate level reached 60 mg/dl and, unless remedial measures were taken, ventricular fibrillation followed. The administration of sodium citrate at rates of 2.5–12 mg/kg per min led to a significant decrease in cardiac output, stroke volume, left ventricular work, mean and systolic aortic pressures, and left ventricular pressure (Corbascio and Smith, 1967).

Although the injection of calcium reverses the toxic effects of citrate it appears that the signs observed are not due solely to the absence of ionized calcium, but are in part due to other effects of citrate. Thus the administration of blood rendered hypocalcaemic by passage across a cation-exchange resin does not produce circulatory derangements as severe as those caused by citrated blood (Nakasone *et al.* 1954). As described below, the low pH and raised plasma potassium concentration of citrated blood may contribute to its toxicity.

Soulier (1958) reported that blood is sometimes found to be incoagulable following massive infusions of citrated blood and that coagulability can be restored *in vitro* by the addition of calcium. A case of this kind with virtually no ionized calcium in the plasma was investigated by Aggeler *et al.* (1967) who suggested that the diminished coagulability might be due partly to deficiency of Factor VIII and platelets, and that the fact that there was no cardiac standstill suggested that there was probably enough calcium to promote normal clotting had other factors been normal.

From data described above, it may be concluded that, in adults, signs of citrate toxicity are likely to develop when blood is transfused at the rate of 1 litre in 10 min and that the toxic effects can be minimized by giving calcium, e.g. 10 ml 10% calcium gluconate for every litre of citrated blood. When even higher rates of transfusion have to be used, it has been recommended that larger amounts of calcium should be given. For example, Firt and Hejhal (1957) recommended that when citrated blood was going to be given at rates up to 500 ml/min, 10 ml 10% calcium gluconate should be given immediately before transfusion, and a further 15 ml i.v. (into another vein) after the first 100 ml, and a further 10 ml after each subsequent 500 ml.

When calcium gluconate is used the dose of the material must be almost four times greater than when calcium chloride is used. Thus the mol. wt. of calcium gluconate is 448 and that of calcium chloride 111; each of the molecules contains one atom of calcium (at. wt. 40) so that the amount of calcium (by weight) in calcium gluconate is 9% but in calcium chloride 37%.

Fatal cardiac arrest, apparently due to calcium overdosage, was reported by Wolf *et al.* (1970). A child who had been transfused with 1250 ml citrated blood in 20 h following cardiac surgery received a total of about 2 g calcium (2 ml 10% $CaCl_2$ with each 50 ml blood). Serum calcium was approximately 50 mg/dl at the end of the transfusion.

Factors that increase citrate toxicity

Impaired liver function. In patients with liver disease or with mechanical obstruction to the hepatic circulation, the rapid administration of citrate is much more likely to produce toxic effects. Bunker *et al.* (1955) found that when citrated blood was infused at a rate of 500 ml in 15 min the plasma citrate concentration rose above 0.5 mmol/l in almost all patients with liver disease, but in only 50% of normal subjects. In five patients with severe liver disease or with mechanical obstruction to the hepatic circulation, the calculated concentration of ionized calcium was 0.6 mmol/l or less, compared with the normal value of 1.0 mmol/l. A concentration of 0.6 mmol/l must be regarded as very dangerous in view of the fact that at a concentration of 0.5 mmol/l the isolated frog's heart stops beating (McLean and Hastings, 1934) and the clotting time of blood is prolonged (Stefanini, 1950).

Bunker *et al.* (1955) found that in patients with citric acid intoxication it was difficult to predict the appropriate dose of calcium; they recommended that if transfusion had to be given to patients likely to develop this syndrome, that is to say patients with liver disease or with mechanical obstruction to the hepatic circulation, packed cells rather than whole citrated blood should be used.

Ludbrook and Wynn (1958) found a considerable rise in plasma citrate in four patients undergoing operations and they concluded that the administration of citrate was particularly dangerous in patients in whom the liver circulation was impaired as, for example, in those undergoing operations in which hepatic circulation was temporarily interfered with. They also considered that hypothermia increased the risk of citrate intoxication.

Acid load in massive blood transfusion
Citrated blood becomes progressively more acid on storage. Nevertheless, in war casualties, who were initially profoundly hypotensive and severely acidotic following massive transfusions of 3-week-old blood, acid–base status returned almost to normal during transfusion provided that blood loss was arrested, even though no alkali was administered (Collins *et al.* 1971).

Potassium toxicity
Since most transfusions are given with citrate, it is more realistic to consider the combined effects of potassium and citrate rather than of potassium alone.

When red cells are stored in the cold the potassium content of the red cells decreases and that of the plasma increases. Normally, red cells contain approximately 100 mmol potassium per litre (of packed cells) and plasma contains 4–5 mmol/l.

In whole blood mixed with CPDA-1 solution, extracellular K increases from an initial level of 4.2 mmol/l to 27.3 mmol/l after 35 d; in red cell concentrates prepared from CPDA-1 blood, extracellular K increases from 5.1 to 78.5 mmol/l in the same period. The amount of plasma in a unit of CPDA-1 blood is approximately 300 ml and in the corresponding red cell concentrate, 70 ml. Thus, the total potassium load (extracellular) of a unit of whole blood stored for 35 d is 8.2 mmol and that of a red cell concentrate is 5.5 mmol (Moore *et al.* 1981). The rate of increase in plasma K in blood stored with ACD is slightly greater; for example, the total extracellular K in a unit stored for 28 d was 10.2 mmol (Loutit *et al.* 1943).

In blood which has been irradiated, the level of extracellular potassium is increased; see Chapter 9.

Miller *et al.* (1954a) found that, whereas in infants transfused with blood stored for less than 1 week serum potassium concentration did not change significantly, in infants transfused with blood stored for 9–21 d (with a concentration in the citrate-plasma of approximately 15 mmol/l) the infants' serum potassium concentration rose to 8 mmol/l in two cases; no ECG changes were observed.

Campbell (1955) measured changes in plasma potassium concentration during exchange transfusion in 36 infants, using donor blood with a plasma potassium concentration of approximately 30 mg/dl (7.5 mmol/l). There was a tendency for the concentration to increase during exchange transfusion, mean values being 4.0–4.5 mmol/l at the beginning and 5.5–6.0 mmol/l after the exchange of 500 ml. A few samples, mostly from infants who showed signs of collapse or who actually died shortly after the samples were taken, had concentrations of 8 or 9 mmol/l.

It is known that in humans marked ECG changes occur when the plasma potassium concentration reaches about 8 mmol/l and that in conditions in which the plasma potassium level is thought to be the immediate cause of death, levels of approximately 10 mmol/l are found (Hoff *et al.* 1941; Stewart *et al.* 1948). When the plasma potassium concentration is found to be raised after collapse has occurred it seems possible that the rise in potassium concentration is a consequence rather than a cause of the collapse; in dogs immediately after respiratory arrest there is a rapid agonal rise in serum potassium (Winkler and Hoff, 1943).

As stated above, in subjects treated with citrated blood it is artificial to consider the toxic effects of potassium and citrate separately because it is known that they reinforce one another. This was demonstrated by Baker *et al.* (1957) on the isolated heart and by Taylor *et al.* (1961) during exchange transfusions in rabbits.

In the experiments of Taylor *et al.*, 10 ml amounts of blood were withdrawn and replaced within 1 min, to a total of 60 or even 100 ml/kg. The blood used had a slightly higher citrate concentration than citrated blood used in normal blood transfusion practice. Fresh blood was used, but in some experiments potassium was added to bring the plasma potassium concentration to about 25 mmol/l (equivalent to 3- or 4-week-old stored blood). When citrated blood without added potassium was exchanged, there was only one death among ten rabbits, but when blood with added potassium was used 15 of 19 rabbits died. The figures for heparinized blood were: without added potassium, none of 13 died and with added potassium, two of 15 died. The common mode of death was ventricular fibrillation. These figures show how dangerous is the combination of citrate and a raised potassium concentration, and also that a raised potassium concentration alone is relatively harmless. It should be emphasized that the rate of exchange transfusion in these experiments was considerably greater than the rate employed in exchange transfusion in infants; that the amounts of citrate and, even more, of potassium that were injected were considerably greater than the amounts involved in exchange transfusion in infants; and that rabbits are more susceptible to citrate toxicity than are humans.

Apart from the special circumstances in which large amounts of blood are rapidly infused, potassium toxicity need be considered only when transfusing patients whose plasma potassium concentration is already raised, e.g. anuric patients with extensive wounds involving muscle.

Ammonia in stored blood

Fresh blood contains only about 100 μg/dl ammonia but this may increase in blood stored for 3 weeks to about 900 μg/dl; it has been suggested that this amount of ammonia may make it undesirable to give large amounts of stored blood to patients with liver failure (Spear *et al.* 1956).

TRANSFUSION OF EXTRANEOUS MATTER

Air embolism

When blood was commonly taken into glass bottles and the pumping of air into the bottle was a well-recognized means of accelerating the flow of blood, and when rubber tubing and glass drip chambers were in use, providing possibilities of air leaks, air embolism was a very real hazard of transfusion, e.g. Schmidt and Kevy (1958) described an episode in which a blood donor became severely ill after receiving 60–80 ml air i.v.

The introduction of plastic bags which contain no air, and of plastic administration sets which have no junctions through which air can leak, has almost eliminated the possibility of introducing air during transfusion. Nevertheless, there are still a few ways in which at least small amounts of air can be introduced into patients' veins during transfusion. For example, air can be introduced at the beginning of the transfusion by failing to expel air from the transfusion tubing, or can be introduced into the giving line when changing from one bag to another. Although the introduction of a few bubbles of air into a patient is harmless, the introduction of large amounts should be avoided.

Particulate matter

Aggregates in stored blood

In blood mixed with either ACD or heparin, aggregates of leucocytes and platelets up to 200 μm in diameter form during storage (Swank, 1961). In ACD the formation of these aggregates begins within 24 h of taking the blood and the aggregates are always very marked by 8–10 d. In heparin, formation begins within 2 h and the changes are marked by 8 h. The presence of these particles was demonstrated by measuring the screen filtration pressure (SFP), i.e. the pressure needed to force blood at a constant rate through a microfilter with a pore size of 20 μm. The aggregates could be removed by passing stored blood through pyrex glass wool although not by passing it through a nylon filter of pore size 200 μm.

In blood stored at 4–6 °C with ACD, microaggregates formed during the first week consist almost entirely of platelets; it is only subsequently that granulocytes begin to disintegrate (Solis *et al.* 1974).

In the studies of the formation of aggregates in stored blood the most commonly used method has been to measure the SFP and it has often been assumed that the formation of aggregates of platelets and leucocytes is the most important determinant of SFP. On the other hand, it has been shown that the formation of fibrin is an important determinant of SFP and that, furthermore, the source of fibrin is predominantly platelet fibrinogen rather than plasma fibrinogen. In experiments in which platelet-rich serum was stored, fibrin formation was observed in the absence of plasma fibrinogen (Marshall *et al.* 1975a).

In blood stored with ACD or CPD there is little increase in SFP during the first 5 d but then there is a sharp increase, coinciding with the onset of fibrin formation as seen by scanning electron microscopy (Marshall *et al.* 1975a). After 4–8 d storage, SFP was found to be substantially higher in CPD blood than ACD blood by Wright and Sanderson (1974). Similarly, during the first week of storage greater formation of microaggregates was found in CPD solution than in ACD by Marshall *et al.* (1975a), although at 14 and 21 d there were no differences.

In standard administration sets the nylon filter has a pore size of 170 μm. There is some evidence that debris which can pass through such a filter is harmful to recipients (see below). Several different filters have therefore been designed to hold back particles down to a size of 20–40 μm. From comparative tests on four widely used filters the following conclusions were reached: the Bentley filter (PFS-127) was readily occluded by more than 1 unit of blood and was therefore considered to be impractical. The Swank (IL-200) was the most effective in removing microaggregates, but with this filter fragments of Dacron wool were observed in filtered blood. The Fenwal (4-C2417) was the next most effective. The Pall (Ultipore) allowed the fastest rate of flow but was less effective in removing microaggregates. The Fenwal filter, which was the preferred one, reduced the screen filtration pressure of 14-day-old blood from 565 to 29 N (Marshall *et al.* 1975b).

Macroaggregates weighing up to 9 g have been observed in red cell concentrates stored with saline–adenine–glucose–mannitol solution (Robertson *et al.* 1985). The aggregates were composed of leucocytes and platelet debris, together with some fibrin. Macroaggregate formation was halved by using less centrifugal force during the preparation of the concentrates and was further reduced by the use of an additive solution containing citrate.

The separation of the buffy coat from red cell concentrates, which results in removal of more than 80% of the platelets and more than 60% of the leucocytes, as expected, reduces aggregate formation (Prins *et al.* 1980).

Clinical importance of microaggregates in stored blood

In patients who have received a massive transfusion of blood, hypoxia commonly develops and the degree of hypoxia appears to be related to the volume of blood transfused. A possible cause is pulmonary microembolism due to debris in stored blood (McNamara *et al.* 1970). A study by Reul *et al.* (1974) appeared to support this conclusion. In a series of severely traumatized patients given massive transfusions some degree of pulmonary insufficiency developed in seven of 17 patients transfused with an average of about 19 units through standard filters (pore size 170 μm) compared with only two of 27 subjects who received an average of 18 units through filters with a pore size of 40 μm. Although this evidence is suggestive, the patients in the two series were not strictly comparable, and there is other evidence which casts substantial doubt on the role of microaggregates in causing pulmonary insufficiency. For example, in an experimental study in baboons, oligaemic shock was induced and the animals were then resuscitated with large amounts of blood stored for 16–21 d, after which they were given an exchange transfusion with stored blood equivalent to twice their blood volume. It was shown that the stored blood used contained aggregates similar to those found in human stored blood. Blood was administered through standard filters of pore size 170 μm. There were no detectable changes in lung function and there was no rise in pulmonary–arterial pressure. Sections of lungs examined by electron microscopy showed no evidence of pulmonary emboli (Tobey et al. 1974).

In patients dying from pulmonary failure following wounding and massive transfusion (65 and over 100 units in two cases) it may be impossible to demonstrate pulmonary microemboli. The conclusion appears to be that although particulate emboli from stored blood may contribute to pulmonary failure following traumatic shock and transfusion, their role is probably minor (Bredenberg, 1977). A study of casualties in Vietnam led to a similar conclusion, namely that differences in pulmonary function related to the type of injury exceeded differences associated with transfusion (Collins et al. 1978). Furthermore, in a randomized prospective study, results in two groups each of 20 patients undergoing abdominal aortic surgery were compared. Patients were transfused with 6–7 units of blood stored for 10–11 d, either through a standard filter (170 μm) or through a microaggregate filter (40 μm). No difference in post-operative function was found between the two groups (Virgilio et al. 1977).

The passage of blood through microaggregate filters may actually induce particle formation. With fresh blood or with blood stored for not more than 10 d the number of particles was found to be greater after than before filtration (Eisert and Eckert, 1979).

There is now little support for the practice of using microaggregate filters, although leucocyte depletion filters are used to prevent sensitization to leucocyte antigens (see Chapter 13).

Accidental loss of plastic tubes into veins
Many instances have been recorded. Taylor and Rutherford (1963) reported a case in which part of a plastic tube was lost into an arm vein. They concluded that it was in the right atrium and was causing no symptoms. Bennett (1963) reported the disappearance of 10 cm of plastic catheter into a vein without apparent ill effect; he referred to six previous publications with eight recorded cases; in one, the catheter was found in the pulmonary artery of a patient who had died from pulmonary embolism. In two cases a 'lost catheter' was successfully recovered — in one instance from the right atrium.

In many of the reported accidents the catheter has been severed during attempts to withdraw it through a needle; that is to say the bevel of the needle has cut it in two. This accident can be avoided by using the type of i.v. catheter in which the catheter fits over the outside of the needle.

Fragments of skin

Small fragments of skin (visible to the naked eye) are commonly taken into the lumen of the needle when the skin is punctured; using needles with an internal diameter of 0.30–0.75 mm (SWG 18 to 24), fragments are found after about two-thirds of punctures (Gibson and Norris, 1958). If skin fragments are injected into animals i.v. they can sometimes be found in pulmonary vessels and if injected subcutaneously dermoid cysts may result. Nevertheless, no ill effects from this cause have yet been reported in humans.

Toxic substances in plastic

In early investigations on the use of plastic containers for blood storage some batches of plastic appeared to have an adverse effect on red cell preservation (Strumia *et al.* 1955; 1959; Donohue and Finch, 1957). It became a requirement in the USA that all batches of plastic should be tested for their effect on red cell survival. So far as is known, the great majority of the tests failed to show any adverse effect whatever. Nevertheless, plastic used in blood transfusion equipment contains at least one potentially harmful substance, so that in retrospect it seems unfortunate that estimation of red cell viability, which is most inconvenient and subject to variables which are difficult to control, was ever chosen as a routine test for the presence of toxic substances.

Polyvinyl chloride (PVC) plastic as used in blood transfusion equipment contains plasticizers and stabilizers. According to Gullbring (1964) the common plasticizers are: dioctyl phthalate (most commonly added to soft polyvinyl chloride), trioctyl phthalate, and dioctyl sebacate and adipate (used with soft vinyl polymers). The 'stabilizers' used are: mild alkalis, fatty acid salts, ethylene oxide compounds and organic compounds of lead, barium, cadmium and tin.

Animal experiments have shown that some batches of PVC tubing liberate a substance or substances capable of: (1) arresting the isolated rat's heart (Meijler and Durrer, 1959); (2) killing minnows (Roggen *et al.* 1964); and (3) damaging mammalian cells cultured *in vitro* (Gullbring *et al.* 1964; Roggen *et al.* 1964).

Phthalates

The plasticizer di-2-ethylhexylphthalate (DEHP) dissolves readily in lipids and can be found in lipid extracts of plasma which has been stored (as blood) in ordinary plastic packs (Marcel and Noel, 1970). The level of DEHP in the plasma increases with time, reaching 5–7 mg/dl at 21 d; moreover, in transfused patients significant amounts of plasticizer are found in the tissues, the largest amounts being in abdominal fat (Jaeger and Rubin, 1970). In a study carried out in infants, those who had died from necrotizing enterocolitis following umbilical catheterization with PVC tubes were found to have significantly higher amounts of DEHP in their tissues than those who had not been catheterized (Hillman *et al.* 1975).

Monoethylhexylphthalate (MEHP) is at least as toxic as DEHP and should be measured as well as DEHP in assessing the potential toxicity of phthalates in extracts (Vessman and Reitz, 1978). One great advantage of fractionating fresh plasma rather than outdated plasma is that the former contains far smaller amounts of phthalates. MEHP (as contrasted with DEHP) has a particular affinity for albumin and, since the conversion of DEHP to MEHP may continue even in frozen plasma, it is desirable to prepare albumin from fresh rather than stored plasma (Cole *et al.* 1981).

From a series of reviews published in an 'International Form' (*Vox Sang.* 1978, **34**, 244) it can be concluded that metabolic processes account for the elimination of more than 50% of infused DEHP during the 8 h after infusion and that, furthermore, there is no definite evidence that DEHP administered in blood or blood products produces any adverse effects in humans.

DEHP, at a concentration of 0.4 mg/dl, was found to be lethal to chick embryo beating hearts in tissue culture (Jaeger and Rubin, 1970). Although DEHP seems to be only mildly toxic in animals (including humans), it is highly toxic in plants (see Hardwick and Cole, 1986). Neither DEHP nor its two major metabolites MEHP and ethylhexanol are mitogenic in rats (De Angelo and Garrett, 1983; Kornburst *et al.* 1984).

Ethylene oxide

Sensitization to ethylene oxide gas (used for sterilizing plastic equipment), associated with the formation of IgE antibodies, has been demonstrated in patients developing acute hypersensitivity reactions during haemodialysis (Nicholls, 1986) and in donors during thrombapheresis (Leitman *et al.* 1986). In the latter subjects symptoms and signs were predominantly ocular.

THROMBOPHLEBITIS

According to McNair and Dudley (1959), '. . . if an infusion is run into a peripheral vein by way of a needle, metal cannula or short length of plastic tubing, sooner or later a painful inflammatory condition will develop, spreading proximally from the tip of the needle; the vein progressively thromboses. . .'.

Duration of infusion

In a trial of the relative effects of plastic and rubber tubing, no case of thrombophlebitis was observed in infusions lasting less than 12 h; beyond that time the incidence rose rapidly and the incidence was almost twice as high with rubber as with plastic, e.g. at 48 h, rubber 82%, plastic 48% (Medical Research Council, 1957).

According to a recent review, the average survival of infusions has increased progressively over the years and is now 2–4 d (Hecker, 1992). Infusion failure, defined as failure of an infusion site to function while needed, is due most commonly to phlebitis and to extravasation. The latter is sometimes due to rupture of the wall of the vein by the tip of the needle or cannula. However, it seems more often to be due to leakage through the hole in the wall of the vein made at the time of entering the vein; extravasation then occurs only if the vein constricts or becomes blocked (see Heckler, 1992).

Septic thrombophlebitis

Septic phlebitis of cannulated veins may be a grave complication of treatment. In a series of patients with burns, it was considered that as a cause of fatal septicaemia infection introduced via a cannulated vein was as important as infection derived from the burn wound itself (Foley, 1969). In a series in which indwelling plastic catheters were cultured, those which had been *in situ* for less than 48 h were always sterile, but those which had been left in for longer were often contaminated (Druskin and Siegel,

1963). In another series, catheters which had been *in situ* for 3 or 4 d were examined. When the distal 5 cm was cultured, 53 of 118 samples were positive; in about half the cases the organisms were the same as those on the skin of the patient; about 10% of the patients had positive blood cultures (Banks *et al.* 1970).

In some circumstances, venous catheters have to be inserted for protracted periods, e.g. for long-term i.v. feeding or for giving a series of platelet transfusions. For this purpose special catheters of non-irritant material have been designed, e.g. the Hickman catheter. Rigorous precautions have to be taken against infection. Insertion of the catheter must be carried out as a surgical procedure, i.e. by a surgeon in an operating theatre. The catheter is 'tunnelled back' under the skin in such a way that the external opening is as far away as possible from the site of entry into the vein. Once inserted, the catheter must be handled as little as possible.

Prophylaxis of infusion failure
Measures which have proved succcessful are buffering of solutions, and the addition to infusions of heparin, corticosteroids or glyceryl trinitrate (see Hecker, 1992).

TRANSFUSION HAEMOSIDEROSIS

One litre of blood contains about 500 mg iron, whereas the daily excretion of iron from the body is only about 1 mg. Thus if numerous transfusions are given to a patient who is not bleeding, the amount of iron in the body is much increased. The association of multiple blood transfusions with haemosiderosis was first recognized by Kark (1937) whose patient had received more than 290 transfusions over a period of 9 years.

In patients who have received relatively few transfusions and in whom serum transferrin is not fully saturated, iron liberated from senescent red cells is taken up by the MPS, where it is relatively harmless. However, even after the transfusion of as few as 10–15 units of blood, transferrin is almost saturated (Ley *et al.* 1982). Following further transfusions, iron is deposited in parenchymal cells, causing widespread tissue damage (see review by Marcus and Huehns, 1985). Moreover, in chronic dyshae-mopoietic anaemias for which patients receive regular transfusions, excess iron is absorbed from the gut and transported via the portal vein to hepatocytes with resultant interference with hepatic function.

Iron can be removed from the body by giving injections of desferrioxamine (DFA), but even when 500 mg is given daily by i.m. injection, serious iron overload is not prevented and there is failure of growth and sexual development (Modell, 1975). When DFA is given by constant subcutaneous injection, it is very much more effective, so that it is actually possible to obtain a net excretion of iron in patients receiving regular transfusion therapy. In some patients with thalassaemia the net iron excretion has been in excess of 8 g per year (Propper *et al.* 1977).

An oral chelating agent, L1, has recently been tested. Single doses of 45–62 mg/kg in patients loaded with iron resulted in the excretion of 10–70 mg iron. Doses of this order appear to be sufficient to reduce the iron load of patients and maintain serum ferritin levels of 1000–2000 μg/l. However, some disturbing side-effects were noted in a multicentre trial, and issues of toxicity will have to be resolved before L1 replaces desferrioxamine (Kontoghiorghes, 1991).

CHAPTER 16

INFECTIOUS AGENTS TRANSMITTED BY TRANSFUSION

Most deaths caused by blood transfusion are due to the transmission of viruses, bacteria or protozoa. The agents responsible share the following characteristics: prolonged persistence in the blood stream, giving rise to carrier or latent states; causation of diseases with long incubation periods; the ability to cause asymptomatic infections; stability in stored blood and, in many cases, in plasma fractions. Ideally, blood for transfusion should be tested for the presence of all those agents that are prevalent in a given population and which, if transmitted, can cause serious disease in the recipient. Tests suitable for mass screening of blood donations are available for most of the infectious agents capable of causing significant morbidity in recipients; however, most tests do not detect all infectious donors. The chance of becoming a carrier of a particular agent varies widely in different populations and the risk of transmitting the agent concerned can be reduced by appropriate selection of donors. For example, the risk of transmitting malaria in non-endemic areas can be minimized by excluding donors from areas in which the disease is endemic, and the risk of transmitting human immunodeficiency virus (HIV) can be greatly reduced by asking sexually promiscuous persons and intravenous drug users not to give blood ('self-exclusion', sometimes referred to as 'self-deferral').

Infectious agents which are present only in cells (e.g. malaria parasites) can be transmitted by all blood components except cell-free plasma. On the other hand, those viruses that are present in plasma (e.g. hepatitis B virus (HBV)) can be transmitted by cell-free plasma and by plasma fractions. HIV can be transmitted by blood cells or plasma.

Some infectious agents (e.g. cytomegalovirus (CMV), human T-lymphotropic virus (HTLV), *Treponema pallidum*) are transmitted more easily by fresh or relatively fresh blood components, but other agents (HBV, HIV) are very stable in stored, and even in frozen, blood or plasma.

The realization that HIV, the agent of the acquired immune deficiency syndrome (AIDS), can be transmitted by blood transfusion has led to an enormous expansion of most aspects of microbiology in blood transfusion. The number of publications and scientific meetings dealing with the microbiological aspects of blood transfusion now by far exceeds those dealing with all other aspects of blood transfusion.

Screening assays for microbiological agents (Fig. 16.1)

Blood donations are routinely screened in most countries for HBsAg, HIV and syphilis. In a large number of countries all blood donations are now screened for hepatitis C virus (HCV) antibodies and in some, test are also made for alanine aminotransferase (ALT) and anti-HBc, the 'surrogate' markers of non-A, non-B hepatitis. In a few countries such as Japan, the USA, France and some Caribbean countries donations are also screened for HTLV antibodies. In most Central and South American countries donations are also screened for *T. cruzi* antibodies. In Austria, blood donations are screened for neopterin as a non-specific marker of inflammation (Hönlinger *et al.* 1988) and in some South American countries, such as Colombia, blood is screened for brucellosis. In several countries a proportion of blood units are tested for CMV antibodies to supply CMV seronegative blood to selected recipients. (The terms seronegative and seropositive are often used to describe the absence or presence of antibody, and the term seroconversion to describe the change from seronegative to seropositive.) Screening tests for malaria antibodies are being developed, to be used in countries where the disease is not endemic. In addition, in some transfusion services blood donations are screened for anti-HBV, anti-varicella zoster, anti-tetanus, anti-rabies and anti-CMV for the provision of immune plasma used in the manufacture of specific immunoglobulins.

With such a wide range of tests, the need to develop specific and sensitive assays amenable to mass screening and automation has become apparent. Transfusion services are faced with the conflict between increasing the specificity of assays to protect donors from false-positive results and at the same time increasing sensitivity to protect recipients from the risk of acquiring infections by transfusion of donations which have given false-negative results. It is difficult to achieve a balance in view of the

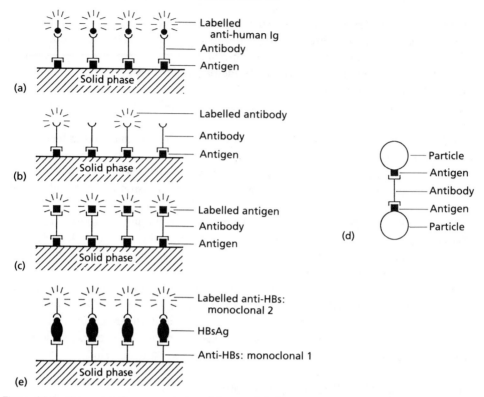

Figure 16.1 Diagrammatic representation of the antiglobulin enzyme-linked immunosorbent assay (ELISA) (a), the competitive ELISA (b), the sandwich ELISA (c), the sandwich particle assay (d) and the monoclonal sandwich ELISA (e). For an explanation of these assays, see text.

number of tests necessary to increase the safety of the blood supply in different countries. More than 10–15% of blood donations are discarded in many countries in addition to the rejection of a similar number of donors before they are bled (personal observations, MC). These losses have a major impact on blood transfusion services, many of which are now struggling to meet demands. An added complication is the number of blood components that must be held in quarantine while initially positive screening tests are repeated; even in fully computerized transfusion services, the possibility of mistakes with the consequent release of the wrong units increases with the number of units held.

Except in detecting HBsAg, all routine screening assays are for the detection of antibody. The confirmation of antigen assays by neutralization of reactivity using specific antibody is much more reliable than the 'confirmatory' techniques available for antibody assays. The principles for the majority of the most commonly used screening assays are described briefly below. Details of the assays, their automation and computerization can be found in several recent reviews (Barbara, 1989a; Barbara and Contreras, 1990; Dodd, 1991).

Passive haemagglutination or particle agglutination
Standardized antigen or antibody is used to coat tanned red cells or particles such as gelatin or latex. If the specific, complementary antibody or antigen is present in the

serum under investigation, the red cells or particles will agglutinate. Nucleated avian red cells tend to sediment faster. This type of assay is usually performed in U- or V-well microplates which can be centrifuged to enhance agglutination. The assay is also amenable to automation in blood grouping machines. If antibodies are used to coat the cells for agglutination by antigen in the serum under investigation, the term 'reverse passive agglutination' is used.

Antiglobulin enzyme-linked immunosorbent assay (ELISA)

Standardized antigen (for example HIV antigen) is linked to a solid phase in the form of beads, the wells of microplates or dipsticks, etc. If antibody (for example anti-HIV) is present in the test sample (donor's serum), which is generally diluted according to the manufacturer's instructions, it will adhere to the solid phase. The coated wells or beads are then washed; if antibodies are present, they will be detected with an enzyme-linked human antiglobulin reagent which will in turn be detected by the appropriate chromogenic substrate (Fig. 16.1a). The antigens can be: (a) disrupted microbial agents with different grades of purity and of contamination with cells used for culture; (b) recombinant polypeptides obtained by molecular genetics; or (c) synthetic antigens. The enzymes most widely used are horseradish peroxidase and alkaline phosphatase. The sensitivity of the ELISA can be enhanced with biotin–avidin or biotin–streptavidin, or by amplification through the addition of NADP, alcohol dehydrogenase and diaphorase.

Antiglobulin radioimmunoassay (RIA)

The basic principles are the same as for ELISA; the only difference is that the label for the antiglobulin is a radioisotope, i.e. ^{125}I.

Chemiluminescence assays

Again, this is similar to an ELISA but here the horseradish peroxidase reacts with luminol in the presence of an enhancer to produce light emission.

Competitive ELISA or RIA

Known antigen (for example HIV-1) is linked to the solid phase and any antibody in the serum will compete for binding with enzyme-labelled or radiolabelled antibody (Fig. 16.1b). The more antibody in the sample, the weaker the enzyme reaction available to colour the substrate, or the weaker the radioactive signal. Hence, in a competitive assay, the weaker the reaction, the larger is the amount of antibody present, whereas in the antiglobulin assay, the stronger the reaction, the larger is the amount of antibody present.

Sandwich ELISA or RIA

Antigen molecules coat the solid phase as in the antiglobulin ELISA and any antibody present in the test sample will be detected by the reaction with labelled antigen (Fig. 16.1c). For the detection of viral antigen, two types of monoclonal antibodies can be used in 'one-step' assays, reacting with different epitopes of the antigen to avoid blocking the sites which attach the antibody onto the solid phase (Fig. 16.1e).

Sandwich particle assay
Particles in suspension are coated with several molecules of antigen. When antibody is present in the test sample, the particles agglutinate (Fig. 16.1d).

Screening assays: conclusion
If any donor's serum is found to give a positive reaction with a screening assay, the test should be repeated in duplicate and, if at least one of the repeat tests is found positive, a sample from the blood pack should be tested. The original sample should also be tested with a 'supplementary' or, ideally, with a 'confirmatory' assay using a different methodology to that used in the screening assay. The most definitive type of confirmation is that used for HBsAg and consists of neutralization or inhibition of the antigen–antibody reaction by a well-authenticated anti-HBs.

Western blot
Lysed viral or recombinant antigens are subjected to electrophoresis in sodium dodecyl sulphate (SDS) polyacrylamide gel. The viral polypeptides are separated by migration on the gel according to their molecular weight. The polypeptide pattern on the gel is transferred ('blotted') on to nitrocellulose paper which is dried and cut into strips. Dilutions of the serum samples found to be positive in screening assays are incubated with the strips; if antibodies to HIV antigens are present, they will combine with different and precise sections of the strip carrying the specific polypeptides. As in any other antiglobulin assay, the strips are washed and antigen–antibody reactions are detected by an appropriately labelled antiglobulin reagent. Antiglobulin is usually labelled with enzyme and a positive reaction is detected by the reaction of the enzyme with its substrate. Antibodies to defined polypeptides can be detected according to the position of the bands on the strip. Criteria of a positive reaction should be well defined for each agent for which Western blot is used as the confirmatory test. Unfortunately, contaminating proteins from viral lysates may travel to positions which are the same as those of specific viral antigens and may sometimes bind to crossreacting antibodies, leading to false-positive reactions.

Recombinant-immunoblot assay (RIBA)
This assay is used for confirmation of HCV antibodies; recombinant antigens on a nitrocellulose strip react with specific antibodies when present in test sera.

Polymerase chain reaction (PCR)
This is a technique which makes it possible to amplify a short specific sequence of viral deoxyribonucleic acid (DNA) in a sample (target sequence in Fig. 16.2); amplification of more than a million copies can be achieved in a few hours (Mullis and Faloona, 1987). Ribonucleic acid (RNA) viruses can also be used after treatment with reverse transcriptase. For PCR it is essential to know the sequence of bases flanking the target DNA region. Two specific short fragments of synthetic DNA (oligonucleotide primers) are then synthesized to match (hybridize) the sequences at either end of the target from the 5′ end (Fig. 16.2). The first primer is a copy of the end of the coding strand and the second primer, a copy of the end of the non-coding homologous strand. DNA polymerase is essential in PCR for the synthesis of the complementary strand of a DNA

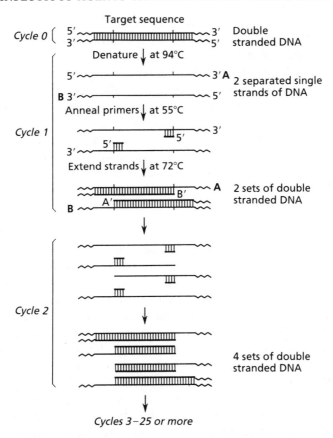

Figure 16.2 The polymerase chain reaction (PCR). A fragment of double-stranded DNA has the specific gene sequence for amplification flanked by two vertical lines. The two DNA strands separate (heat denaturation) and are then allowed to reassociate (anneal) with their primers (dark bars) that mark the ends of the target sequence. The primers then synthesize two new chains complementary to the original strands starting from the 5′ end in the presence of *Taq* polymerase and the four deoxyribonucleotide triphosphates. Each cycle doubles the DNA and is repeated 25–35 times with a final enrichment of the target sequence of 10^5–10^6.

sequence in the presence of the appropriate primers and deoxyribonucleotide triphosphates (dNTP). A thermostable polymerase enzyme from the bacillus *Thermus aquaticus* (*Taq*) has simplified the procedure considerably since it is relatively unaffected at the denaturation temperature of 94°C and does not need to be replenished at each cycle (Saiki *et al.* 1988). The PCR mixture contains the specimen under study, excess oligonucleotide primers, *Taq* polymerase and abundant dNTPs as well as electrolytes such as Mg^{2+}. The binding of the primers to the flanking sequences of the target DNA (annealing) is possible after separation of the two strands of DNA by melting at 94°C and cooling at 40–55°C. At its optimal temperature of 70–75°C, the *Taq* polymerase will stimulate the synthesis of complementary DNAs (extension) to the coding and non-coding strands starting from the annealed primers in the 5′ to 3′ direction. The whole process of melting, cooling, reassociation or annealing and synthesis takes 2–3 min and is repeated cyclically. Since more than 30 cycles are undertaken per procedure, the target DNA becomes amplified exponentially because the new strands, as well as the old ones, become templates for the excess primers (Fig. 16.2). The end result is that the target DNA sequence is amplified 10^5–10^6 times in just a few hours. PCR cycling has been automated using microprocessor-controlled heating blocks. The major problems with PCR relate to the specificity of the oligonucleotide primers and to the possibility of amplification of non-target sequences which can occur especially in contaminated samples. Cross-contamination with foreign DNA during PCR assays is by far the greatest problem because the contaminating DNA can also be amplified. Details of the PCR technique can be found in Williams and Sullivan (1991) and Schochetman and George (1992). For its clinical applications, see Weatherall (1991).

HEPATITIS B VIRUS

Viral hepatitis, acquired from the donor, remains one of the commonest serious, and also one of the commonest lethal, complications of blood transfusion.

The discovery in 1968 (see below) that the viraemic phase of serum hepatitis (hepatitis B) could be recognized serologically led to the expectation that all infectious donors could be detected and post-transfusion hepatitis (PTH) eliminated. In fact, the transmission of HBV by transfusion is now almost completely preventable, but a few infections due to HBV, until recently accounting for 5–10% of PTH, are transmitted by blood donations that are negative for HBsAg with currently available screening tests (Shih *et al.* 1986; J.A.J Barbara, personal communication). In the 1970s and 1980s most cases of PTH were due to then uncharacterized agents named 'non-A, non-B' agents, but in 1988 a new virus, named HCV, was defined by molecular genetics, and it is now possible to screen blood donations for the vast majority of agents transmitting PTH.

HBV-associated antigens and antibodies

An enormously important step in the control of the spread of HBV was taken with the discovery, in serum, of an antigen associated with the disease. Initially, the relationship was not appreciated and the antigen—first recognized in the serum of an Australian aborigine, hence the provisional name 'Australia antigen'—appeared to have an association with acute leukaemia (Blumberg *et al.* 1965). However, it was not long before the association with hepatitis was realized (Blumberg *et al.* 1968; Prince, 1968). Australia antigen is now known to be unassembled viral coat, or surface antigen (HBsAg). Electron microscopy of concentrated serum containing HBsAg reveals so-called Dane particles of diameter 42 nm (Dane *et al.* 1970) which are now known to be the complete HB virus; they are made up of an inner protein core (HBc) containing partially double-stranded DNA with a single-stranded region of variable length and DNA polymerase, surrounded by an outer coat of HBsAg (Fig. 16.3). HBsAg is shed into the plasma in large quantities in the form of spheres and sometimes rods (diameter 18–22 nm); it can be readily detected by immunoassays with anti-HBs. Antibodies to the surface antigen and the core antigen are known respectively as anti-HBs and anti-HBc. HBeAg is a soluble antigen (though also particle associated), found only in some sera containing HBsAg. P19, the major polypeptide in the core of HBV, carries the antigenic determinants of HBcAg and HBeAg (Takahashi *et al.* 1981).

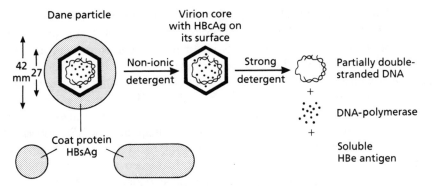

Figure 16.3 The virus (Dane particle) of hepatitis B and its constituents.

In the partially double-stranded DNA, the long (L –) strand is of fixed length whilst the length of the short strand (S +) is variable. The circular HBV genome is about 3200 nucleotides long. The L (–) strand carries virtually all the protein capacity of HBV in four open reading frames (ORF) termed S/pre-S, C, P and X which overlap one another. The S/pre-S region codes for the envelope proteins and is divided into: (i) the *S* gene coding for the major protein, HBsAg, 226 amino acids long, carrying the 'a' immuno-dominant determinant, with allelic variations for *d/y* and *w/r* (see below); (ii) the *pre-S2* region, coding for the pre-S2 antigen, a very immunogenic sequence of 55 amino acids, resistant to denaturation, which elicits neutralizing antibodies and, together with the major protein, codes for the middle protein, a glycoprotein 281 amino acids long; (iii) the *pre-S1* region coding for a variable sequence of 108–119 amino acids, depending on the subtype, which is essential for recognition of hepatocyte receptors and, together with the *S* gene and the *pre-S2* region, codes for the large envelope protein of HBV. The *C* region codes for the core protein and the *P* region for the DNA polymerase; the function of the *X* gene is still unknown (Tiollais *et al.* 1988).

Subtypes of HBV
All HBV strains have one antigenic determinant *a* in common which may be of *d* or *y* subtypes: the subtypes (*ad* and *ay*) have a further determinant which may be either *w* or *r*. The subtypes are useful in epidemiological studies since their distribution varies geographically and in different sections of a community, e.g. in the UK, homosexual HBsAg carriers are usually of the *ad* subtype and drug addicts *ay* (see Barbara, 1983).

HBsAg carriers
The prevalence of HBsAg varies considerably in different parts of the world and exceeds 15% in some populations in Africa, South-East Asia, China and Latin America, In some countries such as the USA in which the disease is not endemic, donors with a history of hepatitis after the age of 10 years are permanently debarred from donation because of the high likelihood that the hepatitis was caused by HBV or HCV (AABB, 1990). Donors found positive for HBsAg are, of course, debarred from blood donation. Soon after the introduction of testing for HBsAg, the frequency of positive results in

volunteer donors giving blood for the first time was about 0.1%, both in the UK (Wallace *et al.* 1972) and in the USA (Cherubin and Prince, 1971). In paid donors the frequency of HBsAg-positive donors was about ten times greater than in volunteer donors (Walsh *et al.* 1970; Cherubin and Prince, 1971). In donors with previously negative tests who give blood on subsequent occasions, the frequency of a positive test for HBsAg is very low; in one series in north London the frequency was one in 60 000; almost all the positive tests were due to acute infections in young men (Barbara and Briggs, 1981). In north London, before 1984, the frequency of HBsAg-positivity in donors giving blood for the first time was 0.2%; the figure fell to 0.07% after donors with a high risk of contracting HIV infection had been asked not to give blood (Barbara, 1989b). Of approximately 2 million blood donations collected in 1982 in England, Wales and Northern Ireland, 261 new donors and 90 previously tested donors were found to be HBsAg positive; corresponding figures for 1987 were 161 and 25 (D. Howell and J. Mortimer, personal communication).

In north London up to 1983, about 85% of the HBsAg-positive donations detected by screening were from long-term HBsAg carriers; the remainder came from donors with acute HBV infections (Barbara, 1983). It is known that a donor can transmit HBV after having had a positive test for HBsAg for as long as 19 years (Zuckerman and Taylor, 1969). It has been estimated that carriers clear their HBsAg at a rate of about 1.7% per annum (Sampliner *et al.* 1979; Barbara, 1983); when HBsAg is eventually lost, it is replaced by anti-HBs as a marker of immunity.

More than 70% of apparently healthy British blood donors who are found to be HBsAg positive have a normal liver function, as judged by serum aspartate transaminase (AST) and aminotransferase (ALT) levels (Barbara *et al.* 1978). In a Dutch series a similar figure was observed: in the 30% with abnormal liver function tests (LFTs), when the tests remained abnormal over a period of time, moderate to severe liver disease, as judged histologically, was present in eight of nine cases. All carriers of HBV were found to be either HBeAg positive (21%) or anti-HBe positive (79%). Abnormal LFTs were found significantly more often in HBeAg-positive carriers than in anti-HBe-positive carriers (Reesink *et al.* 1980). In one other series a small proportion of carriers were negative both for HBeAg and anti-HBe (Barbara *et al.* 1978). In countries where HBV is endemic, the proportion of HBsAg carriers who are HBeAg positive is higher.

Immunosuppression may cause recrudescence of latent HBV; in patients in whom anti-HBc was the only detectable HBV marker before immunosuppression, HBsAg was shown to appear after immunosuppressive therapy (Nagington *et al.* 1977). Activation of latent HBV may be mistaken for PTH in leukaemic patients or in patients with AIDS receiving blood component therapy.

Anti-HBs
Anti-HBs develops in most people who recover from hepatitis B infection: the presence of the antibody in the plasma prevents further infection with HBV. Before the introduction of measures to exclude from donation subjects at risk of HIV infection, the frequency of anti-HBs in blood donors in north London was found to be about 2% (Tedder *et al.* 1980a). The frequency of anti-HBs in multiply-transfused patients such as haemophiliacs is very high, and has become even higher now that it is recommended that these patients should all be vaccinated.

Anti-HBc

Anti-HBc is found in all persons who have been infected with HBV. It can first be detected during the incubation period, after the appearance of HBsAg, and persists thereafter. In acute infection, high levels of IgM anti-HBc have been found which persist for 3–4 months and are then replaced by IgG anti-HBc. High titres of IgG anti-HBc can be found in carriers who may sometimes also have low levels of IgM anti-HBc (see below). During the recovery phase of acute hepatitis B, anti-HBc may be present in the absence of HBsAg and anti-HBs. Donations taken at this time ('window' period) can transmit HBV (Hoofnagle *et al.* 1978). In a small proportion of carriers, only anti-HBc can be detected in the plasma; such subjects may transmit HBV by transfusion.

HBeAg and anti-HBe

HBeAg is a marker of infectivity associated with the presence of large numbers of Dane particles, found during the incubation period and the acute phase of clinical hepatitis B; anti-HBe develops during recovery. HBsAg carriers initially have HBeAg in their blood together with a high level of HBsAg. This phase may last for a variable period, sometimes measured in years. Approximately 20% of HBsAg-positive blood donors in the UK have HBeAg (Dow *et al.* 1980; Harrison *et al.* 1985), compared with 50% in Mediterranean countries (Lieberman *et al.* 1983). The HBeAg-positive phase is followed by a second phase in which anti-HBe replaces HBeAg, with HbsAg often falling to lower levels. Although infectivity is greatly reduced during this second phase, blood transfusion can still transmit HBV (D. S. Dane, personal communication). Some HBV mutants that are incapable of synthesizing HBeAg have been shown to induce fulminant hepatitis (see section on HBV variants).

DNA polymerase

This is a marker of viraemia. Biochemical assays for the detection of DNA polymerase have been developed but are not suitable for mass screening of blood donors. The assay is not as sensitive as that for detecting HBV-DNA.

Serum HBV-DNA

Molecular hybridization techniques and PCR for the detection of HBV-DNA in serum are the most sensitive methods for detecting HBV-infectious subjects. HBV-DNA has been detected in 8–12% of healthy Chinese people who were positive only for anti-HBc or anti-HBs, and also in some healthy Chinese with no HBV markers (Pao *et al.* 1991; see also Jackson, 1991). However, others have suggested that in HBsAg carriers IgM anti-HBc is an even more sensitive marker of infectivity (Tassopoulos *et al.* 1986). Although in general there is a good correlation between the presence of HBeAg and HBV-DNA in serum (Karayiannis *et al.* 1985), HBeAg has been reported in the absence of HBV-DNA (Krogsgaard *et al.* 1985; Govindarajan *et al.* 1986) and *vice versa* (Thiers *et al.* 1988; Vaudin *et al.* 1988; Carman *et al.* 1989).

It is unlikely that PCR for HBV-DNA will replace assays for HBsAg because only about one-third of HBsAg-positives have HBV-DNA by PCR (Editorial, 1991; Pao *et al.* 1991). With regard to screening of blood donors for HBV-DNA, the number of extra infectious donors detected would be minimal in countries with a low prevalence for

HBsAg such as the UK (less than one in 5000) and the USA (one in 2500). Whether screening Chinese blood donors (HBsAg prevalence of 25%) for HBV-DNA would be of value, when an automated test becomes available, is another matter (Jackson, 1991).

Pre-S2 antigen and antibody
Expression of pre-S2 on HBsAg correlates with active liver disease and viral replication whereas the appearance of anti-pre-S2 is essential for recovery from HBV infection (Budkowska *et al.* 1988).

Screening tests for HBsAg in blood donations
The fact that such large amounts of HBsAg are shed into plasma by HBV has made it relatively easy to devise immunoassays suitable for mass screening for this virus. This shedding does not occur with other viruses such as HCV or HIV.

The first test used to screen blood donations was immunodiffusion, and this was superseded by counter-immunoelectrophoresis or endimmuno-osmophoresis (EIOP). Reverse passive haemagglutination (RPHA), a more sensitive and rapid method, was soon developed: red cells coated with anti-HBs are agglutinated by sera containing HBsAg. Immunoradiometric assays, ELISA and enhanced luminescence assays have proved significantly more sensitive than RPHA, detecting less than 0.25 ng HBsAg/ml serum. However, taking the mol. wt. of HBsAg as 3×10^6, 0.25 ng is equivalent to 5×10^7 particles/ml so that a negative ELISA test is compatible with the presence of as many as $2.0–5 \times 10^7$ antigen particles/ml (L.R. Overby, personal communication). Immunoassays involving fluorescence labelling and enzyme amplification assays are potentially more sensitive than RIA and ELISA and may eventually replace them (for a review with references and details of tests for HBsAg, see Barbara, 1983). It is, however, unlikely that complete success in the prevention of PTH due to HBV will be achieved solely by screening for HBsAg, considering the very small size of the sample tested compared with the volume of plasma transfused.

The sensitivities of EIOP, RPHA and RIA or ELISA for the detection of HBsAg are approximately 1000, 10–100 and less than 0.5 ng/ml serum, respectively. Increasing the sensitivity of screening tests does not increase proportionately the number of donors found to be HBsAg positive. For example, at the North London Blood Transfusion Centre, for every 100 HBsAg positives by EIOP, 140 would be found by a sensitive RPHA and 154 by RIA (Barbara, 1983). Thus, increasing the sensitivity of the test by more than 1000 times increases the number of HBsAg-positive donors detected by a factor of less than 2.

Immunoassays are available for the simultaneous detection of HBsAg and anti-HBs. Several monoclonal HBs antibodies directed against the *a* antigen, common to all HBV subtypes, have been produced and used in sensitive screening assays. However, mutations in the *S* region of HBV have led to *a*-deficient 'escape' mutants which could not be detected by assays based on anti-*a* (Carman *et al.* 1990). These mutants are not neutralized by anti-HBs *in vivo* or *in vitro*. In addition, if polyclonal assays based on anti-*ad* are used and the mutating virus was originally *ay*, infectious donors will be missed.

In the UK, the current requirement is that all blood donations should be tested for HBsAg by an assay with a minimum sensitivity of 1 British Standard Unit (BSU)/ml

(UKBTS/NIBSC, 1990). The BSU has now been adopted as the International Standard Unit (ISU, shortened to iu) and is approximately equal to 1 ng HBsAg/ml. Because of the ready availability of several commercial assays for HBsAg based on monoclonal antibodies, which can detect as little as 0.25 ng/ml or less in under 2 h (Ronalds *et al.* 1989), the minimum sensitivity requirement in the UK will soon be revised to 0.5 iu/ml (0.5 ng/ml). As stated above, it is unlikely that this requirement for increased sensitivity will lead to the destruction of many more HBsAg-positive donations in the UK because the number of acute HBV infections, with low levels of HBsAg, has declined considerably since the introduction of measures for self-exclusion of potential donors at risk of HIV infection. Before self-exclusion seven or eight acute HBV infections were detected on screening 200 000 blood donations per year at the North London Blood Transfusion Centre; since self-exclusion, only one or two acute infections per year have been detected (Barbara, 1989b). When the results of testing are required urgently, for example on occasional platelet concentrates, RPHA may be considered even though its sensitivity is lower (provided that the donor has been tested on a previous occasion and found to be HBsAg negative by RIA or ELISA). Blood should not be released for transfusion until the test for HBsAg has shown to be negative.

It has been suggested that testing for anti-HBc should replace the routine testing of blood donations for HBsAg (Smilovici *et al.* 1984). However, there is ample evidence to show that testing solely for anti-HBc would not detect highly infectious HBsAg-positive donors early in acute infections (Barbara *et al.* 1984; Couroucé *et al.* 1985). Whether screening of blood donations for anti-HBc, in addition to HBsAg, is needed to prevent transmission of HBV by 'HBsAg-negative, anti-HBc positive' donors, as well as to help in the detection of donors at risk of sexually transmitted diseases, is another matter.

Transmission of HBV
HBV is spread by transfusions of infected blood, plasma or coagulation factor concentrates. In a wider context, HBV can be transmitted in many other ways: by sexual contact; by accidental puncture of the skin by infected needles ('needle-stick'), of which many instances are known (see Barbara, 1983); by the use of shared syringes and needles by drug addicts; by contaminated needles used in acupuncture, dentistry or tattooing; by the sharing of razors and toothbrushes; by close contact between children leading to cross-infection, presumably by blood (e.g. biting) and observed especially in endemic areas with a high incidence of HBeAg-positive carriers; and by transmission from mother to infant, especially if the mother is HBeAg positive.

In PTH due to the transmission of HBV by blood or blood components, the mean incubation period was found to be 63 d (range 30–150 d) by Gocke (1972) and 73 d (range 39–107 d) by Prince (1975).

Washing of red cells does not eliminate the risk of transmission of HBV. It has been shown that when blood is only lightly contaminated with HBV and the red cells are then washed, or frozen with glycerol and washed, small volumes of red cell suspensions, though apparently HBsAg negative, can still transmit HBV to chimpanzees (Alter *et al.* 1978) or to humans (Rinker and Galambos, 1981).

Methods of inactivating viruses in blood products
Despite the routine testing of donated blood for HBsAg, the transmission of HBV, as

well as HCV and delta agent (see below), in fractionated products obtained from large pools of plasma from thousands of donors was until recently a major complication of blood transfusion. The fractions obtained at an early stage of the cold-ethanol fractionation process, i.e. fibrinogen, Factor VIII and Factor IX (or prothrombin complex concentrate) in which complete virions (i.e. Dane particles) were readily demonstrable, carried a high risk of transmitting hepatitis. The majority of severe haemophiliacs treated with Factor VIII concentrates had serological evidence of past HBV infection and up to 12% of them became carriers of HBsAg (Stehr-Green et al. 1991). NANBH used to be transmitted frequently by both Factor VIII and prothrombin factor concentrates (Wyke et al. 1979; Craske, 1982). Concentrates prepared from plasma from paid donors carried the highest risk of transmitting hepatitis but Factor VIII and IX concentrates prepared only from volunteer donors were not completely free from risk (Fletcher et al. 1983). Plasma fractions obtained later in fractionation, i.e. immunoglobulins and albumin, are either devoid of intact virus particles or are depleted of most intact infectious HBV particles (Trepo et al. 1978; Iwarson et al. 1985). As described below, the transmission of HBV and NANBH by immunoglobulin prepared by Cohn fractionation (see Chapter 14) and its current modifications, or by albumin, is virtually unknown, although there are exceptional reports of NANBH following the i.v. administration of Ig, prepared by Cohn fractionation and passed through a Sephadex G25 column.

Although methods of inactivating viruses in blood products were being investigated before 1982, the realization that HIV could be transmitted to haemophiliacs by Factor VIII concentrates accelerated progress in the development of methods of viral inactivation. Several procedures have been explored successfully including heat treatment of concentrates in the wet or dry state, a combination of β–propiolactone and ultraviolet (UV) irradiation, a combination of a solvent and a detergent and immunosorbent procedures for purification of the clotting factors (for references, see Gomperts, 1986; Cuthbertson et al. 1991). Combinations of these methods seem to give even safer products. One of the major problems of most viral inactivation methods is the low yield of clotting factors in the final product. The efficacy of viral inactivation methods can be assessed in vitro in tissue cultures infected with model viruses (cultures of hepatitis viruses are not available) or in vivo in chimpanzees. However, the only means of properly assessing the potential infectivity of plasma products is through carefully conducted clinical trials in patients who have not previously received blood or blood products. Considerably more data on viral infectivity are available from patients with haemophilia A treated with Factor VIII subjected to inactivation than from patients with haemophilia B (see Cuthbertson et al. 1991).

The methods currently in use for viral inactivation are as follows (for details, see Cuthbertson et al. 1991).

Pasteurization consists in heating blood products in solution at 60°C for 10 h, in the presence of a stabilizer to protect Factor VIII or IX. Unfortunately, stabilizers cause a loss of yield of 30–40% and they also stabilize viruses against heat. A mixture of sucrose and glycine has been used as a stabilizer with great reduction of infectivity but the removal of the stabilizer from the product is complicated and costly. Although the initial clinical trials reported no cases of transmission of HBV, NANBH or HIV by pasteurized Factor VIII (Schimpf *et al.* 1987), transmission of HBV was later reported in two patients (Brackmann and Egli, 1988).

Dry heat treatment. Heating of lyophilized coagulation factor concentrates has partially or totally inactivated contaminant viruses, depending on the temperature used, the time of heat treatment, the composition of the product, the freezing and freeze-drying methods, and the residual moisture content of the final product. Trials on unimmunized patients treated with Factor VIII or Factor IX heated at 80°C for 72 h have shown absence of transmission of NANBH, HBV and HIV (Colvin *et al.* 1988; Ludlum *et al.* 1989). On the other hand, Factor VIII heated at 60°C for 30 or 72 h has transmitted hepatitis (Colombo *et al.* 1985; Preston *et al.* 1985). The advantages of dry heat at 80°C for 72 h are the very good yield and good solubility characteristics of the coagulation factor concentrates and the fact that the process is carried out in the sealed final container, with no possibility of cross-contamination (McIntosh *et al.* 1987; Cuthbertson *et al.* 1991).

Steam treatment of freeze-dried concentrates at 60°C for 10 h under a pressure of 1200 mbar. Although it has been shown that HIV can be inactivated by this process, HBV has been transmitted to non-immune patients (Mannucci *et al.* 1988; Cuthbertson *et al.* 1991).

Heat treatment of Factor VIII mixed with an organic solvent. Factor VIII has been mixed with chloroform or with *n*-heptane and heated at 60°C; both products have transmitted NANBH (Mannucci *et al.* 1985a; Kernoff *et al.* 1987).

Solvent–detergent treatment does not require heat and relies on the fact that the viruses transmitted by fractionated plasma products which cause the main morbidity have a lipid envelope. The method uses the non-volatile solvent, tri-(*n*-butyl) phosphate (TNBP), in combination with a detergent such as sodium deoxycholate. The process is carried out at 20–30°C and can be applied to the majority of plasma products that carry a risk of viral transmission. The solvent–detergent mixture is removed at the end of the procedure by precipitation of the product or by chromatography. No cases of hepatitis or HIV transmission have been reported after the administration of solvent–detergent-treated products (Horowitz *et al.* 1988; see Cuthbertson *et al.* 1991). The main disadvantage of this method is its failure to inactivate non-lipid-coated viruses such as parvovirus (Edwards *et al.* 1987; Prince *et al.* 1987) and HAV (Mannucci, 1992).

β-propiolactone and UV irradiation at 254 nm. The process proved effective for Factor IX but not for Factor VIII (Stephan, 1989). The main disadvantages of this method are the carcinogenic effect of β-propiolactone and the considerable loss of yield of Factor IX (see Cuthbertson *et al.* 1991).

Risk of HBV transmission by blood products
Factor VIII purified with monoclonal antibodies should also be submitted to viral inactivation procedures because the purification process is not able to remove all viral contaminants from the product (see Cuthbertson *et al.* 1991).

As shown above, HBV is more resistant to methods of viral inactivation than HIV and HCV. Now that the majority of patients with haemophilia have been immunized with HBV vaccine, it is difficult to assess, in clinical trials, the efficacy of methods of inactivating HBV.

Up to 50% of haemophiliacs treated with Factor VIII concentrates who are HBsAg positive have antibodies to hepatitis delta virus (HDV) (Rizzetto et al. 1982; Rosina et al. 1985). No data are available on the effectiveness of methods for inactivating HDV.

The most effective way of preventing the development of HBV infection in haemophiliacs likely to receive coagulation factor concentrates is to immunize them in early life with HBV vaccine, subcutaneously (Eddleston, 1990). Sexual and household contacts of haemophiliacs should also be vaccinated.

The majority of therapeutic immunoglobulins are manufactured by cold-ethanol fractionation (see Chapter 14), although small volumes of Ig for intravenous use (i.v. Ig) are manufactured in some places by a special chromatographic process. When obtained by cold-ethanol fractionation, the Ig fraction contains significant amounts of ethanol. Whether the final product is destined for i.m. or i.v. use will depend on the methods used for ethanol removal and formulation of the final product (Cuthbertson et al. 1987). In general, products for i.m. use are freeze-dried to remove the ethanol whereas ethanol removal from i.v. Ig requires gentler processes such as gel chromatography and ultrafiltration to prevent the formation of aggregates (Cuthbertson et al. 1991).

Ig for i.m. use has a very good safety record (Finlayson, 1979) but there are a few reports of transmission of HBV which have been attributed to manufacturing defects (for references, see Cuthbertson et al. 1991) and there are no reports of transmission of NANBH or HIV by i.m. Ig although the number of clinical trials with this product is minimal (WHO, 1983; Iwarson et al. 1985).

The manufacture of i.v. Ig involves various steps, depending on the manufacturer, after ethanol removal to reduce the levels of vasoactive substances and anti-complementary activity. Some of these steps may have antiviral effects. However, despite all these processes, there are reports of at least 44 cases of transmission of NANBH by i.v. Ig, including five deaths from fulminant hepatitis in patients with agammaglobulinaemia (see Dodd et al. 1992). The rate and severity of transmission have varied with different commercial products, some products causing only mild hepatitis by isolated batches (Williams et al. 1989) and other products causing severe hepatitis by more than one batch (Lever et al. 1984; Bjorkander et al. 1988). In one report, NANB PTH occured in all of 12 patients with agammaglobulinaemia who received i.v. Ig. Patients who received i.m. Ig from the same plasma pool did not develop NANBH (Lever et al. 1984). In this series, and in two others in which patients developed NANBH after i.v. Ig, at least half of the patients showed evidence of progressive liver disease (Ochs et al. 1985, 1986; Webster and Lever, 1986; Weiland et al. 1986). A large number of patients in East Germany acquired NANB PTH in 1979 from an infectious batch of anti-Rh D Ig (Durkop et al. 1989).

Although it is known that the viruses in blood products are distributed mainly to non-immunoglobulin fractions during cold-ethanol fractionation and that ethanol can inactivate lipid-coated viruses, the above reports of PTH have led manufacturers to investigate the possibility of adding viral inactivation methods to the preparation of i.v.

Ig (see Cutherbertson *et al.* 1991). Ig prepared for i.v. use by ultrafiltration of a cold-ethanol fraction II treated by the 'pH 4–mild pepsin' method and freeze-dried (Leen *et al.* 1986) appears to be safer and yields a better product (Lever and Webster, 1987), although an occasional batch transmitted mild NANBH shown to be due to HCV (Williams *et al.* 1989). The solvent–detergent method has been used at the New York Blood Center in the manufacture of HIV hyperimmune globulin (Horowitz, 1989).

Currently available methods of viral inactivation in blood products are being improved and some are being used in combination with others. Methods being tested include γ-irradiation, a combination of UV light and psoralens (a method which has also been tried experimentally for blood components; see Alter *et al.* 1988), visible light and haematoporphyrin; ozone treatment; treatment with long-chain fatty acids such as sodium oleate or with phenanthroline–cuprous iron complex (for references, see Cuthbertson *et al.* 1991).

HBV transmitted by HBsAg-negative donors

Using radioimmunoassay or ELISA, as little as 0.1–0.25 ng HBsAg/ml can be detected in blood (see above). However, carriers with even subliminal levels can transmit HBV by blood transfusion; serum from patients which was negative for all HBV serological markers, but positive for HBV-DNA by PCR, transmitted hepatitis B to two chimpanzees (Thiers *et al.* 1988). Moreover, fulminant hepatitis was reported in eight recipients of units of blood negative for HBsAg; analysis of the HBV-DNA showed that point mutations in the pre-core region resulted in the inability to synthesize HBsAg although HBcAg elicited high levels of anti-HBc in the infectious donors (Kojima *et al.* 1991).

In acute infections there are two periods when HBsAg may be undetectable although the subject can transmit HBV: (1) during the early stages of the incubation period when neither HBsAg nor anti-HBc may be detectable (see following paragraph in small type); and (2) during a later stage when HBsAg can no longer be detected although anti-HBs has not yet become detectable ('diagnostic window'); in this phase anti-HBc, and often anti-HBe, can be detected (Tedder *et al.* 1980b). Increasing the sensitivity of screening assays for HBsAg beyond 0.25 ng/ml might lead to an increase in the number of false positives with very few extra real positives, estimated at one or two more per 100 HBsAg-positive donors. However, testing all blood donations for anti-HBc as well as for HBsAg might further decrease the incidence of HBV infection by transfusion. In several countries, routine screening of blood donations for anti-HBc has become mandatory, not only with the object of decreasing the incidence of HBV PTH but mainly to decrease the risk of transmitting NANB PTH and as a safety net for identifying donors at risk of acquiring HIV infection. It has been estimated that 20% of donors with anti-HBc have 'anti-HBc only' and can transmit HBV despite being HBsAg negative. In the UK, with a prevalence of approximately 0.5–0.7% donors with anti-HBc in 2.2 million donations collected annually and assuming 50% false positives, at least 1100 donors would be 'anti-HBc only' at the time screening is introduced. Although it is known that some donations found positive for anti-HBc and negative for anti-HBs can transmit HBV, it is not known what proportion of such units are infectious (J. A. Barbara and MC, personal observations).

Transmission of HBV from a subject in the early stages of the incubation period was described by Rinker and Galambos (1981). In an experiment (not originally related to transmission of HBV), the donor's blood was given to 32 volunteers at a time when it was HBsAg negative. At some time between 36 and 76 d later the donor became HBsAg positive. Of the 32 subjects who received the donor's blood (at a time when he was HBsAg negative) 19 became HBsAg positive and 14 of these developed various degrees of hepatitis. A further nine of the 32 subjects developed anti-HBs.

Serological findings in relation to an attack of HBV hepatitis

In persons exposed to HBV, HBsAg appears first in the incubation period, followed by anti-HBc. HBV-DNA, DNA polymerase, HBeAg and pre-S2 antigen also appear during the incubation period. In acute clinical hepatitis B, HBsAg reaches a peak at the onset of symptoms and then declines during the illness and convalescence, disappearing from the blood in most subjects after a period which varies from a week to several months. Clinical hepatitis B can be a serious disease with approximately 1–3% of acute cases presenting as fulminant hepatitis and 5–10% of infected subjects developing chronic hepatitis, many of whom later die from liver cirrhosis or hepatocellular carcinoma (WHO, 1983; Zuckerman, 1990). Subjects who recover have anti-HBs, anti-HBc and anti-pre-S2 in their plasma. The carrier state most commonly develops after asymptomatic infections (Tedder et al. 1980b), especially if infection is acquired in infancy. A study of children from Senegal showed that 80% of infants infected in the first 6 months of life became carriers compared with 15% of children infected between the ages of 2 and 3 years (Coursaget et al. 1987). In the UK, where acute HBV infections occur mainly in young adults, about 5% of those infected become carriers (Barbara, 1983). In countries where infections are common in infancy and childhood, the proportion of infected individuals who become carriers is higher (Sobeslabsky, 1987) as is the proportion of carriers who, as adults, develop primary hepatocellular carcinoma, a major cause of death in the developing world. Part of the HBV genome is incorporated in the cellular DNA of the hepatoma (Popper, 1988; see Zuckerman, 1990).

Management of HBsAg-positive subjects

If a blood donor is found, on screening, to have a positive test for HBsAg, the following steps should be taken: (1) a specific neutralization test should be performed (Cameron and Briggs, 1980); if this is positive, (2) a sample from the donated unit should be retested both in the transfusion centre and in a reference laboratory, which may also test for other HBV markers (e.g. total and IgM anti-HBc) to decide whether the subject is a carrier or has an acute infection; (3) a follow-up sample should be obtained; if tests are persistently positive the subject should be classified as a carrier, counselled with reference to his or her infectivity and permanently debarred from being a blood donor; (4) LFTs should be performed; if they are abnormal the subject should be advised to consult a physician. Subjects who have had an acute infection and have developed unequivocal anti-HBs can be readmitted as blood donors 1 year after recovery.

A survey carried out by Alter (1975) indicated that carriers of HBsAg are not commonly a danger to those with whom they come into ordinary social contact (excluding sexual contact). However, a few instances have been reported in which infected health-care workers have transmitted HBV to their patients while carrying out invasive surgical or dental procedures. Twelve such outbreaks involving 91 HBV-infected surgical patients who acquired the infection from 11 surgeons and one perfusion technician were reported in England, Wales and Northern Ireland between 1975 and 1990 (Heptonstall, 1991). It has been recommended that the staff of transfusion laboratories should be tested for HBsAg and that those who are found to be positive should not assist in the preparation by an open process of blood or blood components intended for clinical use (Report of NHS Advisory Group, 1975). In carriers of HBsAg, viral replication as revealed by the presence of HBeAg and HBV-DNA in serum is a useful index of infectivity. However, there are patients with severe liver disease who have HBV-DNA but no detectable HBeAg. These HBeAg-negative variants are due to point mutations in the pre-core region which prevent the synthesis of HBeAg (Carman et al. 1989; Harrison and Zuckerman, 1992).

A study of HBsAg-positive blood donors in the UK between 1971 and 1981 identified 2880 men and 1054 women who were traced until 1986. It was shown that male carriers had a significantly higher risk of dying from hepatocellular carcinoma or of acquiring chronic liver disease than the general population (Hall et al. 1988).

Protection against HBV by antibody
Subjects whose serum contains anti-HBs are protected from HBV infection (Grady and Lee, 1975; Seeff et al. 1977). The administration of immunoglobulin prepared from the small proportion of donors with relatively potent anti-HBs was found to reduce the risk of hepatitis in subjects accidentally exposed to HBV infection compared with a control group treated with standard immunoglobulin, i.e. prepared from random donors (Grady and Lee, 1975). Standard immunoglobulin prepared, for example, from donors in the USA, contains too low a titre of anti-HBs to be of value in the prophylaxis of hepatitis B (Seeff et al. 1977).

The major indication for hepatitis B immunoglobulin (HB Ig) is following a single acute exposure to HBV, as when blood known or strongly suspected to contain HBsAg is accidentally inoculated, ingested orally or splashed on to open wounds or mucous membranes of non-immune subjects. In such cases HB Ig should be given in a dose of approximately 600 iu (for adults) as soon as possible after exposure; the subject should also be vaccinated. When appropriate, a further dose should be given 1 month later (Deinhardt and Zuckerman, 1985). Newborn infants in endemic areas should also be given HB Ig (see below).

HBV vaccine
Two types of HBV vaccine are available and have proven to be safe, immunogenic and efficacious; the first was derived from plasma of carriers as a source of surface antigen and the other is a recombinant DNA product synthesized in yeast (Szmuness et al. 1980; Eddleston, 1990; Zuckerman, 1990). Protective antibodies develop in 80–97% of subjects receiving the full immunization course. Protection conferred by either type of vaccine may not be permanent and, in a proportion of subjects, lasts no longer than 2–5 years or even less; reinforcing doses are needed to prevent HBV infection. Individuals with levels of anti-HBs below 10 iu/l are susceptible to infection but it is not clear whether previous immunization helps to prevent the development of the carrier state (Eddleston, 1990; Zuckerman, 1990).

It has been estimated that there are 300 million carriers of HBV in the world (Eddleston, 1990). In areas where HBV is endemic, it has been recommended that subjects at risk should be immunized; infants born to HBeAg-positive mothers should be treated with HB Ig, as well as with vaccine (Ip *et al.* 1989). In addition, patients requiring multiple transfusions of blood or blood products, such as patients with haemophilia or thalassaemia and those in need of renal dialysis, as well as health-care workers and medical or dental students exposed to blood, should also be immunized. Staff in transfusion services are at no increased risk of acquiring HBV infection (Hanson and Polesky, 1985).

HBV variants

Occasional cases of hepatitis may be caused by variants of HBV which fail to react in conventional screening tests for HBsAg. Sera found negative for HbsAg on routine screening with polyclonal antibodies but positive with monoclonal antibody as well as positive for HBV-DNA, were shown to transmit hepatitis to HBV-immune chimpanzees (Wands *et al.* 1986). Other HBV mutants have arisen by point mutations in the pre-core region of the genome; some have caused fulminant hepatitis (Kosaka *et al.* 1991; Liang *et al.* 1991) and others have been found in survivors of fulminant hepatitis or in asymptomatic contacts (Carman *et al.* 1991). The majority of these pre-core mutants do not synthesize HBeAg, which requires intact pre-core and core regions. Hence, there are patients with severe liver disease who have HBV-DNA but no HBeAg in their serum. In such patients there may be continuous viral replication despite the presence of anti-HBe (Tong *et al.* 1990).

In subjects injected with HBV vaccine, the neutralizing antibody is directed against the *a* determinant of HBsAg. Point mutations have given rise to 'escape mutants' of HBV with *a* epitopes that are not neutralized by anti-HBs. If immunized subjects are infected with these mutants, they will have a variant HBsAg in addition to anti-HBs in their plasma (Carman *et al.* 1990; Harrison and Zuckerman, 1992).

HBsAg-positivity in patients with low levels of HBV-DNA and absence of anti-HBc has been attributed to an HBV-related virus, HBV2 with an improved ability for non-sexual, non-parenteral transmission (Coursaget *et al.* 1987; Echevarría *et al.* 1991). However, others have suggested that these unusual findings are not due to an HBV variant but to an impaired immune response to the wild-type HBV (Harrison and Zuckerman, 1992).

Hepatitis delta virus (HDV)

This agent, found originally in northern Italians, occurs only in HBsAg-positive subjects because it requires HBV as a 'helper' virus; delta is a defective RNA virus of low mol. wt. coated by HBsAg (Tiollais *et al.* 1981). The agent multiplies in the liver and is transmitted by blood and body fluids; the commonest mode of transmission is parenteral inoculation, thus explaining the association with intravenous drug addiction (Smedile *et al.* 1982; Rizzetto, 1983; Shattock *et al.* 1985). Anti-HDV has been found in the plasma of infected subjects in Europe, Australia, Asia and America; in the USA it is found in 3.8% of blood donations positive for HBsAg (CDC, 1984) but it is found only very rarely in British blood donors (Tedder *et al.* 1982). Superinfection of a carrier of HBsAg with HDV is associated with a chronic course of the delta infection in

70–90% of cases and with an increase in severity of the underlying chronic hepatitis (Smedile *et al.* 1982; Monjardino and Saldanha, 1990). Simultaneous infection with HBV and HDV in a previously healthy subject tends to be followed by clearance of both HDV and HBV, although in some instances fulminant hepatitis or a more severe acute course has been reported (Shattock *et al.* 1985; Reynes *et al.* 1989; Fagan and Williams, 1990). In HDV infection the delta antigen is present in liver and serum; viral RNA and anti-HDV can also be found in serum.

Screening for HBsAg in blood donors minimizes but does not abolish the risk of PTH delta in HBsAg-positive recipients (Rosina *et al.* 1985). The simultaneous presence of HDV and HBeAg in the absence of detectable HBsAg has been reported (Shattock *et al.* 1985). It has been suggested that HBsAg carriers should be given blood derivatives prepared from a single donor or from small pools.

HDV has been transmitted not only by blood and fresh blood components but also by coagulation factor concentrates (Purcell *et al.* 1985).

NON-A, NON-B HEPATITIS AND HEPATITIS C VIRUS

Non-A, non-B hepatitis (NANBH)

By 1988, three distinct hepatitis viruses had been well characterized: hepatitis A virus (HAV), HBV and HDV. The term NANBH was given to those cases of hepatitis in which the above three agents, as well as CMV, Epstein–Barr virus (EBV) and toxic substances, had been excluded as aetiological agents. Two forms of NANBH were recognized: enteric or epidemic, and parenteral. The agent of the enteric form, recently named HEV, is a 27–32 nm virus particle that can be isolated from faeces; it has been responsible for waterborne epidemics of hepatitis occurring mainly in tropical and sub-tropical countries with low standards of sanitation where it is also responsible for about 50% of cases of sporadic hepatitis. HEV infection is clinically similar to the self-limiting hepatitis A except for the high mortality rate of HEV infection in pregnant women and a lower rate of secondary transmission. HEV has been cloned recently (Reyes *et al.* 1990). Parenteral transmission of HEV has not been reported (Purcell and Ticehurst, 1988). Although parenteral NANBH differs in several respects from typical hepatitis B, the two forms cannot be differentiated solely on clinical grounds.

NANB PTH

After the introduction of routine screening of blood donations for HBsAg, parenteral NANBH accounted for the vast majority of cases of PTH. About 80–90% of cases of NANB PTH are subclinical with no jaundice in the acute phase. Symptomatic disease is usually mild and self-limiting. Hence, the true incidence of this disease can be determined only by prospective serial LFTs, especially estimates of transaminases, in patients transfused with blood components and some fractionated plasma products such as Factors VIII and IX. By convention, NANB PTH is diagnosed when, between 2 and 26 weeks after transfusion, in a patient with a normal ALT level before transfusion, the ALT level rises above 2.5 times the upper limit of normal (ULN) and is more than two times the ULN on a further sample taken within 3 weeks, and known viral or chemical causes of hepatitis have been excluded (Aach *et al.* 1981; Alter *et al.* 1981; Reesink and van der Poel, 1989). ALT fluctuations seem to be characteristic of NANBH both in the acute and chronic phase (see Alter, 1985). Until recently, in the developed world, NANB PTH was the most common infectious disease transmitted by blood transfusion, with a higher incidence in recipients in the USA (7–12%), southern Europe (e.g. Italy 17.8%) and Japan (18.1%) than in northern and middle Europe (Netherlands 2.3%; UK 0.5%) and Australia (1.7%) (Reesink and van der Poel, 1989; Dienstag, 1990; Contreras *et al.* 1991; Japanese Red Cross Non-A, Non-B Hepatitis Research Group, 1991). Interest in preventing this disease was prompted by reports that 40–50% of subjects with NANB PTH developed chronic hepatitis, as judged by persistent or fluctuating elevations in ALT levels, with 20% progressing to cirrhosis and, in a few cases, to hepatocellular carcinoma (Dienstag and Alter, 1986; Reesink and van der Poel, 1989; Hopf *et al.* 1990). A review of 102 patients who underwent liver biopsies for clinically diagnosed chronic NANB PTH showed that 41 had chronic active hepatitis (CAH) and 20 had cirrhosis, five of whom died (Dienstag, 1983). Since, in the USA before the early 1980s, 7% of transfusion recipients developed NANB PTH, cirrhosis following transfusion would be expected to have developed in at least 1.4% of recipients of blood. However, the data are based on biopsies from a very small collection of patients and, the figures do not take into consideration the fact that 50% of blood is transfused to patients who die shortly after transfusion due to their underlying disease (Alter, 1988).

The contribution that NANB PTH makes to chronic liver disease varies in different parts of the world, although this has not been studied in most countries. In Spain, chronic hepatitis and cirrhosis after transfusion are not unusual (Esteban *et al.* 1990), but in the USA (as mentioned above) and in northern Europe there are no reports of large numbers of previously transfused patients with chronic liver disease; in the UK chronic liver disease after blood transfusion has been found to be uncommon (Wood *et al.* 1989). In Africa, where all forms of viral hepatitis have a high prevalence, a history of a previous blood transfusion is relatively uncommon in patients with NANBH (Ayoola, 1988). In Japan, on the other hand, where the incidence of NANBH PTH is very high, blood transfusion accounts for nearly 50% of chronic NANBH and cirrhosis. The time lag from blood transfusion to chronic hepatitis was 13.6 years, to cirrhosis 17.8 years and to hepatocellular carcinoma 23.4 years (Kiyosawa *et al.* 1982). In another survey, 48 of 119 and 37 of 92 patients with cirrhosis or hepatocellular carcinoma had a history of blood transfusion in the previous 9–53 years (Nishioka, 1990).

Transmission of NANBH by blood derivatives
NANBH has been transmitted by the full range of blood components, including washed red cells which had been previously frozen (Haugen, 1979). Before the introduction of methods of viral inactivation NANBH had been shown to be transmitted also by clotting factor concentrates.

Chronic liver disease is a worldwide problem in haemophiliacs treated with clotting factor concentrates; the disease is mild in most haemophiliacs although a proportion of patients develop severe CAH and liver cirrhosis; in five different series, 5–11% of patients died from chronic end-stage liver disease (see Alter, 1988). Chronic persistent hepatitis is more aggressive in these patients than in other recipients, progressing more rapidly to CAH and cirrhosis (Triger and Preston, 1990). Fortunately, current methods of viral inactivation of clotting factor concentrates (see above) have abolished the risk of transmission of NANBH (for references, see Barbara and Contreras, 1991a).

Indirect ('surrogate') markers to detect carriers of NANBH

For many years the search for the agent or agents of NANBH and for serological tests to identify infectious patients and donors was unsuccessful. Such tests failed to distinguish between clinically proven infectious and non-infectious serum samples (see Dienstag, 1990). An association between the results of non-specific tests for 'surrogate markers' and infectivity in blood donors was also looked for and two candidate markers were proposed: raised ALT levels and the presence of anti-HBc.

Following large prospective studies in the USA by two groups, the Transfusion Transmitted Virus Study (TTVS) group and the National Institutes of Health (NIH) group both reported that the incidence of NANB PTH was almost three times greater among recipients of anti-HBc-positive blood compared with recipients of anti-HBc-negative blood (Stevens et al. 1984; Koziol et al. 1986). Although 70–88% of anti-HBc-positive blood donations were not associated with PTH, it was estimated that the exclusion of anti-HBc-positive donors would have prevented 30–43% of the cases of NANB PTH, at a cost of losing 4–8% of donors. Alter (1988) pooled the data of these two prospective studies in the USA with a more recent similar study in Germany (Sugg et al. 1988) where donors with raised ALT levels had already been excluded; overall 2049 recipients were followed up with a 14.5% incidence of hepatitis after receiving at least one unit of anti-HBc-positive blood compared with 5.6% when all units were negative for anti-HBc. From these results, it was predicted that exclusion of donors with anti-HBc would eliminate 28% of cases of NANBH. Alter pointed out that these predictions had not been tested and that efforts should be made where possible to carry out prospective controlled studies of the value of the costly screening of blood donations for surrogate markers. Such a study was done in Spain where no statistically significant difference in the incidence of NANB PTH was found between recipients of unscreened blood and recipients of blood negative for anti-HBc and with normal ALT levels (Esteban et al. 1990).

Both of the USA studies quoted above found that raised ALT levels in blood donors were associated with a significantly increased incidence of NANB PTH in the recipients. It was concluded that although 60–70% of donors with a high ALT level do not transmit PTH, exclusion of blood with abnormal ALT levels might prevent 30% of cases of PTH, at the cost of losing 1.5–3% of blood donors. Incidentally, of 96 donors with chronically raised ALT levels, 45% were considered to have NANBH; most of the rest were obese or admitted to a high consumption of alcohol (Alter, 1985).

The two USA groups concluded that anti-HBc was the best available marker for NANBH and that the donor population identified showed relatively little overlap with the population with raised ALT levels (Stevens et al. 1984; Koziol et al. 1986). The highest incidence of NANB PTH in the two studies occurred in recipients of blood which was both positive for anti-HBc and had a raised ALT (not necessarily involving the same unit of blood).

In 1981, the NIH introduced ALT testing and the exclusion of all blood donations with a high ALT level; the incidence of NANB PTH in the following 3 years, both in patients and in untransfused controls, did not change when compared with the 2 years before ALT testing was introduced (Alter, 1985). Nevertheless, in 1986 the American Association of Blood Banks (AABB) introduced compulsory testing of all blood donations for ALT and anti-HBc (AABB, 1991). No randomized controlled trials of the effect of testing blood donors for ALT levels and anti-HBc have ever been performed in the USA (Alter, 1985) and it is now impossible to undertake them. Blood centres are faced with the prospect of having to reject large numbers of donors, most of whom are not carriers of NANBH agents. In fact, 4–6% of blood donations in the USA are discarded because of abnormal surrogate markers (Dodd, 1991). It will be impossible to determine the real value of screening blood donations for surrogate markers in the USA because these tests were adopted only in the late 1980s. At this time, self-exclusion for HIV infection and screening for HIV antibodies started in blood trans-fusion services, measures which by themselves significantly reduced the incidence of PTH (Dienstag, 1990). In addition, the incidence of NANBH in general has decreased in the USA in recent years (M. Alter, quoted by Dodd, 1991). Before the introduction of self-exclusion of donors for risk factors for HIV, the minimum carrier rate of NANBH virus in volunteer blood donors in the USA was estimated to be 1.6% and in commercial blood donors 5.4% (Blum and Vyas, 1982), with approximately 7–12% of recipients of blood developing PTH (Alter, 1985). After the introduction of measures to abolish the transmission of HIV by transfusion and before the introduction of screening of blood donations for anti-HBc and ALT, the incidence of PTH in the USA decreased to around an estimated 1% (Alter, 1989). However, despite the introduction of screening for anti-HCV (see below) compulsory screening of blood donations for surrogate markers still prevails in the USA.

Although measures to eliminate the risk of HIV infection by blood transfusion have reduced the incidence of NANB PTH in most countries, PTH still remained a significant problem in the late 1980s, with an incidence of about 10% of recipients in countries such as Spain and Japan (Esteban *et al.* 1990; Katayama *et al.* 1990).

Hepatitis C virus (HCV)

The numerous attempts to identify the agent of NANBH provided some useful information: the disease could be transmitted to chimpanzees and it was shown that the agent had a diameter of 30–60 nm, revealed by filtration studies, and was chloroform sensitive, suggesting a small lipid-coated virus. In general, the agent did not achieve high concentrations in plasma of infected chimpanzees (Bradley *et al.* 1985; for references, see Dienstag, 1990).

Isolation and characterization of HCV by cloning

A fruitful association between the group of Bradley, at the Centers for Disease Control (CDC) in Atlanta, with experience of an attested source of NANBH material infectious for chimpanzees, and the group of Houghton at Chiron with expertise in molecular genetics, led, in 1988, to the identification of the agent responsible for most cases of NANB PTH (Choo *et al.* 1989).

A large volume of highly infectious plasma from a chimpanzee was submitted to extensive ultracentrifugation to obtain viral nucleic acid in the pellet. The nucleic acid was denatured and complementary DNA (cDNA) was synthesized from DNA and RNA with random primers of reverse transcriptase. The cDNA library was inserted into the cloning bacteriophage λgt11 and the cDNA-encoded polypeptides were expressed in *Escherichia coli*. The polypeptides were screened with the serum from a patient with chronic NANBH for approximately 10^6 clones expressing polypeptides, leading to the identification of a positive 155 base-pair cDNA named clone 5-1-1. Using clone 5-1-1, a larger overlapping clone 81 was isolated from the same cDNA library and it was shown that clones 5-1-1 and 81 hybridized with total RNA extracted from the liver of an infected chimpanzee and with total nucleic acid extracted from pellets of plasma from highly infectious chimpanzees. The clones are derived from a single-stranded RNA with an estimated size of 5000–10 000 nucleotides. The cDNA containing clone 5-1-1 has one continuous translational ORF. The ORF was inserted into a plasmid and expressed in *E. coli* as a fusion polypeptide with superoxide dismutase (SOD) which facilitates the expression of foreign proteins; total bacterial lysates were used in immunoblot assays to screen for antibodies in sera from patients with chronic NANBH and in sera from routine blood donors. Serum from the original patient that identified clone 5-1-1, as well as seven of 11 sera from patients with chronic NANBH and serum from four infected chimpanzees, reacted with the SOD/5-1-1 (PS5) fusion polypeptide. Sera from ten routine blood donors and from chimpanzees infected with HAV or HBV failed to react with PS5. A radioimmunoassay based on PS5 was used to screen sera from NANBH-infected chimpanzees and from well-characterized patients with NANBH, revealing that PS5 is closely associated with NANBH.

The blood borne agent of NANBH was termed HCV for hepatitis C virus. The above results showed convincingly that cloning of an infectious agent is possible without its prior isolation and characterization (Choo *et al.* 1989). The virus has still not been visualized.

Proof that HCV is the main agent of NANB PTH
The same group that cloned HCV developed a specific RIA for the detection of HCV antibodies using a recombinant polypeptide cloned in yeast. Clone 5-1-1 was used as a hybridization probe to the original cDNA library, and it was possible to isolate three overlapping clones that have one common ORF encoding part of the HCV protein. This ORF was expressed at high levels in yeast as a fusion polypeptide with SOD. It contained 363 amino acids and was named C-100-3. Soluble, purified C-100-3 was the antigen coating the wells of microplates in the RIA used initially for blind testing of a panel of well-characterized NANB PTH sera collected by Alter's group over several years at the NIH in Bethesda. The panel had been used to test the discriminating ability of previous assays claiming to be specific for NANB PTH. A strong association was seen between PTH and the development of anti-HCV in tests on stored samples from prospectively followed transfusion recipients and their donors. All 15 well-characterized patients with chronic NANBH developed antibodies compared with only three of five patients with acute resolving NANBH (Alter *et al.* 1989a). In addition, HCV antibodies were detected in six of seven sera infectious for NANBH in chimpanzees; the only negative serum came from a patient in the acute phase of NANB PTH. Anti-HCV was observed in ten patients with chronic NANBH acquired by transfusion in the USA who developed the antibody during their illness; in nine of these ten prospectively studied cases of PTH, at least one matched donor had HCV antibody. In general, antibodies developed within 6 months of transfusion although in one case they were detectable only at 12 months. HCV antibodies were also found in 80% of patients with chronic NANBH in Japan and Italy, but in only 15% of acute resolving NANBH infections although they were found in 58% of USA patients with 'sporadic'

NANBH, with no history of parenteral exposure. The RIA was negative in the controls which included patients and chimpanzees with hepatitis A or B, non-viral liver disease and normal subjects. The authors concluded that HCV is the major cause of NANBH throughout the world (Kuo *et al.* 1989). Further studies in several countries have confirmed this, but the existence of other agents capable of causing a small proportion of cases of NANBH cannot be excluded.

Structure of HCV

Since its original description, a great deal of knowledge on HCV has accumulated; its genome consists of a 9401-nucleotide, linear, single, positive-stranded RNA containing one large ORF which encodes only one viral polyprotein precursor of 3010 or 3011 amino acids. After translation, the polyprotein is cleaved into several viral proteins (Kato *et al.* 1990; Choo *et al.* 1991; Ogata *et al.* 1991; Takamizawa *et al.* 1991) (Fig. 16.4). HCV has been classified in the family of Flaviviridae which also contains the Flaviviruses (e.g. yellow fever and Dengue virus) and Pestiviruses (e.g. bovine viral diarrhoea virus) (Miller and Purcell, 1990). It has been proposed that the HCV structural proteins are cleaved from the N-terminal of the polyprotein precursor whilst non-structural proteins are cleaved from the C-terminal section (Choo *et al.* 1990). The structural proteins include the 17–19 kD core protein (nucleocapsid) and two envelope proteins, E1 (glycoprotein 33/35) and E2/NS1 (gp 72). The non-structural proteins, involved in replication and membrane binding, comprise the NS2 to NS5 regions (Takeuchi *et al.* 1990; Choo *et al.* 1991; Weiner *et al.* 1991) (Fig. 16.4).

At least three, and possibly four, HCV genomes can be distinguished by comparison of the nucleotides of cDNA clones from plasma samples of different patients: 'HCV-1', comparable to the original USA prototype (Choo *et al.* 1991), 'HCV J-1/K-1', comparable to the Japanese prototype, and 'HCV K-2', a second Japanese isolate (Enomoto *et al.* 1990). A different genome was reported in Scotland (Chan *et al.* 1991). There may well be numerous HCV serotypes worldwide but their clinical relevance is unclear (Bradley, 1991). The high mutation rate of the genome is as expected for RNA viruses, and HCV isolates from different geographical locations differ in nucleotide and amino

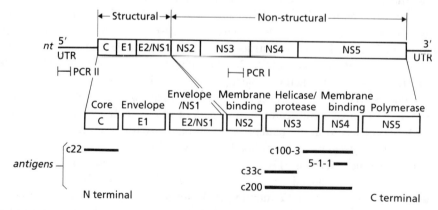

Figure 16.4 The hepatitis C virus (HCV) genome and HCV antigens. Adapted from a diagram provided by Ortho Diagnostics. For an explanation of the abbreviations, see text

acid homology for various regions of the genome (Simmonds *et al.* 1990), with the envelope regions showing the greatest heterogeneity. This envelope variation may reflect the adaptation of HCV to different hosts or the result of immunological selection. A highly conserved and untranslated region (UTR) of 324–341 nucleotides at the 5′ end has proved particularly useful for diagnostic cDNA–PCR assays (Han *et al.* 1991; Ogata *et al.* 1991). At the 3′ end there is a non-coding sequence of 54 bases (see Fig. 16.4).

Screening and confirmatory assays for HCV antibodies

The first commercial assays available for clinical diagnosis and screening of blood donors for HCV antibodies were antiglobulin ELISAs based on the c100-3 (or c100) antigen expressed in yeast as a fusion polypeptide with SOD. A great deal of data soon became available from several studies in different countries, with the new assay for HCV antibodies showing a positive correlation with NANB PTH (Alter *et al.* 1989b). In addition, HCV antibody assays in haemophiliacs showed that whereas anti-HCV was present in all of 17 patients who had been transfused at some stage with untreated clotting factor concentrates, it was present in none of 28 patients who had received only cryoprecipitate and, or, factor concentrates subjected to viral inactivation procedures (Skidmore *et al.* 1990). Similar data were reported by other groups (for references, see Barbara and Contreras, 1991a). However, data from Spain showed that 64% of haemophiliacs had HCV antibodies and that half of those without antibody had raised levels of ALT, sometimes associated with CAH, raising the possibility that other agents are involved in the aetiology of chronic liver disease of haemophiliacs (Esteban *et al.* 1989). On the other hand, it has been suggested that some haemophiliacs with chronic liver disease may lack anti-HCV and still be infected with HCV as evidenced by PCR, or that they may have cleared the virus rapidly (Garson *et al.* 1990b; Simmonds *et al.* 1990). It has also been shown that uninactivated Factor VIII with low or undetectable levels of HCV can be infectious (Simmonds *et al.* 1990).

It was soon realized that more than 60% of reactive sera gave false positive reactions for anti-HCV when screening populations at low risk of HCV infection, such as blood donors (van der Poel *et al.* 1990; Weiner *et al.* 1990a). The number of false positives was even greater in African sera, attributed in part, to their high Ig content (Alter *et al.* 1989b). If blood donors are to be barred from future donations on the basis of microbiological assays, it is important that those who really have HCV antibodies should be excluded. Hence, in the absence of confirmatory assays, means of identifying 'true' positives, such as a concurrent elevation of ALT levels, a significant increase in the optical density of that sample and persistence of anti-HCV in further samples were investigated (Morgan *et al.* 1990; Stevens *et al.* 1990). However, in Europe, the vast majority of donors with HCV antibodies seem to lack surrogate markers for NANBH (Alter *et al.* 1989b), although in The Netherlands a strong correlation was found between raised ALT levels and HCV antibodies in donors responsible for the transmission of NANB PTH (van der Poel *et al.* 1989a).

The first ELISAs ('first generation') had a sensitivity of 60–80% in donor screening for the prevention of NANB PTH but a poor sensitivity in the early stages of infection with NANBH (Alter *et al.* 1989a; Esteban *et al.* 1990; Contreras *et al.* 1991). The limited sensitivity of the assay could be attributed to the absence of antigens other than c100-3 which is encoded by only 12% of the viral genome (van der Poel, 1991; see Fig. 16.4). In addition, the positive predictive value (i.e. the ability of donations positive for anti-HCV to cause NANBH or to stimulate the appearance of anti-HCV in recipients) of the first generation ELISA varied in different countries according to the incidence of NANB PTH, being of the order of 80% in Spain and Japan, but below 20% in countries with a low incidence of NANB PTH such as The Netherlands, the UK and France (for a discussion, see Barbara and Contreras, 1991b). In addition, in PTH the time for appearance of anti-HCV may be as short as 6 weeks and as long as 1 year; HCV immunization can be missed since antibodies can be detectable for only a short time (Esteban *et al.* 1989; Kuo *et al.* 1989).

The first confirmatory assay was available from Ortho Diagnostics in the form of an RIBA which included on a nitrocellulose strip, the c100 antigen expressed in yeast, the 5-1-1 antigen expressed in *E. coli* and SOD. Confirmation consisted of a positive reaction with both HCV antigen bands (Weiner *et al.* 1990a). RIBA positivity was associated with cases of NANB PTH and 'culprit donors' from previous prospective studies (Ebeling *et al.* 1990; van der Poel *et al.* 1990; Contreras *et al.* 1991). However, RIBA could only be considered a supplementary assay and the antigens were not different from those present in the ELISA (c100-3 embraces the 5-1-1 sequence). In addition, RIBA was less sensitive than the ELISAs used in screening (van der Poel *et al.* 1990). An improved assay, '4-RIBA', now called RIBA II, was developed by the Chiron group which added two recombinant antigens to the two original ones another non-structural antigen, c33c derived from NS3, and a structural one, derived from the C region, encoding for the nucleocapsid and named c22 (Fig. 16.4). The presence of two or more bands is required for a confirmed positive result; a single band is considered 'indeterminate'. This RIBA II showed improved sensitivity for the detection of patients with NANB PTH and chronic NANBH and was able to distinguish infectious donors amongst those testing positive by ELISA; in fact only about 10% of subjects found positive by c100-3 ELISA were confirmed positive by RIBA II (Ebeling *et al.* 1990; Marcelling *et al.* 1991; van der Poel *et al.* 1991b). A good correlation was found between RIBA II positivity and PCR positivity (Follett *et al.* 1991).

Research groups other than Chiron have been able to clone HCV, derived from human sources, and have produced structural and non-structural antigens (Arima *et al.* 1989; Garson *et al.* 1990a). However, due to patent restrictions, the use of such clones has been limited.

Further supplementary assays are available; the first one called 'Matrix' was developed by Abbott. It consists of approximately the same antigens as those in RIBA II in a semi-quantitative dot-blot assay for HCV antibodies (Mimms *et al.* 1990). The second confirmatory assay is the 'Liatek HCV' from Innogenetics which seems to confirm as positive the same samples as those confirmed by RIBA II but with fewer indeterminate results (Boudart *et al.* 1992).

A 'second-generation' antiglobulin ELISA for anti-HCV, named c200 ELISA, incorporated into the solid phase c33c, which added to c100-3, made up the larger c200 polypeptide, and also the c22 structural antigen (Fig. 16.4). This improved ELISA has shown increased sensitivity, with antibodies to c22 and c33c being detectable 16–42 d earlier than the appearance of antibodies with the first ELISA; the improved test also has better predictive value. Of 111 anti-HCV-negative patients who developed NANB

PTH in a prospective study carried out in the USA between 1976 and 1979, 51 had anti-HCV by first-generation assays and an additional 16 (total 60%) had anti-HCV by the second-generation ELISA (Aach *et al.* 1991). An ELISA based on synthetic peptides derived from genomic regions encoding structural capsid proteins as well as non-structural proteins was shown to have increased specificity and sensitivity for the detection of HCV antibodies (Hosein *et al.* 1991). Second-generation ELISAs have been developed by Ortho, Abbott and UBI. However, with current serological tests, it is still not possible to discriminate between infectious and immune anti-HCV-positive donors and, in any case, such a difference may not exist.

IgM anti-HCV, mainly anti-core, was detected for an average of 8.1 weeks in 13 of 15 patients with NANB PTH by a dot-blot Matrix immunoassay for the detection of IgM antibodies against core, NS-3 and NS-4 antigens. Nine of these patients had IgM anti-HCV only in the early stages of disease; in five patients late IgM was also detected. The duration of acute-phase IgM was very short in some patients and in general did not precede the IgG response; it is therefore unlikely that tests for IgM will narrow the 'window' period between infection and the appearance of IgG anti-HCV (Clemens *et al.* 1992).

Polymerase chain reaction for the detection of HCV-RNA

As stated above, HCV is not found in high concentrations in the serum of infected humans and chimpanzees where titres are estimated at approximately 10^2–10^4 HCV particles/ml serum (Choo *et al.* 1989; Weiner *et al.* 1990a). PCR has therefore become essential for the detection of viral antigen and infectivity, especially in the case of HCV where cell culture assays are not available. However, PCR cannot detect immunity in the absence of virus and it is therefore an incomplete tool for confirmation of HCV antibodies (Garson *et al.* 1991). On the other hand, HCV-RNA may be detectable by PCR in the absence of HCV antibodies (Simmonds *et al.* 1990; Zanetti *et al.* 1990). Because HCV is an RNA virus, cDNA is obtained by reverse transcription before amplification. The first fragment to be used for PCR was from the non-structural NS3 region (PCR fragment I in Fig. 16.4) but false-negative results can occur due to the nucleotide variation of this region between different HCV isolates (Garson *et al.* 1990c; Weiner *et al.* 1990b). Sensitivity and specificity of PCR can be improved by using 'nested' primers for a second round of DNA amplification (Garson *et al.* 1990a, b). Different patterns of HCV viraemia, including transient, persistent and recurrent, have been observed in haemophiliacs. Viraemia has occurred as shortly as 2 weeks after infusion of Factor VIII (Garson *et al.* 1990b). A second, more sensitive, PCR was developed using a fragment from the highly conserved 5' UTR of the HCV genome (fragment II in Fig. 16.4) (Garson *et al.* 1991; Han *et al.* 1991; Inchauspe *et al.* 1991). The higher sensitivity of the fragment II PCR compared with fragment I PCR was proven when testing stored serum in parallel with quick-frozen plasma samples from 12 blood donors who tested positive by c100 ELISA and by 4-RIBA (van der Poel, 1991). Fresh plasma samples from 11 of these donors were positive by HCV 5' UTR PCR compared with eight positives by NS3 PCR. Nested PCR using a set of primers for the more conserved NS4 region of the HCV genome proved to be more sensitive for the detection of HCV-RNA in patients and chimpanzees than nested PCR using NS3 region primers. HCV-RNA was the only marker of infection detected in the early phases of primary HCV infection in patients with NANB PTH followed up for 10–14 years; its disappearance was correlated with resolution of NANBH of the acute, self-limited type. In contrast, HCV antibodies were first detected 12–14 weeks after transfusion, did not necessarily remain at a high level in all patients with chronic NANBH or could remain present in the circulation of patients with acute, self-limited hepatitis despite the clearance of HCV-RNA (Farci *et al.* 1991). For HCV-cDNA-PCR it is important that plasma samples are snap frozen within 2 h of collection and kept at – 70°C until needed for testing; the original serum samples used for screening and antibody confirmation will give unreliable results in PCR (van der Poel, 1991; Busch and Wilber, 1992). It is therefore impossible to decide whether all the reports on PCR performed on stored serum samples from previous studies of NANB PTH are valid (Busch and Wilber, 1992; Farci *et al.* 1992). Regrettably, prospective studies of NANB PTH in those countries in which donors are screened for HCV antibodies can no longer be made.

Screening sera from blood donors and patients for HCV antibodies

In numerous countries blood donations are now screened routinely for HCV antibodies. Initially, when first-generation ELISAs were used, the prevalence of HCV antibodies in blood donations, as judged solely by reactivity on retesting, ranged from 0.2% to 1.73% around the world. It is difficult to understand why countries with a very different rate of NANB PTH, such as the UK and Spain, have rather similar prevalences of anti-HCV in blood donors and why Japan, with such a high rate of NANB PTH, has a relatively low prevalence of anti-HCV (Alter *et al.* 1989a; Barbara and Contreras 1991a).

Although screening assays for HCV antibodies have improved considerably since the discovery of the agent in 1989, they still give a significant number of false-positive reactions. In fact, in the UK, 0.3–0.45% of blood donations give repeatably positive results on screening with second-generation ELISAs and fewer than 20% of these samples (i.e. 0.05–0.06% of all donations) are confirmed as positive by RIBA II; approximately 20% of ELISA-positive samples are 'RIBA II indeterminate' and more than 60% are negative (H.H. Gunson, personal communication). A similar pattern of confirmation with RIBA II and with Liatek is seen in the west of France (Boudart *et al.* 1992). The majority (80–90%) of RIBA II-positive samples are also positive when tested by PCR and an additional small number of RIBA II indeterminates, mainly amongst those found to be c22 strongly positive, are also positive by PCR (Follett *et al.* 1991; R.S Tedder and J.A.J. Barbara, personal communications). The pattern of confirmation is not different when the Matrix dot-blot immunoassay is used on samples found to be repeatably reactive by first-generation ELISA; of 167 511 Australian blood donors, 0.78% were repeatably positive by ELISA, with 59% of these found to be negative by Matrix and the remainder, positive or indeterminate. PCR on selected samples from confirmed positive or indeterminate donations suggests a prevalence of 0.25% of donors potentially infectious for HCV (Allain *et al.* 1991). In addition, there are reports of infectious patients in whom HCV antibody cannot be detected (Farci *et al.* 1991). Screening assays with a better specificity are needed to reduce the number of false-positive results on ELISA screening with the consequent need for large numbers of expensive supplementary and confirmatory assays. Nevertheless, in countries with a high prevalence of NANBH, screening of blood donations for HCV antibodies has reduced significantly the incidence of post-transfusion NANBH. In Japan, in patients who had received 1–10 units of blood, NANB PTH decreased from 4.9% before the introduction of HCV screening to 1.9% after screening; corresponding figures for patients transfused with 11–20 units were 16.3% and 3.3% (Japanese Red Cross Non-A, Non-B Hepatitis Research Group, 1991).

In most countries in the developed world donations are screened routinely for HCV antibodies, but policies for screening donors of plasma for fractionation differ in different countries. In France and the UK, plasma donors are screened and treated in the same way as blood donors (Habibi and Garretta, 1990), whereas in the USA its is argued that the depletion of HCV antibodies from the plasma pools for fractionation might interfere with the balance of factors that make viral inactivation procedures effective (Finlayson and Tankersley, 1990). These different policies do not seem to affect the safety of plasma products since no transmission of HCV was reported after the introduction of modern methods of viral inactivation in blood products even before the introduction of screening for anti-HCV and despite the presence of HCV antibodies in products such as i.v. Ig (Skidmore et al. 1990; Dodd et al. 1992). In Australia, i.v. Ig manufactured from plasma screened for HCV antibodies was shown to be at least as safe as i.v. Ig made from plasma unscreened for anti-HCV (Schiff and Kemp, 1991).

Epidemiology of HCV
The natural modes of transmission of HCV have not been clearly defined. Heterosexual transmission does not seem to be as significant for HCV as it is for HBV and HIV but it does occur at different rates in different areas (Alter et al. 1989c; Melbye et al. 1990). In several countries, a strong association has been found between the presence of anti-HCV and i.v. drug abuse (Esteban et al. 1989; Barbara and Contreras 1991a; McLennan et al. 1992). The prevalence of HCV antibodies in homosexuals is much lower than the prevalence of anti-HBc and anti-HIV (Esteban et al. 1989). Vertical transmission from mother to child is not as common as with HBV and in a large number of HCV seropositive subjects the source of infection cannot be identified. It is not known whether reinfection with HCV is possible (Simmonds et al. 1990).

In Japan, results from two cohorts of patients with chronic liver disease collected between 1958 and 1989 supported a causal relationship between HCV and hepatocellular carcinoma (HCC). Of 231 patients with chronic hepatitis, cirrhosis or HCC classified as NANBH, 90% had HCV antibodies whereas of 125 patients with similar clinical disease due to HBV, only 6–35% had anti-HCV. Of the patients in the NANBH group with anti-HCV, 33–52% gave a history of previous transfusion. The mean intervals between transfusion and the diagnosis of HCV-related chronic hepatitis, cirrhosis and HCC were 10, 21.2 and 29 years. In two cases the interval between transfusion and HCC was 60 years (Kiyosawa et al. 1990). The same association between HCC and HCV antibodies has been reported in Spain (Bruix et al. 1989) and Italy (Colombo et al. 1989).

Anti-HCV was found in 23 of 50 children with leukaemia who developed chronic liver disease; the children were followed up for 1–12.6 years, and those with persistent HCV antibodies had more severe chronic liver disease (Locasciulli et al. 1991).

Overall, screening for HCV antibodies, including confirmation, counselling of donors and loss of donors and donations is at least five times more expensive than screening for HIV antibodies at the present time (see Barbara and Contreras, 1991a,b).

The studies of HCV antibodies in blood donors and especially in several prospective series of NANB PTH have shown that HCV is the major cause of non-A, non-B, non-D, non-E, hepatitis. It is not known whether any other agents are responsible for those cases of NANBH that are negative for HCV antibodies.

Frequency of post-transfusion hepatitis

Anicteric cases of PTH are commoner than icteric cases. For example, in a study reported from the USA in which 2204 patients were followed and in which PTH was diagnosed in 241 patients, the disease was icteric in less than one-fifth of the cases (Seeff *et al.* 1977). It follows that repeated sampling of recipients is necessary if all cases are to be detected and that only prospective studies are likely to give a true indication of the frequency of PTH. At a time when paid blood donors were still being used and before tests for HBsAg had been introduced, the incidence of PTH in the USA was 33% (Alter, 1985). Following the introduction of testing, in 14 prospective studies in the USA the overall frequency of hepatitis in patients receiving HBsAg-negative blood from volunteer donors was between 4% and 13% compared with 1–2% in untransfused patients (Alter, 1985); between 89% and 100% of cases were believed to be due to NANB virus (Blum and Vyas, 1982).

In the UK the incidence of PTH is substantially lower than in the USA. In the only recent study available, 387 patients who had been transfused during surgery were tested for ALT and HCV antibodies every fortnight for the first 3 months and then monthly for a further 3 months with 229 patients tested also at 12 months. Only one of the 387 patients showed biochemical evidence of acute post-transfusion NANBH after exclusion of non-viral causes. HCV antibodies, confirmed by RIBA and PCR, developed in this patient (Contreras *et al.* 1991).

In some relatively recent prospective studies of PTH, mainly in patients undergoing surgery, estimates varied from 2% or less in Australia, The Netherlands, Finland and the UK (Cossart *et al.* 1982; van der Poel *et al.* 1989a; Contreras *et al.* 1991; van der Poel, 1991) to 44% in Japan (for references, see Alter, 1985; Esteban *et al.* 1990; Japanese Red Cross Non-A, Non-B Hepatitis Research Group, 1991); the proportion of cases attributed to NANBH varied from 78% to 100%.

The introduction of screening of blood donations for HCV antibodies has reduced the incidence of NANB PTH considerably. However, some cases of PTH due to HBV, and probably to HCV, still occur and these are generally caused by transfusion of blood from donors in the early or late stages of HBV infection at a time when tests for HBsAg, or HCV antibodies, are negative. The role of 'non-A, non-B, non-C' agents in post-transfusion hepatitis seems to be minimal at present.

HEPATITIS A VIRUS

HAV, the infectious agent of epidemic hepatitis which is transmitted by the faecal–oral route, causes only transient viraemia and does not cause a carrier state; it is an extremely unusual cause of PTH. In 14 published series, relating to transfusions given to about 9000 subjects, not a single case of PTH due to HAV was observed (see review by Blum and Vyas, 1982). Transmission of HAV, leading to the development of PTH, can occur only in special circumstances (Seeberg *et al.* 1981; Barbara *et al.* 1982a;

Hollinger *et al.* 1983; Sheretz *et al.* 1984; Azimi *et al.* 1986). Thus, in cases where hepatitis A has followed the transfusion of blood, concentrated red cells or fresh-frozen plasma, the donor has been in the early stages of incubating the disease when there is a period of transient viraemia lasting 7–10 d. PTH due to HAV occurs only when the recipient is susceptible to HAV and when, if other units are transfused, they are devoid of anti-HAV which would otherwise neutralize the virus (Hollinger *et al.* 1983). In London 21% of donors are immune to HAV whereas almost all subjects in the developing world have been infected by the age of 10 years (J.A. Barbara, personal communication; Purcell and Ticehurst, 1988). A single unit of blood transmitted HAV to 11 infants in a neonatal intensive care unit (Noble *et al.* 1984). Acute infection with HAV is most readily recognized by the finding of specific IgM antibodies to the virus.

Recently, an unusual outbreak of transfusion-transmitted HAV occurred in 41 Italian haemophiliacs. The source of infection seems to have been Factor VIII concentrate from a local plasma fractionation plant. HAV, with a non-lipid envelope, would be resistant to the solvent–detergent method used for viral inactivation (Mannucci, 1992).

In general, normal Ig for i.m. use contains enough anti-HAV to protect travellers to areas endemic for HAV. If the anti-HAV levels decline in normal Ig, a good source of anti-HAV are donors with a history of jaundice, for example, in London 80% of such donors have anti-HAV (J.A. Barbara, personal communication). When the HAV vaccine becomes widely available, there will be no need to protect frequent travellers with normal Ig (see Zuckerman *et al.* 1991).

HUMAN IMMUNODEFICIENCY VIRUSES

Retroviruses and blood transfusion

Until 1980, retroviruses had never been suspected to be a cause of human disease, let alone a cause of transfusion-transmitted infection. However, rapid advances in molecular biology and recombinant DNA technology led to the discovery of the first human retrovirus, human T-lymphotropic virus type I (HTLV-I) (Poiesz *et al.* 1980). The second (and least common) human retrovirus, HTLV-II, was originally isolated from a patient with hairy T-cell leukaemia but has not been shown to be pathogenic in humans (Kalyaranaman *et al.* 1982). Knowledge of the existence of these prototype retroviruses encouraged workers to look for a human retrovirus as the aetiological agent of AIDS. HIV, initially named LAV or HTLV-III, the agent responsible for AIDS, was discovered in 1983 (Barré-Sinoussi *et al.* 1983). The latest human retrovirus to be isolated, HIV-2 (LAV-2), is also associated with AIDS. Numerous isolates of the different human retroviruses have been reported (for references, see Blattner *et al.* 1985; Wong-Staal *et al.* 1987; Tedder and Weiss, 1990).

Retroviruses owe their name to their ability to reverse the normal sequence of events in macromolecular synthesis; they are RNA viruses which, after entering host cells and losing their envelope, use 'reverse transcriptase' (RNA-dependent DNA polymerase) together with cell-derived RNA as a primer, to transcribe a double-stranded DNA copy of the single-stranded viral RNA genome. The DNA copy enters the nucleus and is permanently integrated as a DNA provirus into the DNA of the host cells (mainly lymphocytes but also monocytes, macrophages and other cells); the provirus remains latent and replicates as an integral part of the host genome. The synthesis of new viral proteins and viral messenger RNA is programmed by proviral DNA and mediated by host enzymes. The virus consists of two identical molecules of single-stranded RNA, in a protein core containing several molecules of reverse transcriptase and cell-derived molecules. The core is surrounded by an envelope consisting of virally encoded glycoproteins (gp) and host-derived lipids which are acquired when the newly assembled viruses bud out through the cell membrane. The progeny viruses will then infect other cells within the same host (Zack and Chen, 1991).

All retroviruses contain three main structural genes: the *gag* gene codes for different mol. wt. proteins which are integral to the nuclear core; the *pol* gene codes for reverse transcriptase; and the *env* gene specifies the envelope glycoproteins. The primary products of these three genes are larger parent polypeptides which can be enzymatically split into smaller peptides. Human retroviruses, especially HTLV-I and -II, have regions of homology between them (see Blattner *et al.* 1985; Wong-Staal and Gallo, 1985; Jeffries, 1986). Retroviruses are composed of 60–70% protein, 30–40% lipid (confined to the envelope), 2–4% carbohydrate and 1% RNA. The proteins are immunogenic. The integrity of the envelope is essential for infectivity and, due to its high lipid content, retroviruses are very sensitive to detergents and organic solvents.

Human retroviruses all share a tropism for lymphocytes inducing fusion and giant cell formation *in vitro* and impairing their function *in vivo*. To enter the cell they bind to cell receptors for the retroviral glycoproteins. The receptor for HIV has been identified as CD4 on helper T lymphocytes, macrophages and other cells. The receptor for HTLV-I and -II is still unknown. All human retroviruses code for a small crossreactive major core protein, p 24/25, and have similar modes of transmission, i.e. sexual, congenital and by blood or blood product inoculation (Wong-Staal and Gallo, 1985).

HIV-1 and HIV-2

The virus which is the causative agent of AIDS was originally described as LAV (lymphadenopathy associated virus) by Montagnier's group (Barré-Sinoussi *et al.* 1983; Vilmer *et al.* 1984) and as HTLV-III by Gallo's group which succeeded in culturing the virus in large quantities in continuously replicating T4 cell lines (Popovic *et al.* 1984). This virus, together with the visna virus, belongs to the Lentivirinae subfamily of the Retroviridae family. HTLV-I and -II belong to the Oncovirinae subfamily. In contrast to the proliferative effect induced by HTLV-I, HIV was found to induce premature death of its host cells and to replicate rapidly (Gallo *et al.* 1984). HIV has also been called AIDS-related retrovirus (ARV) and immuno-deficiency-associated virus (IDAV). HIV has a great propensity for genetic variability, especially within the *env* gene coding for the major external glycoprotein (Wain-Hobson *et al.* 1985; Wong-Staal *et al.* 1985) which carries the epitopes which seem to react with the scarce viral neutralizing antibodies.

A second distinct retrovirus named HIV-2 (LAV-2) was isolated later from West African patients with AIDS and AIDS-related complex (ARC) and from two homosexual men in France. Although this new virus is also lymphotropic, cytotoxic and neurotropic, and shares epitopes of the core and *pol* proteins with the original HIV (HIV-1), its nucleotide identity with HIV-1 isolates is only 40–50%. The main differences between HIV-1 and -2 lie within the envelope nucleotides and proteins. HIV-2 has closer sequence identity with the simian retrovirus SIV (Clavel *et al.* 1986; Brucker *et al.* 1987; Brun-Vezinet *et al.* 1987; Hughes and Corrah, 1990).

The *env* gene of HIV-1 codes for a major precursor polyprotein p 85. This protein becomes heavily glycosylated to form the exterior glycoprotein gp160, which is processed into gp120 and gp41 by a viral protease (Wong-Staal and Gallo, 1985). Gp41 is a transmembrane protein which anchors gp120 in the membrane and it is this protein which has specific amino acid domains for binding to the CD4 molecule on target cells, allowing the entry of the virus into the cell (Fig. 16.5; Weiss 1990; Zack and Chen, 1991). The gp41 protein is also important for syncytial fusion of cells. The transmembrane glycoprotein of HIV-2, gp130–105, awaits more accurate chemical definition (Brun-Vezinet *et al.* 1987). There is no crossreactivity between the envelope glycoproteins of HIV-1 and -2. The *gag* gene of HIV 1 codes for the large precursor protein of 55 kD, p55, which is enzymatically cleaved into the smaller fragments p24, which is phosphorylated, p17 and p15 (Veronese *et al.* 1988). The p24 protein encloses the two strands of RNA and the reverse transcriptase. The antigen p17 encircles the viral core and is attached to the fatty acid myristate. Myristoilation appears to be required for infectivity (Bryant and Ratner, 1990). The *gag* proteins p9 and p7, derived from p15, surround the two strands of RNA and form part of the core. p24 and p17 share epitopes with the less well-defined HIV-2 core proteins, p26 and p16 (Brun-Vezinet *et al.* 1987). The *pol* gene product of HIV-1 are derived from the large precursor molecule Pr 180 *gag–pol* and comprise reverse transcriptase, viral integrase and viral protease, the last-named being responsible for cleaving both the large Pr 180 *gag–pol* and the p55 *gag* precursor into the core proteins (for details, see Weiss, 1990; Schochetman, 1992).

The cell membrane protein CD4 is the receptor for HIV (Dalgleish *et al.* 1984). The HIV envelope glycoprotein gp120 binds specifically to CD4-bearing cells and interacts with gp41 for virus–cell and cell–cell fusion events with the formation of syncytia between infected and uninfected cells. Penetration of HIV into the cell occurs by fusion of the viral and cellular membranes. Once the virus is in the cytoplasm, its partial uncoating activates its reverse transcriptase which converts RNA into double-stranded DNA. The DNA, with the aid of integrase, is then integrated as provirus into the host DNA (for details, see Weiss, 1990; Schochetman, 1992). There are other, though less

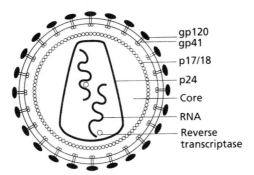

gp120
gp41
p17/18
p24
Core
RNA
Reverse
transcriptase

Figure 16.5 Structure of HIV-1: schematic representation of HIV-1 in cross-section. The two identical single strands of RNA are each associated with a reverse transcriptase. The *gag* proteins p24 and p17/18 form the viral core. The membrane consists of a lipid bilayer containing the transmembrane glycoprotein gp41 and the external gp120, with affinity for CD4 receptors.

efficient, routes for entry of HIV into cells; antibody-coated HIV can adhere to monocytes and macrophages via Fc receptors and possibly via complement receptors (see Weiss, 1990).

The absence of significant amounts of gp120 neutralizing antibodies which could inhibit the binding to CD4, and the fact that the virus, once it enters susceptible cells, either remains latent or establishes 'factories' of progeny virus in the infected host, means that all subjects who are shown to be infected with HIV should be assumed to have persistent infection and hence to be infectious to others (Jeffries, 1986; Schochet-man, 1992). The cells most susceptible to HIV infection, carrying significant amounts of CD4 receptors, are T-helper lymphocytes, macrophages, monocytes, megakaryo-cytes and some bone marrow stem cells. Cells carrying low levels of CD4, such as the epidermal Langerhans' cells, dendritic cells and certain cells of the central nervous system, are also susceptible. There are also cells such as glial cells, colorectal and fetal brain cells which are susceptible to HIV infection despite their lack of CD4 receptors (Takeda *et al.* 1988; Levy, 1989).

Course of HIV infection (Fig. 16.6)

For the first few days after infection, no markers of HIV can be detected in blood. Viraemia follows for a period of several weeks, when HIV and p24 antigen can be detected in serum. During this period, about one-third of patients develop an acute, flu-like or mononucleosis-like syndrome. Two to 4 months after sexually-transmitted infection, and 1–2 months after transfusion-transmitted infection, in more than 95% of HIV-infected subjects, a wide range of antibodies to the structural *env*, *gag* and *pol* viral proteins develop, mostly IgG with some IgA and transient IgM at the start of the immune response (Horsburgh *et al.* 1989; Seligmann, 1990). The period between infection and the development of anti-HIV, the 'window' period, has not been as clearly defined after sexual exposure as it has after blood transfusion because the precise date of infection is usually unknown (Seligmann, 1990). There is some controversy regarding the length of the window period in some HIV-infected homo-sexual men. Incidentally, as applied to HIV, window period means the interval between infection and the appearance of anti-HIV; as applied to HBV, it means the

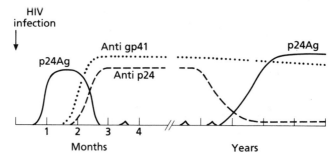

Figure 16.6 Sequence of events following HIV infection; data kindly supplied by J. P. Allain and Abbott Laboratories, USA. Episodes of weak antigenaemia occuring later than about 3 months, and before the strong antigenaemia which occurs after several years, have been added to the original figure.

interval between the disappearance of HBsAg and the appearance of anti-HBs. A significant number of sexual partners of patients with AIDS or ARC and of individuals at high risk of HIV infection were shown to have fluctuating HIV p24 antigenaemia for 6–14 months and for 7–34 months before developing anti-HIV (Ranki *et al.* 1987). On the other hand, another prospective study of similar individuals failed to show prolonged window periods since no evidence could be found of p24 antigenaemia or positive viral cultures long before the appearance of HIV antibodies (Groopman *et al.* 1988). But a further prospective study showed convincingly, by virus culture confirmed by detection of proviral DNA by PCR, that prolonged window periods can in fact occur in homosexual men. HIV-1 was isolated from 31 samples from 133 homosexual men involved in high-risk sexual activities; 27 of these 31 had remained HIV seronegative for 36 months and the remaining four men developed anti-HIV within 11–17 months of a positive virus culture (Imagawa *et al.* 1989). Although it is not known whether these subjects with fluctuating viraemia before the development of antibody have enough infectious virions to transmit HIV, or whether some of them have abortive infections (Imagawa and Detels, 1991), these findings of prolonged window periods are potentially of great importance in the prevention of transfusion-transmitted HIV infection and emphasize the need to exclude from blood donation those subjects who are at risk of HIV infection.

As soon as anti-p24 develops, p24 antigenaemia disappears; however, anti-genaemia reappears in the late stages of AIDS and it may reappear intermittently during the asymptomatic phase of infection, which may last for more than 10 years. Levels of all HIV antibody specificities are usually very high during the asymptomatic period but it is not known which antibodies combat infection and which enhance disease progression. Although some correlation has been found between high levels of neutralizing antibodies (mainly anti-gp120) and better clinical outcome (Robert-Guroff *et al.* 1988), protective humoral and cellular immune responses to HIV are either poor or short-lived (Seligmann, 1990). Disease develops when the CD4 helper cells have almost completely disappeared, leading to a collapse of the immune system and spread of HIV with signs of disease in multiple organs; anti-p24 declines or disappears and p24 antigen reappears at this stage. The rest of the antibodies also decline, with the exception of anti-gp41. In African patients, due to the very high levels of anti-p24, progression to AIDS may not be signalled by p24 antigenaemia and anti-p24 may not disappear (Baillou *et al.* 1987). CD4 T-cell depletion leads to progressive immunological unresponsiveness to foreign stimuli with increased susceptibility to opportunistic infections (e.g. *Pneumocystis carinii*, CMV, atypical mycobacteria) and malignancies such as Kaposi's sarcoma and lymphomas (Mawle and McDougal, 1991). More than 90% of infected subjects have viraemia, detectable at any stage of the disease with modern technology (Coombs *et al.* 1989). The disease is almost invariably fatal.

Unfortunately, the progress in defining prognostic indicators for disease progression has not advanced as rapidly as the development of screening tests for anti-HIV. The most reliable test for clinical progression so far has been the number of CD4 T-helper cells. Other indicators are reappearance of the p24 antigen, a decrease in the level of p24 antibodies, an increase in the level of viraemia and circulating HIV-infected lymphocytes, and raised levels of β_2-microglobulin (Horsborough, 1992).

Epidemiology of HIV infection and spread of AIDS

AIDS was first described in the USA in 1981 in young, previously healthy, homosexual men, It soon became clear that AIDS was spreading rapidly not only in the USA but also in Europe in those groups of the population at high risk of acquiring HIV infection, namely, homosexual men and promiscuous heterosexual individuals, intravenous drug abusers, haemophiliacs treated with Factor VIII concentrate and babies born to infected mothers. In 1982 there were 1304 cases of AIDS reported in the USA and the figures had risen to 161 073 by the end of December 1990 (CDC, 1991a). In the UK, the corresponding figures were three and 4098 (CDR, 1986; 1991). By January 1992, approximately 450 000 cases of AIDS had been reported to the World Health Organization (WHO) from over 150 countries, but WHO estimated that close to 1.5 million cases of AIDS might have occurred by then in adults worldwide. The number of children with AIDS acquired perinatally was estimated to be 500 000 worldwide, with more than 90% of cases in sub-Saharan Africa. The cumulative global total of AIDS cases by 1992 is estimated at 2 million. By January 1992, 9–11 million adults (more than 1 million in the USA alone) were estimated to have been infected with HIV and about 1 million infants to have been infected perinatally (WHO, 1992). It is expected that most of those infected will eventually develop AIDS; in fact about 60% of adults infected with HIV are expected to develop AIDS within 12–13 years of infection.

The epidemiology of AIDS appears to be quite different in sub-Saharan Africa, where heterosexual transmission is common, with a male to female ratio of 1 : 1.2 in infected subjects (WHO, 1992). Other important modes of transmission of HIV in tropical Africa are vertical from mother to infant and through blood transfusion (10% or less of infections), in addition to some transmission by contaminated needles used for injections, or instruments used in scarification (Fleming, 1990; WHO, 1992). There are several million HIV-infected people in tropical Africa, in the area from Gabon to the east coast and from Uganda to Zimbabwe, with the highest prevalence in densely populated areas of central Africa. An annual incidence of 550–1000 AIDS cases per million population was reported in Kinshasa, Zaïre in 1984–85 and it is estimated that this figure could now be as high as 2500 per million in some urban areas of central Africa (Fleming, 1990). In cities of central Africa the frequency of anti-HIV in female prostitutes can be as high as 90%; in pregnant women attending antenatal clinics the frequency is 5% (Fleming, 1990). Other countries in which the HIV epidemic is progressing considerably more rapidly in the heterosexual population than in others include Thailand, India, Brazil and some countries in Central America and the Caribbean (WHO, 1992).

HIV-2 is more restricted in its geographical distribution; it is concentrated mainly in west Africa from the Cape Verde Islands to Benin (e.g. Gambia, Guinea Bisau) with limited spread to those countries in western Europe historically associated with west Africa (Fleming, 1990). Cases of HIV-2 infection have also been reported in east Africa, Asia, Latin America and North America (WHO, 1992). In several west African countries, the frequency of HIV-1 and HIV-2 infections is very similar. In the USA, up to 1991, the prevalence of HIV-2 infection and AIDS caused by HIV-2 has been very limited. HIV-2 may be less virulent than HIV-1; the median survival time after diagnosis in patients with AIDS caused by HIV-2 was found to be considerably longer than in patients with AIDS caused by HIV-1 (Brun-Vezinet *et al.* 1987; Weiss, 1990). In children, AIDS caused by HIV-2 is more likely to be due to transmission by blood transfusion than perinatal transmission (Poulsen *et al.* 1989). Nevertheless, both serotypes have the same modes of transmission and AIDS caused by either is indistinguishable; both HIV-1 and HIV-2 must be excluded from blood donations.

Transmission of HIV by blood transfusion

The first reports of AIDS in three haemophiliacs treated with Factor VIII concentrate appeared in 1982 (CDC, 1982). The first reported case of transfusion-associated AIDS (TAA) was in an 18-month-old infant who had been transfused repeatedly at birth (Amman *et al.* 1983). By 1984, 38 cases of AIDS had been reported in patients with no risk factors other than a history of transfusion. Nineteen of the patients were adults who, during the previous 5 years, had received blood components derived from unpooled donations. In those cases in which all the donors could be followed up, an individual in a 'high-risk' group could always be identified (Curran *et al.* 1984). It was subsequently shown in an enlarged study of 194 patients, that in most cases the high risk donor was anti-HIV positive. In those few cases where the high-risk donor lacked anti-HIV, another donor had it (Peterman *et al.* 1985). A total of 157 525 cases of AIDS was reported in the USA by the end of 1990, and 5371 of these (3.4%) were attributed to the transfusion of blood or blood products. The median incubation period, estimated as the time from exposure by transfusion to diagnosis of AIDS, is shorter than in HIV infection unrelated to transfusion and has been estimated to be 34 months in adults and 22 months in children (Peterman, 1987), although more recent estimates are longer with a median of 7–8 years for adults and 3–5 years for children (Rogers and Schochetman, 1991). As time passess, AIDS cases with longer incubation periods will become evident and the mean incubation period may continue to rise. It has been predicted that 50% of subjects infected with HIV by transfusion will develop AIDS within 7 years compared with 33% of subjects infected by other routes (Ward *et al.* 1989).

The transmission of HIV by transfusion has been confirmed by virus isolation and serological studies on recipients and their implicated donors (Feorino *et al.* 1985; Jaffe *et al.* 1985). Since the first reports, the number of cases of TAA in the USA has risen rapidly. By the end of 1991, out of a total of 206 392 cases of AIDS, there were 6060 adults and 472 infants or children who had acquired the disease by transfusion of blood or blood products, representing 2.99% and 13.60% of the total cases in adults and children respectively (CDC, 1992). Obviously, the chances of transmission of HIV by blood transfusion have now almost completely disappeared in countries without major heterosexual spread and where donor education, encouragement of self-exclusion and screening for HIV antibodies have been established since 1985. Nevertheless, in many countries in tropical Africa and in Thailand, the HIV epidemic is spreading so rapidly amongst heterosexuals that subjects may well give blood in the window period of infection, without realizing that they may be infected (Fleming, 1990; Chiewslip *et al.* 1991; Isarangkura *et al.* 1992).

HIV has been transmitted by whole blood, cellular components, plasma and clotting factor concentrates (Curran *et al.* 1985), indicating that infectious virus is present in the plasma as well as in cellular fractions of blood. Follow-up studies have shown that more than 95% of patients receiving blood or blood components from anti-HIV positive donors have become infected (Ward *et al.* 1987). It has also been shown that the risk of AIDS and the incubation period between transfusion of HIV infected units and the development of AIDS is related to the clinical course in the donor; higher number of AIDS cases and shorter incubation periods were observed if the donors developed AIDS shortly after donation, as opposed to donors who remained asymptomatic (Ward *et al.* 1989). The same study showed that the risk of acquiring AIDS in blood transfusion recipients was related to the number of transfusions, with those developing AIDS receiving larger numbers of transfusions than those recipients who remained asymptomatic after developing anti-HIV. The difference may be explained by the immunosuppressive effects of transfusion (see Chapter 13), by the transmission of other viruses by blood transfusion, or by the fact that the underlying disease in the recipient was more severe (Smith, 1991), No association between AIDS and the administration of albumin preparations, immunoglobulins, antithrombin III or hepatitis B vaccine has been reported (see Desmyter, 1986; Melbye, 1986; Morgenthaler, 1989; Cuthbertson *et al.* 1991). Furthermore, when HIV is added to plasma and the plasma is then fractionated by the cold-ethanol process, HIV does not appear in the Ig fraction (Morgenthaler, 1989).

When a patient develops AIDS following transfusion of blood or a blood derivative, all other recipients of material from the same donation must be followed up as well as recipients of previous donations (if necessary back to 1977) and subsequent blood donations from the same subject. The same considerations apply when a donor develops AIDS, or some other AIDS-related condition, or is found to be anti-HIV positive but asymptomatic at some time after giving blood, when recipients not only of the most recent donation but of previous donations should be investigated. These investigations on recipients of previous donations from donors in whom anti-HIV has only recently been detected have been called 'look-back' programmes. It is recommended by some that all recipients who were transfused before 1985, when screening for HIV antibodies in blood donations was introduced, should be tested for anti-HIV in order to try to slow down the progression to AIDS in seropositive subjects and prevent further transmissions (Kühnl *et al.* 1989).

TAA in infants, and AIDS in infants and children in general, has a shorter incubation period than in adults and, although the pathophysiology of HIV infection is similar to that in adults, many of the clinical manifestations of the disease are different, c.g. lack of dementia, higher incidence of interstitial pneumonitis, etc. (Rogers and Schochetman, 1992). Infants born to anti-HIV-positive mothers who become infected perinatally and infants transfused during the first years of life have the shortest median incubation period, (less than 5 years), and usually develop AIDS in the first year of life. The increased susceptibility of infants to AIDS is possibly due to their immature immune system, and the larger viral load relative to body size. Transfusion accounts for a large proportion of AIDS in children mainly because some of the risk factors for adults, such as sexual activity and i.v. drug abuse, are non-existent in children. The characteristics of children with TAA reflect the child population more likely to need transfusions: premature babies, and children with haemophilia, thalassaemia, and sickle cell anaemia, etc. In the USA, of 2734 children with AIDS, 250 (9.1%) infections were transfusion-associated with 138 (5.0% of the total) occurring in children with coagulation factor deficiencies (CDC, 1991a).

Since the number of individuals infected by transfusion of HIV-positive blood before 1985 is unknown, and since the incubation period from infection to the development of disease is also unknown, it is difficult to estimate the number of patients who will die from TAA within the next few years (Peterman *et al.* 1987; Kalbfleisch and Lawless, 1989; Smith, 1991). In the USA, considering that more than 50% of transfusion recipients die from their underlying disease within 1 year of transfusion and that subjects infected with HIV by blood transfusion will develop AIDS within 8 years, it has been estimated that approximately 15 000 cases of TAA will be reported among transfusion recipients aged 13–69 years. The proportion of patients with TAA amongst subjects over 59 years of age and in children is higher when compared with patients with AIDS in general, correlating with the fact that old people are more likely to require transfusions and that children with AIDS include a high proportion of haemophiliacs (Smith, 1991).

In tropical Africa, the transmission of HIV by blood transfusion is still an important source of infection. The main reasons for an alarmingly high rate of transmission, reported to be up to 10% of all cases, are: (1) the high demands for blood for inpatients with severe anaemia and haemorrhage, mainly in obstetrics, gynaecology and paediatrics; (2) the very high prevalence of HIV infection amongst the donor population, which can be as high as 20%; (3) the fact that the risk of HIV infection is not confined to a minority of the population who can be requested to refrain from blood donation; and (4) the inability of many laboratories to test for HIV antibodies or to perform and control the tests properly. The patient groups at greatest risk of acquiring HIV-1 or -2 by blood transfusion in tropical Africa are children with malaria and anaemia, patients with sickle cell anaemia (120 000 infants with sickle cell disease are born each year in Africa), anaemic antenatal patients, women with severe obstetric haemorrhage, and trauma victims (for references, see Fleming, 1990; WHO, 1992).

Anti-HIV as a marker of infection
There is no convenient and sufficiently sensitive test which can be used to detect the virus itself for screening blood donations; techniques for viral isolation are very complex and cannot be used in routine laboratories. However, as stated above, HIV antibodies to various viral proteins usually become detectable in the serum of infected subjects within 2–4 months of infection and persist thereafter. Detectable levels of anti-HIV are also seen in most patients with AIDS or ARC suggesting that HIV antibodies offer little protection. Since in most cases antibodies coexist with the virus, anti-HIV acts as a marker of infectivity. Consequently, a test for anti-HIV offers a suitable indirect method for screening donations for HIV. The finding of persistent HIV in the majority of high-risk donors implicated retrospectively in TAA (Peterman *et al.* 1985) provided further justification for the use of anti-HIV testing in excluding HIV-infected blood donations.

Transfusion-associated AIDS and haemophilia
The risk of transmitting HIV, like that of transmitting other agents by transfusion, increases arithmetically with the numbers of donations which are pooled as a source of blood products. Since HIV is present in plasma as well as in cells of HIV-infected people, the transfusion of untreated coagulation factor concentrates carries a risk of

transmitting HIV. In the USA, the average patient with severe haemophilia is treated each year with Factor VIII from five to ten different batches, each made from 2500 to 22 500 plasma donations (see Curran *et al.* 1985). It is not surprising that the incidence of AIDS cases in haemophiliacs who were treated with Factor VIII concentrates in the period up to 1985 has been increasing steadily (heat treatment of clotting factor concentrates started on a large scale in most countries in 1985; see below).

Although AIDS was first reported in three haemophiliacs in 1982, studies of serum samples stored from as far back as 1968 have shown that the first cases of the development of anti-HIV in haemophiliacs occcurred in 1978 in the USA and in 1981 in the UK (Evatt *et al.* 1983; Machin *et al.* 1985; Ragni *et al.* 1986). The prevalence of HIV seropositivity and of AIDS varies from one haemophilia centre to another depending on the source, volume and type of concentrate used. The volume is a reflection of the number of different donations used in the manufacture of concentrates; the number of exposures to the same batch reflects the dose-size of the inoculum (Madhok and Forbes, 1990). In a study of 13 haemophilia centres in western Europe, Canada and Australia involving 2370 patients with haemophilia A and 434 patients with haemophilia B, the overall incidence of anti-HIV was 53.6% (CDC, 1987). The percentage of haemophiliacs infected with HIV in different countries has varied from 4% to more than 60%, with the higher rates in those countries using mainly concentrates from plasma imported from the USA. Some batches of Factor VIII concentrate from European plasma have also transmitted HIV (see Madhok and Forbes, 1990). A clear correlation was also found between the severity of haemophilia and HIV seropositivity (UK Haemophilia Centre Directors, 1986; see also Melbye, 1986; Kühnl *et al.* 1989). Haemophiliacs treated before 1985 with cryoprecipitate alone have shown a low risk of HIV infection (CDC, 1985; Ragni *et al.* 1986; UK Haemophilia Centre Directors, 1986).

There is a significantly higher incidence of anti-HIV in haemophilia A than in haemophilia B patients (Evatt *et al.* 1984; Mannucci *et al.* 1985b; Melbye, 1986; Ragni *et al.* 1986; UK Haemophilia Centre Directors, 1986). The difference may be due partly to the uneven partitioning of HIV in infected plasma during fractionation, HIV going to the cryoprecipitate fraction (see Morgenthaler, 1989; Madhok and Forbes, 1990). The source of plasma used for fractionation is also partly responsible for this difference; in many countries all the Factor IX is prepared locally whereas at least part of the Factor VIII is imported from the USA. Approximately 70% of patients in the USA with haemophilia A and 35% with haemophilia B developed HIV antibodies before the introduction of methods for viral inactivation in blood products (CDC, 1987b). In a multicentre study on haemophiliacs treated in the UK between 1980 and 1984, 896 (44%) of 2025 patients with haemophilia A were positive for anti-HIV; 20 (6%) of 324 patients with haemophilia B and 11 (5%) of 215 patients with von Willebrand's disease were seropositive. In addition, 59% of patients with severe haemophilia A were anti-HIV positive compared with 23% and 9% of moderately and mildly affected patients, respectively (UK Haemophilia Centre Directors, 1986; see also Melbye, 1986). Although a large number of severe haemophiliacs in the UK were treated up to 1983 with unheated Factor VIII concentrate imported from the USA, the incidence of anti-HIV in haemophiliacs in the UK is much lower than in countries such as Germany, Spain and the USA where the frequency of anti-HIV ranges between 68%

and 94% (Gurtler, 1984; Kitchen *et al.* 1984; 1985). On the other hand, in Groningen in The Netherlands only one of 18 severe haemophiliacs treated with commercial Factor VIII concentrates between 1978 and 1983 developed HIV antibodies (van der Meer *et al.* 1986). It was postulated at one stage that anti-HIV-positive haemophiliacs with anti-HIV might be 'immunized' to HIV, but this does not seem to be the case since it has been possible to isolate the virus from virtually all such patients (Jackson *et al.* 1988a).

A prospective multi-centre study in the USA, which concentrated on 319 patients in whom the dates of development of anti-HIV were known, showed that the rate of incidence of AIDS after the development of anti-HIV was directly related to age. The 8-year cumulative rates for the incidence of AIDS ranged from 13.3% for ages 1–17 years to 26.8% for ages 18–24 and to 43.7% for ages 35–70. It was suggested that younger haemophiliacs may have a better tolerance to severe immune deficiency partly because they are exposed to fewer other infections than adults (Goedert *et al.* 1989). This report showed that older anti-HIV-positive patients with haemophilia have a similar risk of developing AIDS to that of anti-HIV-positive homosexuals but that younger haemophiliacs have a clearly lower risk. The reason for the discrepancy in risk of developing AIDS between children who become infected with HIV by blood transfusion (see above, Rogers and Schochetman, 1992) and children with haemophilia remains unknown.

The absence of HIV antibodies in some haemophiliacs known to have received HIV-infected Factor VIII may be due to the injection of a low dose of virus, low virulence of the virus, clearance of the virus by the host's immune mechanisms (unlikely) or to loss of HIV antibody. Exceptional cases of loss of HIV antibody have been reported in prospectively followed homosexual men from whom it was also impossible to isolate the virus although HIV provirus was still detectable in three out of four of these subjects (Farzadegan *et al.* 1988). Other isolated cases of loss of HIV antibody have been reported (for references, see Madhok and Forbes, 1990).

In general, haemophiliacs who have been treated with blood products tend to have immunological abnormalities such as alterations of the T4 : T8 cell ratios (Lederman *et al.* 1983; Menitove *et al.* 1983) regardless of their HIV antibody status. It is not known whether these abnormalities may contribute to the development of disease in HIV-infected patients. Cumulative data from several reports do not support a direct correlation between intensity of exposure to Factor VIII concentrates and the presence or severity of the immune defect (Levine *et al.* 1985; Madhok and Forbes, 1990). An association has been found in haemophiliacs between the HLA A1-B8-DR3 haplotype and predisposition to HIV 1 infection (Steel *et al.* 1988).

Prevention of transfusion-transmitted HIV infection

As mentioned above, certain groups of people are far more likely to have AIDS than others. To recapitulate, these high-risk groups include men who have had sexual contact with other men since 1977, intravenous drug abusers, people living in tropical Africa, prostitutes, haemophiliacs who have received 'unsafe' clotting factor concentrates and the sexual partners of people in all these groups. Measures to exclude such subjects from blood donor panels are the most important means of preventing the spread of AIDS by transfusion and hence the spread of the disease to the population outside the high-risk groups. Obviously, this statement applies to areas where there are defined high-risk groups such as countries in Europe, North America and Australasia. The year 1977 was chosen because the first clinical cases of AIDS in the USA were diagnosed retrospectively as far back as 1978 (Jaffe *et al.* 1985) and it appears that AIDS arose at the same time in Africa and the USA (Francis and Quinn, 1987).

Self-exclusion ('self-deferral') of donors

In countries where heterosexual transmission is not the main cause of HIV spread, prospective blood donors must be made aware that some subjects are far more likely than others to be infected with HIV and that if they belong to any of these high-risk groups they should not give blood. Those who have given blood in the past and realize that they are in a high-risk group may not wish to withdraw from blood donation since this may be to admit to their friends or family that they belong to a high-risk group. Accordingly, a procedure should be established by transfusion services to allow donors to indicate confidentially that their blood should not be used for transfusion (Contreras *et al.* 1985; Pindyck *et al.* 1985; NIH, 1986). In New York, an indication of the public response to the donor education campaign has been the reduced number of young male donors (Pindyck *et al.* 1985). Similarly, in London, there has been a significant decrease in the incidence of acute hepatitis B amongst blood donors (Contreras and Barbara, 1985). The number of cases of TAA has not increased at the same rate as AIDS in the population as a whole and, in particular, has not increased as rapidly as AIDS in the homosexual population. These results suggest that self-exclusion by donors is a valuable safeguard. However, direct tests to detect carriers of HIV are also essential.

Routine screening for anti-HIV in blood donors

In most countries, screening tests for anti-HIV on all blood donations are now compulsory; the principal function of these tests is to identify the small number of infected blood donors belonging to high-risk groups who, despite education campaigns, fail to exclude themselves or who do not realize that they may be infected. The purpose of the tests is clearly to protect the recipients. If a positive result is obtained on screening, in order to safeguard the donor, additional tests for anti-HIV using independent methods must be used to confirm or refute the diagnosis of HIV infection (see Dodd, 1986). Two types of serological screening tests are at present in use for anti-HIV 1 (Barbara, 1987); an ELISA antiglobulin test, of which several versions have been developed in the USA and France (see Dodd, 1986), and a competitive inhibition ELISA developed in the UK (Cheingsong-Popov *et al.* 1984; Mortimer *et al.* 1985). Screening assays for the combined detection of HIV 1 and 2 are available as antiglobulin and sandwich assays (see Fig. 16.1).

The first antiglobulin tests for anti-HIV used disrupted purified virus as antigen and contained viral protein together with some non-viral components, such as HLA-DR antigens from host cells used for viral culture, which could become incorporated in the viral coat when it buds out from the cell. With such preparations false-positive results occurred if the serum being tested contained antibodies to the contaminating antigens. False-positive results of this kind are less likely to occur with current screening assays which use mostly antigens derived from recombinant DNA technology or from direct chemical synthesis (see Barbara, 1991).

When a positive result is obtained in a screening assay, the test should be repeated using the original sample tested and, in addition, a sample from the corresponding unit of donated blood. If both these tests are negative the unit can be released for issue, but if one or both of the repeated tests are positive, the unit of blood should be withdrawn and samples referred to a reference laboratory for confirmatory testing. Only if these confirmatory tests are positive should the donor be notified of the result (and a further sample taken for reconfirmation). In areas of high prevalence in the heterosexual population such as tropical Africa, it has been recommended that a different screening assay, using an alternative methodology, should constitute confirmation of positive screening results. This approach would be economical and would obviate the problems of false positivity in standard confirmatory assays caused by crossreacting antibodies stimulated by other infections in people from Africa (Fleming, 1990). For a review of different formats of screening assays for anti-HIV, see Barbara (1991).

Although there is some crossreactivity between antibodies to core and other antigens of HIV-1 and HIV-2, currently available tests for anti-HIV-1 should not be relied upon to detect anti-HIV-2. Crossreactivity for HIV-2 is of the order of 80% with antiglobulin ELISAs used for the detection of HIV-1 antibodies but it is only 30% with competitive ELISAs for HIV-1. Nevertheless when screening of blood donations for HIV-2 is considered to be necessary, assays using a combination of synthetic or recombinant HIV-1 and -2 antigens have proved very suitable (Barbara, 1991b). Such combined assays are available in the form of antiglobulin ELISA or sandwich ELISA (see p. 713) and are used routinely in countries such as the UK and France. Contrary to the fears of some, the range of antibodies detected is not diminished and the sensitivity for HIV 1 antibodies has improved in these combined assays with a consequent beneficial reduction in the length of the window period.

Confirmatory tests
Confirmation of positive screening assays for antibodies is not as clear-cut as the confirmation of assays for antigen screening tests, e.g. tests for HBsAg. Screening tests for antigen are confirmed by neutralization with known specific antibody, but antibody reactivity cannot be confirmed in a similar way and alternative tests for antibody have to be used; such tests should be called supplementary rather than confirmatory (Barbara, 1991).

In the USA, the confirmatory test of choice is the Western blot (or immunoblot) which is a more analytical type of antiglobulin test, capable of identifying antibodies to virus-specific polypeptides (for details, see Dodd, 1986). It has been recommended by the American Red Cross that a Western blot should be considered positive for anti-HIV if antibodies to at least one product of each of the three structural genes, *gag*, *env* and *pol* are detected. The criterion for HIV seropositivity used by the CDC in the USA is that antibodies to at least two of the p24, gp41, and gp120/160 antigens should be present (see Dodd, 1991). If only one of these bands is found on testing a sample from a donor who is not in a high-risk group, the donor should not be confirmed as positive but put in an indeterminate category pending clarification. The donor should be retested 3–6 months later before a definitive diagnosis of HIV infection with the subsequent notification and counselling are considered. In the USA it has been found that only 5% of donors with indeterminate results in Western blot are confirmed as true anti-HIV positives and most of these are amongst donors with isolated bands to *gag* peptides (for references see Dodd, 1991). Since the principles of the antiglobulin ELISA and of the Western blot are essentially the same, it is questionable whether Western blot should be the supplemental assay of choice for antiglobulin-based screening assays. However, no major problems have been encountered with this approach in the USA; of donations found repeatably reactive on screening, when tested by Western blot, 60–80% are negative, 10–20% are postitive and 10–20% have indeterminate patterns. The absence of bands in the Western blot is a clear indication that the donor does not have HIV antibodies (Dodd, 1991).

In the UK the majority of reference laboratories use combinations of two or more confirmatory tests, with or without Western blotting. If possible, the confirmatory test should use a different principle from that which has been used in screening. The following confirmatory tests have been used: competitive radioimmunoassay (COM-PRIA); competitive ELISA (when screening is by antiglobulin assays); radioimmunopre-cipitation (RIPA), which detects antibodies to radiolabelled native viral antigens; immunofluorescence which detects antibodies against normal cells and cells infected with HIV; G antibody capture (GAC) assay which captures a cross-section of IgG antibodies through anti-gamma coating the solid phase and anti-HIV is then probed with HIV antigen which, if bound, can be detected using an enzyme-labelled (GACE) or a radiolabelled (GACRIA) anti-IgG. More specialized tests have also been used but mainly for clinical diagnosis. PCR assays can detect one copy of HIV provirus amongst 100 000 negative cells.

For the definitive differentiation between antibodies to HIV-1 and -2, Western blot may help, since the pattern of binding is different for antibodies to the two viruses. But more specific assays are required, such as the 'Pepti-Lav 1,2', a blot assay in which specific peptides, carrying immunodominant epitopes for HIV-1 and HIV-2 glycopro-teins, are fixed on to membranes (see Barbara and Contreras, 1990). Competitive assays specific for anti-HIV-1 and HIV-2 or DNA amplification by PCR are also useful in the differential diagnosis of HIV-1 and HIV-2 infections (Nusbacher and Naiman, 1989).

Newer screening tests for HIV antibodies continue to be developed using mono-clonal antibodies, recombinant and synthetic peptides, novel labels (e.g. colloidal gold plus protein A), new assay formats (e.g. chemiluminescence) and new instrumentation (for details, see Barbara and Contreras, 1990).

False-negative results
Due to the great genetic variability of HIV, leading to variation in antigenic structure, there is a theoretical possibility that current tests could give weakly positive results with some strains of the virus (Dodd, 1986). Some subjects infected with HIV may make only anti-p24 and no detectable anti-gp41 and, as a consequence, give negative results by some ELISA screening tests (Schupbach *et al.* 1985). Such false-negative results are unlikely to occur with current assays which use several HIV epitopes in one test.

A further source of false-negative results in conventional screening techniques may be the absence of IgG anti-HIV in the early stages of infection; in some subjects IgM anti-HIV may persist for several months prior to the development of IgG anti-HIV

(Bedaraida *et al.* 1986). Competitive assays may be more likely to detect IgM anti-HIV than antiglobulin assays, which are designed for IgG antibodies.

Prevalence of HIV antibodies in different populations

The prevalence of anti-HIV in blood donors in the USA has been found to be significantly higher than in European countries (see Melbye, 1986) but it has decreased significantly since the introduction of screening in 1985. In the first year of screening, more than 3000 blood donations were confirmed positive for HIV antibodies in the USA, giving an approximate prevalence of 27 per 100 000 donations collected by the American Red Cross. Due to the elimination of anti-HIV-positive subjects from the panel of repeat donors, the prevalence of donors with HIV antibodies per 100 000 donors has decreased substantially in subsequent years, being of the order of 16.6 in 1986 and 12.8 in 1987 and in 1988. As in other countries of the Western world, first-time donors have had a much higher rate of seropositivity than those who have given blood before: 51.7 compared with 23.1 in 1985, and 24.6 compared with seven per 100 000 donors in 1988. The current frequency of approximately 10 per 100 000 is 40-fold lower than would be expected in a random sample of the US population and is considerably lower than that seen in military recruits and randomly tested newborn infants (see Dodd, 1991). The rate of seropositivity is much higher in paid plasma donors; seven HIV positives were found out of 35 000 plasma donors attending centres located outside high prevalence areas (Stramer *et al.* 1989).

In the UK, since the introduction of screening for HIV antibodies in 1985 and up to November 1991, a total of 16 774 503 donations have been tested for HIV antibodies and 208 donors have been confirmed positive, giving an overall prevalence of 1.2 per 100 000 donations. The prevalence in new donors is significantly higher, at four in 100 000. Although screening by the combined assay for HIV-1 and -2 antibodies started in the first half of 1990, only one donor has been found to have HIV-2 antibodies. In the majority of donors interviewed, a recognized risk activity for HIV infection could be identified. The figures have been low since the introduction of screening: they were 2.2 and 2.1 per 100 000 donations in 1985 and 1986, decreased substantially to 0.9 in 1987 and 1988, but rose moderately to 1.4 and 1.2 in 1989 and 1990, respectively (H. Gunson and V. Rawlinson, personal communication).

The frequencies of anti-HIV among blood donors for the rest of Europe are also very low, with countries such as Sweden, Norway, Denmark, W. Germany, Switzerland, Belgium and The Netherlands showing prevalence rates similar to the UK. Countries in southern Europe such as Spain, Greece, France and Italy have reported higher prevalence rates of 20 in 100 000 donations collected in 1988 (Gunson, 1990).

Donors who are confirmed positive for HIV antibodies should be counselled and referred to specialized centres for follow-up. Counselling should be performed by specially trained staff; it will not only help the donor to obtain long-term supportive care and to prevent further spread but will also aid transfusion services to understand which groups of the population who are HIV seropositive still come forward to donate (Hewitt and Moore, 1989; Lefrère *et al.* 1992). Donor education and selection methods can then be modified accordingly (Busch *et al.* 1991).

Figures from sub-Saharan Africa have been very different from those above; for example, in the rural population of Zaïre the frequency of anti-HIV positive donors was about 12% (Kestens *et al.* 1985) and in Zambia 18.4% (Melbye *et al.* 1986). With the vast numbers of HIV-infected subjects in tropical Africa (WHO, 1992), all the above considerations on self-exclusion, confirmation and follow-up pale into insignificance; the whole problem of prevention of HIV transmission, 10% of which is accounted for by transfusion, is a major public health dilemma.

Tests for HIV antigen

There are three situations in which the presence of HIV in the absence of anti-HIV has been reported:

1 Very rarely, HIV has been isolated from patients or healthy subjects without detectable anti-HIV (see, for example Salahuddin *et al.* 1984 and Pahwa *et al.* 1986).

2 Anti-HIV, especially anti-p24, may become undetectable before the onset of AIDS (see Fig. 16.6) as well as in the terminal stages of the disease (Schupbach *et al.* 1985; Weber *et al.* 1987). As stated above, loss of anti-HIV in apparently healthy subjects has also been reported.

3 HIV has been transmitted by blood from seronegative donors just prior to the development of anti-HIV (Raevsky *et al.* 1986; Crawford *et al.* 1987; Ward *et al.* 1988; Cohen *et al.* 1989; Irani *et al.* 1991). The period between infection and the appearance of demonstrable antibody usually lasts for 6–8 weeks but can be as long as 11 months (Allain *et al.* 1986). Antigen can be detected for part of the initial antibody-negative viraemic phase but some newer tests for anti-HIV may shorten the window period and may also be positive when HIV antigen first appears (Lelie *et al.* 1989). In one of the cases of transmission of HIV by transfusion of seronegative blood, HIV antigen was shown to be present in high titre (as well as anti-p24 by Western blot) in the serum sample stored frozen at the time of donation (Irani *et al.* 1991).

As shown in Fig 16.6, antigen tests are positive for only part of the initial antibody-negative viraemic phase; in some subjects antigen can be detected as early as 2 weeks after infection, persisting for between 3 weeks and 3 months, and is no longer detectable when anti-p24 appears in the serum although it may reappear intermittently during the asymptomatic phase. Later, antigen may reappear with a loss of anti-p24 (see Fig. 16.6). This reappearance is associated with the development of AIDS or ARC (Schupbach *et al.* 1985; Weber *et al.* 1987). Of 52 asymptomatic subjects with anti-HIV, only 15% were found to be antigen positive (Paul *et al.* 1986). In a study of 40 haemophiliac patients who became anti-HIV positive, HIV antigen could be detected in stored samples from nine before anti-HIV developed and was detected at some time in an additional five patients (Allain *et al.* 1986). In the same study it was also found that anti-gp41 could be detected, using a sensitive competitive immunoassay, weeks or months before routine antibody screening tests became positive.

Tests for HIV antigen, based on sandwich ELISA (see Fig. 16.1) using anti-HIV on the solid phase to capture antigen and labelled anti-HIV to detect any HIV antigen present, are now available for large-scale screening. The tests are very sensitive and confirmation is possible by specific neutralization (Barbara, 1991; Dodd, 1991). Currently, antigen tests are of most value in monitoring the clinical course of HIV infection and the response of AIDS patients to therapy; they would not increase the safety of the blood supply if added to donor screening for anti-HIV in countries in Europe, North America and Australasia. In a multi-centre study in the USA, more than 500 000 donations were screened for p24 antigen. Five donors were confirmed positive, all of whom were also positive for anti-HIV and for HIV by PCR (Alter *et al.* 1990). In a second study, when samples from male donors with particular demographic characteristics in the USA were selected from a library of sera stored in 1984–85 and tested, none was found to have p24 as the sole marker of HIV infection (Busch *et al.* 1990). Altogether, it was estimated that the equivalent of 1.5 million donations had been screened in both studies in the USA and no donor who was negative for HIV antibodies was found to be p24 antigen positive (Busch *et al.* 1991). Similar results had been reported from Germany and Austria where more than 600 000 donors had been screened and none found positive for the p24 antigen in the absence of HIV antibodies (Backer *et al.* 1987; Kühnl *et al.* 1989). From the above studies it has been concluded that screening donations for HIV p24 antigen would have negligible effects on the safety of blood transfusion, especially now that the sensitivity of screening assays for HIV antibodies has improved considerably and when measures to exclude donors in high-risk groups have also improved (Busch *et al.* 1991).

In countries where there are defined risk groups for HIV infection, HBc antibodies might serve as surrogate markers for HIV infection. In France, it has been estimated that 37% of donations in the window period, i.e. infectious but anti-HIV negative, could be eliminated by anti-HBc screening (Le Pont *et al.* 1990). This approach seems to be more efficient than screening for HIV antigen; several countries screen blood donations routinely for anti-HBc.

In areas where the rate of heterosexual transmission is rapidly accelerating, it is impossible to exclude subjects at risk and the possibility of infected subjects giving blood during the window period is considerable. In such areas, screening for p24 antigen might be able to limit the spread of HIV infection by blood transfusion. However, testing for HIV antigen is expensive and should not replace tests for HIV antibodies. In Thailand, recipients have been infected by transfusion of blood that was negative for HIV antibody and possibly positive for antigen (Chiewslip *et al.* 1991; Isarangkura *et al.* 1992).

Inactivation of HIV in blood products
In spite of careful selection of donors and screening of all blood donations for anti-HIV, there is always a danger of failing to detect an occasional donor infected with the virus. Clotting factor concentrates obtained from pooled plasma derived from at least 10 000 donors are obviously far more likely to be infected than any single unit. It has been estimated that since the introduction of screening of blood donations for HIV antibodies, between 1 in 100 000 and 1 in 1 000 000 plasma donations received by plasma fractionators are infected with HIV (Cuthbertson *et al.* 1991).

Fortunately, due to the lipid component of its envelope, HIV is inactivated by the appropriate heat, chemical or physical treatments or combinations of treatments described above for HBV. Because HBV is more resistant to inactivation than HIV, any method used to inactivate HBV in fractionated blood products will also be efficient in the inactivation of HIV. There are several factors that contribute to the viral safety of current plasma products: (1) donor selection and screening; (2) manufacturing processes such as fractionation (viruses migrate selectively with certain fractions);

purification (adsorption, chromatography), freeze-drying and ethanol treatment have been shown to reduce the viral load; (3) specific treatments aimed at viral inactivation (Morgenthaler, 1989; Cuthbertson *et al.* 1991). Transmission of HIV by untreated coagulation factor concentrates has shown that although the first two approaches help they cannot be totally relied upon to prevent viral transmission.

Pasteurized Factor VIII and Factor IX, as well as albumin, have not been reported to transmit HIV (Schimpf *et al.* 1987; Mannucci *et al.* 1988; Cuthbertson *et al.* 1991).

Dry-heat treatment at high temperatures (80°C) for long periods (72 h) has been reported to kill HIV efficiently, with no transmissions reported by clotting factor concentrates treated in this way. Eighteen cases of confirmed HIV transmission by heat-treated Factor VIII had been reported to the Centers for Disease Control in the USA by January 1988 (CDC, 1988). A few more cases are being investigated. Ten of the 18 reports were associated with plasma collected before the introduction of screening for HIV antibodies. All eight cases associated with plasma screened for anti-HIV had been treated at 60°C for 30 h or less. As stated above in the section on hepatitis, the time used for treatment was considered too short and the temperature too low, and this method of heat treatment has been abandoned.

Dry-heat treatment at raised moisture level (steam treatment of freeze-dried plasma products under high pressures) has proved to be efficient for the inactivation of HIV (see Cuthbertson *et al.* 1991).

Solvent–detergent treatment of blood products inactivates HIV due to disruption of its lipoprotein envelope. No cases of HIV transmission or of the development of anti-HIV have been reported in haemophiliacs injected with solvent–detergent-treated Factor VIII (Horowitz *et al.* 1988; Horowitz, 1989).

β-propiolactone used in conjunction with ultraviolet irradiation at a wave length of 254 nm has been used in the manufacture of Factor IX. No patients with haemophilia B treated with this product have become infected with HIV (Stephan, 1989).

Intramuscular and intravenous immunoglobulins have not been reported to transmit HIV (Morgenthaler, 1989).

From the above it can be concluded that it is extremely unlikely that HIV can survive any of the kinds of heat treatment or chemical treatment currently employed by manufacturers of coagulation factor concentrates (McDougal *et al.* 1985; Petricciani *et al.* 1985; Gomperts, 1986; Morgenthaler, 1989; Cuthbertson *et al.* 1991).

Current risk of transmission of HIV by transfusion

Cases of transfusion-associated AIDS (TAA) will continue to occur among subjects who received blood before the policies of education and self-exclusion of donors and testing of blood donations for anti-HIV were introduced. Application of these measures and maintenance of stable donor panels, consisting mainly of donors who give blood repeatedly, cannot be expected to eliminate the risk of HIV transmission entirely but should reduce it to a very low level. In the UK it has been estimated that 3.2 per million blood donations could have been false-negative for anti-HIV in 1986; this figure would have decreased to 1.1 per million in 1987 (Hickman *et al.* 1988). With the improved sensitivity of current assays and the very low prevalence rate of HIV antibodies in the donor population, it is estimated that less than one in 1 000 000 units transfused in 1991 may have been infectious.

In the USA, where the prevalence of HIV infection and the frequency of anti-HIV-positivity amongst blood donors is much higher than in the UK, the risks of transmitting HIV infection through blood transfusion are also higher. Estimates of risk have been decreasing steadily since 1985; a 30% decrease in risk per year was estimated from 1985 to 1987, with an estimated 131 infectious units transfused in 1987 (Cumming et al. 1989). It has been suggested that this downward trend will continue (Smith, 1991). The risk of having 131 HIV infectious units gives a risk of one in 153 000 units transfused; since the average patient in the USA is transfused with 5.4 units, the risk of HIV infection would have been one in 28 000 patients transfused in 1987 (Cumming et al. 1989). The same authors estimated that the number of infectious units undetected in 1988 decreased to 87. Up to November 1990, 14 cases of TAA acquired by the transfusion of tested blood had been reported to the Centers for Disease Control (Smith, 1991); many more cases of TAA acquired before the introduction of screening for anti-HIV have been reported.

HUMAN T-CELL LEUKAEMIA VIRUSES TYPES I AND II

HTLV-I and -II

The human T-cell leukaemia virus type I, HTLV-I, was the first human retrovirus described; it was found to be associated with conditions misdiagnosed as mycosis fungoides and Sézary syndrome but later recognized as variants of adult T-cell leukaemia/lymphoma (ATLL) by Gallo's group (Poiesz et al. 1980; Gallo et al. 1981). The virus was subsequently shown to be identical with adult T-cell leukaemia virus (ATLV) (Yoshida et al. 1982; Watanabe et al. 1984). HTLV-I is associated with a chronic degenerative demyelinating neurological disease called tropical spastic paraparesis (TSP), known in Japan as HTLV-associated myelopathy (HAM) (Vernant et al. 1987; Román and Osame, 1988). HLTV has also been associated sporadically with TSP, polymyositis and Kaposi's sarcoma (for references, see Lemaire et al. 1991). The association of TSP, but not ATLL, with transfusion has been reported (see below). A high incidence of HTLV antibodies has been found in patients infested by *Strongyloides stercoralis* (Nakada et al. 1984) but this association may be coincidental or may be due to immunosuppression by HTLV, and its significance is unknown (Sandler et al. 1991; Taguchi et al. 1991).

HTLV-I and -II are retroviruses belonging to the category oncoviruses and are able to induce polyclonal proliferation of T lymphocytes *in vitro* and *in vivo* (Zack and Chen, 1991). Like the lentiviruses HIV-1 and -2, these viruses are lymphotropic and neurotropic, and they have the essential structural genes *gag* (group antigen), *pol* (reverse transcriptase) and *env* (envelope) in addition to regulatory genes. In HTLV-I, the *gag* gene codes for the structural proteins p55/24/19; *pol* codes for a protein of approximately 100 kD, and *env* codes for glycoproteins gp61/46/21. In HTLV-II the structural proteins are very similar to those in HTLV-I with a high degree of crossreactivity; *gag* encodes the polypeptides p53/24/19; *pol* a protein of approximately 100 kD; and *env* codes for the glycoproteins gp61/46/21 (Williams and Sullivan, 1991).

Areas endemic for HTLV have been found, particularly in south-west Japan with prevalences as high as 15% (Maeda et al. 1984; Blattner et al. 1986) and in the

Caribbean with a 1–8% prevalence (Clark *et al.* 1985); and in regions of Central and South America (Levine, 1990; Williams and Sullivan, 1991) and in parts of sub-Saharan Africa (Gessain *et al.* 1986; Williams and Sullivan, 1991). Populations in these areas show different prevalence rates for anti-HTLV-I, as do emigrants from these regions (Sandler *et al.* 1991; Williams and Sullivan, 1991). It has been estimated that more than 1 million Japanese people are healthy carriers of HTLV-I (Williams and Sullivan, 1991). Carriers of HTLV have also been found in the USA, especially in Florida and states on the Pacific, and in France, UK, The Netherlands and many other countries. The prevalence in blood donors has been reported as 1.6 in 10 000 in the USA (CDC, 1990), 1 in 10 000 in France (Coste *et al.* 1990) and 0.5 in 10 000 in The Netherlands and London (van der Poel *et al.* 1989b; Brennan *et al.* 1992). However, it seems that only a small proportion of antibody-positive subjects develop leukaemia or TSP.

HTLV-II, the second human retrovirus to be discovered, is closely related to HTLV-I and it is difficult to differentiate between these two viruses in the routine laboratory. Most studies of prevalence of HTLV antibodies have not differentiated between HTLV-I and II and, at present, the worldwide distribution of these two viruses is not known in any detail (Williams and Sullivan, 1991). There is a high prevalence of HTLV-II amongst i.v. drug abusers and their sexual contacts in the USA and other countries (Lee *et al.* 1989; Kwok *et al.* 1990). A high proportion of the HTLV-II-positive subjects without a history of i.v. drug abuse in the USA have been Hispanics and American Indians (see Hjelle *et al.* 1990; Sandler *et al.* 1991). No firm association between HTLV-II and any disease has been found so far and, although the virus was first found in a patient with hairy T-cell leukaemia (Kalyanaram *et al.* 1982) and subsequently in other T-cell malignancies, viral RNA expression has not been found in malignant cells (Manns and Blattner, 1991). Of 21 HTLV-II-infected i.v. drug abusers, four had an absolute lymphocytosis and three of these showed an increase in CD8 + T lymphocytes (Rosenblatt *et al.* 1990).

HTLV-I and -II are thought to transform T cells (mainly CD4 +) by one of two mechanisms: (i) by *trans* activation of cellular genes involved in growth control via the *tax* gene; or (ii) by direct mitogenic stimulation of the cells by the virus or its products (see Zack and Chen, 1991). The mechanism by which excessive proliferation or malignant transformation of T cells occurs, or neurological degeneration occurs in some HTLV-I-positive subjects, is not clearly understood. There seems to be an association between immunosuppression in HTLV-I carriers and the subsequent development of ATLL (Taguchi *et al.* 1991). ATLL associated with viral infection is rare even in endemic areas (estimated lifetime risk of 2–5% in anti-HTLV-I-positive subjects infected in the neonatal period) and may have a latent period of 20 or more years (see Murphy *et al.* 1989). All of 18 patients with ATLL in Kyushu were found to have anti-HTLV-I (Lee *et al.* 1985). The lifetime risk for people who acquire HTLV-I infection later in life (e.g. by blood transfusion) is unknown but there is some evidence that genetic predisposition and environmental factors may play a role. The incubation period for TSP can be shorter, with a latency of 18 weeks to 8 years, and a lifetime risk of 0.25% for anti-HTLV-positive subjects (Osame *et al.* 1990).

HTLV and blood transfusion

The main modes of transmission of HTLV-I are by sexual contact and from mother to infant by breast-feeding (Blattner et al 1986; Kajiyama et al. 1986). Mothers with higher titres of HTLV antibodies are at greater risk of transmitting the virus to their infants; if mothers refrain from breast-feeding or if the milk is freeze-thawed or heated at 56°C for 30 min, transmission of HTLV-I is prevented (Ando et al. 1986; Yamato et al. 1986; Hino et al. 1987). Transmission from mother to fetus has been reported from culture studies of cord blood lymphocytes; viral antigen was detected in the lymphocytes of two of 40 cord blood samples from HTLV-I-positive mothers (Satow et al. 1991). The virus has been transmitted by transfusion of cellular elements of blood but not by cell-free components or by blood products (Okochi and Sato, 1985). Antibodies are usually first detectable 14–30 d after transfusion, although the interval may be as long as 98 d (see Inaba et al. 1989; Gout et al. 1990; Williams and Sullivan, 1991). Of 85 recipients of anti-HTLV-I-positive cellular blood components in Japan, 53 (62%) developed specific antibodies 3–6 weeks after transfusion; IgM antibodies were present only in the early stages, while IgG antibodies persisted at high titres through-out the period of follow-up (see Okochi and Sato, 1985). In another report storage of blood appeared to decrease the risk of HTLV transmission; platelets and red blood cells under 6 d old had a transmission rate of 80% (Sullivan et al. 1991). The efficiency of transmission decreased with the age of the cellular blood components, with 79.2% of recipients of blood stored for 1–5 d developing antibodies compared with 63.6% if stored for 6–10 d and 55% for 11–16 d (Okochi and Sato, 1989). It was possible to clone cells carrying ATL antigens from some antibody-positive recipients (Sato and Okochi, 1986). Of eight recipients of cellular blood components from an anti-HTLV-I-positive donor, two developed anti-HTLV-I after transfusion (Fretz et al. 1991). In a retrospective study in the USA, of 118 recipients of cellular components from donors who were subsequently found to be anti-HTLV-positive, 17 developed anti-HTLV giving a transmission rate of 14.4%, which is much lower than the Japanese rate. However, the authors point out that this is a minimum estimate of infectivity since it was assumed that all HTLV seropositive donors were infected at the time of donation, which in some cases was as long as 6 years before. It was suggested that the lower transmission rate in the USA study could be attributed to the likelihood of a greater viral load in Japanese carriers due to the high rate of perinatal transmission.

Although no case of ATLL due to transfusion-transmitted HTLV-I has been documented (Okochi and Sato, 1985), there are reports directly associating a history of blood transfusion with HTLV-associated myelopathy (HAM) or TSP and showing that a high proportion, sometimes as high as 39%, of patients with TSP have a history of blood transfusion (Petz et al. 1989; Cartier et al. 1990; Engel et al. 1990; Gout et al 1990; Osame et al. 1990). The time lag between transfusion and the development of TSP can be as short as 18 weeks and as long as 8 years (Osame et al. 1986; Gout et al. 1990). The factors leading to TSP in patients who acquire HTLV-I by transfusion are unknown; immunosuppression might contribute but genetic factors might also play a role. Of two heart transplant recipients who became infected with HTLV after blood transfusion from the same infectious donor, only one developed TSP (Fretz et al. 1991).

Screening tests for HTLV antibodies
Several HTLV screening assays are available, mostly ELISAs, although a gelatin particle

agglutination test is manufactured in Japan and has been used extensively. The specificity and sensitivity of most of the available screening assays are comparable, ranging from 98.4% to 100% and from 93.2% to 100%, respectively (Kline *et al.* 1991). Recently, assays of apparently good specificity and sensitivity which combine HIV 1 and 2 and HTLV-I and -II have become available but they have not been tried in large-scale donor screening (McAlpine *et al.* 1992). Some assays use semi-purified viral antigens and lysates of the virus obtained from T-cell cultures, while others use recombinant antigens. However, the source of the antigens does not seem to affect significantly the sensitivity or specificity of the assays, except that ELISAs in which whole disrupted virus is used seem to be less sensitive for the detection of HTLV-II (Wiktor *et al.* 1991). None of the available screening assays is able to differentiate between anti-HTLV-I and -II because of crossreactivity due to the 75% homology of amino acid sequences between the two viruses (Rosenblatt *et al.* 1986). In addition, many asymptomatic carriers have low levels of antibody in their plasma. The majority of samples found to be repeatably reactive in one assay will not be reactive in another screening assay (Shih *et al.* 1990; McAlpine *et al.* 1992) and will not be positive in the confirmatory assays available, such as Western blot (protein immunoblot), RIPA, competitive assays, antibody capture radioimmunoassay and PCR (White, 1988; Lillehoj *et al.* 1990; McAlpine *et al.* 1992; Tosswill *et al.* 1992). Western blot was shown to be more sensitive for the detection of antibodies to the core (*gag*) proteins p24 and p19, but recently Western blots have been loaded with more envelope glycoprotein, improving the sensitivity of the assay for envelope antibodies (Lemaire *et al.* 1991). At least one *env* and one *gag* band should be present in the Western blot for confirmation of the presence of HTLV antibodies (WHO, 1990). RIPA, though more lengthy and laborious, was shown to be more sensitive than Western blot for the detection of antibody to the more immunogenic envelope antigens of HTLV-I. When frozen serum samples stored from a previous prospective study of PTH were tested, only those units of blood found positive for HTLV antibodies by Western blot and RIPA transmitted HTLV-I to recipients (Shih *et al.* 1990). Only specialized reference laboratories have the range of tests and expertise to enable them to confirm the presence of anti-HTLV and to distinguish samples with antibodies to HTLV-I from those with antibodies to HTLV-II. It has been recommended, for those countries where both viruses are prevalent, that discrimination between HTLV-I and -II should be done after the presence of anti-HTLV has been confirmed (McAlpine *et al.* 1992). Synthetic antigens have been introduced into immunoblots and other discriminatory assays (Chen *et al.* 1990) and this has reduced the need to use RIPA and PCR for distinguishing between HTLV-I and -II. Despite this array of confirmatory tests, there is still a significant proportion of sera that are repeatably reactive by ELISA but not confirmed or which are reported as indeterminate by the reference laboratory or are confirmed as positive by the reference laboratory but cannot be defined as HTLV-I or -II.

In areas such as Kyushu and Okinawa in Japan, where HTLV-I is endemic and transfusion contributes to the risk of ATLL in the population by providing sources of secondary natural infection, there is a good case for screening blood donations for anti-HTLV-I. It has been shown that the presence of HTLV antibodies correlates with infectivity and with integrated HTLV provirus in the host's cells (see Williams and

Sullivan 1991). Compulsory screening of blood donations for anti-HTLV was introduced throughout Japan in November 1986 (Inaba *et al.* 1989) and the rate of HTLV
seroconversion in recipients of blood in areas of high HTLV prevalence decreased from
53.6% and 8.3% before screening, to 0.9%, 0.15% and even 0% after the introduction
of screening (Kamihira *et al.* 1987; Inaba *et al.* 1989; Nishimura *et al.* 1989).

The risk of HTLV-I transmission by blood transfusion in non-endemic areas will
depend on the number of immigrants from endemic areas and on the incidence of
antibody-positive donors. Selective screening of donors from endemic areas would not
eliminate the low risk of transmission of HTLV by transfusion in countries such as the
USA, France and the UK because sexual partners of carriers from endemic areas or of
i.v. drug abusers can acquire the virus as may transfusion recipients (CDC, 1990a; Coste
et al. 1990; Brennan *et al.* 1992). Sexual transmission from males to females is
significantly more efficient than from females to males (see Williams and Sullivan, 1991).

Universal screening of blood donations for anti-HTLV was introduced in December
1988 in the USA and in July 1991 in France. Other countries, such as the UK, have
not introduced screening for this agent in view of its low prevalence in the donor
population and the high cost of screening to prevent disease in a very small number of
recipients of blood.

During the first 13 months of anti-HTLV screening in the USA, starting in
December 1988, 9.2 million blood donations were screened by the American Red
Cross (ARC) and the Council of Community Blood Centers. A total of 9230 donations
(0.1%) were repeatably reactive by ELISA and 1506 (0.016%) were confirmed as
anti-HTLV-I or -II positive, i.e. only 16.3% of donations which were repeatably reactive
were confirmed as anti-HTLV positive. By March 1990 only 0.04% of donations were
repeatably reactive and fewer than 0.01% were confirmed as anti-HTLV positive
(Sandler *et al.* 1991). The highest incidence of anti-HTLV was found in the states in the
Pacific region. The prevalence of anti-HTLV was higher in females than in males and
was higher in Blacks, Hispanics and Asian than in Whites. Other risk factors were
Japanese or Caribbean ancestry or sexual contact with people from Japan or the
Caribbean, i.v. drug abuse or sexual contact with i.v. drug users. PCR studies on
mononuclear cells from the first 136 ARC donors confirmed as anti-HTLV positive
showed that 56 (41%) were infected with HTLV-I; 57 (42%) with HTLV-II; three (2%)
with both viruses; and 20 (15%) had no evidence of HTLV infection, probably reflecting
the finding that only a small proportion of mononuclear cells in the circulation of
seropositive subjects are infected with the virus. Donors with anti-HTLV-I were from
Japan or the Caribbean or had a history of sexual contact with people therefrom.
HTLV-II-positive donors had a history of i.v. drug abuse or sexual contact with i.v.
drug abusers. Of the donors with a history of transfusion, about half were infected with
HTLV-I and half with HTLV-II. However, since it is not known whether HTLV-II causes
disease and tests that distinguish HTLV-I from HTLV-II are not routinely available in
the USA, the CDC recommends that anti-HTLV-positive donors are counselled as if
they are infected with HTLV-I and asked not to donate blood or organs, not to share
needles and not to breast-feed infants (CDC, 1990b; Sandler *et al.* 1991).

Since the introduction of routine screening of blood donations for HTLV antibodies
in France, the incidence of anti-HTLV-positive donors has been similar to that found in

the UK, i.e. one in 17 000, and the majority of positive donors who have been contacted have come from regions of high prevalence such as the Caribbean or Africa (B. Habibi, personal communication).

CYTOMEGALOVIRUS (CMV)

Characteristics of the virus and of CMV infection

CMV is a large, enveloped, double-stranded DNA, herpes virus which is cell associated and is also found free in plasma and secretions. CMV has a direct cytopathic effect on the cells it enters, leading to neutropenia, some depression of cellular immunity and inversion of T-cell subset ratios, with a consequent increase in susceptibility to bacterial, fungal and protozoal infections (Ho, 1982; Grumet, 1984); in immuno-suppressed patients CMV infection can lead to parenchymal damage, e.g. pneumonitis.

CMV can cause primary acute clinical and subclinical infections; it can also cause chronic subclinical infections when it is shed in saliva and, or, urine; finally, it can remain latent in a large proportion of infected subjects. The presence of anti-CMV does not guarantee immunity. In subjects with antibody, CMV infection may be reactivated or the subject may become reinfected with exogenous strains of CMV. Primary CMV infection is generally more severe than reinfection or reactivation. CMV antibody-positive subjects may infect others with CMV by sexual contact, breast-feeding, transplacental transmission or transfusion (see Ho, 1982; Rock and Quinnan, 1982; Tegtmeier, 1986). Hence, as in HIV infection, specific antibody is a marker of potential infectivity although only a relatively small proportion of subjects with anti-CMV seem to be infectious.

The term recurrent infection has been coined to embrace both reactivation and reinfection, in view of the difficulty of distinguishing between them routinely. However, if necessary, donor viral DNA can be distinguished from recipient viral DNA by restriction enzyme analysis (Glazer *et al.* 1979). In routine work the diagnosis of recurrent infection is limited to demonstrating a four-fold increase in antibody titre or the presence of IgM anti-CMV. In immunosuppressed patients serological tests cannot be relied upon for a diagnosis of CMV partly because the patients do not make antibody and partly because any anti-CMV detected may have been derived from transfused blood. Viral culture is impractical due to the slow growth of the virus *in vitro*. On the other hand, immunofluorescence techniques to detect viral antigen using monoclonal antibodies on biopsies or bronchial washings provide results within hours (see Griffiths, 1984). Other techniques to detect viral antigen, e.g. involving ELISA or the detection of viral DNA, are under investigation.

The consequences of CMV infection and in particular of transfusion-transmitted CMV infection depend largely on whether or not the recipient is immunocompetent.

Prevalence of anti-CMV

The frequency of subjects with anti-CMV varies widely in different populations: it is lower (30–80%) in developed than in developing countries, where the figure may reach 100% (Krech, 1973 ; Preiksaitis, 1991). The prevalence of anti-CMV is correlated with age and poverty (see Lamberson, 1985; Tegtmeier, 1986). The frequency of anti-CMV-positive donors may vary widely within a given country, e.g. 25% in southern California and 70% in Nashville, Tennessee (Grumet, 1984; Tegtmeier, 1986).

Transmission of CMV by transfusion

The transmission of CMV by blood transfusion was first reported by Kääräinen *et al.* (1966). It is now known that CMV is one of the infectious agents most frequently transmitted by transfusion. The pathogenesis of transfusion-transmitted CMV infection is not clearly understood; it is assumed that CMV is transmitted in most cases in a latent, particulate state only by cellular blood components (especially granulocyte concentrates) and that the virus is reactivated from white cells after transfusion. Hence, host as well as donor factors are involved in CMV infection (Tegtmeier, 1989; Preiksaitis, 1991). CMV has been isolated from the mononuclear and polymorphonuclear cells of patients with acute infections. The specific cell type responsible for carrying the virus has not been identified, although mononuclear cells are the favourite candidates as hosts of CMV in latent infection (Rook and Quinnan, 1982). Fresh blood appears more likely than stored blood to transmit CMV infection although no controlled studies have been carried out (Tegtmeier, 1986). It has been estimated that 3–12% of units have the potential to transmit CMV (Adler, 1984), although most authors have reported a carrier rate of only 1–3.5% (see Tegtmeier, 1986). At present there is no easy way of identifying infectious subjects; viral excretion is a good index of infectivity but it is not practicable to test for it at blood collection clinics. Donors with IgM anti-CMV appear to be more likely than others to transmit CMV (Lamberson *et al.* 1984).

Transfusion-transmitted CMV infection in immunocompetent subjects

Some 30% of anti-CMV-negative recipients undergoing cardiac surgery involving transfusion develop infection, as shown by virus isolation or the development of anti-CMV. In addition, some anti-CMV-positive patients develop recurrent infection. In almost all cases the infection is asymptomatic. Of patients who develop a primary or recurrent CMV infection following transfusion, fewer than 10% develop a mononucleosis-like syndrome. This syndrome, originally described as the post-perfusion syndrome but now referred to as the post-transfusion syndrome, appears 3–6 weeks after transfusion. Common features include fever, exanthema, hepatosplenomegaly, enlargement of lymph nodes and the presence in peripheral blood of atypical lymphocytes resembling those found in infectious mononucleosis (Foster, 1966). Recovery is usually complete. The development of atypical lymphocytes due to post-transfusion CMV infection should be distinguished from the development of atypical lymphocytes 1 week after transfusion as a response to allogeneic lymphocytes (see Chapter 13).

Consequences of transfusion in patients with impaired immunity

In immunosuppressed patients, or in fetuses and premature infants whose immune systems are immature, CMV infections, especially primary infections, may cause severe disease which can be fatal.

1 *The fetus in utero.* Following maternal primary CMV infection, the fetus becomes infected in 30–40% of cases: about 5–10% of infected infants develop sequelae such as mental retardation, hearing loss or chorioretinitis (Ho, 1982: Stagno *et al.* 1986).

2 *Premature infants.* The risk of serious CMV infection is high when the infant's birth-weight is less than about 1300 g and when its mother is anti-CMV negative. In two large prospective studies, 25–30% of infants with these risk factors, transfused with a total of 50 ml or more of blood, some of which was anti-CMV positive, acquired CMV infection and 25% of these infants died. Infants transfused with anti-CMV-negative blood did not develop CMV infection (Yeager *et al.* 1981: Adler *et al.* 1983). A lower incidence of CMV infection has been reported from two other centres: in infants weighing less than 1500 g born to anti-CMV-negative mothers and transfused with blood, some of which was anti-CMV positive, only 7–9% developed infection (Smith *et al.* 1984: Tegtmeier *et al.* 1984). All reports agree that clinically significant anti-CMV infection in newborn infants develops only when the infant is premature and of low birth-weight, when the mother lacks anti-CMV and when anti-CMV-positive blood is transfused (Tegtmeier 1986).

3 *Bone marrow transplant recipients* frequently develop primary or recurrent CMV infections which may be fatal (see Tegtmeier, 1986). CMV infection (mainly pneumonitis) is in fact the commonest cause of death following the transplantation of allogeneic marrow (Meyers *et al.* 1986). Since CMV itself can cause immunodeficiency and since infections are so much more severe in immunosuppressed subjects, it is very important that CMV infections should not be misdiagnosed as graft-rejection episodes; if the wrong diagnosis is made and immunosuppresive therapy is increased, CMV infection may become disseminated (The, 1984). In a prospective randomized trial of 97 anti-CMV-negative patients, 57 received anti-CMV-negative marrow: 32 of the 57 received anti-CMV-negative blood components and only one of these developed a CMV infection; of the 25 who received blood components unscreened for anti-CMV, eight developed CMV infection. Among the 40 recipients of anti-CMV-positive bone marrow the rate of CMV infection was no lower in those who received only anti-CMV-negative blood components (Bowden *et al.* 1986).

Granulocyte concentrates carry the greatest risk of transmitting CMV infection (Winston *et al.* 1980; Hersman *et al.* 1982).

4 *Renal transplant recipients* are at high risk of primary or recurrent CMV infection; the main source of infection lies in the transplanted kidney (see Tegtmeier, 1986). In anti-CMV-negative recipients of a kidney from an anti-CMV-negative donor, blood transfusion plays a significant role in CMV transmission (Rubin *et al.* 1985).

5 *Heart and heart–lung transplant recipients* may develop severe primary CMV infection which can lead to opportunistic infections with fungi or bacteria. In anti-CMV-negative recipients the main sources of infection are anti-CMV-positive transplanted organs or organ blood donor units (Preiksaitis *et al.* 1983; M. Yacoub, personal communication). If both donor and recipient are anti-CMV negative, blood transfusion is a major source of CMV disease; infection can be prevented by the use of anti-CMV-negative red cells and platelets (Freeman *et al.* 1990). If a heart or heart–lung from a donor with CMV antibodies is transplanted to an anti-CMV-negative recipient, prophylactic administration of specific CMV hyperimmune i.v. IgG seems to lessen the severity of CMV disease (Freeman *et al.* 1990), although others feel that there is little scientific evidence to support the use of hyperimmune CMV Ig in prophylaxis (P. Griffiths, personal communication, 1991).

6 *Following splenectomy due to trauma*, patients receiving massive transfusion may develop serious CMV infections (Baumgartner *et al.* 1982; Drew *et al.* 1982).

7 *Haemophiliacs infected with HIV*, and especially those with AIDS, if anti-CMV negative may acquire severe primary CMV infection by transfusion (Jackson *et al.* 1988b; Sayers *et al.* 1992).

8 *Liver transplant recipients* should also be considered, especially if they are children or pregnant women. Now that smaller amounts of blood and blood components are needed in liver transplantation, it has been possible to give only anti-CMV-negative blood and platelets to anti-CMV-negative recipients of anti-CMV-negative grafts.

Prevention of transfusion-transmitted CMV infection
As described above, the only subjects who are at risk of severe primary CMV infections are anti-CMV-negative patients with impaired immunity. Steps to prevent the transmission of CMV by transfusion are justified only in patients who are at risk of severe primary CMV infections, are anti-CMV negative and have impaired immunity. Even in these patients, although the morbidity caused by CMV infection is high, the role of transfusion in the transmission of CMV has been demonstrated in only a very few properly controlled studies (Tegtmeier, 1989; Preiksaitis, 1991). In a recent controlled trial in the USA, transfusion-transmitted CMV infection was prevented in anti-CMV-negative recipients of anti-CMV-negative bone marrow transplants by the use of anti-CMV-negative blood components. However, the use of anti-CMV-negative blood components did not improve survival in bone marrow transplant recipients and might have been associated with an increase in Gram-negative septicaemia (Miller *et al.* 1991). Although CMV infection in patients with major trauma may delay recovery from severe bacterial infection, transfusion does not seem to play a major role in CMV transmission in such cases (Curtsinger *et al.* 1989). It must be remembered that if all anti-CMV-positive donors were to be rejected, most donor panels would be halved.

When red cells alone are required, frozen-deglycerolysed red cells or filtered white-cell depleted red cells can be transfused since they have been shown not to transmit CMV (Tegtmeier, 1986; Gilbert *et al.* 1989; De Witte *et al.* 1990; Sayers *et al.* 1992). It is unlikely that γ-irradiated blood components have a decreased risk of CMV transmission since the radiation dose needed to inactivate viruses would damage cells and platelets (see Wagner *et al.* 1991). Platelet concentrates can also be depleted of white cells by centrifugation or by special filtration (see Chapter 13), thus avoiding the risk of CMV transmission (de Graan-Hentzen *et al.* 1989; Murphy *et al.* 1989). The only method of avoiding the transmission of CMV infection which applies to the transfusion of all blood components, including granulocyte concentrates, is to use anti-CMV-negative donations found by screening.

In areas where most donors are anti-CMV positive it will be difficult to find enough anti-CMV-negative donations but since most recipients will also be anti-CMV positive the demands for CMV-free blood will be low. Where the frequency of anti-CMV-positive donors does not exceed 70% it is difficult but not impossible to supply anti-CMV-negative blood components, especially platelet concentrates, for transfusion to well-defined categories of anti-CMV-negative patients (see above). Once a large number of donors has been screened, donations from anti-CMV-negative subjects can be specially selected and after retesting can be used for patients with an increased risk of CMV disease. Anti-CMV-negative whole blood, red cells and platelets are supplied routinely by the North London Blood Transfusion Centre; on average, 600–1000 blood donations, out of a total of 4000–5000, are screened weekly for CMV antibodies by ELISA to meet demands.

Other, still experimental, methods of preventing CMV infection in high-risk patients receiving many transfusions are the i.v. administration of anti-CMV immunoglobulin (Condie and O'Reilly, 1984) and active immunization (Balfour, 1983). It is unlikely that either of these two approaches will be effective due to the biology of the virus (P. Griffiths, personal communication). The risk of transmitting CMV infection by transfusion to premature infants of low birth-weight could be diminished by reducing the amount of blood taken in sampling and thus reducing the transfusion requirements.

Tests for anti-CMV

Although in the past the standard diagnostic reference test has been complement fixation, this test is too complex for routine donor screening. Several tests for IgG anti-CMV or IgG plus IgM anti-CMV are available and have been shown to be adequate for the provision of CMV-free blood. The tests include haemagglutination, indirect immunofluorescence, solid-phase fluorescence immunoassay, ELISA and particle agglutination; although the last proved the most convenient for blood donor screening (Dodd, 1984, Tegtmeier, 1986; Barbara *et al.* 1987), it is not as convenient, in its current form, as ELISA for automated testing and reading.

OTHER VIRUSES

Epstein–Barr virus (EBV)

Infection with EBV, which like CMV is a herpes virus, is endemic throughout the world. EBV can cause primary symptomatic infection (infectious mononucleosis) but most commonly causes asymptomatic infection followed by latent infection (Henle and Henle, 1985). In most countries more than 90% of blood donors have neutralizing anti-EBV which coexists with latent virus in B lymphocytes of peripheral blood and lymph nodes. At least one in 10^7 circulating lymphocytes of carriers harbour EBV genomes (Rocchi *et al.* 1977) but post-transfusion EBV infection is a rare occurrence, and symptomatic infection is even rarer. The virus is found in three of every 10^4 peripheral lymphocytes during acute infection. The majority of susceptible recipients are young children: even in them, the chance of acquiring EBV infection following the transfusion of anti-EBV-positive blood is minimal, due to the donor's neutralizing antibodies which persist in the circulation for longer than the EBV-infected lymphocytes. In a study of 25 EBV-antibody-negative patients aged from 3 months to 15 years, transfused with 1–11 units of blood stored for not more than 4 d, only one developed EBV antibodies and this patient had no symptoms (G. Fleisher, quoted by Henle and Henle, 1985).

Of five patients transfused during cardiac bypass who were initially free from EBV antibody, four produced antibody post-operatively which persisted at a maximum level for many months. Two of the four patients had concomitant CMV infection and no heterophil antibodies; one developed transient fever and the other hepatitis. Only one of the four patients developed an infectious mononucleosis-like syndrome with heterophil antibodies (Gerber *et al.* 1969).

Although most cases of 'post-transfusion syndrome' are due to CMV (see above), two adult patients who were anti-EBV negative before transfusion developed post-transfusion syndrome due to EBV (McMonigal *et al.* 1983).

In a survey of approximately 800 patients, fewer than 8% lacked EBV antibody before transfusion and only 5% of these developed antibody following transfusion. No clinical illness or disturbance of liver function was noted in these patients (Medical Research Council, 1974b). Possibly, the discrepancy between these observations and those of Gerber *et al.* (1969) may have been related to the fact that fresh blood was used in the last-named series.

Post-transfusion infectious mononucleosis (IM) is seen only rarely in anti-EBV-negative immunocompetent patients; it usually occurs when only a single unit of blood or blood component, obtained from the donor during the incubation phase of IM, is given within 4 d of collection, the point being that when more than 1 unit is transfused, one of the units is certain to contain anti-EBV (Henle and Henle, 1985). In the reported cases the donors have developed symptoms of IM 2–17 d after blood donation; the incubation period in recipients has been 21–30 d (Solem and Jörgensen, 1969; Turner *et al.* 1972). Transfusion-transmitted EBV infection with symptomatic IM has occasionally been reported in patients transfused for splenectomy (see Henle and Henle, 1985).

Post-transfusion EBV infections may contribute to the development of lymphomas in severely immunosuppressed patients such as graft recipients, T-lymphocyte suppression would allow EBV-infected B lymphocytes to outlive the passively transfused antibodies and to proliferate (Marker *et al.* 1979; Hanto *et al.* 1983; Henle and Henle, 1985).

Due to the rarity of clinically important EBV infection and in view of the high carrier rate, screening of blood donations for EBV antibodies is not recommended. The current recommendation in the UK, of 2 years deferral from blood donation for subjects who have had IM, does not seem to have any scientific basis.

Other herpes viruses

Herpes simplex and Herpes varicella zoster have never been shown to be transmitted by blood transfusion; viraemia occurs only during primary infections, which usually occur in childhood (Henle and Henle, 1985).

HHV-6 is a newly characterized human herpes virus, originally named HBLV (human B-lymphotropic virus) due to its ability to infect freshly isolated B cells. The virus was found in patients with various lymphoproliferative disorders. It is now known that HHV-6 can infect monocytes, macrophages, T cells and megakaryocytes (Ablashi *et al.* 1987). The virus is cytopathic for selected T-cell lines. Infection is acquired usually within the first year of life and the virus was found to be ubiquitous in blood donors when tested in London and the USA (Briggs *et al.* 1988; Saxinger *et al.* 1988).

Serum parvovirus-like virus (SPLV), or B19 virus

The association of this virus with blood transfusion was discovered by chance: a reagent used for screening blood donations for HBsAg by EIOP was found to give false-positive reactions with sera from nine healthy blood donors and two patients. The sera happened to contain SPLV, identified by immune electron microscopy. Thirty per cent of adults tested had anti-SPLV (Cossart *et al.* 1975). Parvovirus antigenaemia was found to be transient; the frequency in London was one in 40 000 blood donors. A virus named 'Aurillac', also found when screening donors in Paris, in 1972, was later found to be identical to SPLV (Couroucé *et al.* 1984); the antibody was found in 25.3% of blood donors. Parvovirus can precipitate aplastic crises in children with sickle cell anaemia (Pattison *et al.* 1981) and in patients with other types of haemolytic anaemia, through a specific cytotoxic effect on erythroblasts (see Young and Mortimer, 1984). In fact, SPLV infection seems to be the main cause of aplastic crises in chronic haemolytic anaemias and can sometimes reveal an undiagnosed haemolytic anaemia, in particular hereditary spherocytosis (Lefrère *et al.* 1986). B19 virus was found to be the agent of erythema infectiosum or '5th disease' (Anderson *et al.* 1983), and has also caused arthritis, purpura (Pattison, 1987), hydrops fetalis and spontaneous abortion (Anand *et al.* 1987). SPLV is a very small, single-stranded DNA virus with a protein coat but no lipid envelope. The period of antigenaemia lasts for only 1–2 weeks, persistence is unlikely, and SPLV is rarely transmitted by the transfusion of blood (Couroucé *et al.* 1984) or, more commonly, of Factor VIII concentrates (Mortimer *et al.* 1983). The lack of a lipid envelope and the fact that it can achieve extremely high concentrations in plasma, at least 10^{12} virus particles per millilitre, make B19 resistant to several of the viral inactivation procedures used for plasma products (Cuthbertson *et al.* 1991). Contamination of clotting factor concentrates with parvovirus is particularly undesirable for HIV-infected haemophiliacs in view of the association of parvovirus with aplastic anaemia in such patients (Crocchiolo *et al.* 1988).

Creutzfeld–Jacob disease (CJD)

CJD has never been transmitted to humans by blood transfusion. Transmission to mice by intracerebral inoculation of a crushed blood clot obtained at necropsy from a patient with the disease has been reported (Tateishi, 1985). CJD was also transmitted from buffy coats of affected patients by intracerebral inoculation into guinea pigs (Manuclidis *et al.* 1985). Although viraemia can occur in patients with CJD, current criteria for the selection of blood donors ensure that demented subjects as well as people who have received growth hormone derived from pituitary extracts are excluded from blood donations (WHO, 1989; Contreras and Barbara, 1991).

BACTERIA

Treponema pallidum

From a review of the literature, Hartmann and Schøne (1942) concluded that the incubation period in transfusion syphilis varies from 4 weeks to 4.5 months, averaging 9–10 weeks, and that the recipient usually exhibits a typical secondary eruption. They also concluded that even donors with latent syphilis can transmit the infection.

Transfusion syphilis was once a serious problem; nowadays cases are very rare in the Western world. The chief reasons for the decline seem to be the almost universal practice of storing blood at low temperatures before using it for transfusion and the decline in the prevalence of syphilis in many countries since the advent of penicillin. Other factors that have probably contributed to the decline in transfusion syphilis are the administration of antibiotics to a large proportion of patients requiring transfusion and, lately, the exclusion of sexually promiscuous subjects from blood donation.

In citrated blood stored for more than 72 h at 4–6°C sphirochaetes are unlikely to survive (Bloch, 1941; Turner and Diseker, 1941); slightly longer survival, namely 6 d, was found by Selbie (1943). There is a close relationship between the number of treponemes added to donor blood and the survival times of *T. pallidum* determined by a sensitive assay in rabbits; in blood heavily contaminated with spirochaetes (1.3×10^6 and 2.5×10^7 per ml blood), surviving treponema were found at 120 h (Garretta *et al.* 1977; van der Sluis *et al.* 1985).

Several tests are available to screen blood donations for syphilis, such as the automated reagin test (ART), rapid plasma reagin test (RPR), venereal disease research laboratory slide technique (VDRL) and the *Treponema pallidum* haemagglutination assay (TPHA). The VDRL is a quantitative reagin test. Non-specific reagin tests detect antibody to lipoidal antigen and are insufficiently sensitive as screening tests for syphilis. A specific and much more sensitive test is the TPHA (Barbara *et al.* 1982b; Chadwick, 1984), although a newly developed ELISA has an even greater sensitivity, especially for primary infection (Young *et al.* 1992). Samples found to be positive by TPHA should be checked with a reagin test and the likely positives sent to a reference laboratory for confirmation by more specific tests such as the fluorescent treponemal antibody absorption test (FTA-ABS).

There is no general agreement regarding the need for screening of blood donations (Bove *et al.* 1981) and there is no mandatory requirement to screen blood donations in Europe (Commission of the European Communities, 1991). Serological tests cannot prevent all cases of transfusion syphilis in view of the fact that in early primary syphilis, when spirochaetaemia is most prominent, serological tests and particularly reagin tests are frequently negative. In addition, a proportion of prospective blood donors with a positive reagin test (a test still used in many transfusion centres) are 'biological false positives' (BFPs), and have never been infected with *T. pallidium*. BFPs can be transient or chronic, the former usually unexplained or due to recent bacterial, viral infections or vaccinations. Chronic BFPs are sometimes associated with drug addiction, paraproteinaemias or autoimmune diseases such as systemic lupus erythematosus (Csonka, 1983).

At the present time, it seems best to continue testing blood donations for syphilis (but using a specific test), for the following reasons: (1) the incidence of syphilis has been gradually increasing throughout the world, although the prevalence in the developed world is not nearly as high as it was in the first half of this century and there are indications that, at least in the UK, the incidence is now decreasing sharply (Editorial, 1987); (2) increasing demands for fresh blood components, especially platelets, fresh frozen plasma and blood for exchange transfusion in newborn infants, increase the risk of the transmission of syphilis (Chambers *et al.* 1969; Soendjojo *et al.* 1982; Risseew-Appel and Kothe, 1983); (3) screening helps to exclude donors who are in high-risk groups for HIV and HBV infection; (4) the cost of screening by TPHA is relatively low; (5) recipients of infected blood may have aborted syphilis due to incomplete antibiotic therapy; (6) even after antibody first becomes detectable ('early latent seropositive stage') spirochaetes may be present in the blood; (7) it may be important to demonstrate that a positive test in a transfusion recipient is due to antibody acquired passively from the donor, as otherwise the recipient may be wrongly suspected of having syphilitic infection, although passively acquired antibody never remains detectable for more than 20 d after transfusion (Ravitch et al. 1949); (8) in certain countries (e.g. USA) screening is still a legal requirement.

Every donation found positive in the screening test should have confirmatory tests even if confirmatory tests on previous donations from the same subject have been negative. In the USA, units that are positive in a screening test but have not been confirmed as positive can be issued for transfusion provided that they are labelled with the results of the screening and confirmatory tests. Donors who give plasma for fractionation ('source plasma') should be screened for syphilis on the day of the first medical examination and every 4 months thereafter. Since syphilis is not transmitted by plasma products, there is no requirement to label units intended for fractionation with the test results and retrieval of blood products containing plasma with positive tests for syphilis is not recommended. Since December 1990, as an additional measure to broaden the exclusion criteria for donors at risk of HIV infection by sexual transmission, the Food and Drug Administration (FDA) has ruled that those blood and plasma donors who give a history of infection or treatment for syphilis or gonorrhoea in the last 12 months should be deferred from blood donation and requalified if after 12 months they have a negative screening test. Requalification also applies to donors who are positive on confirmatory tests or who have a positive screening test with no additional test result. For donors with confirmed positive tests, written evidence of adequate treatment for syphilis should also be obtained. If a screening test for syphilis is positive on an autologous donation, the unit should have two labels: 'For Autologous Use Only' and 'Biohazard'. The patient's physician should be informed in writing of the results before transfusion (FDA, 1991b).

In countries with a high incidence of syphilis, if fresh blood is given, 2 megaunits of penicillin G or its equivalent should be injected into recipients (Bruce-Chwatt, 1985). In endemic areas, subjects who have had non-venereal trepanomatosis such as yaws or pinta, caused by T. pallidum pertenus or T. pallidum carateum, will also give a positive screening test for syphilis, caused by T. pallidum. Serological tests cannot distinguish between venereal and non-venereal trepanomatosis and the only means of distinguishing between syphilis, yaws and pinta is by clinical and epidemiological characteristics (Perine, 1983).

Brucella abortus

This organism is known to survive for months in stored blood and there are several reports of blood transfusion-transmitted symptomatic infection, mainly in children and splenectomized patients (Wood, 1955; see also Tabor, 1982). Antibody-positive donors are common in Mexico, Greece, Spain and in some rural areas of the USA although transfusion-transmitted brucellosis has not been reported in the USA. Infected donor blood has very low concentrations of brucella and hence poses only a small threat except in immunosuppressed patients (Fernandez *et al.* 1981; for references, see Tabor, 1982).

After an incubation period ranging from 6 d to 4 months, recipients of infected blood may develop undulant fever, headache, chills, excessive sweating, muscle pains and fatigue. There may be hepatosplenomegaly, lymphadenopathy, leucopenia and arthritis and, very rarely, complications such as purpura, encephalitis or endocarditis (Tabor, 1982).

In view of the chronic nature of the disease, persons with a history of brucellosis should not be used as donors. Unfortunately, however, 80% of infections are asymptomatic. It has been recommended that in areas with a very high prevalence of brucellosis, subjects with brucella agglutinin titres of 1 in 1000 or greater should be excluded from blood donation (Tabor, 1982), although most subjects with high-titre brucella antibodies do not transmit infection by transfusion (Fernandez *et al.* 1981). It seems that the only reasonable way of preventing the transmission of brucella by transfusion in areas where brucellosis is endemic is to exclude from blood donation all subjects with a history of the disease within the previous 2 years.

Miscellaneous

Lyme disease

The organism responsible for this disease is *Borrelia burgdorferi*, a tick-borne spirochaete whose primary reservoir is the white-footed mouse. Humans are infected in the nymphal stage of the cycle and white-tailed deer are infected during the second year of life of the tick. Most cases of Lyme disease have been reported in the USA but thousands of cases have also been reported in Europe.

The disease has three stages: in the acute stage of erythema migrans, a skin rash starting at the site of the tick bite spreads locally and it is often accompanied by 'flu-like symptoms'. If this stage is not treated promptly with antibiotics, the second stage progresses to disseminated infection with cardiovascular and neurological manifestations. In the third stage, arthritis develops.

Although no cases of transmision of *B. burgdorferi* by blood transfusion have been reported so far, transmission is theoretically possible. The spirochaete has been isolated and cultured from blood as old as 14 d from a few symptomatic patients in the primary stage of infection. However, since spirochaetaemia occurs in symptomatic patients and is of low intensity and of short duration, it is unlikely that infectious donors will come forward to give blood (for details see Popovsky, 1990; Westphal, 1991b).

Four transfusion recipients of blood components from a donor who gave blood between the disappearance of erythema migrans and the second stage of the disease were studied; none of the recipients showed signs of disease or developed antibodies against *B. burgdorferi* (Halkier-Sørensen *et al.* 1990).

Mycobacterium leprae

This organism is known to have been inadvertently transfused to two patients from a donor incubating leprosy, without apparent harm. *M. leprae* has also been injected i.v. into human volunteers without the recipients becoming infected, although the period of follow-up is not known (see Tabor, 1982).

Rickettsia rickettsii

Rickettsiosis (Rocky Mountain spotted fever) has been reported to have been transmitted by blood from a donor incubating the disease who subsequently died (Wells *et al.* 1978). The rarity of the transmission of rickettsiosis by blood transfusion is explained by the fact that patients are too ill to give blood when rickettsiae are in the blood stream (Tabor, 1982).

Exogenous and various endogenous bacteria and bacterial products contaminating stored blood or blood components

Bacteria may infect blood or blood components, in one of the following ways:

1 They may contaminate solutions or equipment which are to be used for transfusions but which have not yet been sterilized. After sterilization the solutions or equipment may remain contaminated with heat-stable bacterial products (pyrogens) capable of producing febrile reactions when they are introduced into the circulation (see Chapter 15).

2 In contaminated equipment or solutions such as hydroxyethyl starch used in leucapheresis, they may survive 'sterilization' or may even contaminate solutions which have previously been sterilized. Both 1 and 2 are now very rare in view of the strict adherence of blood pack manufacturers to Good Manufacturing Practice regulations.

3 Bacteria originating from skin flora, such as *Staphylococcus epidermidis*, *Micrococcus* species, *Sarcina* species and diphtheroids, may gain entrance to the blood pack during venesection, especially if the site of venepuncture is scarred. It is virtually impossible to disinfect the deeper layers of the skin and a skin plug often enters the blood pack upon collection (see Puckett, 1986b).

4 Bacteria in the environment (*Pseudomonas* species, *Flavobacterium* species, *Bacillus* species) may gain entrance to blood components through minute lesions in the packs, during collection or processing in open systems (Puckett, 1986b).

5 The ports of packs of cryoprecipitate or fresh frozen plasma may become contaminated, if not protected by a secondary plastic bag, during thawing in water baths contaminated with *Pseudomonas* (e.g. *P. cepacia*, *P. aeruginosa*).

6 Bacteria circulating in the blood of an apparently healthy donor suffering from asymptomatic bacteraemia may proliferate in red cell components stored at 4°C or in platelet concentrates stored at room temperature. Bacteraemia in donors may be chronic and low grade as in the case of the incubation or convalescence periods of salmonella, *Yersinia enterocolitica* or *Campylobacter jejuni* infections, or acute and transient as occurs within the first few hours after dental extractions when the organisms involved are usually *Streptococcus viridans*, *Bacteroides* species and, more rarely, *Staphylococcus aureus* (for details, see Goldman and Blajchman, 1991).

Contamination of blood with live bacteria is very uncommon: the use of disposable plastic packs with multiple satellite bags makes it possible to use a virtually closed system, and the introduction of sterile docking devices has increased the safety of processing blood components. Even when blood does become contaminated, storage at 4 ± 2°C inhibits the growth of most likely contaminants.

Random tests for bacterial growth in blood components or on donor skin

When units of blood which have been stored for 2–3 weeks are cultured, very few are found to be contaminated, even when the cultures are kept at 22°C to favour the growth of psychrophilic organisms. Bacteria are usually prevented from growing by the bactericidal properties of blood (see Puckett, 1986b). The commonest organisms isolated from units of whole blood have been pseudomonads, coliforms and achromobacters (all Gram-negative), although flavobacteria have also been isolated. Gram-positive bacteria have only rarely been isolated from units of blood (for references, see Mollison *et al.* 1987). The range of positive cultures from routine platelet concentrates has varied from 0% to 10%. Positive cultures from frozen-deglycerolized red cells have been much lower: 0–0.2% from red cells cultured 2–3 weeks after collection and 0.14–0.5% at their expiry date (see Goldman and Blajchman, 1991). These variations may be a reflection of the different conditions in each study such as storage temperature of the blood component, storage time before sampling, volume of sample used for the culture, culture medium used and culture incubation temperature. Fewer than ten micro-organisms per millilitre of blood component were found in a significant proportion of positive cultures; such low concentrations may be undetected if the volume of sample used for the culture is too small. On the other hand, it is possible that some of the samples were contaminated during culture and that a positive culture does not always reflect contamination of the unit in question. Moreover, some of the organisms, such as diphtheroids, isolated from cultures of blood components are of low pathogenicity and have not been implicated in reports of post-transfusion septicaemia or endotoxic shock. Even when a pathogenic organism is isolated, the recipient of that contaminated unit may be receiving appropriate antibiotics for the underlying condition and may come to no harm (for details and references, see Puckett, 1986b; Mollison *et al.* 1987; Goldman and Blajchman, 1991). In one very extensive survey, in which approximately 2500 units of red cells and an equal number of platelet concentrates were sampled annually, over a 10-year period the mean rates of positive cultures were 0.3% and 0.4%, respectively (Goldman and Blajchman, 1991). The number of reports of patients with septicaemia or endotoxic shock following transfusion is very much lower than the number expected from reports of positive bacterial cultures of blood components.

A study of skin swabs taken from the arms of 782 donors which were cultured on to heated blood agar and then subcultured, showed that non-fermentative Gram-negative rods were found on 11.7% of donors, *Pseudomonas* species were found on 1.0% and *P. fluorescens* on 0.3% (Puckett *et al.* 1992).

Some properties of organisms which grow in stored blood
Organisms isolated from stored blood are usually Gram-negative rods capable of using citrate (Pittman, 1953); many strains of organisms isolated from contaminated stored blood produce clotting by consuming citrate (Braude *et al.* 1952; Pittman, 1953). Blood that is heavily contaminated with organisms is not necessarily haemolysed. Among bacteria isolated from stored blood, 25% produce no haemolysis (Braude *et al.* 1952). Many organisms that grow in stored blood are psychrophilic, that is to say, they grow preferentially in the cold.

Unless blood is heavily contaminated with organisms, microscopic examination is an unreliable method of detecting infection. Walter *et al.* (1957) added serial dilutions of an inoculum of a coliform organism to blood and found that when 24×10^5

organisms per ml were present they could be detected readily but that 24×10^4 per ml could be detected only with difficulty since on the average only one organism was found in every 100 fields examined. On the other hand, when 0.3 ml of the material was cultured for 24 h, contamination could be detected when the number of organisms was as low as 24 per ml.

The effect of antibiotics on bacteria in stored blood has been investigated. Chlortetracycline, oxytetracycline and polymyxin B in concentrations as low as 10 mg in 500 ml blood (i.e. 20 μg/ml) would all prevent the inocula of either cold-growing or warm-growing bacteria from multiplying in human blood either in the cold or at room temperature. Nevertheless, there are several reasons why the routine addition of antibiotics to stored blood cannot be recommended. First, antibiotics cannot be autoclaved and would therefore have to be added later, and this addition might itself introduce infection. Second, no antibiotics are effective against all organisms. Third, there is the risk of immunizing patients to particular antibiotics or of inducing a hypersensitivity reaction in a patient already immunized.

Importance of maintaining refrigeration
After the first 24 h or so of storage the maintenance of strict refrigeration at a temperature of 4°C becomes essential. When a patient is to be given several units of blood, only one should be taken to the bedside at a time; the others must remain in a refrigerator until the last possible moment.

When blood has to be transported for any considerable distance the use of refrigerated containers is essential. In properly designed insulated boxes with ice inserts, blood can be kept below 10°C for as long as 48 h. Modern containers designed to be connected to a power supply of any voltage have been used by the British Army to transport blood abroad and in field hospitals. They can keep the temperature of 72 units of blood controlled at 4 ± 2°C for as long as there is a power supply (M. Thomas and R. Jones, personal communication). Some transfusion centres routinely keep blood at approximately 20°C for up to 24 h after collection before it is processed. The storage at room temperature does not seem to affect the yields of Factor VIII in plasma subsequently frozen and fractionated, nor the shelf-life of platelets or red cells (Pietersz *et al.* 1989b; Högman *et al.* 1991a). Leucocytes in fresh blood have a bactericidal effect for a few hours after collection and before processing into blood components with removal of the buffy coats. From experiments in which defined numbers of colony forming units of different bacteria were added to fresh blood, it was shown that leucocytes have a clearing effect on bacteria which varies according to the bacterial species: *Staphylococcus epidermidis* and *Escherichia coli* were cleared more readily than *S. aureus*, which was engulfed by the leucocytes and then released after causing cell death. The clearing effect of leucocytes required a few hours, sometimes as long as 24 h. It was also shown that some Gram-negative bacteria were killed by plasma factors, presumably antibodies and complement. Some anaerobic bacteria such as *Propionibacterium* species did not grow in stored blood, regardless of the presence or absence of white cells. *Yersinia enterocolitica* was cleared temporarily, to reappear within a few hours, but if leucocytes were removed from the blood after 5 h, the units remained sterile. Hence, it was concluded that leucocytes had a potent clearing effect on bacteria contaminating fresh blood and that it might be unwise to remove them during or immediately after collection. Although some bacteria are killed intracellularly, others kill the cells, which then disintegrate releasing the bacteria (Högman et al. 1991a,b).

Limitation of storage period

In general, as stated above, blood or red cells contaminated with bacteria do not become dangerous until they have been stored for a few days and usually for more than 1 week.

Any preparations of red cells, leucocytes or platelets that have been prepared by an 'open' method, e.g. red cells which have been thawed after storage in the frozen state with glycerol and subsequently washed, must be kept refrigerated and discarded if not used within 24 h.

An exception is made for platelets, for which storage at room temperature is optimal. As described in Chapter 14, with some permeable plastics platelet viability is well maintained at room temperature for up to 7 d. Nevertheless, in view of reports of bacterial contamination (e.g. Buchholtz et al. 1971) it has been recommended that the storage period should be limited to 5 d (FDA, 1986). Using virtually closed systems and permeable plastic containers, platelets collected by apheresis have a shelf-life of 5 d.

Effect of transfusing bacterially contaminated blood

Shock following the injection of bacteria is presumably due, as a rule, to bacterial toxins although an immune reaction between naturally occurring antibodies and bacteria may also produce ill effects. The transfusion of contaminated blood may produce immediate collapse, followed by profound shock and hyperpyrexia; haemorrhagic phenomena due to disseminated intravascular coagulation are common; in a series of 25 cases, mortality was 58% (Habibi et al. 1973b).

A review of more than 30 reports of post-transfusion sepsis due to contaminated red cells, platelets or a few other blood components showed that septic shock developed in many cases and that the overall mortality rate was 26%. Common signs and symptoms reported were fever, chills, vomiting, tachycardia and hypotension, often during the transfusion, but sometimes developing a few hours later. In the case of Pseudomonas cepacia, septicaemia or wound infection developed several days or weeks after transfusion (Goldman and Blajchman, 1991).

In the USA, the incidence of fatalities due to the transfusion of bacterially contaminated blood components has increased in recent years; the increase has been attributed largely to contaminated platelet concentrates stored at 20–24°C. Of all deaths associated with blood transfusion during the 3 years from 1976 to 1978, 4% were attributed to bacterial contamination. Corresponding figures for the 10 years between 1976 and 1985 and for the 3-year period 1986 to 1988 were 7% and 10%. Of the nine deaths in the period 1986–88, seven were attributed to contaminated platelet concentrates (Sazama, 1990; Goldman and Blajchman, 1991). In the UK, of 16 reports of severe transfusion reactions due to bacterial contamination in the 5 years between 1986 and 1990, nine proved to be fatal and only one of these fatalities was attributed to a contaminated platelet concentrate (R. Mitchell, personal communication).

Bacteria contaminating different blood components
The type of bacterial contaminant depends largely on the type of blood component:
1   *Red cells* involved in cases of bacterial infection have been contaminated mainly with *Pseudomonas fluorescens*, *P. putida* and *Yersinia enterocolitica*.

   Y. enterocolitica is a Gram-negative aerobic rod that grows well in stored blood at 4°C, uses citrate as a source of energy and, due to its lack of siderophores, requires iron to grow well, making red cell concentrates an ideal culture medium. *Yersinia* produces endotoxin and does not cause haemolysis so that bacterial growth cannot easily be seen by simple visual inspection. Transfusion of blood from donors with subclinical *Yersinia* bacteraemia can cause fatal septicaemia, especially in immunosuppressed patients.

   Between April 1987 and the end of February 1991, eight fatalities associated with the transfusion of red cells contaminated with bacteria were reported to the FDA; seven of these were due to *Y. enterocolitica*. During the same period, ten cases of *Y. enterocolitica* caused by contaminated red cell transfusions were reported to the FDA, and three cases were reported in France, one in Belgium and one in Australia. The patients developed fever and hypotension within 50 min of the start of transfusion. In the ten cases that occurred in the USA, the blood had been stored in the cold for a mean of 33 d (range 25–42 d). The bacteria proliferate after a lag period of 10–20 d. Questioning of blood donors for a recent history of gastrointestinal upset would not help to prevent transmission since a high proportion of implicated donors would not be excluded from donation; moreover, approximately 1–13% of the current total donor population in the USA would be excluded. Reducing the shelf-life of red cell units to under 25 d would reduce the availability of red cells in the USA. Testing units older than 25 d for endotoxin and micro-organisms might be the simplest measure to reduce or eliminate the risk of *Y. enterocolitica* bacteraemia and endotoxic shock (for a report and references, see CDC, 1991b). Although the reports of septicaemia due to *Yersinia* are rare, the numbers have increased in the past 10 years. If patients are taking antibiotics, infection by blood contaminated with *Yersinia* can be asymptomatic (Jacobs *et al.* 1989).
2   *Platelet concentrates* stored at 20–24°C have caused fatal bacterial sepsis when contaminated with any of several Gram-negative or -positive organisms such as staphylococci, streptococci, *Serratia* species, flavobacteria and salmonellae (Goldman and Blajchman, 1991). One (paid) thrombapheresis donor with subclinical *Salmonella cholerae suis* osteomyelitis transmitted septicaemia to seven patients (Rhame *et al.* 1973). Bacterial proliferation is more likely to occur after prolonged storage of platelet concentrates at room temperature; of nine deaths due to post-transfusion septicaemia recorded by the FDA between 1980 and 1983, six were due to contaminated platelet concentrates (Heal *et al.* 1987b).
3   *Cryoprecipitates and fresh frozen plasma* can become contaminated with *P. cepacia* and *P. aeruginosa* during thawing in contaminated water baths (see Goldman and Blajchman, 1991).

Investigations following the suspected transfusion of infected blood
Any blood remaining in the container should be cultured at various temperatures, including 4°C and 20°C, in appropriate culture media. A negative culture excludes the possibility that the blood was heavily infected at the time of transfusion. A positive

culture does not enable one to say with certainty whether the blood was contaminated before the transfusion or became contaminated during or after transfusion, or upon sampling. Techniques to exclude contamination upon sampling have been described (see Puckett, 1986a). It might be thought that if the blood remaining in a container had been left at room temperature for 24 h after having been entered, it would be useless to culture it, since it would inevitably be infected but, if left sealed in a clean place, such blood is usually sterile or at most lightly contaminated. The likelihood of contamination is greater if, after transfusion, packs are left in sinks.

In fatal cases, blood for culture should be collected from the body (e.g. by cardiac puncture) as soon as possible after death. Pittman (1953) found that when blood contaminated with a coli-aerogenes bacterium had been transfused, cultures collected were usually positive, although when pseudomonads were concerned blood collected at autopsy was sterile. Tests for endotoxin should also be carried out, especially when the culture from the patient's blood is negative.

MALARIA

Transmission of malaria by blood transfusion

Malaria can be transmitted by the transfusion of any blood component likely to contain even small numbers of red cells; platelet and granulocyte concentrates, fresh plasma and cryoprecipitate have all been incriminated. An inoculum containing as few as ten parasites can cause *Plasmodium vivax* malaria (Bruce-Chwatt, 1972).

Despite intensive eradication programmes, the prevalence of malaria in tropical and subtropical countries is extremely high, with about 300 million cases reported each year and more than 1 million annual fatalities attributed to malaria in tropical Africa (Wyler, 1983).

Malaria parasites of all species can remain viable in stored blood for at least 1 week (Hutton and Shute, 1939). Cases of *P. falciparum* malaria have been transmitted by blood stored for 14 d (Grant *et al.* 1960) and for 19 d (de Silva *et al.* 1988). It seems that malaria parasites survive longer in blood stored in adenine-containing solutions (WHO, 1986). In reviewing nearly 2000 cases of transfusion malaria due to *P. malariae*, it was noted that in the great majority of cases the blood had been stored for less than 5 d and that cases following the transfusion of blood stored for 2 weeks were very rare (Bruce-Chwatt, 1974). The parasites survive well in frozen blood (see Kark, 1982). Plasma which has been frozen or fractionated has never been known to transmit malaria.

In non-malarious countries, mainly because of delay in diagnosis, post-transfusion malaria has a relatively high fatality rate; it can be particularly serious in pregnant women and in splenectomized or immunosuppressed patients (Kark, 1982; Bruce-Chwatt, 1985).

Transfusion-transmitted malaria usually responds to conventional drug therapy; primaquine is not indicated because the parasites are confined to circulating red cells. In severe cases in which the diagnosis has been delayed and in fulminant cases, the patient may benefit from exchange transfusion in the period before anti-malarial drugs have had time to become effective (Yarrish *et al.* 1982; Kramer *et al.* 1983; Files *et al.* 1984).

The red cells in a kidney transplant and in a bone marrow transplant have been known to transmit *P. falciparum* malaria (Kark, 1982; Dharmasena and Gordon-Smith, 1986). The plasmodia can also be transmitted by transplacental passage.

Frequency of post-transfusion malaria
Estimates of the frequency of post-transfusion malaria vary from less than 0.2 cases per million units of blood transfused in non-endemic countries to 50 or more cases per million in some endemic countries (Bruce-Chwatt, 1985). In countries where malaria is non-endemic the frequency of reported transfusion malaria is relatively low, e.g. in the UK eight cases in 50 years; in the USA 26 cases in 10 years from 1972 to 1981; and in France 110 cases in 20 years (Bruce-Chwatt, 1985), although between 1980 and 1986 only 14 cases were observed (B. Genetet, personal communication). On the other hand, nine cases of transfusion-transmitted malaria were reported in the USA to the Centers for Disease Control in 1982 although only 11 cases in the following 4 years (Westphal, 1991b). In many malarious areas, the frequency of post-transfusion malaria is unknown, due to lack of reporting.

Frequency with which the different parasites are involved
In the period 1950–72, *P. malariae* was responsible for about 50% of cases of transfusion malaria and *P. vivax* for 20% (Bruce-Chwatt, 1974). In the period 1973–80 a global survey showed that there was a big relative increase of cases due to *P. vivax* which, with a few cases of *P. ovale*, accounted for 42% of all cases; cases due to *P. malariae* fell to 38% whereas those due to *P. falciparum* increased four-fold (Bruce-Chwatt, 1982). In over half the cases reported, the species involved was not identified. The relative increase in cases due to two of the parasites has been attributed to the failure of donors from highly endemic areas to comply with rules laid down by transfusion services (Guerrero *et al.* 1983; Shulman *et al.* 1984). The simultaneous transmission of two different strains of malaria (*P. falciparum* and *P. malariae*) by transfusion has been described (Aymard *et al.* 1980).

Incubation period
The incubation period of transfusion malaria depends on the numbers and strain of plasmodia transfused, on the host, and on the use of anti-malarial prophylaxis; with *P. falciparum* and *P. vivax* it is between 1 week and 1 month, but with *P. malariae* it may be many months (Bruce-Chwatt, 1974).

Period for which donors remain infectious
P. falciparum infections, prevalent in west Africa, are usually eliminated within 1 year but have been known to persist for as long as 5 years after the last exposure to infected mosquitoes (Guerrero *et al.* 1983). *P. falciparum* transmitted from asymptomatic blood donors can cause fulminant infection and death in an already ill, non-immune recipient in whom the diagnosis, being unexpected, is usually delayed. *P. vivax* infections, prevalent in the Indian subcontinent, may relapse for up to 2.5 years after infection but only very rarely after more than 3 years. With *P. ovale* a clinical attack may occur up to 4 years after returning from an endemic area. In immune carriers who have lived in endemic areas for most of their lives, *P. falciparum* or *P. vivax* may

reappear long after the limits given above. *P. malariae* infections persist for longer than those of any of the other malaria parasites; transmission of malaria has been known to occur up to 46 years after the last exposure to infection (Miller, 1975).

Rules to prevent transmission of malaria in non-endemic areas
In non-endemic areas there are various regulations concerning eligibility of potential blood donors who have visited endemic areas (WHO, 1989; AABB, 1990; UK BTS/NIBSC, 1992). These regulations are not always consistent with each other and can be confusing. Two different approaches have been adopted; in the USA reliance is placed solely on the deferral of subjects who have been in endemic areas, whereas in Europe deferral and testing for malaria parasites can be combined.

All donor clinics should have an up-to-date WHO map showing the areas endemic for malaria together with an alphabetical list of the countries.

In the USA, those who normally live in a non-endemic area but have travelled in an area considered to be endemic for malaria may be accepted as regular blood donors 6 months after returning to a non-malarious area, provided that they have had no symptoms and have not taken anti-malarial drugs. Prospective donors who have had malaria are deferred for 3 years after the cessation of therapy or after leaving the malarial area if they have been asymptomatic meanwhile (WHO, 1989; AABB, 1990).

The Council of Europe has recommended that individuals born or brought up in endemic areas may be accepted as donors of whole blood 3 years after their arrival in a non-endemic area provided that an approved immunological test has given a negative result. Others, for example travellers, can be accepted as blood donors 6 months after their return if they have been afebrile and have not taken anti-malarial prophylaxis; those who have had febrile illnesses may be accepted if an antibody test is negative at 6 months. Although a proportion of antibody-positive subjects are non-infectious and are thus unnecessarily rejected, application of these procedures makes it possible to use 75–90% of units of blood from donors returning from malarious areas to France, the UK and Belgium (Brasseur and Bonneau, 1981; Soulier, 1984; Wells and Ala, 1985; R. Masure, personal communication).

The foregoing rules will not prevent the occasional transmission of *P. malariae* and, especially, of *P. vivax*. With the object of excluding donors who are potentially infected with *P. vivax*, the new regulations in the UK exclude for 1 year donors who have returned from endemic areas and have had no previous exposure which may have rendered them immune.

Donations to be used for the preparation of plasma for fractionation may be accepted from donors who do not meet the above criteria.

Tests to detect carriers
When blood films are examined by simple microscopy, a density of less than 100 parasites per microlitre of blood cannot be detected, although a unit from a donor whose blood contained even one parasite per microlitre would contain about half a million parasites (Bruce-Chwatt, 1985).

The indirect fluorescent antibody test or ELISA offers a good chance of detecting latent malarial infection (Deroff *et al.* 1982; Voller and Draper, 1982). ELISA is more suitable for large-scale screening in the blood transfusion service and its specificity is improving with the use of chromogenic substrates (WHO, 1985). A commercial ELISA for malarial antibodies is undergoing trial in the UK. Ideally, potential carriers who volunteer as blood donors in non-malarious areas should be screened for malaria antibodies using a test covering three homologous antigens. However, only *P. falciparum* is readily available for *in vitro* tests; although there is some degree of cross-reactivity between the different strains of malaria parasites it is not known how valuable a test based on the use of *P. falciparum* would be in a country like Mexico where none of the 44 cases of transfusion malaria reported in 5 years were due to this strain (Olivares-Lopez *et al.* 1985).

Sensitive tests, using monoclonal antibodies, are being developed for use in endemic areas for detection of parasites in red cells, and soluble antigens and antibodies in plasma (Soulier, 1984; Prou, 1985). In a study in blood donors in Chandigarh, India, a comparison of different screening techniques for malaria carriers showed that a test for malaria antigen, using monoclonal antibodies, had good sensitivity and specificity. The test was considerably more sensitive than the direct examination of blood films (Choudhury *et al.* 1991). Donors with a positive antigen test were treated with the appropriate anti-malarial drugs and were eligible to donate 3 months after treatment when the malarial antigen test had become negative (Choudhury *et al.* 1988).

Serological tests for malarial antibodies and tests for malarial antigens are useful in the identification of donors implicated in cases of transfusion-transmitted malaria in non-endemic countries when blood films are negative. These tests will also help in the diagnosis of cases of transfusion-transmitted malaria with persistently negative blood films (CDC, 1983).

Prevention of transfusion malaria in malarious countries

In countries such as Nigeria, Zambia and Papua New Guinea, where up to 10% of donors have plasmodia detectable by simple microscopy, the contribution of blood transfusion to the overall problem of the transmission of malaria is negligible. In such countries, the transmission of malaria to the recipient can be prevented by giving anti-malarial treatment to donor or recipient.

Officer (1945) injected blood containing some 300 million malaria parasites into each of five healthy volunteers. All volunteers were given anti-malarial treatment after transfusion and none developed malaria.

Prophylactic treatment of donors with chloroquine seems to be effective in preventing the transmission of malaria but must be given for at least 48 h before donation. Alternatively, a single dose of chloroquine (up to 1500 mg) may be given orally to the recipient 24 h before, or immediately after, transfusion. Ideally, further doses of at least 300 mg per week should be given for 1 month (see reviews by Bruce-Chwatt, 1974; 1985). Unfortunately, due to the emergence of chloroquine-resistant strains of *P. falciparum*, treatment of donors or recipients with chloroquine is not as successful as it used to be and sulfadoxine with pyrimethamine or mefloquine have to be used in addition to chloroquine for subjects (excluding children and pregnant women) from areas of chloroquine resistance (PHLS Malaria Ref. Lab., 1983). It has been suggested that a single-dose treatment of recipients with quinghaosu, the extract of *Artemisia annua*, might be effective in areas of resistant malaria (see Wells and Ala, 1985). Since transfusion-induced malaria does not involve extra-erythrocytic stages, it does not relapse after appropriate treatment (Bruce-Chwatt, 1985). It has been suggested that the addition of chloroquine to the anticoagulant in the collection bag to a final concentration of 20–50 mg/l would eliminate even resistant strains of *P. falciparum* (White, 1987).

TRYPANOSOMA CRUZI

In Latin America, where 16–18 million people are infected with *T. cruzi*, blood transfusion is a frequent cause of the transmission of Chagas' disease. Infection is prevalent in poor rural areas with mud huts and thatched roofs, where it is transmitted to humans, usually in childhood, by triatomid bugs. The second most important mode of transmission is by blood transfusion. Treatment of acute infection cures 50–90% of patients but most acute infections are subclinical and untreated individuals remain infected throughout life. Depending on the country, between 5% and 40% of untreated patients may develop serious chronic complications such as cardiomyopathy, megaoesophagus, megacolon, etc., 10 or more years after infection (Marsden, 1984; Schmuñis, 1991).

In chronic infection, antibodies can be detected by complement fixation, direct or indirect haemagglutination, immunofluorescence or ELISA (see Schmuñis, 1991). ELISA appears to be more sensitive than indirect immunofluorescence and haemagglutination (Magnaval *et al.* 1985). Although tests for antibody are positive in about 95% of chronic cases and in 50% of acute cases, they are often negative during the first few months of infection (see Wolfe, 1975). At least 50% of those infected have parasitaemia and are thus likely to be able to transmit infection by blood transfusion (Cerisola *et al.* 1972). Parasitaemia is diagnosed by allowing triatomid bugs to suck the patient's blood and then examining the insects for infestation ('xenodiagnosis'). Most Latin American countries test part, but not all, of their blood donations for *T. cruzi* antibodies; the frequency of a positive test amongst donors varies from about 0.3% to 28% and is as high as 62% in parts of Bolivia (see Schmuñis, 1991). Due to migration to urban areas and to the existence of paid donors, antibody-positive donors are often found in cities with no vectors. When blood from an antibody-positive donor is transfused, the incidence of infection in recipients is between 12% and 18% and can be as high as 50% (Schmuñis, 1991). The parasites of Chagas' disease survive well in stored blood, and blood stored for over 10 d can still be infectious (Cerisola *et al.* 1972). *T. cruzi* can be transmitted by plasma as well as by whole blood; the parasite survives in plasma which has been frozen at –20°C for 24 h but it does not resist lyophilization (see Schmuñis, 1991; Wendel and Gonzaga, 1992). The addition of 125 mg of crystal (gentian) violet to a unit of stored blood kills the parasites after storage at 4°C for 24 h without damaging the red cells. Blood treated with gentian violet causes no obvious toxic reaction in the recipient but it can cause minor side-effects and rouleaux formation of the red cells. Artificial light and sodium ascorbate accelerate the effect and reduce the dose of gentian violet required to kill the parasites. Gentian violet has been reported to have mutagenic effects *in vitro* (for references see Schmuñis, 1991; Wendel and Gonzaga, 1992). Several antibiotics (e.g. amphotericin B tetracycline derivatives) are known to kill *T. cruzi* in blood but their application to blood transfusion needs to be tested (Hammond *et al.* 1984).

Migration from Latin America is mainly to North America; it has been estimated that there are 100 000 people infected with *T. cruzi* living in the USA. Chagas' disease acquired by blood transfusion has been reported in the USA and Canada (see Schmuñis, 1991). In countries non-endemic for Chagas' disease, prospective donors who have lived in poor rural areas in Latin America should be debarred from donation, unless shown to be negative for *T. cruzi* antibodies.

Other parasites

Toxoplasma gondii

There is a wide geographical variation in the prevalence of toxoplasma antibodies amongst blood donors: in the USA 20–80% may be antibody positive and, of these, about 18% have IgM anti-toxoplasma, a marker of active infection. *T. gondii* has been isolated from donors' blood up to 4 years after the onset of infection; entry of parasites into the blood occurs for only a few weeks but since *T. gondii* is an obligate intracellular parasite it persists in the white cells for a long time; it can survive storage at 4°C for 4–7 weeks (see Tabor, 1982).

Leucocyte transfusions from donors with high levels of toxoplasma antibodies, sometimes partly IgM, have transmitted severe acute toxoplasmosis to immunosuppressed patients (Siegel *et al.* 1971; see also Tabor, 1982). The prevalence of toxoplasma antibodies was found to be six times higher in multi-transfused thalassaemic patients than in an age-matched control population; in another study antibodies were not found more commonly in transfused thalassaemic patients (see Tabor, 1982). Since the risk of severe transfusion-acquired toxoplasmosis is confined to immunosuppressed patients transfused with leucocyte concentrates, it seems appropriate to collect leucocytes only from donors without toxoplasma antibodies. A panel of donors negative for toxoplasma antibodies is available at the North London Blood Transfusion Centre for leucapheresis and for the provision of granulocyte concentrates for premature babies.

Babesia microti

This tick-borne protozoan is limited to the north-eastern coast of the USA, Wisconsin and Minnesota. The parasite survives for more than 14 d in stored blood. The appearances in blood films resemble those of malaria. The diagnosis is confirmed by testing for babesia antibodies and by inoculation of hamsters with the patient's blood. Although the disease is normally mild and frequently asymptomatic, in splenectomized or immunosuppressed subjects it is usually rapidly fatal. In two splenectomized patients infected by transfusion (one by a platelet concentrate from an infected subject), exchange transfusion, using whole blood, brought about control of the condition (Jacoby *et al.* 1980; Cahill *et al.* 1981). Exchange transfusion is not always effective but the combination of clindamycin and quinine seems to eradicate the parasite from most immunosuppressed patients (Smith *et al.* 1986). It has been recommended that subjects from endemic areas who have had a recent febrile illness or those with high levels of babesia antibodies should be excluded from blood donation (see Bruce-Chwatt, 1985).

Microfilariae

Microfilariae of five common species have been shown to persist in the circulation of infected subjects for years and to survive in stored blood (*Wuchereria bancrofti* can survive for 3 weeks); hence microfilariae can be transmitted to transfusion recipients. Three varieties of filariae can cause disease in humans: *Brugia malayi* in South-East Asia, *Loa loa* in Africa and *W. bancrofti* in southern Asia, tropical Africa and some tropical areas of Latin America. However, blood transfusion-transmitted microfilariae never reach the adult stage in non-endemic areas because of the absence of the vector insect necessary for the second passage to humans. Recipients of infected blood usually have no symptoms although they may occasionally experience acute inflammation of the spleen, lymph nodes or lungs, sometimes with tropical pulmonary eosinophilia; alternatively, they may develop fever, headache and rash as a hypersensitivity response to the dead microfilariae. Signs and symptoms are self-limited and so is the survival of microfilariae in transfusion recipients (see Tabor, 1982; Westphal, 1991b).

Leishmaniasis

Visceral leishmaniasis or kala-azar is caused by *Leishmania donovani* and transmitted by the bite of sand-flies in China, India and the eastern Mediterranean. The leishmania multiplies in the mononuclear phagocyte system and clinical disease transmitted by blood transfusion has been reported in transplant recipients and in newborn infants. When present in blood, the parasite has been found in large mononuclear cells and granulocytes (for details, see Shulman and Appleman, 1990).

African trypanosomiasis (sleeping sickness) has rarely been transmitted by transfusion; references are given by Wolfe (1975) and Tabor (1982).

APPENDICES

TABLE

APPENDIX 1

Preparation of platelet concentrates

From platelet-rich plasma (PRP)

The method used at the North London Blood Transfusion Centre (Valerie Mijovic, personal communication), which yields $0.72 \pm 0.3 \times 10^{11}$ platelets per concentrate with minimal lymphocyte and granulocyte contamination ($0.032 \pm 0.02 \times 10^9$ and $0.009 \pm 0.004 \times 10^9$ cells, respectively), is as follows: blood is collected into Fenwal multi-unit (triple) bags containing the normal amount of CPD-A. The bags are centrifuged at $1611\,g$ for 3 min; the PRP is transferred into a plastic satellite bag (PL-146 for 3 days' storage or PL-732 for 5–7 days' storage) and is centrifuged at $1850\,g$ for 7 min; the platelet-poor plasma is transferred to the third satellite bag and frozen for issue as fresh-frozen plasma (FFP), leaving 50 ml of residual plasma with the platelets. The platelet concentrate is left undisturbed for 1 h to allow the platelets to disaggregate spontaneously. The platelet pellet is then resuspended in the 50 ml of residual plasma, by gentle manual agitation. The unit of blood is kept at room temperature from the time of collection onwards and all procedures are carried out at room temperature. Constant gentle mixing is essential to maintain viability of platelets stored at 22°C (Slichter and Harker, 1976b).

From buffy coat

The method developed at the Amsterdam Blood Bank, which yields $79 \pm 8\%$ of the platelets, with a leucocyte count in the concentrate of $13 \pm 7 \times 10^6$, is as follows: blood is taken into the collecting bag of a quadruple blood bag system (for example, Terumo, Fenwal, NPBI) with CPD as an anticoagulant. The bag is then stored in a 'cooling unit' containing butane-1,4-diol in such a way that the collecting bag is in contact with the unit. The temperature of the blood is reduced to 22°C in 2 h. The blood is then stored at ambient temperature for 16–20 h, during which time the temperature of the blood remains at 22°C. This storage is important because without it the buffy coat is likely to contain platelet aggregates. The blood is then centrifuged for 10 min at 3600 r.p.m. in a Beckman JFM centrifuge with the shielded six-place JS 4.2 rotor. The plasma is pressed into an empty satellite bag and the buffy coat into the 300 ml bag which is the second in the row of four. The saline-adenine-glucose-mannitol (SAG-M) solution in the fourth bag is then added to the red cells and 30 ml of plasma is returned to the bag containing the buffy coat. The bags with the red cells and the plasma are then detached. The buffy coat is mixed gently with the plasma and once more centrifuged at 22°C for 6 min at 1250 r.p.m. The PRP is then slowly transferred to the bag which originally contained the SAG-M solution. Inserts can be made in the oval cups of the Beckman JGM centrifuge so that four sets of bags can be centrifuged per cup (Pietersz et al. 1987).

APPENDIX 2

Estimation of red cell volume, using ^{99m}Tc, ^{111}In and ^{51}Cr

Although ^{51}Cr has far the lowest rate of elution from red cells, ^{99m}Tc and ^{111}In should be used in preference for estimating red cell volume: first, because of their far lower radiotoxicity, and second, because the rate of elution is not of great importance when samples are being taken over a period of less than 1 h after injecting labelled red cells.

Labelling with ^{99m}Tc
^{99m}Tc-pertechnetate is obtained from a molybdenum generator; ^{99m}Tc has a $T_{1/2}$ of 6.0 h but ^{99}Mo (the generator) has a $T_{1/2}$ of 72 h. Pertechnetate will not bind firmly to red cells (actually, to Hb) unless it is first reduced; labelling is accomplished by first treating the cells with a very small amount of a stannous compound and then incubating the cells with ^{99m}Tc-pertechnetate. In 5 min at room temperature red cells take up approximately 95% of the added ^{99m}Tc (Smith and Richards, 1976). The optimal amount of Sn (as $SnCl_2$) to use with heparinized red cells is 0.02 µg per ml red cells (Jones and Mollison, 1978). This amount can conveniently be added using commercially available vials (Technescan PYP, supplied by Amersham International). These vials contain 3.4 mg $SnCl_2$ (with pyrophosphate) in 5 ml saline; 1 ml of the solution is added to 500 ml saline; addition of 0.1 ml of the diluted solution to red cells from 10 ml heparinized blood gives the required ratio of tin to red cells. The red cells should be washed once in saline before being incubated for 5 min with the tin. Alternatively, red cells can be treated with tin *in vivo* by injecting an ampoule of the stannous compound 30 min before withdrawing a sample of red cells for labelling with ^{99m}Tc.

Red cells which have been treated with tin are incubated at room temperature with 25 µCi (0.9 MBq) ^{99m}Tc, then washed once in saline before being made up to a convenient volume (e.g. 20 ml) for injection. They should be kept on ice until injected. (For further details, see Jones and Mollison, 1978; ICSH, 1980c.)

The loss of ^{99m}Tc from the red cells during the 60 min after reinjection into the circulation has been found to be about 4% (Smith and Richards, 1976; Jones and Mollison, 1978); variable loss rates have been reported in the first 24 h, e.g. about 50% (Atkins et al. 1985), 33% (Holt et al. 1983) and about 23% as judged by the ratio of ^{99m}Tc to ^{51}Cr in surviving red cells (Marcus et al. 1987).

Labelling with ^{111}In

^{111}In has a $T_{1/2}$ of 2.8 d. For red cell labelling a chelating agent must be used: oxine, acetylacetone and tropolone have been found to be equally suitable (Aubuchon and Brightman, 1989). In 11 subjects in whom red cells were labelled using oxine on one occasion and tropolone on another, with both methods uptake exceeded 96%; during the first 15 min after injection of the labelled cells, there was a loss of 3–4% of the label but there was no further loss at 60 min; loss in the first 24 h was 10–13%.

Details of the tropolone method were as follows: tropolone was dissolved in saline to a concentration 0.1 mg/ml and pH adjusted to 7.4 with 0.1 NaOH. 100 μCi (3.7 MBq) ^{111}InCl$_3$ were mixed with 40 μl of the tropolone solution and allowed to stand for 20 min; 4 ml of red cells were then added and left at room temperature for 20 min. Fifteen millilitres of a mixture of ACD and saline (1 : 7) were added and the cells were separated by centrifugation. After three washings in saline the cells were ready for injection (Aubuchon and Brightman, 1989).

Labelling with ^{51}Cr

Radioactive chromium is obtained as sodium chromate (Na$_2$^{51}CrO$_4$) with a specific activity which may be as high as 200 μCi (7.4 MBq)/μg Cr. It is convenient to dilute the stock in 9 g/l sodium chloride solution and then to put suitable amounts into ampoules which are sealed and autoclaved. ^{51}Cr has a half-life of 27.7 d and if the ampoules are to be used over a period of several weeks the amounts placed in them must be increased to take account of this. For the estimation of red cell volume the amount of ^{51}Cr added should be such that the patient receives no more than 0.2 μCi (7.4kBq)/kg. The amount of ^{51}Cr actually added to the red cells must be greater than this by about 25% since only about 90–95% of the ^{51}Cr will be taken up by the red cells and part of the final suspension must be retained as a standard.

The added Na$_2$^{51}CrO$_4$ should be in a volume of at least 0.2 ml. The amount of red cells labelled should be such that the dose of chromium does not exceed 2 μg/ml red cells.

When Na$_2$^{51}CrO$_4$ is added to blood, the rate of uptake by the red cells is more rapid at pH 6.8–7.0 than at physiological pH (Ebaugh et al. 1953; Mollison, 1961b, p. 63), is approximately three times more rapid at 37°C than at 22°C, and is more rapid when the ^{51}Cr is added to packed red cells than when it is added to the same red cells suspended in their own plasma (Mollison and Veall, 1955). In practice, if the ^{51}Cr is added to packed red cells from ACD blood, uptake will exceed 90% after 15 min at room temperature.

Obtain blood by venepuncture and add 10 ml to 1.5 ml ACD (NIH-A, see Appendix 8). Centrifuge the citrated blood at 1000–1500 g for 5–10 min. Remove and discard the supernatant plasma, taking care not to remove any red cells. However, if the leucocyte count is greater than $25 \times 10^9/l$, also remove and discard the buffy coat. Add the ^{51}Cr sodium chromate solution slowly and with continuous gentle mixing to the packed red cells. Allow the mixture to stand at room temperature for 15 min or place it in a water-bath at 37°C for 10 min. Wash the labelled cells twice in 4–5 volumes of isotonic saline.

Standards

A volume (e.g. 3 ml) of the washed, labelled red cell suspension should be set aside for the preparation of standards; one in 100 dilutions are suitable and should be prepared in duplicate.

Injection of labelled red cells

Several methods of injecting a known amount of cells can be used. For example, a pre-calibrated syringe, known to deliver a certain volume, can be used. Alternatively, the syringe can be weighed before and after injection and the exact volume injected can be calculated as:

$$\frac{\text{weight of suspension injected}}{\text{specific gravity of suspension}}$$

Assuming that packed red cells have an Hb concentration of 34 g/dl and a specific gravity of 1.097, the specific gravity of the suspension can be deduced from the Hb concentration of the suspension as:

$$1.000 + \left[\left(\frac{\text{Hb concentration of suspension (g/dl)}}{(34 \text{ g/dl})}\right) \times (1.097 - 1.000)\right]$$

Blood samples

Normally, a blood sample should be taken about 10 min after injection, but when it is suspected that mixing will not be complete in 10 min, as for example in a patient with gross splenomegaly, the sample should be taken at 60 min instead. Corrections to apply for elution of ^{99m}Tc and ^{111}In can be deduced from data given above; with ^{51}Cr, no correction is necessary since the loss in the first 60 min is not more than 0.5% (Mollison, 1961a).

The packed cell volume (PCV) of the 10- or 60-min sample is determined in duplicate and duplicate volumes (e.g. 2 ml) are pipetted into vials, together with duplicate volumes of each of two dilutions of the standard. Saponin is added to each vial and the samples are counted in a gamma counter; when possible, 10 000 counts are recorded for each sample.

In determining the PCV, the spun haematocrit, preferably using Wintrobe's tubes and applying appropriate corrections for trapped plasma (Chaplin and Mollison, 1952) remains the most accurate method (ICSH, 1980a).

For further details of estimating red cell volume (RCV), see ICSH (1980b,c).

Formula for estimating red cell volume

$$RCV \, (ml) = \frac{\text{total counts injected}}{\text{counts per ml red cells at zero time}}$$

For example, suppose a one in 100 dilution of the injection suspension has a counting rate of 1100 per min and 20 ml of suspension have been injected, so that the total counts injected $= 20 \times 100 \times 1100$, or 2.2×10^6/min, and that a blood sample taken 10 min after injection has a PCV of 0.45 (after correction for trapped plasma) and a counting rate of 460 per min, so that counts per min per ml at zero time are

$$\left(460 \times \frac{100}{45}\right) \times \frac{100}{98.5}, \quad \text{or} \quad 1.04 \times 10^3$$

then

$$RCV = \frac{2.2 \times 10^6}{1.04 \times 10^3} = 2100 \, ml$$

APPENDIX 3

Estimation of plasma volume

Use of ^{125}I-labelled albumin
In preparing a dilution of 'stock' ^{125}I-albumin for injection it is best to add the labelled albumin to a few millilitres (e.g. 7 ml) of heparinized plasma obtained from the subject whose plasma volume is to be estimated. Dilution of labelled albumin in a large volume of saline should be avoided as there would then be a risk of loss of protein by adsorption on to glass surfaces. However, the mixture of labelled albumin and plasma can be diluted with saline to a convenient volume such as 25 ml, of which 20 ml can be injected into an arm vein.

In diluting an aliquot of the injection solution for counting as a standard, the injection solution may either be diluted in saline to which bovine albumin has been added to give a final concentration of at least 0.05% or alternatively may be diluted in saline containing 1% detergent to prevent the adsorption of protein on to glass.

Following injection of the labelled albumin, blood samples should be taken at 10, 20 and 30 min; the concentration of the label at zero time is determined by extrapolating a line fitted to the points (ICSII, 1980c). Plasma volume is given by the expression: total c.p.m. injected (i.e. c.p.m./ml of standard × dilution of standard × volume of labelled albumin injected) divided by c.p.m./ml of recipient's plasma at zero time. There is evidence that in a wide variety of disease states, measurements with labelled albumin overestimate blood volume, presumably due to extra loss of albumin from the circulation (Strumia *et al.* 1968; Valeri *et al.* 1973).

APPENDIX 4

Derivation of blood volume from red cell volume or plasma volume
If the haematocrit (PCV) of blood in peripheral veins (H_v) were representative of the

blood in the whole circulation, blood volume could be derived from RCV as RCV $\times$ 1/H_v and from plasma volume (PV) as PV $\times$ 1/(1 – H_v). In fact, the haematocrit of blood in the whole body, H_B, is lower than H_v, the ratio H_B/H_v being about 0.91 (Chaplin *et al.* 1953). Accordingly, BV = RCV $\times$ 1/($H_v \times$ 0.91) or PV $\times$ 1/(1 –[$H_v \times$ 0.91]).

In subjects with splenomegaly, the ratio H_B/H_v is increased and may exceed 1.1 (Fudenberg *et al.* 1961). For other references, see Mollison *et al.* 1987.

APPENDIX 5

Prediction of normal blood volume from height and weight
Prediction of blood volume from height (H) and weight (W) cannot be highly accurate, partly because no allowance is made for variation in the ratio of fat, with a blood content of 11–22 ml/kg, to lean body mass, with a blood content of 92 ml/kg. The effect of this variation can be reduced by using formulae in which the subject's height is cubed (Allen *et al.* 1956). Slight improvements on predictions from these formulae, obtained by 'computer correction' (Nadler *et al.* 1962), were as follows:

$$\text{For men} \qquad BV = 0.3669\,H^3 + 0.03219\,W + 0.6041$$

$$\text{For women} \qquad BV = 0.3561\,H^3 + 0.03308\,W + 0.1833$$

Tables 1a and 1b are based on these formulae which were derived from measurements of plasma volume (using ^{131}I-labelled albumin) and haematocrit on 92 men and 63 women. The standard error of estimates was found to be about 0.4 litres. Similarly, in a series in which the BV of 38 men was deduced from RCV (estimated with ^{51}Cr) and compared with the values obtained by Nadler *et al.*, the standard deviation of the estimates was 0.5 litres (Mollison, 1972a, p. 86). In one obese subject, measured BV was more than 1 litre less than the predicted value and in one muscular subject was 1 litre more than the predicted value.

APPENDIX 6

Estimation of red cell survival using [51]Cr

Autologous or presumably compatible allogeneic red cells
Red cells are labelled exactly as described in Appendix 2 except that the amount of ^{51}Cr must be increased, e.g. when survival is to be followed for as long as a month, about 0.8 μCi (30 kBq)/kg will be needed.

Blood samples should be taken at 10 min and 24 h, and three further samples should be taken between days 2 and 7; thereafter, at least two further samples should be taken each week for the duration of the study.

Interpretation of results. Uncorrected Cr results, as counts/g Hb or counts/ml red cells, should first be plotted on semi-logarithmic paper and a straight line fitted to them by eye so as to determine the $T_{50}Cr$. (Strictly speaking, the points cannot be fitted by a straight line since the disappearance curve is not an exponential (see Chapter 9), but for the present purpose the error is not serious.) If the $T_{50}Cr$ is within normal

Table 1(a)   Table of predicted normal blood volumes in men (from Nadler *et al.* 1962)

Weight		Height							
		1.52	1.58	1.63	1.68	1.73	1.78	1.83	1.88 (m)
(kg)	(lb)	60	62	64	66	68	70	72	74 (in)
45.4	100	3365	3500	3643	3795	3957	4129	4311	4503
49.9	110	3512	3646	3789	3941	4103	4275	4457	4649
54.5	120	3658	3792	3935	4088	4250	4422	4603	4796
59.0	130	3804	3938	4082	4234	4396	4658	4750	4942
63.5	140	3951	4085	4228	4380	4542	4714	4896	5088
68.0	150	4097	4231	4374	4527	4689	4860	5042	5235
72.5	160	4243	4377	4521	4673	4835	5007	5189	5381
77.0	170	4389	4524	4667	4819	4981	5153	5335	5527
81.6	180	4536	4670	4813	4966	5128	5299	5481	5673
86.2	190	4682	4816	4959	5112	5274	5446	5627	5820
90.7	200	4828	4963	5106	5258	5420	5592	5774	5966
95.3	210	4975	5109	5252	5405	5566	5738	5920	6112
99.8	220	5121	5255	5398	5551	5713	5885	6066	6295
103.4	230	5267	5402	5545	5697	5859	6031	6213	6405
108.9	240	5414	5548	5692	5843	6005	6177	6359	6551
113.4	250	5560	5694	5837	5990	6152	6323	6505	6698
118.0	260	5706	5840	5984	6136	6298	6470	6652	6844
122.5	270	5852	5987	6130	6282	6444	6616	6798	6990
127.0	280	5999	6133	6276	6429	6591	6762	6944	7136
131.6	290	6145	6279	6423	6575	6737	6909	7091	7283
136.1	300	6291	6426	6569	6721	6883	7055	7237	7429
140.6	310	6438	6572	6715	6868	7030	7201	7383	7575

limits, i.e. about 25–37 d, the interpretation is that red cell survival has not been shown to be abnormal and nothing further should be done. If the $T_{50}Cr$ is less than 25 d the estimates are corrected for Cr elution using the correction values given in Table 9.1 on p. 384. The values are now plotted on semi-logarithmic and linear graph paper and the best straight-line fits determined by a least-squares fitting procedure. When the best fit is obtained with a semi-logarithmic plot, mean red cell life span is given by the time taken for survival to fall to 37%. When the best fit is obtained with a linear plot, mean life span is given by the point at which the line cuts the time axis (Dornhorst, 1951). If it is not obvious by simple inspection which plot gives the best fit, a statistical fitting criterion can be applied to decide which one to use. If the data are not fitted well on either a semi-logarithmic or a linear plot, one can use only the first few points, plotted on linear paper, to obtain the initial slope (ICSH, 1971).

Estimation of survival of red cells known to be, or suspected of being, incompatible
As described in Chapter 10, when an estimate of the survival of incompatible red cells is being made, and red cell volume is not determined using a second red cell label, the

Table 1(b). Table of predicted normal blood volumes in women (from Nadler *et al.* 1962)

Weight		Height							
		1.52	1.58	1.63	1.68	1.73	1.78	1.83	1.88 (m)
(kg)	(lb)	60	62	64	66	68	70	72	74 (in)
36.2	80	2646	2776	2915	3036	3220	3387	3564	3750
40.8	90	2796	2927	3066	3214	3371	7537	3714	3901
45.4	100	2947	3077	3216	3364	3521	3688	3864	4052
49.9	110	3097	3227	3366	3514	3671	3838	4015	4201
54.5	120	3247	3378	3517	3665	3822	3989	4165	4352
59.0	130	3398	3528	3667	3815	3972	4139	4315	4502
63.5	140	3548	3678	3817	3695	4123	4289	4466	4652
68.0	150	3698	3829	3968	4116	4273	4440	4616	4803
72.5	160	3849	3979	4118	4266	4423	4590	4766	4953
77.0	170	3999	4129	4268	4416	4574	4740	4917	5103
81.6	180	4150	4280	4419	4567	4724	4891	5067	5254
86.2	190	4300	4430	4569	4717	4874	5041	5217	5404
90.7	220	4450	4581	4719	4867	5025	5191	5368	5554
95.3	210	4601	4731	4870	5018	5175	5342	5518	5705
99.8	220	4751	4881	5020	5168	5325	5492	5669	5855
103.4	230	4901	5032	5171	5318	5476	5642	5819	6005
108.9	240	5052	5182	5321	5469	5626	5793	5969	6156
113.4	250	5202	5332	5471	5619	5776	5943	6120	6306
118.0	260	5352	5483	5622	5770	5927	6093	6270	6457
122.5	270	5503	5633	5772	5920	6077	6244	6420	6607
127.0	280	5653	5783	5922	6070	6227	6394	6571	6757
131.6	290	5803	5934	6073	6221	6378	6544	6721	6908

first sample should be taken at 3 min and further samples should be taken at suitable intervals (see p. 438 and pp. 479–480).

APPENDIX 7

Red cell survival methods based on antigenic differences between donor and recipient

Differential agglutination or haemolysis
When transfused red cells are present in the circulation of a recipient it may be possible to recognize them serologically either: (1) indirectly, i.e. by their failure to be agglutinated by a serum which agglutinates the recipient's red cells (e.g. when group O red cells have been transfused to a group A recipient they may be recognized by their failure to be agglutinated by anti-A); or (2) directly, i.e. by their being agglutinated by a serum that fails to agglutinate the recipient's red cells (e.g. when group M red cells have been transfused to a group N recipient they may be recognized by their reaction with anti-M serum).

Indirect differential agglutination. If quantitative estimates are required, agglutination of the recipient's red cells must be virtually complete; the number of cells remaining unagglutinated should not exceed $10 \times 10^9/l$. The importance of using potent antisera cannot be overstated.

Technique of indirect differential agglutination. (Based on Dacie and Mollison, 1943.) One volume (approximately 0.2 ml) of a one in 50 dilution of blood is mixed with 1 volume of antiserum in a small test tube. The mixture is left at room temperature for about 1 h and then centrifuged (150 g) for 1 min to pack the cells. The tube is tapped to break up the agglutinated mass into a few fragments. The process of centrifugation and resuspension is repeated once or twice more. Then, after waiting a few moments for the large agglutinates to settle to the bottom of the tube, a drop of the supernatant suspension is transferred to a haemocytometer for counting. Provided that really good agglutination is obtained, as indicated by a pre-transfusion count of 10×10^9 unagglu-tinated cells or less per litre, the error of the method is determined mainly by the number of red cells counted; for further details see Mollison (1961b, p. 140).

The use of the AutoAnalyzer for quantitative differential agglutination was de-scribed by Szymanski *et al.* (1968).

Indirect differential haemolysis. Potent haemolytic anti-A or anti-B sera can be used to produce virtually complete lysis of A or B red cells and the unhaemolysed cells can then be counted as in differential agglutination. Alternatively, the unhaemolysed cells can be washed free of Hb and the remaining cells then lysed with distilled water, following which the amount of Hb can be determined photometrically. In the technique described by Mayer and D'Amaro (1964), 0.05 ml of the recipient's blood is mixed with 0.5 ml anti-A (from a group O subject previously immunized with hog A substance) and 0.5 ml of fresh O serum is added as a source of complement. After incubating the mixture at 37°C for 30 min the unhaemolysed red cells (group O) are washed four times in saline and then lysed and estimated as cyanmethaemoglobin.

Direct differential agglutination. Recognition of the survival of foreign red cells by directly agglutinating them, using a serum which does not react with the recipient's own red cells, is valuable chiefly in the investigation of suspected incompatibility. For example, usc may be made of chance differences in MN group between donor and recipient and it may then be possible to say whether or not the circulation of the recipient contains a considerable proportion of transfused cells. This method was used by Wiener and Peters (1940) in investigating the first cases in which anti-Rh D was identified as a cause of incompatibility in blood transfusion. The technique is the same as that of the indirect method until the point is reached where a drop of the mixture has to be placed on the red cell counting chamber. At this point it is important to obtain a representa-tive drop of free cells and clumps, rather than to try, as in the indirect method, to avoid taking up any clumps. If moderate or large agglutinates are present, their number and size can be assessed and recorded, e.g. 'scattered clumps of 20 to 30 cells'. By comparing the appearances with mixtures containing known proportions of agglutin-able cells, semi-quantitative results can be obtained. With potent antisera, 'foreign' red cells can be detected when they comprise only 0.5% of the total number present.

The indirect antiglobulin test can be used for the direct identification of Rh D-positive red cells in the circulation of a D-negative subject; a suspension of red cells is incubated with anti-D and the cells are then washed and mixed with antiglobulin serum. D-positive red cells can be detected when they constitute not less than 0.3–1.0% of the total population.

The mixed antiglobulin reaction was used by Jones and Silver (1958) to detect a very small proportion of foreign red cells which they referred to as the 'minor population'. The technique which they recommended was as follows: approximately 0.25 ml of a suspension of D-negative red cells containing one in 10 000 or less D-positive red cells is incubated for 30 min with anti-D; the cells are then washed four times and incubated for 5 min with 0.25 ml of antiglobulin serum; the cells are washed again four times, then mixed with washed, D-sensitized ('detector') red cells and finally examined for the presence of agglutinates. A modification of this method (rosetting test) is described on p. 548.

Combined indirect and direct method using ^{51}Cr

The following method has been used for obtaining quantitative estimates of the survival of group A red cells inadvertently transfused to a group O recipient (see Fig. 11.7 on p. 530). The method could also be used to obtain quantitative estimates of the survival of group O red cells transfused to a group A (or B) recipient.

Red cells from 0.1 ml blood are labelled with 20 μCi (0.7 MBq) ^{51}Cr; saline is added to the washed, labelled cells to provide an approximately 2% suspension. The following mixtures are prepared in vials suitable for counting in a gamma counter, using potent anti-A and suitably diluted (e.g. 1 in 5) guinea-pig serum as complement:

1 *Test.* 0.5 ml cell suspension + 0.5 ml anti-A + 0.1 ml complement.
2 *One hundred per cent lysis.* 0.5 ml cell suspension + 0.6 ml distilled water + 'pinch' of dry saponin.
3 *Blank.* 0.5 ml cell suspension + 0.5 ml EDTA-treated anti-A + 0.1 ml EDTA-treated complement.
4 *Control of anti-A potency.* 0.5 ml 2% ^{51}Cr-labelled A cells + 0.5 ml anti- A + 0.1 ml complement.

The tubes are incubated at 37°C for 30 min, then mixed and centrifuged. The supernatants are taken off as completely as possible, transferred to counting vials and counted together with the cell residues. The percentage of A cells (as Hb) in (1) is given by (counts in supernatant of (1) – counts in supernatant of (3)) divided by (counts in (2)). The percentage of O cells present in (1) is given by (counts in cell residue of (1)) divided by (counts in (2)). In (4), virtually all counts (99% or more) should be in the supernatant.

APPENDIX 8

Solutions for red cell preservation

Citrate–phosphate–dextrose (CPD)

Trisodium citrate (dihydrate)	26.30 g
Citric acid (monohydrate)	3.27 g
Sodium dihydrogen phosphate (monohydrate)	2.22 g
Dextrose (monohydrate)	25.50 g
Water to	1 litre

Sixty-three millilitres of this solution (pH 5.6–5.8) are mixed with 450 ml whole blood (or, at some centres, with 420 ml). (This solution is almost identical to 'CPD 5' of Gibson *et al.* 1957.)

Citrate–phosphate–dextrose–adenine (CPDA-1)

Trisodium citrate (dihydrate)	26.30 g
Citric acid (monohydrate)	3.27 g
Sodium dihydrogen phosphate (monohydrate)	2.22 g
Dextrose (monohydrate)	31.8 g
Adenine	0.275 g
Water to	1 litre

14 ml to be added to each 100 ml blood.

In *CPDA-2* the amount of dextrose is increased to 44.6 g and that of adenine to 0.55 g.

Acid–citrate–dextrose A (ACD A, NIH-A)
The most widely used ACD solution has the following composition:

Trisodium citrate (dihydrate)	22.0 g
Citric acid (monohydrate)	8.0 g
Dextrose (monohydrate)	24.6 g
Water to	1 litre

67.5 ml of this solution (pH 5.0–5.1) are mixed with 450 ml of blood.

ACD B (NIH-B)
This solution is sometimes used in plasma exchange (see Chapter 1):

Trisodium citrate (dihydrate)	13.2 g
Citric acid (monohydrate)	4.8 g
Dextrose	14.7 g
Water to	1 litre

Saline–adenine–glucose–mannitol (SAGM)

Sodium chloride	8.77 g
Dextrose (monohydrate)	8.99 g
Adenine	0.169 g
Mannitol	5.25 g
Water to	1 litre

100 ml of this solution (pH 5.7) are added to packed red cells (approximately 200 ml) from 450 ml blood.

Adenine–dextrose solution (Adsol)

Sodium chloride	9.0 g
Dextrose (monohydrate)	22.0 g
Adenine	0.27 g
Mannitol	7.5 g
Water to	1 litre

100 ml of this solution (pH 5.6) are added to packed red cells (approximately 200 ml) from 450 ml blood.

Glycerol solutions for storage of red cells (slow freezing)

Storage for later transfusion. A standard CPD unit of blood, stored at 4°C for not more than 5 d, is centrifuged at 3630 g for 10 min; plasma is squeezed out of the bag, the bag is weighed and the net weight of red cells deduced. With continuous mixing an appropriate volume of a solution containing 6.2 mmol/l glycerol is added in stages (e.g. 300 ml when the weight of packed red cells is 151–230 g). The bag is centrifuged, the supernatant is expressed and the red cells then stored at -80°C. When needed, the unit is thawed in a water-bath at 37°C and the red cells washed free of glycerol, using a Haemonetics Model 115 cell washer or similar instrument; (slightly modified from Valeri *et al.* 1981b).

Storage for blood grouping tests. A convenient solution is 'glycigel', which is made up as follows: 62.9 ml glycerol are placed in a graduated cylinder and distilled water is added to 100 ml. After adding 0.9 g NaCl, the solution is warmed; 2.5 g gelatin are then added and warming continued until the gelatin has liquefied. After adding 0.3 g EDTA, 0.25–1.0 ml quantities are placed in 2 ml evacuated blood sample tubes and the tubes stored at 1–6°C. For storage, an equal volume of washed red cells is added to a volume of glycigel. For other details see Chapter 8.

Removal of glycerol by washing in hypertonic solutions. Red cells which have been equilibrated with about 3.0 mol/l glycerol (approximately 30% w/v) are first centriguged and the supernatant discarded. The red cells are then washed first in 12% v/v glycerol in 5% trisodium citrate, then in 5% v/v glycerol in 5% trisodium citrate, and finally in saline (MacDonald and Marsh, 1958). This method gives too much lysis if the red cells have been stored with glycerol concentrations of the order of 4.5 mol/l. For such cells the following method has been used successfully:

The red cells are first washed in 10% (v/v) glycerol in 5% trisodium citrate, then in 1.6% (v/v) glycerol in 5% trisodium citrate, and finally in saline. There should be very little lysis at any stage, provided that the solutions used are buffered to about pH 7.

Removal of glycerol by dialysis. A convenient method is to place a few millilitres of the thawed glycerolized red cells in a length of dialysis tubing and then place the tubing in saline for 30–60 min (Weiner, 1961). Lysis can be minimized by dialysis against a citrate–phosphate solution (e.g. the one described by Mollison *et al.* 1958), rather than saline and, after dialysis, giving the cells one wash in citrate–phosphate before washing them in saline. Provided that dialysis is allowed to continue for 60 min and the concentration of glycerol in the original red cell mixture does not exceed 30% (w/v), there should be very little lysis.

Glycerol solutions for storage of red cells (rapid freezing)

Storage for later transfusion. In the method described by Krijnen *et al.* (1968), red cells and plasma are first separated and the plasma is frozen or freeze-dried. The packed red cells are then mixed with a glycerol–sorbitol–saline solution giving a final glycerol concentration of about 20% w/v, transferred to a stainless steel container and frozen in 2.5–3.0 min by placing the container in liquid nitrogen. The cells are rapidly thawed in a water-bath at 40°C and washed, in a final suspension volume of 500 ml, first with a solution containing 160 g sorbitol and 8 g NaCl/l, and then twice with 9 g NaCl/l; the cells can then be resuspended in their original plasma.

Storage for blood grouping tests. Glycerolized red cells prepared as above may be aspirated into special PVC straws, 135 mm long, 4 mm in diameter, capacity about 1.5 ml, as described by Bouilenne *et al.* (1965). The filled straws are placed in a Union Carbide-3-2-biological freezer and cooled at the maximum rate. A faster cooling rate obtained by plunging the straws directly into liquid nitrogen gives very poor results. If a special freezer is not available, the cooling rate can be reduced by placing the straws on a piece of styrofoam floating on liquid nitrogen. The blood samples are thawed by shaking them manually in a water-bath kept at 37°C. Glycerol is removed as described in the preceding paragraph (Krijnen *et al.* 1968).

A method that is convenient when large volumes of red cells are needed to provide cell panels is described briefly in Chapter 8.

APPENDIX 9

Acid-elution method for the detection of fetal red cells
(Betke and Kleihauer, 1958)
From whole fresh blood, mixed with anticoagulant, spread ordinary films on glass slides and allow them to dry in air for not longer than 60 min. Fix the films in 80%

ethanol for 5 min. Rinse with tap water and dry. (The films can be left at this stage for up to 2 d in a refrigerator.)

The films are now placed in the following buffer:

$$26.6 \text{ ml } 0.2 \text{ mol/l } Na_2HPO_4$$
$$73.4 \text{ ml } 0.1 \text{ mol/l citric acid}$$

In making up the buffer, anhydrous Na_2HPO_4 should be used; the final pH should be 3.3.

The buffer must be warmed to 37°C before the slides are put (vertically) into it; the slides should be moved up and down from time to time; 15 min should be allowed for elution. The slides are now washed in tap water, stained with acid haematoxylin for 3 min and finally with erythrosine (0.3% solution in water) for 30 sec.

For variations of the original method, see Sebring (1984).

Quantitation

Apart from research purposes, quantitative estimates of transplacental haemorrhage (TPH) are required in two circumstances: first, in screening the blood of D-negative women to detect a TPH that is believed to be too large to be covered by the prophylactic dose of anti-D which is being administered and, second, in cases in which a relatively large TPH is detected, to provide an estimate of the size of the TPH and thus determine the dose of anti-D which may be expected to suppress Rh D immunization.

In making quantitative estimates of the size of TPH by the acid-elution method, the density of red cells on the film which is being scanned must be known, i.e. the average number of red cells in a given area. Each laboratory can determine this for itself by counting the average number of adult red cells per high-power field and determining the area of the high-power field from the expression πr^2, r being determined by means of a micrometer scale placed on the stage of a microscope. In one survey (Mollison, 1972b) the density was found to vary from 1.2 to 13.4×10^3 cells per mm^2; it is suggested that a density of $5.0 \times 10^3/mm^2$ should be aimed at.

In order to draw quantitative conclusions from the average number of red cells seen per low-power field, the area of the low-power field must be determined. Again, this is done by reading a micrometer scale under the low power of the microscope to determine 'r'. Most observers have found that a low-power field with an area of approximately 0.8 mm^2 is convenient. When the density of adult red cells is 5000 per mm^2, the number or red cells per low-power field will be 4000.

As discussed in Chapter 12 the size of TPH (as millilitres of fetal red cells) in the mother's circulation can be deduced approximately from the formula:

$$\frac{2400}{\text{number-ratio, adult to fetal red cells}}$$

When the purpose of examining a film for fetal red cells is simply to ensure that not more than a certain number is present, it is evidently unnecessary, when very few cells are seen, to determine the number precisely. As an example, suppose the object is to ensure that the size of TPH does not exceed 4 ml, corresponding to one fetal red cell for every 600 adult cells (see above). Assume that the low-power field usually contains 4000 adult red cells (based on experience of actual counts in the laboratory concerned) but that as a safety factor it is supposed the average number might fall as low as 2400. The average number of fetal red cells expected per low-power field with a TPH of 4 ml is then four. Using tables giving the confidence limits for a Poisson variable (Pearson and Hartley, 1954), the maximum number of cells that can be seen in a given number of low-power fields without arousing the suspicion that the actual number present exceeds an average of four can be determined. For example, if five fields are scanned, the maximum number of cells that can be seen without arousing the suspicion that the average number present is 20 or more is nine at the $P = 0.01$ level and 12 at the 0.05 level (Mollison, 1972b).

APPENDIX 10

Technique of exchange transfusion in newborn infants, using the umbilical vein
The essential equipment required is a plastic catheter, a multi-way tap and a 20 ml syringe (10 ml for a premature infant). The plastic catheter required is one with side openings at its distal end and with a female luer fitting at its proximal end (as originally introduced for intragastric feeding). A commercially available exchange transfusion tray is often used. The multi-way tap makes it possible to draw blood from the infant into the syringe, to discard the blood into a sterile empty vessel, then to draw blood from a donor unit into the syringe and inject this into the infant.

The umbilical vein and surrounding skin are swabbed with disinfectant in the normal way and the area is covered with sterile towels. The umbilicus is cut across about 1.5 cm from the abdominal wall; a clamp should be available in case there is profuse bleeding from the vein. If, as is usual, it does not bleed at all, it can be identified as a large patulous vessel which contrasts with the two smaller, tightly contracted arteries. The wall of the vein is seized with a pair of fine artery forceps and the catheter is introduced into the vein and pushed gently upwards. If it sticks at the level of the abdominal wall it can usually be persuaded to advance by pulling the stump of the cord downwards. When the catheter has been introduced for about 8 cm its advance may be blocked by the wall of the portal arch. By a little manipulation it can usually be persuaded to pass through the ductus venosus and, at about 4″ (10 cm), to enter the vena cava. However, it is not essential to pass a catheter as far as this to carry out an exchange transfusion. Even at a distance of 5–8 cm, a good flow of blood can often be obtained.

After the first 48 h or so of life, it becomes increasingly difficult to pass a catheter into the stump of the umbilical vein because of drying and shrivelling and the formation of clots in the vein. Nevertheless, if the cord is kept covered with a saline dressing it is usually possible to catheterize the umbilical vein at any time during the first week of life.

Other aspects of exchange transfusion are discussed in Chapter 12.

REFERENCES

Order of references

References are arranged alphabetically according to the surname of the first (or only) author, and then by date of publication. The author's initials are not taken into account. Date order applies whatever the number of authors. For example, Allen, T.H. and others (1956) precedes Allen, F.H. (1966).

Page numbers

Last (in addition to first) page numbers are given only for references from 1979 onwards.

AABB (1989) AABB makes recommendations regarding directed donations and graft-versus-host disease. *AABB News Briefs*, **12**, 1–2.

AABB (1990) *Technical Manual*, 10th edn. Amer. Assoc. Blood Banks, Arlington, VA.

AABB (1991) *Standards for Blood Banks and Transfusion Services*, 14th edn. Amer. Assoc. Blood Banks, Arlington, VA.

Aach, R.D., Szmuness, W., Mosley, J.W., Höllinger, F.B., Kahn, R.A., Stevens, C.E., Edwards, Virginia M. and Werch, J. (1981) Serum alanine aminotransferase of donors in relation to the risk of non-A, non-B hepatitis in recipients: the transfusion-transmitted viruses study. *New Engl. J. Med.* **304**, 989–994.

Aach, R.D., Stevens, Cladd, E., Höllinger, F.B., Mosley, J.W., Peterson, D.A., Taylor, Patricia, E., Johnson, Rhonda, G., Barbosa, L.H. and Nemo, G.J. (1991) Hepatitis C virus infection in post-transfusion hepatitis. An analysis with first- and second-generation assays. *New Engl. J. Med.* **325**, 1325–1329.

Aas, K.A. and Gardner, F.H. (1958) Survival of blood platelets labeled with chromium[51]. *J. clin. Invest.* **37**, 1257.

Abbott, D. and Hussain, S. (1970) Intravascular coagulation due to inter-donor incompatibility. *Canad. Med. Assoc. J.* **103**, 752.

Abdalla, S. and Weatherall, D.J. (1982) The direct antiglobulin test in *P. falciparum* malaria. *Brit. J. Haemat.* **51**, 415–425.

Abe, T., Morimoto, C., Toguchi, T., Kiyotaki, M., Takenchi, T., Koide, J., Asakura, H., Tsuchiya, M. and Homma, M. (1983) Functional differences of anti-T-cell antibody in patients with systemic lupus erythematosus and ulcerative colitis. *Scand. J. Immunol.* **18**, 521–530.

Abel, J.J., Rowntree, L.G. and Turner, B.B. (1914) Plasma removal with return of corpuscles. *J. Pharmacol. exp. Ther.* **5**, 625.

Abelson, Neva M. and Rawson, A.J. (1959) Studies of blood group antibodies. II. Fractionation of Rh antibodies by anion-cation cellulose exchange chromatography. *J. Immunol.* **83**, 49.

Abelson, Neva M. and Rawson, A.J. (1961) Studies of blood group antibodies. V. Fractionation of examples of anti-B, anti-A, B, anti-M, anti-P, anti-Jk[a], anti-Le[a], anti-D, anti-CD, anti-K, anti-Fy[a] and anti-Good. *Transfusion*, **1**, 116.

Abilgaard, U. (1984) Biological action and clinical significance of antithrombin III. *Haematologia*, **17**, 77–79.

Ablashi, D.V., Salahuddin, S.Z., Josephs, S.F., Imam, F., Lusso, P., Gallo, R.C., Hung, C., Lemp, J. and Markham, P.D. (1987) HBLV (or HHV-6) in human cell lines (Letter). *Nature (Lond.)*, **329**, 207.

Abrahamsen, A.F. (1970) Survival of ^{51}Cr-labelled autologous and isologous platelets as differential diagnostic aid in thrombocytopenic states. *Scand. J. Haemat.* **7**, 525.

Abramson, N. and Schur, P.H. (1972) The IgG subclasses of red cell antibodies and relationship to monocyte binding. *Blood*, **40**, 500.

Ackerman, B.D., Dyer, Geraldine Y. and Leydorf, Mary M. (1970) Hyperbilirubinemia and kernicterus in small premature infants. *Pediatrics*, **45**, 968.

Ackerman, R. and Terasaki, P. (1974) Capping of granulocyte membrane antigens. *Tissue Antigens*, **4**, 429.

Ackroyd, J.F. (1954) The role of sedormid in the immunological reaction that results in platelet lysis in sedormid purpura. *Clin. Sci.* **13**, 409.

Adams, W.E., Thornton, T.F., Allen, J.G. and Gonzalez, D.E. (1944) Danger and prevention of citrate intoxication in massive transfusions of whole blood. *Ann. Surg.* **120**, 656.

Adams, J., Broviac, M., Brooks, W., Johnson, N.R. and Issitt, P.D. (1971) An antibody, in the serum of a Wr(a +) individual, reacting with an antigen of very high frequency. *Transfusion,* **11**, 290.

Adamson, J. and Hillman, R.S. (1968) Blood volume and plasma protein replacement following acute blood loss in normal man. *J. Amer. med. Assoc.* **205**, 609.

Adinolfi, M., Polley, Margaret J., Hunter, Denise A. and Mollison, P.L. (1962) Classification of blood-group antibodies as β_2M or gamma globulin. *Immunology,* **5**, 566.

Adinolfi, M., Daniels, Christine and Mollison, P.L. (1963) Evidence that 'normal incomplete cold antibody' is not a gamma globulin. *Nature (Lond.),* **199**, 389.

Adinolfi, M. (1965a) Some serological characteristics of the normal incomplete cold antibody. *Immunology,* **9**, 31.

Adinolfi, M. (1965b) Anti-I in normal newborn infants. *Immunology,* **9**, 43.

Adinolfi, A., Mollison, P.L., Polley, Margaret J. and Rose, Jane M. (1966) γA blood group antibodies. *J. exp. Med.* **123**, 951.

Adinolfi, M. and Zenthon, Joanna (1984) Complement in infant and maternal sera. *Reviews in Perinatal Medicine,* **5**, 61–94.

Adinolfi, M. (1986) Recurrent habitual abortion. HLA sharing and deliberate immunization with partner's cells; a controversial topic. *Hum. Reproduction,* **1**, 45–48.

Adler, S.P., Chandrika, T., Lawrence, L. and Baggett, J. (1983) Cytomegalovirus infections in neonates acquired by blood transfusions. *Pediat. infect. Dis.* **2**, 114–118.

Adler, S.P. (1984) International forum: Transfusion transmitted CMV infections. *Vox Sang.* **46**, 387–414.

Adner, P.L. and Sjölin, S. (1957) Unexpected blood group incompatibility revealed by Cr^{51}-labelled red cells. *Scand J Clin. Lab. Invest.* **9**, 265.

Adner, P.L., Foconi, S. and Sjölin, S. (1963) Immunization after intravenous injection of small amounts of ^{51}Cr-labelled red cells. *Brit. J. Haemat.* **9**, 288.

Adner, M.M., Fisch, G.R., Starobin, S.G. and Aster, R.H. (1969) Use of "compatible" platelet transfusion in treatment of congenital isoimmune thrombocytopenic purpura. *New Engl. J. Med.* **280**, 244–247.

Advani, H., Zamor, J., Judd, W.J., Johnson, C.L. and Marsh, W.L. (1982) Inactivation of Kell blood group antigens by 2-amino-ethylisothiouronium bromide. *Brit. J. Haemat.* **51**, 107–115.

Aggeler, P.M., Perkins, H.A. and Watkins, H.B.

(1967) Hypocalcemia and defective hemostasis after massive blood transfusion. Report of a case. *Transfusion,* **7**, 35.

Agote, L. (1915) Nuevo procedimiento para la transfusión de sangre. *An. Inst. Clin. Méd. (B. Aires),* **1**.

Agranenko, V.A. and Maltseva, I.Yu. (1990) Cadaveric blood transfusion. *Transfusion Today,* **5**, 11.

Agre, P. and Cartron, J-P. (1991a) Biochemistry and molecular genetics of Rh antigens, in *Molecular Immunohaematology,* ed A.E.G. Kr. von dem Borne. Baillière's Clinical Haematology, **4**, 793–819.

Agre, P. and Cartron, J-P. (1991b) Molecular biology of the Rh antigens. *Blood,* **78**, 1–5.

Aho, K. and Christian, C.L. (1966) Studies of incomplete antibodies. 1. Effect of papain on red cells. *Blood,* **27**, 662.

Ahmed, K.Y., Nunn, G., Brazier, D.M., Bird, G.W.G. and Crockettt, R.E. (1987) Haemolytic anemia resulting from autoantibodies produced by the donor's lymphocytes after renal transplantation. *Transplantation,* **34**, 163–164.

Ahn, J.H., Rosenfield, R.E. and Kochwa, S. (1987) Low ionic antiglobulin tests. *Transfusion,* **27**, 125–133.

Ahrons, S. (1971) HL-A antibodies: Influence on the human foetus. *Tissue Antigens,* **1**, 129.

Aird, I. and Bentall, H.H. (1953) A relationship between cancer of stomach and the ABO blood groups. *Brit. Med. J.* **i**, 799.

Åkerblom, O., de Verdier, C.-H., Finnson, M., Garby, L., Högman, C.F. and Johansson, S.G.O. (1967) Further studies on the effect of adenine in blood preservation. *Transfusion,* **7**, 1.

Åkerblom, O., de Verdier, C.-H., Garby, L. and Högman, C. (1968) Restoration of defective oxygen-transport function of stored red clood cells by addition of inosine. *Scand. J. Clin. Lab. Invest.* **21**, 245.

Åkerblom, O. and Ericson, Å. (1971) Effects of inosine, pyruvate and inorganic phosphate on the 2, 3 DPG level in fresh and stored erythrocytes. *VIth International Symposium on Structure and Function of Erythrocytes, Berlin,* 1970.

Åkerblom, O. and Kreuger, A. (1975) Studies on citrate-phosphate-dextrose (CPD) blood supplemented with adenine. *Vox Sang.* **29**, 90.

Akeroyd, J.H. and O'Brien, W.A. (1958) Survival of group AB red cells in a group A recipient. *Vox Sang.* **3**, 330.

Albrey, J.A., Vincent, E.E.R., Hutchinson, J., Marsh, W.L., Allen, F.H., Gavin, June and Sanger, Ruth (1971) A new antibody, anti-Fy3, in the Duffy blood group system. *Vox Sang.* **20**, 29–35.

Alderman, E.M., Fudenberg, H.H. and Lovins, R.E. (1980) Binding of immunoglobulin classes to subpopulations of red blood cells separated by density-gradient centrifugation. *Blood*, **55**, 817–822.

Alderman, E.M., Fudenberg, H.H. and Lovins, R.E. (1981) Isolation and characterization of an age-related antigen present on senescent human red blood cells. *Blood*, **58**, 341–349.

Alevi, J.B. and 10 others (1977) A randomized clinical trial of granulocyte transfusions for infection in acute leukemia. *New Engl. J. Med.* **296**, 706.

Al-Jawad, S.T., Keenan, P. and Kholeif, S. (1985) Incidence of ABO haemolytic disease in a mixed Arab population. *Saudi med. J.* **7**, 41–45.

Allain, J.P., Laurian, Y., Paul, Deborah A. and Senn, D. (1986) Serological markers in early stages of human immunodeficiency virus infection in haemophiliacs. *Lancet*, **ii**, 1233–1236.

Allain, J-P., Coghlan, P.J., Kenrick, K.G., Whitson, K., Keller, A., Cooper, G.J., Vallari, D.S., Delaney, S.R. and Kuhns, Mary, C. (1991) Prediction of hepatitis C virus infectivity in seropositive Australian blood donors by supplemental immunoassays and detection of viral RNA. *Blood*, **78**, 2462–2468.

Allan, C.J., Lawrence, R.D., Shih, S.C., Williamson, K.R., Sweat, M.A. and Taswell, H.F. (1972) Agglutination of erythrocytes freshly washed with saline solution. Four saline-auto-agglutinating sera. *Transfusion*, **12**, 306.

Allan, D., Billah, M.M., Finean, J.B. and Michell, R.H. (1976) Release of diacylglycerol-enriched vesicles from erythrocytes with increased intracellular [Ca^{2+}]. *Nature (Lond.)*, **261**, 58.

Allan, J. and Garratty, G. (1980) Positive direct antiglobulin tests in normal blood donors, in *Abstracts, 16th Congr. Int. Soc. Blood Transfus.*, Montreal.

Allan, J.C., Bruce, M. and Mitchell, R. (1990) The preservation of red cell antigens at low ionic strength. *Transfusion*, **30**, 423–426.

Allen, F.H. jr, Diamond, L.K. and Vaughan, V.C. III (1950) Erythroblastosis fetalis. VI. Prevention of kernicterus. *Amer. J. Dis. Child.* **80**, 779.

Allen, F.H. jr, Diamond, L.K. and Niedziela, Bevely (1951) A new blood-group antigen. *Nature (Lond.)*, **167**, 482

Allen, T.H., Peng, M.T., Chen, K.P., Huang, T.F., Chang, C. and Fang, H.S. (1956) Prediction of blood volume and adiposity in man from body weight and cube of height. Prediction of total adiposity from skinfolds and the curvilinear relationship between external and internal adiposity. Similarity of vital capacity in terms of body weight less adiposity in both sexes. *Metabolism*, **5**, 328, 346, 353.

Allen, F.H. jr (1957) Induction of labor in the management of erythroblastosis fetalis. *Quart. Rev. Pediat.* **12**, 1.

Allen, F.H. and Lewis, Sheila J. (1957) Kp^a(Penney), A new antigen in the Kell blood group system. *Vox Sang.* **2**, 81.

Allen, P.Z. and Kabat, E.A. (1958) Persistence of circulating antibodies in human subjects immunized with dextran, levan and blood group substances. *J. Immunol.* **80**, 495.

Allen, F.H. jr and Tippett, P.A. (1958) A new Rh blood type which reveals the Rh antigen G. *Vox Sang.* **3**, 321.

Allen. F.H. and Warshaw, A.L. (1962) Blood group sensitization. A comparison of antigens K1 (Kell) and c (hr'). *Vox Sang.* **7**, 222.

Allen, F.H. jr, Rosenfield, R.E. and Adebahr, Margot E. (1963) Kidd and Duffy blood typings without Coombs serum. Adaptation of the Auto-Analyzer haemagglutination system. *Vox Sang.* **8**, 698.

Allen, J.C. and Kunkel, H.G. (1963) Antibodies to genetic types of gamma globulin after multiple transfusions. *Science*, **139**, 418.

Allen, J.C. and Kunkel, H.G. (1966) Antibodies against γ globulin after repeated blood transfusions in man. *J. clin. Invest.* **45**, 29.

Allen, F.H. jr, Issitt, P., Degnan, T., Jackson, Valerie, Reihart, J., Knowlin, R. and Adebahr, M. (1969) Further observations on the Matuhasi-Ogata phenomenon. *Vox Sang.* **16**, 47.

Alperin, J.B., Riglin, H., Branch, D.R., Gallagher, M.T. and Petz, L.D. (1983) Anti-M causing delayed hemolytic transfusion reaction. *Transfusion*, **23**, 322–324.

Alter, A.A. and Rosenfield, R.E. (1964a) B$_x$: subtype of B. *Blood*, **23**, 600.

Alter, A.A. and Rosenfield, R.E. (1964b) The nature of some subtypes of A. *Blood*, **23**, 605.

Alter, H.J. (1975) Hepatitis B surface antigen and the health care professions, in *Transmissible Disease and Blood Transfusion*, eds T.J. Greenwalt and G.A. Jamieson. Grune & Stratton, New York.

Alter, H.J., Tabor, E., Meryman, H.T., Hoofnagle, J.H., Kahn, R.A., Holland, P.V., Geretyn, R.J. and Barker, L.F. (1978) Transmission of hepatitis B virus infection by transfusion of frozen-deglycerolized red blood cells. *New Engl. J. Med.* **298**, 637.

Alter, H.J., Purcell, R.H., Holland, P.V., Alling, D.W. and Koziol, D.E. (1981) Donor transaminase and recipient hepatitis: impact on blood transfusion services. *J. Amer. med. Assoc.* **246**, 630-634.

Alter, H.J. (1985) Post-transfusion hepatitis: clinical features, risk and donor testing, in *Infection, Immunity and Blood Transfusion*, eds R.Y. Dodd and L.F. Barker, pp. 47–61. A.R. Liss, Inc. New York.

Alter, H.J. (1988) Transfusion-associated non-A,

non-B hepatitis: the first decade, in *Viral Hepatitis and Liver Disease*, ed A.J. Zuckerman, pp. 537–542. Alan R. Liss, New York.

Alter, H.J., Creagan, R.P., Morel, Phyllis, A., Wiesehahn, G.P., Dorman, B.P., Corash, L., Smith, G.C., Popper, H. and Eichberg, J.W. (1988) Photochemical decontamination of blood components containing hepatitis B and non-A, non-B virus. *Lancet*, **ii**, 1446–1450.

Alter, M.J. (1989) Disease transmissions: The relationship of blood transfusion to other modes of transmission, in *Autologous Blood Transfusions. Principles, Policies and Practices*. eds V.D. Fairchild, N.R. Holland and A.R. Lyons, pp. 4–6. American Blood Commission, Alexandria, VA.

Alter, H.J., Purcell, R.G., Shih, J.W., Melpolder, Jacqueline, C., Houghton, M., Choo, Q-L. and Kuo, G. (1989a) Detection of antibody to hepatitis C virus in prospectively followed transfusion recipients with acute and chronic non-A, non-B hepatitis. *New Engl. J. Med.* **321**, 1495–1500.

Alter, H.J., Alter, M., Barbara, J., Colombo, M., Hanson, P., Houghton, M., Krauledat, P., Polito, A. and Tegtmeier, G. (1989b) *Proc. 1st Int. Symp. Hepatitis C Virus*, Rome 1989.

Alter, M.J., Coleman, P.J., Alexander, W.J., Kramer, E., Miller, J.K., Mandel, E., Hadler, S.C. and Margolis, H.S. (1989c) Importance of heterosexual activity in the transmission of hepatitis B and non-A, non-B hepatitis. *J. Amer. med. Assoc.* **262**, 1201–1205.

Alter, H.J. and 12 others (1990) Prevalence of human immunodeficiency virus type 1 p24 antigen in U.S. blood donors — an assessment of the efficacy of testing in donor screening. *New Engl. J. Med.* **323**, 1312–1317.

Altschule, M.D. and Freidberg, A.S. (1945) Circulation and respiration in fever. *Medicine (Baltimore)*, **24**, 403.

Alves de Lima, L.M., Berthier, M.E., Sad, W.E., Dinapoli, J., Johnson, C.L. and Marsh, W.L. (1982) Characterization of an anti-Di^a antibody causing hemolytic disease in a newborn infant. *Transfusion*, **22**, 246–247.

Alving, Barbara M., Hojima, Y., Pisano, J.J., Bobby, L., Mason, M.S., Buckingham, R.E. jr, Milton, M., Mozen, Ph.D. and Finlayson, J.S. (1978) Hypotension associated with prekallikrein activator (Hageman-factor fragments) in plasma protein fraction. *New Engl. J. Med.* **299**, 66.

Alving, Barbara M., Tankersley, D.L., Mason, B.L., Rossi, Françoise, Aronson, D.L. and Finlayson, J.S. (1979) Vasoactive enzymes in immunoglobulin preparations, in *Immunoglobulins: Characteristics and Use of Intravenous Preparations*, eds Barbara M. Alving and J.S.

Finlayson. U.S. Government Printing Office, Washington, D.C.

AMA (American Medical Association) (1973) *General Principles of Blood Transfusion*, revised edn, eds T.J. Greenwalt *et al.* American Medical Association, Chicago.

Amberson, W.R., Flexner, J., Steggarda, F.R., Mulder, A.G., Tendler, M.J., Pankratz, D.S. and Lang, E.P. (1934) On the use of Ringer-Locke solutions containing hemoglobin as a substitute for normal blood in animals. *J. cell. comp. Physiol.* **5**, 359.

Amberson, W.R., Jennings, Joyce, J. and Rhode, C.M. (1949) Clinical experience with hemoglobin-saline solutions. *J. appl. Physiol.* **I**, 469.

Ambriz, R., Muñoz, R., Pizzuto, J., Quintanar, Elisa, Morales, M. and Agustin, A. (1987) Low-dose autologous in vitro opsonised erythrocytes. *Arch. intern. Med.* **147**, 105–108.

Ambrus, M. and Bajtai, G. (1969) A case of an IgG-type cold agglutinin disease. *Haematologia*, **3**, 225.

Ames, A.C. and Lloyd, R.S. (1964) A scheme for the ante-natal prediction of ABO haemolytic disease of the newborn. *Vox Sang.* **9**, 712.

Amman, A.J., Cowan, M.J., Wara, D.M., Weintrub, P., Dritz, S., Goldman, H. and Perkins, H.A. (1983) Acquired immunodeficiency in an infant: possible transmission by means of blood products. *Lancet*, **i**, 956–957.

Anand, Aditi, Gray, Elizabeth S., Brown, T., Clewley, J.P. and Cohen, B.J. (1987) Human parvovirus infection in pregnancy and hydrops fetalis. *New Engl. J. Med.* **316**, 183–186.

Andersen, T. (1936) Über die Ursache der Isohaemagglutinationshemmung in frischem, unverdünnten Seren. *Klin. Wschr.* **15**, 152.

Andersen, J. (1958) Modifying influence of the secretor gene on the development of the ABH substance. *Vox Sang.* **3**, 251.

Andersen, Elsebeth, Bashir, Helen and Archer, G.T. (1981) Modification of the platelet suspension immunofluorescence test. *Vox Sang.* **40**, 44–47.

Anderson, C., Hunter, J., Zipursky, A, Lewis, M. and Chown, B. (1963) An antibody defining a new blood group antigen, Bu^a. *Transfusion*, **3**, 30.

Anderson, B.R. and Terry, W.D. (1968) Gamma G4-globulin antibody causing inhibition of clotting Factor VIII. *Nature (Lond.)*, **217**, 174.

Anderson, R.R., Holliday, R.L., Driedger, A.A., Lefcoe, M., Reid, B. and Sibbald, W.J. (1979) Documentation of pulmonary capillary permeability in the adult respiratory distress syndrome accompanying human sepsis. *Amer. Rev. respir. Dis.* **119**, 869–877.

Anderson, C.B., Sicard, G.A. and Etheredge, E.E. (1982) Pretreatment of renal allograft recipients with azathioprine and donor specific blood products. *Surgery*, **92**, 315–321.

Anderson, M.J., Jones, S.E., Fisher-Hoch, S.P., Lewis, E., Hall, S.M., Bartlett, C.L.R. Cohen, B.J., Mortimer, P.P. and Pereira, M.S. (1983) Human parvovirus, The cause of erythema infectiosum (fifth disease)? *Lancet*, **i**, 1378.

Anderson, H.J., and Patel, S. (1984) Red cell phenotyping using hexadi-methrine bromide (Polybrene) in a microplate system. *Transfusion*, **24**, 353–356.

Anderson, C.B., Tyler, J.D., Sicard, G.A., Anderman, C.K., Rodey, G.E. and Etheredge, E.E. (1985a) Renal allograft recipient pretreatment with immunosuppression and donor-specific blood. *Transplant. Proc.* **17**, 1047–1050.

Anderson, H.J., Aubuchon, J.P., Draper, E.K. and Ballas, S.K. (1985b) Transfusion problems in renal allograft recipients. Anti-lymphocyte globulin showing Lutheran system specificity. *Transfusion*, **25**, 47–50.

Anderson, B.V. and Tomasulo, P.A. (1988) Current autologous transfusion practices. Implication for the future. *Transfusion*, **28**, 394–396.

Anderson, C.L. (1989) Human IgG Fc receptors. *Clin. Immunol. Immunopath.* **53**, S63–71.

Anderson, K.C. and Weinstein, H.J. (1990) Transfusion-associated graft-versus-host disease. *New. Engl. J. Med.* **323**, 315–319.

Anderson, N.A., Tandy, A., Westgate, J., Raymond, S., Kumpel, B., Hadley, A. and Fraser, I.D. (1990) Haemolytic disease of the newborn caused by anti-k (Abstract). *Transfus. Med.* **1**, Suppl. 1, 58.

Anderson, G., Gray, L.S. and Mintz, P.D. (1991a) Red cell survival studies in a patient with anti-Tc^a. *Amer. J. clin. Path.* **95**, 87–90.

Anderson, K.C. Gorgone, Barbara C., Wahlers, Elizabeth, Cook, Jane, Barrett, Barbara and Andersen, Janet (1991b) Preparation and utilization of leukocyte poor apheresis platelets. *Transfus. Sci.* **12**, 163–170.

Andersson, M., Bohme, J., Andersson, C., Moller, E., Thorsby, E., Rask, L. and Peterson, P.A. (1984) Genomic hybridization with class II transplantation antigen cDNA probes as a complementary technique in tissue typing. *Hum. Immunol.* **11**, 57–69.

Andersson, B., Porras, O., Hanson, L.Å., Lagergård, T. and Svanborg-Edén, C. (1986) Inhibition of attachment of *Streptococcus pneumoniae* and *Haemophilus influenzae* by human milk and receptor oligosaccharides. *J. infect Dis.* **153**, 232–237.

Ando, Y., Nakano, S., Saito, K., Shimamoto, I., Ichiko, M., Toyama, T. and Hinuma, Y. (1986) Prevention of HTLV-I transmission through the breast milk by a freeze-drying process. *Jap. J. Cancer Res.* (Gann) **77**, 974–977.

Andorka, D.W., Arosemena, Annette and Harris, J.L. (1974) Neutralization *in vivo* of Lewis antibodies. Report of two cases. *Amer. J. Clin. Path.* **62**, 47.

André, A., Dreyfus, B., Salmon, CH. and Malassenet, R. (1952) Les donneurs universels dangereux. Recherches sur les causes d'immunisation contre l'antigène A. *Rev. Hémat.* **7**, 604.

André, C., Lambert, R., Bazin, H. and Heremans, J.F. (1974) Interference of oral immunization with the intestinal absorption of heterologous albumin. *Eur. J. Immunol.* **4**, 701.

André, C., Heremans, J.F.. Vaerman, J.P. and Cambiaso, C.L. (1975) A mechanism for the induction of immunological tolerance by antigen feeding: antigen–antibody complexes. *J. exp. Med.* **142**, 1509.

Andresen, P.H. (1947) Blood group with characteristic phenotypical aspects. *Acta path. microbiol. scand.* **24**, 616.

Andresen, P.H. (1948) The blood group system L. A new blood group L$_2$. A case of epistasy within the blood groups. *Acta path. microbiol. scand.* **25**, 728.

Andresen, P.H. and Jordal, K. (1949) An incomplete agglutinin related to the L-(Lewis) system. *Acta. path. microbiol. scand.* **26**, 636.

Andresen, P.H. and Henningsen, K. (1951) The Lewis blood group system and the X-system in 5 tables. *Acta haemat. (Basel)*, **5**, 123.

Andreu, C., Doinel, C., Cartron, J.P. and Mativet, S. (1979) Induction of Tk polyagglutination by bacteroides fragilis culture supernatants. Associated modifications of ABH and Ii antigens. *Rev. franç. Transfus. Immunohémat.* **22**, 551–561.

Andreu, G. and 13 others (1988) Prevention of HLA immunization with leucocyte-poor packed cells and platelet concentrates obtained by filtration. *Blood*, **72**, 964–969.

Andreu, G., Boccaccio, C., Lecrubier, C., Fretault, J., Coursaget, J., Leguen, J.P., Oleggini, M., Fournell, J.J. and Samama, M. (1990) Ultraviolet irradiation of platelet concentrates: feasibility in transfusion practice. *Transfusion*, **30**, 401–406.

Andrews, A.T., Zinigewski, C.M., Bowman, H.S. and Reihart, Judith K. (1976) Transfusion reaction with pulmonary infiltration associated with HLA-specific leukocyte antibodies. *Amer. J. clin. Path.* **66**, 483.

Angelini, G., de Preval, C., Gorski, J. and Mach B. (1986) High-resolution analysis of the human HLA-DR polymorphism by hybridization with sequence-specific oligonucleotide probes. *Proc. nat. Acad. Sci. USA*, **83**, 4489–4493.

Angevine, C.D., Andersen, B.R. and Barnett, E.V. (1966) A cold agglutinin of the IgA class *J. Immunol.* **96**, 578.

Anstee, D.J. (1980) Blood group MNSs-active sialoglycoproteins of the human erythrocyte membrane, in *Immunobiology of the Erythrocyte*, eds S.G. Sandler, J. Nusbacher and M.S. Schanfield. *Progress in clinical and biological Research*, **43**, 67–98. Alan R. Liss, New York.

Anstee, D.J. (1981) The blood group MNSs-active sialoglycoproteins. *Semin. Hemat.* **18**, 13–31.

Anstee, D.J., Mawby, W.J. and Tanner, M.J. (1982) Structural variations in human erythrocyte sialoglycoproteins, in *Membranes & Transport, a critical review*, ed A. Martonosi. Plenum Press, New York.

Anstee, D.J., Ridgwell, K., Tanner, M.J.A., Daniels, G.L. and Parsons, S.F. (1984) Individuals lacking the Gerbich blood group antigen have alterations in the human erythrocyte membrane sialoglycoproteins β and γ. *Biochem. J.* **221**, 97–104.

Antin, J.H., Smith, B.R., Holmes, Wendy and Rosenthal, D.S. (1988) Phase I/II study of recombinant human granulocyte-macrophage colony-stimulating factor in aplastic anemia and myelodysplastic syndrome. *Blood*, **72**, 705–713.

Antman, Karen S. and 9 others (1988) Effect of recombinant human granulocyte-macrophage colony-stimulating factor on chemotherapy-induced myelosuppression. *New Engl. J. Med.* **319**, 593–598.

Aoki, N., Naito, K. and Yoshida, N. (1978) Inhibition of platelet aggregation by protease inhibitors. *Blood*, **52**, 1–12.

Arcara, P.C., O'Conner, M.A. and Dimmette, R.M. (1969) A family with three Jk(a – b –) members (Abstract). *Transfusion*, **9**, 282.

Archer, G.T., Cooke, B.R., Mitchell, K. and Parry, P. (1969) Hyper-immunisation des donneurs de sang pour la production des gammaglobulines anti-Rh(D). *Rev. Franç. Transfus.* **12**, 341.

Arcilla, Minerva B. and Sturgeon, P. (1973) Studies on the secretion of blood group substances. II. Observations on the red cell phenotype Le (a – b – x –). *Vox Sang.* **25**, 72.

Arcilla, Minerva B. and Sturgeon, P. (1974) Le^x, the spurned antigen of the Lewis blood group system. *Vox Sang.* **26**, 425.

Argiolu, F., Diana, G., Arnone, M., Batzella, M.G., Piras, P. and Cao, A. (1990) High-dose intravenous immunoglobulin in the management of autoimmune hemolytic anemia complicating thalassemia major. *Acta haemat.* **83**, 65–68.

Arima, T., Shimomura, H., Nakajima, T., Kanai, K., Nagashima, H. and Tsuji, T. (1989) Detection of hepatitis C infection (Abstract 531). *Proc. Int. Symp. on Non-A, Non-B Hepatitis*, Tokyo, p. 55.

Armitage, P. and Mollison, P.L. (1953) Further analysis of controlled trials of treatment of haemolytic disease of the newborn. *J. Obstet. Gynaec. Brit. Emp.* **60**, 605.

Armstrong, R.F., Secker Walker, J, St. Andrew, D., Cobbe, S.M., Lincoln, J.C.R. and Cohen, S. (1978) Continuous monitoring of mixed venous oxygen tension in cardio-respiratory disorders. *Lancet*, **ii**, 632–634.

Armstrong, Sylvia S., Weiner, Edith, Garner, S.F., Urbaniak, S.J. and Contreras, Marcela (1987) Heterogeneity of monoclonal anti-Rh(D): an investigation using ADCC and macrophage binding assays. *Brit J. Haemat.* **66**, 257–262.

Arndt, P. and Garratty, G. (1988) Evaluation of the optimal incubation temperature for detecting certain IgG antibodies with potential clinical significance. *Transfusion*, **28**, 210–213.

Aronson, D.L. and Menache, D. (1987) Thrombogenicity of Factor IX complex: *in vivo* investigation. *Joint IABS CSL Symposium on Standardization in Blood Fractionation including Coagulation Factors*, Melbourne 1986. Div. Biol. Standard, S. Karger, Basel.

Aronstam, A., Arblaster, P.G., Rainsford, S.G., Turk, P., Slattery, M., Alderson, M.R., Hall, D.E. and Kirk, P.J. (1976) Prophylaxis in haemophilia: a double-blind controlled trial. *Brit. J. Haemat.* **33**, 81.

Arturson, G. (1961) Capillary permeability in burned and non-burned areas in dogs. *Acta chir. scand.* Suppl. 274, 55.

Arturson, G. and Westman, M. (1976) Survival of rats subjected to acute anaemia at different levels of erythrocyte 2,3-diphosphoglycerate. *Scand. J. clin. Lab. Invest.* **35**, 745.

Ash, R.C. and 17 others (1990) Successful allogeneic transplantation of T-cell-depleted bone marrow from closely HLA-matched unrelated donors. *New Engl. J. Med.* **322**, 485–494.

Ashby, Winifred (1919) The determination of the length of life of transfused blood corpuscles in man. *J. exp. Med.* **29**, 267.

Aster, R.H. and Jandl, J.H. (1964) Platelet sequestration in man. II. Immunological and clinical studies. *J. clin. Invest.* **43**, 856.

Aster, R.H. (1965) Effect of anticoagulant and ABO incompatibility on recovery of transfused human platelets. *Blood*, **26**, 732.

Aster, R.H. (1966) Pooling of platelets in the spleen: role in the pathogenesis of 'hypersplenic' thrombocytopenia. *J. clin. Path.* **45**, 645.

Astrup, J. and Kornstad, L. (1977) Presence of anti-c in the serum of 42 women giving birth to c positive babies: serological and clinical findings. *Acta obstet. gynec. scand.* **56**, 185.

Atchley, W.A., Bhagavan, N.V. and Masouredis, S.P. (1964) Influence of ionic strength on the reaction between anti-D and D positive red cells. *J. Immunol.* **93**, 701.

Athkabhira, S. and Chiewsilp, P. (1978) Neutralization of Lewis antibodies *in vivo*. *Commun. 17th Congr. Int. Soc. Hemat.*, Paris.

Atichartakarn, V., Chiewsilp, P., Ratanasirivanich P. and Stabunswodgan, S. (1985) Autoimmune haemolytic anemia due to anti-B autoantibody. *Vox Sang.* **49**, 301–303.

Atkins, H.L., Srivastava, S.C., Meinken, G.E. and Richards, P. (1985) Biological behaviour of erythrocytes labelled *in vivo* and *in vitro* with technetium-99m. *J. nucl. Med. Technol.* **13**, 136–139.

Atkinson, J.P. and Frank, M.M. (1974a) Studies on the *in vivo* effects of antibody. Interaction of IgM antibody and complement in the immune clearance and destruction of erythrocytes in man. *J. clin. Invest.* **54**, 339.

Atkinson, J.P. and Frank, M.M. (1974b) Complement-independent clearance of IgG-sensitized erythrocytes: inhibition by cortisone. *Blood*, **44**, 629.

Aubert, E.F., Boorman, Kathleen E. and Dodd, Barbara E. (1942a) The agglutinin-inhibiting substance in human serum. *J. Path. Bact.* **54**, 89.

Aubert, E.F., Boorman, Kathleen E., Dodd, Barbara E. and Loutit, J.F. (1942b) The universal donor with high titre iso-agglutinins; the effect of anti-A iso-agglutinins on recipients of group A. *Brit. med. J.* **i**, 659.

Aubuchon, J.P., Davey, R.J., Estep, T. and Miripol, J. (1984) Effect of the plasticizer di-2-ethylhexyl phthalate on survival of stored red cells (Abstract). *Transfusion*, **24**, 422.

Aubuchon, J.P. and Popovsky, M.A. (1988) Autologous donor safety in non-hospital programs (Abstract). *Transfusion*, **28**, 345.

Aubuchon, J.P. (1989) Autologous transfusion and directed donations: current controversies and future directions. *Transfus. Med. Rev.* **3**, 290–306.

Aubuchon, J.P. and Brightman, A. (1989) Use of Indium-111 as a red cell label. *Transfusion*, **29**, 143–147.

Auerswald, V.W., Bodis-Wollner, I., Kiesewetter, E., Mickerts, D. and Speiser, P. (1967) Zur Frage der Antikörperbildung Erwachsener gegen Gm nach wiederholter parenteraler Zufuhr von homologem Gammaglobulin. *Wien. Med. Wschr.* **117**, 1006.

Auguste, C. (1934) Sur le pouvoir anticomplementaire du sérum humain. *C.R. Soc. Biol. (Paris)*, **116**, 770.

Avent, N.D., Ridgwell, K., Mawby, W.J., Tanner, M.J.A., Anstee, D.J. and Kumpel, B. (1988) Protein-sequence studies of Rh-related polypeptides suggest the presence of at least two groups of proteins which are associated in the human red-cell membrane. *Biochem. J.* **256**, 1043–1046.

Avoy, D.R., Canuel, M.L., Otton, B.M. and Mileski, E.B. (1977) Hemoglobin screening in prospective blood donors: A comparison of methods. *Transfusion*, **17**, 261.

Avoy, D.R., Ellisor, S.S., Nolan, N. Jean, Cox, R.S. jr, Franco, J.A., Harbury, Christina B., Schrier, S.L. and Pool, Judith G. (1978) The effect of delayed refrigeration on red cells, platelet concentrates and cryoprecipitable AHF. *Transfusion*, **18**, 160.

Avoy, D.R., Toy, P., Reid, M.E. and Ellisor, S.S. (1980) Reactivity of red cells from patients with diabetes mellitus with a dextrose-dependent panagglutinin (Abstract). *Transfusion*, **20**, 629.

Avoy, D.R. (1981) Delayed serum sickness-like transfusion reactions in a multiply transfused patient. *Vox Sang.* **41**, 239–244.

Avoy, D.R. (1990) Transfusion-associated graft-versus-host disease in non-immunocompromised hosts. *Transfusion*, **30**, 849.

Awdeh, Z.L. and Alper, C.A. (1980) Inherited structural polymorphism of the fourth component of human complement. *Proc. nat. Acad. Sci. USA*, **77**, 3576–3580.

Axelrod, F.B., Pepkowitz, S.H. and Goldfinger, D. (1988) An assessment of patients currently participating in an autologous blood program: are we overcollecting autologous blood? (Abstract). *Transfusion*, **28**, 595.

Ayland, Judith, Horton, M.A., Tippett, Patricia and Waters, A.H. (1978) Complement binding anti-D made in a D^u variant woman. *Vox Sang.* **34**, 40.

Aylward, F.X., Mainwaring, B.R.S. and Wilkinson, J.F. (1940) Effects of some preservatives on stored blood. *Lancet*, **i**, 685.

Aymard, J.P., Vinet, E., Lederlin, P., Witz, F., Colomb, J.N. and Herbeuval, R. (1980) Paludisme post-transfusionnel: un cas de double infestation à *Plasmodium falciparum* et *Plasmodium malariae*. *Rev. franç. Transfus. Immunohémat.* **23**, 491–493.

Ayoola, E.A. (1988) Viral hepatitis in Africa, in *Viral Hepatitis and Liver Disease*, ed A.J. Zuckerman, pp. 161–169. Alan R. Liss, New York.

Azimi, P.H., Roberto, R.R., Guralnik, J., Livermore, T., Hoag, Silvija, Hagens, Shirley and Lugo, Nelia (1986) Transfusion-acquired hepatitis A in a premature infant with secondary nosocomial spread in an intensive care nursery. *Amer. J. Dis. Child.* **140**, 23–27.

Bach, P. and Hirschhorn, K. (1964) Lymphocyte interaction: a potential histocompatibility test *in vitro*. *Science*, **143**, 813–815.

Bach, F.H. and Voynow, N.K. (1966) One-way stimulation in mixed leukocyte cultures. *Science*, **153**, 545.

Backacs, T., Totpal, K., Ringwald, G. and Yefenof, E. (1988) Comparison of monocyte and complement mediated haemolysis of human A_1 erythrocytes: the relationship between antibody, target and effector concentrations in the induction of lysis. *J. clin. Lab. Immunol.* **25**, 53–58.

Backer, U., Weinauer, F., Gathof, G. and Eberle, J. (1987) HIV antigen screening in blood donors (Letter). *Lancet*, **ii**, 177–180.

Bacon, N., Patten, E. and Vincent, J. (1991) Primary immune response to blood group antigens in burned children. *Immunohematology*, **7**, 8–11.

Badakere, S.S., Joshi, S.R, Bhatia, H.M., Desai, P.K., Giles, C.M. and Goldsmith, K.L.G. (1973) Evidence for a new blood group antigen in the Indian population. *Indian J. med. Res.* **61**, 563–564.

Badakere, S.S., Parab, B.B. and Bhatia, H.M. (1974) Further observations on the In^a (Indian) antigen in Indian populations. *Vox Sang.* **26**, 400–403.

Badet, J., Ropars, C., Cartron, J.P., Doinel, C. and Salmon, C. (1976) Groups of α-D-galactosyltransferase activity in sera of individuals with normal B phenotype. II. Relationship between transferase activity and red cell agglutinability. *Vox Sang.* **30**, 105.

Badet, J. Ropars, C. and Salmon, C. (1978) α-N-acetyl-D-glactosaminyl- and α-D-galactosyltransferase activities in sera of *cis* AB blood group individuals. *J. Immunogenet.* **5**, 221.

Baillou, A., Barin, F., Allain, J-P., Petat, E., Kocheleff, P., Kadende, P. and Goudeau, A. (1987) Human immunodeficiency virus antigenemia in patients with AIDS and AIDS-related disorders: a comparison between European and central African populations. *J. infect. Dis.* **156**, 830–833.

Bailly, P., Sondag, D., Chevaleyre, J., Piquet, Y., Vezon, G. and Cartron, J.P. (1986) Monoclonal antibodies directed against the human P blood group glycolipid antigen (Abstract) *19th Congr. Int. Soc. Blood Transfus.*, Sydney, p. 503.

Bain, Barbara, Vas, Magdalene R. and Lowenstein, L. (1964) The development of large immature mononuclear cells in mixed leukocyte cultures. *Blood*, **23**, 108.

Bain, B.J. and England J.M. (1975) Normal haematological values: sex difference in neutrophil count. *Brit. med. J.* i 306.

Baker, J.B.E., Bentall, H.H., Dreyer, B. and Melrose, D.G. (1957) Arrest of isolated heart with potassium citrate. *Lancet*, **ii**, 555.

Baker, N., Kickey, K. and Koplin, B. (1988) A blood center and a major medical center: a team effort in bleeding high risk autologous donors (Abstract). *Transfusion*, **28**, 59S.

Baldwin, M.L., Barrasso, C., Ness, P.M. and Garratty, G. (1983a) A clinically significant erythrocyte antibody detectable only by ^{51}Cr survival studies. *Transfusion*, **23**, 40–44.

Baldwin, W.M., Claas, F.H.J., Paul, L.C., Springer, T.A., Hendriks G.F.J., Van Es, L.A., and Van Rood, J.J. (1983b) All monocyte antigens are not expressed on renal endothelium. *Tissue Antigens*, **21**, 254–259.

Baldwin, M.L., Ness, P.M., Barrasso, C., Kickler, T.S., Drew, H., Tsan, M.F. and Shirley, R.S. (1985) *In vivo* studies of the long-term ^{51}Cr red cell survival of serologically incompatible red cell units. *Transfusion*, **25**, 34–38.

Baldwin, J., Pence, H.L., Karibo, J.M. and Massey, E.N. (1991) C1 esterase inhibitor deficiency: three presentations. *Ann. Allergy*, **67**, 107.

Balfour, H.H. jr (1983) Cytomegalovirus disease. Can it be prevented? *Ann. intern. Med.* **98**, 544–546.

Balgairies, E. and Christiaens, L. (1937) Elévation du taux des isoagglutinines sériques sous l'influence de stimulations immunitaires spécifiques (vaccination triple associée). *C.R. Soc. Biol. (Paris)*, **126**, 31.

Ballas, S.K. and Sherwood, W.C. (1977) Rapid *in vivo* destruction of Yt(a+) erythrocytes in a recipient with anti-Yt^a. *Transfusion*, **17**, 65.

Ballas, S.K., Clark, Margaret R., Mohandas, Narla, Colfer, H.F., Caswell, M.S., Bergren, M.O., Perkins, H.A. and Shohet, S.B. (1984) Red cell membrane and cation deficiency in Rh_{null} syndrome. *Blood*, **63**, 1046–1055.

Ballas, S.K., Dignam, C., Harris, M. and Marcolina, M.J. (1985) A clinically significant anti-N in a patient whose red cells were negative for N and U antigens. *Transfusion*, **25**, 377–380.

Ballem, Penny J., Buskard, N.A., Décary, Francine and Doubroff, P. (1987a) Posttransfusion purpura secondary to passive transfer of anti- $P1^{A1}$ by blood transfusion. *Brit. J. Haemat.* **66**, 113–114.

Ballem, Penny J., Segal, G.M., Stratton, J.R., Gernsheimer, T., Adamson, J.W. and Slichter, Sherill (1987b) Mechanisms of chronic autoimmune thrombocytopenic purpura: evidence of both impaired platelet production and increased platelet clearance. *J. clin Invest.* **80**, 33–40.

Ballowitz, Leonore, Beck, C., Eibs, G. and Winter, U. (1981) Rh Antikörper in kommerziellen Immunoglobulin-Konzentrat. *Monatschr. Kinderheilk.* **129**, 537–540.

Bangham, D.R., Kirkwood, T.B.L., Whybrow, G., Hughes-Jones, N.C. and Gunson, H.H. (1978) International collaborative study of assay of anti-D (anti-Rho) immunoglobulin. *Brit. J. Haemat.* **38**, 407.

Banks, D.C., Cawdrey, H.M., Yates, D.B., Harries, M.G. and Kidner, P.H. (1970) Infection from intravenous catheters. *Lancet*, **i**, 443.

Barandun, S., Büchler, H. and Hässig, A. (1956) Das Antikörpermangelsyndrom: agammalobulinämie. *Schweiz. Med. Wschr.* **86**, 33.

Barandun, S., Kistler, P., Jeunet, F. and Isliker, H. (1962) Intravenous administration of human γ-globulin. *Vox Sang.* **7**, 157.

Barandun, S. and Isliker, H. (1986) Development of immunoglobulin preparations for intravenous use. *Vox Sang.* **51**, 157–160.

Barbara J.A.J., Mijovic, Valerie, Cleghorn, T.E., Tedder, R.S. and Briggs, Moya (1978) Liver enzyme concentrations as a measure of possible infectivity in chronic asymptomatic carriers of hepatitis B. *Brit. Med. J.* **2**, 1600–1602.

Barbara, J.A.J. and Briggs, Moya (1981) Follow-up of HBsAg-positive donors to determine the proportion undergoing acute infections (Abstract). *Transfusion,* **21**, 605–606.

Barbara J.A.J., Howell, D.R., Briggs, Moya and Parry, J.V. (1982a) Post-transfusion hepatitis A (letter). *Lancet*, **i**, 738.

Barbara J.A.J., Salker, R., Lalji. F. and Mochnaty, P. (1982b) TPHA compared with cardiolipin tests for serological detection of early primary syphilis. *J. clin. Path.* **35**, 1394–1395.

Barbara, J.A.J. (1983) *Microbiology in Blood Transfusion.* John Wright, Bristol.

Barbara J.A.J., Tedder, R.S. and Briggs, Moya (1984) Anti-HBc testing alone not a reliable blood donor screen (Letter). *Lancet*, **i**, 346.

Barbara, J.A.J. (1987) Current anti-LAV/HTLV-III screening methods (and some of their problems), in *AIDS: The Safety of Blood and Blood Products,* eds J.C. Petricciani, I.D. Gust, P.A. Hoppe and H.W. Krijnen, pp. 157–170. John Wiley & Sons Ltd. U.K.

Barbara J.A.J., Moulsdale, H., Brown, S., Griffiths, P.D., Berry, M.J. and Contreras, Marcela (1987) Modified latex agglutination test for anticytomegalovirus, suitable for pretransfusion screening. *J. clin. Path.* **40**, 115–116.

Barbara, J.A.J. (1989a) Defining the information flow in the transfusion-microbiology laboratory, in *Automation in Blood Transfusion,* eds C. Th. Smit Sibinga, P.C. Das and C.F. Högman, pp. 91–96. Kluwer Academic, Boston.

Barbara, J.A.J. (1989b) Detection of hepatitis B surface antigen. *Serodiagnosis and Immunotherapy in Infectious Disease,* **3**, 363–365.

Barbara, J.A.J. and Contreras, M. (1990) Microbiological screening of blood donations, in *Blood Transfusion: The Impact of New Technologies,* ed Marcela Contreras. *Baillière's Clinical Haematology,* **3**, 339–354.

Barbara, J.A.J. (1991) Screening blood donors for retroviruses. *J. biomed. Sci.* **2**, 45–56.

Barbara, J.A.J. and Contreras, Marcela (1991a) Non-A, non-B hepatitis and the anti-HCV assay. *Vox Sang.* **60**, 1–7.

Barbara, J.A.J. and Contreras, M. (1991b) Posttransfusion NANBH in the light of a test for anti-HCV. *Blood Rev.* **3**, 234–239.

Barclay, G.R., Greiss, M.A. and Urbaniak, S.J. (1980) Adverse effect of plasma exchange on anti-D production in rhesus immunization owing to removal of inhibitory factors. *Brit. Med. J.* **ii**, 1569.

Barcroft, H., Edholm, O.G., McMichael, J. and Sharpey-Schafer, E.P. (1944) Post-haemorrhagic fainting: study by cardiac output and forearm flow. *Lancet,* **i**, 489.

Barker, Joan M. (1982) Serological comparison of a hybridoma anti-C3d with commercial antiglobulin reagents. *Transfusion,* **22**, 507–510.

Barnes, R.M.R., Duguid, Jennifer K.M., Roberts, Freda M., Risk, Janet M., Johnson, P.M., Finn, R., Hardy, Joan, Napier, J.A.F. and Clarke, C.A. (1987) Oral administration of erythrocyte membrane antigen does not suppress anti-Rh(D) antibody responses in humans. *Clin. exp. Immunol.* **67**, 220–226.

Barnstable, C.J., Jones, E.A. and Crumpton, M.J. (1978) Isolation, structure and genetics of HLA-A, -B, -C and -DRw (Ia) antigens. *Brit. med. Bull.* **34**, 241.

Barnwell, J.W. Nichols, M.E. and Rubinstein, P. (1989) *In vitro* evaluation of the role of the Duffy blood group in erythrocyte invasion by *Plasmodium vivax. J. exp. Med.,* **169**, 1795–1802.

Barr, Mollie and Glenny, A.T. (1945) Some practical applications of immunological principles. *J. Hyg. (Lond.),* **44**, 135.

Barr, Mollie and Llewellyn-Jones, M. (1953) Some factors influencing the response of animals to immunization with combined prophylactics. *Brit. J. exp. Path.* **34**, 12.

Barré-Sinoussi, F. and 11 others (1983) Isolation of a T-lymphotrophic retrovirus from a patient at risk of acquired immune deficiency syndrome (AIDS). *Science,* **220**, 868–871.

Barrie, Jean V. and Quinn, M.A. (1985) Selection of donor red cells for fetal intravenous transfusion in severe haemolytic disease of the newborn (Letter). *Lancet,* **i**, 1327–1328.

Barrowcliffe, T.W., Johnson, E.A. and Thomas, D. (1978) Antithrombin III and heparin. *Brit. med. Bull.* **34**, 143–150.

Barss, Vanessa A., Doubilet, P.M., St. John-Sutton, M., Cartier, M.S. and Frigoletto, F.D. (1987) Cardiac output in a fetus with erythroblastosis fetalis: assessment using pulsed Doppler. *Obstet. Gynec.* **70**, 442–444.

Barss, Vanessa A. and 9 others (1988) Management of isoimmunised pregnancy by use of intravascular techniques. *Amer. J. Obstet. Gynec.* **159**, 932–937.

Bartsch, F.K. (1972) Fetale Erythrozyten im mütterlichen Blut und Immunprophylaxe der

Rh-Immunisierung. Klinische und experimentelle Studie. *Acta obstet. gynec. Scand. Suppl.* 20.

Bass, L.S., Rao, A.H., Goldstein, J. and Marsh, W.C. (1983) The Sd-antigen and antibody: biochemical studies on the inhibitory property of human urine. *Vox Sang.* **44**, 191–196.

Bass, H., Trenchard, P.M. and Mustow, M.J. (1985) Microwave-thawed plasma for cryoprecipitate production. *Vox Sang.* **48**, 65–71.

Basta, M., Langlois, P.F., Marques, Marisa, Frank, M.M. and Fries, L.F. (1989a) High-dose intravenous immunoglobulin modifies complement-mediated *in vivo* clearance. *Blood,* **74**, 326–333.

Basta, M., Kirshbom, P., Frank, M.M. and Fries, L.F. (1989b) Mechanism of therapeutic effect of high-dose intravenous immunoglobulin. *J. clin. Invest.* **84**, 1974–1981.

Basta, M., Fries, L.F. and Frank. M.M. (1991) High doses of intravenous Ig inhibit *in vitro* uptake of C4 fragments onto sensitized erythrocytes. *Blood,* **77**, 376–380.

Bastian, J.F., Williams, R.A., Ornelas, W., Tani, Patricia and Thompson, L.F. (1984) Maternal isoimmunisation resulting in combined immunodeficiency and fatal graft-versus-host disease in an infant. *Lancet,* **i**, 1435–1437.

Batson, H.C., Jayne, Martha and Brown, Martha (1950) Preservation of Rh agglutinating antiserum with sodium azide. *J. Lab. clin. Med.* **35**, 297.

Bauer, D.C. and Stavitsky, A.B. (1961) On the different molecular forms of antibody synthesized by rabbits during the early response to a single injection of protein and cellular antigens. *Proc. nat. Acad. Sci. USA,* **47**, 1667.

Baumgarten, A., Kruchok, A.H. and Weirich, F. (1976) High frequency of IgG anti-A and -B antibody in old age. *Vox Sang.* **30**, 253.

Baumgartner, J.D., Glauser, M.P., Burgo-Black, A.L., Black, R.D., Pyndiah, N. and Chiolero, R. (1982) Severe cytomegalovirus infection in multiply transfused, splenectomised, trauma patients. *Lancet,* **ii**, 63–66.

Bautista, A.P., Buckler, P.W., Towler H.M.A., Dawson, A.A. and Bennett, B. (1984) Measurement of platelet life-span in normal subjects and patients with myeloproliferative disease with indium oxine labelled platelets. *Brit.J. Haemat.* **58**, 679–687.

Baxter, C.R. and Shires, G.T. (1968) Physiologic response to crystalloid resuscitation of severe burns. *Ann. N. Y. Acad. Sci.* **150**, 874.

Baxter, C.R. (1974) Fluid volume and electrolyte changes of the early postburn period. *Clinics in Plastic Surgery,* **1**, (4) 693–709.

Bayliss, W.M. (1919) Intravenous injection to replace blood. *Spec. Rep. Ser. med. Res. Cttee. (Lond.),* No. 25.

Bayliss, W.M. (1920) Is haemolysed blood toxic? *Brit. J. exp. Path.* **1**, 1.

BCSH/BBTS (British Committee for Standarisation in Haematology/British Blood Transfusion Society Working Party) (1990) Guidelines for microplate techniques in liquid-phase blood grouping and antibody screening. *Clin. lab. Haemat.* **12**, 437–460.

Beal, R.W. (1972) Vaso-vagal reactions in blood donors. *Med. J. Aust.* **2**, 757.

Beal, R. and Van Aken, W.G. (1992) Gift or good? A contemporary examination of the voluntary and commercial aspects of blood donation. *Vox Sang.* in press.

Beard, M.E.J., Pemberton, J., Blagdon, J. and Jenkins, W.J. (1971) Rh immunization following incompatible blood transfusion and a possible long-term complication of anti-D immunoglobulin therapy. *Med. Genetics,* **8**, 317.

Beardsley, D.S., Spiegel, J.E., Jacobs, M.M., Handin, R.I. and Lux, I.V.S.E. (1984) Platelet membrane glycoprotein IIIa contains target antigens that bind anti-platelet antibodies in immune thrombocytopenias. *J. clin. Invest.* **74**, 1701–1707.

Beardsley, D.S., Ho, J.S. and Moulton, T. (1987) A new platelet specific antigen on glycoprotein V. *Blood,* **70**, Suppl. 347a.

Beardsley, D.S. (1989) Platelet autoantigens, in *Platelet Immunobiology*, eds T.J. Kunicki and J.N. George. J.P. Lippincott, Philadelphia.

Bearn, A.G. and Litwin, S.D. (1978) Deficiencies of circulating enzymes and plasma proteins, in *The Metabolic Basis of Inherited Disease*, 4th edn., eds S.B. Stanbury, J.B. Wyngaarden and D.S. Fredrickson. McGraw Hill, New York.

Beattie, K.M. and Zuelzer, W.W. (1965) The frequency and properties of pH-dependent anti-M. *Transfusion,* **5**, 322.

Beattie, K.M. and Zuelzer, W.W. (1968) A serum factor reacting with acriflavin causing an error in ABO cell grouping. *Transfusion,* **8**, 254.

Beattie, K.M., Seymour, D.S. and Scott, A. (1971) Two further examples of acriflavin antibody causing ABO cell typing errors. *Transfusion,* **11**, 107.

Beattie, K.M. and Castillo, S. (1975) A case report of a hemolytic transfusion reaction caused by anti-Holley. *Transfusion,* **15**, 476.

Beattie, K.M., Ferguson, S.J., Burnie, K.L., Barr, R.M., Urbaniak, S.J. and Atherton, P.J. (1976) Chloramphenicol antibody causing interference in antibody detection and identification tests (Abstract). *Transfusion,* **16**, 174.

Beattie, K.M. (1980) Control of the antigen-antibody ratio in antibody detection/compatibility tests. *Transfusion,* **20**, 277–284.

Beatty, P.G. and 10 others (1985) Marrow transplantation from related donors other than

HLA-identical siblings. *New Engl. J. Med.* **31**, 765–771.

Beaumont, J.L., Lorenzelli, L., Delplanque, B., Zittoun, R. and Homberg, J.C. (1976) A new serum liproprotein-associated erythrocyte antigen which reacts with a monoclonal IgM. The stored human red blood cell SHRBC antigen. *Vox Sang.* **30**, 36.

Bechdolt, S., Schroeder, Linda K., Samia, Concepcion and Schmidt, P.J. (1986) *In vivo* hemolysis of deglycerolized red blood cells. *Arch. Path. lab. Med.* **110**, 344–345.

Beck, M.L., Haines, R.F. and Oberman, H.A. (1971) Unexpected serologic findings following lung homotransplantation. *Commun. Amer. Assoc. Blood banks*, Chicago.

Beck, M.L., Hicklin, B. and Pierce, S.R. (1976a) Unexpected limitations in the use of commercial antiglobulin reagents. *Transfusion*, **16**, 71.

Beck, M.L., Edwards, R.L., Pierce, S.R., Hicklin, B.L. and Bayer, W.L. (1976b) Serologic activity of the fatty acid dependent antibodies in albumin-free systems. *Transfusion*, **16**, 434.

Beck, M.L., Myers, M.A., Moulds, J., Pierce, S.R., Hardman, J., Wingham, J. and Bird, G.W.G. (1978) Coexistent Tk and VA polyagglutinability. *Transfusion*, **18**, 680.

Beck, M.L., Marsh, W.L., Pierce, S.R., Dinapoli, J., Oyen, R. and Nichols, M.E. (1979) Auto-anti Kp^b associated with weakened antigenicity in the Kell blood group system: a second example. *Transfusion*, **19**, 197–202.

Beck, M.L., Rachel, Jane M., Sinor, L.T. and Plapp, F.V. (1984) Semi-automated solid phase adherence assays for pre-transfusion testing. *Med. Lab. Sciences*, **41**, 374–381.

Beck, M.L., Sinor, L.T., Rachel, Jane M. and Plapp, F.V. (1985) Solid-phase ABO blood grouping using saliva. *Med. Lab. Sciences*, **42**, 86–87.

Becker, T., Panzer, S., Maas, D., Kiefel, V., Sprenger, R., Kirschbaum, M. and Mueller-Eckhardt, C. (1985) High-dose intravenous immunoglobulin for post-transfusion purpura. *Brit. J. Haemat.* **61**, 149–155.

Becker, T., Kuenzlen, E., Salama, A., Mertens, R., Kiefel, V., Weiss, H., Lampert, F., Gaedicke, G. and Mueller-Eckhardt, C. (1986) Treatment of childhood idiopathic thrombocytopenic purpura with Rhesus antibodies (anti-D). *Eur. J. Pediat.* **147**, 166–169.

Bedaraida, G., Cambie, G., D'Agostino, F., Ronsivalle, M.G., Berto, E., Grisi, M.E. and Magni, E. (1986) HIV IgM antbodies in risk groups who are seronegative on ELISA testing. *Lancet*, **ii**, 570–571.

Beer, A.E., Semprini, A.E., Ziaoyu, Z. and Quebbeman, J.F. (1985) Pregnancy outcome in human couples with recurrent spontaneous abortions; HLA antigen profiles; HLA antigen sharing; female serum MLR blocking factors; and paternal leukocyte immunization. *Exp. clin. Immunogenet.* **2**, 137–153.

Belcher, E.H. and Harriss, Eileen (1959) Studies of red cell life span in the rat. *J. Physiol. (Lond.)*, **146**, 127.

Bell, C.A., Zwicker, H. and Rosenbaum, D.L. (1973a) Paroxysmal cold hemoglobinuria (P.C.H.) following mycoplasma infection: Anti-I specificity of the biphasic hemolysin. *Transfusion*, **13**, 138.

Bell, C.A., Zwicker, H. and Nevius, D.B. (1973b) Nonspecific warm hemolysins of papain-treated cells: Serologic characterization and transfusion risk. *Transfusion*, **13**, 207.

Bell, A.J., Mufti, G.J. and Hamblin, T.J. (1983) Complications of constructing arteriovenous-grafts and fistulae for plasma exchange. *Apheresis Bull.* **1**, 92–95.

Bell, Karen and Gillon, J. (1990) Erythropoietin and preoperative blood donation (Letter). *New Engl. J. Med.* **322**, 1158.

Bell, A.B., Kurczynski, E.M. and Bergman, C. (1990) Inhibitors to monoclonal antibody purified Factor VIII. *Lancet*, **ii**, 638.

Belzer, F.O., Kountz, S.L. and Perkins, H.A. (1971) Red cell cold autoagglutinins as a cause of failure of renal transplantation. *Transfusion*, **11**, 422.

Benacerraf, B. (1981) Role of MHC gene products in immune regulation. *Science*, **212**, 1229–1238.

Benbassat, J., Groen, J.J., Heiman-Hollander, E. and Leibovitz, Z. (1966) The influence of packing, stagnation and isoagglutination on glucose utilization, glutathione and cation content of human blood cells *in vitro*. *Clin. Sci.* **20**, 51.

Benesch, R. and Benesch, Ruth E. (1967) The influence of organic phosphates on the oxygenation of hemoglobin. *Fed. Proc.* **26**, 673.

Benesch, Ruth, E. and Benesch, R. (1969) Interaction of red cell organic phosphates with hemoglobin. *Försvarsmedicin*, **5**, 154.

Benesch, R.E., Benesch, R., Renthal, R.D. and Maeda, N. (1972) Affinity labeling of the polyphosphate binding site of hemoglobin. *Biochemistry*, **11**, 3675.

Bengtson, J.P., Backman, L., Stenqvist, O., Heideman, M. and Bengtsson, A. (1990) Complement activation and reinfusion of wound drainage blood. *Anesthesiology*, **73**, 376–380.

Ben-Ismail, R., Rouger, P., Carme, B., Gentilini, M. and Salmon, C. (1980) Comparative automated assay of anti-P$_1$ antibodies in acute hepatic distomiasis (fascioliasis) and in hydatidosis. *Vox Sang.* **38**, 165–168.

Ben-Izhak, C., Slechter, Y. and Tatorsky, I. (1985) Significance of multiple types of antibodies on red blood cells of patients with positive direct antiglobulin test: a study of monospecific antiglobulin reagents in 85 patients. *Scand. J. Haemat.* **35**, 102–108.

Bennett. P.J (1963) The use of intravenous plastic catheters. *Brit. med. J.,* **ii,** 1252.

Bensinger, T.A., Metro, J. and Beutler, E. (1975) *In vitro* metabolism of packed erythrocytes stored in CPD-adenine. *Transfusion,* **15**, 135.

Bensinger, T.A., Chillar, R.K. and Beutler, E. (1977) Prolonged maintenance of 2, 3-DPG in liquid blood storage: use of an internal CO_2 trap to stabilize pH. *J. Lab. clin. Med.* **89**, 498.

Bensinger, W.I., Baker, D.A., Buckner, C.D., Clift, R.A. and Thomas, E.D. (1981) Immunoadsorption for removal of A and B bloodgroup antibodies. *New Engl. J. Med.* **304**, 160–162.

Bentall, H.H., Smith, Bianca, Omeri, M.A., Melrose, D.G. and Allwork, Sally (1964) Blood loss after cardiopulmonary bypass. *Lancet,* **ii,** 277.

Bentley, S.A., Glass, H.I., Lewis, S.M. and Szur, L. (1974) Elution correction in ^{51}Cr red cell survival studies. *Brit. J. Haemat.* **26**, 179.

Berg, E.M., Fasting, S. and Sellevold, O.F.M. (1991) Serious complications with dextran-70 despite hapten prophylaxis. *Anaesthesia,* **46**, 1033–1035.

Bergentz, S.-E. (1978) Dextran in the prophylaxis of pulmonary embolism. *World Surg.* **2**, 19–25.

Bergvalds, Helena, Stock, Anne and McClure, P.D. (1965) A further example of anti-Yt^a. *Vox Sang.* **10**, 627.

Berk, P.D., Bloomer, H.R., Howe, R.B. and Berlin, N.I. (1970) The life span of the red blood cell as determined with labeled bilirubin, in *Formation and Destruction of Blood Cells,* p. 91. J.B. Lippincott, Philadelphia.

Berkan, E.M. and Orlin, J.B. (1980) Use of plasmapheresis and partial plasma exchange in the management of patients with cryoglobulinemia. *Transfusion,* **20**, 171–178.

Berkman, S.A., Lee, M.L. and Calc, R.P.G. (1990) Clinical uses of intravenous immunoglobulins. *Ann. intern. Med.* **112**, 278–292.

Berkow, S.G. (1931) Value of surface-area proportions in the prognosis of cutaneous burns and scalds. *Amer. J. Surg.* **11**, 315.

Berkowitz, R.L., Chitkara, Usha, Wilkins, Isabelle A., Lynch, Lauren, Plosker, H. and Bernstein, H.H. (1988) Intravascular monitoring and management of erythroblastosis fetalis. *Amer. J. Obstet. Gynec.* **158**, 783–795.

Berlin, N.I., Lawrence, J.H. and Lee, Helen C. (1954) The pathogenesis of the anemia of chronic leukemia: measurement of the life-span of the red blood cell with glycine-2-C^{14}. *J. Lab. clin. Med.* **44**, 860.

Berlin, N.I. and Berk, P.D. (1981) Quantitative

aspects of bilirubin metabolism for hematologists. *Blood,* **57**, 983–999.

Berndt, M.C., Chong, B.H., Bull, Helen A., Zola, H. and Castaldi, P.A. (1985) Molecular characterization of quinine/quinidine drug-dependent antibody platelet interaction using monoclonal antibodies. *Blood,* **66**, 1292–1301.

Bernini, L., Latte, B., Siniscalco, M., Piomelli, S., Spada, U., Adinolfi. M. and Mollison, P.L. (1964) Survival of ^{51}Cr-labelled red cells in subjects with thalassaemia-trait or G6PD deficiency or both abnormalities. *Brit. J. Haemat.* **10**, 171.

Berry-Dortch, S., Woodside, C.H. and Boral, L.I. (1985) Limitations of the immediate spin crossmatch when used for detecting ABO incompatibility. *Transfusion,* **25**, 176–178.

Bertolini, F., Rebulla, P., Riccardi, D., Cortellaro, M., Ranzi, M.L. and Sirchia, G. (1989) Evaluation of platelet concentrates prepared from buffy coats and stored in a glucose-free crystalloid medium. *Transfusion,* **29**, 605–609.

Betke, K. and Kleihauer, E. (1958) Fetaler und bleibender Blutfarbstoff in Erythrozyten und Erythroblasten von menschlichen Feten und Neugeborenen. *Blut.* **4**, 241.

Bettaieb, A., Fromont, P., Rodet, M., Godeau, B., Duedari, N. and Bierling, P. (1991) Br^b, a platelet alloantigen involved in neonatal alloimmune thrombocytopenia. *Vox Sang.* **60**, 230–234.

Betteridge, A. and Watkins, W.M. (1985) Variant forms of alpha-2-L fucosyltransferase in human submaxillary glands from blood group ABH 'secretor' and 'non-secretor' individuals. *Glycoconjugate J.* **2**, 61–78.

Bettigole, R., Harris, Jean P., Tegoli, J. and Issitt, P.D. (1968) Rapid *in vivo* destruction of Yt(a+) red cells in a patient with anti-Yt^a. *Vox Sang.* **14**, 143.

Beutler, E. (1957) The glutathione instability of drug-sensitive red cells. A new method for the *in vitro* detection of drug sensitivity. *J. Lab. clin. Med.* **39**, 84.

Beutler, E. and Duron, Olga (1965) Effect of pH on preservation of red cell ATP. *Transfusion,* **5**, 17.

Beutler, E. and Wood, L. (1969) The *in vivo* regeneration of red cell 2, 3-diphosphoglyceric acid (DPG) after transfusion of stored blood. *J. Lab. clin. Med.* **74**, 300.

Beutler, E., Meul, A. and Wood L.A. (1969) Depletion and regeneration of 2, 3-diphosphoglyceric acid in stored red blood cells. *Transfusion,* **9**, 109.

Beutler, E. and Wood, L.A. (1972) Preservation of red cell 2, 3-DPG and viability in bicarbonate-containing medium: the effect of blood-bag permeability. *J. Lab. clin. Sci.* **80**, 723.

Beutler, E. (1974) Experimental blood preservatives for liquid storage, in *The Human Red Cell in Vitro*, eds T.J. Greenwalt and G.A. Jamieson. Grune and Stratton, New York.

Beutler, E. and West, Carol (1979) The storage of hard-packed red blood cells in citrate-phosphate-dextrose (CPD) and CPD-adenine (CPDA-1). *Blood*, **54**, 280–284.

Beutler, E., Kuhl, Wanda and West Carol (1982) The osmotic fragility of erythrocytes after prolonged liquid storage and after reinfusion. *Blood*, **59**, 1141–1147.

Beutler, E. and West, C. (1984) Measurement of the viability of stored red cells by the single-isotope technique using ^{51}Cr. *Transfusion*, **24**, 100–104.

Beutler, E. and West, Carol (1985) Measurement of the viable Adsol-preserved human red cells (Letter). *New Engl. J. Med.* **312**, 1392.

Beutler, E. (1988) Isolation of the aged. *Blood Cells*, **14**, 1–5.

Bevan, A., Hammond, W. and Clarke, R.L. (1970) Anti-P_1 associated with liver-fluke infection. *Vox Sang.* **18**, 188.

Bevan, P.C., Seaman, Muriel, Tolliday, B. and Chalers, D.G. (1985) ABO haemolytic anaemia in transplanted patients. *Vox Sang.* **49**, 42–48.

Bharucha, Z.A., Joshi, S.R. and Bhatia, H.M. (1981) Hemolytic disease of the newborn due to anti-Le^b. *Vox Sang.* **41**, 36–39.

Bhende, Y.M, Despande, C.K, Bhatia, H.M, Sanger, Ruth, Race, R.R., Morgan, W.T.J. and Watkins, Winifred M. (1952) A 'new' blood-group character related to the ABO system. *Lancet*, **i**, 903.

Bidstrup, B.P., Royston, D. Taylor, K.M. and Sapsford, R.N. (1988) Effect of aprotinin on need for blood transfusion in patients with septic endocarditis having open-heart surgery (Letter). *Lancet*, **i**, 366–367.

Bier, O.G., Leyton, G., Mayer, M.M. and Heidelberger, M. (1945) A comparison of human and guinea-pig complements and their component fractions. *J. exp. Med.* **81**, 445.

Bierman, H.R., Marshall, G.J., Kelly, K.H. and Byron, R.L. jr. (1962) Leucopheresis in man. II. Changes in circulating granulocytes, lymphocytes and platelets in the blood. *Brit. J. Haemat.* **8**, 77.

Biggs, Rosemary (1974) Jaundice and antibodies directed against Factors VIII and IX in patients treated for haemophilia or Christmas disease in the United Kingdom. *Brit. J. Haemat.* **26**, 313.

Binder, L.S., Ginsberg, V. and Harmel, M.H. (1959) A six-year study of incompatible blood transfusions. *Surg. Gynec. Obstet.* **108**, 19.

Bird, G.W.G. (1952) Relationship of the blood sub-groups A_1, A_2 and A_1B, A_2B to haemagglutinins present in the seeds of *Dolichos biflorus*. *Nature (Lond.)*. **170**, 674.

Bird, G.W.G. (1959) Haemagglutinins in seeds. *Brit. med. Bull.* **15**, 165.

Bird, G.W.G. (1964) Anti-T in peanuts. *Vox Sang.* **9**, 748.

Bird, G.W.G. and Wingham, June (1970a) Agglutinins for antigens of two different human blood group systems in the seeds of *Moluccella laevis*. *Vox Sang.* **18**, 235.

Bird, G.W.G. and Wingham, June (1970b) N-Acetylneuraminic (sialic) acid and the human blood group antigen structure. *Vox Sang.* **18**, 240.

Bird, G.W.C., Shinton, N.K. and Wingham, June (1971) Persistent mixed-field polyagglutination. *Brit. J. Haemat.* **21**, 443.

Bird, G.W.G. and Wingham, June (1972) Tk: a new form of red cell polyagglutination. *Brit. J. Haemat.* **23**, 759.

Bird, G.W.G., and Wingham, June (1973) Anti-I autoantibody acting preferentially in albumin. *Vox Sang.* **25**, 162.

Bird, T. and Stephenson, J. (1973) Acute haemolytic anaemia associated with polyagglutinability of red cells. *J. clin. Path.* **26**, 868.

Bird, G.W.G., McEvoy, M.W. and Wingham, June (1975) Acute haemolytic anaemia due to IgM penicillin antibody in a 3-year-old child: a sequel to oral penicillin. *J. clin. Path.* **28**, 321.

Bird, G.W.G. and Wingham, June (1976) The action of seed and other reagents on HEM-PAS erythrocytes. *Acta haemat.* **55**, 174.

Bird, G.W.G., Wingham, June, Pippard, M.J., Hoult, J.G. and Melikian, V. (1976a) Erythrocyte membrane modification in malignant disease of myeloid and lymphoreticular tissues. I. Tn-polyagglutination in acute myelocytic leukaemia. *Brit. J. Haemat.* **33**, 289.

Bird, G.W.G., Wingham, June, Martin, A.J., Richardson, S.G.N., Cole, A.P., Wayne, R.W. and Savage, B.F. (1976b) Idiopathic non-syphilitic paroxysmal cold haemoglobinuria in children. *J. clin. Path.* **29**, 215.

Bird, G.W.G., Wingham, June, Chester, G.H., Kidd, P. and Payne, R.W. (1976c) Erythrocyte membrane modification in malignant disease of myeloid and lymphoreticular tissues. II. Erythrocyte 'mosaicism' in acute erythroleukaemia. *Brit. J. Haemat.* **33**, 295.

Bird, G.W.G., Battey, Diana A., Greenwell, Pamela, Mortimer, C.W., Watkins, Winifred M. and Wingham, June (1976d) Case report: further observations of the Birmingham chimaera. *J. med. Genet.* **13**, 70.

Bird, G.W.G. (1977) Erythrocyte polyagglutination, in CRC *Handbook Series in Clinical Laboratory Science, Section D: Blood Banking*, eds T.J. Greenwalt and E.A. Steane, vol. 1, p. 443. CRC Press, Inc., Cleveland, U.S.A.

Bird, G.W.G. and Wingham, June (1977a) Erythrocyte autoantibody with unusual specificity. *Vox Sang.* **32**, 280.

Bird, G.W.G. and Wingham, June (1977b) Anti-N antibodies in renal dialysis patients. *Lancet*, **i**, 1218.

Bird, G.W.G. (1978a) The application of lectins to some problems in blood group serology. *Rev. franç. Transfus. Immunohémat.* **21**, 103.

Bird, G.W.G. (1978b) Significant advances in lectins and polyagglutinable red cells. *15th Congr. Int. Soc. Blood Transfus.*, Paris, 1978.

Bird, G.W.G., Wingham, June, Beck, M.L., Pierce, S.R., Oates, G.D. and Pollock, A. (1978) Th, a 'new' form of erythrocyte polyagglutination (Letter). *Lancet*, **i**, 1215.

Bird, G.W.G. (1980) Lectins and red cell polyagglutinability: history, comments and recent developments, in *Polyagglutination, A Technical Workshop*. Amer. Assoc. Blood Banks, Washington, D.C.

Bird, G.W.G. and Wingham, J. (1980) Anti-A autoantibodies with unusual properties in a patient on renal dialysis. *Immunol. Commun.* **9**, 155–159.

Bird, G.W.G. (1981) Lectins. *Lab-Lore*, **9**, 683–684.

Bird, G.W.G. and Wingham, June (1981) *Vicia cretica*: a powerful lectin for T- and Th- but not Tk- or other polyagglutinable erythrocytes. *J. clin. Path.* **34**, 69–70.

Bird, C.W.G. (1982) Clinical aspects of red blood cell polyagglutinability of microbial origin, in *Blood Groups and other Red Cell Surface Markers in Health and Disease*, ed C. Salmon. Masson Publishing, New York.

Bird, G.W.G., Wingham, June, Seger, R. and Kenny, A.B. (1982) Tx, a 'new' red cell cryptantigen exposed by pneumococcal enzymes. *Rev. franç. Transfus. Immunohémat.* **25**, 215–216.

Bird, G.W.G. and Wingham, June (1983) 'New' lectins for the identification of erythrocyte cryptantigens and the classification of erythrocyte polyagglutinability: *Medicago disciformis* and *Medicago turbinata. J. clin. Path.* **36**, 195–196.

Bird, G.W.G., Wingham, J. and Richardson, S.G.N. (1985) Myelofibrosis, autoimmune haemolytic anaemia and Tn-polyagglutinability. *Haematologia*, **18**, 99–103.

Birgegård, G., Högman, C., Johansson, A., Killander, A., Simonsson, B. and Wide, L. (1980) Serum ferritin in the regulation of iron therapy in blood donors. *Vox Sang.* **38**, 29–35.

Birndorf, N.L. and Lopas, H. (1970) The effect of red cell stroma free hemoglobin solution on renal function in monkeys. *J. appl. Physiol.* **29**, 573.

Birndorf, N.L., Lopas, H. and Robboy, S.J. (1971) Disseminated intravacular coagulation and renal failure. Production in the monkey with autologous red blood cell stroma. *Lab. Invest.* **25**, 314.

Biro, G.P. (1982) Comparison of acute cardiovascular effects and oxygen-supply following haemodilution with dextran, stroma-free haemoglobin solution and fluorocarbon suspension. *Cardiovasc. Res.* **16**, 194–204.

Biro, C.P., White, F.C., Guth, B.D., Breisch, E.A. and Bloor, C.M. (1987) The effect of hemodilution with fluorocarbon or dextran on regional myocardial flow and function during acute coronary stenosis in the pig. *Amer. J. cardiovasc. Path.*, **1**, 99–114.

Bishop, G.J. and Krieger, Vera I. (1969) The timing of rhesus immunization and the prevention of antibody response using anti-Rh immune globulin. *Austral. N.Z. J. Obstet. Gynaec.* **9**, 228.

Bjerrum, O.J. and Jersild, C. (1971) Class-specific anti-IgA associated with severe anaphylactic transfusion reactions in a patient with pernicious anaemia. *Vox Sang.* **21**, 411.

Bjørkander, J., Cunningham, Rundles, C., Lundin, P., Olsson, R., Söderström, R. and Hanson, L.A. (1988) Intravenous immunoglobulin prophylaxis causing liver damage in 16 of 77 patients with hypogammaglobulinaemia or IgG subclass deficiency. *Amer. J. Med.* **84**, 107–111.

Bjorkman, P.J., Saper, M.A., Samraoui, B., Bennet, W.S., Strominger, J.L. and Wiley, D.C. (1987a) Structure of the human class I histocompatibility antigen, HLA-A2. *Nature (Lond.)*, **329**, 506–511.

Bjorkman, P.J., Saper, M.A., Samraoui, B., Bennet, W.S., Strominger, J.L. and Wiley, D.C. (1987b) The foreign antigen binding site and T cell recognition regions of class I histocompatibility antigens. *Nature (Lond.)*, **329**, 512–518.

Blackburn, G.K. (1976) Massive fetomaternal haemorrhage due to choriocarcinoma of the uterus. *J. Pediat.* **89**, 680.

Blacklock, H.A., Prentice, H.G., Evans, J.P.M., Knight, C.B.T., Gilmore, M.J.M.L., Hazlehunt, G.R.P., Ma, D.D.F. and Hoffbrand, A.V. (1982) ABO incompatible bone-marrow transplantation; removal of red blood cells from donor marrow avoiding recipient antibody depletion. *Lancet*, **ii**, 1061–1064.

Blackwell, C.C., Jóndsóttir, K., Hanson, M., Todd, W.T.A., Chaudhuri, A.K.R., Mathew, B., Brettle, R.P. and Weir D.M. (1986) Nonsecretion of ABO antigens predisposing to infection by *Neisseria meningitidis* and *Streptococcus pneumoniae. Lancet*, **ii**, 284–285.

Blaese, R.M. and Culver, K.W. (1991) Progress towards the application of gene therapy, in

Clinical and Basic Science Aspects of Immunohematology, ed S.J. Nance. Amer. Assoc. Blood Banks, Arlington, VA.

Blanchard, D., Huet, M., Marcus, D., Salmon, C. and Cartron, J.P. (1984) Blood group Cad specific components of the human red cell membrane. *Abstracts, 18th Congr. Int. Soc. Blood Transfus., Munich, p. 221.*

Blanchard, Dominique, Piller, F., Gillard, B., Marcus, D. and Cartron, J-P. (1985) Identification of a novel ganglioside on erythrocytes with blood group Cad specificity. *J. biol. Chem.*, **260**, 7813–7817.

Blanchard, D., Bloy, C., Hermand, P., Cartron, J-P., Saboori, A., Smith, B.L. and Agre, P. (1988) Two-dimensional iodopeptide mapping demonstrates erythrocyte Rh D, c and E polypeptides are structurally homologous but nonidentical. *Blood*, **72**, 1424–1427.

Blanchette, V.S., McCombie, N.E. and Rock, G. (1985a) Factors that influence lymphocyte yields in lymphocytapheresis. *Transfusion*, **25**, 242–245.

Blanchette, V.S., Dunne, J., Steele, D., McPhail, S., Sklar, S., Algom, D., Richter, M.A. and Rock, G. (1985b) Immune function in blood donors following short-term lymphocytapheresis. *Vox Sang.* **49**, 101–109.

Blanchette, V.S. and Turner, C. (1986) Treatment of acute idiopathic thrombocytopenic purpura. *J. Pediat.* **108**, 326–327.

Blanchette, V., Andrew, Maureen, Perlman, M., Ling, Emily and Ballin, A.M.I. (1989) Neonatal autoimmune thrombocytopenia: role of high-dose intravenous immunoglobulin G therapy. *Blut*, **59**, 139–144.

Bland J.H.L Laver, M.B. and Lowenstein, E. (1972) Hypotension due to 5 per cent plasma protein fractions (Letter). *New. Engl. J. Med.* **286**, 109.

Blank, J.P., Sheagren, T.G., Vajaria, J., Mangurten, H.H., Benawra, R.S. and Puppla, B.L. (1984) The role of rbc transfusion in the premature neonate. *Amer. J. Dis. Child.* **138**, 831–833.

Blatt, P.M., White, G.C., II, McMillan, C.W., Webster, W.P., Kingdon, H.S., Zeitler, K.D., Taylor, R.D., Braunstein, K.M. and Roberts, H.R. (1982) The treatment of hemorrhage in hemophiliacs with anti-Factor VIII antibodies, in *Safety in Transfusion Practices*. College of American Pathologists, Skokie, Illinois.

Blattner, W.A., Saxinger, C.W. and Gallo, R.C. (1985) HTV-I, the prototype human retrovirus: epidemiologic features, in *Infection, Immunity and Blood Transfusion*, eds R.Y. Dodd and L.F. Barker, pp. 223–243. A.R. Liss, New York.

Blattner, W.A., Nomura, A., Clark, J.W., Ho, G.Y.F., Nakao, Y., Gallo, R. and Robert-

Guroff, M. (1986) Modes of transmission and evidence for viral latency from studies of human T-cell lymphotropic virus type I in Japanese migrant populations in Hawaii. *Proc. nat. Acad. Sci. USA*, **83**, 4895–4898.

Blazar, B.R. and 9 others (1989) *In vivo* effect of recombinant human granulocyte/macrophage colony-stimulating factor in acute lymphoblastic leukemia patients receiving purged autografts. *Blood*, **73**, 849–857.

Bleeker, W.K., van Rosevelt, R.F., Ufkes, J.G.R., Loos, J.A., van Mourik, J.A. and Bakker, J.C. (1982) Hypotensive effects of plasma protein fraction. *J. Lab. clin. Med.* **100**, 540–547.

Bloch, O. (1941) Loss of *Treponema pallidum* in citrated blood at 5°C. *Bull. Johns Hopk. Hosp.* **68**, 412.

Blood Transfusion Task Force (1991) Microplate techniques in liquid phase blood grouping and antibody screening, in *Standard Haematology Practice*, ed B.E. Roberts, pp. 164–188. Blackwell Scientific Publishers, Oxford.

Bloy, C., Blanchard, D., Dahr, W., Beyrouther, K., Salmon, C. and Cartron, J.P. (1988) Determination of the N-terminal sequence of human red cell Rh(D) polypeptide and demonstration that the Rh(D), (c) and (E) antigens are carried by distinct polypeptide chains. *Blood*, **72**, 661–666.

Bloy, C., Hermand, P., Cherif-Zahar, B., Sonneborn, H. and Cartron, J-P. (1990) Comparative analysis by two-dimensional iodopeptide mapping of the RhD protein and LW glycoprotein. *Blood*, **75**, 2245.

Blum, H.E. and Vyas, G.N. (1982) Non-A, non-B hepatitis: a contemporary assessment. *Haematologia*, **15**, 162–183.

Blumberg, B.S., Alter, H.J. and Visnich, S. (1965) A new antigen in leukemia sera. *J. Amer. med. Assoc.* **191**, 541.

Blumberg, B.S., Sutnick, A.I. and London, W.T. (1968) Hepatitis and leukaemia: their relation to Australia antigen. *Bull. N.Y. Acad. Med.* **44**, 1566.

Blumberg, N., Cowles, J., Blumenfeld, O. and Spitalnik, S. (1982) Anti-M sera bind to NN red cells and NN glycophorin A (Abstract). *Transfusion*, **22**, 420.

Blumberg, N., Peck, Kathy, Ross, Karen and Avila, E. (1983) Immune response to chronic red blood cell transfusion. *Vox Sang.* **44**, 212–217.

Blumberg, N., Masel, Debra, Mayer, Th., Horan, P. and Heal, Joanna (1984a) Removal of HLA-A, B antigens from platelets. *Blood*, **63**, 448–450.

Blumberg, N., Ross, K., Avila, E. and Peck, K. (1984b) Should chronic transfusions be matched for antigens other than ABO and $Rh_0(D)$? *Vox Sang.* **47**, 205–208.

Blumberg, N., Triulzi, D.J. and Heal, J.M. (1990) Transfusion-induced immunomodulation and its clinical consequences. *Transfus. Med. Rev.* **4**, Suppl. 1, 24–35.

Blundell, J. (1818) Experiments on the transfusion of blood by the syringe. *Med.-Chir. Trans.* **9**, 56.

Blundell, J. (1824) *Researches Physiological and Pathological.* E. Cox and Son, London.

Blundell, J. (1829) A successful case of transfusion. *Lancet,* i, 431.

Bockstaele, D.R., Berneman, Z.N., Muylle, L., Coledergent, J. and Peetermans, M.E. (1986) Flow cytometric analysis of erythrocytic D antigen density profile. *Vox Sang.* **51**, 40–46.

Bode, A.P. and Miller, D.T. (1985) Storage of platelet concentrates for 15 days in novel anticoagulants (Abstract). *Transfusion,* **25**, 461.

Bode, A.P. and Miller, D.T. (1988) Preservation of *in vitro* function of platelets stored in the presence of inhibitors of platelet activation and a specific inhibitor of thrombin. *J. Lab. clin. Med.* **111**, 118–124.

Bode, A.P. and Miller, D.T. (1989) The use of thrombin inhibitors and aprotinin in the preservation of platelets stored for transfusion. *J. Lab. clin. Med.* **113**, 753–758.

Bode, A.P., Holme, S., Heaton, A.W. and Swanson, M.S. (1991) Extended storage of platelets in an artificial medium with the platelet activation inhibitors prostaglandin E1 and theophylline. *Vox Sang.* **60**, 105–112.

Bodemann, H.H., Rieger, A., Bross, K.J., Schroter-Urban, H. and Lohr, G.W. (1984) Erythrocyte and plasma ferritin in normal subjects, blood donors and iron deficiency anaemia patients. *Blut,* **48**, 131–137.

Bodensteiner, D.C. (1989) A flow cytometric technique to accurately measure post-filtration white blood cell counts. *Transfusion,* **29**, 651–653.

Bodensteiner, D.C. (1990) Leukocyte depletion filters: a comparison of efficiency. *Amer. J. Hemat.* **35**, 184–186.

Bodmer, Julia, Bodmer, W., Heyes, Judith, So, A., Tonks, S. Trowsdale, J. and Young, J. (1987) Identification of HLA-DP polymorphism with DPα and DPβ probes and monoclonal antibodies: correlation with primed lymphocyte typing. *Proc. nat. Acad. Sci. USA,* **84**, 4596–4600.

Bodmer, W.F. and 9 others (1988) Nomenclature for factors of the HLA system, 1987. *Vox Sang.* **55**, 119–127.

Bodmer, Julia G. and 13 others (1991) Nomenclature for factors of the HLA system, 1990. *Vox Sang.* **61**, 146–155.

Bodmer, Julia, C. and 14 others (1992) Nomenclature for factors of the HLA system. *Tissue Antigens,* **39**, 161–173.

Boizard, Bernadette and Wautier, J.L. (1984) Lek[a], a new platelet antigen absent in Glanzmann's thrombasthenia. *Vox Sang.* **46**, 47–54.

Bolin, R.B., Chevey, B.A., Smith, D.J., Gildengorin, V. and Shigekawa, R. (1982) An *in vivo* comparison of CPD and CPDA-2 preserved platelet concentrates after an 8-hour preprocess hold of whole blood. *Transfusion,* **22**, 491–495.

Bonilla, Mary A. and 12 others (1989) Effects of recombinant human granulocyte colony-stimulating factor on neutropenia in patients with congenital agranulocytosis. *New Engl. J. Med.* **320**, 1574–1580.

Boon, J.C., Jesch, F. and Messmer, K. (1977) Intravascular persistence of hydroxyethyl starch in man. *Eur. surg. Res.* **8**, 497.

Boorman, Kathleen E., Dodd, Barbara E. and Mollison P.L. (1945a) Iso-immunisation to the blood-group factors A, B and Rh. *J. Path. Bact.* **57**, 157.

Boorman, Kathleen E., Dodd, Barbara E. and Morgan, W.T.J. (1945b) Enhancement of the action of immune haemagglutinins by human serum. *Nature (Lond.),* **156**, 663.

Boorman, Kathleen E., Dodd, Barbara E., Loutit, J.F. and Mollison, P.L. (1946) Some results of transfusion of blood to recipients with 'cold' agglutinins. *Brit. Med. J.* i, 751.

Booth, P.B., Dunsford, I., Grant, Jean and Murray, S. (1953) Haemolytic disease in first-born infants. *Brit med. J.* ii, 41.

Booth, P.B., Plaut, Gertrude, James, J.D., Ikin, Elizabeth W., Moores, Phyllis, Sanger, Ruth and Race, R.R. (1957) Blood chimerism in a pair of twins. *Brit. Med. J.* i, 1456.

Booth, P.B., Jenkins, W.J. and Marsh, W.L. (1966) Anti-I[T]: A new antibody of the I blood-group system occurring in certain Melanesian sera. *Brit J. Haemat.* **12**, 341.

Booth, P.B. (1970) Anti-I[T]P$_1$: an antibody showing a further association between the I and P blood group system. *Vox Sang.* **19**, 85.

Booth, P.B. and McLoughlin, K. (1972) The Gerbich blood group system, especially in Melanesians. *Vox Sang.* **22**, 73.

Booth, P.B., Serjeantson, S., Woodfield, D.G. and Amato, D. (1977) Selective depression of blood group antigens associated with hereditary ovalocytosis among Melanesians. *Vox Sang.* **32**, 99.

Boral, L.I. and Henry, J.B. (1977) The type and screen: a safe alternative and supplement in selected surgical procedures. *Transfusion,* **17**, 163.

Bordet, J. (1909) *Studies in Immunity.* p. 512. Chapman & Hall, London.

Bork, K. and Witzke, G. (1989) Long-term prophylaxis with C1-inhibitor (C1 INH) concentrate in patients with recurrent angioedema caused by hereditary and acquired C1-inhibitor deficiency. *J. Allergy clin. Immunol.* **83**, 677–682.

Borst-Eilers, E. (1972) Rhesusimmunisatie: onstaan en preventie. MD Thesis. University of Amsterdam.

Borun, E.R., Fuguetoa, W.G. and Perry, S.M. (1957) The distribution of Fe[59] tagged human erythrocytes in centrifuged specimens as a function of cell age. *J. clin. Invest.* **36**, 676.

Bothwell, T. and Finch C.A. (1962) *Iron Metabolism.* Churchill, London.

Böttiger, L.E. and Molin, L. (1968) Turnover of [131]I- and [125]I -labelled haptoglobin in man. *Acta med. scand.* **184**, 187.

Boudart, D., Lucas, J-C., Adjou, Chantal and Muller, J-Y. (1992) HCV confirmatory testing of blood donors (Letter). *Lancet,* **i**, 372.

Boughton, B.J., Chaskraverty, R., Baglin, T.P., Simpson, A., Galvin, G., Rose, R. and Rohlova, B. (1988) The treatment of chronic idiopathic thrombocytopenia with anti-D(Rh$_0$) immunoglobulin; its effectiveness, safety and mechanism of action. *Clin. lab. Haemat.* **10**, 275–284.

Boughton, B.J., Chakravertyy, R.K., Simpson, A. and Smith, N. (1990) The effect of anti-Rh$_0$ and non-specific immunoglobulins on monocyte Fc receptor function: the role of high molecular weight IgG polymers and IgG subclasses. *Clin. lab. Haemat.* 12, 17–23.

Bouillenne J.D., André, A., Brocteur, J. and Otto-Servais, Monique (1965) Application à la conservation d'hématies-test d'une technique utilisée en insémination artificielle (méthode des paillettes). *Proc. 10th Congr. Europ. Soc. Haemat.,* Strasbourg, 1965, Part II, p. 1497.

Bove, J.R. and Ebaugh, F.G. jr (1958) The use of diisopropylfluorophosphate[32] for the determination of *in vivo* red cell survival and plasma cholinesterase turnover ratio. *J. Lab. clin. Med.* **51**, 916.

Bove, J.R. (1968) Delayed complications of transfusion. *Connecticut Medicine,* **32**, 36.

Bove, J.R., Holburn, A.M. and Mollison, P.L. (1973) Non-specific binding of IgG to antibody-coated red cells (the 'Matuhasi-Ogata phenomenon'). *Immunology,* **25**, 793.

Bove, J.R. (1978) In International Forum. Which is the factual basis, in theory and clinical practice, for the use of fresh frozen plasma? *Vox Sang.* **35**, 428.

Bove, J.R., Chateau, H., Kluge, S., Roelcke, F., Menke, H.E. and Muller, F. (1981) Does it make sense for blood transfusion services to continue the time-honored syphilis screening with cardiolipin antigen? International forum. *Vox Sang.* **41**, 183–192.

Bowden, R.A., Sayers, M., Flournoy, N., Newton, B., Banaji, M., Thomas, E.D. and Meyers, J.D. (1986) Cytomegalovirus immune globulin and seronegative blood products to prevent primary cytomegalovirus infection after marrow transplantation. *New Engl. J. Med.* **314**, 1006–1010.

Bowell, P.J., Wainscot, J.S., Peto, T.E.A. and Gunson, H.H. (1982) Maternal anti-D concentrations and outcome in rhesus haemolytic disease of the newborn. *Brit. med. J.* **285**, 327–329.

Bowell, P.J. (1984) Reproducibility studies on the automated anti-D quantitation method: preliminary report on the UK Quality Control Studies. *Plasma Therap. Transfus. Technol.* **5**, 73–80.

Bowell, P.J., Allen, D.L. and Entwistle, C. (1986a) Blood group antibody screening tests during pregnancy. *Brit. J. Obstet. Gynaec.* **93**, 1038, 1043.

Bowell, P.J., Brown, S.E., Dike, A.E. and Inskip, M.J. (1986b) The significance of anti-c alloimmunization in pregnancy. *Brit. J. Obstet. Gynaec.* **93**, 1044–1048.

Bowell, P.J., Inskip, M.J. and Jones, M.N. (1988) The significance of anti-C sensitization in pregnancy. *Clin. lab. Haemat.* **10**, 251–255.

Bowley, C.C. and Dunsford, I. (1949) The agglutinin anti-M associated with pregnancy. *Brit med. J.* **ii**, 681.

Bowley, A.R., Gordon, I. and Ross, D.W. (1984) Computer-controlled automated reading of blood groups using microplates. *Med. Lab. Sciences,* **41**, 19–28.

Bowman, H.S., Brason, F.W., Mohn, J.F. and Lambert, R.M. (1961) Experimental transfusion of donor plasma containing blood-group antibodies into compatible normal human recipients. II. Induction of isoimmune haemolytic anaemia by a transfusion of plasma containing exceptional anti-CD antibodies. *Brit J. Haemat.* **7**, 130.

Bowman, J.M. and Pollock, Janet M. (1965) Amniotic fluid spectrophotometry and early delivery in the management of erythroblastosis fetalis. *Pediatrics,* **35**, 815.

Bowman, H.S., Marsh, W.L., Schumacher, H.R., Oyen, R. and Reihart, J. (1974) Auto anti-N immunohemolytic anemia in infectious mononucleosis. *Amer. J. clin. Path.* **61**, 465.

Bowman, H.S. (1976) Effectiveness of prophylactic Rh immunosuppression after transfusion with D-positive blood. *Amer. J. Obstet. Gynec.* **124**, 80.

Bowman, J.M., Chown, B., Lewis, Marion and Pollack, Janet (1978) Rh-immunization during pregnancy, antenatal prophylaxis. *Canad. med. Assoc. J.* **118**, 623.

Bowman, J.M. and Pollack, Janet M. (1980) Haemolysis of donor red cells at fetal transfusion due to catheter trauma. *Lancet,* **ii**, 1190.

Bowman, J.M., Friesen, A.D., Pollack, Janet M.

and Taylor, Wilma E. (1980) WinRho: Rh immune globulin prepared by ion exchange for intravenous use. *Canad. med. Assoc. J.* **123**, 1121–1125.

Bowman, J.M. (1983) Blood group immunization in obstetric practice. *Current problems in Obstetrics and Gynecology*, **7**, 4–61.

Bowman, J.M. (1984) Controversies in Rh prophylaxis, in *Hemolytic Disease of the Newborn*, ed G. Garratty, pp. 67–85. Amer. Assoc. Blood banks, Arlington, VA.

Bowman, J.M. and Pollock J.M. (1984) Reversal of Rh immunization. Fact or fancy? *Vox Sang.* **47**, 209–215.

Bowman, J.M., Lewis, Marion and De Sa, D.J. (1984) Hydrops fetalis caused by massive maternofetal transplacental haemorrhage. *J. Pediat.* **104**, 769–772.

Bowman. J.M., and Pollock, J.M. (1985) Transplacental fetal hemorrhage after amniocentesis. *Obstet. gynec.* **66**, 749–754.

Bowman, J.M. and Pollock, J.M. (1987) Failures of intravenous Rh immune globulin prophylaxis; an analysis of the reasons for such failures. *Transfus. Med. Rev.* **1**, 101–112

Bowman, J.M., Harman, F.A., Manning, C.R. and Pollock, J.M. (1989) Erythroblastosis fetalis produced by anti-k. *Vox Sang.* **56**, 187–189.

Bowman, J.M. (1990) Treatment options for the fetus with alloimmune hemolytic disease. *Transfus. Med. Rev.* **4**, 191–207.

Boyan, C.P. and Howland, W.S. (1963) Cardiac arrest and temperature of bank blood. *J. Amer. med. Assoc.* **183**, 58.

Boyan C.P. (1964) Cold or warmed blood for massive transfusions. *Ann. Surg.* **160**, 282.

Boycott, A.E. and Oakley, C.L. (1933) The regulation of marrow activity: experiments on blood transfusion and on the influence of atmospheres rich in oxygen. *J. Path. Bact.* **36**, 205.

Boyd, W.C. and Reguera. R.M. (1949) Hemagglutinating substances for human cells in various plants. *J. Immunol.* **62**, 333.

Boyd, W.C., Everhart, D.L. and McMaster, Marjorie H. (1958) The anti-N lectin of *Bauhinea purpurea. J. Immunol.* **81**, 414.

Boyd, W.C. (1963) The lectins: their present status. *Vox Sang.* **8**, 1.

Boyd, W.C., Brown, Rebecca and Boyd, L.G. (1966) Agglutinins for human erythrocytes in molluscs. *J. Immunol.* **96**, 301.

Boyden, S.V. (1951) The adsorption of proteins on erythrocytes treated with tannic acid and subsequent hemagglutination by anti-protein sera. *J. exp. Med.* **93**, 107.

Boyland, I.P., Mufti. G.F. and Hamblin, T.J. (1982) Delayed haemolytic transfusion reaction caused by anti-Fy^b in a splenectomized patient (Letter). *Transfusion*, **22**, 402.

Boylston, A.W., Gardner, B., Anderson, R.L. and

Hughes-Jones, N.C. (1980) Production of human IgM anti-D in tissue culture by EB virus transformed lymphocytes. *Scand. J. Immunol.* **12**, 355–358.

Bracey, A.W., Klein, H.G., Chambers, S. and Corash, L. (1983) *Ex vivo* selective isolation of young red blood cells using the IBM-2991 Cell Washer. *Blood*, **61**, 1068–1071.

Brackmann, H.H. and Egli, H. (1988) Acute hepatitis B infection after treatment with heat-inactivated Factor VIII concentrate. *Lancet*, **ii**, 967.

Brackmann, H H., Scharrer, Inge, Kernoff, B A. and The Kogenate^T_M Study Group (1991) Clinical efficacy of recombinant Factor VIII (r FVIII) in prophylaxis and treatment of bleeding episodes in hemophiliacs. *Thrombos. Haemostas.* Abstract 183.

Bradley, B.A., Edwards, J.M., Durm, D.C. and Calne, R.Y. (1972) Quantitation of mixed lymphocyte reaction by gene dosage phenomenon. *Nature (Lond.).* **240**, 54.

Bradley, D.W., McCaustland, Karen, A., Cook, E.H., Schable, C.A., Ebert, J.W. and Maynard, J.E. (1985) Posttransfusion non-A, non-B hepatitis in chimpanzees. Physicochemical evidence that the tubule-forming agent is a small, enveloped virus. *Gastroenterology*, **88**, 773–779.

Bradley, D.W. (1991) HCV: current status and issues for the future. *Proc. 3rd Int. Symp. on HCV*, p. 34. Strasbourg

Brake, J.M. and Deindoerfer. F.H. (1973) Preservation of red blood cell 2, 3-diphosphoglycerate in stored blood containing dihydroxyacetone. *Transfusion*, **13**, 84.

Branch, D.R. and Petz, L.D. (1980) A new reagent having multiple applications in immunohematology (Abstract). *Transfusion*, **20**, 642.

Branch, D.R. and Petz, L.D. (1982) A new reagent (ZZAP) having multiple applications in immunohematology. *Amer. J. clin. Path.* **78**, 161–167.

Branch, D.R., Muensch, H.A., Sy Siok Hian, Anita L. and Petz, L.D. (1983) Disulfide bonds are a requirement for Kell and Cartwright (Yt^a) blood group antigen integrity. *Brit. J. Haemat.* **54**, 573–578.

Branch, D.R. and Gallagher, M.T. (1985) The importance of CO_2 in short-term monocyte-macrophage assays (Letter). *Transfusion*, **25**, 399.

Branch, D.R., Sy Siok Hian, Anita, L. and Petz, L.D. (1985) Unmasking of Kx antigen by reduction of disulphide bonds on normal and McLeod red cells. *Brit J. Haemat.* **59**, 505–512.

Brand, Anneke, Sintnicolaas, K., Claas, F.H.J. and Eernisse, J.G. (1986) ABH antibodies causing platelet transfusion refractoriness. *Transfusion*, **26**, 463–366.

Brand, Anneke, Claas, F.H.J., Voogt, P.J., Wasser, M.N.J.M. and Eernisse, J.G. (1988) Alloimmunization after leukocyte depleted multiple random donor platelet transfusions. *Vox Sang.* **54**, 160–166.

Brandt, S.J. and 9 others (1988) Effects of recombinant human granulocyte-macrophage colony-stimulating factor on hematopoietic reconstitution after high-dose chemotherapy and autologous bone marrow transplantation. *New Engl. J. Med.* **318**, 869–876.

Brasseur, Ph. and Bonneau, J.C. (1981) Le paludisme transfusionnel: risque, prevention et coût. *Rev. franç. Transfus. Immunohemat.* **24**, 597–608.

Bratteby, L.-E. and Wadman, B. (1968) Labelling of red blood cells *in vitro* with small amounts of di-iso-propyl-fluorophosphonate (DF^{32}P). *Scand. J. clin. Lab. Invest.* **21**, 197.

Bratteby, L.-E, Garby, L., Groth, T., Schneider, W. and Wadman, B. (1968a) Studies on erythro-kinetics in infancy. XIII. The mean life span and the life span frequency function of red blood cells formed during foetal life. *Acta. paediat. Scand.* **57**, 311.

Bratteby, L.-E., Garby, L. and Wadman, B. (1968b) Studies on erytho kinetics in infancy. XII. Survival in adult recipients of cord blood red cells labelled *in vitro* with di-isopropyl-fluorophosphonate (DF^{32}P). *Acta. paediat. scand.* **57**, 305.

Braude, A.I., Sandford, J.P., Bartlett, J.E. and Mallery, O.T. jr (1952) Effects and clinical significance of bacterial contaminants in transfused blood. *J. Lab. clin. Med.* **39**, 902.

Brazier, D.J., Gregor, Z.J., Blach, R.K., Porter, J.B. and Huehns, E.R. (1986) Retinal detachment in patients with proliferative sickle cell retinopathy. *Transact. ophthalmol. Soc. U.K.* **105**, 100–105.

Brecher, M.E., Moore S.B. and Taswell, H.F. (1988) Minimal exposure transfusion: a new approach to homologous blood transfusion. *Mayo Clin. Proc.* **63**, 903–905.

Brecher, M.E., Moore, S.B., Reisner, Rebecca K., Rakela, J. and Krom, R.A.F. (1989) Delayed hemolysis resulting from anti-A$_1$ after liver transplantation. *Amer. J. clin. Path.* **91**, 232–235.

Brecher, M.E., Moore, S.B. and Letendre, L. (1990) Posttransfusion purpura: the therapeutic value of Pl^{A1}-negative platelets. *Transfusion*, **30**, 433–435.

Bredenberg, C.E. (1977) In International Forum. Does a relationship exist between massive blood transfusions and the adult respiratory distress syndrome? etc. *Vox Sang.* **32**, 311.

Brendel, W.L., Issitt, P.D., Moore, R.E., Lenes, B.A., Zeller, D.J., Tse, T.P. and Atkins, W. (1985) Temporary reduction of red cell Kell system antigen expression and transient production of anti-Kp^b in a surgical patient. *Biotest Bulletin*, **2**, 201–206.

Brendemoen, O.J. (1950) Further studies of agglutination and inhibition in the Le^a-Le^b system. *J. Lab. clin. Med.* **36**, 335.

Brendemoen, O.J. (1952a) A cold agglutinin specifically active against stored red cells. *Acta path. microbiol. Scand.* **31**, 574.

Brendemoen, O.J. (1952b) Some factors influencing Rh immunization during pregnancy. *Acta path. microbiol. scand.* **31**, 579.

Brendemoen, O.J. and Aas, K. (1952) Hemolytic transfusion reaction probably caused by anti-Le^a. *Acta med. scand.* **141**, 458.

Brennan, M. (1991) Fibrin glue. *Blood Reviews*, **5**, 204–244.

Brennan, Mary, T., Runganga, Judith, Barbara, J.A.J. and Contreras, Marcela (1992) The prevalence of anti-HTLV in North London blood donors (Abstract). *HTLV Symposium*, Montpellier, France.

Brettler, D.B., Forsberg, A.D., Levine, P.H., Petillo, J., Lamon, K. and Sullivan, S.L. (1989) Factor VIII: concentrate purified from plasma using monoclonal antibodies: human studies. *Blood*, **73**, 1859–1863.

Breuning, M.H., van den Berg-Loonen, Petronella M., Bernini, L.F., Bijlsma, J.B., van Loghem, Erna, Meera Khan, P. and Nijenhuis, L.E. (1977) Localization of HLA on the short arm of chromosome 6. *Human Genet.* **37**, 131–139.

Brewer, G.J., Tarlov, A.R. and Kellermeyer, R.W. (1961) The hemolytic effect of primaquine. XII. Shortened erythrocyte life span in primaquine-sensitive male Negroes in the absence of drug administration. *J. Lab. clin. Med.* **58**, 217.

Briggs, M., Fox, J. and Tedder, R.S. (1988) Age prevalence of antibody to human herpesvirus 6 (Letter). *Lancet*, i, 1058–1059.

Brigham, K.L., Bowers, R.E. and McKeen, C.B. (1981) Methylprednisolone prevention of increased vascular permeability following endotoxemia in sheep. *J. clin. Invest.* **67**, 1103–1110.

Brittingham, T.E. and Chaplin, H. jr (1957) Febrile transfusion reactions caused by sensitivity to donor leukocytes and platelets. *J. Amer. med. Assoc.* **165**, 819.

Brittingham, T.E. and Chaplin, H. jr (1961) The antigenicity of normal and leukemic human leukocytes. *Blood*, **17**, 139.

Britton, L.W., Eastland, D.T., Dziuban, S.W., Foster, E.D., McIlduff, J.B., Canavan, T.E. and Older, T.M. (1989) Predonated autologous blood use in elective cardiac surgery. *Ann. thorac. Surg.* **47**, 529–532.

Brockhaus, M., Magnani, J.L., Blaszczyk,

Magdalena, Steplewski, S., Koprowski, Hilary, Karlsson, K.-A., Larson, G. and Ginsburg, V. (1981) Monoclonal antibodies directed against the human Le^b blood group antigen. *J. biol. Chem.* **256**, 13 223–13 225.

Brocteur, J., Francois-Gerard, C., André, A., Radermecker, M,. Bruwier, M. and Salmon, J. (1975) Immunization against avian proteins. *Haematologia*, **9**, 43.

Brody, N.I., Walker, J.G. and Siskind. G.W. (1967) Studies on the control of antibody synthesis: interaction of antigenic competition and suppression of antibody formation by passive antibody on the immune response. *J. exp. Med.* **126**, 81.

Brojer, E., Merry, A.H. and Zupanska, B. (1989) Rate of interaction of IgG1 and IgG3 sensitized red cells with monocytes in the phagocytosis assay. *Vox Sang.* **56**, 101–103.

Broman, B. (1944) The blood factor Rh in man. *Acta paediat. (Uppsala)*, **31**, Suppl. 2, p. 128.

Bronchud, M.H. and 10 others (1988) *In vivo* and *in vitro* analysis of the effects of recombinant human granulocyte colony-stimulating factor in patients. *Brit. J. Cancer*, **58**, 64–69.

Bronson, W.R. and McGinniss, M.H. (1962) The preservation of human red blood cell agglutinogens in liquid nitrogen: study of a technic suitable for routine blood banking. *Blood*, **20**, 478.

Brooks, D.E. (1973) The effect of neutral polymers on the electrokinetic potential of cells and other charged particles. IV. Electrostatic effects in dextran-mediated cellular interaction. *J. colloid Interface Sci.* **43**, 714.

Brooks, D.E. and Seaman, G.V.F. (1973) The effect of neutral polymers on the electrokinetic potential of cells and other charged particles. I Models for the zeta potential increase. *J. colloid Interface Sci.* **43**, 670.

Brouet, J.C., Vainchenker, W., Blanchard, Dominique, Testa, U. and Cartron, J-P. (1983) The origin of human B and T cells from multipotent stem cells: a study of the Tn syndrome. *Eur. J. Immunol.* **13**, 350–352.

Brouwers H.A.A., Overbeeke, M.A.M., Gemke. R.J.B.J., Maas, C.J., van Leeuwen, E.F. and Engelfriet, C.P. (1987) Sensitive methods for determining subclasses of IgG anti-A and anti-B in sera of blood-group-O women with a blood-group-A or -B child. *Brit. J. Haemat.* **66**, 267–70.

Brouwers, H.A.A., Overbeeke M.A.M Huiskes, E., Bos, M.J.E., Ouwehand, W.H. and Engelfriet, C.P. (1988a) Complement is not activated in ABO-haemolytic disease of the newborn. *Brit. J. Haemat.* **68**, 363–366.

Brouwers, H.A.A., Overbeeke, M.A.M., van Ertbruggen, I., Schaasberg, W., Alsbach, G.P.J., van der Heiden, C., van Leeuwen, E .F. Stoop,

J.W. and Engelfriet, C.P. (1988b) What is the best predictor of the severity of ABO haemolytic disease of the newborn? *Lancet*, **ii**, 641–644.

Brown, I.W. jr and Hardin, H.F. (1953) Recovery and *in vivo* survival of human red cells. *Arch. Surg.* **66**, 267.

Brown, I.W. jr and Smith, W.W. (1958) Hematologic problems associated with the use of extra-corporeal circulation for cardiovascular subjects. *Ann. intern. Med.* **49**, 1035.

Brown, D.L. and Cooper, A.G. (1970) The *in vivo* metabolism of radioiodinated cold agglutinins of anti-I specificity. *Clin. Sci.* **38**, 175.

Brown, D.L., Lachmann, P.J. and Dacie, J.V. (1970) The *in vivo* behaviour of complement-coated red cells: studies in C6-deficient, C3-depleted and normal rabbits. *Clin. exp. Immunol.* **7**, 401.

Brown, E. (1983) Studies in splenectomy pp. 213–14, in Immunoglobulin G Fc receptor-mediated clearance in autoimmune diseases, M.M. Frank, moderator. *Ann. intern. Med.* **98**, 206–18.

Brown, J.H., Jardetsky, T., Saper, M.A., Samraoui, B., Bjorkman, P.J. and Wiley, D.C. (1988) A hypothetical model of the foreign antigen binding site of class-II histocompatibility molecule. *Nature (Lond.)*, **332**, 845–850.

Brozović, B. (1984): International forum: How much plasma, relative to his body weight, can a donor give over a certain period without a continuous deviation of his plasma protein metabolism in the direction of plasma protein deficiency? *Vox. Sang.* **47**, 435–436.

Brozović, B. and McShine, R.L. (1991) Platelet counting and function testing, in *Coagulation and Blood Transfusion*, eds C. Th. Smit Sibinga, P.C. Das and P.M. Mannuci. *Developments in Hematology and Immunology*, **26**. Kluwer Academic Publishers, Dordrecht, Boston, London.

Brubaker, D.B. and Romnie, C.M. (1988) The *in vitro* evaluation of two filters (Erypur and Imugard IG 500) for white cell-poor platelet concentrates. *Transfusion*, **18**, 383–385.

Bruce, M. and Mitchell. R. (1981) The LOX antigen: A new chemically-induced red cell antigen. *Med. Lab. Sciences*, **38**, 177–186.

Bruce, M., Watt, A.H., Gabra, G.S. and Mitchell, R. (1985) Rh null with anti-Rh29 complicating pregnancy: the first example in the United Kingdom. *Commun. Brit. Blood Transfus. Soc.* Oxford.

Bruce, M., Watt, A.H., Hare, W., Blue, A. and Mitchell R. (1986) A serious source of error in antiglobulin testing. *Transfusion*, **26**, 177–181.

Bruce, M., Watt, A., Gabra, G.S., Mitchell, R., Lakhesar, D. and Tippett, P. (1988) LKE red cell antigen and its relationship to P_1 and P^k: serological study of a large family. *Vox Sang.* **55**, 237–240.

Bruce-Chwatt, L.J. (1972) Blood transfusion and tropical disease. *Trop. Dis. Bull.* **69**, 825.

Bruce-Chwatt, L.J. (1974) Transfusion malaria. *Bull. Wld. Hlth. Org.* **50**, 337.

Bruce-Chwatt, L.J. (1982) Transfusion malaria revisited. *Trop. Dis. Bull.* **79**, 827–840.

Bruce-Chwatt, L.J. (1985) Transfusion associated parasitic infections, in *Infection, Immunity and Blood Transfusion*, eds R.Y.Dodd and L.F. Barker, pp. 101–125. Alan R. Liss, New York.

Brucker, G., Brun-Vezinet, F., Rosenheim, M., Rey, M.A., Katlama, C. and Gentilini, M. (1987) HIV-2 infection in two homosexual men in France. *Lancet.* i, 223.

Bruix, J. and 11 others (1989) Prevalence of antibodies to hepatitis C virus in Spanish patients with hepatocellular carcinoma and hepatic cirrhosis. *Lancet*, ii, 1004–1006.

Brun-Vezinet, F. and 10 others (1987) Lymphadenopathy-associated virus type 2 in AIDS and AIDS related complex. Clinical and virological features in four patients. *Lancet*, i, 128–132.

Brummelhuis, H.G.J. (1980) Preparation of Cl esterase inhibitor and its clinical use. *Proc. Joint Meeting of the 18th Congr. Int. Soc. Hemat. and 16th Congr. Int. Soc. Blood Transfus.* Montreal, Canada.

Bryant, M.L. and Ratner, L. (1990) Myristoylation-dependent replication and assembly of human immunodeficiency virus 1. *Proc. nat. Acad. Sci. USA*, **87**, 523–527.

B.S.I. (1972) BS4843, sterile intravenous cannulae for single use. British Standards Institution, London.

Bucala, R., Kawakami, M. and Cerani, A. (1983) Cytotoxicity of a perfluorocarbon blood substitute to macrophages in vitro. *Science*, **220**, 965–967.

Buchbinder, L. (1933) The blood grouping of *Macacus rhesus*, including comparative studies of the antigenic structure of the erythrocytes of man and *Macacus rhesus*. *J. Immunol.* **25**, 33.

Buchholz, D.H., Young, Viola M., Friedman, N.R., Reilly, J.A. and Mardiney, M.R. jr (1971) Bacterial proliferation in platelets stored at room temperature. *New Engl. J. Med.* **285**, 429.

Buchholz, D.H. and Bove, J.R. (1975) Unusual response to ABO incompatible blood transfusion. *Transfusion*, **15**, 577.

Buchholz, D.H., Porten, J.H., Menitove, J.E., Rzad, L., Buleger, R.R., Aster, R.H. and Smith, J. (1983) Description and use of the CS-3000 blood cell separator for single donor platelet collection. *Transfusion*, **23**, 190-196.

Buchholz, D.H., Porten, J.H., Grode, G., Lin, A.T., Smith, J., Barber, T., Brda, J. and Kozar, J. (1985) Extended storage of single-donor platelet concentrate collected by a blood separator. *Transfusion*, **25**, 557–562.

Buchholz, D. and 9 others (1989) Red blood cell storage studies in a citrate-plasticized polyvinyl chloride container. *Transfusion*, **29**, Suppl. 8S.

Buckley, Rebecca, H., Dees, Susan, C. and O'Fallon, W.M. (1968) Serum immunoglobulins: 1. Levels in normal children and in uncomplicated allergy. *Pediatrics*, **41**, 600.

Buckner, D., Graw, R.G. jr, Eisel, R.J., Henderson, E.S. and Perry, S. (1969) Leukapheresis by continuous flow centrifugation (CFC) in patients with chronic myelocytic leukaemia (CML). *Blood*, **33**, 353.

Budd, J.L., Wiegers, Susan E. and O'Hara, J.M. (1985) Relapsing post-transfusion purpura. A preventable disease. *Amer. J. Med.* **78**, 361–362.

Budin, P. (1875) A quel moment doit-on pratiquer la ligature du cordon ombilical? *Progr. méd. (Paris)*, **3**, 750. (see also (1876), **4**, 2 and 36.)

Budkowska, A., Dubreuil, P. and Pillot, J. (1988) Prognostic value of Pre S2 epitopes of hepatitis B virus and anti-Pre S2 response evaluated by monoclonal assays, in *Viral Hepatitis and Liver Disease*, ed A.J. Zuckerman, pp. 287–289. Alan R. Liss, New York.

Bueno, R., Garratty, G. and Postoway, N. (1981) Elution of antibody from red blood cells using xylene - a superior method. *Transfusion*, **21**, 157–162.

Buffaloe, G.W., Erickson, R.R. and Dau, P.C. (1983) Evaluation of a parallel plate membrane plasma exchange system. *J. clin. Apheresis*, **1**, 86–94.

Bukowski, R.M., Hewlett, J.S., Reimer, R.R., Groppe, C.W., Weick, J.K. and Livingston, R.B. (1981) Therapy of thrombotic thrombocytopenic purpura: an overview. *Semin. Thrombos. Hemostas.* **7**, 1–8.

Bull, J.P., Ricketts, C., Squire, J.R., Maycock, W.d'A., Spooner, S.J.L., Mollison, P.L. and Paterson, J.C.S. (1949b) Dextran as a plasma substitute. *Lancet*, i, 134.

Bull, J.P. (1954) Shock caused by burns and its treatment. *Brit. med. Bull.* **10**, 9.

Bull, J.P. and Jackson, D.M. (1955) Unpublished observations cited by Squire J.R., Bull, J.P., Maycock, W.d'A. and Richetts, C.R. (1955) Dextran. Its properties and use in medicine. pp. 63–65. Blackwell Scientific Publications, Oxford.

Bunker, J.P., Stetson, J.B., Coe, R.C., Grillo, H.C. and Murphy, Anna J. (1955) Citric acid intoxication. *J. Amer. med. Assoc.* **157**, 1361.

Bunn, F.H., Esham, W.T. and Bull, R.W. (1969a) The renal handling of hemoglobin. I. Glomerular filtration. *J. exp. Med.* **129**, 909.

Bunn, H.F., May, M.H., Kocholaty, W.F. and Shields, C.E. (1969b) Hemoglobin function of stored blood. *J. clin. Invest.* **48**, 311.

Burgstaler, E.A., Pineda, A.A. and Ellefson, R.D. (1980) Laboratory study. Removal of plasma liproproteins from circulating blood with a heparin-agarose column. *Mayo Clin. Proc.* **55**, 180–184.

Burkart, P., Rosenfield, R.E., Hsu, T.C.s., Wong, K.Y., Nusbacher, J., Shaikh, S.H. and Kochwa, S. (1974) Instrumented PVP-augmented antiglobulin tests. I. Detection of allogeneic antibodies coating otherwise normal erythrocytes. *Vox Sang.* **26**, 289.

Burkart, P.T. and Hsu, T.C.S. (1979) IgM cold-warm hemolysins in infectious mononucleosis. *Transfusion*, **19**, 535–538.

Bürki, U., Degnan, T.J. and Rosenfield, R.E. (1964) Stillbirth due to anti-U. *Vox Sang.* **9**, 209.

Burks, A.W., Sampson, H.A. and Buckley, R.H. (1986) Anaphylactic reactions after gamma globulin administration in patients with hypogammaglobulinemia. *New Engl. J. Med.* **314**, 560–564.

Burnet, F.M. and Fenner, F. (1949) *The Production of Antibodies*, 2nd edn. Macmillan, Melbourne.

Burnie, Katherine L. (1965) The recovery of red cells from blood samples stored in liquid nitrogen. *Canad. J. med. Technol.* **27**, 179.

Burnie, Katherine (1973) Ii antigens and antibodies. *Canad. J. med. Technol.* **35**, 5.

Burnouf, T., Constans, J., Clerc, A., Descamps, J., Martinache, L. and Goudemand, M. (1987) Biochemical and biological properties of an α_1 antitrypsin concentrate. *Vox Sang.* **52**, 291–297.

Burnouf, T. Michalski, C., Coudemand, M., and Huart, J.J. (1989) Properties of a highly purified human plasma factor IX:c therapeutic concentrate prepared by conventional chromatography. *Vox Sang.* **57**, 225–232.

Burns, Linda J., Westberg, M.W., Burns, C.F., Klassen, L.W., Goeken, Nancy E., Ray, T.L. and MacFarlane, D.E. (1984) Acute graft-versus-host disease resulting from normal donor blood transfusion. *Acta haemat.* **71**, 270–276.

Burrows. L. and Tartter, P. (1982) Effects of blood transfusion on colonic malignancy recurrence rate (Letter). *Lancet*, **ii**, 662.

Burton, Marie S. and Mollison, P.L. (1968) Effect of IgM and IgG iso-antibody on red cell clearance. *Immunology*, **14**, 861.

Busch, M.P. and 9 others (1990) Screening of selected male blood donors for p24 antigen of human immunodeficiency virus type 1. *New Engl. J. Med.* **323**, 1308–1312.

Busch, M.P., Mosley, J.W., Alter, H.J. and Epstein, J.S. (1991) Case of HIV-1 transmission by antigen-positive, antibody-negative blood (Letter). *New Engl. J. Med.* **325**, 1175.

Busch, M.P. and Wilber, J.C. (1992) Hepatitis C virus replication (Letter). *New Engl. J. Med.* **326**, 64–65.

Bush, M., Sabo, B., Stroup, M. and Masouredis, S.P. (1974) Red cell D antigen sites and titration scores in a family with weak and normal D^u phenotypes inherited from a homozygous D^u mother. *Transfusion*, **14**, 433.

Bussel, A., Benbunan, M., Boiron, M. and Bernard. J. (1976) Prélèvement de leucocytes de leucémie myeloide chronique par sedimentation. *Nouv. Rev. franç. Hémat.* **16**, 106.

Bussel, A., Sitthy, X. and Reviron, J. (1982) Aspects technologiques et complications des échanges plasmatiques. *Rev. franç. Transfus. Immunohémat.* **25**, 547–576.

Bussel, J., Lalezari, P., Hilgartner, M., Partin, J., Fikrig, S., Malley, J.O. and Barandum, S. (1983) Reversal of neutropenia with intravenous gammaglobulin in autoimmune neutropenia of infancy. *Blood*, **62**, 398–400.

Bussel, J.B., Goldman, A., Imbach, P. Shulman, I. and Hilgartner, M.W. (1985) Treatment of acute idiopathic thrombocytopenia of childhood with intravenous infusions of gammaglobulin. *J. Pediat.* **106**, 886–900.

Bussel, J., Berkowitz, R., McFarland, J., Lynch, L. and Chitkara, U. (1988) In-utero platelet transfusion for alloimmune thrombocytopenia. *Lancet*, **ii**, 1307–1308.

Button, L.N., Dewolf, W.C., Newburger, P.E., Jacobson, M.S. and Kevy, S.V. (1981) The effect of irradiation on blood components. *Transfusion*, **21**, 419–426.

Byrnes, J.J. and Khurana, M. (1977) Treatment of thrombotic thrombocytopenic purpura with plasma. *New Engl. J. Med.* **297**, 1386.

Byrnes, J.J., Moake, J.L., Klug, P. and Periman, P. (1990) Effectiveness of the cryosupernatant fraction of plasma in the treatment of refractory thrombotic thrombocytopenic purpura. *Amer. J. Hemat.* **34**, 169–174.

Bystryn, J.-C., Graf, M.W. and Uhr, J.W. (1970) Regulation of antibody formation by serum antibody. II. Removal of specific antibody by means of exchange transfusion. *J. exp. Med.* **132**, 1279.

Caballero, C., Vekemans, M., Lopez del Campo, J.G. and Robyn C. (1977) Serum alpha-fetoprotein in adults, in women during pregnancy, in children at birth, and during the first week of life: a sex difference. *Amer, J. Obstet. Gynec.* **127**, 384.

Cabrol, I, Gandjbakhch, I., Pavie, A., Cabral, A.,

Mattei, M.F., Leger, P., Chonette, G. and Aupetit, B. (1987) Heart and heart–lung transplantation. *Transplant. Proc.* **29**, 103–112.

Cáceres, E. and Whittembury, G. (1959) Evaluation of blood losses during surgical operations. Comparison of the gravimetric method with the blood volume determination. *Surgery*, **45**, 681.

Cahill, K.M., Benach, J.L., Reich, L.M., Bilmes, E., Zins, J.H., Siegel, F.P. and Hochweis, S. (1981) Red cell exchange: treatment of babesiosis in a splenectomized patient. *Transfusion*, **21**, 193–198.

Caine, M.E. and Mueller-Heubach. (1986) Kell sensitization in pregnancy. *Amer. J. Obstet. Gynec.* **154**, 85–90.

Cairo, M.S., Worcester, C. and Rucker, R. (1987) Role of circulating complement and polymorphonuclear leukocyte transfusion in treatment and outcome in critically ill neonates with sepsis. *J. Pediat.* **110**, 935–941.

Cairo, M.S. (1989) Neutrophil transfusions in the treatment of neonatal sepsis. *Amer. J. pediat. Hematol. Oncol.* **11**, 227–234.

Calabrese, L.H., Clough, J.D., Krakauer, R.S. and Hoeltge, G.A. (1980) Plasmapheresis therapy of immunologic disease. *Cleveland Clin. Quart.* **47** 53–72.

Callender, Shelia T.E., Powell, E.O. and Witts, L.J. (1945a) The life-span of the red cell in man. *J. Path. Bact.* **57**, 129.

Callender, Shelia, Race, R.R. and Paykoç, Z.V. (1945b) Hypersensitivity to transfused blood. *Brit. med. J.* **ii**, 83.

Callender, Shelia T.E. and Race R.R. (1946) A serological and genetical study of multiple antibodies formed in response to blood transfusion by a patient with lupus erythematosus diffusus. *Ann. Eugen. (Camb.)* **13**, 102.

Callender, Shelia T.E., Powell, E.O. and Witts, L.J. (1947) Normal red cell survival in men and women. *J. Path. Bact.* **59**, 519.

Callender, Shelia T.E., Nickel, J.F. and Moore, C.V. (1949) Sickle-cell disease: studied by measuring the survival of transfused red blood cells. *J. Lab. clin. Med.* **34**, 90.

Calne, R.Y., Sells, R.A., Pena, J.R., Davis, D.R., Millard, P.R., Herbertson, B.M., Binors, R.M. and Davies, D.A.L. (1969) Induction of immunological tolerance by porcine liver grafts. *Nature (Lond.),* **292**, 840–842.

Calvelli, T.A. and Rubinstein, A. (1986) Intravenous gamma-globulin in infants with acquired immunodeficiency syndrome. *Pediat. infect. Dis.* **5**, 207–210.

Cameron, G.L. and Staveley, J.M. (1957) Blood group P substance in hydatid cyst fluids. *Nature (Lond.),* **179** 147.

Cameron, C., Dunsford, I., Sickles, Gretchen R., Cahan, A., Sanger, Ruth and Race, R.R. (1959) Acquisition of a B-like antigen by red blood cells. *Brit. Med J.* **ii**, 29.

Cameron, C.H. and Briggs, Moya (1980) Confirmation of specificity by neutralisation in immun-ora diometric assay for hepatitis B surface antigen. *J. virol. Methods*, **1**, 113–116.

Campbell, W.A.B. (1955) Potassium levels in exchange transfusion. *Arch. Dis. Childh.* **30**, 513.

Campbell, D.A., Swartz, R.D., Waskerwitz, J.A., Haines, R.F. and Turcotte, J.G. (1982) Leukoagglutination with interstitial pulmonary edema. A complication of donor-specific transfusion. *Transplantation*, **34**, 300–301.

Camussi, G., Tetta, C. and Caligaris-Cappio, F.C. (1979) Detection of immune complexes on the surface of polymorphonuclear neutrophils. *Int. Arch. Allergy appl. Immunol.* **58**, 135–139.

Cant, B. and Flamand, C. (1967) The albumin anti-globulin test. *Canad. J. med. Technol.* **29**, 101.

Caplan, S.N., Berkan, E.M. and Babior, B.M. (1977) Cytotoxins against a granulocyte antigen system: detection by a new method employing cytochalasin B-treated cells. *Vox Sang.* **33**, 206.

Capon, S.M., Sacher, R.A. and Deeg, H.J. (1990) Effective ultraviolet irradiation of platelet concentrates in Teflon bags. *Transfusion*, **30**, 678–681.

Capra, J.D., Dowling, P.M., Cook, S. and Kunkel, H.G. (1969) An incomplete cold-reactive γ G antibody with i specificity in infectious mononucleosis. *Vox Sang.* **16**, 10.

Card, R.T., Mohandas, N. and Mollison, P.L. (1983) Relationship of post-transfusion viability to deformability of stored red cells. *Brit. J. Haemat.* **53**, 237–240.

Carman, W.F., Jacyna, M.R., Hadziyannis, S., Karayiannis, P., McGarvey, M.J., Makris, A. and Thomas, H.C. (1989) Mutation preventing formation of hepatitis e antigen in patients with chronic hepatitis B virus infection. *Lancet*, **ii**, 588–591.

Carman, W.F., Zanetti, A.R., Karayiannis, P., Waters, J., Manzillo, G., Tanzi, E., Zuckerman, A.J. and Thomas, H.C. (1990) Vaccine induced escape mutant of hepatitis B virus. *Lancet*, **ii**, 325–329.

Carman, W.F., Fagan, E.A., Hadziyannis, S., Karayiannis, P., Tassopoulos, N.C, Williams, R. and Thomas, H.C. (1991) Association of a precore variant of hepatitis B virus with fulminant hepatitis. *Hepatology*, **14**, 219–222.

Carmen, R.A. and 10 others (1988) Five-week red cell storage with preservation of 2,3 DPG. *Transfusion*, **28**, 157–161.

Carpentier, M. and Meersseman, F. (1956) Considération sur le traitement, à propos d'un cas d'isoimmunisation gravidique vis-à-vis du facteur A. *Bull. Soc. roy. belge. Gynéc. Obstet.* **26**, 374.

Carrel, A. (1902) La technique operatoire des anastomoses vasculaires et la transplantation des visceres. *Lyon Med.* **98**, 862.

Carstairs, K.C., Breckenridge, A., Dollery, C.T. and Worlledge, Sheila (1966) Incidence of a positive direct Coombs test in patients on α-methyldopa. *Lancet*, **ii**, 133.

Cartier, L., Araya, F., Castillo, J.L., Verdugo, R., Mora, C., Gajdusek, D. and Gibbs, C. (1990) HTLV-I retrovirus in Chile: a study in 140 neurological patients. *Rev. med. Chile*, **118**, 622–628

Cartron, J.P., Gerbal, A., Hughes-Jones, N.C. and Salmon, C. (1974) 'Weak A' phenotypes. Relationship between red cell agglutinability and antigen site density. *Immunology*, **27**, 723.

Cartron, J.P. (1976) Étude quantative et thermodynamique des phénotypes érythrocytaires 'A faible'. *Rev. franç. Transfus. Immunohémat.* **19**, 35.

Cartron, J.P., Andreu, G., Cartron, J., Bird, G.W.G., Salmon, C. and Gerbal, A. (1978) Demonstration of T-transferase deficiency in Tn-polyagglutinable blood samples. *Eur. J. Biochem.* **92**, 111.

Cartron, J.F. and Nurden, A.T. (1979) Galactosyltransferase and membrane abnormality in human platelets from Tn-syndrome donors. *Nature (Lond.)*, **282**, 621–623.

Cartron, J.P., Blanchard, D., Nurden, A.T., Cartron, C., Rahuel, C., Lee, D., Vainchenker, W., Testa, U. and Rochant, H. (1981) Tn syndrome: a disorder affecting red cell, platelet and granulocyte cell surface components, in *Blood Groups and other Red Cell Surface Markers in Health and Disease*, ed C. Salmon, Masson Publishing, USA.

Cartron, J.-P., Colin, Y., Kudo, S. and Fukuda, M. (1990) Molecular genetics of human erythrocyte sialoglycoproteins glycophorins A,B,C and D, in *Blood Cell Biochemistry*, ed J.R. Harris. **1**, pp. 299–335. Plenum Press, New York.

Cartwright, G.E., Athens, J.W. and Wintrobe, M.M. (1964) The kinetics of granulopoiesis in normal man. *Blood*, **24**, 780.

Case, R.B., Sarnoff, S.J., Waithe, P.E. and Sarnoff, L.C. (1953) Intra-arterial and intravenous blood infusions in hemorrhagic shock. Comparison of effects on coronary blood flow and arterial pressure. *J. Amer. med. Assoc.* **152**, 208.

Case, J. (1976) Albumin autoagglutinating phenomenon as a factor contributing to false positive reactions when typing with rapid slide-test reagents. *Vox Sang.* **30**, 441.

Case, J. (1982) Potentiators of agglutination, in *A Seminar on Antigen-Antibody Reactions Revisited*, ed Carol A. Bell. Amer. Assoc. Blood Banks, Arlington. VA.

Cash, J.D. (1991) High potency Factor VIII concentrates: value not proved? *Brit. med. J.* **303**, 633–634.

Cassell, Mona and Chaplin, H. jr (1961) Changes in the recipient's plasma hemoglobin concentration after transfusion with stored blood. *Transfusion*, **1**, 23.

Castella, A., Labarge, B.P., Lanenstein, K.J. and Davey, F.R. (1983) Autoanti-A_1 antibody in a patient with metastatic carcinoma. *Transfusion*, **23**, 339–341.

Castellanos, A. (1937) La transfusión de globulós. *Arch. Med. infant.* **6**, 319.

Castino, F., Friedman, L.I. and Wiltbank, T.B. (1981) Plasma separation by membrane filtration, in *Plasma Exchange Therapy*, eds H. Borberg and P. Reuther, pp. 11–19. G. Thieme Verlag.

Cattaneo, M., Gringeri, A., Capitanio, Anna M., Santagostino, Elena and Mannucci, P.M. (1989) Anti-D immunoglobulin for treatment of HIV-related immune thrombocytopenic purpura (Letter). *Blood*, **73**, 357.

Cavill, I., Trevett, D., Fisher, J. and Hoy, T. (1988) The measurement of the total volume of red cells in man: a non-radioactive approach using biotin. *Brit. J. Haemat.* **70**, 491–493.

Cazal, P., Monis, M., Caubel, J. and Brives, J. (1968) Polyagglutinabilité héréditaire dominante: antigène privé (Cad) correspondant à un anticorps public et à une lectine de *Dolichos biflorus*. *Rev. franç. Transfus.* **11**, 209.

Cazal, P., Monis, M. and Bizot, M. (1971) Les antigènes Cad et leurs rapports avec les antigènes A. *Rev. franç. Transfus.* **14**, 321.

Cazzola, M. and Ascari, E. (1986) Red cell ferritin as a diagnostic tool. *Brit J. Haemat.* **62**, 209–213.

CDC, see Centers for Disease Control.

Celano, M.J., Levine, P. and Lange, S. (1957) Studies on eluates from Rhesus and human A_0 red cells. *Vox Sang.* **2**, 375.

Celano, M.J. and Levine, P. (1967) Anti-LW specificity in autoimmune acquired hemolytic anemia. *Transfusion.* **7**, 265.

Centers for Disease Control (1982) *Pneumocystis carinii* pneumonia among persons with haemophilia A. *MMWR*, **31**, 365–367.

Centers for Disease Control (1983) Transfusion malaria: serologic identification of infected donors — Pennsylvania, Georgia. *MMWR*, **32**, 222–229.

Centers for Disease Control (1984) Delta hepatitis — Massachusetts. *MMWR*, **33**, 493–494.

Centers for Disease Control (1986) Safety of therapeutic immune globulin preparations with respect to transmission of human T-lymphotropic virus type III/lymphadenopathy-associated virus infection. *MMWR*, **35**, 231–233.

Centers for Disease Control (1987a) Survey of non-US haemophilia treatment centers for HIV seroconversion following therapy with heat treated factor concentrates. *MMWR*, **36**, 121–124.

Centers for Disease Control (1987b) Human immunodeficiency virus infection in the United States. *MMWR*, **36**, 801–804.

Centers for Disease Control (1988) Safety of therapeutic products used for hemophilia patients. *MMWR*, **37**, 441–444.

Centers for Disease Control (1990a) HIV/AIDS Surveillance Report. *MMWR*, **34**, 1–18.

Centers for Disease Control (1990b) Human T-lymphotropic virus type I screening in volunteer blood donors — United States, 1989. *MMWR*, **39**, 915–924.

Centers for Disease Control (1991a) HIV/AIDS Surveillance Report. Jan. 1991, Atlanta.

Centers for Disease Control (1991b) Update: *Yersinia enterocolitica* bacteremia and endotoxin shock associated with red blood cell transfusions — United States, 1991. *MMWR*, **40**, 176–178.

Centers for Disease Control (1992) HIV/AIDS. Surveillance Report. *MMWR*, **9**.

CDR, *see* Communicable Disease Report.

Ceppellini, R. (1955) On the genetics of secretor and Lewis characters: a family study. *Prac. 5th Congr. Int. Soc. Blood Transfus.*, Paris.

Ceppellini, R., Dunn, L.C. and Turri. M. (1955) An interaction between alleles at the Rh locus in man which weakens the reactivity of the Rh$_0$ factor (D^u). *Proc. nat. Acad. Sci. USA*, **41**, 283.

Ceppellini, R.. Dunn, L.C. and Innella, F. (1959) Immunogenetica. II. Analisi genetica formale dei caratteri Lewis con particolare riguardo alla natura epistatica della specificità serologica Le^b. *Folia hered. path. (Milano)* **8**, 261.

Cerilli, G.J., Brasile, L., Gazoulis, T. and DeFrancis, M.E. (1981) Clinical significance of anti-monocyte antibody in kidney transplant recipients. *Transplantation*, **32**, 495–497.

Cerilli, G.J., Brasile, L., Clarke, J. and Gazoulis, T. (1985) The vascular endothelial cell-specific antigen system: three years' experience in monocyte cross-matching. *Transplant. Proc.* **17**, 567–570.

Cerisola, J.A., Rabinovich, A., Alvarez, M., Di Corleto, C.A. and Pruneda, J. (1972) Enfermedad de Chagas y la transfusión de sangre. *Bol. Ofic. Sanit. Panamer.* **73**, 203–206.

Chadwick, K. (1984) An evaluation of some commonly used screening tests for syphilis for use in routine blood banking. *J. Acad. Med. Lab. Sci.* **6**, 9–18.

Chambers, R.W., Foley, H.T. and Schmidt, P.J. (1969) Transmission of syphilis by fresh blood components. *Transfusion*, **9**, 32–34.

Champlin, R.E., Nimer, S.D., Ireland, P., Oette, D.H. and Golde, D.W. (1989) Treatment of refractory aplastic anemia with recombinant granulocyte-macrophage colony-stimulating factor. *Blood*, **73**, 694–699.

Champneys, Dr. (1880) in Discussion of paper by A.E. Schäfer, *Obstet. Transact.* **21**, 346.

Chan, P.C.Y. and Deutsch, H.F. (1960) Immunochemical studies of human serum Rh agglutinins. *J. Immunol.* **85**, 37.

Chan, S-W, Simmonds, P., McOmish, Fiona, Yap, P-L, Mitchell, R., Dow, B. and Follett, E. (1991) Serological responses to infection with three different types of hepatitis C virus (Letter). *Lancet*, ii, 1391.

Chandeysson, P.L., Flye, M.W., Simpkins, S.M. and Holland, P.V. (1981) Delayed hemolytic transfusion reaction caused by anti-P$_1$ antibody. *Transfusion*, **21**, 77–82.

Chan-Shu, S.A. and Blair, O. (1979) A new method of antibody elution from red blood cells. *Transfusion*, **19**, 182–185.

Chanutin, A. (1967a) The effect of the addition of adenine and nucleosides at the beginning of storage on the concentrations of phosphates of human erythrocytes during storage in acid-citrate-dextrose and citrate-phosphate-dextrose. *Transfusion*, **7**, 120.

Chanutin, A. (1967b) Effect of storage of blood in ACD-adenine-inorganic phosphate plus nucleosides on metabolic intermediates of human red cells. *Transfusion*, **7**, 409.

Chanutin, A. and Curnish, R.R. (1967) Effect of organic and inorganic phosphates on the oxygen equilibrium of human erythrocytes. *Arch. Biochem. Biophys.* **121**, 96.

Chaplin, H. jr and Mollison, P.L. (1952) Correction for plasma trapped in the red cell column of the hematocrit. *Blood*, **7**, 1227.

Chaplin, H. jr, Crawford, Hal, Cutbush, Marie and Mollison, P.L. (1952) The effects of a phenothiazine derivative (RP3300) on red cell preservation. *J. clin. Path.* **5**, 9.

Chaplin, H. jr, Mollison, P.L. and Vetter, H. (1953) The body/venous hematocrit ratio: its constancy over a wide hematocrit range. *J. clin. Invest.* **32**, 1309.

Chaplin, H. jr, Crawford, Hal, Cutbush, Marie and Mollison, P.L. (1954) Post-transfusion survival of red cells stored at −20°C. *Lancet*, i, 852.

Chaplin, H. jr and Chang, Estelle (1955) *In vitro* comparison of the effects of four different preservative solutions on single donor blood with special emphasis on rate of flow. *J. Lab. Clin. Med.* **46**, 234.

Chaplin, H. jr, Crawford, Hal, Cutbush, Marie and Mollison, P.L. (1956a) The preservation of red cells at −79°C. *Clin. Sci.* **15**, 27.

Chaplin, H. jr, Wallace, Mary G. and Chang, Estelle (1956b) A study of iso-agglutinin and hemolysin screening procedures for universal donors. *Amer. J. clin. Path.* **26**, 721.

Chaplin, H. jr, Schmidt, P.J. and Steinfeld, J.L. (1957) Storage of red cells at sub-zero temperatures, further studies. *Clin. Sci.* **16**, 651.

Chaplin, H. jr (1959) Studies on the survival of incompatible cells in patients with hypogammaglobulinemia. *Blood*, **14**, 24.

Chaplin, H. jr and Cassell, Mona (1962) The occasional fallibility of *in vitro* compatibility tests. *Transfusion*, **6**, 375.

Chaplin, H. jr (1969) Packed red blood cells. *New. Engl. J. Med.* **281**, 364.

Chaplin, H. jr (1973) Clinical usefulness of specific antiglobulin reagents in autoimmune hemolytic anemias, in *Progress in Hematology*, ed E.B. Brown, vol. VIII. Grune & Stratton, New York.

Chaplin, H. and Torke, N. (1978) Use of radio-labeled antibodies for detection of C3d bound to anti-Rh(D) coated red blood cells. *Commun. 17th Congr. Int. Soc. Hematol. and 15th Congr. Int Soc. Blood Transfus.*, Paris.

Chaplin, H. (1979) Special problems in transfusion management of patients with autoimmune hemolytic anemia, in *A seminar on Laboratory Management of Hemolysis*, Amer. Assoc. Blood Banks, Washington, D.C..

Chaplin, H., Nasongkla, M. and Monroe, M.C. (1981) Quantitation of red blood cell-bound C3d in normal subjects and random hospitalized patients. *Brit J. Haemat.* **48**, 69–78.

Chaplin, H. and Hoffmann, L. (1982) Radioimmunoassay evaluation of anti-C3d activity in broad spectrum commercial antiglobulin reagents. A three year study. *Transfusion*, **22**, 6–11.

Chaplin, H., Coleman, Margaret E. and Monroe, Martha C. (1983) *In vivo* instability of red-blood-cell-bound C3d and C4d. *Blood*, **62**, 965–971.

Chaplin, H. jr (1984) Editorial retrospective. Frozen red cells revisited. *New Engl. J. Med.* **311**, 1696–1698.

Chaplin, H., Hunter, V.L., Rosche, M.E. and Shirey, R.S. (1985) Long-term *in vivo* survival of Rh(D)-negative donor red cells in a patient with anti-LW. *Transfusion*, **25**, 39–43.

Chaplin, H., Hunter, V.L., Malecek, A.C., Kilzer, F. and Rosche, M.E. (1986) Clinically significant allo-anti-I in an I-negative patient with massive hemorrhage. *Transfusion*, **26**, 57–61.

Chapman, R.G., Reitberg, W.A.H. and Dough-

erty, S. (1977) Effect of initial storage at room temperature on human red blood cell ATP, 2,3-DPG and viability. *Transfusion*, **17**, 147.

Chapman, J., Murphy, M.F. and Waters, A.H. (1982) Chronic cold haemagglutinin disease due to an anti-M like autoantibody. *Vox Sang.* **42**, 272–277.

Charache, S. and Moyer, Martha A. (1982) Treatment of patients with sickle cell anemia—another view, in *Advances in the Pathophysiology, Diagnosis and Treatment of Sickle Cell Disease*, ed R.B. Scott, *Progress in Clinical and Biological Research*, **98**, 73–81. Alan R. Liss, New York.

Charache, S. (1983) Sickle cell disease, in *Current Therapy in Haematology—Oncology 1983–84*, eds M.C. Brain and P.B. McCulloch. pp. 44–48. C.V. Mosby, St. Louis.

Charlton, R.K. and Zmijewski, C.M. (1970) Soluble HL-A7 antigen: localization in the β-lipoprotein fraction of human serum. *Science*, **170**, 636.

Chattoraj, A., Gilbert, R. jr and Josephson, A.M. (1968a) Immunologic characterization of anti-H isohemagglutinins. *Transfusion*, **8**, 368.

Chattraj, A., Gilbert, R. jr and Josephson, A.M. (1968b) Serological demonstration of fetal production of blood group isoantibodies. *Vox Sang.* **14**, 289.

Chauffard, M.A. and Vincent, C. (1909) Anémie grave avec hemolysines dans le sérum; ictère hémolysinique. *Ser. Med. (Paris)*, **28**, 345.

Chavez, G.F., Mulinare, J. and Edmonds, L.D. (1991) Epidemiology of Rh hemolytic disease of the newborn in the United States. *J. Amer. med. Assoc.* **265**, 3270–3274.

Chavin, S.J., Siegel, D.M., Rocco, T.A. and Olson, J.P. (1988) Acute myocardial infarction during treatment with an activated prothrombin complex concentrate in a patient with Factor VIII deficiency and Factor VIII inhibitor. *Amer. J. Med.* **85**, 245–273.

Cheingsong-Popov, R., Weiss, R.A., Dalgleish, A., Tedder, R.S., Shanson, D. and Jeffries, D.J. (1984) Prevalence of antibody to human T-lymphocyte virus type III in AIDS and AIDS-risk patients in Britain. *Lancet*, **2**, 477–480.

Chen, Y.A., Lee, T., Wiktor, S.Z., Shaw, G.M., Murphy, E.L., Blattner, W.A. and Essex, M. (1990) Type-specific antigens for serological discrimination of HTLV-I and HTLV-II infection. *Lancet*, **ii**, 1153.

Cheng, M.S. and Lukomskyj, Luba (1989) Lewis antibody following a massive blood transfusion. *Vox Sang.* **57**, 155–156.

Chenoweth, D.E. (1981) Complement activation during cardiopulmonary by-pass (Letter). *New Engl. J. Med.* **305**, 51.

Chenoweth, D.E., Cooper, S.W., Hugli. T.E.,

Stewart. R.W., Blackstone, E.H. and Kirklin, J.W. (1981) Complement activation during cardiopulmonary bypass: evidence for generation of C3a and C5a anaphylatoxins. *New Engl. J. Med.* **304**, 497–503.

Cherif-Zahar, B., Bloy, C., Le Van Kim, Caroline, Blanchard, Dominique, Bailly, P., Hermand, Patricia, Salmon, C., Cartron, J-P. and Colin, Y. (1990) Molecular cloning and protein structure of a human blood group polypeptide. *Proc. nat. Acad. Sci. USA*, **87**, 6243–6247.

Cherubin, C.E. and Prince, A.M. (1971) Serum hepatitis specific antigen (SH) in commercial and volunteer sources of blood. *Transfusion*, **11**, 25.

Chessin, L.N. and McGinniss, Mary H. (1968) Further evidence for the serologic association of the O (H) and I blood groups. *Vox Sang.* **14**, 194.

Chien, S. and Kung-Ming, J. (1973) Ultrastructure basis of the mechanism of rouleaux formation. *Microvasc. Res.* **5**, 155.

Chiewsilp, P. Isarangkura, P. Pookasem, A. Iamsilp, W. Khamenkhetkran, M. and Stabunswadigan, S. (1991) Risk of transmission of HIV by seronegative blood (Letter). *Lancet*, **ii**, 1341.

Childs, R.A., Feizi, T., Fukuda, M. and Hakomori, S.-I. (1978) Blood-group-I activity associated with band 3, the major intrinsic membrane protein of human erythrocytes. *Biochem. J.* **173**, 333.

Chiroco, G., Rondini, G., Plenbani, A., Chiara, A., Massa, M. and Ugazio, A.G. (1987) Intravenous gammaglobulin therapy for prophylaxis of infection in high-risk neonates. *J. Pediat.* **110**, 437–442.

Chodirker, W.B. and Tomasi, T.B. (1963) γ globulin: quantitative relationships in human serum and non-vascular fluid. *Science*, **142**, 1080.

Choo, Q-L., Kuo, G., Weiner, Amy J., Overby, Lacy R., Bradley, D.W. and Houghton, M. (1989) Isolation of a cDNA clone derived from a blood-borne non-A, non-B viral hepatitis genome. *Science*, **244**, 359–361.

Choo, Q-L., Weiner, A.J., Overby, L.R., Kuo, G., Houghton, M. and Bradley, D.W. (1990) Hepatitis C virus: the major causative agent of viral non-A, non-B hepatitis. *Brit. med. Bull.* **46**, 423–441.

Choo, Q-L. and 13 others (1991) Genetic organization and diversity of the hepatitis C virus. *Proc. nat. Acad. Sci. USA*, **88**, 2451–2455.

Chorpenning, F.W. and Hayes, J.C. (1959) Occurrence of the Thomsen-Friedenreich phenomenon *in vivo*. *Vox Sang.* **4**, 210.

Choudhury, N., Jolly, J.G., Mahajan, R.C., Dubey, M.L., Kalra, A. and Ganguly, M.K. (1988) Selection of blood donors in malaria-endemic countries. *Lancet*, **ii**, 972.

Choudhury, N., Jolly, J.G., Mahajan, R.C., Ganguly, N.K., Dubey, M.L. and Agnihotri, S.K. (1991) Malaria screening to prevent transmission by transfusion: an evaluation of techniques. *Med. Lab. Sci.* **48**, 206–211.

Chown, B. (1944) A rapid, simple and economical method for Rh agglutination. *Amer. J. Clin. Path.* **14**, 144.

Chown, B. and Lewis, Marion (1946) Further experiences with the slanted capillary method for the Rh typing of red cells. *Canad. med. Assoc. J.* **55**, 66.

Chown, B. (1949) Never transfuse a woman with her husband's blood. *Canad. med. Assoc. J.* **61**, 419.

Chown, B. and Lewis, Marion (1951) The slanted capillary method of rhesus blood-grouping. *J. clin. path.* **4**, 464.

Chown, B. (1954) Anaemia from bleeding of the foetus into the mother's circulation. *Lancet*, **i**, 1213.

Chown, B. (1955) On a search for rhesus antibodies in very young foetuses. *Arch. Dis. Childh.* **30**, 237.

Chown, B., Kaita, H., Lewis, Marion, Roy, R.B. and Wyatt, L. (1963) A 'D-positive' man who produced anti-D. *Vox Sang.* **8**, 420.

Chown, B., Kaita, H., Lowen, B. and Lewis, M. (1971) Transient production of anti-LW by LW-positive people. *Transfusion*, **11**, 220.

Chown, B., Lewis, Marion, Hiroko, K. and Lowen, Bonnie (1972) An unlinked modifier of Rh blood groups: effects when heterozygous and when homozygous. *Amer. J. hum. Genet.* **24**, 623.

Christensen, B.E. (1971) Effects of an enlarged splenic erythrocyte pool in chronic lymphocytic leukaemia. *Scand. J. Haemat.* **8**, 92.

Christensen, R.D. and Rothstein, G. (1980) Exhaustion of mature marrow neutrophils in neonates. *J. Pediat.* **96**, 316–318.

Christensen, R.D., Rothstein, G., Austoll. H. and Bybee, B. (1982) Granulocyte transfusions in neonates with bacterial infection, neutropenia and depletion of mature marrow neutrophils. *Pediatrics*, **70**, 1–6.

Christian, R.M., Stewart, W.B., Yuile, C.L., Ervin, D.M. and Young, L.E. (1951) Limitation of hemolysis in experimental transfusion reactions related to depletion of complement and isoantibody in the recipient. *Blood*, **6**, 142.

Christie, D.J., Pulkrabek, Shelley, Putnam, J.L., Slatkoff, M.L. and Pischel, K.D. (1991) Posttransfusion purpura due to an alloantibody reactive with glycoprotein Ia/IIa (anti-HPA-5b). *Blood*, **12**, 2785–2789.

Chudwin, D.S., Ammann, A.J., Wara, Diane W., Cowan, M.J. and Phibbs, R.H. (1982) Post-transfusion syndrome. Rash, eosinophilia and thrombocytopenia following intrauterine and exchange transfusion. *Amer. J. Dis. Child.* **136**, 612–614.

Ciavarella, D. (1989) Blood processors and cell separators. *Transfus. Sci.* **10**, 165–184.

Cimo, P.L. and Aster, R.H. (1972) Post-transfusion purpura. Successful treatment by exchange transfusion. *New Engl. J. Med.* **287**, 290.

Cines, D.C., Dusak, B., Tomaski, A., Mennati, M. and Schreiber, A.D. (1982) Immune thrombocytopenia and pregnancy. *New Engl. J. Med.* **306**, 826–831.

Claas, F.H.J., Paul, L.C., van Es, L.A. and van Rood, J.J. (1980) Antibodies against donor antigens on endothelial cells and monocytes in eluates of rejected kidney allografts. *Tissue Antigens*, **15**, 19–24.

Claas, F.H.J., Smeenk R.J.T., Schmidt, R., van Steenbrugge, G.J. and Eernisse, J.G. (1981) Alloimmunization against the MHC antigens after platelet transfusions is due to contaminating leukocytes in the platelet suspension. *Exp. Hemat.* **9**, 84–89.

Clancey, M., Bond, S. and Van Eys, J. (1972) A new example of anti-Lan and two families with Lan-negative members. *Transfusion*, **12**, 106–108.

Clark, D.A., Dessypris, E.N., Jenkins, D.E. and Krantz, S.B. (1984) Acquired immune-hemolytic anemia associated with IgA erythrocyte coating: investigations of hemolytic mechanisms. *Blood*, **64**, 1000–1005.

Clark, J. and 9 others (1985) Seroepidemiologic studies of human T-cell leukemia/lymphoma virus type I in Jamaica. *Int. J. Cancer*, 36, 37–41.

Clarke, T.W. (1949) The birth of transfusion. *J. Hist. Med.* **4**, 337.

Clarke. R., Topley, Elizabeth and Flear, C.T.G. (1955) Assessment of blood loss in civilian trauma. *Lancet*, **i**, 629.

Clarke, C.A., McConnell, R.B. and Sheppard, P.M. (1960) A genetical study of the variations in ABH secretion. *Ann. hum. genet.* **24**, 295.

Clarke, C.A., Donohoe W.T.A., McConnell, R.B., Woodrow, J.C., Finn, R., Krevans, J.R., Kulke, W., Lehane, D. and Sheppard, P.M. (1963) Further experimental studies on the prevention of Rh haemolytic disease. *Brit. med. J.* **i**, 979.

Clarke, Sir Cyril and Whitfield, A.G.W. (1979) Deaths from rhesus haemolytic disease in England and Wales in 1977: accuracy of records and assessment of anti-D prophylaxis. *Brit med. J.* **i**, 1665–1669.

Clarke, C.A., Mollison, P.L. and Whitfield, A.G.W. (1985) Deaths from rhesus haem-

olytic disease in England and Wales in 1982 and 1983. *Brit. med. J.* **291**, 17–19.

Clarke, C.A. and Mollison. P.L. (1989) Deaths from Rh haemolytic disease of the fetus and newborn, 1977–87. *J. roy. Coll. Phycns.* **23**, 181–184.

Clausen, H., Levery, S.B., Nudelman, S., Tsuchiya, S. and Hakomori, S. (1985) Repetitive A epitope (Type 3 chain A) defined by blood group A_1-specific antibody TH-1: chemical basis of qualitative A_1 and A_2 distinction. *Proc. nat. Acad. Sci. USA*, **82**, 1119–1203.

Clavel, F. and 12 others (1986) Isolation of a new human retrovirus from West African patients with AIDS. *Science*, **233**, 343–346.

Clay, Mary E. and Kline, W.E. (1985) Detection of granulocyte antigens and antibodies, in *Current Concepts in Transfusion Therapy*. Amer. Assoc. Blood Banks, Arlington, VA.

Cleghorn, T.E. (1960) The frequency of the Wr^a, By and M^g blood group antigens in blood donors in the South of England. *Vox Sang.* **5**, 556.

Cleghorn, T.E. (1966) A memorandum on the Miltenberger blood groups. *Vox Sang.* **11**, 219.

Clemens, J.M., Taskar, S., Chau, K., Vallari, D., Shih, J. W-K., Alter, H.J., Schleicher, J.B. and Mimms, L.T. (1992) IgM antibody response in acute hepatitis C viral infection. *Blood*, **79**, 169–172.

Cline, M.J. and Berlin, N.I. (1962) Red blood-cell life span using DFP^{32} as a cohort label. *Blood*, **19**, 715.

Cline, M.J. and Berlin, N.I. (1963a) The red cell chromium elution rate in patients with some hematologic disease. *Blood*, **21**, 63.

Cline, M.J. and Berlin, N.I. (1963b) Simultaneous measurement of the survival of two populations of erythrocytes with the use of labelled diisopropylfluorophosphate. *J. Lab. clin. Med.* **61**, 249.

Cline, M.J. and Berlin, N.I. (1963c) An evaluation of $DF^{32}P$ and ^{51}Cr as methods of measuring red cell life span in man. *Blood*, **22**, 459.

Coates, P., Bateson, E.A.J., England, J., Chettey, M. and Brozovic, B. (1992) Recovery and survival of human autologous platelets labelled with ^{111}Indium following cryopreservation with glycerol. *Transfus. Med.*, submitted.

Cockshott, W.P., Thompson, G.T., Howlett, Lois J. and Seeley, Elizabeth T. (1982) Intramuscular or intralipomatous injections. *New Engl. J. Med.* **307**, 356–368.

Cohen, J.A. and Warringa, Mia G.P.J. (1954) The fate of P^{32} labelled diisopropylfluorophosphonate in the human body and its use as a labelling agent in the study of the turnover of blood plasma and red cells. *J. clin. Invest.* **33**, 459.

Cohen, S. and Freeman, T. (1960) Metabolic heterogeneity of human γ-globulin. *Biochem. J.* **76**, 475.

Cohen, Flossie and Zuelzer, W.W. (1964) Identification of blood group antigens by immunofluorescence and its application to the detection of the transplacental passage of erythrocytes in mother and child. *Vox Sang.* **9**, 75.

Cohen, Flossie and Zuelzer, W.W. (1967) Mechanisms of isoimmunization. II. Transplacental passage and postnatal survival of fetal erythrocytes in heterospecific pregnancies. *Blood*, **30**, 796.

Cohen, M.A. and Oberman, H.A. (1970) Safety and long-term effects of plasmapheresis. *Transfusion*, **10**, 58.

Cohen, D.W., Garratty, G., Morel, P. and Petz, L.D. (1979) Autoimmune hemolytic anemia associated with IgG autoanti-N. *Transfusion*, **19**, 329–331.

Cohen, Hannah and Kernoff, P.B.A. (1990) plasma, Plasma products, and indications for their use. *Brit. med. J.* **300**, 803–806.

Cohen, N.D. and 10 others (1989) Transmission of retroviruses by transfusion of screened blood in patients undergoing cardiac surgery. *New Engl. J. Med.* **320**, 1172–1176.

Cohn, E.J., Oncley, J.L., Strong, L.E., Hughes, W.L. jr and Armstrong, H.S. jr (1944) Chemical, clinical and immunological studies on the products of human plasma fractionation. I. The characterization of the protein fractions in human plasma. *J. clin. Invest.* **23**, 417.

Cohn, E.J., Tullis, J.L., Surgenor, D.M., Batchelor, W.H. and D'Hont, M.D. (1951) Biochemistry and biomechanics of blood collection, processing and analyzing of human blood and other tissues. Address presented before the National Academy of Science, Yale University, New Haven.

Cole, R.S., Tocchi, M., Wye, E., Villeneuve, D.C. and Rock, G. (1981) Contamination of commercial blood products by di-2-ethylhexyl phthalate and mono-2-ethylhexyl phthalate. *Vox Sang.* **40**, 317–322.

Coles, S.M., Klein, H.G. and Holland, P.V. (1981) Alloimmunization in two multitransfused patient populations. *Transfusion*, **21**, 462–466.

Colin, Y., Cherif-Zahar, B., Le van Kim, Raynal, Virgina, van Huffel, Veronique and Cartron, J-P. (1991) Genetic basis of the Rh-D positive and Rh-D negative blood group polymorphism as determined by Southern analysis. *Blood*, **78**, 1–6.

Colledge, Katherine I., Pezzulich, Marisa and Marsh, W.L. (1973) Anti-Fy5, an antibody disclosing a probable association between the Rhesus and Duffy blood group genes. *Vox Sang.* **24**, 193.

Collins, J.O., Sanger, Ruth, Allen, F.H. and Race, R.R. (1950) Nine blood-group antibodies in a single serum after multiple transfusions. *Brit. med. J.* **i**, 1297.

Collins, J.A., Simmons, R.L., James, P.M., Bredenberg, C.E., Anderson, R.W. and Heisterkamp, C.A. III (1971) Acid-base status of seriously wounded combat casualties. II. Resuscitation with stored blood. *Ann. Surg.* **173**, 6.

Collins, J.A., James, P.M., Bredenberg, C.E., Anderson, R.W., Heisterkamp, C.A. and Simmons, R.L. (1978) The relationship between transfusion and hypoxemia in combat casualties. *Ann. Surg.* **188**, 513.

Collins, J.A. (1980) Abnormal hemoglobin–oxygen affinity and surgical hemotherapy, in *Surgical Hemotherapy*, eds J.A. Collins and P. Lundsgaard-Hansen, *Bibl. Haemat.* **46**. S. Karger, Basel.

Collins. J.A. (1987) Recent developments in the area of massive transfusion. *World J. Surg.* **11**, 75–81.

Collins, D.R., Entwistle, C.C., Feldman, P.A., Winkelman, L., Evans, H and Sims, G.E.C. (1989) Fractionation of plasma derived from the Baxter Autopheresis-C and Haemonetics PCS. *Transfus. Sci.* **10**, 295–300.

Collins, S.H. (1990) Production of secreted proteins in yeast, in *Protein Production by Biotechnology*, ed T.J.R. Harris, pp. 61–77. Elsevier, Oxford.

Colman, R.W., Chang, L.K., Murkherji, B. and Sloviter, H.A. (1980) Effects of a perfluoro erythrocyte substitute on platelets *in vitro* and *in vivo*. *J. Lab. clin. Med.* **75**, 553–562.

Colombo, M., Mannucci, P.M., Carnelli, V., Savidge, G.F., Gazengel, C. and Schimpf, K. (1985) Transmission of non-A, non-B hepatitis by heat-treated Factor VIII concentrate. *Lancet*, **ii**, 1–4.

Colombo, M., Kuo, G., Choo, Q.L., Donato, M.F., Del Nino, E., Tommasini, M.A., Dioguardi, N. and Houghton, M. (1989) Prevalence of antibodies to hepatitis C virus in Italian patients with hepatocellular carcinoma. *Lancet*, **ii**, 1006–1008.

Colvin, B.T., Rizza, C .R. and the Study Group of the UK Haemophilia Centre Directors (1988) Effect of dry-heating of coagulation factor concentrates at 80°C for 72 hours on transmission of non-A, non-B hepatitis. *Lancet*, **ii**, 814–816.

Combined Study (1966) Prevention of Rh-haemolytic disease: results of the clinical trial. A combined study from centres in England and Baltimore. *Brit. med. J.* **2**, 907.

Combs, M.R., Telen, M.J., Hall, S.E. and Rosse W.F. (1990) A case report: IgG autoanti-N as a cause of severe autoimmune hemolytic anemia. *Immunohematology* **6**, 83.

Commission of the European Communities (1991) *Medicinal Products Derived from Human Blood and Plasma*, pp. 40–56. Brussels.

Communicable Disease report (1986) Acquired immune deficiency syndrome, p. 4. United Kingdom.

Communicable Disease Report (1991) AIDS and HIV-1 antibody reports — United Kingdom: Dec. 1990. 1, 13.

Condie, R.M. and O'Reilly, R.J. (1984) Prevention of cytomegalovirus infection by prophylaxis with an intravenous, hyperimmune, native unmodified cytomegalovirus globulin: randomised trial in bone marrow transplant recipients. *Amer. J. Med.* 76, 134–141.

Connell, G.E. and Painter, R.H. (1966) Fragmentation of immunoglobulin during storage. *Canad. J. Biochem.* 44, 371.

Consensus Conference (1988) Perioperative red blood cell transfusion. *J. Amer. med. Assoc.* 260, 2700–2703.

Constantoulakis, M., Kay, H.E.M., Giles, Carolyn M. and Parkin, Dorothy M. (1963) Observations on the A_2 gene and H antigen in foetal life. *Brit. J. Haemat.* 9, 63.

Constantoulis, N.C., Paidoussis, M. and Dunsford, I. (1955) A naturally occurring anti-S agglutinin. *Vox Sang. (O.S.)* 5, 143.

Conte, D., Brunelli, Lucia, Bozzani, A., Tidone, Laura, Quatrini, M. and Bianchi, P.D. (1983) Erythrocytapheresis in idiopathic haemochromatosis. *Brit. Med. J.* 286, 939.

Contreras, Marcela, Stebbing, Birgit, Blessing, Margaret and Gavin, June (1978) The Rh antigen Evans. *Vox Sang.* 34, 208–211.

Contreras, Marcela, Amitage, Susan, Daniels, G.L. and Tippett, Patricia (1979a) Homozygous D. *Vox Sang.* 36, 81–84.

Contreras, Marcela, Barbolla, A., Lubenko, A. and Armitage, Susan E. (1979b) The incidence of antibodies to low frequency antigens (LFA) in plasmapheresis donors with hyperimmune Rh antisera. *Brit. J. Haemat.* 41, 413.

Contreras, Marcela and Mollison, P.L. (1981) Failure to augment primary Rh immunization using a small dose of 'passive' IgG anti-Rh. *Brit. J. Haemat.* 49, 371–381.

Contreras, Marcela and Mollison, P.L. (1983) Rh immunization facilitated by passively-administered anti-Rh? *Brit. J. Haemat.* 53, 153–159.

Contreras, Marcela, Armitage, Susan E. and Hewitt, Patricia E. (1983a) Response to immunization with A and B human glycoproteins for the procurement of blood grouping reagents. *Vox Sang.* 47, 224–235.

Contreras, Marcela, Hazlehurst, G.R. and Armitage, Susan E. (1983b) Development of auto-anti-A_1 antibodies following alloimmu-

nization in an A_2 recipient. *Brit. J. Haemat.* 55, 657–663.

Contreras, Marcela, Gordon, H. and Tidmarsh, Elizabeth (1983c) A proven case of maternal alloimmunization due to Duffy antigens in donor blood used for intrauterine transfusion (Letter). *Brit. J. Haemat.* 53, 355–356.

Contreras, Marcela and Barbara. J.A.J. (1985) Acquired immune deficiency syndrome and blood transfusion. *J. Hosp. Infect.* 6, Suppl. C, 27–34.

Contreras, Marcela, Hewitt, Patricia E., Barbara, J.A.J. and Mochnaty, P.Z. (1985) Blood donors at risk of transmitting the acquired immune deficiency syndrome. *Brit. Med. J.* 290, 749–750.

Contreras, Marcela, De Silva, Mahes, Teesdale, Phyllis and Mollison, P.L. (1987) The effect of naturally occurring Rh antibodies on the survival of serologically incompatible red cells. *Brit. J. Haemat.* 65, 475–478.

Contreras, Marcela and Knight, R.C. (1989) The Rh-negative donor. *Clin. lab. Haemat.* 11, 317–322.

Contreras, Marcela and Barbara, J. (1991) Jakob–Creutzfeldt disease and blood transfusion (Letter). *Brit. Med. J.* 302, 1148–1149.

Contreras, Marcela, Barbara, J.A.J., Anderson, Catherine, C., Ranasinghe, E., Moore, Christine, Brennan, Mary. T., Howell, D.R., Aloysius, Sriyani, Yardumian, Anne (1991) Low incidence of non-A, non-B posttransfusion hepatitis in London confirmed by hepatitis C virus serology. *Lancet,* i, 753–757.

Coombs, R.R.A., Mourant, A.E. and Race, R.R. (1945) A new test for the detection of weak and 'incomplete' Rh agglutinins. *Brit. J. exp. Path.* 26, 255.

Coombs, R.R.A., Mourant, A.E. and Race, R.R. (1946) *In vivo* iso-sensitization of red cells in babies with haemolytic disease. *Lancet,* i, 264.

Coombs, R.W., Collier. Ann, C., Allain, J-P., Nikora, Beverley, Leuther, M., Gjerset, C.F. and Corey, L., (1989) Plasma viremia in human immunodeficiency virus infection. *New Engl. J. Med.* 321, 1626–1631.

Coon, J., Weinstein, R.S. and Sammers, J. (1982) Blood group precursor T antigen expression in human urinary bladder carcinoma. *Amer. J. clin. Path.* 77, 692–699.

Cooper, A.G., Hoffbrand, A.V. and Worlledge, S.M. (1968) Increased agglutinability by anti-i of red cells in sideroblastic and megaloblastic anaemia. *Brit. J. Haemat.* 15, 381.

Cooper, A.G. and Brown, D.L. (1971) Haemolytic anaemia in the rabbit following the injection of human anti-I cold agglutinin. *Clin. exp. Immunol.* 9, 99.

Cooper, A.G. and Brown, M.C. (1973) Serum i

antigen: a new human blood group glycoprotein. *Biochem. biophys. Res. Commun.* **55**, 297.

Cooper, M.R., Heise, E., Richards, F., Kaufmann, J. and Spurr, C.L. (1975) A prospective study of histocompatible leucocyte and platelet transfusions during chemotherapeutic induction of acute myeloblastic leukaemia, in *Leucocytes: Separation, Collection and Transfusion*, eds J.M. Goldman and R.M. Lowenthal. Academic Press, New York.

Cooper, R.A. (1977) Abnormalities of cell-membrane fluidity in the pathogenesis of disease. *New Engl. J. Med.* **297**, 371.

Cooper, B., Tishler, P.V., Atkins, L. and Breg, W.R. (1979) Loss of Rh antigen associated with acquired Rh antibodies and a chromosome translocation in a patient with myeloid metaplasia. *Blood*, **54**, 642–647.

Cooper, D.K.C. (1990) A clinical survey of cardiac transplantation between ABO blood group-incompatible recipients and donors. *Transplant. Proc.* **22**, 1457.

Cooperative Group for the Study of Immunoglobulin in Chronic Lymphocytic Leukemia (1988) Intravenous immunoglobulin for the prevention of infection in chronic lymphocytic leukemia. A randomized, controlled clinical trial. *New Engl. J. Med.* **319**, 902–907.

Copplestone, J.A. (1990) Fetal platelet counts in thrombocytopenic pregnancy (Letter). *Lancet*, **ii**, 1375.

Corash, L.M. (1978) Platelet heterogeneity: relationship between density and age, in *The Blood Platelet in Transfusion Therapy*, eds T.J.Greenwalt and C.A.Jamieson. Alan R. Liss, New York.

Corash, L., Klein, H., Deisseroth, A., Shafer, Brenda, Rosen, S., Beman, Joann, Griffith, Patricia and Nienhuis, A. (1981) Selective isolation of young erythrocytes for transfusion support of thalassemia major patients. *Blood*, **57**, 599–606.

Corbascio, A.N. and Smith, N.T. (1967) Hemodynamic effects of experimental hypercitremia. *Anesthesiology*, **28**, 510.

Corcoran, Patricia A., Allen, F.H., Lewis, Marion and Chown, B. (1961) A new antibody, anti-Ku (anti-Peltz) in the Kell blood-group system. *Transfusion*, **1**, 181.

Cordell, Ruth A., Yalon, V.A., Cigahn-Haskell, Carla, McDonough, B.P. and Perkins, H.A. (1986) Experience with 11,916 designated donations. *Transfusion*, **26**, 485–486.

Corsetti, J.P., Cowles, J.W., Cox, M.T. and Blumberg, N. (1988) A rapid and accurate single-drop modification of the acid-elution technique for detecting fetomaternal hemorrhage. *Vox Sang.* **54**, 39–42.

Cory, H.T., Yates, A.D., Donald, A.S.R., Watkins, W.M. and Morgan, W.T.J. (1974) The nature of the human blood group P_1 determinant. *Biochem. biophys. Res. Commun.* **61**, 1289.

Cosgrove, D.M., Loop, F.D. and Lytle, B.W. (1981) Blood conservation in cardiac surgery. *Cardiovasc. Clinics*, **12**, 165–175.

Cossart, Y.E., Field, A.M., Cant, B. and Widdows, D. (1975) Parvovirus-like particles in human sera. *Lancet*, **i**, 72–73.

Cossart, Y.E., Kirsh, S. and Ismay, S.L. (1982) Post-transfusion hepatitis in Australia. *Lancet*, **i**, 208–213.

Costa Ferreira, H., Cardim, W.H. and Mellone, O. (1960) Fototerapia. Novo recurso terapeutico na hiperbilirrubinemia do recem-nascido. *J. de Pediat.* **25**, 347–391.

Coste, J., Lemaire, J.M., Barin, F. and Couroucé, A.M. (1990) HTLV I/II antibodies in French blood donors (Letter). *Lancet*, **i**, 1167–1168.

Costea, N., Schwartz, R., Constantoulakis, M. and Dameshek, W. (1962) The use of radioactive antiglobulin for the detection of erythrocyte sensitization. *Blood*, **20**, 214.

Costea, N., Yakulis, V. and Heller, P. (1966) Light chain heterogeneity of anti-I and anti-i antibodies. *Fed. Proc.* **25**, 373.

Costea, N., Yakulis, V.J. and Heller, P. (1972) Inhibition of cold agglutinins (anti-I) by *M. pneumoniae* antigens. *Proc. Soc. exp. Biol. (N.Y.)*, **139**, 476.

Cotter, J. and McNeal, W.J. (1938) Citrate solution for preservation of fluid blood. *Proc. Soc. exp. Biol. (N.Y.)*, **38**, 751.

Council of Europe (1984) Meeting report of the Committee of Experts on Blood Transfusion and Immunohaematology.

Counts, R.B., Haisch, C., Simmon, T.L., Maxwell, N.G., Heimbach, D.M. and Caprico, C.J. (1979) Hemostasis in massively transfused trauma patients. *Ann. Surg.* **190**, 91–99.

Couroucé, Anne-Marie, Ferchal, F., Morinet, F., Pérol, Y., Drouet, J., Muller, A. and Soulier, J.P. (1984) Parvovirus (SPLV) et antigène Aurillac. *Rev. franç. Transfus. Immunohémat.* **27**, 5–19.

Couroucé, Anne-Marie, Drouet, J. LeMarrec, N., Drouet, A. and Soulier, J.P. (1985) Blood donors positive for HBsAg and negative for anti-HBc antibody. *Vox Sang.* **49**, 26–33.

Coursaget, P., Yvonnet, B., Chotard, J., Vincelot, P., Saar, M., Diouf, C., Chiron, J.P. and Diop-Mar, I. (1987) Age- and sex-related study of hepatitis B virus chronic carrier state in infants from an endemic area (Senegal). *J. med. Virol.* **22**, 1–5.

Cox, M.T., Shells, l., masel, D. and Blumberg, N. (1991) Fetal hydrops due to anti-B (Abstract). *Transfusion*, **31**, Suppl. 29S.

Craske, J. (1982) The epidemiology of Factor VIII and IX associated hepatitis in the U.K., in *Unresolved Problems in Haemophilia*, eds

C.D. Forbes and G.D.O. Lowe. pp. 5–14. MTP Press, Lancaster.

Crawford, Hal, Cutbush, Marie and Mollison, P.L. (1953a) Hemolytic disease of the newborn due to anti-A. *Blood*, **8**, 620.

Crawford, Hal, Cutbush, Marie and Mollison, P.L. (1953b) Specificity of incomplete 'cold' antibody in human serum. *Lancet*, **i**, 566.

Crawford, Hal, Cutbush, Marie and Mollison, P.L. (1954) Preservation of red cells for blood-grouping tests. *Vox Sang. (O.S.)*, **4**, 149.

Crawford, Hal and Mollison, P.L. (1955) Reversal of electrolyte changes in stored red cells after transfusion. *J. Physiol. (Lond.)*, **129**, 639.

Crawford, M.N., Greenwalt, T.J., Sasaki, T., Tippett, P.A., Sanger, R. and Race, R.R. (1961) The phenotype Lu(a–b) together with unconventional Kidd groups in one family. *Transfusion*, **1**, 228.

Crawford, M.N., Gottman, F.E. and Gottman, C.A. (1970) Microplate system for routine use in blood bank laboratories. *Transfusion*, **10**, 258–263.

Crawford, D.H., Barlow, M.J., Harrison, J.F., Winger, L. and Huehns, E.R. (1983) Production of human monoclonal antibody to Rhesus D antigen. *Lancet*, **i**, 386–388.

Crawford, M.N. (1987) A review of micromethods for Blood Bank laboratories. *Lab. Med.* **18**, 149–152.

Crawford, R.J., Mitchell, R., Burneti, A.K. and Follett. E.A.C. (1987) Who may give blood? *Brit. med. J.* **294**, 572.

Crawford, Mary N. (1988) The Lutheran blood group system: serology and genetics, in *Blood Group Systems: Duffy. Kidd and Lutheran*. Amer. Assoc. Blood Banks, Arlington, VA.

Crawford, M.N., Wolford, F.E., Pilkington, P.M. and Lugo, J. (1988a) Identification of antibodies on microplates. *Immunohematology*, **4**, 11–12.

Crawford, D.H., Azim, T., Daniels, G.L. and Huehns, E.R. (1988) Monoclonal antibodies to the Rh D antigen, in *Progress in Transfusion Medicine*, ed J.D. Cash. pp. 175–197, Churchill Livingstone, Edinburgh.

Cream, J.J. (1968) Prednisolone-induced granulocytosis. *Brit. J. Haemat.***15**, 259.

Cregan, P., Donegan, E. and Gotelli, G. (1991) Hemolytic transfusion reaction following autologous frozen and washed red cells. *Transfusion*, **31**, 172–175.

Creger, W.P., Choy, S.H. and Rantz, L.A. (1951) Experimental determination of the hypersensitive diathesis in man. *J. Immunol.* **66**, 445.

Cremer, R.J., Perryman, P. and Richards, D.H. (1958) Influence of light on the hyperbilirubinaemia of infants. *Lancet*, **i**, 1094.

Crile, G.W. (1909) *Hemorrhage and Transfusion: an Experimental and Clinical Research*. D. Appleton and Company, New York and London.

Cripps, C.M. (1968) Rapid method for the estimation of plasma haemoglobin levels. *J. clin. Path.* **21**, 110.

Crispen, J. (1976) Immunosuppression of small quantities of Rh-positive blood with MICRhoGAM in Rh-negative male volunteers, in *Proceedings of Symposium on Rh Antibody Mediated Immunosuppression*. Ortho Research Institute, Raritan, New Jersey.

Crocchiolo, P.R., Lizioli, A. and Leopardi, O. (1988) HIV and aplastic anaemia (Letter). *Lancet*, **ii**, 109.

Crome, Patricia and Mollison, P.L. (1964) Splenic destruction of Rh-sensitized, and of heated red cells. *Brit. J. Haemat.* **10**, 137.

Crookston, J.H., Crookston, Marie C., Burnie, Katherine L., Francombe, W.H., Dacie, J.V., Davis, J.A. and Lewis, S.M. (1969a) Hereditary erythroblastic multinuclearity associated with a positive acidified-serum test: a type of congenital dyserythropoietic anaemia. *Brit. J. Haemat.* **17**, 11.

Crookston, J.H., Crookston, Marie C. and Rosse, W.F. (1969b) Red cell membrane abnormalities in hereditary erythroblastic multinuclearity (Abstract). *Blood*, **34**, 844.

Crookston, Marie C., Tilley, Christine A. and Crookston, J.H. (1970) Human blood chimaera with seeming breakdown of immune tolerance. *Lancet*, **ii**, 1110.

Crookston, J.H. and Crookston, M.C. (1982) HEMPAS: clinical, hematologic and serologic features, in *Blood Groups and Other Red Cell Surface Markers in Health and Disease*, ed C. Salmon. Masson Publishing U.S.A., New York.

Crosby, W.H. and Dameshek, W. (1951) The significance of hemoglobinuria and associated hemosiderinuria, with particular reference to various types of hemolytic anemia. *J. Lab. clin. Med.* **38**, 3.

Crosby, W.H. and Stefanini, M. (1952) Pathogenesis of the plasma transfusion reaction with especial reference to the blood coagulation system. *J. Lab. clin. Med.* **40**, 374.

Crosby, W.H. and Furth, F.W. (1956) A modification of the benzidine method for measurement of hemoglobin in plasma and urine. *Blood*, **11**, 380.

Croucher, Betty E.E., Scott, J.G. and Crookston, J.H. (1962) A further example of anti-Lu^b. *Vox Sang.* **7**, 492.

Croucher, Betty E.E., Crookston, Marie C. and Crookston, J.H. (1967) Delayed transfusion reactions simulating auto-immune haemolytic anaemia. *Vox Sang.* **12**, 32.

Croucher, Betty, E.E. (1979) Differential diagnosis of delayed transfusion reaction, in *A Seminar on Laboratory Management of Hemolysis*. Amer. Assoc. Blood Banks, Las Vegas.

Crowley, L.V., Rice, J.D. and Breen, Mary (1957) High titred anti-M iso-agglutinins in human blood: their detection and significance in blood banking and transfusion therapy. *Amer. J. clin. Path.* **28**, 481.

Crowley, J.P. Skrabut, E.M. and Valeri, C.R. (1974) Immunocompetent lymphocytes in previously frozen washed red cells. *Vox Sang.* **26**, 513–517.

Crowley, Mary, Kayo, I. and Steinman, R.M. (1990) Dendritic cells are the principal cells in mouse spleen bearing immunogenic fragments of foreign proteins. *J. exp. Med.* **172**, 383–386.

Cruz, W.O. and Junqueira, P.C. (1952) Resistance of reticulocytes and young erythrocytes to the action of specific hemolytic serum. *Blood*, **7**, 602.

Csonka, G.W. (1983) Syphilis, in *Oxford Textbook of Medicine*, eds D.J. Weatherall, J.G.G. Ledingham and D.A. Warrell, pp. 5.277–5.292. Oxford University Press, Oxford.

Cuatrecasas, P. and Aufinsen, C.B. (1971) Affinity chromatography, in *Methods in Enzymology*, ed W.B. Jakoby, **22**, 345. Academic Press, New York.

Cugno, M., Nuijens, J., Hack, E., Eerenberg, A., Frangi, D., Agostoni, A. and Cicardoi, M. (1990) Plasma levels of C1 inhibitor complexes and cleaved C1 inhibitor in patients with hereditary angioneurotic edema. *J. clin. Invest.* **85**, 1215–1220.

Culliver, H.A. and Penington, D.G. (1979) Mechanisms of vasomotor reactions in the use of SPPS. *Vox Sang.* **36**, 201–207.

Cumberland, G.D., Titford, M. and Riddick, L. (1991) Demonstration of a fatal hemolytic transfusion reaction using immunoperoxidase techniques. *Amer. J. forensic Med. Path.* **12**, 250–251.

Cumming, P.D., Wallace, E.L., Schorr, J.B. and Dodd, R.Y. (1989) Exposure of patients to human immunodeficiency virus through the transfusion of blood components that test antibody-negative. *New Engl. J. Med.* **321**, 941–946.

Cummings, Elizabeth, Pisciotto, Patricia and Roth, G. (1984) Normal survival of Rh₀(D) negative, LW(a+) red cells in a patient with allo-anti-LWª. *Vox Sang.* **46**, 286–290.

Cunningham, F.G. and Pritchard, J.A. (1979) Prophylactic transfusions of normal red cells during pregnancies complicated by sickle cell hemoglobinopathies. *Amer. J. Obstet. Gynec.* **135**, 994–1003.

Cunningham, C.C. and Lind, S.E. (1989) Apparent response of refractory post-transfusion

purpura to splenectomy. *Amer. J. Hemat.* **30**, 112–113.

Curran, J.W. and 19 others (1984) Acquired immunodeficiency syndrome (AIDS) associated with transfusions. *New Engl. J. Med.* **310**, 69–75.

Curran, J.W., Jaffe, H.W., Peterman, T.A. and Allen, J.R. (1985) Epidemiologic aspects of acquired immunodeficiency syndrome (AIDS) in the United States: cases associated with transfusions, in *Infection, Immunity and Blood Transfusion*, eds R.Y. Dodd and L.F. Barker, pp. 259–269. Alan R. Liss Inc. New York.

Currie, M.S., Rustagi, P.K., Wojcieszak, Roslyn, Ziolowski, Lynn, Ross, G.D. and Logue, G.L. (1988) Effect of antigen site and complement receptor status on the rate of cleavage of C3c antigen from cell bound C3b. *Blood*, **71**, 786–790.

Curtain, C.C. (1969) Anti-I agglutinins in non-human sera. *Vox Sang.* **16**, 161.

Curtsinger, L.J., Cheadle, W.G., Hershman, M.J., Cost, Karen, and Polk, H.C. (1989) Association of cytomegalovirus infection with increased morbidity is independent of transfusion. *Amer. J. Surg.* **158**, 606–611.

Cutbush, Marie and Mollison, P.L. (1949) Haemolytic transfusion reaction due to anti-S. *Lancet*, **ii**, 102.

Cutbush, Marie, Mollison, P.L. and Parkin, Dorothy M. (1950) A new human blood group. *Nature (Lond.)*, **165**, 188.

Cutbush, Marie and Chanarin, I. (1956) The expected blood-group antibody anti-Luᵇ. *Nature (Lond.)*, **178**, 855.

Cutbush, Marie, Giblett, Eloise R. and Mollison, P.L. (1956) Demonstration of the phenotype Le(a+b+) in infants and in adults. *Brit. J. Haemat.* **2**, 210.

Cutbush, Marie and Mollison, P.L. (1958) Relation between characteristics of blood-group antibodies *in vitro* and associated patterns of red cell destruction *in vivo*. *Brit. J. Haemat.* **4**, 115.

Cuthbertson, B., Perry, R.J., Foster, P.R., Reid, K.G., Crawford, R.J and Yap, P.L. (1987) The viral safety of intravenous immunoglobulin. *J. Infect.* **15**, 125–133.

Cuthbertson, B., Reid, K.G. and Foster, P.R. (1991) Viral contamination of human plasma and procedures for preventing virus transmission by plasma products. *Blood Separation and Plasma Fractionation*, ed J.R. Harris, pp. 385–435. Wiley-Liss, New York.

Cuttner, J., Holland, J.F., Norton, L., Ambinder, E., Button, G. and Meyer, R.J. (1983) Therapeutic leukapheresis for hyperleukocytosis in acute myelocytic leukemia. *Med. pediat. Oncol.* **11**, 76–78.

Czer, L, Bateman, T., Gray, R., Raymond, M.,

Chaux. A., Marloff, J. and Stewart, M. (1985) Prospective trial of DDAVP in treatment of severe platelet dysfunction and hemorrhage after cardiopulmonary bypass (Abstract). *Circulation*, **72**, Suppl. 3, section III, 130.

Dacie, J.V. and Firth, D. (1943) Blood transfusion in noctural haemoglobinuria. *Brit. Med. J.* **i**, 626.

Dacie, J.V. and Mollison, P.L. (1943) Survival of normal erythrocytes after transfusion to patients with familial haemolytic anaemia (acholuric jaundice). *Lancet*, **i**, 550.

Dacie, J.V. (1949) Diagnosis and mechanism of hemolysis in chronic hemolytic anemia with nocturnal hemoglobinuria. *Blood*, **4**, 1183.

Dacie, J.V. (1950) Occurrences in normal human sera of 'incomplete' forms of 'cold' autoantibodies. *Nature (Lond.)*, **166**, 36.

Dacie, J.V. and de Gruchy, G.C. (1951) Autoantibodies in acquired haemolytic anaemia. *J. clin. Path.* **4**, 253.

Dacie, J.V. (1954) *The Haemolytic Anaemias, Congenital and Acquired, Part II. The Autoimmune Haemolytic Anaemias*. Churchill, London.

Dacie, J.V. and Cutbush, Marie (1954) Specificity of auto-antibodies in acquired haemolytic anaemia. *J. clin. Path.* **7**, 18.

Dacie, J.V., Crookston, J.H. and Christenson, W.N. (1957) 'Incomplete' cold antibodies: role of complement in sensitization to antiglobulin serum by potentially haemolytic antibodies. *Brit. J. Haemat.* **3**, 77.

Dacie, J.V. (1962) *The Haemolytic Anaemias, Congenital and Acquired, Part II. The Auto-Immune Haemolytic Anaemias*, 2nd edn. Churchill, London.

Dacie, J.V. (1967) *The Haemolytic Anaemias, Congenital and Acquired, Part III. Secondary or Symptomatic Haemolytic Anaemias* 2nd edn. Churchill, London.

Dacie, J.V. and Worlledge, Sheila M. (1969) Auto-immune hemolytic anemias, in *Progress in Hematology, VI.* eds. E.B. Brown and C.V. Moore, p. 82. Grune & Stratton, New York.

Daffos, F., Capella-Pavlovsky, M. and Forrestier, F. (1985) Fetal blood sampling during pregnancy with use of a needle guided by ultrasound: a study of 606 consecutive cases. *Amer. J. Obstet. Gynec.* **153**, 655–660.

Daffos, F., Forestier, F., Kaplan, Cecile and Cox, W. (1988) Prenatal diagnosis and management of bleeding disorders with fetal blood sampling. *Amer. J. Obstet. Gynec.* **158**, 939–946.

Dahlén, S.E., Björk, J., Hedqvist, P., Arfors, K.E., Hammarström, S., Linogren, J.Å. and Samuelsson, B. (1981) Leukotrienes promote plasma leakage and leukocyte adhesion in postcapillary venules: *in vivo* effects with relevance to the acute inflammatory response. *Proc. nat. Acad. Sci. USA*, **78**, 3887–3891.

Dahr, P. (1941) Über im Menschenserum natürlich vorkommendes anti-M Agglutinin. *Klin. Wschr.* **20**, 1273.

Dahr, W., Uhlenbruck, G., Gunson, H.H. and van der Hart, M. (1975) Molecular basis of Tn-polyagglutinability. *Vox Sang.* **29**, 36.

Dahr, W., Uhlenbruck, G., Leikola, J. and Wagstaff, W. (1978) Studies on the membrane glycoprotein defect of En(a−) erythrocytes: III. N-terminal amino-acids of sialoglycoproteins from normal and En(a−) erythrocytes. *J. Immunogenet.* **5**, 117.

Dahr, W., Gielen, W., Beyreuther, K. and Krüger, J. (1980a) Structure of the Ss blood group antigens. I. Isolation of Ss-active glycopeptides and differentiation of the antigens by modification of methionine. *Hoppe-Seyler's Z. Physiol. Chem.* **361**, 145–152.

Dahr, W., Beyreuther, K., Steinbach, H., Gielen, W. and Krüger, J. (1980b) Structure of the Ss blood group antigens. II. A methionine/threonine polymorphism within the N-terminal sequence of the Ss glycoprotein. *Hoppe-Seyler's Z. Physiol. Chem.* **361**, 895–906.

Dahr, W., Lichthardt, D. and Roelcke, D. (1981a) Studies on the sites of the monoclonal anti-Pr and -Sa cold agglutinins. *Protides biol. Fluids*, **29**, 365–368.

Dahr, W., Metaxas-Bühler, M., Metaxas, M.N. and Gallasch, E. (1981b) Immunochemical properties of M^g erythrocytes. *J. Immunogenet.* **8**, 79–87.

Dahr, W. (1986) Immunochemistry of sialoglycoproteins in human red blood cell membranes, in *Recent Advances in Blood Group Biochemistry*, eds V. Vengelen-Tyler and W.J. Judd, pp. 23–52. Amer. Assoc. Blood Banks, Arlington, V.A.

Dahr, W., Kordowicz, M., Moulds, J. Gielen, W., Lebeck, L. and Krüger, J. (1987) Characterization of the Ss sialoglycoprotein and its antigens in Rh_{null} erythrocytes. *Blut*, **54**, 13–24.

Dahr, W. (1992) The Miltenberger subsystem of the MNSs blood group system. Review and outlook. *Vox Sang.* **62**, 129–135.

Dale, R.E., Lindop, M.J., Farman, J.V. and Smith, M.E. (1986) Auto-transfusion, an experience of seventy-six cases. *Ann. roy. Coll. Surg. Engl.* **68**, 295–297.

Dale, G.L. and Norenberg, S.L. (1990) Density fractionation of erythrocytes by Percoll-hypaque results in only a slight enrichment for aged cells. *Biochim. biophys. Acta*, **1036**, 183–187.

Dalgleish, A.G., Beverley, P.C.L., Clapham, P.R., Crawford, D.H., Greaves, M.F. and Weiss, R.A. (1984) The CD4 (T4) antigen is an essential component of the receptor for the AIDS retrovirus. *Nature (Lond.)*, **312**, 763–767.

Daly, P.A., Schiffer, C.A., Aisner, J. and Wiernik, P.H. (1980) Platelet transfusion therapy. One-hour posttransfusion increments are valuable in predicting the need for HLA-matched preparations. *J. Amer. Med. Assoc.* **243**, 435–438.

Dameshek, W. and Schwartz, S.D. (1938) The presence of hemolysins in acute hemolytic anemia; preliminary note. *New Engl. J. Med.* **218**, 75.

Dancey, J.T., Deubelbeiss, K.A., Harker, L.A. and Finch, C.A. (1976) Neutrophil kinetics in man. *J. clin. Invest.* **58**, 705.

Dane, D.S., Cameron, C.H. and Briggs, M. (1970) Virus-like particles in serum of patients with Australia-antigen associated hepatitis. *Lancet*, i, 695–698.

Daneshvar, A. (1988) Fluid replacement after blood donation: implications for elderly and autologous blood donors. *Maryland med. J.* **37**, 787–791.

Daniels, G.L., Judd, W.J., Moore, B.P.L., Neitzer, G., Ouellet, P., Plantos, M. and Verrette, S. (1982) A 'new' high frequency antigen Erª. *Transfusion*, **22**, 189–193.

Daniels, G.L. (1984) Studies on anti-H reagents. *Rev. franç. Transfus. Immunohémat.* **27**, 603–612.

Daniels, G.L., Shaw, M.A., Judson, P.A., Reid, M.E., Anstee, D.J., Colpitts, P., Cornwall, S., Moore, B.P.L. and Lee, S. (1986) A family demonstrating inheritance of the Leach phenotype: a Gerbich-negative phenotype associated with elliptocytosis. *Vox Sang.* **50**, 117–121.

Daniels, G.L., Reid, M.E., Anstee, D.J., Beattie, K.M. and Judd, W.J. (1988) Transient reduction in erythrocyte membrane sialoglycoprotein *β* associated with the presence of elliptocytes. *Brit. J. Haemat.* **70**, 477–481.

Daniels, G. (1989) Cromer-related antigens — blood group determinants on decay-accelerating factor. *Vox Sang.* **56**, 205–211.

Daniels, G.L., Le Pennec, P.Y., Rouger, Salmon, C. and Tippett, P. (1991) The red cell antigens Auª and Auᵇ belong to the Lutheran system. *Vox Sang.* **60**, 191–192.

Dankbar, D.T., Blake, B.E., Pierce, S.R. and Beck, M.L. (1986) Comparison of anti-K reactivity using saline and LISS tests (Abstract). *Transfusion*, **26**, 549.

Danpure, H.J., Osman, S. and Peters, A.M. (1990) Labelling autologous platelets with ¹¹¹In tropolonate for platelet kinetic studies: limitations imposed by thrombocytopenia. *Eur. J. Haemat.* **45**, 223–230.

Darke, C., Street, J., Sargeant, C. and Dyer, P.A. (1983) HLA-DR antigens and properdin factor B allotypes in responders and non-responders to the Rhesus-D antigen. *Tissue Antigens*, **21**, 333–335.

Darnborough, J., Firth, R., Giles, Carolyn M., Goldsmith, K.L.G. and Crawford, Mary N. (1963) A 'new' antibody anti-Luªub and two further examples of the genotype Lu(a–b–). *Nature (Lond.)*, **198**, 796.

Darnborough, J., Dunsford, I. and Wallace, Josephine, A. (1969) The Enª antigen and antibody: a genetical modification of human red cells affecting their blood grouping reactions. *Vox Sang.* **17**, 241.

Dausset, J. and Vidal, G. (1951) Accidents de la transfusion chez des receveurs de groupe A ayant reçu du sang de groupe O—rôle de la vaccination par l'anatoxine diphtérique et tétanique. *Sang.* **22**, 478.

Dausset, J. and Nenna, A. (1952) Présence d'une leuco-agglutinine dans le sérum d'un cas d'agranulocytose chronique. *C.A. Soc. Biol. (Paris)*, **146**, 1539.

Dausset, J. (1953) Immuno-hématologie des plaquettes et des leucocytes. *Presse méd.* **61**, 1533.

Dausset, J. (1954) Leuco-agglutinins. IV. Leuco-agglutinins and blood transfusion. *Vox Sang. (O.S.)*, **4**, 190.

Dausset, J. and Brécy, H. (1957) Identical nature of the leucocyte antigens detectable in monozygotic twins by means of iso-leuco-agglutinins. *Nature (Lond.)*, **180**, 1430.

Dausset, J. (1958) Iso-leuco-anticorps. *Acta Haemat.* **20**, 156.

Dausset, J. and Colombani, J. (1959) The serology and the prognosis of 128 cases of autoimmune hemolytic anaemia. *Blood*, **14**, 1280.

Dausset, J., Moullec, J. and Bernard, J. (1959) Acquired hemolytic anemia with polyagglutinability of red blood cells due to a new factor present in normal human serum (anti-Tn). *Blood*, **14**, 1079.

Davenport, R.D., Strieter, R.M., Standiford, T.J. and Kunkel, S.L. (1990) Interleukin-8 production in red blood cell incompatibility. *Blood*, **76**, 2439–2442.

Davey, M.G., Campbell, A.L. and James, J. (1969) Some consequences of hyperimmunization to the rhesus (D) blood group antigen in man (Abstract). *Proc. Aust. Soc. Immunol.*, Adelaide, Dec. 1969.

Davey, M.G. (1976a) Epidemiology of failures of Rh immune globulin and ABO protection, in *Proceedings of Symposium on Rh Antibody Mediated Immunosuppression*. Ortho Research Institute, Raritan, New Jersey.

Davey, M.G. (1976b) Antenatal administration of anti-Rh: Australia 1969–1975, in *Proceedings of Symposium on Rh Antibody Mediated Immunosuppression*. Ortho Research Institute, Raritan, New Jersey.

Davey, R.J., O'Gara, C. and McGinniss, M.H. (1979) Incompatibility *in vitro* and *in vivo* demonstrated only with saline-suspended red cells. *Vox Sang.* **36**, 301–306.

Davey, R.J., Gustafson, M. and Holland, P.V. (1980) Accelerated immune red cell destruction in the absence of serologically detectable alloantibodies. *Transfusion*, **20**, 348–353.

Davey, R.J. and Simpkins, S.S. (1981) ^{51}Chromium survival of Yt(a+) red cells as a determinant of the *in vivo* significance of anti-Yt^a. *Transfusion*, **21**, 702–705.

Davey, R.J., Rosen, S.R. and Holland, P.V. (1982) *In vitro* thermal characteristics of anti-Le^b antibodies as predictors of their *in vivo* significance. *Abstracts, 17th Congr. Int. Soc. Blood Transfus.* Budapest.

Davey, R.J., Lenes, B.L., Casper, A.J. and Demets, D.I. (1984) Adequate survival of red cells from units 'undercollected' in citrate-phosphate-dextrose-adenine-one. *Transfusion*, **24**, 319–322.

Davidsohn, I. (1938) Isoagglutinin titers in serum disease, in leukemias, in infectious mononucleosis and after blood transfusions. *Amer. J. clin. Path.* **8**, 179.

Davidsohn, I., Lee, C.L. and Takashi, T. (1963) Hepatic infarcts in mice injected with anti-erythrocytic serum. *Arch. Path.* **76**, 398.

Davidson, L.T., Merritt, Katherine T. and Weech, A.A. (1941) Hyperbilirubinemia in the newborn. *Amer. J. Dis. Child.* **61**, 958.

Davies, J.W.L. and Fisher, Mary R. (1958) Red cell and total blood volume changes following a minor operation. *Clin. Sci.* **17**, 537.

Davies, Sally C., McWilliam, A.C., Hewitt, Patricia E., Devenish, A. and Brozovic, Milica (1986) Red cell alloimmunization in sickle cell disease. *Brit. J. Haemat.* **63**, 241–245.

Dawson, R.B. jr, Kocholaty, W.F. and Gray, J.L. (1970) Hemoglobin function and 2,3-DPG levels of blood stored at 4 C in ACD and CPD: pH effect. *Transfusion*, **10**, 299.

Dawson, R.B., Ellis, T.J. and Hershey, R.T. (1976) Blood preservation. XVI. Packed red cell storage in CPD-adenine. *Transfusion*, **16**, 179.

Day, D., Perkins, H.A. and Sams, B. (1965) The minus minus phenotype in the Kidd system. *Transfusion*, **5**, 315.

De Angelo, A.B. and Garrett, C.T. (1983) Inhibition of development of preneoplastic lesions in the livers of rats fed a weakly carcinogenic environmental contaminant. *Cancer Letters*, **20**, 199–205.

Derelle, G.D., Gillam, G.L. and Tauro, G.P. (1977) A case of hydrops fetalis due to foetomaterno haemorrhage. *Aust. paediat. J.* **13**, 131.

DeBruin, H.G., De Leur-Ebeling, I. and Aaij, C. (1983) Quantitative determination of the number of FITC molecules bound per cell in immuno-fluorescence flow cytometry. *Vox Sang.* **45**, 373–377.

Décary, F. and 14 others (1984) An investigation of nonhemolytic transfusion reactions. *Vox Sang.* **46**, 277–285.

Décary, Francine, L'Abbé, D., Tremblay, L. and Chartrand, P. (1991) The immune response to the HPA-1a antigen: association with HLA-DRw52a. *Transfus. Med.* **1**, 55–63.

DeCesare, W.R., Bove, J.R. and Ebaugh, E.G. jr (1964) The mechanism of the effect of iso- and hyperosmolar dextrose-saline solutions on *in vivo* survival of human erythrocytes. *Transfusion*, **4**, 237.

Deeg, H.J., Aprile, J., Graham, T.C., Appelbaum, F.R. and Storb, R. (1986) Ultraviolet irradiation of blood prevents transfusion-induced sensitization and marrow graft rejection in dogs. *Blood*, **76**, 537–539.

Deeg, H.J., Aprile, J., Starb, R., Graham, T.C., Hackman, R., Appelbaum, F.R. and Schuering, F. (1988) Functional dendritic cells are required for transfusion-induced sensitization in canine marrow graft recipients. *Blood*, **71**, 1138–1140.

Deeg, H.J. (1989) Transfusion with a tan. Prevention of allosensitization by ultraviolet irradiation. *Transfusion*, **29**, 450–455.

Degnan, T.J. and Rosenfield, R.E. (1965) Hemolytic transfusion reaction associated with poorly detectable anti-Jk^a. *Transfusion*, **5**, 245.

De Graan-Hentzen, Y.C.E. and 9 others (1989) Prevention of primary cytomegalovirus infection in patients with hematologic malignancies by intensive white cell depletion of blood products. *Transfusion*, **29**, 757–760.

Deinhardt, F. and Zuckerman, A.J. (1985) Immunization against hepatitis B: report on a WHO meeting on viral hepatitis in Europe. *J. med. Virol.* **17**, 209–217.

Dekkers, H.J.N. (1939) The fate of the transfused red blood cells. *Acta. med. scand.* **99**, 587.

De Korte, D., Gouwerok, C.W.N., Fijnheer, R., Pietersz, Ruby N.I. and Roos, D. (1990) Depletion of dense granule nucleotides during storage of human platelets. *Thrombos. Haemostas.* **63**, 275–278.

De la Barrera, S., Fainboim, L., Lugo, S., Picchio, G.R., Muchinik, G.R. and de Bracco M.M.E. (1987) Anti-class II antibodies in AIDS patients and AIDS-risk groups. *Immunology*, **62**, 599–604.

De Lange, Gerda, G. (1988) *Monoclonal Antibodies against Human Immunoglobulin Allotypes*. Ph.D. Thesis, University of London.

Dellagi, K., Brouet, J.C., Schenmetzler, Claudine and Praloran, V. (1981) Chronic hemolytic anemia due to a monoclonal IgG cold agglutinin with anti-Pr specificity. *Blood*, **57**, 189–191.

Delmas-Marsalet, Y., Chateau, G., Foissac-Gegoux, P. and Goudemand, M. (1967) Accident transfusionnel par iso-anticorps naturels de spécificité anti-N. *Transfusion (Paris)*, **4**, 369.

Delmas-Marsalet, Y., Parquet-Gernez, A., Bauters, F. and Goudemand, M. (1969) Anémies hémolytiques dues á la plasmathérapie chez les hémophiles. *Rev. franç. Transfus.* **12**, 351.

De Man, A.J.M. and Overbeeke, Marijke A.M. (1990) Evaluation of the polyethylene glycol antiglobulin test for detection of red blood cell antibodies. *Vox Sang.* **58**, 207–211.

DeMarsh, Q.B., Windle, W.F. and Alt, H.L. (1942) Blood volume of newborn infants in relation to early and late clamping of the umbilical cord. *Amer. J. Dis. Child.* **63**, 1123.

Demling, R.H., Manohar, M. and Will, J.A. (1980) Response of the pulmonary microcirculation to fluid loading after hemorrhagic shock and resuscitation. *Surgery*, **87**, 552–559.

Demling, R.H. (1990) Pathophysiological changes after cutaneous burns and approach to initial resuscitation, in *Acute Management of the Burned Patient*, ed J.A.J. Martyn, pp. 12–24. W.B. Saunders, Philadelphia.

DeNatale, A., Cahan, A., Jack, J.A., Race, R.R. and Sanger, Ruth (1955) V, A 'new' Rh antigen, common in Negroes, rare in white people. *J. Amer. med. Assoc.* **159**, 247.

Denborough, M.A. and Downing, H.J. (1969) The incidence of anti-A and anti-B isoagglutinins in cord blood and maternal saliva. *Brit. J. Haemat.* **16**, 111.

Denborough, M.A., Downing, H.J. and Doig, A.G. (1969) Serum blood group substances and ABO haemolytic disease. *Brit. J. Haemat.* **16**, 103.

Denegri, J.F., Nangi, A.A., Sinclair, Margaret and Stillwell, Gail (1983) Autoimmune haemolytic anaemia due to immunoglobulin G with anti-Sd^x specificity. *Acta Haemat.* **69**, 19–22.

Denis, J. (1667–8) Letter to the Publishers. *Phil. Trans.* **32**, 617.

DePalma, L. and Luban N.L.C. (1990) Autologous blood transfusion in pediatrics. *Pediatrics*, **85**, 125–128.

DePalma, L., Criss, V.R., Roseff, S.D. and Luban, N.L.C. (1991) Formation of alloanti-E in an 11 week old infant. *Transfusion*, **31**, Suppl. 52S.

Department of Health (1989) *Guidelines for the Blood Transfusion Services in the United Kingdom.* HMSO, London.

De Rie, M.A., van der Plas-van Dalen, C.M., Engelfriet, C.P. and von de Borne, A.E.G.Kr. (1985) The serology of febrile transfusion reactions. *Vox Sang.* **49**, 126–134.

Dern, R.J., Gwinn, R.P. and Wiorkowski, J.J. (1966) Studies on the preservation of human blood. Variability in erythrocyte storage characteristics among healthy donors. *J. Lab. clin. Med.* **67**, 955.

Dern, R.J., Brewer, G.J. and Wiorkowski, J.J. (1967) Studies on the preservation of human blood. II. The relationship of erythrocyte adenosine triphosphate levels and other *in vitro* measures to red cell storage ability. *J. Lab. clin. Med.* **69**, 968.

Dern, R.J. (1968) Studies on the preservation of human blood. III. The posttransfusion survival of stored and damaged erythrocytes in healthy donors and patients with severe trauma. *J. Lab. clin. Med.* **71**, 254.

Dern, R.J. (1970) Double label studies of the poststorage viability of erythrocytes in trauma patients, in *Modern Problems of Blood Preservation*, eds W. Spielmann and S. Seidl. Gustav Fischer, Stuttgart.

Dern, R.J., Wiorkowski, J.J. and Matsuda, T. (1970) Studies on the preservation of human blood. V. The effect of mixing anticoagulated blood during storage on the poststorage erythrocyte survival. *J. Lab. clin. Med.* **75**, 37.

Deroff, P., Regner, M., Simitzis, A.M., Boudon, A. and Saleun, J.P. (1982) Screening of blood donors likely to transmit falciparum malaria. *Rev. franç. Transfus. Immunohémat.* **25**, 3–10.

Descamps-Latscha, Béatrice, Golub, R.M., Guyen, A.T. and Feuillet-Fieux, Marie-Noëlle (1983) Monoclonal antibodies against T-cell differentiation antigens initiate stimulation of monocyte/macrophage oxidative metabolism. *J. Immunol.* **131**, 2500–2507.

De Silva, Mahes and Contreras, Marcela (1985) Pooled cells versus individual screening cells in pre-transfusion testing. *Clin. lab. Haemat.* **7**, 369–373.

De Silva, Mahes, Contreras, Marcela and Mollison, P.L. (1985) Failure of passively administered anti-Rh to prevent secondary Rh responses. *Vox Sang.* **48**, 178–180.

De Silva, Mahes, Contreras, Marcela and Barbara, J. (1988) Two cases of transfusion-transmitted malaria (TTM) in the UK (Letter). *Transfusion*, **28**, 86.

Desjardins, L., Blajchman, M.A., Chintu, C., Gent, M. and Zipursky, A. (1979) The spectrum of ABO hemolytic disease of the new born infant. *J. Pediat.* **95**, 447–449.

Desmyter, J. (1986) AIDS and blood transfusion. *Vox Sang.* **51**, Suppl. 1, 21.

Devenish, A., Burslem, M.F., Morris, R. and Contreras, M. (1986) Serologic characteristics of a further example of anti-Xg^a and the frequency of Xg^a in North London blood donors. *Transfusion*, **26**, 426–427.

DeVenuto, F. and Zegna, A. (1983) Preparation

and evaluation of pyridoxalated-polymerized human hemoglobin. *J. Surg. Res.* **34**, 205–212.

De Verdier, C.-H., Garby, L., Killander, J., Hjelm, M. and Högman, C.F. (1963) The relation between the age of red cells labelled with radio-iron and haemolysis induced by mechanical trauma and rapid freezing-thawing. *Vox Sang.* **8**, 660.

De Verdier, C.-H., Högman, C., Garby, L. and Killander, J. (1964a) Storage of human red blood cells. II. The effect of pH and of the addition of adenine. *Acta physiol. Scand.* **60**, 141.

De Verdier. C.-H., Garby, L., Hjelm, M., Högman, C. and Eriksson, A. (1964b) Adenine in blood preservation: Post-transfusion viability and biochemical changes. *Transfusion*, **4**, 331.

De Verdier, C.-H., Finnson, M., Garby, L., Högman, C.F., Johansson, S.G.O. and Åkerblom, O. (1966) Experience of blood preservation in ACD adenine solution. *Proc. 10th Congr. Europ. Soc. Haemat.*, Strasbourg, 1965.

De Verdier, C.-H., Garby, L., Högman, C.F. and Åkerblom, O. (1969) Maintenance of a normal oxygen transport function of stored red blood cells. *Försvarsmedicin*, **5**, 244.

De Verdier, C.-H., Åkerblom, O, Garby, L. and Högman, C. (1970) Methods to preserve the concentration of 2,3-diphosphoglycerate and ATP in stored blood, in *Modern Problems of Blood Preservation*, eds W. Spielmann and S. Seidl. Gustav Fischer, Stuttgart.

De Vetten, M.P. and Agre, P. (1988) The Rh polypeptide is a major fatty acid acylated erythrocyte membrane protein. *J. biol. Chem.* **263**, 18 193–18 196.

Devereaux, S., Linch, D.C., Gribben, J.G., McMullan, A., Patterson, K. and Goldstone, A.H. (1989) GM-CSF accelerates neutrophil recovery after autologous bone marrow transplantation for Hodgkin's disease. *Bone Marrow Transplant*, **4**, 49–54.

Devey, M.E. and Voak, D. (1974) A critical study of the IgG subclasses of Rh anti-D antibodies formed in pregnancy and in immunized volunteers. *Immunology*, **27**, 1073.

Devine, Dana V. and Rosse, W.F. (1984) Identification of platelet proteins that bind alloantibodies. *Blood*, **64**, 1240–1245.

De Vries, L.S., Connell, J., Bydder, G.M., Dubowitz, L.M.S., Rodeck, C.H., Mibashan, R.S. and Waters, A.H. (1988) Recurrent intracranial haemorrhage *in utero* in an infant with alloimmune thrombocytopenia. *Brit. J. Obstet. Gynaec.* **95**, 299–302.

De Waal, L.P., van Dalen, Carla M., Engelfriet, C.P. and von dem Borne, A.E.G.Kr. (1986) Alloimmunization against the platelet-specific Zw^a antigen, resulting in neonatal thrombocytopenia or posttransfusion purpura, is as-sociated with the supertypic DRw52 antigen including DR3 and DRw6. *Hum. Immunol.* **17**, 45–54.

De Wit, D.C. and Borst-Eilers, Els (1968) Failure of anti-D immunoglobulin injection to protect against rhesus immunization after massive foeto-maternal haemorrhage. Report of 4 cases. *Brit. med. J.* **i**, 152.

De Wit, D.C. and van Gastel, C. (1969) Red cell age and susceptibility to immune haemolysis. *Scand. J. Haemat.* **6**, 373.

De Wit, D.C. and van Gastel, C. (1970) Haemolysis in cold agglutinin disease: the role of C′ and cell age in red cell destruction. *Brit. J. Haemat.* **18**, 557.

De Witte, T., Schattenberg, A., van Dijk, B.A., Galama, J., Olthuis, H. van der Meer, J.W.W. and Kunst, V.A.J.M. (1990) Prevention of primary cytomegalovirus infection after allogeneic bone marrow transplantation by using leukocyte-poor random blood products from cytomegalovirus-unscreened blood-bank donors. *Transplantation*, **50**, 964–967.

Dharmasena, Finella and Gordon-Smith, E.C. (1986) Transmission of malaria by bone marrow transplantation. *Transplantation*, **42**, 228.

Diamond, L.K. and Denton, R.L. (1945) Rh agglutination in various media with particular reference to the value of albumin. *J. Lab. clin. Med.* **30**, 821.

Diamond, L.K. (1947) Erythroblastosis foetalis or haemolytic disease of the newborn. *Proc. roy. Soc. Med.* **40**, 546.

Diamond, L.K. and Allen, F.H. (1949) Rh and other blood groups. *New Engl. J. Med.* **241**, 867.

Diamond, W.J., Brown, F.L. jr, Bitterman, P., Klein, H.G., Davey, R.J. and Winslow, R.M. (1980) Delayed hemolytic transfusion reaction presenting as sickle-cell crisis. *Ann. intern. Med.* **93**, 231-234.

Diamond, Betty, A., Yelton, D.E. and Scharff, M.D. (1981) Monoclonal antibodies. *New Engl. J. Med.* **304**, 1344-1349.

Dienst, A. (1905) Das Eklampsiegift. *Zbl. Gynäk.* **29**, 353 and 651.

Dienstag J.L. (1983) Non-A, non-B hepatitis I. Recognition, epidemiology and clinical features. *Gastroenterology*, **85**, 439–462.

Dienstag, J.L. and Alter, H.J. (1986) Non-A, non-B hepatitis: evolving epidemiologic and clinical perspective. *Semin. Liver Dis.* **6**, 67–81.

Dienstag, J.L. (1990) Hepatitis non-A, non-B: C at last. *Gastroenterology*, **99**, 117–1180.

Diepenhorst, P., Sprokholt, R. and Prins, H.K. (1972) Removal of leukocytes from whole blood and erythrocyte suspensions by filtration through cotton wool. I. Filtration technique. *Vox Sang.* **23**, 308.

Diepenhorst, P. and Engelfriet, C.P. (1975) Removal of leukocytes from whole blood and erythrocyte suspensions by filtration through cotton wool. V. Results after transfusion of 1,820 units of filtered erythrocytes. *Vox Sang.* **29**, 15.

Dietrich, W., Spannagl, M., Jochum, M., Wendt, P., Schramm, W., Barankay, A., Sabening, F. and Richter, J.A. (1990) Influence of high-dose aprotinin treatment on blood loss and coagulation patterns in patients undergoing myocardial revascularisation. *Anesthesiology*, **73**, 1119–1126.

Dike, G.W.R., Griffiths, D., Bidwell, E., Snape, T.J. and Rizza, C.R. (1980) A Factor VII concentrate for therapeutic use. *Brit. J. Haemat.* **45**, 107–118.

DiMinno, G., Silver, M.J. and Murphy, S. (1982) Stored human platelets retain full aggregation potential in response to pairs of aggregating agents. *Blood*, **59**, 563–568.

Dinapoli, J.B., Nichols, M.E., Marsh, W.L., Warren, D. and Mayer, K. (1977) Hemolytic transfusion reaction caused by IgG anti-P₁. *Commun. Amer. Assoc. Blood Banks*, Atlanta.

Dinarello, C.A., Cannon, J.G., Wolff, S.M., Bernheim, H.H., Beutler, B., Cerami, A., Figari, Irene S., Palladino, A. jr and O'Connor, J.V. (1986) Tumor necrosis factor (cachectin) is an endogenous pyrogen and induces interleukin-1. *J. exp. Med.* **163**, 1433–1451.

Dinsmore, R.E., Reich, Lilian M., Kapoor, Neena, Gulati, S., Kirkpatrick, Dahlia, Flomenberg, N. and O'Reilly. R.J. (1983) ABH incompatible bone marrow transplantation: removal of erythrocytes by starch sedimentation. *Brit. J. Haemat.* **54**, 441–449.

Djordjevich, L. and Miller, I.F. (1980) Synthetic erythrocytes from lipid encapsulated hemoglobin. *Exp. Hemat.* **8**, 584–592.

Dobbs Joan, Prutting, D.L., Adebahr, Margot E., Allen, F.H. jr and Alter, A.A. (1968) Clinical experience with three examples of anti-Ytᵃ. *Vox Sang.* **15**, 217.

Dobson, Aileen and Ikin, Elizabeth W. (1946) The ABO blood groups in the United Kingdom: frequencies based on a very large sample. *J. Path. Bact.* **58**, 221.

Dodd, B.E. and Eeles, D.A. (1961) Rh antibodies detectable only by enzyme technique. *Immunology*, **4**, 337.

Dodd, Barbara E. and Wilkinson, P.C. (1964) A study on the distribution of incomplete rhesus antibodies among the serum immunoglobulin fractions. *J. exp. Med.* **120**, 45.

Dodd, Barbara E., Lincoln, P.J. and Boorman, Kathleen E. (1967) The cross-reacting antibodies of group O sera: immunological studies and a possible explanation of the observed facts. *Immunology*, **12**, 39.

Dodd, L.G., McBride, J.H., Gitnick, G.L., Howanitz, P.J. and Rodgerson, D.O. (1992) Prevalence of non-A, non-B hepatitis/hepatitis C virus antibody in human immunoglobulins. *Amer. J. clin. Path.* **97**, 108–113.

Dodd, R.Y. (1984) International forum: Transfusion-transmitted CMV infections. *Vox Sang.* **46**, 387–414.

Dodd, R.Y. (1986) Testing for HTLV-III/LAV, in *AIDS*, eds J.E. Menitove and J. Kolins, pp. 55–78. Amer. Assoc. Blood Banks, Arlington, VA.

Dodd, R.Y. (1991) Donor testing and its impact on transfusion-transmitted infection, in *Transfusion Transmitted Infections*, eds D.M. Smith and R.Y. Dodd, pp. 243–269. ASCP, Chicago.

Dodd, L.G., McBride, J.H., Gitnick, G.L., Howanitz, P.J. and Rodgerson, D.O. (1992) Prevalence of non-A, non-B hepatitis/hepatitis C virus antibody in human immunoglobulins. *Amer. J. clin. Path.* **97**, 108–113.

Doinel, C., Ropars, C. and Salmon, C. (1976) Quantitative and thermodynamic measurements on I and i antigens of human red blood cells. *Immunology*, **30**, 289.

Doinel, C., Andreu, G., Cartron, J.P., Salmon, C. and Fukuda, M.N. (1980) Tk polyagglutination produced *in vitro* by an endo-beta-galactosidase. *Vox Sang.* **38**, 94–98.

Donahue, R.P., Bias, Wilma, Renwick, J.H. and McKusick, V.A. (1968) Probable assignment of the Duffy blood group locus to chromosome 1 in man. *Proc. nat. Acad. Sci. USA*, **61**, 949.

Donahue, R.E. and 16 others (1988) Human IL-3 and GM-CSF act synergistically in stimulating hematopoiesis in primates. *Science*, **241**, 1820–1823.

Donohue, D.M., Motulsky, A.G., Giblett, Eloise R., Pirzio-Biroli, G., Viranuvatti, V. and Finch, C.A. (1955) The use of chromium as a red cell tag. *Brit. J. Haemat.* **1**, 249.

Donohue, D.M. and Finch, C.A. (1957) An animal assay method for the measurement of post-transfusion survival of stored blood. *Vox Sang.* **2**, 369.

Dooley, S.W. jr, Castro, K.G., Hutton, M.D., Mullan, R.J., Polder, J.A. and Snider, D.E. jr. (1990) Guidelines for preventing the transmission of tuberculosis in health care settings, with special focus on HIV-related issues. *MMWR*, **39**, 1–29.

Dooren, Marion C., Kuijpers, R.W.A.M., Joekes, Elizabeth C., Huiskes, Elly, Goldschmeding, Roel, Overbeeke, Marijke A.M., von dem Borne, A.E.G. Kr., Engelfriet, C.P.E. and Ouwehand, W.H. (1992a) Protection against immune haemolytic disease of newborn infants by maternal monocyte-reactice IgG alloantibodies (anti-HLA-DR). *Lancet*, **i**, 1067–1070.

Dooren, Marion C., Kuijpers, R.W.A.M., Goldschmeding, R., Verhoeven, A.J., Hack, C.E., von dem Borne, A.E.G.Kr., Engelfriet, C.F. and Ouwehand, W.H. (1992b) Adult respiratory distress syndrome after administration of an experimental intravenous gammaglobulin concentrate with a high titre of monocyte-reactive IgG antibodies. *Lancet*, submitted.

Dorf, M.E., Eguro, S.Y., Cabrera, G.. Yunis, E.J., Swanson, J. and Amos, D.B. (1972) Detection of cytotoxic non-HL-A antisera. I. Relationship to anti-Le^a. *Vox Sang.* **22**, 447.

Dorner, Irene M., Parker, C.W. and Chaplin, H. jr (1968) Autoagglutinin developing in a patient with acute renal failure. Characterization of the autoagglutinin and its relation to transfusion therapy. *Brit. J. Haemat.* **14**, 383.

Dorner, I., Moore, J.A. and Chaplin, H. jr (1974) Combined maternal erythrocyte autosensitization and materno-fetal Jk^a incompatibility. *Transfusion*, **14**, 212.

Dornhorst, A.C. (1951) The interpretation of red cell survival curves. *Blood*, **6**, 1284.

Douglas, R., Rowthorne, N.V. and Schneider, J.V. (1985) Some quantitative aspects of the human monocyte erythrophagocytosis and rosette assays. *Transfusion*, **25**, 535–539.

Dow, B.C., MacVarish, I., Barr, A., Crawford, R.J. and Mitchell, R. (1980) Significance of tests for HBeAg and anti-HBe in HBsAg positive blood donors. *J. clin. Path.* **33**, 1106–1109.

Downie, D.M., Madin, D.F. and Voak, D. (1977) An evaluation of salmon anti-B reagent in manual and automated blood grouping. *Med. Lab. Sciences*, **34**, 319.

Doxiadis, I. and Grosse-Wilde H. (1989) Typing for HLA class I gene products using plasma as a source. *Vox Sang.* **56**, 196–200.

Drachmann, O. and Hansen, K.B. (1969) Haemolytic disease of the newborn due to anti-s. *Scand. J. Haemat.* **6**, 93.

Drew, W.L. and Miner, R.C. (1982) Transfusion-related cytomegalovirus infection following noncardiac surgery. *J. Amer. med. Assoc.* **247**, 2389–2391.

Dreyfus, Marie, Magny, J.F., Bridey, Françoise, Schwarz, H.P., Planché, C., Dehan, M. and Tchernia, G. (1991) Treatment of homozygous protein C deficiency and neonatal purpura fulminans with a purified protein C concentrate. *New Engl. J. Med.* **325**, 1565–1568.

Druskin, M.S. and Siegel, P.D. (1963) Bacterial contamination of indwelling intravenous polyethylene catheters. *J. Amer. med. Assoc.* **185**, 966.

Dube, V.E., House, R.F. jr, Moulds, J. and Polesky, H.F. (1975) Hemolytic anemia caused by auto anti-N. *Amer. J. Clin. Path.* **63**, 828.

Dube, V.E., Zoes, C. and Adesman, P. (1977) Caprylate dependent autoanti-e. *Vox Sang.* **33**, 359.

Ducos, J., Ruffie, J. Colobies, P., Marty, Y. and Ohayon, E. (1965) I antigen in leukaemia patients. *Nature (Lond.)*, **208**, 1329.

Dudgeon, L.S., Panton, P.N. and Ross, E.A. (1909) The action of splenotoxic and haemolytic sera on the blood and tissues. *Proc. roy. Soc. Med.* **2**, Part III, Path. Section, 64.

Dugoujon, J.M., De Lange, Gerda G., Blancher, Antoine, Alie-Daram, Simone and Marty, Yvonne (1989) Characterization of an IgG2, G2m(23) anti-Rh-D antibody *Vox Sang.* **57**, 133–136.

Duguid, Jennifer, Winkelman, L., Feldman, P. and Brady, Anna-Maria (1989) The effect of citrate anticoagulants on apheresed plasma. *Transfus. Sci.* **10**, 287–293.

Duhm, J. Deuticke, B. and Gerlach, E. (1971) Complete restoration of oxygen transport function and 2,3-diphosphoglycerate concentration in stored blood. *Transfusion*, **11**, 147.

Duke, W.W. (1911) The relation of blood platelets to hemorrhagic diseases. Description of a method for determining the bleeding time and coagulation time and report of three cases of hemorrhagic disease relieved by transfusion. *J. Amer. med. Assoc.* **55**, 1185.

Dumaswala, U. and Greenwalt, T.J. (1984) Human erythrocytes shed exocytic vesicles *in vivo*. *Transfusion*, **24**, 490–497.

Dunbar, R.W., Price, Karen A. and Cannarella, C.F. (1974) Microaggregate blood filters: effects on filtration time, plasma haemoglobin, and fresh blood platelet counts. *Anaesth. Analg.* **53**, 577.

Dunn, M.J. (1970) The effects of transport inhibitors of sodium outflux and influx in red blood cells: evidence for exchange diffusion. *J. clin. Invest.* **49**, 1804.

Dunsford, I., Bowley, C.C., Hutchinson, A.M., Thompson, Joan S., Sanger, Ruth and Race, R.R. (1953) A human blood-group chimera. *Brit. med. J.* **ii**, 81.

Dunsford, I. (1954) The Wright blood group system. *Vox Sang.* **4**, 160.

Dunsford, I. and Bowley, C.C. (1955) *Techniques in Blood Grouping*. Oliver & Boyd, Edinburgh.

Dunsford, I. (1962) A new Rh antibody-anti-CE. *Proc. 8th Congr. Europ. Soc. Haemat.*, Vienna, 1961.

Dunstan, R.A., Simpson, M.B. and Rosse, W.F. (1984) Erythrocyte antigens on human platelets. Absence of the Rhesus, Duffy, Kell, Kidd, and Lutheran antigens. *Transfusion*, **24**, 243–246.

Dunstan, R.A. and Simpson, M.B. (1985) Heterogeneous distribution of antigens on human platelets demonstrated by fluorescence flow cytometry. *Brit. J. Haemat.* **61**, 603–609.

Dunstan, R.A., Simpson, M.B. and Borowitz, M. (1985a) Absence of ABH antigens on neutrophils. *Brit. J. Haemat.* **60**, 651–657.

Dunstan, R.A., Simpson, M.B. and Rosse, W.F. (1985b) Presence of P blood group antigens on human platelets. *Amer. J. clin. Path.* **83**, 731–735.

Dunstan. R.A., Simpson, M.B., Knowles, R.W. and Rosse, W.F. (1985c) The origin of ABH antigens on human platelets. *Blood*, **65**, 615–619.

Dunstan, R.A. (1986a) Status of major red cell blood group antigens on neutrophils, lymphocytes and monocytes. *Brit. J. Haemat.* **62**, 301–309.

Dunstan, R.A. (1986b) The expression of ABH antigens during *in vitro* megakaryocyte maturation: origin of heterogeneity of antigen density. *Brit. J. Haemat.* **62**, 587–593.

Du Pan, R.M., Wenger, P., Koechli, S., Scheidegger, J.J. and Roux, T. (1959) Étude du passage de la γ- globuline marquée à travers le placenta humain. *Clin. Chim. Acta.* **4**, 110.

Duquesnoy, R.J., Filip, D.J., Rodney, G.E., Rimm, A.A. and Aster, R.H. (1977) Successful transfusion of platelets "mismatched" for HLA antigens to alloimmunized thrombocytopenic patients. *Amer. J. Hemat.* **2**, 219–226.

Duquesnoy, R.J., Anderson, A.J., Tomasulo, P.A. and Aster, R.H. (1979) ABO compatibility and platelet transfusions of alloimmunized thrombocytopenic patients. *Blood*, **54**, 595–599.

Durandy, Anne, Fischer, A. and Griscell, C. (1981) Dysfunctions of pokeweed mitogen-stimulated T and B lymphocyte responses induced by gammaglobulin therapy. *J. clin. Invest.* **67**, 867–877.

Duran-Suarez, J.R., Martin-Vega, C., Argelagues, E., Asset, L., Ribera, A. and Triginer, J. (1981) Red cell I antigen as immune complex receptor in drug-induced hemolytic anemias. *Vox Sang.* **41**, 313–315.

Durkop, J., Roggendorf, M., Wiese, M., Lorbeer, B., Dittmann, S., Glathe, H. and Deinhardt, F. (1989) Antibodies to hepatitis C virus (HCV) in acute and chronic parenterally transmitted hepatitis non-A, non-B (HNANB) (Abstract). *Proc. 1st Int. Meeting on Hepatitis C Virus*, Rome.

Durocher, J.R., Payne, R.C. and Conrad, M.E. (1975) Role of sialic acid in erythrocyte survival. *Blood*, **45**, 11.

Dutcher, Janice P., Schiffer, C.A., Aisner, J. and Wiernik, P.H. (1980) Alloimmunization following platelet transfusion: the absence of a dose response relationship. *Blood*, **57**, 395–398.

Dutcher, J. P., Schiffer, C.A. and Johnston, G.S. (1981a) Rapid migration of [111]indium-labeled granulocytes to sites of infection. *New Engl. J. Med.* **304**, 586–589.

Dutcher, Janice P., Schiffer, C.A., Aisner, J. and Wiernik, P.H. (1981b) Long-term follow-up of patients with leukemia receiving platelet transfusion: identification of a large group of patients who do not become alloimmunized. *Blood*, **58**, 1007–1011.

Dwyer, J.M., Wade, M.J. and Katz, A.J. (1981) Removal of thymic-derived lymphocytes during pheresis procedures. *Vox Sang.* **41**, 287–294.

Dybkjaer, E. and Elkjaer, P. (1964) The use of heated blood in massive blood replacement. *Acta anaesth. Scand.* **8**, 271.

Dybkjaer, E. (1967) Anti-E antibodies disclosed in the period 1960-1966. *Vox Sang.* **13**, 446.

Dyer, P.A. and 12 others (1989) Evidence that matching for HLA antigens significantly increases transplant survival in 1001 renal transplants performed in the north-west region of England. *Transplantation*, **48**, 131–135.

Dzik, W.H. and Blank, J. (1986) Accelerated destruction of radiolabelled red cells due to anti-Colton[b]. *Transfusion*, **26**, 246–248.

Dzik, W.H. (1988) Perioperative blood salvage, in *NIH Consensus Development Conference: Perioperative red cell transfusion.*

Dzik, W.H. and Sherburne, B. (1990) Intraoperative blood salvage: medical controversies. *Transfus. Med. Rev.* **4**, 208–235.

Eadie, G.S. and Brown, I.W. jr (1955) The potential life-span and ultimate survival of fresh red blood cells in normal healthy recipients as studied by simultaneous ^{51}Cr tagging and differential hemolysis. *J. Clin. Invest.* **34**, 629.

Eastlund, T., McGrath, Patricia C., Britten, A. and Propp, R. (1989) Fatal pulmonary transfusion reaction to plasma containing donor HLA antibody. *Vox Sang.* **57**, 63–66.

Eaton, B.R., Morton, J.A., Pickles, Margaret M. and White, K.E. (1956) A new antibody, anti-Yt[a], characterizing a blood group of high incidence. *Brit. J. Haemat.* **2**, 333.

Ebaugh, F.G. jr, Emerson, C.P. and Ross, J.F. (1953) The use of radioactive chromium 51 as an erythrocyte tagging agent for the determination of red cell survival *in vivo*. *J. clin. Invest.* **32**, 1260.

Ebaugh, F.G. jr and Beekin, W.L. (1959) Quantitative measurement of gastro-intestinal blood loss. II. Determination of 24-hour fecal blood loss by a chemical photospectrometric technique. *J. Lab. clin. Med.* **53**, 777.

Ebaugh, F.G., Valentine, W.N. and McIntyre, O.R. (1964) The effect on in vivo ^{51}Cr red cell survival of chromate inhibition of glutathione reductase. *Commun. 10th Congr. Int. Soc. Haemat.*, Stockholm.

Ebeling, F., Naukkarinen, R. and Leikola, J. (1990) Recombinant immunoblot assay for hepatitis C virus antibody as predictor of infectivity (Letter). *Lancet*, i, 982–983.

Ebert, R.V., Stead, E.A. and Gibson, J.G. (1941) Response of normal subjects to acute blood loss, with special reference to the mechanism of restoration of blood volume. *Arch. intern. Med.* **68**, 578.

Ebert, R.V. and Emerson, C.P. (1946) A clinical study of transfusion reactions. The hemolytic effect of group O blood and pooled plasma containing incompatible isoagglutinins. *J. clin. Invest.* **25**, 627.

Echevarria, J.M., Leon, P., Domingo, C.J., Lopez, J.A., Echevarria, J.E., Contreras, G. and Fuertes, A. (1991) Characterization of HBV2-like infections in Spain. *J. med. Virol.* **33**, 240–247.

Economidou, Joanna (1966) A study of the reactions between certain human blood group antigens and their respective antibodies with special reference to the ABO system. Ph.D. Thesis, London University.

Economidou, Joanna, Hughes-Jones, N.C. and Gardner, Brigitte (1967a) Quantitative measurements concerning A and B antigen sites. *Vox Sang.* **12**, 321.

Economidou, Joanna, Hughes-Jones, N.C. and Gardner, B. (1967b) The functional activities of IgG and IgM anti-A and anti-B. *Immunology*, **13**, 227.

Economidou, Joanna, Hughes-Jones, N.C. and Gardner, B. (1967c) The reactivity of subunits of IgM anti-B. *Immunology*, **13**, 235.

Economidou, Joanna, Constantoulakis, M., Augoustaki, Olga and Adinolfi, M. (1971) Frequency of antibodies to various antigenic determinants in polytransfused patients with homozygous thalassaemia in Greece. *Vox Sang.* **20**, 252.

Eddleston, A. (1990) Modern vaccines. Hepatitis. *Lancet*, i, 1142–1145.

Editorial (1986) Adult respiratory distress syndrome. *Lancet*, i, 301–302.

Editorial (1987) AIDS. *Lancet*, i, 175.

Editorial (1988) Complement activation in plasma exchange. *Lancet*, ii, 1464–1465.

Edwards J.M., Moulds, J.J. and Judd, W.J. (1982) Chloroquine dissociation of antigen-antibody complexes. A new technique for typing red blood cells with a positive direct antiglobulin test. Transfusion, **22**, 59–61.

Edwards, C.A., Piet, M.P.J., Chin, S. and Horowitz, B. (1987) Tri(n-butyl) phosphate/detergent treatment of licensed therapeutic and experimental blood derivatives. *Vox Sang.* **52**, 53–59.

Edwards-Moulds, J. and Kasschau, M. (1986) A mechanism by which Jk(a – b –) red cells resist lysis in 2 M urea (abstract). *Transfusion*, **26**, 561.

Eernisse, J.G. and van Rood, J.J. (1961) Erythrocyte survival time determinations with the aid of DF^{32}P. *Brit. J. Haemat.* **7**, 382.

Eernisse, J.G. and Brand, A. (1981) Prevention of platelet refractoriness due to HLA antibodies by administration of leukocyte-poor blood components. *Exp. Hemat.* **9**, 77–83.

Ehlenberger, A.G. and Nussenzweig, V. (1977) The role of membrane receptors for C3b and C3d in phagocytosis. *J. exp. Med.* **145**, 357.

Ehrlich, P. and Sachs, H. (1905) *Collected Studies on Immunity*, p.209. John Wiley & Sons, New York.

Eicher C.A., Wallace, M.E., Frank, S. and De Jongh, D.S. (1978) The Lui elution: a simple method of antibody elution. *Transfusion*, **18**, 647.

Eijsvoogel, V.P., van Rood, J.J., du Toit, Ernette D. and Schellekens, P.Th.A. (1972) Position of a locus determining mixed lymphocyte reaction distinct from the known HLA loci. *Eur. J. Immunol.* **2**, 413–419.

Einhorn, M.S., Granoff, D.M., Nahm, M.H., Quinn, A. and Shackleford, Penelope G. (1987) Concentration of antibodies in paired maternal and infant sera. (1987) *J. Pediat.* **111**, 783–788.

Eisen, H.N. and Karush, F. (1949) The interaction of purified antibody with homologous hapten. Antibody valency. *J. Amer. Chem. Soc.* **71**, 363.

Eisen, H.N. and Siskind, G.W. (1964) Variations in affinities of antibodies during the immune response. *Biochemistry*, **3**, 996.

Eisenstaedt, R.S., Glanz, K. and Smith, D.C. (1988) Underutilization of autologous transfusion: attitudinal survey among transfusion centers (Abstract). *Transfusion*, **28**, 53S.

Eisert, W.G. and Eckert, G. (1979) Current problems and results in testing microaggregate filters. *Vox Sang.* **37**, 310-320.

Ejby-Poulsen, P. (1954a) Experimentally produced polyagglutinability (T-transformation of erythrocytes *in vivo*) in guinea pigs infected with pneumococci. *Nature (Lond.)*, **173**, 82.

Ejby-Poulsen. P. (1954b) Haemolytic anaemia produced experimentally in the guinea pig by T-transformation of the erythrocytes *in vivo* with purified concentrated enzyme. *Nature (Lond.)*, **174**, 929.

Eklund, J. and Nevanlinna, H.R. (1971) Immunosuppression therapy in Rh-incompatible transfusion. *Brit med. J.* iii, 623.

Eklund, J. and Nevanlinna, H.R. (1973) Rh prevention: a report and analysis of a national programme. *J. med. Genet.* **10**, 1.

Eklund, J. (1978) Prevention of Rh immunization in Finland. A national study, 1969–1977. *Acta paed. Scand.* Suppl. 274.

Eklund, J., Hermann, M., Kjellman, H. and Pohja, Paula (1982) Turnover rate of anti-D IgG injected during pregnancy. *Brit. med. J.* **284**, 854–855.

Eldon, K. (1955) Simultaneous ABO and Rh groupings on cards in the laboratory or at the bedside. *Danish med. Bull.* **2**, 33.

Elliot, Margaret, Bossom, Edith, Dupuy, Mary Edith and Masouredis, S.P. (1964) Effect of ionic strength on the serologic behaviour of red cell isoantibodies. *Vox Sang.* **9**, 396.

Ellis, M.I., Hey, E.N. and Walker, W. (1979) Neonatal death in babies with Rhesus iso-immunization. *Quart. J. Med. (N.S.)*, **48**, 211–225.

Ellisor, S.S., Reid, M.E., Day, T.O., Swanson, J., Papenfus, L. and Avoy, D.R. (1983) Autoantibodies mimicking anti-Jk^b plus anti-Jk3 associated with autoimmune haemolytic anaemia in a primipara who delivered an unaffected infant. *Vox Sang.* **45**, 53–59.

Ellory, J.C. and Tucker, Elizabeth M. (1969) Stimulation of the potassium transport system in low potassium type sheep red cells by a specific antigen-antibody reaction. *Nature (Lond.)*, **222**, 477.

Elson, C.J and Bradley, J. (1970) Human peripheral blood leucocytes forming rosettes with rhesus (D) isoantigen. *Lancet*, **i**, 798.

Emerson, T.E. (1989) Pharmacology of aprotinin and efficacy during cardiopulmonary bypass. *Cardiovasc. Drug Rev.* **7**, 127–140.

Engel, W.K., Hanna C.J. and Misra, A.K. (1990) HTLV-I-associated myelopathy (Letter). *New Engl. J. Med.* **323**, 552.

Engelfriet, C.P., von dem Borne, A.E.G.Kr., von dem Giessen, M., Beckers, Do and van Loghem, J.J. (1968a) Autoimmune haemolytic anaemias. I. Serological studies with pure anti-immunoglobulin reagents. *Clin. exp. Immunol.* **3**, 605.

Engelfriet, C.P., von dem Borne, A.E.G.Kr., Moes, Mieke and Van Loghem, J.J. (1968b) Serological studies in autoimmune haemolytic anaemia. *Bibl. Haemat.* **29**, 473.

Engelfriet, C.P., Beckers, Do, von dem Borne, A.E.G.Kr., Reynierse, E. and van Loghem, J.J. (1972a) Haemolysins probably recognising the antigen p. *Vox Sang.* **23**, 176.

Engelfriet, C.P., von dem Borne, A.E.G.Kr., Beckers, Th.A.P., Reynierse, E. and van Loghem, J.J. (1972b) Autoimmune haemolytic anaemias. V. Studies on the resistance against complement haemolysis of red cells of patients with chronic cold agglutinin disease. *Clin. exp. Immunol.* **2**, 255.

Engelfriet, C.P. (1976) C4 and C3 on red cells coated in *vivo* and in *vitro*, in *The Nature and Significance of Complement Activation*. Ortho Research Institute, Raritan, New Jersey.

Engelfriet, C.P. (1978) Unpublished observations cited in the 7th edn. of this book.

Engelfriet, C.P., von dem Borne, A.E.G.Kr., van der Meulen, F.W., Fleer, A., Roos, D. and Ouwehand, W.H. (1981) Immune destruction of red cells, in *A Seminar on Immune-Mediated cell Destruction*. Amer. Assoc. Blood Banks, Chicago.

Engelfriet, C.P., Beckers, Th.A.P., van 'T Veer, M.B., von dem Borne, A.E.G.Kr. and Ouwehand, W.H. (1982) Recent advances in immune haemolytic anaemia, in *Recent Advances in Haematology*, ed S.R. Hollan, pp. 235–251. Akademia Kiado, Budapest.

Engelfriet, C.P., Tetteroo, P.A.T., van der Veen J.P.W., Werner, W.F., van der Plas-van Dalen, Carla and von dem Borne, A.E.G.Kr. (1984a) Granulocyte-specific antigens and methods for their detection, in *Advances in Immunology: Blood Cell Antigens and Bone Marrow Transplantation, Progress in Clinical and Biological Research*, eds J. McCullough and S.G. Sandler, pp. 121–154. Alan R. Liss, New York.

Engelfriet, C.P., Holburn, A.M., Leikola, J. and Lothe, F. (1984b) The production of anti-human globulin reagent for use in immuno-haematology. W.H.O. and League of Red Cross Societies, Lab/84.8.

Engelfriet, C.P. and Voak, D. (1987) International reference polyspecific anti-human globulin reagents. *Vox Sang.* **43**, 241–247.

Engelfriet, C.P., Overbeeke, Marijke A.M. and Voak. D. (1987) The anti-globulin test (Coombs test) and the red cell, in *Progress in Transfusion Medicine*, ed J.D. Cash, Vol. 2. Churchill Livingstone, Edinburgh.

Engelfriet, C.F. and Ouwehand, W.H. (1990) ADCC and other cellular bioassays for predicting the clinical significance of red cell alloantibodies, in *Blood Transfusion: the Impact of New Technologies*, ed Marcela Contreras. *Ballière's Clinical Haematology*, **3**, 321–337.

Enomoto, N., Takada, A., Nakao, T. and Date, T. (1990) There are two major types of hepatitis C virus in Japan. *Biochem. biophys. Res. Comm.* **170**, 1021–1025.

Epstein, W.V. (1965) Specificity of macroglobulin antibody synthesized by the normal human fetus. *Science*, **148**, 1591.

Erichson, R.B., Viles, H., Grann, V. and Zeigler, Zella (1978) Posttransfusion purpura. *Arch. intern. Med.* **138**, 998.

Eriksson, S. (1989) Replacement therapy in α_1-

antitrypsin deficiency. *J. intern. Med.* **225**, 69–72.

Ervin, D.M. and Young, L.E. (1950) Dangerous universal donors. I. Observations on destruction of recipient's A cells after transfusion of group O blood containing high titer of A antibodies of immune type not easily neutralizable by soluble A substance. *Blood*, **5**, 61.

Ervin, D.M., Christian, R.M. and Young, L.E. (1950) Dangerous universal donors. II. Further observations on the in *vivo* and *in vitro* behaviour of isoantibodies of immune type present in group O blood. *Blood*, **5**, 553.

Eschbach, J.W. jr, Epstein, R.B., Burnell, J.M. and Thomas, E.D. (1965) Physiologic observations in human cross circulation. *New Engl. J. Med.* **273**, 997.

Eschbach, J.W., Korn, D. and Finch, C.A. (1977) ^{14}C cyanate as a tag for red cell survival in normal and uremic man. *J. Lab. clin. Med.* **89**, 823.

Eschbach, J.W., Egrie, J.C., Downing, M.R., Browne, J.K. and Adamson, J.W. (1987) Correction of the anemia of end stage renal disease with recombinant human erythropoietin: results of a combined phase I and II clinical trial. *New. Engl. J. Med.* **316**, 73.

Eschbach, J.W. and 24 others (1989a) Recombinant human erythropoietin in anemic patients with end-stage renal disease. *Ann. intern. Med.* **111**, 992–1000.

Eschbach, J.W., Kelly, M.R., Haley, N. Rebecca, Abels, R.I. and Adamson, J.W. (1989b) Treatment of the anemia of progressive renal failure with recombinant human erythropoietin. *New Engl. J. Med.* **321**, 158–163.

Eska, Patricia L. and Grindon, A.J. (1974) The high frequency of anti-Bg^a. *Brit. J. Haemat.* **27**, 613.

Esteban, J.I. and 13 others (1989) Hepatitis C virus antibodies among risk groups in Spain. *Lancet*, **ii** 294–297.

Esteban, J.I. and 10 others (1990) Evaluation of antibodies to hepatitis C virus in a study of transfusion associated hepatitis. *New Engl. J. Med.* **323**, 1107–1112.

Estep, T.N., Pedersen, R.A., Miller, Theresa J. and Stupar, Kathleen R. (1984) Characterization of erythrocyte quality during the refrigerated storage of whole blood containing di-(2-ethylhexyl) phthalate. *Blood*, **64**, 1270–1276.

Etges, C.C., Callicoat, P.A. and Smith, D.M. jr (1982) A polybrene microplate technique for large-scale red cell typing (Abstract). *Transfusion*, **22**, 429.

Etzler, M.E. and Kabat, E.A. (1970) Purification and characterization of a lectin (plant hemagglutinin) with blood group A specificity from *Dolichos biflorus*. *Biochemistry*, **9**, 869.

Evans, E.I., James G.W. and Hoover, M.J. (1944) Studies in traumatic shock. II. The restoration of blood volume in traumatic shock. *Surgery*, **15**, 420.

Evans, R.S. and Duane, Rose (1949) Hemolytic anemias; recent advances in diagnosis and treatment. *Calif. Med.* **70**, 1.

Evans, E.I., Purnell, O.J.. Robinett, R.W. and Martin, M. (1952) Fluid and electrolyte requirements in severe burns. *Ann. Surg.* **135**, 804–807.

Evans, R.S., Bingham, Margaret and Weiser, R.S. (1963a) A hemolytic system associated with enteritis in rabbits. II. Studies on the survival of transfused cells. *J. Lab. clin. Med.* **62**, 569.

Evans, R.S., Turner, Elizabeth and Bingham, Margaret (1963b) Studies of ^{131}I tagged Rh antibody of D specificity. *Vox Sang* **8**, 153.

Evans, R.S., Turner, Elizabeth and Bingham, Margaret (1965) Studies with radio-iodinated cold agglutinins of ten patients. *Amer. J. Med.* **38**, 378.

Evans, R.S., Turner, Elizabeth and Bingham, Margaret (1967) Chronic hemolytic anaemia due to cold agglutinins: the mechanism of resistance of red cells to C' hemolysis by cold agglutinins. *J. clin. Invest.* **46**, 1461.

Evans, R.S., Turner, Elizabeth, Bingham, Margaret and Woods, R. (1968) Chronic hemolytic anemia due to cold agglutinins. II. The role of C' in red cell destruction. *J. clin. Invest.* **47**, 691.

Evans, W.H and Mage, M. (1978) Development of surface antigen during maturation of bone marrow neutrophil granulocytes. *Exp. Hemat.* **6**, 37–42.

Evans, R.T., MacDonald, Rosemary and Robinson, Angela (1980) Suxamethonium apnoea associated with plasmapheresis. *Anaesthesia*, **35**, 198–201.

Evatt, B.L. and 10 others (1983) Antibodies to human T-cell leukemia virus-associated membrane antigens in hemophiliacs: evidence for infection before 1980. *Lancet*, **ii**, 698.

Evatt, B.L., Ramsey, R.B., Lawrence, D.N., Zyla, L.D. and Curran, J.W. (1984) The acquired immunodeficiency syndrome in patients with hemophilia. *Ann. intern. Med.* **100**, 499.

Ewald, R.A., Williams, J.H. and Bowden, D.H. (1961) Serum complement in the newborn. An investigation of complement activity in normal infants and in Rh and AB hemolytic disease. *Vox Sang.* **6**, 312.

Eylar, E.N., Madoff, M.A., Brody, O.V. and Oncley, J.L. (1962) The contribution of sialic acid to the surface charge of the erythrocyte. *J. biol. Chem.* **237**, 1992.

Eyster, M. Elaine and Jenkins, D.E. (1970) γG erythrocyte autoantibodies: comparison of in *vivo* complement coating and *in vitro* 'Rh' specificity. *J. Immunol.* **105**, 221.

Facer, C.A., Bray, R.S. and Brown, J. (1979) Direct Coombs antiglobulin reactions in Gambian children with *Plasmodium falciparum* malaria. I. Incidence and class specificity. *Clin. exp. Immunol.* **35**, 119–127.

Fagan, E.A. and Williams, R. (1990) Fulminant viral hepatitis. *Brit. med. Bull.* **46**, 462–480.

Fagge, C.H. and Pye-Smith, P.H. (1891) *Textbook of the Principles and Practice of Medicine*, Vol. 2, p. 648. J. & A. Churchill, London.

Fairley, N.H. (1940) The fate of extracorpuscular circulating haemoglobin. *Brit. med. J.* **ii**, 213.

Fairley, N.H. (1941) Methaemalbumin. Part I. Clinical aspects. Part II. Its synthesis, chemical behaviour and experimental production in man and animals. *Quart. J. Med.* **10**, 95.

Falk, J.S., Lindblad, G.T.O. and Westman, B.T.M. (1972) Histopathological studies on kidneys from patients treated with large amounts of blood preserved with ACD-adenine. *Transfusion*, **12**, 376.

Falk, R.J. and Jeunette, J.Ch. (1988) Antineutrophil cytoplasmic autoantibodies with specificity for myeloperoxidase in patients with vasculitis and idiopathic necrotizing and crescentic glomerulonephritis. *New Engl. J. Med.* **318**, 1651–1657.

Falterman, C.G. and Richardson, Joan (1980) Transfusion reaction due to unrecognized ABO hemolytic disease of the newborn infant. *J. Pediat.* **97**, 812–814.

Fantus, B. (1937) The therapy of the Cook County Hospital, ed B. Fantus. *J. Amer. med. Assoc.* **108**, 128.

Farci, Patrizia, Alter, H.J., Wong, Doris, Miller, R.H., Shih, J.W., Jett, B. and Purcell, R.H. (1991) A long-term study of hepatitis C virus replication in non-A, non-B hepatitis. *New Engl. J. Med.* **325**, 98–104.

Farci, Patrizia, Alter, H.J., Wong, Doris, Miller, R.H., Shih, J.W., Jett, Betsy and Purcell, R.H. (1992) Hepatitis C virus replication (Letter). *New Engl. J. Med.* **326**, 65–66.

Farman, J.V. and Powell, D. (1969) The performance of disposable venous catheters, needles and cannulae. *Brit. J. hosp. med. Equipment Suppl.* 37–45.

Farmer, Martha C. and Gaber, B.P. (1984) Encapsulation of haemoglobin in phospholipid vesicles: surrogate red cells *in vitro* and *in vivo* (Abstract). *Biophys. J.* **45**, 201a.

Farrow, Susan P. (1967) Effects of infusion of various colloid solutions upon the circulatory volumes of rabbits. M.Sc. Thesis, University of Birmingham, England.

Farrow, S.P. (1977) Comparative effects of dextran and plasma protein solutions. *Burns*, **3**, 202.

Farzadegan H. and 10 others (1988) Loss of human immunodeficiency virus type 1 (HIV-1) antibodies with evidence of viral infection in asymptomatic homosexual men. *Ann. intern. Med.* **108**, 785–790.

Fassbinder, W., Seidl, S. and Koch, K.M. (1978) The role of formaldehyde in the formation of haemodialysis-associated anti-N-like antibodies. *Vox Sang.* **35**, 41.

Faulstick, D.A., Lowenstein, J. and Yiengst, M.J. (1962) Clearance kinetics of haptoglobin-hemoglobin complex in the human. *Blood*, **20**, 65.

FDA (Food and Drugs Administration) (1986) Guidelines for reducing the maximum platelet storage period.

FDA (Food and Drugs Administration) (1991a) Points to consider in the safety evaluation of hemoglobin-based oxygen carriers. *Transfusion*, **31**, 369–371.

FDA (Food and Drugs Administration) (1991b) Clarification of FDA recommendations for donor deferral and product distribution based on the results of syphilis testing. Dec. 12. Bethesda, Md.

Feest, T.G. (1976) Low molecular weight dextran: a continuing cause of acute renal failure. *Brit. med. J.* **ii**, 1275.

Fehr, J., Hofman, V. and Kappeler, U. (1982) Transient reversal of thrombocytopenia in idiopathic thrombocytopenic purpura by high-dose intravenous gamma globulin. *New Engl. J. Med.* **306**, 1254–1258.

Fein, A., Grossman, R.F., Jones, J.G., Overland, E., Pitts, L., Murray, J.F. and Straub, N.C. (1979) The value of edema fluid protein measurement in patients with pulmonary edema. *Amer. J. Med.* **67**, 32–38.

Feinstein, A., Munn, E.A. and Richardson, N.E. (1971) The three-dimensional conformation of M and A globulin molecules. *Ann. N.Y. Acad. Sci.* **190**, 104.

Feinstein, D.I. (1988) Treatment of disseminated intravascular coagulation. *Semin. Thrombos. Hemostas.* **14**, 351–362.

Feizi, Ten and Marsh, W.L. (1970) Demonstration of I-anti-I interaction in a precipitin system. *Vox Sang.* **18**, 379.

Feizi, Ten, Kabat, E.A., Vicari, G., Anderson, B. and Marsh, W.L. (1971) Immunochemical studies on blood groups. XLVII. The I antigen complex–precursors in the A, B, H, Le^a and Le^b, blood group system—hemagglutination-inhibition studies. *J. exp. Med.* **133**, 39.

Feizi, Ten (1977) Immunochemistry of the Ii blood group antigens, in *Human Blood Groups*, eds J.F. Mohn, R.W. Plunkett, R.K. Cunningham and R.M. Lambert, pp. 164-171. S. Karger, Basel.

Feizi, Ten, Childs, R.A., Watanabe, K. and Hakomori, S. (1979) Three types of blood group I specificity among monoclonal anti-I autoantibodies revealed by analogues of a branched erythrocyte glycolipid. *J. exp. Med.* **149**, 975–980.

Feizi, Ten (1980a) Structural and biological aspects of blood group I and i antigens on glycolipids and glycoproteins. *Rev. franç. Transfus. Immunohémat.* **23**, 563–577.

Feizi, Ten (1980b) The monoclonal antibodies of cold agglutinin syndrome. *Med. Biol.* **58**, 3, 123-127.

Feizi, T. (1981) The blood group Ii system: a carbohydrate antigen system defined by naturally occurring monoclonal or oligoclonal autoantibodies of man. *Immunol. Commun.* **10**, 127–156.

Fellous, M., Gerbal, A., Thessier, C., Frezal, J., Dausset, J. and Salmon, C. (1974) Studies on the biosynthetic pathway of human P erythrocyte antigens using somatic cells in culture. *Vox Sang.* **26**, 516–536.

Feo, C. and Mohandas, N. (1977) Clarification of role of ATP in red-cell morphology and function. *Nature (Lond.),* **265**, 166.

Feorino, P.M. and 15 others (1985) Transfusion-associated acquired immunodeficiency syndrome. Evidence for persistent infection in blood donors. *New Engl. J. Med.* **312**, 1293–1296.

Fernandez, M.N., Daza, R.M., Orden, B., Royo, G., Sanjuan, I., Cabrera, R., Zabala, P. and Barolla, L. (1981) Anticuerpos a Brucela en donantes de sangre. *Sangre,* **26**, 360–366.

Ferrara, G.B., Tosi, R.M., Azzolina, G., Carinati, G. and Longo, A. (1974) HL-A unresponsiveness induced by weekly transfusions of small aliquots of whole blood. *Transplantation,* **17**, 194.

Ferrara, G.B., Strelkauskas, A.J., Longo, Anna, McDowell, Joan, Yunis, E.J. and Schlossman, S.F. (1979) Markers of human T-cell subsets identified by allo-antibodies. *J. Immunol.* **123**, 1272–1277.

Ferrara, A., Macarthur, J.D., Wright, H.K., Modlin, I.M. and McMillen, M.A. (1990) Hypothermia and acidosis worsen coagulopathy in the patient requiring massive transfusion. *Amer. J. Surg.* **160**, 575–578.

Ferreira, A., Rodriguez, Maria C.C., Lopez-Trascasa, Margarita, Salcedo, Dora P. and Fontan, G. (1988) Anti IgA antibodies in selective IgA deficiency and in primary immunodeficient patients treated with globulin. *Clin. Immunol. Immunopath.* **47**, 199–207.

Ferrer, Z., Wright, J., Moore, B.P.L. and Freedman, J. (1985) Comparison of a modified manual hexadimethrine bromide (Polybrene) and a low-ionic-strength solution antibody-detection technique. *Transfusion,* **25**, 145–148.

Fijnheer, R., Pietersz, Ruby N.I., de Korte, D. and Roos, D. (1989) Monitoring of platelet morphology during storage of platelet concentrates. *Transfusion,* **29**, 36–40.

Fijnheer, R., Modderman, P.W., Veldman, W.H., Ouwehand, W.H., Nieuwenhuis, H.K., Roos, D. and de Korte, D. (1990a) Detection of platelet activation with monoclonal antibodies and flow cytometry: changes during platelet storage. *Transfusion,* **30**, 20–25.

Fijnheer, R., Pietersz, Ruby N.I., Huijgens, P.C., de Korte, D., Roos, D. and Reesink, H.W. (1990b) Beneficial effect of pre-transfusion warming of platelets prepared from buffy coats. *Lancet,* **i**, 1524.

Fijnheer, R., Veldman, H.A., van den Eertwegh, A.J.M., Gouwerok, C.W.N., Homburg, C.H.E., Boomgaard, M.N., de Korte, D. and Roos, O. (1991) *In vitro* evaluation of buffy-coat-derived platelet concentrates stored in a synthetic medium. *Vox Sang.* **60**, 16–22.

Filatov, A.N. and Kartasevskij, N. (1934) The transfusion of red cells. *Soviet Surgery.*

Filatov, A. and Kartasevskij, N. (1935) Die Transfusion von menschlichem Blutplasma als blutstillendes Mittel. *Zentralbl. f. Chirurg.* **8**, 441.

Filatov, A.N. (1937) (Abstract). *Int. Abstracts Surg.* **66**, 500.

Files, J.C., Case, C.J. and Morrison, F.S. (1984) Automated erythrocyte exchange in fulminant falciparum malaria. *Ann. intern. Med.* **100**, 396–397.

Finch, C.A. (1972) In International Forum. Which measures should be taken in order to prevent iron deficiency in blood donors? *Vox Sang.* **23**, 238.

Finch, C.A., Cook, J.D., Labbe. R.F. and Culala, Maria (1977) Effect of blood donation on iron stores as evaluated by serum ferritin. *Blood,* **50**, 441–447.

Finch, C.A. and Huebers, H.A. (1987) Maintenance of normal iron balance. *Haematologia,* **20**, 225–228.

Finke, J., Heimpel, H., Hoffman, G. and Keiderling, W. (1965) Vergleichende Untersuchungen zur Bestimmung der Erythrozytenlebenszeit mit Cr^{51} und DFP^{32} beim Menschen. *Nucl. Med. (Amst.),* **4**, 349.

Finlayson, J.S. (1979) Immune globulins. *Semin. Thromb. Haemostas.* **6**, 44–74.

Finlayson, J.S. and Tankersley, D.L. (1990) Anti-HCV screening and plasma fractionation: the case against. *Lancet,* **335**, 1274.

Finn, R. (1960) in Report of the Liverpool Medical Institution. *Lancet,* **i**, 526.

Finn, R., Clarke, C.A., Donohoe, W.T.A, McConnell, R.B., Sheppard, P.M., Lehane, D.

and Kulke, W. (1961) Experimental studies on the prevention of Rh haemolytic disease. *Brit. med. J.* **i**, 1486.

Finn. R., Harper, D.T., Stallings, S.A. and Krevans, J.R. (1963) Transplacental hemorrhage. *Transfusion*, **3**, 114.

Finne, J. (1980) Identification of the blood-group ABH-active glycoprotein components of human erythrocyte membrane. *Eur. J. Biochem.* **104**, 181-189.

First International Workshop on Red Cell Monoclonal Antibodies (1987) *First International Workshop on Monoclonal Antibodies against Human Red Blood cells and Related Antigens*, Paris, eds Ph. Rouger, D. Anstee and Ch. Salmon. *Rev. franç. Transfus. Immunohémat.* **30**, no. 5.

Firt, P. and Hejhal, L. (1957) Treatment of severe haemorrhage. *Lancet*, **ii**, 1132.

Fischer, H., Fritsche, W. and Argenton, H. (1958) Die Bedeutung des Properdinsystems für den normalen und gesteigerten Blutzellabbau. *Klin. Wschr.* **36**, 411.

Fischer, K. (1961) *Morbus Haemolyticus Neonatorum im ABO-System*. Georg Thieme Verlag, Stuttgart.

Fischer, K. (1964) Immunhämatologische und klinische Befunde bei einem Transfusions-Zwischen-fall infolge Gm (a)-Antikörperbildung. *Commun. 10th Congr. Int. Soc. Blood Transfus.*, Stockholm.

Fischer, A., Durandy, Anne, De Villartay, J.-P., Vilmer, E., Le Deist, Francoise, Gerota, Ilona and Griscelli, C. (1986) HLA-haploidentical bone marrow transplantation for severe combined immunodeficiency using E rosette fractionation and cyclosporine. *Blood*, **67**, 444–449.

Fisher, R.A. and Race, R.R. (1946) Rh gene frequencies in Britain. *Nature (Lond.)*, **157**, 48.

Fisher, G.A. (1983) Use of the manual polybrene test in the routine hospital laboratory. *Transfusion*, **23**, 151–154.

Fisher, M., Chapman, J.R., Ting, A. and Morris, P. (1985) Alloimmunization to HLA antigens following transfusion with leucocyte-poor and purified platelet suspensions. *Vox Sang.* **49**, 331–335.

Fisher, E.S. (1990) Reduction of Lutheran antibody reactions with polyethylene glycol, *Abstracts ISBT and AABB Joint Congress*, Los Angeles, Scientific Section, 611.

Fisk, R.T. and Foord, A.G. (1942) Observations on the Rh agglutinogen of human blood. *Amer. J. clin. Path.* **12**, 545.

Fitzsimmons, J.M. and Morel, P.A. (1979) The effects of red blood cell suspending media on haemagglutination and the antiglobulin test. *Transfusion*, **19**, 81–85.

Flanagan, C.J. and Mitoma, T.F. (1958) Clumping (false agglutination) of blood from the umbilical cord. *Amer. J. clin. Path.* **29**, 337.

Fleer, A., van Schaik, M.L.J., von dem Borne, A.E.G.Kr. and Engelfriet, C.P. (1978) Destruction of sensitized erythrocytes by human monocytes in vitro: effects of cytochalasin B, hydrocortisone and colchicine. *Scand. J. Immunol.* **8**, 515.

Fleetwood, P. and McNeill, O. (1990) Quality assurance of anti-D quantitation. *Transfusion Med.* Suppl. 1, 44.

Fleig, C. (1910) Les eaux minérales. Milieux vitaux. Sérothérapie artificielle et balnéothérapie tissulaire par leur injection dans l'organisme. *Académie des Sciences et Lettres de Montpellier. Mémoires de la Section de Médecine*, 2^E Série, **3**, 1.

Fleming, A.F. (1990) AIDS in Africa, in *Haematology in HIV Disease*, ed Christine Costello. *Baillière's Clinical Haematology*, **3**, 177–206.

Fletcher, J.L. and Zmijewski, C.M. (1970) The first example of auto-anti-M and its consequences in pregnancy. *Int. Arch. Allergy*, **37**, 586.

Fletcher, G., Cooke, B.R. and McDowall, J. (1971) Attempts to immunize Rh(D) negative volunteers against the D antigen. *Proc. 2nd Mtg. Asian & Pac. Divn. Int. Soc. Haemat.*, Melbourne, p. 69.

Fletcher, M.L., Trowell, J.M., Craske, J., Pavier, K. and Rizza. C.R. (1983) Non-A, non-B hepatitis after transfusion of Factor VIII in infrequently treated patients. *Brit. med. J.* **287**, 1754–1757.

Flick, M.R., Peel, A. and Staub, N.C. (1981) Leukocytes are required for increased lung microvascular permeability after microembolization in sheep. *Circulation Res.* **48**, 344–351.

Floss, A.M., Strauss, R.G., Goeken, N. and Knox, L. (1986) Multiple transfusions fail to provoke antibodies against blood cell antigens in human infants. *Transfusion*, **26**, 419–422.

Florey, J.W. and Jennings M.A. (1941) The effects of massive injections of blood, plasma and serum into normal cats. Unpublished report to the Medical Research Council.

Florio P.H.L., Stewart, Mabel and Mugrage, E.R. (1943) The effect of freezing on erythrocytes. *J. Lab. clin. Med.* **28**, 1486.

Foconi, S. and Sjölin, S. (1959) Survival of Cr^{51}labelled-red cells from newborn infants. *Acta paediat.* (Uppsala), **48**, Suppl. 117, 18.

Foley, F.D. (1969) The burn autopsy. Fatal complications of burns. *Amer. J. clin. Path.* **52**, 1.

Follett, E.A.C. Dow, B.C., McOmish, F., Lee Yap, P. Hughes, W., Mitchell, R. and Simmonds, P. (1991) HCV confirmatory testing of blood donors (Letter). *Lancet*, **ii**, 1024.

Fong, S.W., Qaqundah, B.Y. and Taylor, W.F. (1974) Developmental patterns of ABO iso-agglutinins in normal children correlated with the effects of age, sex and maternal isoagglutinins. *Transfusion*, **14**, 551.

Ford, J.M., Lucey, J.J Cullen, M.H., Tobias, J.S. and Lister, T.A. (1976) Fatal graft-versus-host disease following transfusion of granulocytes from normal donors. *Lancet*, **ii**, 1167.

Forestier, Francois, Daffos, F., Galacteaos, F., Bardakjian, Josiane, Rainaut, Martine and Beuzard, Y. (1986) Hematological values of 163 normal fetuses between 18 and 30 weeks gestation. *Pediat. Res.* **20**, 342–346.

Forslid, J., Hed, J. and Stendahl, O. (1985) Erythrocyte enhancement of C3b-mediated phagocytos is by human neutrophils *in vitro*: a combined effect of the erythrocyte complement receptors CR1 and erythrocyte scavengers to reactive oxygen metabolites (ROM). *Immunology*, **55**, 97–103.

Forssman, J. (1911) Die Herstellung hochwertiger spezifischer Schafhämolysine ohne Verwendung von Schafblut. Ein Beitrag zur Lehre von heterologer Antikörperbildung. *Biochem. Z.* **37**, 78.

Foster, K.M. (1966) Post-transfusion mononucleosis. *Aust. Ann. Med.* **15**, 305.

Fowler, R. jr, Schubert, W.K. and West, C.D. (1960) Acquired partial tolerance to homologous skin grafts in the human infant at birth. *Ann. N.Y. Acad. Sci. USA*, **87**, 403.

Frame, Marion and Mollison, P. L. (1969) Charge differences between human IgG isoantibodies associated with specificity. *Immunology*, **16**, 277.

Frame, Marion, Mollison, P.L. and Terry, W.D. (1970) Anti-Rh activity of human γG4 proteins. *Nature (Lond)* **225**, 641.

Franciosi, R., Awer, Erica and Santana, M. (1967) Interdonor incompatibility resulting in anuria. *Transfusion*, **7**. 297.

Francis, Betty J. and Hatcher, D.E. (1966) MN blood types. The S-s-U+ and the M_2 phenotypes. *Vox Sang.* **11**, 213.

Francis, H.L. and Quinn, T.C. (1987) AIDS in Africa, in *Current Topics in AIDS*, ed A.J. Pinching, pp. 262–285. John Wiley and Sons, Chichester.

François–Gérard, C., Brocteur, J. and André, A. (1980) Turtledove: a new source of P_1-like material cross-reacting with the human erythrocyte antigen. *Vox Sang.* **39**, 141–148.

Frank, M. M., Hamburger, M.I., Lawley, T.J., Kimberly, R.P. and Plotz, P.H. (1979) Defective Fc-receptor function in lupus erythematosus. *New Engl. J. Med.* **300**, 518–523.

Frank, L. and Massaro, D. (1980) Oxygen toxicity. *Amer. J. Med.* **69**, 117.

Franklin, E.C. and Kunkel, H.G. (1958) Comparative levels of high molecular weight (19S) gamma globulin in maternal and umbilical cord sera. *J. Lab. clin. Med.* **52**, 724.

Franks, D. and Coombs, R.R.A. (1969) General aspects of heterophil antibody systems, in *Infectious Mononucleosis*, eds R.L.Carter and H.G. Penman. Blackwell Scientific Publications, Oxford.

Fraser, I.D. and Tovey, G.H. (1976) Observations on Rh iso-immunisation: past, present and future. *Clin. Haemat.* **5**, 149.

Fraser, R.H., Munro, A.C., Williamson, A.R., Barrie, E.K., Hamilton, E.A. and Mitchell, R. (1982) Mouse monoclonal anti-N. I. Production and serological characterisation. *J. Immunogenet.* **9**, 295–301.

Fraser, R. H., Inglis, G., Mackie, A., Munro, A.C., Allan, E.K., Mitchell, R., Sonneborn, H.H. and Uthemann, H. (1985) Mouse monoclonal antibodies reacting with M blood group-related antigens. *Transfusion*, **25**, 261–266.

Fratantoni, J.C. and French, J.E. (1980) International Forum. Which are the principal established or potential risks for donors undergoing cytapheresis procedures and how can they be prevented? *Vox Sang.* **39**, 174–176.

Frazer, W.F. and Fowweather, F.S. (1942) Tetany in blood donors. *Brit. med. J.* **i**, 759.

Freda, V.J., Wiener, A.S. and Gordon, Eve B. (1957) An unsuspected source of ABO sensitization. *Amer. J. Obstet. Gynec.* **73**, 1148.

Freda, V.J. and Gorman J.G. (1962) Current concepts. Antepartum management of Rh haemolytic disease. *Bull. Sloane Hosp. Women, N.Y.* **8**, 147.

Freda, V.J., Gorman, J.G. and Pollack, W. (1964) Successful prevention of experimental Rh sensitization in man with an anti-Rh gamma$_2$-globulin antibody preparation: a preliminary report. *Transfusion*, **4**, 26.

Freda, V.J., Gorman, J.G. and Pollack, W. (1966) Rh factor: prevention of immunization and clinical trial on mothers. *Science*, **151**, 828.

Freda, V.J., Gorman, J.G., Galen, R.S. and Treacy, N. (1970) The threat of Rh immunization from abortion. *Lancet*, **ii**, 147.

Frederick, J., Hunter, J., Greenwell, P., Winter, K. and Gottschall, J.L. (1985) The A^1B genotype expressed as A_2B on the red cells of individuals with strong B gene-specific transferases. *Transfusion*, **25**, 30–33.

Freedman, J., Masters, Carol A., Newlands, Marion and Mollison, P.L. (1976) Optimal conditions for the use of sulphydryl compounds in dissociating red cell antibodies. *Vox Sang.* **30**, 231.

Freedman, J. and Newlands, Marion (1977) Autoimmune haemolytic anaemia with the unusual combination of both IgM and IgG autoantibodies. *Vox Sang.* **32**, 61.

Freedman, J., Newlands, M. and Johnson, C.A. (1977) Warm IgM anti-I^T causing autoimmune haemolytic anaemia. *Vox Sang.* **32**, 135.

Freedman, J. (1979) False-positive antiglobulin tests in healthy subject and in hospital patients. *J. clin. Path.* **32**, 1014–1018.

Freedman, J., Massey, A., Chaplin, H. and Monroe, M.C. (1980) Assessment of complement binding by anti-D and anti-M antibodies employing labelled antiglobulin antibodies. *Brit. J. Haemat.* **45**, 309–318.

Freedman, J., Blanchette, V., Hornstein, A., Farkas, S., Milner, A., Adams, M., Lim, F.C., Garvey, M.B. and Hannach B. (1991) White cell depletion of red cell and pooled randomdonor platelet concentrates by filtration and residual lymphocyte subset analysis. *Transfusion*, **31**, 433–440.

Freeman, R., Gould, F.K. and McMaster, A. (1990) Management of cytomegalovirus antibody negative patients undergoing heart transplantation. *J. clin. Path.* **43**, 373–376.

Freiesleben, E. and Knudsen, E.E. (1957) A human incomplete immune anti-M, in *P.H. Andresen, Papers in Dedication of his 60th Birthday*, p. 26. Munksgaard, Copenhagen.

Freiesleben, E. and Jensen, K.G. (1959) An antibody specific for washed red cells. *Commun. 7th Congr. Europ. Soc. Haemat.*, London, Abstract 330.

Freiesleben, E. and Jensen, K.G. (1961) Haemolytic disease of the newborn caused by anti-M. The value of the direct conglutination test. *Vox Sang.* **6**, 328.

Freireich, E.J., Judson, G. and Levin, R.H. (1965) Separation and collection of leukocytes. *Cancer Research*, **25**, 1516–1520.

Frenz, G., Doniadis, I., Vögeler, U. and Grosse-Wilde, H. (1989) HLA class I biochemistry: definition and frequency determination of subtypes by one-dimensional isoelectric focusing and immunoblotting. *Vox Sang.* **56**, 190–196.

Fretz, C., Jaulmes, D., Jordan, G., Fournel, J.J., Jullien, A.M., Gout, O., Gluckman, J.C., and De The, G. (1991) HTLV-I transmission and myelopathy induced by blood transfusion (Letter). *Transfusion*, **31**, 379.

Friedenreich, V. (1930) *The Thomsen Hemagglutination Phenomenon.* Levin and Munksgaard, Copenhagen.

Friedenreich, V. (1931) Ueber die Serologie der Untergruppen A$_1$ und A$_2$. *Z. Immun.-Forsch.* **71**, 283.

Friedenreich, V. (1936) Eine bisher unbekannte Blutgruppeneigenschaft. *Z. Immun.-Forsch.* **89**, 409.

Friedman, B.A., Schork, M.A., Mocniak, J.L. and Oberman, H.A. (1975) Short-term and long-term effects of plasmapheresis on serum proteins and immunoglobulins. *Transfusion*, **15**, 467.

Friedman, B.A. (1979) Analysis of surgical blood use in United States hospitals with application to the maximum surgical blood order schedule. *Transfusion*, **19**, 268–278.

Friedman, J.M. and Aster, R.H. (1985) Neonatal alloimmune thrombocytopenic purpura and congenital porencephaly in two siblings associated with a "new" maternal anti-platelet antibody. *Blood*, **65**, 1412–1415.

Frigoletto, F.D., Greene, M.F., Benaceraff, Beryl R., Barss, Vannessa A., van't Veer, M.B. and Saltzman, D.H. (1986) Ultrasonographic fetal surveillance in the management of the isoimmunized pregnancy. *New Engl. J. Med.* **315**, 430–432.

Frim, J. and Mazur, P. (1980) Approaches to the cryopreservation of human granulocytes. *Cryobiology*, **17**, 282–286.

Frommel, D., Grob, P.J., Masouredis, S.P. and Isliker, H.C. (1967) Studies on the mechanism of immunoglobulin binding to red cells. *Immunology*, **13**, 501.

Fuchs, F., Freiesleben, E., Knudsen, Else E. and Riis, P. (1956) Determination of foetal bloodgroup. *Lancet*, **i**, 996.

Fudenberg, H.H. and Allen, F.H. jr (1957) Transfusion reactions in the absence of demonstrable incompatibility. *New Engl. J. Med.* **256**, 1180.

Fudenberg, H.H., Kunkel, H.G. and Franklin, E.C. (1959) High molecular weight antibodies. *Acta haemat.* (*Basel*), Fasc. **10**, 522.

Fudenberg, H.H. and German, J.L. (1960) Certain physical and biological characteristics of penicillin antibody. *Blood*, **15**, 683.

Fudenberg, H.H., Baldini, M., Mahoney, J.P. and Dameshek, W. (1961) The body hematocrit/venous hematocrit ratio and the 'splenic reservoir'. *Blood*, **16**, 71.

Fudenberg, H.H. and Fudenberg, Betty R. (1964) Antibody to hereditary human gammaglobulin (Gm) factor resulting from maternalfetal incompatibility. *Science*, **145**, 170.

Fudenberg, H.H., E.R., Franklin, E.C., Meltzer, M. and Frangione, B. (1964) Antigenicity of hereditary human gamma-globulin (Gm) factors—biological and chemical aspects. *Cold Spr. Harb. Symp. quant. Biol.* **29**, 463.

Fujita, T., Inoue, T., Ogawa, Kiyoko, Iida, K. and Tamura, N. (1987) The mechanism of action of decay-accelerating factor (DAF). *J. exp. Med.* **166**, 1221–1228.

Fukuda, M., Fukuda, M.N. and Hakomori, S.-I. (1979) Developmental change and genetic defect in the carbohydrate structure of band 3 glycoprotein of human erythrocye membrane. *J. biol. Chem.* **254**, 3700–3703.

Fullerton, M.W., Philippart, A.I., Sarnaik, Sharada and Lusher, Jeanne M. (1981) Preoperative exchange transfusion in sickle cell anemia. *J. pediat. Surg.* **16**, 297–300.

Furihata, K., Nugent, D.J., Bissonette, A., Aster, R.H. and Kunicki, T.J. (1987) On the association of the platelet-specific alloantigen, Pen^a, with glycoprotein III^a. Evidence for the heterogeneity of glycoprotein III^a. *J. clin. Invest.* **80**, 1624–1630.

Furman, R.A., Hellerstein, H.K. and Startzman, Viola (1951) ECG changes occurring during the course of replacement transfusions *J. Pediat.* **38**, 45.

Furthmayr, H., Metaxas, M.N. and Metaxas-Bühler, M. (1981) M^g and M^c: mutations within the amino-terminal region of glycophorin A. *Proc. nat. Acad. Sci. USA*, **78**, 631–635.

Furuhjelm, U., Myllylä, G., Nevanlinna, H.R., Nordling, S., Pirkola, Anna, Gavin, June, Gooch, Ann, Sanger, Ruth and Tippett, Patricia (1969) The red cell phenotype En(a-) and anti-En^a: serological and physicochemical aspects. *Vox Sang.* **17**, 256.

Furukawa, K., Mattes, M.J. and Lloyd, K.O. (1985) A_1 and A_2 erythrocytes can be distinguished by reagents that do not detect structural differences between the two cell types. *J. Immunol.* **135**, 4090–4094.

Gabrilove, Janice L. and 13 others (1988) Effects of granulocyte colony-stimulating factor on neutropenia and associated morbidity due to chemotherapy for transitional-cell carcinoma of the urothelium. *New Engl. J. Med.* **318**, 1414–1422.

Gabrio, Beverly and Finch, C.A. (1954) Erythrocyte preservation. I. The relation of the storage lesion to *in vivo* erythrocyte senescence. *J. clin. Invest.* **33**, 242.

Gabrio, Beverly W. and Huennekens, F.M. (1955) Nucleoside metabolism of the stored erythrocyte. *Fed. Proc.* **14**, 217.

Gabrio, Beverly W., Hennessey, Marion, Thomasson, Joan and Finch, C.A. (1955a) Erythrocyte preservation. IV. The *in vitro* reversibility of the storage lesion. *J. biol. Chem.* **215**, 357.

Gabrio, Beverly W., Donohue, D.M. and Finch, C.A. (1955b) Erythrocyte preservation. V. Relationship between chemical changes and viability of stored blood treated with adenosine. *J. clin, Invest.* **34**, 1509.

Gabrio, Beverly W., Finch, C.A. and Huennekens, F.M. (1956) Erythrocyte preservation: a topic in molecular biochemistry. *Blood*, **11**, 103.

Gadek, J.E., Hosea, S.W., Gelfand, M.A., Santaella, Maria, Wickerhouser, M., Triantaphyllopoulos, D.C. and Frank, M. (1980) Replacement therapy in hereditary angioedema. Successful treatment of acute episodes of angioedema with partly purified C1 inhibitor. *New Engl. J. Med.* **302**, 542–546.

Gadek, J.E., Klein, H.G., Holland, P.V. and Crystal, R.G. (1981) Replacement therapy of alpha 1-antitrypsin deficiency. Reversal of protease-antiprotease imbalance within the alveolar structures of PiZ subjects. *J. clin. Invest.* **68**, 1158–1165.

Gahmberg, C.G., Jakinen, M. and Andersson, L.C. (1978) Expression of the major sialoglycoprotein (glycophorin) on erythroid cells in human bone marrow. *Blood*, **52**, 379.

Gahmberg, C.G. (1982) Molecular identification of the human $Rh_0(D)$ antigen. *FEBS Letters*, **140**, 93–97.

Gaidulis, Laima, Branch, D.R., Lazar, G.S., Petz, L.D. and Blume, K.G. (1985) The red cell antigens A, B, D, U, Ge, Jk 3 and Yt^a are not detected on human granulocytes. *Brit. J. Haemat.* **60**, 659–668.

Gale, R.P. and Winston, D. (1991) Intravenous immunoglobulin in bone marrow transplantation. *Cancer*, **68**, 1451–1453.

Gallo, R.C., De-The, G.B. and Ito, Y. (1981) Kyoto workshop on some specific recent advances in human tumor virology. *Cancer Res.* **41**, 4738–4739.

Gallo, R.C. and 12 others (1984) Frequent detection and isolation of cytopathic retroviruses (HTLV-III) from patients with AIDS and at risk for AIDS. *Science*, **224**, 500–503.

Gammelgaard, A. (1942) *Om Sjaeldne. Svage A-receptorer* (A_3, A_4, A_5, *og* A_x), Haos Mennesket, Nyt Nordisk Forlag, Copenhagen, English Translation published in 1964 by Walter Reed Army Institute of Medical Research, Washington, DC, USA.

Gane, P., Mollicone, R., Rouger, P. and Oriol, A. (1987a) Inhibition of haemagglutination with synsorbs and salivas of anti-A monoclonal antibodies. *Rev. franç. Transfus. Immunohémat.* **30**, 135 142.

Gane, P., Vellayoudom, J., Mollicone, R., Breimer, M.E., Samuelsson, B.E., Rouger, P., Gerard, G., Le Pendu, J. and Oriol, R. (1987b) Heterogeneity of anti-A and anti-B monoclonal reagents. Agglutination of some weak ABH erythrocyte variants and recognition of synthetic olgosaccharide and tissue antigens. *Vox Sang.* **53**, 117–125.

Ganeval, D., Bournerias, F., Daniel, F., Rozen, J., Homberg, J.C. and Habibi, B. (1978) Hémolyse par anticorps anti-glofénine avec insuffisance rénale aigue. *Nouv. Presse med.* **7**, 3254.

Ganly, P.S., Laffan, M.A., Owen, I. and Hows, J.M. (1988) Auto-anti-Jk^a in Evans' syndrome with negative direct antiglobulin test. *Brit. J. Haemat.* **69**, 537–539.

Gans, R.O.B., Duurkens, V.A.M., van Zundert, A.A. and Hoorntje, S.J. (1988) Transfusion-related acute lung injury. *Intensive Care Med.* **14**, 654–659.

Ganser, A., Völkers, B., Greher, J., Ottmann, O.G., Walther, F., Becher, R., Bergmann, L., Schulz, G. and Hoelzer, D. (1989) Recombinant human granulocyte-macrophage colony-stimulating factor in patients with myelodysplastic syndromes — a phase I/II trial. *Blood*, **73**, 31–37.

Ganzoni, A.M., Oakes, R. and Hillman, R.S. (1971) Red cell ageing *in vivo. J. clin. Invest.* **50**, 1373.

Garby, L. and Noyes, W.D. (1959) Studies on hemoglobin metabolism. I. The kinetic properties of the plasma hemoglobin pool in normal man. *J. clin. Invest.* **38**, 1479.

Garby, L. (1962) Analysis of red-cell survival curves in clinical practice and the use of di-isopropylfluorophosphonate (DF^{32}P) as a label for red cells in man. *Brit J. Haemat.* **8**, 15.

Garby, L. (1970) Annotation: The normal haemoglobin level. *Brit. J. Haemat.* **19**, 429.

Garby, L. and Mollison, P.L. (1971) Deduction of mean red cell life-span from ^{51}Cr survival curves. *Brit. J. Haemat.* **20**, 527.

Gardas, A. (1983) Immunochemistry of blood group I glycolipids, in *Red Cell Membrane Glycoconjugates and Related Genetic Markers*, eds J.P. Carton, P. Rouger and C. Salmon, pp. 117–124. Lib. Arnette, Paris.

Gardner, B., Ghosh, S., Brazier, D.M. and Holburn, A.M. (1983) Quantitative quality control of antiglobulin reagents. *Clin. Lab. Haemat.* **5**, 215–229.

Gardner, B., Anstee, D.J., Mawby, W.J., Tanner, M.J.A. and von dem Borne, A.E.C.Kr. (1991) The abundance and organization of polypeptides associated with antigens of the Rh blood group system. *Transfus. Med.* **1**, 77–85.

Garner, S.F., Devenish, A., Barber, H. and Contreras, M. (1991) The importance of monitoring "enzyme-only" red cell antibodies during pregnancy (Letter). *Vox Sang.* **61**, 219–220.

Garner, S.F., Wiener, E., Contreras, M., Nicolini, U., Kochenour, N., Letsky, E. and Rodeck, C.H. (1992) Mononuclear phagocyte assays, AutoAnalyzer quantitation and IgG subclasses of maternal anti-RhD in the prediction of the severity of haemolytic disease of the fetus before 32 weeks gestation. *Brit. J. Haemat.* **80**, 97–101.

Garratty, G. and Kleinschmidt, Gillian (1965) Two examples of anti-Le^b detected in the sera of patients with the Lewis phenotype Le(a+b–). *Vox Sang.* **10**, 567.

Garratty, G. (1970) The effect of storage and heparin on serum complement activity with particular reference to the detection of blood group antibodies. *Amer. J. clin. Path.* **54**, 531.

Garratty, G., Haffleigh, B., Dalziel, J. and Petz, L.D. (1972) An IgG anti-I^T detected in a caucasian American. *Transfusion*, **12**, 325.

Garratty, G., Petz, L.D., Brodsky, I. and Fudenberg, H.H. (1973) An IgA high-titer cold agglutinin with an unusual blood group specificity within the Pr complex. *Vox Sang.* **25**, 32.

Garratty, G., Petz, L.D., Wallerstein, R.O. and Fudenberg, H.H. (1974) Autoimmune hemolytic anemia in Hodgkin's disease associated with anti-I^T. *Transfusion*, **14**, 226.

Garratty, G. and Petz, L.D. (1975) Drug-induced immune hemolytic anemia. *Amer. J. Med.* **58**, 398.

Garratty, G. and Petz, L.D. (1976) The significance of red cell bound complement components in development of standards and quality assurance for the anti-complement components of antiglobulin sera. *Transfusion*, **16**, 297.

Garratty, G., Petz, L.D. and Hoops, J.K. (1977) The correlation of cold agglutinin titrations in saline and albumin with haemolytic anaemia. *Brit. J. Haemat.* **35**, 587.

Garratty, G., Gattler, M.S., Petz, L.D. and Flannery, E.P. (1979) Immune hemolytic anemia associated with anti-Kell and a carrier state for chronic granulomatous disease. *Rev. franç. Transfus. Immunohémat.* **22**, 529–549.

Garratty, G., Davis, J., Myers, M., Nelson, A. and Pierce, A. (1980) IgG red cell sensitization associated with *in vitro* clotting in patients with ulcerative colitis (Abstract). *Transfusion*, **20**, 646.

Garratty, G., Brunt, O., Greenfield, B., Simon, T., Smith, K., Garner, R. and Horvath, A. (1983) An autoanti-En^a mimicking an alloanti-En^a associated with pure red cell aplasia (Abstract). *Transfusion*, **23**, 408.

Garratty, G., Postoway, N., Nance, S.J. and Brunt, D.J. (1984) Spontaneous agglutination of red cells with a positive direct antiglobulin test in various media. *Transfusion*, **24**, 214–217.

Garratty, G., Prince, H., Arndt, P. and Shulman, I. (1986) *In vitro* IgG production following preincubation of lymphocytes with methyldopa and procainamide. (Abstract). *Blood*, **68**, Suppl. 1, 108a.

Garratty, G. (1990) Flow cytometry; its applications to immunohaematology, in *Blood Transfusion: the Impact of New Technologies*, ed Marcela Contreras. *Baillière's Clinical Haematology*, **3**, 267–287.

Garretta, M., Paris-Hamelin, A. and Vaismam, A. (1977) Syphilis et transfusion. *Rev. franç. transfus. Immunohémat.* **2**, 287–308.

Garson, J.A. and 9 others (1990a) Detection of hepatitis C viral sequences in blood donations by "nested" polymerase chain reaction and prediction of infectivity. *Lancet*, i, 1419–1422.

Garson, J.A., Tuke, P.W., Makris, M., Briggs, M., Machin, S.J., Preston, F.E. and Tedder, R.S. (1990b) Demonstration of viraemia patterns in haemophiliacs treated with hepatitis-C-virus-contaminated Factor VIII concentrates. *Lancet*, ii, 1022–1025.

Garson, J.A., Ring, C., Tuke, P. and Tedder, R.S. (1990c) Enhanced detection by PCR of hepatitis C virus RNA (Letter). *Lancet*, ii, 878–879.

Garson, J.A., Ring, C.J.A. and Tuke, P.W. (1991) Improvement of HCV genome detection with "short" PCR products (Letter). *Lancet*, ii, 1466–1467.

Gascon, O., Zoumbos, N.C. and Young, N.S. (1984) Immunologic abnormalities in patients receiving multiple blood transfusions. *Ann. intern. Med.* 100, 173–177.

Gasser, C. (1945) Akute hämolytische Krisen nach Plasma-Transfusionen bei dystrophis-chtoxischen Säuglingen. *Helv. paediat. Acta*, 1, 38.

Gattegno, Liliane, Bladier, Dominique and Cornillat, P. (1975) Ageing *in vivo* and neuraminidase treatment of rabbit erythrocytes: influence on half-life assessed by ^{51}Cr labelling. *Hoppe-Zeyler's Z. Physiol. Chem.* 356, 391.

Gay, F.P. (1905) Observations on the single nature of haemolytic immune bodies, and on the existence of so-called 'complementoids'. *Zbl. Bakt. (Orig.)*, 39, 172.

Geisen, H.P., Roelcke, D., Rehn, K. and Konrad, G. (1975) Hochtitrige Kälteagglutinine der Spezifität Anti-Pr nach Rötelninfektion. *Klin. Wschr.* 53, 767–772.

Gemke, R.J.B.J., Kanhai, H.H.H., Overbeeke, M.A.M., Maas, C.J., Bennebroek, G., Bernini, L.F., Engelfriet, C.P. and van't Veer, M.B. (1986) ABO and Rhesus phenotyping of fetal erythrocytes in the first trimester of pregnancy. *Brit. J. Haemat.* 64, 689–697.

Genetet, B. and Mannoni, P. (1978) *La Transfusion*. Flammarion, Paris.

Gengozian, N. and McLaughlin, C.L. (1978) Activity induced platelet-bound IgG associated with thrombocytopenia in the marmoset. *Blood*, 51, 1197–1210.

George, V.M., Holme, S. and Moroff, G. (1989) Evaluation of two instruments for non invasive platelet concentrate quality assessment. *Transfusion*, 29, 273–275.

Gerbal, A., Maslet, C. and Salmon, C. (1975) Immunological aspects of the acquired B antigen. *Vox Sang.* 28, 398.

Gerbal, A., Ropars, C., Gerbal, R., Cartron, J.P., Maslet, C. and Salmon, C. (1976a) Acquired B antigen disappearance by *in vitro* acetylation associated with A_1 activity restoration. *Vox Sang.* 31, 64.

Gerbal, A., Lopez, M., Maslet, C. and Salmon, Ch. (1976b) Polyagglutinability associated with the Cad antigen. *Haematologia*, 10, 383.

Gerbase de Lima, M., Wollman, E.E., Lepage, V., Degos, L. and Dausset, J. (1981) Alloantigens expressed on activated human T cells different from HLA-A, B, C and DR antigens. *Immunogenetics*, 13, 529–537.

Gerber, P., Walsh, J.H., Rosenblum, Edith N. and Purcell, R.H. (1969) Association of EB-virus infection with the post-perfusion syndrome. *Lancet*, i, 593.

Gerlini, G., Ottaviano, S., Sbraccia, C. and Carapella, E. (1968) Reattività dell'antigene A_1 e suoi rapporti con la malattia emolitica del neonato da incompatibilità ABO. *Haematologica*, 53, Suppl, 1019.

Gerstner, J.B., Smith, M.J., Davis, K.D., Cimo, P.L. and Aster, R.H. (1979) Posttransfusion purpura: therapeutic failure of PI^{A1}-negative platelet transfusion. *Amer. J. Hemat.* 6, 71–75.

Gesellius, F. (1874) *Zur Thierblut-Transfusion beim Menschen*. St Petersburg and Leipzig.

Gessain, A. and 9 others (1986) HTLV-I and tropical spastic paraparesis in Africa. *Lancet*, ii, 698.

Geyer, R.P. (1975) 'Bloodless' rats through the use of artificial blood substitutes. *Fed. Proc.* 34, 1499.

Ghebrehiwet, B., Silverberg, M. and Kaplan, A.P. (1981) Activation of the classical pathway of complement by Hageman factor fragment. *J. exp. Med.* 153, 665–676.

Gibberd, F.B., Billimoria, J.D., Page, N.G.R. and Retsas, S. (1979) Heredopathia atactica polineuritiformis (Refsum's disease) treated by diet and plasma exchange. *Lancet*, i, 575–578.

Gibble, J.W., Salmon, J.L. and Ness, P.M. (1983) Comparison of antibody elution techniques by enzyme-linked antiglobulin tests. *Transfusion*, 23, 300–304.

Gibbons, D.S., Kano, T. and Edelmann, M. (1986) A terraced microplate system for automated ABO and Rh grouping. *Amer. clin. Prod. Rev.* 5, 42–46.

Giblett, Eloise R., Chase, Jeanne and Crealock, F.W. (1958) Hemolytic disease of the newborn resulting from anti-s antibody. *Amer. J. clin. Path.* 29, 254.

Giblett, Eloise R. (1961) A critique of the theoretical hazard of inter- *vs* intra-racial transfusion. *Transfusion*, 1, 233.

Giblett, Eloise R. (1964) Blood group antibodies causing hemolytic disease of the newborn. *Clin. Obstet. Gynec.* 7, 1044.

Giblett, Eloise R. and Crookston, Marie C. (1964) Agglutinability of red cells by anti-i in patients with thalassaemia major and other haematological disorders. *Nature (Lond.)*, **201**, 1138.

Giblett, Eloise R., Hillman, R.S. and Brooks, Lucy E. (1965) Transfusion reaction during marrow suppression in a thalassemic patient with a blood group anomaly and an unusual cold agglutinin. *Vox Sang.* **10**, 448.

Giblett, Eloise R. (1969) *Genetic Markers in Human Blood*. Blackwell Scientific Publications, Oxford.

Giblett, Eloise R., Klebanoff, S.J., Pincus, Stephanie H., Swanson, Jane, Park, B.H. and McCullough, J. (1971) Kell phenotypes in chronic granulomatous disease: a potential transfusion hazard. *Lancet*, **i**, 1235.

Giblett, Eloise R. (1977) Blood group alloantibodies: an assessment of some laboratory practices. *Transfusion*, **17**, 229.

Gibson, J.G., Murphy, W.P. jr, Scheitlin, W.A. and Rees, S.B. (1956) The influence of extracellular factors involved in the collection of blood in ACD on maintenance of red cell viability during refrigerated storage. *Amer. J. clin. Path.* **26**, 855.

Gibson, J.G., Rees, S.B., McManus, T.J. and Scheitlin, W.A. (1957) A citrate-phosphate-dextrose solution for the preservation of human blood. *Amer. J. clin. Path.* **28**, 569.

Gibson, T. and Norris, W. (1958) Skin fragments removed by injection needles. *Lancet*, **ii**, 983.

Gibson, J.G., Gregory, C.B. and Button, L.N. (1961) Citrate-phosphate-dextrose solution for preservation of human blood. A further report. *Transfusion*, **1**, 280.

Gibson, T. (1979) Providing saline reacting anti-D cell typing reagent. *Clin. lab. Haemat.* **1**, 321–323.

Gilardi, Von A. and Miescher, P. (1957) Die Lebensdauer von autologen und homologen Erythrocyten bei Frühgeborenen und älteren Kindern. *Schweiz. med. Wschr.* **87**, 1456.

Gilbert, Gwendolyn, L., Hayes, Kathleen, Hudson, Irene, L., James, Jennifer, and the Neonatal Cytomegalovirus Infection Study Group (1989) Prevention of transfusion-acquired cytomegalovirus infection in infants by blood filtration to remove leucocytes. *Lancet*, **i**, 1228–1231.

Giles, Carolyn M. (1960) Survey of uses for ficin in blood group serology. *Vox Sang.* **5**, 467.

Giles, Carolyn M. and Metaxas, M.N. (1964) Identification of the predicted blood group antibody anti-Yt^b. *Nature (Lond.)*, **202**, 1122.

Giles, Carolyn M. and Lundsgaard, Anne (1967) A complex serological investigation involving LW. *Vox Sang.* **13**, 406.

Giles, Carolyn M., Darnborough, J., Aspinall, P.

and Fletton, M.W. (1970) Identification of the first example of anti-Co^b. *Brit. J. Haemat.* **19**, 267.

Giles, C.M. (1975) Antithetical relationship of anti-In^a with the Salis antibody. *Vox Sang.* **29**, 73–76.

Giles, C. M., Gedde-Dahl, T. jr, Robson, E.B., Thorsby, E., Olaisen, B., Arnason, A., Kissmeyer-Nielsen, F. and Schreuder, I. (1976) Rg^a (Rodgers) and the HLA region: Linkage and associations. *Tissue Antigens*, **8**, 143.

Giles, Carolyn M. (1977) The identity of Kamhuber and Far antigens. *Vox Sang.* **32**, 269.

Giles, Carolyn M. and Poole, Joyce (1979) Auto-anti-Le^b in the serum of a renal dialysis patient. *Clin. lab. Haemat.* **1**, 239–242.

Giles, C. M. (1980) The LW blood group: a review. *Immunol. Commun.* **9**, 225–242.

Giles, Carolyn M. and Engelfriet, C.P. (1980) Working Party on the Standardization of Antiglobulin Reagents of the ISBT/ICSH Expert Panel on Serology. *Vox Sang.* **38**, 178–179.

Giles, Carolyn M. (1982) Serological activity of low frequency antigens of the MNSs system and reappraisal of the Miltenberger complex. *Vox Sang.* **42**, 256–261.

Giles, Carolyn M. (1985a) 'Partial inhibition' of anti-Rg and anti-Ch reagents. I. Assessment for Rg/Ch typing by inhibition. *Vox Sang.* **48**, 160–166.

Giles, Carolyn M. (1985b) 'Partial inhibition' of anti-Rg and anti-Ch reagents. II. Demonstration of separable antibodies for different determinants. *Vox Sang.* **48**, 167–173.

Giles, C.M. (1989) An update on Rodgers and Chido, the antigenic determinants of human C4. *Immunohematology*, **5**, 1–6.

Gill, T.J., Kunz, H.W., Stechschulte, D.J. and Austen, K.F. (1970) Genetic and cellular factors in the immune response. I. Genetic control of the antibody response to poly Glu^{52} Lys^{33} Tyr^{15} in the inbred rat strains ACI and F344. *J. Immunol.* **105**, 14.

Gillard, B.A., Blanchard D., Bouhours, J-F., Cartron, J-P., Van Kuik, J.A., Kamerling, J.P., Vliegenthart, J.F.G. and Marcus, D.M. (1988) Structure of a ganglioside with Cad blood group antigen activity. *Biochemistry*, **27**, 4601–4606.

Gillespie, E.M. and Gold, E.R. (1960) Weakening of the B-antigen by the presence of A$_1$ as shown by reactions with Fomes fomentarius (anti-B) extract. *Vox Sang.* **5**, 497.

Gilligan, D.R., Altschule, M.D. and Katersky, E.M. (1941) Studies of hemoglobinemia and hemoglobinuria produced in man by intravenous injection of hemoglobin solutions. *J. Clin. Invest.* **20**, 179.

Gilliland, B.C., Baxter, Elizabeth and Evans, R.S.

(1971) Red cell antibodies in acquired hemolytic anemia with negative antiglobulin serum tests. *New Engl. J. Med.* **285**, 252.

Giltay, J.C., Leeksma, O.C., von dem Borne, A.-E.G.Kr. and Van Mourik, J.A. (1988a) Allo-antigenic composition of the endothelial vitronectin receptor. *Blood*, **72**, 230–233.

Giltay, J.C., Brinkman, H.J.M., von dem Borne, A.E.G.Kr. and Van Mourik, J.A. (1988b) Expression of alloantigen Zw^a (or PL^{A1}) on human vascular smooth muscle cells and foreskin fibroblasts. A study on normal individuals and a patient with Glanzmann's thrombasthenia. *Blood*, **74**, 965–970.

Giordano, C.F. and 9 others (1988) Intraoperative autotransfusion in cardiac operations; effect on intraoperative and postoperative transfusion requirements. *J. thorac. cardiovasc. Surg.* **96**, 382–386.

Gitlin, D. and Borges, W.H. (1953) Studies on the metabolism of fibrinogen in two patients with congenital afibrinogenemia. *Blood*, **8**, 679.

Gitlin, D., Kumate, J., Urrusti, J. and Morales, C. (1964) The selectivity of the human placenta in the transfer of plasma proteins from mother to fetus. *J. clin. Invest.* **43**, 1938.

Glaser, E.M. (1949) The effects of cooling and warming on the vital capacity, forearm and hand volume and skin temperature of man. *J. Physiol. (Lond.)*, **109**, 421.

Glaspy, J.A., Baldwin, G.C., Robertson, P.A., Souza, L.M., Vincent, M., Ambersly, J. and Goede, D.W. (1988) Therapy for neutropenia in hairy cell leukemia with recombinant human granulocyte colony-stimulating factor. *Ann. intern. Med.* **109**, 789–795.

Glasser, L., Fiederlein, R.L. and Huestis, D.W. (1985) Liquid preservation of human neutrophils stored in synthetic media at 22°C: Controlled observations on storage variables. *Blood*, **66**, 267–272.

Glasser, L., West, J.H. and Hagood, R.M. (1970) Incompatible fetomaternal transfusion with maternal intravascular lysis. *Transfusion*, **10**, 322.

Glazer, J.P., Friedman, H.M., Grossman, R.A., Starr, S.E., Barker, C.F., Perloff, L.J., Huang, E.S. and Plotkin, S.A. (1979) Live cytomegalovirus vaccination of renal transplant candidates: a preliminary trial. *Ann. intern. Med.* **91**, 676–683.

Gleichmann, H. and Breininger, J. (1975) Over 95% sensitization against allogeneic leukocytes following single massive blood transfusion. *Vox Sang.* **28**, 66.

Glenny, A.T. and Südmersen, H.J. (1921) Notes on the production of immunity to diphtheria toxin. *J. Hyg. (Camb)*, **20**, 176.

Glinz, W., Grob, P.J., Nydegger, U.E., Ricklin, T., Stamin, F., Stobel, D. and Lasance, A. (1985) Polyvalent immunoglobulin for prophylaxis of bacterial infections in polytraumatical patients. *Intensive Care Med.* **11**, 288–294.

Glover, J.L. and Broadie, T.A. (1987) Intraoperative autotransfusion. *World J. Surg.* **11**, 60–64.

Glud, T.K., Rosthy, S., Krogh Jensen, M., Laursen, Benedicte, Grunnet, N. and Jersild, C. (1983) High dose intravenous immunoglobulin for post-transfusion purpura. *Scand. J. Haemat.* **31**, 495–500.

Gmür, J. and 10 others (1983) Delayed alloimmunization using random single donor platelet transfusion: a prospective study in thrombocytopenic patients with acute leukemia. *Blood*, **62**, 473–479.

Gmür, J., Burger, Johanna, Schanz, U., Fehr, J. and Schaffner, A. (1991) Safety of stringent prophylactic platelet transfusion policy for patients with acute leukaemia. *Lancet*, **ii**, 1223–1226.

Göbel, U., Drescher, K.H., Pöttgen, W. and Lehr, H.J. (1974) A second example of anti-Yt^a with rapid *in vivo* destruction of Yt(a+) red cells. *Vox Sang.* **27**, 171.

Gocke, D.J. (1972) A prospective study of post-transfusion hepatitis. The role of Australia antigen. *J. Amer. med. Assoc.* **219**, 1165.

Godzisz, J. (1979) La synthèse des allohémagglutinines naturelles du système ABO chez les enfants sains âgés de 3 mois à 3 ans. *Rev. franç. Transfus. Immunohémat.* **22**, 399–412.

Goedert, J.J. and 19 others (1989) A prospective study of human immunodeficiency virus type 1 infection and the development of AIDS in subjects with hemophilia. *New Engl. J. Med.* **321**, 1141–1148.

Gjörstrup, P. and Watt, R.M. (1990) Therapeutic protein A immunoabsorption. A review. *Tranfus. Sci.* **11**, 281–302.

Gold, E.R., Lockyer, W.J. and Tovey, G.H. (1958) Use of lyophilized formol-treated red cells in blood group serology. *Nature (Lond.)*, **182**, 951.

Gold, E.R., Tovey, G.H., Benney, W.E. and Lewis, F.J.W. (1959) Changes in the group A antigen in a case of leukaemia. *Nature (Lond.)*, **183**, 892.

Gold, E.R. (1964) Observations on the specificity of anti-O and anti-AI sera. *Vox Sang.* **9**, 153.

Gold, E.R. and Fudenberg, H.H. (1967) Chromic chloride: a coupling reagent for passive hemagglutination reactions. *J. Immunol.* **99**, 859.

Goldberg, L.S. and Barnett, E.V. (1967) Mixed γG-γM cold agglutinin. *J. Immunol.* **99**, 803.

Goldberg, L.S. and Fudenberg, H.H. (1968) Warm antibody hemolytic anemia; prolonged remission despite persistent positive Coombs test. *Vox Sang.* **15**, 443.

Golde, D.W., McGinniss, M.N. and Holland, P.V. (1969) Mechanism of the albumin agglutination phenomenon. *Vox Sang.* **16**, 465.

Golde, D.W., Greipp, P.R. and McGinniss, M.H. (1973) Spectrum of albumin autoagglutinins. *Transfusion*, **13**, 1.

Goldfinger, D. and McGinniss, Mary H. (1971) Rh-incompatible platelet transfusions—risks and consequences of sensitizing immunosuppressed patients. *New Engl. J. Med.* **284**, 942.

Goldfinger, D. (1977) Acute hemolytic transfusion reactions—a fresh look at pathogenesis and considerations regarding therapy. *Transfusion*, **17**, 85.

Goldfinger, D., Kleinman, S., Connelly, M., Chaux, A. and Sacks, H.J. (1979) Acute hemolytic transfusion reaction (HTR) with disseminated intravascular coagulation (DIC) and acute renal failure (ARF) due to transfusion of plasma containing Rh antibodies (Abstract). *Transfusion*, **19**, 639–640.

Goldman, J.M., Lowenthal, R.M., Buskard, N.A., Spiers, A.S.D., Th'ng, K.H. and Park, D.S. (1975) Chronic granulocytic leukaemia—selective removal of immature granulocytic cells by leukapheresis. *Series Haemat.* **8**, 28.

Goldman, J.M., Hein, L. and Wright, D.G. (1979) Filtration leukapheresis; review and reevaluation. *Exp. Hemat.* **7**, 1–51.

Goldman, Mindy and Blajchman, M.A. (1991) Blood product-associated bacterial sepsis. *Transfus. Med. Rev.* **5**, 73–83.

Goldman, M., Frame, B., Sincal, D.P. and Blajchman, M.A. (1991) Effect of blood transfusion on survival in a mouse bacterial peritonitis model. *Transfusion*, **31**, 710–712.

Goldschmeding, R., van der Schoot, C. Ellen, Ten Bokkel Huinink, D., Hack, C.E., van den Ende, Marlies E., Kallenberg, C.G.M. and von dem Borne, A.E.G.Kr. (1989) Wegener's granulomatosis autoantibodies identify a novel diisopropyl-fluorophosphate-binding protein in the lysosomes of normal neutrophils. *J. clin. Invest.* **84**, 1577–1587.

Goldschmeding, R., Cohen Tervaert, J.W., Dolman, K.M., von dem Borne, A.E.G.Kr. and Kallenberg, C.G.M. (1991) ANCA: a class of vasculitis-associated autoantibodies against myeloid granule proteins, in *New Aspects of Human Polymorphonuclear Leukocytes*, eds W.H. Horl and P.J. Schollmeyer, pp. 129–138. Plenum Press, New York.

Goldschmeding, R., van Dalen, C. M., Faber, N., Calafat, J., Huizinga, T.W.J., Van Der Schoot, C. E., Clement, L.T. and Von Dem Borne, A.E.G.Kr. (1992) Further characterization of the NB1 antigen as a variably expressed 56–62 kD GPI-linked glycoprotein of plasma membranes and specific granules of neutrophils. *Brit. J. Haemat* **81**, 336–345.

Goldstein, I.M., Eyre, H.J., Terasaki, P.I., Henderson, E.S. and Graw, R.G. jr (1971) Leukocyte transfusions: role of leukocyte alloantibodies in determining transfusion response. *Transfusion*, **11**, 19.

Goldstein, I.J. and Hayes, Coleen E. (1978) Lectins: carbohydrate-binding proteins, in *Advances in Carbohydrate Chemistry and Biochemistry*, eds R.S. Tipson and D. Horton, **35**, 127–340.

Goldstein, I.J., Hughes, R.C., Monsigny, M., Osawa, T. and Sharon, N. (1980) What should be called a lectin? (Letter). *Nature (Lond.)*, **285**, 66.

Goldstein, I.J., Blake, Diane A., Ebisu, S., Williams, T.J. and Murphy, L.A. (1981) Carbohydrate binding studies on the *Bandeiraea simplicifolia* I isolectins. Lectins which are mono-, di-, tri-, and tetravalent for *N*-acetyl-D-galactosamine. *J. biol. Chem.* **256**, 3890–3893.

Goldstein, J., Siviglia, Geraldine, Hurst, Rosa, Lenny, Leslie and Reich, Lilian (1982) Group B erythrocytes enzymatically converted to group O survive normally in A, B, and O individuals. *Science*, **215**, 168–170.

Gomperts, E.O. (1986) Procedures for the inactivation of viruses in clotting factor concentrates. *Amer. Hemat.* **23**, 295–305.

Goodman, N.G. (1934) *Benjamin Rush, Physician and Citizen, 1746–1813*. University of Pennsylvania Press, Philadelphia.

Goodman, H.S. and Masaitis, L. (1964) Binding characteristics of Rh antibodies and their serologic properties. *Vox Sang.* **9**, 6.

Goodman, H.S. and Masaitis, L. (1967) Analysis of the isoimmune response to leucocytes. I. Maternal cytotoxic leucocyte isoantibodies formed during the first pregnancy. *Vox Sang.* **16**, 97.

Goodnouch, L.T. and 14 others (1989) Increased preoperative collection of autologous blood with recombinant human erythropoietin therapy. *New Engl. J. Med.* **321**, 1163–1168.

Goodwin, C.W., Dorethy, J., Lam, V. and Pruitt, B.A. jr (1983) Randomised trial of efficacy of crystalloid and colloid resuscitation on hemodynamic response and lung water following thermal injury. *Ann. Surg.* **197**, 520–529.

Goosens, D., Champonier, F., Rouger, P. and Salmon, C. (1987) Human monoclonal antibodies against blood group antigens. Preparation of a series of stable EBV immortalised B clones producing high levels of antibody of different isotypes and specificities. *J. immunol. Methods*, **101**, 193–200.

Gordon, J. and Murgita, R.A. (1975) Suppression and augmentation of the primary *in vitro* immune response by different classes of antibodies. *Cellular Immunol.* **15**, 392.

Gordon, I. and Ross, D. (1987) Large-scale blood grouping and antibody screening using microplates and an automated reader for ABO and Rh determination, in *The Use of Microplates in Blood Group Serology*, eds R. Knight and G. Poole, pp. 20–25. British Blood Transfusion Society, Manchester.

Gorick, B.D., Thompson, K.M., Melamed, M.D. and Hughes-Jones, N.C. (1988) Three epitopes on the human Rh antigen D recognised by ^{125}I-labelled human monoclonal IgG antibodies. *Vox Sang.* 55, 165–170.

Gorick, B.D. and Hughes-Jones, N.C. (1991) Relative functional binding activity of IgG1 and IgG3 anti-D in IgG preparations. *Vox Sang.* 62 251–254.

Gorski, J., Tosi, R., Strubin, M., Rabourdin-Combe, G. and Mach, B. (1985) Serological and immunochemical analysis of the products of a single HLA-DRα and DRβ chain gene expressed in a mouse cell line after DNA-mediated cotransformation reveals that the β chain carries unknown supertypic specificity. *J. exp. Med.*, 162, 105–117.

Gorski, J., Rollini, P. and Mach, B. (1987) Structural comparison of the genes of two HLA-DR supertypic groups: the loci encoding DRw52 and DRw53 are not truly allelic. *Immunogenetics*, 25, 397–402.

Gorst, D.W., Riches, R.A. and Renton, P.H. (1977) Formaldehyde induced anti-N: a possible cause of renal graft failure. *J. clin. Path.* 30, 956.

Gorst, D.W., Rawlinson, Violet I., Merry, A.H. and Stratton, F. (1980) Positive direct antiglobulin test in normal individuals. *Vox Sang.* 38, 99–105.

Gottlieb, A.M. (1991) History of the first blood transfusion but a fable agreed upon: the transfusion of blood to a Pope. *Transfusion Med. Rev.* 5, 228–235.

Gottschall, J.L., Johnston, V.L., Azod, L., Anderson, A.J. and Aster, R.H. (1984) Importance of white blood cells in platelet storage. *Vox Sang.* 47, 101–107.

Gottsche, B., Salama, A. and Mueller Eckhardt, C. (1990) Autoimmune hemolytic anemia associated with an IgA autoantiGerbich. *Vox Sang.* 58, 211–214.

Goudeman, M. and Salmon, C. (1980) *Immuno-hématologie et Immunogénétique*. Flammarion, Paris.

Goudsmit, R. and van Loghem, J.J. (1953) Studies on the occurrence of leucocyte antibodies. *Vox Sang. (O.S.)* 3, 58.

Gouge, J.J., Boyce, F., Peterson, P. and Marsh, S. (1977) A puzzling problem due to a harmless cold auto-antibody: unpublished observations.

Gould, S.A., Rosen, A.L., Sehgal, L.R., Sehgal,

Hansa L., Langdale, Lorrie A., Frause, L.M., Rice, C.L., Chamberlin, W.H. and Moss, G.S. (1986) Fluosol-DA as a red cell substitute in acute anemia. *New Engl. J. Med.* 314, 1653–1656.

Gould, S.A., Sehgal, L.R., Rosen, A.L., Sehgal, Hansa L. and Moss, G.S. (1990) The efficacy of polymerised pyridoxylated hemoglobin solution as an O_2 carrier. *Ann. Surg.* 291, 394–398.

Gourdin, M.F., Reyes, F., Lejonic, J.L., Mannoni, P., Bretton-Gorius, J. and Dreyfus, B. (1976) L'hétérogénéité de la distribution cellulaire des antigènes A érythrocytaires. Étude au microscope électronique. *Rev. franç. Transfus. Immunohémat.* 19, 55.

Gout, O. and 10 others (1990) Rapid development of myelopathy after HTLV-1 infection acquired by transfusion during cardiac transplantation. *New Engl. J. Med.* 322, 383–388.

Govindarajan, S., DeCock, K.M., Valinluck, B. and Ashcavi, Mary (1986) Serum hepatitis B virus DNA in acute hepatitis B. *Amer. J. clin. Path.* 86, 352–354.

Gower, D.B. and Davidson, W.M. (1963) The mechanism of immune haemolysis. I. The relationship of the rate of destruction of red cells to their age, following the administration to rabbits of an immune haemolysin. *Brit. J. Haemat.* 9, 132.

Grady, G.F. and Lee, V.A. (1975) Prevention of hepatitis from accidental exposure among medical workers. *New Engl. J. Med.* 293, 1067.

Graf, H., Watzinger, U., Ludvik, B., Wagner, A., Hocker, P. and Zweymuller, K.K. (1990) Recombinant human erythropoietin as adjuvant treatment for autologous blood donation. *Brit. med. J.* 300, 1627–1628.

Graham, H.A., Davies, D.M. jr, Tigner, J.A. and Brower, C.E. (1976) Evidence suggesting that trace amounts of C3d are bound to most human red cells (Abstract). *Transfusion*, 16, 530.

Graham, H.A., Hirsch, Heidi F. and Davies, D.M. (1977) Genetic and immunochemical relationships between soluble and cell-bound antigens of the Lewis system, in *Human Blood groups*, eds J.F. Mohn, R.W. Plunkett, R.K. Cunningham and R.M. Lambert, pp. 257–267. S. Karger, Basel.

Graham, H.A. and Williams, A.N. (1978) A genetic model for the inheritance of the P, P_1 and P^k antigens (Abstract). *Transfusion*, 18, 638.

Graham, H.A., Hawk, J.B., Chachowski, R. and Savitz, S.R. (1982) A new approach to prepare cells for the Coombs test (Abstract). *Transfusion*, 22, 408.

Graninger, W., Ramesis, H., Fischer, K.,

Poschmann, A., Bird, G.W.G., Wingham, J. and Neumann, E. (1977a) 'VA', a new type of erythrocyte polyagglutination characterized by depressed H receptors and associated with hemolytic anemia. I. Serological and hematological observations. *Vox Sang.* **32**, 195.

Graninger, W., Poschmann, A., Fischer, K., Schedl-Giovannoni, I., Hörandner, H. and Klaus-Hofer, K. (1977b) 'VA', a new type of erythrocyte polyagglutination characterized by depressed H receptors and associated with hemolytic anemia. II. Observations by immunofluorescence, electron microscopy, cell electrophoresis and biochemistry. *Vox Sang.* **32**, 201.

Grannum, P.A., Copel J.A., Plaxe, S.C., Scioscia, Angela L. and Hobbins, J.C. (1986) *In utero* exchange transfusion by direct intravascular injection in severe erythroblastosis fetalis. *New Engl. J. Med.* **314**, 1431–1434.

Grannum, P.A.T. and Copel, J.A. (1988) Prevention of Rh isoimmunization and treatment of the compromised fetus. *Semin. Perinatol.* **12**, 324–335.

Granström, Martha, Olinder-Nielsen, Ann M., Holmblad, P., Mark, A., Hanngren, K. (1991) Specific immunoglobulin for treatment of whooping cough. *Lancet*, **i**, 33, 1230–1233.

Grant, R.T. and Reeve, E.B. (1951) Observations on the general effects of injury in man, with special reference to wound shock. *Spec. Rep. Ser. med. Res. Coun. (Lond.)*, **277**.

Grant, D.B., Perinpanayagam, M.S., Shute, P.G. and Zeitlin, R.A. (1960) A case of malignant tertian (*Plasmodium falciparum*) malaria after blood-transfusion. *Lancet*, **ii**, 469.

Grant, C.J., Hamblin, T.J., Smith, D.S. and Wellstead, L. (1983) Plasmapheresis in Rh hemolytic disease: the danger of amniocentesis. *Int. J. Artificial Organs*, **6**, 83–86.

Graw, R.G. jr, Buckner, C.D., Whang-Peng, Jacqueline, Leventhal, Brigid G., Krüger, G., Berard, C. and Henderson, E.S. (1970) Complications of bone-marrow transplantation. Graft-versus-host disease resulting from chronic-myelogenous-leukaemia leucocyte transfusions. *Lancet*, **ii**, 338.

Gray, S.J. and Sterling, K. (1950) The tagging of red cells and plasma proteins with radioactive chromium. *J. clin. Invest.* **29**, 1604.

Gray, Margery P. (1964) A human serum factor agglutinating human red cells exposed to lactose. *Vox Sang.* **9**, 608.

Graziano, J.H., Piomelli, S., Seaman, Carol, Wang, T., Cohen, A.R., Kelleher, J.F. jr and Schwartz, E. (1982) A simple technique for preparation of young red cells for transfusion from ordinary blood units. *Blood*, **59**, 865–868.

Green, E.S., Hewitt, P.E. and England, J.M. (1988) Iron depletion in male donors bled at three monthly intervals is not accompanied by changes in haematological parameters. *Abstracts, 20th Congr. Int. Soc. Blood Transfus.* London, p. 124.

Green, C.A., Daniels, G.L., Khalid, G. and Tippett, P. (1990a) Monoclonal anti-S, in *Second International Workshop and Symposium on Monoclonal Antibodies against Human Red Blood Cells and Related Antigens*, eds M.A. Chester, U. Johnson, A. Lundblad, B. Löw, L. Messeter and B. Samuelson, p. 131. Lund, Sweden.

Green, E.D., Curtis, B.R., Issitt, P.D., Gutgsell, N.S., Roelcke, D., Farrar, R.P and Chaplin, H. (1990b) Inhibition of an anti-Pr_1d cold agglutinin by citrate present in commercial red cell preservative solutions. *Transfusion*, **30**, 267–270.

Greenberg, B.R. and Watson-Williams, E.J. (1975) Successful control of life-threatening thrombocytosis with a blood processor. *Transfusion*, **15**, 620.

Greenburg, A.G., Nayashi, R., Siefert, I., Reese, H.S. and Peskin, G.W. (1979) Intravascular persistence and oxygen delivery of pyridoxalated stroma-free hemoglobin during gradations of hypotension. *Surgery*, **86**, 13–16.

Greenbury, C.L., Moore, D.H. and Nunn, L.A.C. (1963) Reaction of 7S and 19S components of immune rabbit antisera with human group A and AB red cells. *Immunology*, **6**, 421.

Greenbury, C.L., Moore, D.H. and Nunn, L.A.C. (1965) The reaction with red cells of 7S rabbit antibody, its sub-units and their recombinants. *Immunology*, **8**, 420.

Greendyke, R.M. and Chorpenning, F.W. (1962) Normal survival of incompatible red cells in the presence of anti-Lu^a. *Transfusion*, **2**, 52.

Greenwalt, T.J. and Sasaki, T. (1957) The Lutheran blood groups: a second example of anti-Lu^b and three further examples of anti-Lu^a. *Blood*, **12**, 998.

Greenwalt T.J., Sasaki, T. and Gajewski, M. (1959) Further examples of haemolytic disease of the newborn due to anti-Duffy (anti-Fy^a). *Vox Sang.* **4**, 138.

Greenwalt, T.J., Gajewski, M. and McKenna, J.L. (1962) A new method for preparing buffy coat-poor blood. *Transfusion*, **2**, 221.

Greenwalt, T.J., Sasaki, T.T. and Steane, E.A. (1967) The Lutheran blood groups: A progress report with observations on the development of the antigens and characteristics of the antibodies. *Transfusion*, **7**, 189.

Greenwalt, T.J., Bryan, Donna J. and Dumaswala, V.J. (1984) Erythrocyte membrane vesiculation and changes in membrane composition during storage in citrate-phosphate-dextrose-adenine-1. *Vox Sang.* **47**, 261–270.

Greenwell, P., Johnson, P.H., Edwards-Moulds, J., Reed, R.M., Moores, P.P., Graham, H.A. and Watkins, W.M. (1986) Association of the human Lewis blood group Le(a−b−c−d−) phenotype with the failure of expression of α-3-L-fucosyltransferase. *Rev. franç. Transfus. Immunohémat.* **29**, 233–249.

Griffith, L.D., Billman, G.F., Daily, P.O. and Lane, T.A. (1989) Apparent coagulopathy caused by infusion of shed mediastinal blood and its prevention by washing of the infusate. *Ann. thorac. Surg.* **47**, 400–406.

Griffiths, P.D. (1984) Diagnostic techniques for cytomegalovirus infection. *Clinics in Haemat.* **13**, 631–644.

Griffiths, H., Brennan, V., Lea, J., Bunch, C. Lee, M. and Chapel, H. (1989) Crossover study of immunoglobulin replacement therapy in patients with low-grade B-cell tumors. *Blood*, **73**, 366–368.

Griggs, R.C. and Harris. J.W. (1961) Susceptibility to immune hemolysis as related to the age of human and dog red blood cells. *Blood*, **18**, 806.

Gronemeyer, P., Chaplin, H., Ghazarian, V., Tuscany, F. and Wilner, G.D. (1981) Hemolytic anemia complicating infectious mononucleosis due to the interaction of an IgG cold anti-i and an IgM cold rheumatoid factor. *Transfusion*, **21**, 715–718.

Groopman, J.E., Mitsuyasu, R.T., Deheo, M., Oette, Dagmar and Golde, D.W. (1987) Effect of recombinant human granulocyte-macrophage colony-stimulating factor on myelopoiesis in the acquired immunodeficiency syndrome. *New Engl. J. Med.* **317**, 593–598.

Groopman, J.E., Caiazzo, Teresa, Thomas, Mary Anne, Ferriani, Roberta, A., Saltzman, S., Moon, Martha, Seage, G., Horsburgh, C.R. and Mayer, K. (1988) Lack of evidence of prolonged human immunodeficiency virus infection before antibody seroconversion. *Blood*, **71**, 1752–1754.

Groopman, J.E., Molina, J.-E. and Scadden, D.T. (1989) Haematopoietic growth factors. Biology and clinical applications. *New Engl. J. Med.* **321**, 1449–1457.

Grossman, J.E., Dewling, R.H., Duy Nguyen, D. and Mosher, D.F. (1980) Response of plasma fibronectin to major body burns. *J. Trauma*, **20**, 967–970.

Grossman, Brenda J., Stewart, Nadina C. and Grindon, A.J. (1988) Increased risk of a positive test for antibody to hepatitis B core antigen (anti-HBc) in autologous blood donors. *Transfusion*, **28**, 283–285.

Grove-Rasmussen, M., Soutter, L. and Marceau, E. (1951) The use of group O donors as 'universal' donors. *Commun. Amer. Assoc. Blood Banks*, Minneapolis.

Grove-Rasmussen, M., Shaw, R.S. and Marceau, E. (1953) Hemolytic transfusion reaction in group-A patient receiving group-O blood containing immune anti-A antibodies in high titer. *Amer. J. clin. Path.* **23**, 828.

Grove-Rasmussen, M. (1964) Routine compatibility testing standards of the AABB as applied to compatibility tests. *Transfusion*, **4**, 200.

Grove-Rasmussen, M. and Huggins, C.E. (1973) Selected types of frozen blood for patients with multiple blood group antibodies. *Transfusion*, **13**, 124.

Grubb, R. and Morgan, W.T.J. (1949) The 'Lewis' blood group characters of erythrocytes and body fluids. *Brit. J. exp. Path.* **30**, 198.

Grubb, R. (1951) Observations on the human group system Lewis. *Acta path. microbiol. scand.* **28**, 61.

Grubb, R. (1956) Agglutination of erythrocytes coated with 'incomplete' anti-Rh by certain rheumatoid arthritic sera and some other sera despite dilution. The existence of human serum groups. *Acta path. microbiol. scand.* **39**, 105.

Grubb, R. and Swahn, B. (1958) Destruction of some agglutinins but not of others by two sulfhydryl compounds. *Acta path. microbiol. scand.* **43**, 305.

Gruber, U.F. (1969) *Blood Replacement*. Springer-Verlag, New York.

Grumbach, A. and Gasser, C. (1948) ABO-inkompatibilitäten und Morbus haemolyticus neonatorum. *Helv. paediat. Acta*, **3**, 447.

Grumet, F.C. (1984) In International Forum: Transfusion-transmitted CMV infections. *Vox Sang.* **46**, 387–414.

Grundbacher, F.J. (1964) Changes in the human A antigen of erythrocytes with the individual's age. *Nature (Lond.)*, **204**, 192.

Grundbacher, F.J. (1967) Quantity of hemolytic anti-A and Anti-B in individuals of a human population: correlations with isoagglutinins and effects of the individual's age and sex. *Z. Immun. Forsch.* **134**, 317.

Grundbacher, F.J. (1976) Genetics of anti-A and anti-B levels. *Transfusion*, **16**, 48.

Guerrero, I.C., Weniger, B.C. and Schultz, M.G. (1983) Transfusion malaria in the United States 1972–1981. *Ann. intern. Med.* **99**, 221–226.

Guest, A.R., Scott, M.L., Smythe, J. and Judson, P.A. (1992) Analysis of the struture and activity of A and A,B immunoglobulin A monoclonal antibodies. *Transfusion*, **32**, 239–245.

Guigner, F., Domy, M., Angue, M., Richaud, P. and Chatelain, P. (1988) Comparison between a solid-phase low-ionic-strength antiglobulin test and conventional low-ionic-strength antiglobulin test: assesment for the screening of antierythrocyte antibodies. *Vox Sang.* 55, 30–34.

Guilbert, Brigitte, Dighiero, G. and Avreamas, S. (1982) Naturally occurring antibodies against nine common antigens in human sera. I. Detection, isolation and characterization. *J. Immunol.* 128, 2779–2787.

Gullbring, B. and Ström, G. (1956) Changes in oxygen-carrying function of human hemoglobin during storage in cold acid-citrate-dextrose solution. *Acta med. scand.* 155, 413.

Gullbring, B., (1964) The use of plastic in blood transfusion equipment with special regard to toxicity problems. *Vox Sang.* 9, 513.

Gullbring, B., Eklund, L.H. and Svartz-Malmberg, G. (1964) Chemical and biological test-methods applied to plastic products used in transfusion equipment. *Vox Sang.* 9, 530.

Gulliksson, H., Shanwell, A., Wikman, A., Reppucci, A.J., Sallander, S. and Uden, A.M. (1991) Storage of platelets in a new plastic container. *Vox Sang.* 61, 165–170.

Gundolf, F. (1973) Anti-A_1Le^b in serum of a person of a blood group A_1h. *Vox Sang.* 25, 411.

Gunson, H.H. (1957) Neonatal anemia due to fetal hemorrhage into the maternal circulation. *Paediatrics*, 20, 3.

Gunson, H.H. and Donohue, W.L. (1957) Multiple examples of the blood genotype C^wD- / C^wD- in a Canadian family. *Vox Sang.* 2, 320.

Gunson, H.H., Stratton, F. and Cooper, D.G. (1970a) Primary immunization of Rh-negative volunteers. *Brit. med. J.* i, 593.

Gunson, H.H., Stratton, F. and Mullard, G.W. (1970b) An example of polyagglutinability due to the Tn antigen. *Brit. J. Haemat.* 18, 309.

Gunson, H.H., Stratton, F. and Phillips, P.K. (1971) The use of modified cells to induce an anti-Rh response. *Brit. J. Haemat.* 21, 683.

Gunson, H.H. and Latham, Valerie (1972) An agglutinin in human serum reacting with cells from Le(a−b−) non-secretor individuals. *Vox Sang.* 22, 344.

Gunson, H.H., Stratton, F. and Phillips, P.K. (1974) The anti-$Rh_0(D)$ responses of immunized volunteers following spaced antigenic stimuli. *Brit. J. Haemat.* 27, 171.

Gunson, H.H., Bowell, P.J. and Kirkwood, T.B.L. (1980) Collaborative study to recalibrate the international reference preparation of anti-D immunoglobulin. *J. clin. Path.* 33, 249–253.

Gunson, H.H., Merry, A.H., Makar, Y., Thomson, E.E. and Carter, A.C. (1983) Five day storage of platelet concentrates. II. *In vivo*-studies. *Clin. lab. Haemat.* 5, 287–294.

Gunson, H. (1990) Transfusion: news from the Council of Europe. *Vox Sang.* 58, 324–327.

Gupte, S.C. and Bhatia, H.M. (1980) Increased incidence of haemolytic disease of the newborn caused by ABO-incompatibility when tetanus toxoid is given during pregnancy. *Vox Sang.* 38, 22–28.

Gurland, H.J., Samtleben, W. and Schmidt, B. (1981) Plasmaperfusion, in *Plasma Exchange Therapy*, eds H. Borger and P. Reuther, pp. 26–29. Georg Thieme Verlag, New York and Stuttgart.

Gürtler, L.G., Wernicke, D., Eberle, J., Zoulec, G., Deinhardt, F. and Schramm, W. (1984) Increase in prevalence of anti-HTLV-III in haemophiliacs. *Lancet*, ii, 1275–1276.

Gustafson, J.E. (1951) Electrocardiographic changes in exchange transfusion. *J. Pediat.* 39, 593.

Gutgsell, N.S., Issitt, P.D., Tomasulo, P.A. and Hervis, L. (1988) Use of the direct enzyme-linked antiglobulin test (ELAT) in patients with unexplained anemia. *Transfusion*, 28, Suppl. 36S.

Habash, Janet, Devenish, A., Macdonald, Susan, Garner, S. and Contreras, Marcela (1991) A further example of anti-Di^b not causing haemolytic disease of the newborn. *Vox Sang.* 61, 77.

Haber, Gladys and Rosenfield, R.E. (1957) Ficin treated red cells for hemagglutination studies, In *P.H. Andresen—Papers in Dedication of his 60th Birthday*, p. 45. Munksgaard, Copenhagen.

Habibi, B., Gerbal, A. and Salmon, C. (1973a) A papain-bromelin-polybrene four-channel Autoanalyzer system for blood group antibody screening. Analysis of 22,912 sera. *Vox Sang.* 25 ,289.

Habibi, B., Kleinknecht, D., Vachon, F., Cavalier, J. and Salmon, C. (1973b) Le choc transfusionnel par contamination bactérienne du sang conservé. Analyse de 25 observations. *Rev. franç. Transfus.* 16, 41.

Habibi, B., Homberg, J.-C., Schaison, G. and Salmon, G. (1974) Autoimmune hemolytic anemia in children. A review of 80 cases. *Amer. J. Med.* 56, 61.

Habibi, B., Avril, J., Fouillade, M.T., Lopez, M., Vaucelle, R. and Salmon, C. (1976) Jk(a−b−) phenotype in a French family. Quantitative evidence for the inheritance of a silent allele (Jk). *Haematologia*, 10, 403–410.

Habibi, B., Tipppett, P., Lebesnerais, M. and Salmon, C. (1979) Protease inactivation of the red cell antigen Xg^a. *Vox Sang.* 36, 367–368.

Habibi, B., Muller, A., Lelong, F., Homberg, J.C., Foucher, M., Duhamel, G. and Salmon, C. (1980) Auto-immunisation érythrocytaire dans la population 'normale'. 63 observations. *Nouv. Presse méd.* 9, 3253–3257.

Habibi, B., Baumelou, A. and Serdaru, M. (1981)

Acute intravascular haemolysis and renal failure due to Teniposide related antibody. *Lancet*, i, 1423–1424.

Habibi, B. (1983) Disappearance of alpha-methyldopa induced red cell autoantibodies despite continuation of the drug. *Brit. J. Haemat.* **54**, 493–495.

Habibi, B. and Lecolier, B. (1983) Inopportunité de la prophylaxie elaborée de l'allo-immunisation transfusionelle contre les globules rouges dans l'insuffisance rénale chronique. *Rev. franç. Transfus. Immunohémat.* **26**, 267–277.

Habibi, B., Basty, Regine, Chodez, Sophie and Prunat, A. (1985) Thiopental related immune hemolytic anemia and renal failure. Specific involvement of red cell antigen I. *New Engl. J. Med. 12*, 353–355.

Habibi, B. and Garretta, M. (1990) Screening and plasma fractionation: the case against. *Lancet*, i, 855–856.

Hach-Wunderle, V., Texidor, D., Zumpe, P., Kuhnl, P. and Scharrer, I. (1989) Anti-A in Factor VIII concentrate: a cause of severe hemolysis in a patient with acquired Factor VIII:C antibodies. *Infusiontherapie*, **16**, 100–101.

Hack, E.C., Voerman, J., Eiselo, B., Keinecke, H.O., Nuijens, J.H., Eerenberg, Anke, J.M., Strack van Schijndel, R.J.M., Delvos, U.D. and Thijs, L.G. (1992) Administration of high doses of C1 inhibitor to five patients with septic shock and its effects on activation of complement and contact systems. *Lancet*, submitted.

Hackmann, T., Gascoyne, R.D., Naiman, S.C., Growe, G.H., Burchill, Linda D., Jamieson, E., Sheps, S.B., Schechter, M.T. and Townsend, G.E. (1989) A trial of desmopressin (1-desamino-8-d-arginine vasopressin) to reduce blood loss in uncomplicated cardiac surgery. *New Engl. J. Med.* **321**, 1437–1443.

Haddad, Sheila A. (1974) A serological study of an O_h woman and her newborn infant. *Canad. J. Med. Technol.* **36**, 373.

Hadley, T.J., David, P.H., McGinniss, M.H. and Miller, L.H. (1984) Identification of an erythrocyte component carrying the Duffy blood group Fy^a antigen. *Science*, **223**, 597–599.

Hadley, T.J., Klotz, F.W. and Miller, L.H. (1986) Invasion of erythrocytes by malaria parasites: a cellular and molecular overview. *Ann. Rev. Microbiol.* **40**, 451–477.

Hadley, A.G., Kumpel, B.M. and Merry. A.H. (1988) The chemiluminescent response of human monocytes to red cells sensitized with monoclonal anti-Rh(D) antibodies. *Clin. lab. Haemat.* **10**, 377–384.

Hadley, A.G. and Kumpel, B.M. (1989) Synergistic effect of blending IgG1 and IgG3 mono-clonal anti-D in promoting the metabolic response of monocytes to sensitised red cells. *Immunology*, **67**, 550–552.

Hadley, A.G., Kumpel, B.M., Leader, K., Merry, A.H., Brojer, E. and Zupanska, B. (1989) An in-vitro assessment of the functional activity of monoclonal anti-D. *Clin. lab. Haemat.* **11**, 47–54.

Hadley, A.C., Kumpel, B.M., Leader, K.A., Poole, G.D. and Fraser, I.D. (1991) Correlation of serological, quantitative and cell-mediated functional assays of maternal antibodies with the severity of haemolytic disease of the newborn. *Brit. J. Haemat.* **77**, 221–228.

Hagen, J., Bjerrum, O.J., Gogstad, G., Korsmo, R. and Solum, N.O. (1982) Involvement of divalent cations in the complex between the platelet glycoproteins IIb and IIIa. *Biochem. biophys. Acta*, **701**, 1–6.

Hahn, P.F., Miller, L.L., Rosbscheit-Robbins, F.S., Bale W.F. and Whipple, G.H. (1944) Peritoneal absorption. Red cells labeled by radio-iron hemoglobin move promptly from the peritoneal cavity into the circulation. *J. exp. Med.* **80**, 77.

Hakomori, S., Watanabe, K. and Laine, R.A. (1977) Glycosphingolipids with blood group A, H and I activity: their status in group A_1 and A_2 erythrocytes and their changes associated with ontogeny and oncogeny, in *Human Blood Groups*, eds J.F. Mohn, R.W. Plunkett, R.K. Cunningham and R.M. Lambert, pp. 150–163. S. Karger, Basel.

Hakomori, S.-I. (1981) Blood group ABH and Ii antigens of human erythrocytes: chemistry, polymorphism, and their developmental change. *Semin. Hemat.* **18**, 39–62.

Hakomori, S. (1984a) Blood group glycolipid antigens and their modifications as human cancer antigens. *Amer. J. clin. Path.* **82**, 635–648.

Hakomori, S.I. (1984b) Monoclonal antibodies directed to cell-surface carbohydrates, in *Monoclonal Antibodies and Functional Cell Lines*, eds R.H. Kennett, K.B. Bechtol and T.J. McKearn, pp. 67 100. Plenum Press, New York and London.

Halbrecht, I. (1951) Icterus precox: further studies on its frequency, etiology, prognosis and the blood chemistry of the cord blood. *J. Pediat.* **39**, 185.

Halima, D., Garratty, G. and Bueno, R.A. (1982a) An apparent anti-Jk^a reacting only in the presence of methylesters of hydroxy-benzoic acid (Abstract). *Transfusion*, **22**, 521–524.

Halima, D., Postoway, N., Brunt, D. and Garratty, G. (1982b) Haemolytic transfusion reactions (HTR) due to a probable anti-C, not detectable by multiple technics (Abstract). *Transfusion*, **22**, 405.

Halkier-Sørensen, L., Kragballe, K., Nedergaard, S.T., Jørgensen, J. and Hansen, K. (1990) Lack of transmission of *Borrelia burgdorferi* by blood transfusion. *Lancet*, **i**, 550.

Hall, A.R. and Boas Hall, M. (1967) *The Correspondence of Henry Oldenburg*, Vol. IV, p. 381. The University of Winsconsin Press.

Hall, A.J., Alveyn C.G., Winter, P.D. and Wright R. (1988) Mortality of hepatitis B-positive blood donors in England and Wales, in *Viral Hepatitis and Liver Disease*, ed A.J. Zuckerman, pp. 192–194. Alan R. Liss, New York.

Halmagyi, D.F.J., Starzecki, B., McRae, J. and Horner, G.J. (1963) The lung as the main target organ in the acute phase of transfusion reaction in sheep. *J. surg. Res.* **3**, 418.

Halpern, B.N., Dreyfus, B. and Bourdon, Gabrielle (1950) Influence favorable sur la conservation du sang des dérivés de la phénothiazine. *Presse méd.* **58**, 1151.

Halverson, G.R., Mabile, R., Santiago, I., Spruell, P., Moulds, M.K., Thurrell, T., Strupp, A.M. and Wolf, C.F.W. (1989) The first reported case of anti-Dombrock[b] causing an acute hemolytic transfusion reaction. *Transfusion*, **29**, Suppl. 48S.

Hamblin, T.J. (1983) Update on plasmapheresis. *Apheresis Bull.* **1**, 10–17.

Hamblin, T.J., Naorose Abidi, S.M., Nee, P.A., Copplestone, A., Mufti, G.J. and Oscier, D.G. (1985) Successful treatment of post-transfusion purpura with high dose immunoglobulins after lack of response to plasma exchange. *Vox Sang.* **49**, 164–167.

Hamblin, T.J. (1991) Interleukin-2 and lymphokine activated killer cells. *Transfus. Sci.* **12**, p 35–42.

Hamilton, H.E., Sheets, R.F. and De Gowin, E.L. (1950) Studies with inagglutinable erythrocyte counts. II. Analysis of mechanism of Cooley's anemia. *J. clin. Invest.* **29**, 714.

Hamilton, H.E., De Gowin, E.L., Sheets, R.F., Janney, C.D. and Ellis, J.A. (1954) Studies with inagglutinable erythrocyte counts. VI. Accelerated destruction of normal adult erythrocytes in pernicious anemia: contribution of hemolysis to the oligocythemia. *J. clin. Invest.* **33**, 191.

Hamilton, H.E., Sheets, R.F. and De Gowin, E.L. (1958) Studies with inagglutinable erythrocyte counts. VII. Further investigation of the hemolytic mechanism in untreated pernicious anemia and the demonstration of a hemolytic property in the plasma. *J. Lab. clin. Med.* **51**, 942.

Hammar, L., Mansson, S., Rohr, T., Chester, M.A., Ginsburg, V., Lundblad, A. and Zopf, D. (1981) Lewis phenotype of erythrocytes and Le[b]-active glycolipid in serum of pregnant women. *Vox Sang.* **40**, 27–33.

Hammarström, S. and Kabat, E.A. (1969) Purification and characterization of a blood-group A reactive hemagglutinin from the snail *Helix pomatia* and a study of its combining site. *Biochemistry*, **8**, 2696.

Hammerschmidt, D.E., Weaver, L. Jean, Hudson, L.H., Craddock, P.R. and Jacob, H.S. (1980) Association of complement activation with elevated plasma-C5a with adult respiratory distress syndrome. *Lancet*, **i**, 947–948.

Hammerström, L. and Smith, C.I.E. (1986) Placental transfer of intravenous immunoglobulin (Letter). *Lancet*, **i**, 681.

Hammond, D.J., Cover, B. and Gutteridge, W.E. (1984) A novel series of chemical structures active in *vitro* against the trypomastigote forms of *Trypanosoma cruzi*. *Transact. roy. Soc. Trop. Med. Hyg.* **78**, 91–95.

Hammond, W.P., Price, T.H., Souza, L.M. and Dale, D.C. (1989) Treatment of cyclic neutropenia with granulocyte colony-stimulating factor. *New Engl. J. Med.* **320**, 1306–1311.

Han, J.H. and 9 others (1991) Characterization of the terminal regions of hepatitis C viral RNA: identification of conserved sequences in the 5′ untranslated region and poly(A) tails at the 3′ end. *Proc. nat. Acad. Sci. USA*, **88**, 1711–1715.

Hanfland, P. (1978) Isolation and purification of Lewis blood group active glycosphingolipids from the plasma of human O Le[b] individuals. *Eur. J. Biochem.* **87**, 161–170.

Hanfland, P. and Graham, H.A. (1981) Immunochemistry of the Lewis blood-group system: partial characterization of Le[a]-, Le[b]- and H-type 1 (Le[dH]) blood-group active glycosphingolipids from human plasma. *Arch. Bio-chem. Biophys.* **210**, 383–395.

Hanfland, P., Kordowicz, Maria, Peter-Katalinic, P., Pfannschmidt, G., Crawford, R.J., Graham, H.A. and Egge, H. (1986) Immunochemistry of the Lewis blood group system: isolation and structures of Lewis-c active and related glycosphingolipids from the plasma of blood group O Le(a–b–) non-secretors. *Arch. Bio-chem. Biophys.* **246**, 655–672.

Hanks, G.E., Cassell, Mona, Ray, R.N. and Chaplin, H. jr (1960) Further modification of the benzidine method for measurement of hemoglobin in plasma. *J. Lab. clin. Med.* **56**, 486.

Hanson, D.G., Vaz, N.M., Maia, L.C.S. and Lynch, J.M. (1979) Inhibition of specific immune response by feeding protein antigens. III. Evidence against maintenance of tolerance to ovalbumin by orally induced antibodies. *J. Immunol.* **123**, 2337–2343.

Hanson, M.R. and Polesky, H.F. (1985) Hepatitis B surveillance in employees of a community blood center. *Transfusion*, **25**, 18–20.

Hanto, D.W., Gajl-Peczalska, K.J., Frizzera, G., Arthur, D.C., Balfour, H.H. jr, McClain, K., Simmons, R.L. and Najarian, J.S. (1983) Epstein-Barr virus (EBV)-induced polyclonal and monoclonal B-cell lymphoproliferative diseases occurring after renal transplantation. *Ann. surg.* **198**, 356–369.

Haradin, A.R., Weed, R.I. and Reed, C.F. (1969) Changes in physical properties of stored erythrocytes: relationship to survival *in vivo*. *Transfusion*, **9**, 229.

Harboe, M., Muller-Eberhard, H.J., Fudenberg, H., Polley, Margaret J. and Mollison, P.L. (1963) Identification of the components of complement participating in the antiglobulin reaction. *Immunology*, **6**, 412.

Harboe, M. (1964) Interactions between ^{131}I trace-labelled cold agglutinin, complement and red cells. *Brit. J. Haemat.* **10**, 339.

Hardaway, R.M. III (1974) Vasoconstrictors vs. vasodilators, in *Treatment of Shock: Principles and Practice*, eds W. Schumer and L.W. Nyhus. Lea & Febiger, Philadelphia.

Hardman, J.T. and Beck, M.L. (1981) Hemagglutination in capillaries: correlation with blood group specificity and IgG subclass. *Transfusion*, **21**, 343–346.

Hardwick, R. and Cole, Rosemary (1986) Plastics that kill plants. *The Garden*, **111**, 264–267.

Hardy, Joan and Napier, J.A.F. (1981) Red cell antibodies detected in antenatal tests on Rhesus positive women in south and mid Wales 1948–1978. *Brit. J. Obstet. Gynaec.* **88**, 91–100.

Harke, H., Thoenies, R., Margraf, I. and Momsen, W. (1976) Der Einfluss verschiedener Plasmaersatzmittel auf Gerinnungssystem und Thrombocytenfunktion während und nach operativen Eingriffen. Vorläufige Ergebnisse einer klinischen Studie. *Anaesthetist*, **25**, 366–373.

Harke, H. and Rahman, S. (1980) Hemostatic disorders in massive transfusion. *Bibl. Haemat.* **16**, 179–188.

Harker, L.A. and Finch, C.A. (1969) Thrombokinetics in man. *J. clin. Invest.* **48**, 963.

Harker, L.A. and Slichter, S.J. (1972) The bleeding time as a screening test for evaluating platelet function. *New Engl. J. Med.* **287**, 155.

Harker, L.A. (1977) The kinetics of platelet production and destruction in man. *Clin. Haemat.* **6**, 671.

Harpaz, N., Flowers, H.N. and Sharon, N. (1975) Studies on B-antigenic sites of human erythrocytes by use of coffee bean α-galactosidase. *Arch. Biochem. Biophys.* **170**, 676.

Harper, P., Bias, W.B., Hutchinson, Judith R. and McKusick, V.A. (1971) ABH secretor status of the fetus: a genetic marker identifiable by amniocentesis. *J. med. Genetics*, **8**, 438.

Harrigan, Celestine, Lucas, C.E., Ledgerwood, Anna M., Walz, D.A. and Mannen, E.F. (1985) Serial changes in primary hemostasis after massive transfusion. *Surgery*, **98**, 836–844.

Harrington, W.J., Minnich, Virginia, Hollingsworth, J.W. and Moore, C.V. (1951) Demonstration of a thrombocytopenic factor in the blood of patients with thrombocytopenic purpura. *J. Lab. clin. Med.* **38**, 1.

Harrington, W.J. (1954) The clinical significance of antibodies for platelets. *Commun. 5th Congr. Int. Soc. Haemat.*, Paris.

Harris, I.M., McAlister, Joan M. and Prankerd, T.A.J. (1957) The relationship of abnormal red cells to the normal spleen. *Clin. Sci.* **16**, 223.

Harris, Jean P., Tegoli, J., Swanson, Jane, Fisher, Natalie, Gavin, June and Noades, Jean (1967) A nebulous antibody responsible for cross-matching difficulties. *Vox Sang.* **12**, 140.

Harris, R. and Zervas, J.D. (1969) Reticulocyte HL-A antigens. *Nature (Lond.)*, **221**, 1062.

Harris, P.A., Roman, G.K., Moulds, J.J., Bird, G.W.G. and Shah. N.G. (1982) An inherited rbc characteristic, NOR, resulting in erythrocyte polyagglutination. *Vox Sang.* **42**, 134–140.

Harris, Teresa, Steiert, Sue, Marsh, W.L. and Berman, L.B. (1986) A Wj-negative patient with anti-Wj (Letter). *Transfusion*, **26**, 117.

Harris, T. (1990) Two cases of autoantibodies that demonstrate mimicking specificity in the Duffy blood group system. *Immunohematology* **6**, 87.

Harrison, J. (1970) The 'naturally occurring' anti-E. *Vox Sang.* **19**, 123.

Harrison, R.A. and Lachmann, P.J. (1980) The physiological breakdown of the third component of human complement. *Mol. Immunol.* **17**, 9–20.

Harrison T.J., Bal, V., Wheeler, E.G., Meacock, T.J., Harrison, J.F. and Zuckerman, A.J. (1985) Hepatitis B virus DNA and e antigen in serum from blood donors in the United Kingdom positive for hepatitis B surface antigen. *Brit. med. J.* **290**, 663–664.

Harrison, C.R., Hayes T.C., Trow, L.L. and Benedetto, A.R. (1986) Intravascular hemolytic transfusion reaction without detectable antibodies: a case report and review of literature. *Vox Sang.* **51**, 96–101.

Harrison, T.J. and Zuckerman, A.J. (1992) Variants of hepatitis B virus. *Vox Sang.* in press.

Harte, P.G., Cooke, A. and Playfair, J.H.L. (1983) Specific monoclonal IgM; a novel and potent adjuvant in murine malaria vaccination. *Nature (Lond.)*, **302**, 256–258.

Hartmann, Grethe (1941) *Group Antigens in Human Organs*. Munksgaard, Copenhagen.

Hartmann, O. and Schøne, R. (1942) Syfilis overført ved blodtransfusion. *Nord. T. milit.-Med.* **45**, 1.

Hartmann, O. and Brendemoen, O.J. (1953) Incidence of Rh antibody formation in first pregnancies. *Acta paediat. (Uppsala)*, **42**, 20.

Hartmann, O. (1957) Blood group A₂B as a 'dangerous' recipient of blood, In *P.H. Andresen—Papers in Dedication of his 60th Birthday*, p. 76. Munksgaard, Copenhagen.

Harvey, W. (1628) *De Motu Cordis*, Frankfurt. See Chap. XII in Translation by K.J. Franklin (1957), Blackwell Scientific Publications, Oxford.

Hasegawa, T., Bergh, O.J., Terasaki, P.I. and Graw, R.G. (1975) Occurrence of granulocyte cytotoxins and agglutinins. *Transfusion*, **15**, 226.

Hasse, O. (1874) *Die Lammblut-transfusion beim Menschen*. St Petersburg and Leipzig.

Hässig, A. and Lundsgaard-Hansen, P. (1978) The procurement of blood plasma for the production of components and derivatives within the frame of an integrated national blood program. *Vox Sang.* **34**, 257–260.

Hässig, A. (1990) Fifty years of Swiss Red Cross Blood Transfusion Service, in *Transfusion in Europe*, eds D. Castelli, B. Genetet, B. Habibi and U. Nydegger. Arnette, Paris.

Hathaway, W.E., Fulginiti, V.A., Pierce, C.W., Githens, J.H., Pearlman, D.S., Muschenheim, F. and Kempe, C.H. (1967) Graft vs. host reaction following a single blood transfusion. *J. Amer. Med. Assoc.* **201**, 1015.

Haugen, R.K. (1979) Hepatitis after the transfusion of frozen red cells and washed red cells. *New Engl. J. Med.* **301**, 393–395.

Haughton, G. and Nash, D.R. (1969) Specific immunosuppression by minute doses of passive antibody. *Transplant. Proc.* **1**, 616.

Hawkey, C.J., Newsom-Davis, J. and Vincent, Angela (1981) Plasma exchange and immunosuppressive drug treatment in myasthenia gravis: no evidence for synergy. *J. Neurol. Neurosurg. Psychiat.* **44**, 469–475.

Hawkins, P., Anderson, S.E., McKenzie, J.L., McLoughlin, K., Beard, M.E.J. and Hart, D.N.J. (1985) Localization of MN blood group antigens in kidney. *Transplant Proc.* **17**, 1697–1700.

Haworth, S.J. and Pusey, C.D. (1983) Plasma exchange in the management of type II mixed cryoglobulinaemia. A case report and review of the literature. *Apheresis Bull.* **1**, 40–45.

Hay, F.C., Hull, M.G.R. and Torrigiani, G. (1971) The transfer of human IgG subclasses from mother to foetus. *Clin. exp. Immunol.* **9**, 355–358.

Hay, C.R.M., Laurian, Y., Verroust, F., Preston, F.E. and Kernoff, P.B.A. (1990) Induction of immune tolerance in patients with hemophilia A and inhibitors treated with porcine VIIIC by home therapy. *Blood*, **76**, 882–886.

Hayashida, Y. and Watanabe, A. (1968) A case of a blood group p Taiwanese woman delivered of an infant with hemolytic disease of the newborn. *Jap. J. legal Med.* **22**, 10.

Haynes, L.L., Tullis, J.L., Pyle, H.M., Sproul, Mary T., Wallach, S. and Turville, W.C. (1960) Clinical use of glycerolized frozen blood. *J. Amer. med. Assoc.* **173**, 1657.

Haynes, Carolyn R., Dorner, I., Leonard, G.L., Arrowsmith, W.R. and Chaplin. H. jr (1970) Persistent polyagglutinability *in vivo* unrelated to T-antigen activation. *Transfusion*, **10**, 43.

Haynes, Carolyn R. and Chaplin, H. jr (1971) An enhancing effect of albumin on the determination of cold hemagglutinins. *Vox Sang.* **20**, 46.

Heal, J.M., Blumberg, N. and Masel, D. (1987a) An evaluation of crossmatching, HLA, and ABO matching for platelet transfusions of refractory patients. *Blood*, **70**, 23.

Heal, Joanna M., Jones, M.E., Forey, Janice, Chaudhry, N.A. and Stricof, Rachel L. (1987b) Fatal *Salmonella* septicemia after platelet transfusion. *Transfusion*, **27**, 2–5.

Heaton, D.C. and Mcloughlin, K. (1982) Jk(a−b−) red cells resist urea lysis. *Transfusion*, **22**, 70–71.

Heaton, W.A., Davis, H.H., Welch, M.J., Mathias, Carla, J., Joist, J.H., Sherman, L.A. and Siegel, B.A. (1979) Indium-III: a new radionuclide label for studying human platelet kinetics. *Brit. J. Haemat.* **42**, 613–622.

Heaton, A., Miripol, J., Aster, R., Hartman, P., Dehart, D., Rzad, L., Grapka, B., Davisson, W. and Buchholz, D.H. (1984) Use of Adsol® preservation solution for prolonged storage of low viscosity AS-1 red blood cells. *Brit. J. Haemat.* **57**, 467–478.

Heaton, A., Keegan, Thais and Holme, S. (1989a) *In vivo* regeneration of red cell 2, 3-diphosphoglycerate following transfusion of DPG-depleted AS-1, AS-3 and CPDA-1 red cells. *Transfusion*, **71**, 131–136.

Heaton, W.A.L., Keegan, T., Holme, S. and Momoda, C. (1989b) Evaluation of ⁹⁹m Technetium/⁵¹Chromium post-transfusion recovery of red cells stored in saline, adenine, glucose, manitol for 42 days. *Vox Sang.* **57**, 37–42.

Heaton, W.A.L., Hanbury, C.M., Keegan, T.E., Pleban, P. and Holme, S. (1989c) Studies with nonradioisotopic sodium chromate I. Development of a technique for measuring red cell volume. *Transfusion*, **29**, 696–702.

Heaton, W.A.L., Keegan, T., Hanbury, C.M.,

Holme, S. and Pleban, P. (1989d) Studies with nonradioisotopic sodium chromate II. Single and double-label $^{52}Cr/^{51}Cr$ posttransfusion recovery estimations. *Transfusion*, 29, 703–707.

Hecker, J.F. (1992) Potential for extending survival of peripheral intravenous infusions. *Brit. med. J.* 304, 619–624.

Heddle, N.M., Blajchman, M.A., Bodner, N. and Sacher, R. (1977) Absence of hemolysis of T-activated red cells following infusion of blood products. *Commun. Amer. Assoc. Blood Banks*, Atlanta.

Heddle, N.M., Kelton, J.G., Turchyn, K.L. and Ali, M.A.M. (1988) Hypergammaglobulinemia can be associated with a positive direct antiglobulin test, a nonreactive eluate, and no evidence of hemolysis. *Transfusion*, 28, 29–33.

Hedin, H., Kraft, D., Richter, W., Scheiner, O. and Devey, M. (1979) Dextran reactive antibodies in patients with anaphylactoid reactions to dextran. *Immunology*, 156, 289–290.

Hedin, H. and Richter, W. (1982) Pathomechanisms of dextran-induced anaphylactoid/anaphylactic reactions in man. *Int. Arch. Allergy appl. Immunol.* 68, 122–126.

Hedley, C.P., Doughty, R.W. and Collins, A.K. (1986) Microplate blood grouping with computer-controlled reading and data interpretation. *Med. Lab. Sciences*, 43, 199–200.

Hedner, U. and Kisiel, W. (1983) Use of human Factor VIIa in the treatment of two haemophilia A patients with high titre inhibitors. *J. clin. Invest.* 71, 1836–1841.

Hedner, U., Glazer, S. and Pingel, K. (1988) Successful use of recombinant Factor VIIa in a patient with severe haemophilia A during synovectomy. *Lancet*, ii, 1193.

Hédon (1902) *Archives de Médecine expérimentale et d'Anatomie pathalogique*, 4, 297.

Heidelberger, M. and Mayer, M.M. (1948) Quantitative studies on complement. *Advanc. Enzymol.* 8, 71.

Heimpel, H., Erdmann, H., Hoffman, G. and Keiderling, W. (1964) Tierexperimentelle Untersu chungen zur Markierung von Erythrozyten mit radioaktivem Diisopropylfluorphosphat (DFP^{32}). *Nucl. Med. (Amst.)*, 4, 32.

Heiner, D.C. and Kevy, S.V. (1956) Visceral larva migrans: report of the syndrome in three siblings. *New Engl. J. Med.* 254, 629.

Heistö, H., Myhre, K., Vogt, E. and Heier, A.-M. (1960) Haemolytic transfusion reaction due to incompatibility without demonstrable antibodies. *Vox Sang.* 5, 538.

Heistö, H., Myhre, Käre, Börresen, W., Vogt, Else and Heier, Anna-Margrethe (1962) Another case of haemolytic transfusion reaction due to incompatibility without demonstrable antibodies. *Vox Sang.* 7, 470.

Heistö, H., Harboe, M. and Godal, H.C. (1965) Warm haemolysins active against trypsinized red cells: occurrence, inheritance, and clinical significance. *Proc. 10th Congr. Int. Soc. Blood Transfus.*, Stockholm.

Heistö, H., van der Hart, Mia, Madsen, Grethe, Moes, Mieke, Noades, Jean, Pickles, M.M., Race, R.R., Sanger, Ruth and Swanson, Jane (1967) Three examples of a new red cell antibody, anti-Co^a. *Vox Sang.* 12, 18.

Heistø, H. (1979) Pretransfusion blood group serology: limited value of the antiglobulin phase of the crossmatch when a careful screening test for unexpected antibodies is performed. *Transfusion*, 19, 761–763.

Helderweirt, G. (1963) Le passage de globules foetaux et maternels à travers le placenta *Ann. Soc. belge Méd. trop.* 43, 575.

Hellings, J.A. (1981) On the structure and function of Factor VIII — von Willebrand factor. *Thesis*, Amsterdam, Rodopi.

Helmerhorst, F.M., van Oss, C.J., Bruynes, E.C.E., Engelfriet, C.P. and von dem Borne, A.E.G.Kr. (1982) Elution of granulocyte and platelet antibodies. *Vox Sang.* 43, 196–204.

Helmerhorst, F.M., Smeenk, R.J.T., Hack, C.E., Engelfriet, C.P. and von dem Borne, A.E.G. KR. (1983) Interference of IgG, IgG aggregates and immune complexes in tests for platelet autoantibodies. *Brit. J. Haemat.* 55, 533.

Hendry, Jessie L. and Sickles, Gretchen R. (1951) Ann. Rep. of Division of Labs. and Res., N.Y. State Dept of Health.

Hendry, P.I.A. and Simmons, R.T. (1955) An example of polyagglutinable erythrocytes, and reference to panagglutination, polyagglutination and autoagglutination as possible sources of error in blood grouping. *Med. J. Aust.* i, 720.

Henle, W. and Henle, Gertrude (1985) Epstein-Barr virus and blood transfusion, in *Infection, Immunity and Blood Transfusion*, eds R.Y. Dodd and L.F. Barker, pp. 201–209. Alan R. Liss, New York.

Henningsen, K. (1949a) A case of polyagglutinable human red cells. *Acta path. microbiol. scand.* 26, 339.

Henningsen, K. (1949b) Investigations on the blood factor P. *Acta path. microbiol. scand.* 26, 639.

Henningsen, K. (1952) *Om Blodtypesystemet P.* (Thesis for the Degree of M.D.) Dansk Videnskabs Forlag A/S, Copenhagen. (Cited by Race and Sanger, 1954.)

Henon, P.R., Butturini, Anna and Gale, R.P. (1991) Blood-derived haematopoietic cell transplants: blood to blood? *Lancet*, i, 337, 961–963.

Henry, Claudia and Jerne, N.K. (1968) Competition of 19*S* and 7*S* antigen receptors in the regulation of the primary immune response. *J. exp. Med.* **128**, 133.

Henry, J.B., Mintz, P. and Webb, M. (1977) Optimal blood ordering for elective surgery. *J. Amer. med. Assoc.* **237**, 451.

Henry, S.M., Dent, Alison, M. and Harding, Yvonne (1990) Detection of an Le^b epitope peculiar to Polynesians, in *Second International Workshop on Monoclonal Antibodies against Human Red Cells and Related Antigens*, eds M.A. Chester, U. Johnson, A. Lundblad, B. Low, L. Messeter and B. Samuelsson, p. 75. Lund, Sweden.

Henson, P.M., Larsen, C.L., Webster, R.O., Mitchell, B.C., Goins, A.J. and Henson, J.E. (1982) Pulmonary microvascular alterations and injury induced by complement fragments: synergistic effect of complement activation, neutrophil sequestration and prostaglandins. *Ann. N.Y. Acad. Sci.* **384**, 300.

Heptonstall, J. (1991) Outbreaks of hepatitis B virus infection associated with infected surgical staff. *CDR*, **1**, 81–85,

Herman, J.H., Jumbeli, M.I., Ancona, R.J. and Kickler, T.S. (1986) *In utero* cerebral hemorrhage in alloimmune thrombocytopenia. *Amer. J. Fed. Hemat. Oncol.* **8**, 312–317.

Herman, J.H., Shirey, R.S., Smith, B., Kickler, T.S. and Ness, P.M. (1987) The activation in congenital hypoplastic anaemia. *Transfusion*, **27**, 253–256.

Herron, R., Hyde, R.D. and Hillier, S.J. (1979) The second example of an anti-Vel autoantibody. *Vox Sang.* **36**, 179–181.

Herron, R., Clark, M., Tate, D, Kruger, A. and Smith, D.S. (1986) Immune haemolysis in a renal transplant recipient due to antibodies with anti-c specificity. *Vox Sang.* **51**, 226–227.

Herron, R., Clark, M. and Smith, D.S. (1987) An autoantibody with activity dependent on red cell age in the serum of a patient with autoimmune haemolytic anaemia and a negative direct antiglobulin test. *Vox Sang.* **52**, 71–74.

Hershko, C., Cook, J.D. and Finch, C.A. (1972) Storage iron kinetics. II. The uptake of hemoglobin iron by hepatic parenchymal cells. *J. Lab. clin. Med.* **80**, 624.

Hershko, C., Gale, R.P., Ho, W. and Fitchen, J. (1980) ABH antigens and bone marrow transplantation. *Brit. J. Haemat.* **44**, 65–73.

Hershko, C., Sonnenblick, M. and Ashkenazi, J. (1990) Control of steroid-resistant autoimmune haemolytic anaemia by cyclosporine. *Brit. J. Haemat.* **76**, 436–437.

Hersman, J., Meyers, J.D., Thomas. E.D., Buckner, C.D. and Clift, R. (1982) The effect of granulocyte transfusions on the incidence of cytomegalovirus infection after allogeneic marrow transplantation. *Ann. intern. Med.* **96**, 149–152.

Herzig, R.H., Poplack, D.G. and Yankee, R.A. (1974) Prolonged granulocytopenia from incompatible platelet transfusions. *New Engl. J. Med.* **290**, 1220.

Herzig. R.H., Herzig, G.P., Graw, R.G. jr, Bull, M.I. and Ray, K.K. (1977) Successful granulocyte transfusion therapy for gram-negative septicemia. *New Engl. J. Med.* **296**, 701.

Hesselvik, R., Brodin, B., Carlsson, C., Cedergren, B., Jorfeldt, L. and Lieden, G. (1987) Cryoprecipitate infusion fails to improve organ function in septic shock. *Crit. Care Med.* **15**, 594–597.

Hesser, S. (1924) Serological studies of human red corpuscles. *Acta med. scand.* Suppl. 9.

Hester, J.P. (1979) Variable anticoagulant (AC) flow rates for plateletpheresis in the dual stage disposable channel (Abstract). *Blood*, **54**, Suppl. **5**, 124a.

Hester, J.P., McCredie, K.B. and Freireich, E.J. (1982) Response to chronic leukapheresis procedures and survival of chronic myelogenous leukaemia patients. *Transfusion*, **22**, 305–307.

Hewitt, W.C. jr, Wheby, M. and Crosby, W.H. (1961) Effect of prednisolone on incompatible blood transfusions. *Transfusion*, **1**, 184.

Hewitt, Patricia, E., MacIntyre, Elizabeth, A., Devenish, A., Bowcock, Stella, J. and Contreras, Marcela (1988) A prospective study of the incidence of delayed haemolytic transfusion reactions following peri-operative blood transfusion. *Brit. J. Haemat.* **69**, 541–544.

Hewitt, Patricia and Moore, Chris (1989) HIV counselling in the National Blood Transfusion Service (Abstract). *Counselling Psychology Quarterly*, **2**, 59–64.

Heyman, B. (1990) Fc-dependent IgG-mediated suppression of the antibody response: fact or artefact? *Scand. J. Immunol.* **31**, 601–607.

Heyns, A. du P., Lötter, M.G., Badenhorst, P.N., van Reenen, O.R., Pieters, H., Minnaar, P.C. and Retief, F.P. (1980) Kinetics, distribution and sites of destruction of ^{111}indium-labelled human platelets. *Brit. J. Haemat.* **44**, 269–280.

Hickman, M., Mortimer, J.Y. and Rawlinson, V.I. (1988). Donor screening for HIV: how many false negatives? (Letter). *Lancet*, **i**, 1221.

Higby, D.J., Cohen, E., Holland, J.F. and Sinks, L. (1974) The prophylactic treatment of thrombocytopenic leukemic patients with platelets: a double blind study. *Transfusion*, **14**, 440.

Higby, D.L., Yates, J.W., Henderson, E.S. and Holland, J.F. (1975) Filtration leukapheresis for granulocyte transfusion therapy: clinical and laboratory studies. *New Engl. J. Med.* **292**, 761.

Hill, Z., Vacl, J., Kalasova, E., Calabkova, M. and Pintera, J. (1974) Haemolytic disease of the newborn in a D^u positive mother. *Vox Sang.* **27**, 92–94.

Hillman, R.S. (1964) Pooled human plasma as a volume expander. *New Engl. J. Med.* **271**, 1027.

Hillman, R.S. and Giblett, Eloise R. (1965) Red cell membrane alteration associated with 'marrow stress'. *J. clin. Invest.* **44**, 1730.

Hillman, Laura S., Goodwin, Sally L. and Sherman, W.R. (1975) Identification and measurement of plasticizer in neonatal tissues after umbilical catheters and blood products. *New Engl. J. Med.* **292**, 381.

Hillman, N.M. (1979) Fatal delayed hemolytic transfusion reaction due to anti-c+E. *Transfusion*, **19**, 548–551.

Hillyer, C.D., Tiegerman, K.O. and Berkman, E.M. (1991) Evaluation of the red cell storage lesion after irradiation in filtered packed red cell units. *Transfusion*, **31**, 497–499.

Hindemann, P. (1966) Experimentelle und klinische Untersuchungen über eine transabdominale Späteinschwemmung fetaler Erythrozyten in den mütterlichen Kreislauf. *Gerburtsh. u. Frauenheilk.* **26**, 1359.

Hino, S., Sugiyama, H., Doi, H., Ishimaru, T., Yamabe, T., Tsuji, Y. and Miyamoto, T. (1987) Breaking the cycle of HTLV-I transmission via carrier mother's milk. *Lancet*, **ii**, 158–159.

Hinz, C.F. jr, Picken, Mary E. and Lepow, I.H. (1961a) Studies on immune human hemolysis. I. The kinetics of the Donath-Landsteiner reaction and the requirements for complement in the reaction. *J. exp. Med.* **113**, 177.

Hinz, C.F. jr, Picken, Mary E. and Lepow, I.H. (1961b) Studies on immune human hemolysis. II. The Donath-Landsteiner reaction as a model system for studying the mechanism of action of complement and the role of C'1 and C'1 esterase. *J. exp. Med.* **113**, 193.

Hinz, C.F. (1963) Serologic and physiochemical characterization of Donath-Landsteiner antibodies from six patients. *Blood*, **22**, 600.

Hirsch, W., Moores, Phyllis, Sanger, Ruth and Race, R.R. (1957) Notes on some reactions of human anti-M and anti-N sera. *Brit. J. Haemat.* **3**, 134.

Hirsch, H.F., Graham, H.A. and Davies, D.M. (1975) The relationship of the Le^c and Le^d antigens to the Lewis, Secretor and ABO systems (Abstract). *Transfusion*, **15**, 521.

Hirsch, H.F. and Graham, H.A. (1980) Adsorption of Le^c and Le^d from plasma onto red blood cells. *Transfusion*, **20**, 474–475.

Hirschman, R.J., Itscoitz, S.B. and Shulman, N.R.

(1970) Prophylactic treatment of factor VIII deficiency. *Blood*, **35**, 189.

Hirszfeld, L. and Dubiski, S. (1954) Untersuchungen über die Struktur der inkompletten Antikörper. *Schweiz. Z. allg. Path.* **17**, 73.

Hjelle, B., Donegan, E., Cruz, J. and Stites, D. (1988) Antibody to c antigen consequent to renal transplantation. *Transfusion*, **28**, 496–498.

Hjelle, B., Scalf, R. and Swenson, S. (1990) High frequency of human T-cell leukemia-lymphoma virus type II infection in New Mexico blood donors: determination by sequence-specific oligonucleotide hybridization. *Blood*, **76**, 450–454.

Ho, M. (1982) *Cytomegalovirus Biology and Infection.* Plenum Press, New York.

Hoak, J.C., Aster, R.H., Fry, G.L., Braschke, J.W., Thompson, J.S. and Parsons, T.J. (1979) Post-transfusion purpura (PTP)—a multifaceted enigma. *Thrombos. Haemostas.* **42**, 256.

Hobsley, M. (1958) Chlorpheniramine maleate in prophylaxis of pyrexial reactions during blood-transfusions. *Lancet*, **i**, 497.

Hočevar, M. and Glonar, L. (1972) Reimmunization of sensitized women. *Vox Sang.* **22**, 532.

Hočevar, M. and Glonar, L. (1974) Rhesus factor immunization, in *The Ljubljana Abortion Study 1971–1973*, ed L. Ardolsek. National Institute of Health Center for Population Research, Maryland, USA.

Hoerlein, A.B. (1957) The influence of colostrum on antibody response in baby pigs. *J. Immunol.* **78**, 112.

Hoff, H.E., Smith, P.K. and Winkler, A.W. (1941) The cause of death in experimental anuria. *J. clin. Invest.* **20**, 607.

Hoffsten, P. and Chaplin, H. jr (1969) Hemolytic transfusion reaction occurring in a patient with acute renal failure. *Blood*, **33**, 234.

Hogan, V.A., Blanchette, V.S. and Rock, G. (1986) A simple method for preparing neocyte-enriched leukocyte-poor blood for transfusion-dependent patients. *Transfusion*, **26**, 253–257.

Högman, C., Killander, J. and Sjölin, S. (1960) A case of idiopathic auto-immune haemolytic anaemia due to anti-e. *Acta paed.* **49**, 270.

Högman, C.F. (1971) Oxygen affinity of stored blood. *Acta anaesth. scand.* Suppl. **45**, 53.

Högman, C.F., Perrault, R., Bergkvist, K., Löw, B. and Messeter, L. (1973) Evaluation of red cell antibody screening and identification, and a study of the reactivity of sera from dextran-infused patients, using different AutoAnalyzer techniques, in *Advances in Automated Analysis, Technicon International Congress, 1972*, **4**, 43, Mediad Inc.

Högman, C.F., Åkerblom, O., Arturson, G., de

Verdier, C.-H., Kreuger, A. and Westman, M. (1974) Experience with new preservatives: summary of the experiences in Sweden, in *The Human Red Cell* in vitro, eds T.J. Greenwalt and G.A. Jamieson. Grune & Stratton, New York.

Högman, C.F., Hedlund, K. and Zetterström, H. (1978a) Clinical usefulness of red cells preserved in protein-poor mediums. *New Engl. J. Med.* **299**, 1377.

Högman, C.F., Hedlund, K., Åkerblom, O. and Venge, P. (1978b) Red blood cell preservation in protein-poor media. I. Leukocyte enzymes as a cause of hemolysis. *Transfusion*, **18**, 233.

Högman, C.F., Åkerblom, O., Hedlund, K., Rosen, I. and Wiklund, L. (1983) Red cell suspensions in SAGM medium. *Vox Sang.* **45**, 217–223.

Högman, C.F., Hornblower, M.L.-S., Flodin, M., Gillberg, C., Meryman, H.T. and Safwenberg, J. (1986) A simple method for high-quality frozen red cells in blood group serology. *Transfusion*, **26**, 434–436.

Högman, C.F., de Verdier, C.H., Eriksson, L. and Sandhagen, B. (1987) Studies on the mechanism of human red cell loss of viability during storage at +4°C *in vitro*. III. Effects of mixing during storage. *Vox Sang.* **53**, 84–88.

Högman, C.F., Gong, J., Eriksson, L., Hambraeus, A. and Johansson, Caroline, S. (1991a) White cells protect donor blood against bacterial contamination. *Transfusion*, **31**, 620–626.

Högman, C.F., Gong, J., Eriksson, L., Hambraeus, Anna, Johansson, Caroline S. (1991b) Transfusion transmitted bacterial infection (TTBI). *Abstracts, 2nd Congr. W. Pacific Region Int. Soc. Blood Transfus.*, Hong Kong.

Högman, C.F., Eriksson, L., Ericson, Å. and Reppucci, A.J. (1991c) Storage of saline-adenine-glucose-mannitol-suspended red cells in a new plastic container: polyvinylchloride plasticized with butyryl-*n*-trihexylcitrate. *Transfusion*, **31**, 26–29.

Holburn, A.M., Cleghorn, T.E. and Hughes-Jones, N.C. (1970) Re-stimulation of anti-D in donors. *Vox Sang.* **19**, 162.

Holburn, A.M., Frame, Marion, Hughes-Jones, N.C. and Mollison, P.L. (1971a) Some biological effects of IgM anti-Rh (D). *Immunology*, **20**, 681.

Holburn, A.M., Cartron, J.-P., Economidou, Joanna, Gardner, Brigitte and Hughes-Jones, N.C. (1971b) Observations on the reactions between D-positive red cells and [125I]-labelled IgM anti-D molecules and subunits. *Immunology*, **21**, 499.

Holburn, A.M. (1973) Quantitative studies with [125I] IgM anti-Le^a. *Immunology*, **24**, 1019.

Holburn, A.M. (1974) IgG anti-Le^a. *Brit. J. Haemat.* **27**, 489.

Holburn, A.M. and Masters, C.A. (1974a) The reactions of IgG and IgM anti-A and anti-B blood group antibodies with [125I]-labelled blood group glycoproteins. *Vox Sang.* **27**, 115.

Holburn, A.M. and Masters, Carole A. (1974b) The radioimmunoassay of serum and salivary blood group A and Le^a glycoproteins. *Brit. J. Haemat.* **28**, 157.

Holburn, A.M. (1976) Radioimmunoassay studies of the cross-reacting antibody of human group O sera. *Brit. J. Haemat.* **32**, 589.

Holburn, A.M. and Prior, Dilys (1984) The UK National Quality Assessment Scheme in blood group serology. Compatibility testing 1981–1982: performance and practice. *Clin. lab. Haemat.* **6**, 325–340.

Holburn, A.M. and Prior, Dilys (1986) The UK National External Quality Assessment Scheme in blood group serology. ABO and D groupings, and antibody screening 1982–1983. *Clin. lab. Haemat.* **8**, 243–256.

Holburn, A.M. and Prior, Dilys (1987) The UK National External Quality Assessment Scheme in blood group serology. Compatibility testing 1983–1984: the influence of variables in test procedures on detection of incomplete antibodies. *Clin. lab. Haemat.* **9**, 33–48.

Holcroft, J.W. and Trunkey, D.D. (1974) Extravascular lung water following hemorrhagic shock in the baboon: comparison between resuscitation with Ringer's lactate and Plasmanate. *Ann. Surg.* **180**, 408–417.

Holguin, M.H., Fredrick, L.R., Bernshaw, N.J., Wilcox, L.A. and Parker, C.J. (1989) Isolation and characterization of a membrane protein from normal human erythrocytes that inhibits reactive lysis of the erythrocytes of paroxysmal nocturnal hemoglobinuria. *J. clin. Invest.* **84**, 7–17.

Holland, P.V. and Wallerstein, R.O. (1968) Delayed hemolytic transfusion reaction with acute renal failure. *J. Amer. med. Assoc.* **204**, 1007.

Holländer, L. (1954) Study of the erythrocyte survival time in a case of acquired haemolytic anaemia. *Vox Sang. (O.S.)*, **4**, 164.

Hollinger, F.B., Khan, N.C., Oefinger, P.E., Yawn, D.H., Schmulen, A.C., Dreesman, G.R. and Melnick, J.L. (1983) Post transfusion hepatitis type A. *J. Amer. med. Assoc.* **250**, 2313–2317.

Hollingsworth, J.W. (1955) Life-span of fetal erythrocytes. *J. Lab. clin. Med.* **45**, 469.

Hollingsworth, J.W., Birend, J.A., Silbert, D.R. and Finch, S.C. (1957) Leukocyte mobilization in normal splenectomized and leukemic rats after replacement transfusions. *J. Lab. clin. Med.* **50**, 36.

Holman, C.A. (1953) A new rare human blood-group antigen. *Lancet*, **ii**, 119.

Holme, S. and Murphy, S. (1983) Platelet storage at 22°C for transfusion: interrelationship of platelet density and size, medium pH and viability after *in vivo* infusion. *J. Lab. clin. Med.* **101**, 161–174.

Holme, S., Heaton, W.A.L. and Courtright, W.L. (1987) Improved *in vivo* and *in vitro* viability of platelet concentrates stored for seven days in a platelet additive solution. *Brit. J. Haemat.* **66**, 233–238.

Holme, S., Bode, A.P. and Heaton, A. (1989a) A combined storage medium (CSM) for storage of platelet and red cell concentrates. *Blood,* **74**, Suppl. 257a.

Holme, S., Heaton, A. and Momoda, G. (1989b) Evaluation of a new, more oxygen-permeable, polyvinylchloride container. *Transfusion,* **29**, 159–164.

Holme, S., Heaton, W.A.L. and Whitley, P. (1990) Platelet storage lesions in second-generation containers: correlation with *in vivo* behavior with storage up to 14 days. *Vox Sang.* **59**, 12–18.

Holmes, L.D., Pierce, S.R. and Beck, M. (1976) Autoanti-Jk^a in a healthy donor (Abstract). *Transfusion,* **16**, 521.

Holohan, T.V., Terasaki, P.I. and Deisseroth, A.B. (1981) Suppression of transfusion related alloimmunization in intensively treated cancer patients. *Blood,* **58**, 122–128.

Holt, P.D.J., Tandy, N.P. and Anstee, D.J. (1977) The screening of blood donors for IgA deficiency: a study of the donor population of South-West England. *J. clin. Path.* **30**, 1007.

Holt, J.T., Spitalnik, S.L., McMican, A.E., Wilson, G. and Blumberg, N. (1983) A technetium-99m red cell survival technique for *in vivo* compatibility testing. *Transfusion,* **23**, 148–151.

Holzgreve, W., Holzgreve, Brigitte and Curry, Cynthia J. (1985) Nonimmune hydrops fetalis: diagnosis and management. *Semin. Perinatol.* **9**, 52–67.

Homburger, H.A., Smith, J.R., Jacob, G.L., Laschinger, C., Naylor, D.H. and Pineda, A.A. (1981) Measurement of anti-IgA antibodies by a two-site immunoradiometric assay. *Transfusion,* **21**, 38–44.

Homi, J., Reynolds, Jennifer, Skinner, Alison, Hanna, Wadia and Serjeant, G. (1979) General anaesthesia in sickle-cell disease. *Brit. med. J.* **i**, 1599–1601.

Honig, C.L. and Bove, J.R. (1980) Transfusion-associated fatalities: review of Bureau of Biologics Reports 1976–78. *Transfusion,* **20**, 653–661.

Hönlinger, M., Reibnegger, G., Schonitzer, D., Wachter, H. (1988) Prevention of post-transfusion infectious complications. *Lancet,* **ii**, 405–406.

Hoofnagle, J.H., Seeff, L.B., Bales, Z.B. and Zimmerman, H.J. (1978) Type B hepatitis after transfusion with blood containing antibody to hepatitis B core antigen. *New Engl. J. Med.* **298**, 1379.

Hopf, U. and 9 others (1990) Long term follow up of posttransfusion and sporadic chronic hepatitis non-A, non-B and frequency of circulating antibodies to hepatitis C virus (HCV). *J. Hepatol.* **10**, 69–76.

Hopkins, J.G. (1910) Phagocytosis of red blood-cells after transfusion. *Arch. intern. Med.* **6**, 270.

Hopkins, D.F. (1969a) The decline and fall of anti-Rh(D). *Brit. J. Haemat.* **17**, 199.

Hopkins, D.F. (1969b) The correlation between IgM anti-D and 'saline agglutination' of D-positive cells by anti-D sera. *Brit. J. Haemat.* **17**, 597.

Hopkins, D.F. (1970a) Saline agglutinating anti-K and anti-k in the apparent absence of IgM antibody. *Brit. J. Haemat.* **19**, 749.

Hopkins, D.F. (1970b) Maternal anti-Rh(D) and the D-negative fetus. *Amer. J. Obstet. Gynec.* **108**, 268.

Hopkins, D.F. (1971) Naturally occurring anti-Rh(E) in one identical twin but not the other. *Lancet,* **ii**, 409.

Hoppe, H.H., Mester, T., Hennig, W. and Krebs, H.J. (1973) Prevention of Rh-immunization. Modified production of IgG anti-Rh for intravenous application by ion exchange chromatography (IEC). *Vox Sang.* **25**, 308.

Höppner, W., Fischer, K., Poschmann, A. and Paulsen, H. (1985) Use of synthetic antigens with the carbohydrate structure of a sialoglycophorin A for the specification of Thomsen-Friedenreich antibodies. *Vox Sang.* **48**, 246–253.

Hornick, C.L. and Karush, F. (1972) Antibody affinity—III. The role of multivalence. *Immuno chemistry,* **9**, 325.

Horowitz, J.D. and Mashford, M.L. (1980a) Purification of a peptide with venoconstrictor and vasodepressor activity, from Cohn fraction III-O of human plasma protein. *Vox Sang.* **38**, 259–265.

Horowitz, J.D. and Mashford, M.L. (1980b) Venoconstrictor activity of some precursor fractions of stable plasma protein solution. *Vox Sang.* **38**, 266–271.

Horowitz, B., Stryker, M.H., Wardman, A.A., Woods, K.R., Gass, J.D. and Drago, J. (1984) Stabilization of red blood cells by the plasticizer, diethylhexylphthalate. *Vox Sang.* **48**, 150–155.

Horowitz, M.S., Rooks, C., Horowitz, B. and Hilgartner, M.W. (1988) Virus safety of solvent/detergent treated anti-haemophilic factor concentrate. *Lancet,* **ii**, 186–189.

Horowitz, B. (1989) Investigations into the application of tri(n-butyl) phosphate/detergent mixtures to blood derivatives, in *Virus Inactivation in Plasma Products*, ed J.J. Morgenthaler, pp. 83–96. S. Karger, Basel.

Horrow, J.C., Hlavacek, J., Strong, M.D., Collier, W., Brodsky, I., Goldman, S.M. and God, I.P. (1990) Prophylactic tranexamic acid decreases bleeding after cardiac operations. *J. thorac. cardiovasc. Surg.* 99, 70–74.

Horsburgh, C.R. and 13 others (1989) Duration of human immunodeficiency virus infection before detection of antibody. *Lancet*, ii, 637–640.

Horsburgh, C.R. (1992) Prognostic indicators for progression of HIV disease, in *AIDS Testing. Methodology and Management Issues*, eds G. Schochetman and J.R. George, pp. 143–151. Springer-Verlag, New York.

Hosein, Barbara, Fang, C.T., Popovsky, M.A., Ye, J., Zhang, M. and Wang, C.Y. (1991) Improved serodiagnosis of hepatitis C virus infection with synthetic peptide antigen from capsid protein. *Proc. nat. Acad. Sci. USA*, 88, 3647–3651.

Hossaini, A.A. (1972) Neutralization of Lewis antibodies *in vivo* and transfusion of Lewis incompatible blood. *Amer. J. clin. Path.* 57, 489.

Høstrup, H. (1963a) A and B blood group substances in the serum of the newborn infant and the foetus. *Vox Sang.* 8, 557.

Høstrup, H. (1963b) The influence of A and B blood group substances on the 7S fractions of anti-A and anti-B. *Vox Sang.* 8, 567.

Høstrup, H. (1964) Influence of foetal A and B blood-group substances on the immunization of pregnant women. *Vox Sang.* 9, 301.

Howard, P.L. and Picoff, R.C. (1972) Another example of anti-M in an M-positive patient. *Transfusion*, 12, 59.

Howard, Jean E. and Perkins, H.A. (1976) Lysis of donor RBC during plateletpheresis with a blood processor. *J. Amer. Med. Assoc.* 236, 289.

Howard, J.E. and Perkins, H.A. (1978) The natural history of alloimmunization to platelets. *Transfusion*, 18, 496.

Howard, D.R. (1979) Expression of T-antigen on polyagglutinable erythrocytes and carcinoma cells: preparation of T-activated erythrocytes, anti-T lectin, anti-T absorbed human serum and purified anti-T antibody. *Vox Sang.* 37, 107–110.

Howard, J.E., Winn, L.C., Gottlieb, C.E., Grumet, F.C., Garratty, G. and Petz, L. (1982a) Clinical significance of the anti-complement component of antiglobulin sera. *Transfusion*, 22, 269–272.

Howard, L., Shulman, S., Sadanandan, S. and

Karpatkin, S. (1982b) Crossed immunoelectrophoresis of human platelet membranes. The major antigen consists of a complex of glycoproteins GPIIb and GPIIIa held together by Ca^{2+} and missing in Glanzmann's thrombasthenia. *J. biol. Chem.* 257, 8331–8336.

Howarth, Shelia and Sharpey-Schafer, E.P. (1947) Low blood pressure phases following haemorrhage. *Lancet*, i, 19.

Howell, Eleanor D. and Perkins, H.A. (1972) Anti-N-like antibodies in the sera of patients undergoing chronic hemodialysis. *Vox Sang.* 23, 291.

Howland, W.S., Bellville, J.W., Zucker, Marjorie B., Bryan, P. and Cliffton, E.E. (1957) Massive blood replacement. V. Failure to observe citrate intoxication. *Surg. Gynec. Obstet.* 105, 529.

Howland, W.S., Jacobs, Rita G. and Goulet, Anita H. (1960) An evaluation of calcium administration during rapid replacement. *Anaesth. Analg.* 39, 557.

Hows, J.M., Chipping, P.M., Palmer, S. and Gordon-Smith, E.C. (1983) Regeneration of peripheral blood cells following ABO-incompatible allogeneic BMT for severe aplastic anaemia. *Brit. J. Haemat.* 53, 145–151.

Hows, Jill, Beddow. K., Gordon-Smith, E., Branch, D.R., Spruce, W., Sniecinski, Irena, Krance, R.A. and Petz, L.D. (1986) Donor derived red blood cell antibodies and immune hemolysis after allogeneic bone marrow transplantation. *Blood*, 67, 177–181.

Hows, D.M. (1990) Annotation: the use of unrelated marrow donors for transplantation. *Brit. J. Haemat.* 76, 1–6.

Hoyer, L.W. and Trabold, Norma C. (1971) The significance of erythrocyte antigen site density. II. Hemolysis. *J. clin. Invest.* 50, 1840.

Hraba, T., Májsky, A., Vitová, Z. and Matoušek, V. (1962) Influence of the mother's blood group on the formation of natural isoagglutinins by the child. *Folia Biol. (Praha)*, 8, 60.

Hsu, T.C.S., Rosenfield, R.E., Burkart, P., Wong, K.Y. and Kochwa, S. (1974a) Instrumented PVP-augmented antiglobulin tests. II. Evaluation of acquired hemolytic anemia. *Vox Sang.* 26, 305.

Hsu, T.C.S., Rosenfield, R.E. and Rubinstein, P. (1974b) Instrumented PVP-augmented antiglobulin tests. III. IgG-coated cells in ABO incompatible babies; depressed hemoglobin levels in type A babies of type O mothers. *Vox Sang.* 26, 326.

Hsu, T.C.S., Jagathambal, K., Sabo, B.H. and Sawitsky, A. (1975) Anti-Holley (Hy): characterization of another example. *Transfusion*, **15**, 604.

Hübener, G. (1925) Untersuchungen über Isoagglutination, mit besonderer Berücksichtigung scheinbarer Abweichungen vom Gruppenschema. *Z. Immun.-Forsch.* **45**, 223.

Huber, H., Lewis, S.M. and Szur, L. (1964) The influence of anaemia, polycythaemia and splenomegaly on the relationship between venous haematocrit and red-cell volume. *Brit. J. Haemat.* **10**, 567.

Huber, H., Polley, Margaret, Linscott, W., Fudenberg, H. and Müller-Eberhard, H. (1968) Human monocytes: distinct receptor sites for the third component of complement and for immunoglobulin G. *Science*, **162**, 1281.

Hubinont, P.O. (1949) Isoimmunization by blood group factors A and B in man. *Brit. med. J.* **ii**, 574.

Huchet, J., Crégut, R. and Pinon, F. (1970) Immuno-globulines anti-D. Efficacité comparée des voies intra-musculaire et intra-veineuse. *Rev. franç. Transfus.* **13**, 231.

Huchet, J., Crégut, R., Pinon, F., Sender, A. and Brossard, Y. (1975) Les hémorragies foeto-maternelles et leur importance dans ia pathologie perinatale. *Rev. franç Transfus. Immunohémat.* **18**, 361.

Huchet, J., Defossez, Y. and Brossard, Y. (1988) Detection of transplacental haemorrhage during the last trimester of pregnancy (Letter). *Transfusion*, **28**, 506.

Huestis, D.W. (1971) In International Forum: What constitutes adequate routine Rh typing on donors and recipients? *Vox Sang.* **21**, 183.

Huestis. D.W., White. R.F., Price, M.J. and Inman, M. (1975) Use of hydroxyethyl starch to improve granulocyte collection in the Latham blood processor. *Transfusion*, **15**, 559.

Huestis, D.W., Price, M.J., White, R.F. and Imman, M. (1976) Leukapheresis of patients with chronic granulocytic leukaemia (CGL), using the Haemonetics blood processor. *Transfusion*, **16**, 255.

Huestis, D.W., Bove, J.R. and Busch, S. (1981) Hemapheresis, in *Practical Blood Transfusion*, 3rd edn. Little Brown, Boston.

Huestis, D.W. (1983a) Technical aspects of cell collection—donor considerations. *Clinics in Oncology*, **2**, 529–547.

Huestis, D.W. (1983b) Mortality in therapeutic haemapheresis (Letter). *Lancet*, **i**, 1043.

Huestis, D.W., Loftus, T.J., Gilcher, R., Lichtiger, B., Rock, G., Price, T.H., Glasser, L., White, R.F. and Robinson, R. (1985) Modified fluid gelatin. An alternative macromolecular agent for centrifugal leukapheresis. *Transfusion*, **25**, 343–348.

Huestis, D.W. (1986a) Therapeutic plasmaphere-sis, in *Progress in Transfusion Medicine*, ed J.D. Cash, **1**, pp. 78–94. Churchill Livingstone. Edinburgh.

Huestis, D.W. (1986b) Complications of therapeutic apheresis, in *Therapeutic Hemapheresis*, eds M. Valbonesi, A. Pineda and J.C. Briggs, pp. 179–186. Wichtig Editore, Milano.

Huestis, D.W. (1989) Risks and safety practices in hemapheresis procedures. *Arch. Path. lab. Med.* **113**, 273–278.

Huggins, C.E., Parker, B.H., Milbury, C.S. and Murtagh, P.B. (1982) "Glycigel"—a practical technique for preservation of small aliquots of red cells (Abstract). *Transfusion*, **22**, 408.

Hughes, A.S.B. and Brozović, B. (1982) Leuco-cyte depleted blood: an appraisal of available techniques. *Brit. J. Haemat.* **50**, 381–386.

Hughes, A. and Corrah, T. (1990) Human immunodeficiency virus type 2 (HIV2). *Blood Rev.* **4**, 158–164.

Hughes-Jones, N.C. and Mollison, P.L. (1956) Interpretation of ^{51}Cr survival curves. *Clin. Sci.* **15**, 207.

Hughes-Jones, N.C., Mollison, P.L. and Robinson, Margaret A. (1957a) Factors affecting the viability of erythrocytes stored in the frozen state. *Proc. roy. Soc. Lond. B*, **147**, 476.

Hughes-Jones, N.C., Mollison, P.L. and Veall, N. (1957b) Removal of incompatible red cells by the spleen. *Brit. J. Haemat.* **3**, 125.

Hughes-Jones, N.C. (1958a) Measurement of red-cell loss from gastro-intestinal tract, using radioactive chromium. *Brit. med. J.* **i**, 493.

Hughes-Jones, N.C. (1958b) Storage of red cells at temperatures between +10°C and −20°C. *Brit. J. Haemat.* **4**, 249.

Hughes-Jones, N.C. and Gardner, Brigitte (1962) The exchange of ^{131}I-labelled lipid and ^{131}I-labelled protein between red cells and serum. *Biochem. J.* **83**, 404.

Hughes-Jones, N.C., Gardner, Brigitte and Telford, Rachel (1962) The kinetics of the reaction between the blood-group antibody anti-c and erythrocytes. *Biochem. J.* **85**, 466.

Hughes-Jones, N.C. (1963) Nature of the reaction between antigen and antibody. *Brit. med. Bull.* **19**, 171.

Hughes-Jones, N.C. and Mollison, P.L. (1963) Clearance by the R.E.S. of 'non-viable red cells', in *Role du système réticulo-endothélial dans l'immunité antibactérienne et antitumorale.* Edition du C.N.R.S., Paris.

Hughes-Jones, N.C., Gardner, Brigitte and Telford, Rachel (1963a) Studies on the reaction between the blood-group antibody anti-D and erythrocytes. *Biochem. J.* **88**, 435.

Hughes-Jones, N.C., Gardner, Brigitte and Telford, Rachel (1963b) Comparison of various methods of dissociation of anti-D, using ^{131}I-labelled antibody. *Vox Sang.* **8**, 531.

Hughes-Jones, N.C., Gardner, Brigitte and Telford, Rachel (1964a) The effect of pH and ionic strength on the reaction between anti-D and erythrocytes. *Immunology*, 7, 72.

Hughes-Jones, N.C., Gardner, Brigitte and Telford, Rachel (1964b) The effect of ficin on the reaction between anti-D and red cells. *Vox Sang.* 9, 175.

Hughes-Jones, N.C., Polley, M.J., Telford, R., Gardner, B. and Kleinschmidt, G. (1964c) Optimal conditions for detecting blood group antibodies by the antiglobulin test. *Vox Sang.* 9, 385.

Hughes-Jones, N.C. (1967) The estimation of the concentration and the equilibrium constant of anti-D. *Immunology*, 12, 565.

Hughes-Jones. N.C., Hughes, M.I.J. and Walker, W. (1967) The amount of anti-D on red cells in haemolytic disease of the newborn. *Vox Sang.* 12, 279.

Hughes-Jones, N.C. and Mollison, P.L. (1968) Failure of a relatively small dose of passively administered anti-Rh to suppress primary immunization by a relatively large dose of Rh-positive red cells. *Brit. med. J.* i, 150.

Hughes-Jones, N.C. and Stevenson, Mary (1968) The anti-D content of IgG preparations for use in the prevention of Rh haemolytic disease. *Vox Sang.* 14, 401.

Hughes-Jones. N.C. (1970) Reactivity of anti-D immunoglobulin G subunits. *Nature (Lond.)*, 227, 174.

Hughes-Jones, N.C. and Gardner, Brigitte (1970) The equilibrium constants of anti-D immunoglobulin preparations made from pools of donor plasma. *Immunology*, 18, 347.

Hughes-Jones, N.C. and Gardner, Brigitte (1971) The Kell system studied with radioactively-labelled anti-K. *Vox Sang.* 21, 154.

Hughes-Jones, N.C., Gardner, Brigitte and Lincoln, P. (1971a) Observations of the number of available c, D, e and E antigen sites on red cells. *Vox Sang.* 21, 210.

Hughes-Jones, N.C., Ellis, M., Ivona J. and Walker, W. (1971b) Anti-D concentration in mother and child in haemolytic disease of the newborn. *Vox Sang.* 21, 135.

Hughes-Jones, N.C., Norley, I. and Hunt, Valerie (1972) Automatic red cell washing machine for quantitative assay of anti-D concentration. *Vox Sang.* 22, 268.

Hughes-Jones, N.C. (1972) The attachment of IgG molecules on the red cell surface. *Haematologia*, 6, 269.

Hughes-Jones, N.C. (1975) Red-cell antigens, antibodies and their interaction. *Clin. Haemat.* 4, 29.

Hughes-Jones, N.C., Green, Elizabeth, J. and Hunt, Valerie, A.M. (1975) Loss of Rh antigen activity following the action of phospholipase A2 on red cell stroma. *Vox Sang.* 29, 184–191.

Hughes-Jones, N.C., Hunt, Valerie A., Maycock, W.d'A., Wesley, E.D. and Vallet, L. (1978) Anti-D immunoglobulin preparations: the stability of anti-D concentrations and the error of the assay of anti-D. *Vox Sang.* 35, 100.

Hughes-Jones N.C. and Ghosh, S. (1981) Anti-D-coated Rh-positive red cells will bind the first component of the complement pathway, C1q. *FEBS Letters*, 128, 318–320.

Hughes-Jones, N.C., Gorick, Barbara D., Miller, N.G.A. and Howard, J.C. (1984) IgG pair formation on one antigenic molecule is the main mechanism of synergy between antibodies in complement-mediated lysis. *Europ. J. Immunol.* 14, 974–978.

Hughes-Jones, N.C. (1986) The classical pathway, in *Immunobiology of the Complement System*, ed G.D. Ross. Academic Press.

Hughes-Jones, N.C., Bloy, C., Gorick, B., Blanchard, D., Doinel, C., Rouger, P. and Cartron, J-P. (1988) Evidence that the c, D and E epitopes of the human Rh blood group system are on separate polypeptide molecules. *Molec. Immunol.* 25, 931–936.

Hughes-Jones, N.C. and Bradley, B.A. (1989) Heterogeneity in the ability of IgG1 monoclonal anti-D to promote lymphocyte-mediated red cell lysis. *Eur. J. Immunol.* 19, 2283–2288.

Hughes-Jones, N.C., Gorick, B.D. and Beale, D. (1990) Multiple epitopes recognised by human monoclonal IgM anti-D antibodies. *Vox Sang.* 59, 112–115.

Huh, Y.O., Liu, F.J., Rogge, Karen, Chakrabarty, Lila, and Lichtiger, B. (1988) Positive direct antiglobulin test and high serum immunoglobulin G values. *Amer. J. clin. Path.* 90, 179–200.

Huizinga, T.W.J., Kerst, J.M., Nuyens, J.H., Vlug, A., von dem Borne, A.E.G. Kr., Roos, D. and Tetteroo, P.A.T. (1989) Binding characteristics of dimeric IgG subclass complexes to human neutrophils. *J. Immunol.* 142, 2359–2364.

Huizinga, T.W.J., Kleijer, Marion, Tetteroo, P.A.T., Roos, D. and von dem Borne, A.E.G.Kr. (1990) Biallelic neutrophil Na-antigen system is associated with a polymorphism on the phospho-inositol-linked Fc-gamma receptor III (CD16). *Blood*, 75, 213–217.

Huizinga, T.W.J., Kuijpers R.W.A.M., Kleijer, Marion, Schulpen, T.W.J., Cuypers, H.T.M., Roos, D. and von dem Borne, A.E.G.Kr. (1991) Maternal genomic neutrophil FcRIII deficiency leading to neonatal isoimmune neutropenia. *Blood* 76, 1927–1932.

Hummel, K. (1962) Quantitative Untersuchungen uber die Bindung von Polyvinylpyrrolidon an die Erythrozytenoberflache. *Blut*, **9**, 215.

Humphrey, J.H. and Dourmashkin, R.R. (1965) Electron microscope studies of immune cell lysis, in *Ciba Foundation Symposium, Complement*, eds G.E.W. Wolstenholme and J. Knight. J. & A. Churchill, London.

Hunt, Beverley, J, Yacoub, M., Amin, Sheela, Devenish, A. and Contreras, Marcela (1988) Induction of red blood cell destruction by graft-derived antibodies after minor ABO mismatched heart and lung transplantation. *Transplantation*, **46**, 246–249.

Hunt, A.F. and Reed, M.I. (1990) Anti-IgA screening and use of IVIG. *Lancet*, **336**, 1197.

Hunter, W. (1884) The demonstration of the life of red blood corpuscles as ascertainable by transfusion. *Proc. roy. Soc. Edinb.* **13**, 849.

Hurdle, A.D.F. and Rosin, A.J. (1962) Red cell volume and red cell survival in normal aged people. *J. clin. Path.* **15**, 343.

Hussey, Ruth and Clarke, C.A. (1991) Deaths from Rh haemolytic disease in England and Wales in 1988 and 1989. *Brit. Med. J.* **303**, 445–446.

Hustin. A. (1914) Principe d'une nouvelle méthode de transfusion. *J. Méd. Brux.* **2**, 436.

Hutchinson, R.M., Sejeny, S.A., Fraser, I.D. and Tovey, G.H. (1976) Lymphocyte response to blood transfusion in man: a comparison of different preparations of blood. *Brit. J. Haemat.* **33**, 105.

Hutchinson, A.A., Drew, J.H., Yu, V.Y.H., Williams, Margaret L., Fortune, D.W. and Beischer, N.A. (1982) Nonimmunologic hydrops fetalis: a review of 61 cases. *Obstet. Gynaec.* **59**, 347–352.

Hutchison, J.L. Freedman, S.O., Richards, B.A. and Burgen, A.S.V. (1960) Plasma volume expansion and reactions after infusion of autologous and non-autologous plasma in man. *J. Lab. clin. Med.* **56**, 734.

Hutchison, J.L and Burgen, A.S.V. (1963) Infusion of non-autologous plasma. Effects of chlorpheniramine, prednisolone and adrenaline. *Brit. med. J.* ii, 904.

Hutchinson, R.E. and 9 others (1989) Beneficial effect of brief pre-transfusion incubation of platelets at 37°C. *Lancet*, ii, 986.

Hutton, E.L. and Shute, P.G. (1939) The risk of transmitting malaria by blood transfusion. *J. trop. Med. Hyg.* **42**, 309.

Hyde, P. and Zucker-Franklin, D. (1987) Antigenic differences between human platelets and megakaryocytes. *Amer. J. Path.* **127**, 349–357.

Hysell, J.K., Gray, J.M., Hysell, J.W. and Beck, M.L. (1975) An anti-neomycin antibody interfering with ABO grouping and antibody screening. *Transfusion*, **15**, 16.

Hysell, J.K., Hysell, J.W., Nichols, M.E., Leonardi, R.G. and Marsh, W.L. (1976) *In vivo* and *in vitro* activation of T-antigen receptors on leukocytes and platelets. *Vox Sang.* **31**, 9.

Ichikawa, Y. (1959) A study of the iso-agglutinin titres in the sera of Australian subjects (white). *Jap. J. med. Sci. Biol.* **12**, 1.

ICSH (International Committee for Standardization in Haematology) (1971) Recommended methods for radioisotope red-cell survival studies. *Brit. J. Haemat.* **21**, 241.

ICSH (International Committee for Standardization in Haematology): Expert Panel on Blood Cell Sizing (1980a) Recommendation for reference method for determination by centrifugation of packed cell volume of blood. *J. clin. Path.* **33**, 1–2.

ICSH (International Committee for Standardization in Haematology) (1980b) Recommended methods for radioisotope red-cell survival studies. *Brit. J. Haemat.* **45**, 659–666.

ICSH (International Committee for Standardization in Haematology) (1980c) Recommended methods for measurement of red-cell and plasma volume. *J. nucl. Med.* **21**, 793–800.

ICSH (International Committee for Standardization in Haematology) (1982) Working party on the standardization of albumin reagents, unpublished report.

Ikeda, H., Mitani, T., Ohnuma, M. and others (1989) A new platelet specific antigen, Nak[a] involved in the refractoriness of HLA-matched platelet transfusion. *Vox Sang.* **57**, 213.

Ikin, Elizabeth, Kay, H.E.M., Playfair, J.H.I. and Mourant, A.E. (1961) P_1 antigen in the human foetus. *Nature (Lond.)*, **192**, 4805.

Ilabaca, P.A., Ochsner, J.L. and Mills, N.L. (1980) Positive end-expiratory pressure in the management of the patient with a postoperative bleeding heart. *Ann. thorac. Surg.* **30**, 281–284

Imagawa, D.T. and 12 others (1989) Human immunodeficiency virus type 1 Infection in homosexual men who remain seronegative for prolonged periods. *New Engl. J. Med.* **320**, 1458–1462.

Imagawa, D. and Detels, R. (1991) HIV-1 in seronegative homosexual men. *New Engl. J. Med.* **325**, 1250–1251.

Imaizumi, A., Suzuki, Y., Sato, H. and Sato, Y. (1985) Protective effects of human gamma-globulin preparation against experimental aerosol infections of mice with *Bordetella pertussis. Vox Sang.* **48**, 18–25.

Imbach, P. and 9 others (1981) High-dose intravenous gammaglobulin for idiopathic thrombocytopenic purpura in childhood. *Lancet*, i, 1228–1231.

Imbach, P. and 9 others (1985) Intravenous immunoglobulin versus oral corticosteroids in acute immune thrombocytopenic purpura in childhood. *Lancet*, **ii**, 464–468.

Inaba, S., Sato, H., Okochi, K., Fukada, K., Takakura, F., Tokunaga, K., Kiyokawa, H. and Maeda, Y. (1989) Prevention of transmission of human T-lymphotrophic virus type 1 (HTLV-1) through transfusion, by donor screening with antibody to the virus. *Transfusion*, **29**, 7–11.

Inchauspe, Genevieve, Abe, K., Zebedee, Suzanne, Nasoff, M. and Prince, A.M. (1991) Use of conserved sequences from hepatitis C virus for the detection of viral RNA in infected sera by polymerase chain reaction. *Hepatology*, **14**, 595–600.

Inglis, G., Bird. G.W.G., Mitchell, A.A.B., Milne, G.R. and Wingham, June (1975a) Erythrocyte polyagglutination showing properties of both T and Tk, probably induced by *Bacteroides fragilis* infection. *Vox Sang.* **28**, 314.

Inglis, G., Bird, G.W.G., Mitchell, A.A.B., Milne, G.R. and Wingham, June (1975b) Effect of *Bacteroides fragilis* on the human erythrocyte membrane: pathogenesis of Tk polyagglutination. *J. clin. Path.* **28**, 964.

Inglis, G., Bird, G.W.G., Mitchell, A.A.B. and Wingham, June (1978) Tk polyagglutination associated with reduced A and H activity. *Vox Sang.* **35**, 370.

Inkster, M., Sherman, L.A., Ahmed, L.A., Benton, M.B. and Gaston, L.W. (1984) Preservation of anti-thrombin III activity in stored whole blood. *Transfusion*, **24**, 57–59.

Inwood, M.J. and Zuliani, B. (1978) Anti-A hemolytic transfusion with packed O cells. *Ann. intern. Med.* **89**, 515–516.

Ip, Henrietta, M.H., Lelie, P.N., Wong, Vivian, C.W., Kuhns, Mary, C. and Reesink, H.W. (1989) Prevention of hepatitis B virus carrier state in infants according to maternal serum levels of HBV DNA. *Lancet*, **ii**, 406–409.

Irani, M.S., Dudley, A.W. and Lucco, L.J. (1991) Case of HIV-1 transmission by antigen-positive, antibody-negative blood (Letter). *New Engl. J. Med.* **325**, 1174–1175.

Isarangkura, P., Mahaphan, W., Chiewsilp, P., Chuansumrit, A. and Hathirat, P. (1992) HIV transmission by seronegative blood components: report of 2 cases. *Vox Sang. in press.*

Isbister, J.P., Ting, Amy and Seeto, K.M. (1977) Development of Rh specific maternal auto-antibodies following intensive plasmapheresis for Rh immunization during pregnancy. *Vox Sang.* **33**, 353.

Iserson, K.V. and Huestis, D.W. (1991) Blood warming: current applications and techniques. *Transfusion*, **31**, 558–571.

Ishimori, T. and Hasekura. H. (1967) A Japanese with no detectable Rh blood group antigens due to silent Rh alleles or deleted chromosomes. *Transfusion*, **7**, 84.

Ishizaka, K., Ishizaka, T., Lee, E.H. and Fudenberg, H.H. (1965) Immunochemical properties of human γA isohemagglutinin. I. Comparisons with γG- and γM-globulin antibodies. *J. Immunol.* **95**, 197.

Ishizaka, T., Tada, T. and Ishizaka, K. (1968) Fixation of C' and C' 1a by rabbit γG- and γM-antibodies with particulate and soluble antigens. *J. Immunol.* **100**, 1145.

Issitt, P.D. (1965) On the incidence of second antibody populations in the sera of women who have developed anti-Rh antibodies. *Transfusion*, **5**, 355.

Issitt, P.D. and Jackson, Valerie A. (1968) Useful modifications and variations of technics in work on I system antibodies. *Vox Sang.* **15**, 152.

Issitt, P.D., Tegoli, J., Jackson, Valerie, Sanders, C.W. and Allen, F.H. jr (1968) Anti-IP$_1$: antibodies that show an association between the I and P blood group systems. *Vox Sang.* **14**, 1.

Issitt, P.D., Issitt, C.H., Moulds, J. and Berman, H.J. (1972) Some observations on the T, Tn and Sd^a antigens and the antibodies that define them. *Transfusion*, **12**, 217.

Issitt, P.D., McKeever, B.G., Moore, V.K. and Wilkinson, S.L. (1973) Three examples of Rh-positive, good responders to blood group antigens. *Transfusion*, **13**, 316.

Issitt, P.D. and Issitt, Charla H. (1975) *Applied Blood Group Serology*. Spectra Biologicals, Oxnard, California.

Issitt, P.D., Pavone, B.G. and Goldfinger, D. (1975) The phenotype En(a–), Wr(a–b–). *Commun. 14th Congr. Int. Soc. Blood. Transfus.*, Helsinki.

Issitt, P.D., Pavone, B.G., Goldfinger, D., Zwicker, J., Issitt, C.H., Tessel, J.A., Kroovand, S.W. and Bell, C.A. (1976a) Anti-Wr^b, and other autoantibodies responsible for positive direct antiglobulin tests in 150 individuals. *Brit. J. Haemat.* **34**, 5.

Issitt, C.H., Duckett, J.B., Osborne, B.M., Gut, J.B. and Beasley, J. (1976b) Another example of an antibody reacting optimally with p red cells. *Brit J. Haemat.* **34**, 19.

Issitt. P.D. (1977) The antiglobulin test and the evaluation of antiglobulin reagents. II. The IgG-anti-IgG and IgA-anti-IgA reactions and the evaluation of anti-IgG. *Advances in Immunohematology*, **4**, No. 5. Spectra Biologicals, Oxnard, California.

Issitt, P.D. and Pavone, Beverly G. (1978) Critical re-examination of the specificity of auto-anti-Rh antibodies in patients with a positive direct antiglobulin test. *Brit. J. Haemat.* **38**, 63.

Issitt, P.D. (1979) *Serology and Genetics of the Rhesus Blood Group System*. Montgomery Scientific Publications, Cincinnati, Ohio.

Issitt, P.D. (1981) *The MN Blood Group System*. Montgomery Scientific Publications, Cincinnati, Ohio.

Issitt, P.D. and Tessel, J.A. (1981) On the incidence of antibodies to the Rh antigens G, rh_i (Ce), C, and C^G in sera containing anti-CD or anti-C. *Transfusion*, **21**, 412–418.

Issitt, P.D., Gruppo, R.A., Wilkinson, Susan L. and Issitt, Charla H. (1982) Atypical presentation of acute phase, antibody-induced haemolytic anaemia in an infant. *Brit. J. Haemat.* **52**, 537–543.

Issitt, P.D., Wilkinson, Susan L. and Gruppo, R.A. (1983) Depression of Rh antigen expression in antibody-induced haemolytic anaemia (Letter). *Brit. J. Haemat.* **53**, 688.

Issitt, P.D. (1985) *Applied Blood Group Serology*, 3rd edn. Montgomery Scientific Publications, Miami, Florida.

Issitt, P.D. (1990) Heterogeneity of anti-U. *Vox Sang.* **58**, 70–71.

Issitt, P.D., Valinsky, J.E., Marsh, W.L., Dinapoli, J. and Gutgsell, N.S. (1990a) In vivo red cell destruction by anti-Lu6. *Transfusion*, **30**, 258–260.

Issitt, P.D., Obarski, G., Hartnett, P.L., Wren, M.R. and Prewitt, P.L. (1990b) Temporary suppression of Kidd system expression accompanied by transient production of anti-Jk3. *Transfusion*, **30**, 46–50.

Ito, K. and 9 others (1988) Change of HLA phenotype in postoperative erythroderma. *Lancet*, **i**, 413–414.

Iwaki, Y., Cecka, J.M. and Terasaki, P.I. (1990) The transfusion effect in cadaver kidney transplants, yes or no. *Transplantation*, **49**, 56–59.

Iwarson, S., Steen, Y., Rybo, G., Hermodsson, S., Antonsson, I. and Vietorisz, A. (1985) Does Cohn-fractionated Rh immune globulin transmit viral hepatitis? *Transfusion*, **25**, 15–17.

Jackson, Valerie A., Issitt, P.D., Francis, Betty J., Garis, Mary Lou and Sanders, C.W. (1968) The simultaneous presence of anti-I and anti-i in sera. *Vox Sang.* **15**, 133.

Jackson, J.B., Sannerud, K.J., Hopsicker, J.S., Kwok, S.Y., Edson, J.R. and Balfour, H.H. (1988a) Hemophiliacs with HIV antibody are actively infected. *J. Amer. med. Assoc.* **260**, 2236–2239.

Jackson, J.B., Englund, E.A., Edson, J.R. and Balfour, H.H. (1988b) Prevalence of cytomegalovirus antibody in hemophiliacs and homosexuals infected with human immunodeficiency virus type 1. *Transfusion*, **28**, 187–189.

Jackson, J.B. (1991) Editorial: polymerase chain reaction assay for detection of hepatitis B virus. *Amer. J. clin. Path.* **95**, 442–444.

Jacobs, J., Jamaer, D., Vandeven, J., Wouters, M., Vermylen, C. and Vandepitte, J. (1989) *Yersinia enterocolitica* in donor blood: a case report and review. *J. clin. Microbiol.* **27**, 1119–1121.

Jacoby, G.A., Hunt, J.V., Kosinski, Katherine S., Demirjian, Z.N., Huggins, C., Etkind, P., Marcus, L.C. and Spielman, A. (1980) Treatment of transfusion-transmitted babesiosis by exchange transfusion. *New Engl. J. Med.* **303**, 1098–1100.

Jacot-Guillarmod, H. and Isliker, H. (1964) Scission réversible des isoagglutinines 19s; études de fixation des subunités. *Vox Sang.* **9**, 31.

Jaeger, R.J. and Rubin, R.J. (1970) Plasticizers from plastic devices; extraction, metabolism, and accumulation by biological systems. *Science*, **170**, 460.

Jaffe, C.F., Atkinson, J.P. and Frank, M.M. (1976) The role of complement in the clearance of cold agglutinin-sensitized erythrocytes in man. *J. clin. Invest.* **58**, 942.

Jaffe, J.P. and Mosher, D.F. (1981) Plasma antithrombin III and plasminogen levels in chronic plasmapheresis. *New Engl. J. Med.* **304**, 789.

Jaffe, H.W. and 10 others (1985) The acquired immunodeficiency syndrome in a cohort of homosexual men: a six-year follow-up study. *Ann. intern. Med.* **103**, 210–214.

Jaffe, J.G., Wohlgelernter, D., Cabin, H., Bowman, L., Decklebaum, L., Remetz, M. and Clemen, M. (1988) Preservation of left ventricular ejection fraction during percutaneous transluminal coronary angioplasty by distal transcatheter coronary perfusion of oxygenated Fluosol-DA 20%. *Amer. Heart J.* **115**, 1156–1164.

Jager, Martine J., Claas, F.H.J., Witvliet, Marian and van Rood, J.J. (1986) Correspondence of the monocyte antigen HMA-1 to the non-HLA antigen 9a. *Immunogenetics*, **23**, 71–78.

Jakobowicz, Rachel, Bryce, Lucy M. and Simmons, R.T. (1949) The occurrence of unusual positive Coombs reactions and M variants in the blood of a mother and her first child. *Med. J. Aust.* **ii**, 945.

Jakobowicz, Rachel, Crawford, Hal, Graydon, J.J. and Pinder, Marjorie (1959) Immunological tolerance within the ABO blood group system. *Brit. J. Haemat.* **5**, 232.

Jakobowicz, Rachel, Simmons, R.T. and Carew, J.P. (1961) Group A blood incompatibility due to the development of apparent anti-A_1 antibodies in a patient of subgroup A_2. *Vox Sang.* **6**, 320.

Jakobowicz, Rachel, Williams, L. and Silberman, F. (1972) Immunization of Rh negative volunteers by repeated injections of very small amounts of Rh positive blood. *Vox Sang.* **23**, 376.

Jakubowski, Ann A., Souza, L., Kelly, Felicia, Fain, Katherine, Budman, D., Clarkson, B., Bonilla, Mary Ann, Moore, M.A.S. and Gabrilove, Janice (1989) Effects of human granulocyte colony-stimulating factor in a patient with idiopathic neutropenia. *New Engl. J. Med.* **320**, 38–42.

James, J., Stiles, P., Boyce, F. and Wright, J. (1976) The HL-A type of Rg(a –) individuals. *Vox Sang.* **30**, 214.

James, P., Rowe, G.P. and Tozzo, G.G. (1988) Elucidation of alloantibodies in autoimmune haemolytic anaemia. *Vox Sang.* **54**, 167–171.

Janatova, Jarmila and Tack, B.F. (1981) Fourth component of human complement: studies of an amine-sensitive site comprised of a thiol component. *Biochemistry*, **20**, 2394–2402.

Jancik, J. and Schauer, R. (1974) Sialic acid—a determinant of the life-time of rabbit erythrocytes. *Hoppe-Seyler's Z. Physiol. Chem.* **355**, 395

Jandl, J.H. (1955) Sequestration by the spleen of red cells sensitized with incomplete antibody and with metallo-protein complexes (Abstract). *J. clin. Invest.* **34**, 912.

Jandl, J.H., Greenberg, M.S., Yonemoto, R.H. and Castle, W.B. (1956) Clinical determination of the sites of red cell sequestration in hemolytic anemias. *J. clin. Invest.* **35**, 842.

Jandl, J.H. and Greenberg, M.S. (1957) The selective destruction of transfused 'compatible' normal red cells in two patients with splenomegaly. *J. Lab. clin. Med.* **49**, 233.

Jandl, J.H. and Simmons, R.L. (1957) The agglutination and sensitization of red cells by metallic cations: interactions between multivalent metals and the red-cell membrane. *Brit. J. Haemat.* **3**, 19.

Jandl, J.H., Jones, A.R. and Castle, W.B. (1957) The destruction of red cells by antibodies in man. I. Observations on the sequestration and lysis of red cells altered by immune mechanisms. *J. clin. Invest.* **36**, 1428.

Jandl, J.H. and Tomlinson, Ann S. (1958) The destruction of red cells by antibodies in man. II. Pyrogenic, leukocytic and dermal responses to immune hemolysis. *J. clin. Invest.* **37**, 1202.

Jandl, J.H. (1960) The agglutination and sequestration of immature red cells. *J. Lab. clin. Med.* **55**, 662.

Jandl, J.H. and Kaplan, M.E. (1960) The destruction of red cells by antibodies in man. III. Quantitative factors influencing the patterns of hemolysis *in vivo. J. clin. Invest.* **39**, 1145.

Jandl, J.H. (1965) Mechanisms of antibody-induced red cell destruction. *Ser. Haemat.* **9**, 35.

Janot, C., Andreu, G., Schooneman, F. and Salmon, Ch. (1979) Association des polyagglutinabilités de types T et B acquis. A propos d'une observation. *Rev. franç. Transfus. Immunohémat.* **22**, 375–385.

Janson, P.A., Jubelirer, S.J., Weinstein, M.J. and Deykin, D. (1980) Treatment of the bleeding tendency in uremia with cryoprecipitate. *New Engl. J. Med.* **303**, 1318–1322.

Japanese Red Cross Non-A, Non-B Hepatitis Research Group (1991) Effect of screening for hepatitis C virus antibody and hepatitis B virus core antibody on incidence of post-transfusion hepatitis. *Lancet*, **ii**, 1040–1041.

Jayne, D.R.W. (1990) New strategies for plasma exchange in systemic vasculitis. *Transfus. Sci.* **11**, 263–269.

Jeanneney, G. and Servantie, L. (1939) Influence du pH et de la nature du citrate de soude employé sur le rapport sodium/potassium du plasma sanguin citraté. *Soc. Biol. Bordeaux*, **130**, 473.

Jeanneney, G. and Ringenbach, G. (1940) *Traité de la Transfusion Sanguine.* Masson et Cie, Paris.

Jeannet, M., Metaxas-Bühler, M. and Tobler, R. (1964) Anomalie héréditaire de la membrane érythrocytaire avec test de Coombs direct positif et modification de l'antigène de groupe N. *Vox Sang.* **9**, 52.

Jeannet, M., Bodmer, J.G., Bodmer, W.F. and Schapira, M. (1972) Lymphocytoxic sera associated with the ABO and Lewis red cell blood groups, in *Histocompatibility Testing.* Munksgaard, Copenhagen.

Jeffries, D. (1986) Virological aspects of AIDS. *Clinics in Immunology and Allergy*, **6**, 627–644.

Jeje, M.O., Blajchmann, M.A., Steeves, K., Horsewood, P. and Kelton, J.G. (1984) Quantitation of red cell-associated IgG using an immunoradiometric assay. *Transfusion*, **24**, 473–176.

Jenkins, G.C., Polley, Margaret J. and Mollison, P.L. (1960a) Role of C'4 in the antiglobulin reaction. *Nature (Lond.)*, **186**, 482.

Jenkins, W.J., Marsh, W.L., Noades, Jean, Tippett, Patricia, Sanger, Ruth and Race, R.R. (1960b) The I antigen and antibody. *Vox Sang.* **5**, 97.

Jenkins, W.J. and Marsh, W.L. (1961) Autoimmune haemolytic anaemia. Three cases with antibodies specifically active against stored red cells. *Lancet*, **ii**, 16.

Jenkins, W.J., Koster, H.G., Marsh, W.L. and Carter, R.L. (1965a) Infectious mononucleosis: an unsuspected source of anti-i. *Brit. J. Haemat.* **11**, 480.

Jenkins, W.J., Marsh, W.L. and Gold, E.R. (1965b) Reciprocal relationship of antigens 'I' and 'i' in health and disease. *Nature (Lond.)*, **205**, 813.

Jenkins, D.E. and Moore, W.H. (1977) A rapid method for the preparation of high-potency auto and alloantibody eluates. *Transfusion*, **17**, 110.

Jennings, E.R. and Hindmarsh, Corinne (1958) The significance of the minor crossmatch. *Amer. J. clin. Path.* **30**, 302.

Jennings, M.L. (1984) Oligomeric structure and the anion transport function of human erythrocyte band 3 protein. *J. membr. Biol.* **80**, 105–117.

Jensen, K.G. and Freiesleben, E. (1962) Inherited positive Coombs' reaction connected with a weak N-receptor (N_2). *Vox Sang.* **7**, 696.

Jensen, K.G., Freiesleben, E. and Sørensen, S.S. (1965) The survival of red cells incompatible with Rh antibodies demonstrable only by enzyme technique. *Commun. 10th Congr. Europ. Soc. Haemat.*, Strasbourg.

Jervell, F. (1924) Untersuchungen über die Lebensdauer des transfundierten roten Blutkörperchen beim Menschen. *Acta path. microbiol. scand.* **1**, 20.

Jochem, E.-M. (1958a) Rôle des streptocoques dans la panhémagglutination et la polyagglutinabilité. *Ann. Inst. Pasteur*, **95**, 756.

Jochem, E.-M. (1958b) Rôle de *Bacillus anthracis* dans la panhémagglutination. *Ann. Inst. Pasteur*, **95**, 760.

Johnson, A.H., Mowbray, J.F. and Porter, K.A. (1975) Detection of circulating immune complexes in pathological human sera. *Lancet*, **i**, 762.

Johnson, M.H., Plett, M.J., Conant, C.N. and Worthington, M. (1978) Autoimmune hemolytic anemia with anti-S specificity (Abstract). *Transfusion*, **18**, 389.

Johnson, C.A., Brown, B.A. and Lasky, L.C. (1985) Rh immunization caused by osseous allograft (Letter). *New Engl. J. Med.* **312**, 121–122.

Johnston, A.O.B. and Clark, R.G. (1972) Malpositioning of central venous catheters. *Lancet*, **ii**, 1395.

Joint Cardiology Committee of the Royal College of Physicians of London and the Royal College of Surgeons of England (1985) Provision of services for the diagnosis and treatment of heart disease in England and Wales. *Brit. Heart. J.* **53**, 477–482.

Joly, H.R. and Weil, M.H. (1969) Temperature of the great toe as an indication of the severity of shock. *Circulation*, **39**, 131.

Jonah, M.M., Carny, E.A. and Rahman, Y.E. (1978) Tissue distribution of EDTA encapsulated within liposomes containing glycolipids or brain phospholipids. *Biochim. Biophys. Acta*, **541**, 321–333.

Jones, A.R., Diamond, L.K. and Allen, F.H. jr (1954a) A decade of progress in the Rh blood-group system. *New Engl. J. Med.* **250**, 283 and 324.

Jones, A.R., Steinberg, A.G., Allen, F.H. jr, Diamond, L.K. and Kriete, B. (1954b) Observations on the new Rh agglutinin anti-f. *Blood*, **9**, 117.

Jones, A.R. and Silver, Sheila (1958) The detection of minor erythrocyte populations by mixed agglutinates. *Blood*, **13**, 763.

Jones, J.H., Kilpatrick, G.S. and Franks, E.H. (1962) Red cell aggregation in dextrose solutions. *J. clin. Path.* **15**, 161.

Jones, J.M., Kekwick, R.A. and Goldsmith, K.L.G. (1969) Influence of polymer on the efficacy of serum albumin as a potentiator of 'incomplete' Rh agglutinins. *Nature (Lond.)*, **224**, 510.

Jones, Jennifer and Mollison, P.L. (1978) A simple and efficient method of labelling red cells with ^{99m}Tc for determination of red cell volume. *Brit. J. Haemat.* **38**, 141.

Jones, R.J., Roe, E.A. and Gupta, J.C. (1980) Controlled trial of pseudomonas immunoglobulin and vaccine in burn patients. *Lancet*, **ii**, 1263–1265.

Jonsson, B. (1936) Zur Frage der heterospezifischen Schwangerschaft. *Acta path. microbiol. scand.* **13**, 424.

Jorda, F.D. (1939) The Barcelona Blood-Transfusion Service. *Lancet*, **i**, 773.

Jordal, K. and Lyndrup, S. (1952) The distribution of C-D and Le^a in 1000 mother-child combinations. *Acta path. microbiol. scand.* **31**, 476.

Jordal, K. (1956) The Lewis blood groups in children. *Acta path. microbiol. scand.* **39**, 399.

Jørgensen, J.R. (1964) Delayed haemolytic transfusion reaction caused by anti-c and anti-E. *Dan. med. Bull.* **11**, 1.

Jørgensen, J. (1975) Foeto-maternal blødning. M.D. Thesis, University of Copenhagen.

Jørgensen, J., Nielsen, M., Laugesen, J. and Stoltenberg, S. (1979) The influence of ionic strength and incubation time on the sensitivity of methods using papainized red cells. *Vox Sang.* **37**, 111–115.

Jørgensen, J., Nielsen, M., Nielsen, C.B. and Normark, J. (1980) The influence of ionic strength, albumin and incubation time on the sensitivity of the indirect Coombs' test. *Vox Sang.* **36**, 186–191.

Jørstad, S., Smeby, L.C., Balstad, T., Wideroe, T.E., Wirum, E., Siegel, J. and Bolso, Marit (1985) Complement activation in single and double filter plasma exchange. *Plasma Ther. Transfus. Technol.* **6**, 111–128.

Joseph, J.I.J., Awer, Erika, Laulicht, Martine and Scudder, J. (1964) Delayed hemolytic transfusion reaction due to appearance of multiple antibodies following transfusion of apparently compatible blood. *Transfusion*, **4**, 367.

Jouvenceaux, A., Adenot, N., Berthoux, F. and Revol, L. (1969) Gamma-globuline anti-D lyophilisée intra-veineuse pour la prévention de l'immunisation anti-Rh. *Rev. franç. Transfus.* **13**, Suppl. 1, 341.

Jouvenceaux, A. (1971) Prévention de l'immunisation anti-Rh. *Rev. franç. Transfus.* **14**, 39.

Joyce, S., Wayne Flye, W. and Mohanakumar, T. (1988) Characterization of kidney cell-specific, non-major histocompatibility complex alloantigen using antibodies eluted from rejected human renal allografts. *Transplantation*, **46**, 362–369.

Judd, W.J. and Jenkins, W.J. (1970) Assay of anti-D using the Technicon AutoAnalyzer and the international standard anti-D typing serum. *J. clin. Path.* **23**, 801.

Judd, W.J., Steiner, E.A., Friedman, B.A. and Oberman, H.A. (1978) Anti-Le^a as an autoantibody in the serum of a Le(a – b +) individual. *Transfusion*, **18**, 436.

Judd, W.J., Issitt, P.D., Pavone, B.G., Anderson, J. and Aminoff, D. (1979a) Antibodies that define NANA-independent MN-system antigens. *Transfusion*, **19**, 12–18.

Judd, W.J., McGuire-Mallory, D., Anderson, K.M., Heath, E.J., Swanson, J., Gray, J.M. and Oberman, H.A. (1979b) Concomitant T- and Tk-activation associated with acquired-B antigens. *Transfusion*, **19**, 293–298.

Judd, W.J., Steiner, E.A. and Cochran, R.K. (1980) Paraben associated auto-anti-Jk^a. Two examples (Abstract). *Transfusion*, **20**, 621.

Judd, W.J., Walter, W.J. and Steiner, E.A. (1981) Clinical and laboratory findings on two patients with naturally-occurring anti-Kell agglutinins. *Transfusion*, **21**, 184–188.

Judd, W.J., Oberman, H.A., Sileniels, Aina and Steiner, E. Ann (1984) Clinical significance of anti-Lan (Letter). *Transfusion*, **24**, 181.

Judd, W.J., Barnes, B.A., Steiner, E.A., Oberman, H.A., Averill, D.B. and Butch, S.H. (1986a) The evaluation of a positive direct antiglobulin test (autocontrol) in pretransfusion testing revisited. *Transfusion*, **26**, 220–224.

Judd, W.J., Wilkinson, S.L., Issitt, P.D., Johnson, T.L., Keren, D.F. and Steiner, E.A. (1986b) Donath–Landsteiner hemolytic anemia due to anti-Pr-like biphasic hemolysin. *Transfusion*, **26**, 423–425.

Judd, W.J., Steiner, Elisabeth A., O'Donnell, D.B. and Oberman, H.A. (1988) Discrepancies in reverse ABO typing due to prozone. How safe is the immediate-spin crossmatch? *Transfusion*, **28**, 334–338.

Judd, W.J. and Steiner, E. Ann (1991) Multiple hemolytic transfusion reactions caused by anti-Do^b (Letter). *Transfusion*, **31**, 477–478.

Judson, P.A. and Anstee, D.J. (1977) Comparative effect of trypsin and chymotrypsin on blood group antigens. *Med. Lab. Sciences*, **34**, 1.

Juji, T., Shibata, Y., Ide, H., Sakakibara, T., Ino, T. and Mori, S. (1989) Post-transfusion graft-versus-host disease in immunocompetent patients after cardiac surgery in Japan (Letter). *New Engl. J. Med.* **321**, 56.

Jungfer. H. (1970) Die Subklassen IgGI, II und III humaner Immunoglobuline G. I. Verteilung von Blutgruppenantikörpern sowie von Gm- und InV-Faktoren auf IgG I, II und III. *Z. Immun.-Forsch.* **139**, 182.

Jungi, T.W. and Barandun, S. (1985) Estimation of the degree of opsonization of homologous erythrocytes by IgG for intravenous and intramuscular use. *Vox Sang.* **49**, 9–20.

Kääriäinen, L., Paloheimo, J., Klemola, E., Mäkelä, T. and Koivuniemi, A. (1966) Cytomegalovirus-mononucleosis: isolation of the virus and demonstration of subclinical infections after fresh blood transfusion in connection with open-heart surgery. *Ann. Med. exp. Fenn.* **44**, 297.

Kaban, B.D., van Buren, C.T., Flechner, S.M., Payne, W.D., Boileau, M. and Kerman, R.H. (1983) Cyclosporine immunosuppression mitigates immunologic risk factors in renal allotransplantation. *Transplant. Proc.* **15**, 2469–2479.

Kabat. E.A. and Berg, D. (1953) Dextran—an antigen in man. *J. Immunol.* **70**, 514.

Kabat, E.A. and Mayer, M.M. (1961) *Experimental Immunochemistry*, 2nd edn. Charles C. Thomas, Springfield, Illinois, U.S.A.

Kabat, E.A. (1973) General features of antibody molecules. Ernest Witebsky Memorial Lecture, in *Specific Receptors of Antibodies, Antigens and Cells*, eds D. Pressman, T.B. Tomasi jr, A.L. Grossberg and N.R. Rose. S. Karger, Basel.

Kafer, E.R. and Collins, Myra, L. (1990) Acute intraoperative hemodilution and perioperative blood salvage. *Anesthesiol. Clinics N. Amer.* **8**, 543–567.

Kahn, R.A., Allen, R.W. and Baldassare, J. (1985a) Alternate sources and substitutes for therapeutic blood components. *Blood*, **66**, 1–12.

Kahn, R.A., Duffy, B.F. and Rode, G.G. (1985b) Ultraviolet irradiation of platelet concentrates abrogates lymphocyte activation without affecting platelet function *in vitro*. *Transfusion*, **25**, 547–550.

Kajiyama, W., Kashiwagi, S., Ikematsum, H., Hayashi, J., Nomura, H. and Okochi, K. (1986) Intrafamilial transmission of adult T cell leukaemia virus. *J. infect. Dis.* **154**, 851–857.

Kalbfleisch, J.D. and Lawless, J.F. (1989) Estimating the incubation time distribution and expected number of cases of transfusion-associated acquired immune deficiency syndrome. *Transfusion*, **29**, 672–676.

Källenius, G., Svenson, S.B., Möllby, R., Cedergren, B., Hultberg, H. and Winberg, J. (1981) Structure of carbohydrate part of receptor on human uroepithelial cells for pyelonephritogenic *Escherichia coli*. *Lancet*, **ii**, 604–606.

Kaltwasser, J.P. (1981) In International Forum: The Hippocratian principle of 'primum nil nocere' demands that the metabolic state of a donor should be normalized prior to a subsequent donation of blood or plasma. How much blood, relative to his body weight, can a donor give over a certain period, without a continuous deviation of iron metabolism in the direction of iron deficiency? *Vox. Sang.* **41**, 336–343.

Kalyanaraman, V.S., Sarngadharan, M.G., Robert-Guroff, M., Miyoshi, I., Blayney, D., Golde, D. and Gallo, R.C. (1982) A new subtype of human T cell leukaemia virus (HTLV-II) associated with a T-cell variant of hairy cell leukaemia. *Science*, **218**, 571–573.

Kamada, N., Davies, H.F.S. and Roser, B. (1981) Reversal of transplantation immunity by liver grafting. *Nature (Lond.)*, **292**, 840–842.

Kamihira, S., Nakashima, S. and Oyakawa, Y. (1987) Transmission of human T cell lymphotropic virus type I by blood transfusion before and after mass screening of sera from seropositive donors. *Vox Sang.* **52**, 43–44.

Kanel, G.C., Davis, I. and Bowman, J.E. (1978) 'Naturally-occurring' anti-K1: possible association with mycobacterium infection. *Transfusion*, **18**, 472.

Kanhai, H.H.H., Gravenhorst, J.B., van't Veer, M.B., Maas, C.J., Beverstock, G.G. and Bernini, L.F. (1984) Chorion villi biopsy in management of severe rhesus isoimmunization (Letter). *Lancet*, **ii**, 157–158.

Kao, K.J. and Scornik, J.C. (1989) Accurate quantitation of the low number of white cells in white cell-depleted blood components. *Transfusion*, **29**, 774–777.

Kaplan, E. and Zuelzer, W.W. (1950) Erythrocyte survival studies in childhood. II. Studies in Mediterranean anaemia. *J. Lab. clin. Med.* **36**, 517.

Kaplan, E. and Hsu, K.S. (1961) Determination of erythrocyte survival in newborn infants by means of Cr^{51}-labelled erythrocytes. *Pediatrics*, **27**, 354.

Kaplan, M.E. and Jandl, J.H. (1961) Inhibition of red cell sequestration by cortisone. *J. exp. Med.* **114**, 921.

Kaplan, C., Niaudet, P., Gagnadoux, M.F., Reznikoff, M.F., Muller, J-Y. and Broyer, M. (1984) Donor-specific blood transfusion and renal graft survival: a 3 year experience in pediatrics, in *Histocompatibility Testing 1984*, eds E.D. Albert, M.P. Baur and W.R. Mayr. Springer-Verlag.

Kaplan, H.S. and Garratty, G. (1985) Predictive value of direct antiglobulin test results. *Diagnostic Med.* **8**, 29–33.

Kaplan, Cecile, Daffos, F., Forestier, F., Cox, W.L., Lyon-Caen, D., Dupuy-Montbrun, N.C. and Salmon, Ch. (1988) Management of allo-immune thrombocytopenia antenatal diagnosis and *in utero* transfusion of maternal platelets. *Blood*, **72**, 340–343.

Kaplan, Cecile, Daffos, F., Forestier, F., Tertian, G., Cahterine, Nicole, Pons, J.C. and Tchernia, Gil (1990) Fetal platelet counts in thrombocytopenic pregnancy. *Lancet*, **ii**, 979–982.

Kaplan, Cecile, Morel-Kopp, M.C., Kroll, H., Kiefel, V., Schlegel, N., Chesnel, N. and Mueller-Eckhardt, C. (1991) HPA-5b (Br^a) neonatal alloimmune thrombocytopenia; clinical and immunological analysis of 39 cases. *Brit. J. Haemat.* **78**, 425–430.

Karayiannis, P., Fowler, M.J.K., Lok, Anna S.F., Greenfield, C., Monjardino, J. and Thomas, H.C. (1985) Detection of serum HBV-DNA by molecular hybridisation. Correlation with HBeAg/anti-HBe status, racial origin, liver histology and hepatocellular carcinoma. *J. Hepatol.* **1**, 99–106.

Karhi, K.K. and Gahmberg, C.G. (1980) Identification of blood group A-active glycoproteins on the human erythrocyte membrane. *Biochem. biophys. Acta*, **622**, 344–354.

Kark, R.M. (1937) Two cases of aplastic anaemia. One with secondary haemochromatosis following 290 transfusions in nine years, the other with secondary carcinoma of the stomach. *Guy's Hosp. Rep.* **87**, 343.

Kark, J.A. (1982) Malaria transmitted by blood transfusion, in *Infectious Complications of Blood Transfusion*, ed E. Tabor, pp. 93–126. Academic Press, New York.

Karle, H. (1969) Destruction of erythrocytes during experimental fever. Quantitative aspects. *Brit. J. Haemat.* **16**, 409.

Karlson, K.E., Garzon, A.A., Shaftan, G.W. and Chu, C.-J. (1967) Increased blood loss associated with administration of certain plasma expanders: Dextran 75, Dextran 40 and hydroxyethyl starch. *Surgery*, **62**, 670.

Karsh, J., Wright, D.G., Klippel, J.H., Decker, J.L., Deisseroth, A.B. and Flye, M.W. (1979) Lymphocyte depletion by continuous flow cell centrifugation in rheumatoid arthritis. *Arthritis Rheum.* **22**, 1055–1059.

Kaslow, R.A., Phair, J.P., Friedman, H.B., Lyter, D., Solomon, R.E., Dudley, J., Polk, B.F. and Blackweiler, B. (1987) Infection with the human immunodeficiency virus: clinical manifestations and their relationship to immune deficiency: a report from the multicenter AIDS Cohort Study. *Ann. intern. Med.* **107**, 474–480.

Kasper, C.K., Graham, J.B., Kernoff, P.B.A., Larrieu, M.J., Rickard, K.A. and Mannucci, P.M. (1989) Hemophilia: state of the art of haematologic care 1988. *Vox Sang.* **56**, 141–144.

Katayama, T., Kikuchi, S. and Tanaka, Y. (1990) Blood screening for non-A, non-B hepatitis by hepatitis C virus antibody assay. *Transfusion*, **30**, 374–376.

Kato, N., Hijikata, M., Ootsuyama, Y., Nakagawa, M., Ohkoshi, S., Sugimura, T. and Shimotohno, K. (1990) Molecular cloning of the human hepatitis C virus genome from Japanese patients with non-A, non-B hepatitis. *Proc. nat. Acad. Sci. USA*, **87**, 9524–9528.

Katz, J. (1969) Transplacental passage of fetal red cells in abortion; increased incidence after curettage and effect of oxytocic drugs. *Brit. med. J.* **4**, 84.

Kawamura, T., Sakagami, K., Haisa, M., Morisaki, F., Takasu, S., Inagaki, M., Oiwa T. and Orita Kunzo. (1989) Induction of anti-idiotypic antibodies by donor-specific blood transfusions. *Transplantation*, **48**, 459–463.

Kaye, D. and Hook, E.W. (1963) The influence of hemolysis on susceptibility to salmonella infection: additional observations. *J. Immunol.* **91**, 518.

Kaye, T., Williams, E.M., Garner, S.F., Leak, M.R. and Lumley, H. (1990) Anti-Sc1 in pregnancy. *Transfusion*, **30**, 439–440.

Kee, D.B. jr. and Wood, J.H. (1984) Rheology of the cerebral circulation. *Neurosurgery*, **15**, 125–131.

Keidan, S.E., Lohoar, Elizabeth and Mainwaring, Dorothy (1966) Acute anuria in a haemophiliac due to transfusion of incompatible plasma. *Lancet*, **i**, 179.

Keith, N.M. (1919) Blood volume in wound shock. *Spec. Rep. Ser. med. Res. Cttee.* (*Lond.*), No. 27.

Kekwick, R.A. and Mackay, Margaret E. (1954) The separation of protein fractions from human plasma with ether. *Spec. Rep. Ser. med. Res. Coun.* (*Lond.*), No. 286.

Keller, A.J. and Urbaniak, S.J. (1978) Intensive plasma exchange on the cell separator: effects on serum immunoglobulins and complement components. *Brit. J. Haemat.* **38**, 531.

Keller, A.J., Chirnside, Ann and Urbaniak, S.J. (1979) Coagulation abnormalities produced by plasma exchange on the cell separator with special reference to fibrinogen and platelet levels. *Brit. J. Haemat.* **42**, 593–603.

Kelton, J.G., Hamid, Colleen, Aker, Sylvia and Blajchman, M.A. (1982a) The amount of

blood group A substance on platelets is proportional to the amount in the plasma. *Blood*, **59**, 980–985.

Kelton, J.G., Inwood, M., Barr, R., Effer, S., Hunter, D., Wilson, W., Ginsburg, D. and Powers, P. (1982b) The prenatal prediction of thrombocytopenia in infants of mothers with clinically diagnosed immune thrombocytopenia. *Amer. J. Obstet. Gynec.* **144**, 449–454.

Kelton, J.G. and 11 others (1984) The relationship among platelet-associated IgG, platelet life span and reticuloendothelial cell function. *Blood*, **63**, 1434–1438.

Kelton, J.G., Smith, J.W., Horsewood, P., Humbert, J.R., Hayward, C.P.M. and Warkentin, T.E. (1990) Gov$^{a/b}$ alloantigen system on human platelets. *Blood*, **75**, 2172–2176.

Kemp, T. (1930) Über den Empfindlichkeitsgrad der Blutkörperchen gegenüber Isohämagglutininen im Föttalleben und im Kindesalter beim Menschen. *Acta path. microbiol. scand.* **7**, 146.

Kendall, A.G. (1976) Clinical importance of the rare erythrocyte antibody anti-Jr^a. *Transfusion*, **16**, 646.

Kennell, C.B. and Muschel, L.H. (1956) Effect of mothers' ABO blood group on isoantibody levels of group O children. *U.S. Armed Forces Med. J.* **7**, 1313.

Kenwright, M.G., Sangster, J.M. and Sachs, J.A. (1976) Development of RhD antibodies after kidney transplantation. *Brit. med. J.* **2**, 151.

Keogh, E.V., North, E.A. and Warburton, M.F. (1948) Adsorption of bacterial polysaccharides to erythrocytes. *Nature* (*Lond.*), **161**, 687.

Kerde, C., Fünfhausen, G., Brunk, Re. and Brunk, Ru. (1960) Über die Gewinnung von hochwertigen Anti-P-Immunserun durch Immunisierung mit Echinokokken-zysten Flüssigkeit. *Z. Immun.-Forsch.* **119**, 216.

Kernoff, P.B.A., Durrant, I.J., Rizza, C.R. and Wright, F.W. (1972) Severe allergic pulmonary oedema after plasma transfusion. *Brit. J. Haemat.* **23**, 777–781.

Kernoff, P.B.A., Lilley, T.P.A. and Tuddenham, E.G.D. (1981) Clinical experience with polyelectrolyte-fractionated porcine Factor VIII concentrate in the treatment of haemophiliacs with antibodies to Factor VIII (Abstract). *Brit. J. Haemat.* **49**, 131–132.

Kernoff, P.B.A., Miller, E.J., Savidge, G.F., Machin, S.J., Dewar, M.S. and Preston, F.E. (1987) Reduced risk of non-A, non-B hepatitis after a first exposure to "wet heated" Factor VIII concentrate. *Brit. J. Haemat.* **67**, 207–211.

Kessinger, A., Armitage, J.O., Landmark, J.D., Smith, D.M. and Weisenburger, D.D. (1988) Autologous peripheral haematopoietic stem cell transplantation restores haematopoietic function following marrow ablative therapy. *Blood*, **71**, 723–727.

Kessinger, Anne and Armitage, J.O. (1991) The evolving role of autologous peripheral stem cell transplantation following high-dose therapy for malignancies (Editorial) *Blood*, **77**, 211–213.

Kessler, G.M. and Sachse, K. (1990) Factor VIII inhibitor associated with monoclonal antibody purified Factor VIII concentrate. *Lancet*, **i**, 1403.

Kevy, S.V., Schmidt, P.J., McGinniss, Mary H. and Workman, W.G. (1962) Febrile, non-hemolytic transfusion reactions and the limited role of leukoagglutinins in their etiology. *Transfusion*, **2**, 7.

Keynes, G. (1949) The history of blood transfusion, in *Blood Transfusion*, ed G. Keynes. John Wright & Sons, Bristol.

Keynes, Sir Geoffrey (1967) Tercentenary of blood transfusion. *Brit. med. J.* **iv**, 410–411.

Khansari, N., Springer, G.F., Merler, E. and Fudenberg, H.H. (1983) Mechanisms for the removal of senescent human erythrocytes from circulation: specificity of the membrane-bound immunoglobulin G, in *Mechanisms of Ageing and Development*, **21**, 49–58. Elsevier Scientific Publishers, Ireland.

Kickler, T.S., Ness, P.M., Herman, J.H. and Bell, W.R. (1986) Studies on the pathophysiology of posttransfusion purpura. *Blood*, **68**, 347–350.

Kickler, T.S., Herman, J.H., Furihata, K., Kunicki, T.J. and Aster, R.H. (1988a) Identification of Bak(b), a new platelet-specific antigen associated with posttransfusion purpura. *Blood*, **71**, 894–898.

Kickler, T.S., Ness, P.M. and Braine, H.G. (1988b) Platelet crossmatching. A direct approach to the selection of platelet transfusions for the alloimmunized thrombocytopenic patient. *Amer. J. clin. Path.* **90**, 69–72.

Kickler, T.S., Bell, W., Drew, H. and Pall, D. (1989) Depletion of white cells from platelet concentrates with a new adsorption filter. *Transfusion*, **29**, 411–414.

Kiefel, V., Santoso, S., Weisheit, M. and Mueller-Eckhardt, Ch. (1987) Monoclonal antibody-specific immobilization of platelet antigen (MAIPA). A new tool for the identification of platelet-reactive antibodies. *Blood*, **70**, 1722–1726.

Kiefel, V., Santoso, S., Katzmann, B. and Mueller-Eckhardt, Ch. (1988) A new platelet-specific alloantigen Br(a). Report on four cases with neonatal alloimmune thrombocytopenia. *Vox Sang.* **54**, 101–106.

Kiefel, V., Santoso, S., Glockner, B., Mayer, W. and Mueller-Eckhardt Ch. (1989a) Post-transfusion purpura associated with an anti-body against an allele of the Bak\u1d43 antigen. *Vox Sang.* **56**, 93–97.

Kiefel, V., Santoso, S., Katzmann, B. and Mueller-Eckhardt, C. (1989b) The Br(a)/Br(b) alloantigen systems on platelets. *Blood*, **73**, 2219–2223.

Kiefel, V., Santoso, S. and Mueller-Eckhardt Ch. (1989c) Autoimmune thrombocytopenic purpura: diversity of glycoprotein specificity of autoantibodies determined with monoclonal antibodies. *Blood*, Suppl. 1, 147a.

Kiefel, V., Slechter, Y., Atias, D., Kroll, H., Santoso, S. and Mueller-Eckhardt, Ch. (1991) Neonatal alloimmune thrombocytopenia due to anti-Br\u1d47 (HPA-5a). Report of three cases in two families. *Vox Sang.* **60**, 244–245.

Kieffer, N., Boizard, B., Didry, D., Wautier, J.L. and Nurden, A.T. (1984) Immunochemical characterization of the platelet-specific alloantigen Lek\u1d43, a comparative study with the Pl\u1d2c\u1d2c alloantigen. *Blood*, **64**, 1212–1219.

Killpack, W.S. (1950) Letter to the Editor. *Lancet*, **ii**, 827.

Kim, B.K., Tanoue, K. and Baldini, M.G. (1974) The shelf-life of previously frozen human platelets. *Proc. Int. Symposium on Blood Platelets*, Istanbul, Turkey.

Kim, B.K., Tanque, L. and Baldini, M.G. (1976) Storage of human platelets by freezing. *Vox Sang.* **30**, 401.

Kim, Y.D. (1980) Immunochemical characteristics of human anti-T antibodies. *Vox Sang.* **39**, 162–168.

Kim, H.C., Barnsley, W. and Sweisfurth, A.W. (1984) Incidence of alloimmunization in multiply transfused pediatric patients (Abstract). *Transfusion*, **24**, 417.

Kim, H.C., Park, C. Lucy, Cowan III, J.H., Fattori, F.D. and August, C.S. (1988) Massive intravascular hemolysis associated with intravenous immunoglobulin in bone marrow transplant recipients. *Amer. J. pediat. Hemat./ Oncol.* **10**, 69–74.

Kim, H.C., McMillan, C.W., White, G.C., Bergman, G.E. and Saidi, P. (1990) Clinical experience of a new monoclonal antibody purified Factor IX: half-life, recovery, and safety in patients with hemophilia B. *Semin. Haemat.* **27**, 30–35.

Kimmel, J.R. and Smith, E.L. (1954) Crystalline papain. I. Preparation, specificity and activation. *J. biol. Chem.* **207**, 515.

King, M.E.E., Breslow, J.L. and Lees, R.S. (1980) Plasma-exchange therapy for homozygous familial hypercholesterolemia. *New Eng. J. Med.* **302**, 1457–1459.

King, J.C. and Sacher, R.A. (1989) Percutaneous umbilical blood sampling, in *Contemporary Issues in Pediatric Transfusion Medicine*, eds

R.A. Sacher and R.G. Strauss, pp. 33–53. Amer. Assoc. Blood Banks, Arlington, VA.

Kiprov, D.D., Busch, D.F., Simpson, D.M., Morand, P.R., Tardelli, G.P., Gallet, J.H., Lippert, R. and Mielke, H. (1984) Antilymphocyte factors in patients with acquired immunodeficiency syndrome, in *Acquired Immune Deficiency Syndrome*, eds M. Gotlieb and J. Goodman, pp. 299–308. Alan R. Liss, New York.

Kirkman, N.N. (1977) Further evidence for a racial difference in frequency of ABO hemolytic disease. *J. Pediat.* **90**, 717.

Kirtland, H.H., Mohler, D.N. and Horwitz, D.A. (1980) Methyldopa inhibition of suppressor-lymphocyte function. *New Engl. J. Med.* **305**, 825–832.

Kiruba, R. and Han, P. (1988) Quantitation of red cell-bound immunoglobulin and complement using enzyme-linked antiglobulin consumption assay. *Transfusion*, **28**, 519–542.

Kissmeyer-Nielsen, F., Bastrup-Madsen, Kirsten and Stenderup, A. (1955) Irregular blood-group antibodies. Incidence and clinical significance. *Dan. med. Bull.* **2**, 202.

Kissmeyer-Nielsen, F. (1960) A further example of anti-Lu^b as a cause of a mild haemolytic disease of the newborn. *Vox Sang.* **5**, 517.

Kissmeyer-Nielsen, F., Jensen, K.B. and Ersbak, J. (1961) Severe haemolytic transfusion reactions caused by apparently compatible red cells. *Brit. J. Haemat.* **7**, 36.

Kissmeyer-Nielsen, F. (1965) Irregular blood group antibodies in 200,000 individuals, *Scand. J. Haemat.* **2**, 331.

Kistler, P. and Nitschmann, H. (1962) Large scale production of human plasma fractions. Eight years experience with the alcohol fractionation procedure of Nitschmann, Kistler and Lergies. *Vox Sang.* **7**, 414–424.

Kitazawa, M. and Ohnishi, Y. (1982) Long term experiment of perfluorochemicals using rabbits. *Virchows Arch.* **398**, 1–10.

Kitchen, L.W., Barin, F., Sullivan, J.L., McLane, M.F., Brettler, D.B., Levine, P.H. and Essex, M. (1984) Aetiology of AIDS-antibodies to human T-cell leukaemia virus (type III) in haemophiliacs. *Nature (Lond.)*, **312**, 367–369.

Kitchen, L.W., Leal, M., Wichman, F., Lissen, E., Ollero, M., Allan, J.S., McLane, M.F. and Essex, M. (1985) Antibodies to HTLV-III in haemophiliacs from Spain. *Blood*, **66**, 1473–1475.

Kiyosawa, K., Akahane, Y., Nagata, A., Koike, Y. and Furata, S. (1982) The significance of blood transfusion in non-A, non-B chronic liver disease in Japan. *Vox Sang.* **43**, 45–52.

Kiyosawa, K. and 10 others (1990) Interrelationship of blood transfusion, non-A, non-B hepatitis and hepatocellular carcinoma: analysis

by detection of antibody to hepatitis C virus. *Hepatology*, **12**, 671–675.

Klarkowski, D.B. (1984) An avid anti-Jk3 antibody detected in a Jk(a – b –) Caucasian propositus: an unusual prenatal finding. *Aust. J. med. lab. Sci.* **5**, 26–28.

Klaassen, R.J.L., Ouwehand, W.H., Huizinga, T.W.J., Engelfriet, C.P. and von dem Borne, A.E.G.Kr. (1990) The Fc-receptor III on cultured human monocytes. Structural similarity with FcRIII of natural killer cells and role in the extracellular lysis of sensitized erythrocytes. *J. Immunol.* **144**, 599–606.

Klaus, G.G.B. (1978) The generation of memory cells. II. Generation of B memory cells with preformed antigen-antibody complexes. *Immunology*, **34**, 643.

Klaus, G.G.B., Humphrey, J.H., Kunkl, Annalisa and Dongworth, D.W. (1980) The follicular dendritic cell: its role in antigen presentation in the generation of immunological memory. *Immunol. Rev.* **53**, 3–59.

Kleihauer, E., Braun, H. and Betke, K. (1957) Demonstration von fetalem Hämoglobin in den Erythrocyten eines Blutausstrichs. *Klin. Wschr.* **35**, 637.

Kleihauer, E. and Betke, K. (1960) Praktische Anwendung des Nachweises von Hb F-haltigen Zellen in fixierten Blutausstrichen. *Internist*, **1**, 292.

Klein, H.G. (1982) Cell separators for red cell exchange, in *Advances in the Pathophysiology, Diagnosis, and Treatment of Sickle Cell Disease*, ed R.B. Scott, *Progress in Clinical and Biological Research*, **98**, 109–116. Alan R. Liss, New York.

Kleine, N. and Heimpel, H. (1965) The early loss of radioactivity in ^{51}Cr survival curves: destruction of cells or loss of the label? *Blood*, **26**, 819.

Kliman, A., Carbone, P.P., Gaydos, L.A. and Freireich, E.J. (1964) Effects of intensive plasmapheresis on normal blood donors. *Blood*, **23**, 647.

Kline, W.E., Press, C., Clay, M.E., McCullough, J.J. and Keashen-Snell, M. (1982) Studies of sera defining a new granulocyte antigen (Abstract). *Transfusion*, **22**, 428.

Kline, R.L., Brothers, T., Halsey, N., Boulos, R., Lairmore, M.D. and Quinn, T.C. (1991) Evaluation of enzyme immunoassays for antibody to human T-lymphotropic viruses type I/II. *Lancet*, **i**, 30–33.

Klingemann, H.G., Shepherd, J.D., Eaves, Connie J. and Eaves, A.C. (1991) The role of erythropoietin and other growth factors in transfusion medicine. *Transfus. Med. Rev.* **1**, 33–47.

Klinman, N.R. and Karush, F. (1967) Equine anti-hapten antibody—V. The nonprecipitability of bivalent antibody. *Immuno-chemistry*, **4**, 387.

Klosters, B.C., Tomar, R.H. and Spera, T.J. (1984) Lymphocytotoxic antibodies in the acquired immune deficiency syndrome (AIDS). *Clin. Immunol. Immunopath.* **30**, 330–335.

Knight, R.J. (1968) Flow rates through disposable intra-venous cannulae. *Lancet*, **ii**, 665–667.

Knowles, R.W., Bai, Y., Daniels, G.L. and Watkins, Winifred (1982a) Monoclonal anti-Type 2 H: an antibody detecting a precursor of the A and B blood group antigens. *J. Immunogenet.* **9**, 69–76.

Knowles, R.W., Bai, Y., Lomas, C., Green, C. and Tippett, Patricia (1982b) Two monoclonal antibodies detecting high frequency antigens absent from red cells of the dominant type of Lu(a – b –) Lu:-3. *J. Immunogenet.* **9**, 353–357.

Knowles, R.W. (1989) Structural polymorphism of the HLA class II α and β chains: summary of the 10th Workshop 2-D gel analysis, in *Immunobiology of HLA*, ed B. Dupont, pp 365–380. Springer-Verlag, New York, Berlin, Heidelberg.

Kobata, A., Grollman, Evelyn F. and Ginsburg, V. (1968) An enzymatic basis for blood type A in humans. *Arch. Biochem. Biophys.* **124**, 609.

Kochwa, S., Rosenfield, R.E., Tallal, L. and Wasserman, L.R. (1961) Isoagglutinins associated with erythroblastosis. *J. clin. Invest.* **40**, 874.

Kochwa, S. and Rosenfield, R.E. (1964) Immunochemical studies of the Rh system. I. Isolation and characterization of antibodies. *J. Immunol.* **92**, 682.

Koepke, J.A., Parks, W.M., Gocken, J.A., Klee, G.G. and Strauss, R.G. (1981) The safety of weekly plateletpheresis: effect on the donors' lymphocyte population. *Transfusion*, **21**, 59–63.

Koerner, K. (1984) Platelet function of room temperature platelet concentrates stored in a new plastic material with high gas permeability. *Vox Sang.* **47**, 406–411.

Kogure, T. and Furukawa, K. (1976) Enzymatic conversion of human group O red cells into group B active cells by α-D-galactosyl-transferases of sera and salivas from group B and its variant types. *J. Immunogenet.* **3**, 147.

Kohan, A.I. and 9 others (1991) Solution of a serious transfusional problem in a patient with antibody to Kp^b (K4). *Vox Sang.* **59**, 216–217.

Kohler, P.F. and Farr, R.S. (1966) Elevation of cord over maternal IgG immunoglobulin: evidence for an active placental IgG transport. *Nature (Lond.)*, **210**, 1070.

Köhler, G. and Milstein, C. (1975) Continuous cultures of fused cells secreting antibody of predefined specificity. *Nature (Lond.)*, **256**, 495.

Koistinen, J. and Sarna, S. (1975) Immunological abnormalities in the sera of IgA-deficient blood donors. *Vox Sang.* **29**, 203.

Koistinen, J. (1975) Selective IgA deficiency in blood donors. *Vox Sang.* **29**, 192.

Koistinen, J. and Leikola, J. (1977) Weak anti-IgA antibodies with limited specificity and non-hemolytic transfusion reactions. *Vox Sang.* **32**, 77.

Kojima, M. and 10 others (1991) Posttransfusion fulminant hepatitis B associated with precore-defective HBV mutants. *Vox Sang.* **60**, 34–39.

Kokkini, G.. Vrionis, G., Liosis, G. and Papaefstathiou, J. (1984) Cold agglutinin syndrome and haemophagocytosis in systemic leishmaniasis. *Scand. J. Haemat.* **32**, 441–445.

Kolb, H.J., Mittermuller, J., Clemm, Ch., Holler, E., Ledderose, G., Brehm, G., Heim, M. and Wilmanns, W. (1990) Donor leukocyte transfusions for treatment of recurrent chronic myelogenous leukaemia in marrow transplant patients. *Blood*, **76**, 2462–2465.

Koller, B.H., Geraghty, D.E., Shimizu, Y., Demars, R. and Orr, H.T. (1988) HLA-E: a novel HLA class I gene expressed in resting T lymphocytes. *J. Immunol.* **141**, 897–904.

Koller, B.H, Geraghty, D.E., Demars, R., Duvick, L., Rich, S.S. and Orr, H.T. (1989) Chromosomal organization of the human major histocompatibility complex class I gene family. *J. exp. Med.* **169**, 469–480.

Konietzko, N., Becker, M. and Schmidt, E.W. (1988) Substitution therapy with alpha-1-Pi in patients with alpha-1-Pi deficiency and progressive pulmonary emphysema. *Dtsch. med. Wschr.* **113**, 369–373.

Konig, A.L., Borner, Ch., Braun, R.W. and Roelcke, D. (1985) Cold agglutinins of anti-Pr$_a$ specificity in rubella embryopathy. *Immunobiology*, **46**, 170.

Kontoghiorghes, G.J. (1991) Oral iron chelation is here (Editorial). *Brit. med. J.* **303**, 1279–1280.

Konugres, A.A., Brown, L.S. and Corcoran, P.A. (1966) Anti-M^A, and the phenotype M^{a}N, of the MN blood group system (a new finding). *Vox Sang.* **11**, 189.

Konugres, Angelyn A. (1978) Transfusion therapy for the neonate, in *A Seminar on Perinatal Blood Banking*. Amer. Assoc. Blood Banks, New Orleans.

Kools, A., Collins, J. and Aster, R.H. (1981) Studies of the ABO antigens of human platelets (Abstract). *Transfusion*, **21**, 615–616.

Korman, A.J., Auffray, C., Schamboeck, A. and Strominger, J.L. (1982) The amino acid sequence and gene organization of the heavy chain of the HLA-DR antigen: homology to immunoglobulins. *Proc. nat. Acad. Sci. USA,* **79**, 6013–6017.

Korn, R.J., Yakulis, V.J., Lemke, C.E. and Chamet, B. (1957) Cold agglutinins in *Listeria monocytogenes* infections. *Arch. intern. Med.* **99**, 573.

Kornbrust, O.J., Barfknecht, T.R., Ingram, P. and Shelburne, J.D. (1984) Effect of di(2-ethylhexyl) phthalate on DNA repair and lipid peroxidation in rat hepatocytes and on metabolic cooperation in chinese hamster V-79 cells. *J. Toxicol. environ. Health,* **13**, 99–116.

Kornstad, L. and Heistö, Helge (1957) The frequency of formation of Kell antibodies in recipients of Kell-positive blood. *Proc. 6th Congr. Europ. Soc. Haemat.,* Copenhagen, p. 754.

Kornstad, L. (1969) Anti-Le^b in the serum of Le(a + b –) and Le(a – b –) persons: absorption studies with erythrocytes of different ABO and Lewis phenotypes. *Vox Sang.* **16**, 124.

Kornstad, L. (1983) New cases of irregular blood group antibodies other than anti-D in pregnancy: frequency and clinical significance. *Acta obstet. gynec. scand.* **62**, 431–436.

Kosaka, Y. and 11 others (1991) Fulminant hepatitis B: induction by hepatitis B virus mutants defective in the precore region and incapable of encoding e antigen. *Gastroenterology,* **100**, 1087–1094.

Kosanke, Joanne (1983) Production of anti-Fy^a in Black Fy(a – b –) individuals. *Red Cell Free Press,* **8**, 4–5.

Koskimies, S. (1980) Human lymphoblastoid cell line producing specific antibody against Rh antigen D. *Scand. J. Immunol.* **11**, 73–77.

Kosmin, M. (1980) Bacteremia during leukapheresis. *Transfusion,* **20**, 115.

Kotilainen, M. (1969) Platelet kinetics in normal subjects and in haematological disorders. *Scand. J. Haemat.* Suppl. 5.

Koutras, G.A., Hattori, M., Schneider, A.S., Ebaugh, F.G. jr and Valentine, W.N. (1964) Studies on chromated erythrocytes. Effect of sodium chromate on erythrocyte glutathione reductase. *J. clin. Invest.* **43**, 323.

Koziol, Deloris E. and 9 others (1986) Antibody to hepatitis B core antigen as a paradoxical marker for non-A, non-B hepatitis agents in donated blood. *Ann. intern. Med.* **104**, 488–495.

Krackmalnicoff, A. and Thomas, D.P. (1983) The stability of factor VIII in heparinized plasma. *Thrombos. Haemostas.* **49**, 224–227.

Kramer, S.L., Campbell, C.C. and Moncrieff, R.E. (1983) Fulminant *Plasmodium falciparum* infection treated with exchange blood transfusion. *J. Amer. med. Assoc.* **249**, 244–245.

Krech, U. (1973) Complement fixing antibodies against cytomegalovirus in different parts of the world. *Bull. WHO,* **49**, 103–106.

Krestin, I.G. (1987) Flow through intravenous cannulae. *Anaesthesia,* **42**, 67–70.

Kreuger, A. and Blombäck, Margareta (1974) Exchange transfusion with frozen blood. *Haemostasis,* **3**, 329–339.

Kreuger, A., Åkerblom, O. and Högman. C.F. (1975) A clinical evaluation of citrate–phosphate–dextrose–adenine blood. *Vox Sang.* **29**, 81.

Kreuger, A. (1976) Adenine metabolism during and after exchange transfusions in newborn infants with CPD-adenine blood. *Transfusion,* **16**, 249.

Kreuger, A. and Åkerblom, O. (1980) Adenine consumption in stored citrate–phosphate–dextrose–adenine blood. *Vox Sang.* **38**, 156–160.

Krevans, J.R. and Jackson, D.P. (1955) Hemorrhagic disorder following massive whole blood transfusions. *J. Amer. med. Assoc.* **159**, 171.

Krevans, J.R., Jackson. D.P., Conley C.L. and Hartmann, R.C. (1957) The nature of the hemorrhagic disorder accompanying hemolytic transfusion reactions in man. *Blood,* **12**, 834.

Krevans, J.R. (1959) *In vivo* behaviour of sickle-trait erythrocytes when exposed to continuous hypoxia. *Clin. Res.* **7**, 203.

Krevans, J.R., Woodrow, J.C., Nosenzo, C. and Finn, R. (1964) Patterns of Rh-immunization. *Commun. 10th Congr. Int. Soc. Haemat.,* Stockholm.

Krijnen, H.W., de Wit, J.J.Fr.M., Kuivenhoven, A.C.J., Loos, J.A. and Prins, H.K. (1964) Glycerol treated human red cells frozen with liquid nitrogen. *Vox Sang.* **9**, 559.

Krijnen, H.W., Kuivenhoven, A.C.J. and de Wit, J.J.F.M. (1968) The preservation of blood cells in the frozen state. *Cryobiology,* **5**, 136.

Krijnen, H.W., Kuivenhoven, A.C.J. and de Wit, J.J.F.M. (1970) The preservation of blood cells in the frozen state, in *Modern Problems of Blood Preservation,* eds W. Spielmann and S. Seidl. Gustav Fischer, Stuttgart.

Krogsgaard, K., Kryger, P., Aldershvile, J., Andersson, P., Brechot, C. and The Copenhagen Hepatitis Acute Programme (1985) Hepatitis B virus DNA in serum from patients with acute hepatitis B. *Hepatology,* **5**, No. 1, 10–13.

Kroll, H., Kiefel, V., Santoso, S. and Mueller-Eckhardt, Ch. (1990) Sr^a, a private platelet antigen on glycoprotein IIIa associated with neonatal alloimmune thrombocytopenia. *Blood,* **76**, 2296–2302.

Kronenberg, H., Kooptzoff, Olga and Walsh, R.J. (1958) Haemolytic transfusion reaction due to anti-Kidd. *Aust. Ann. Med.* **7**, 34.

Kruger, L.M. and Colbert, J.M. (1985) Intra-operative autologous transfusion in children undergoing spinal surgery. *J. pediat. Orthoped.* **5**, 330–332.

Kuehl, G.V., Harkness, D.R., Skrabut, E.M., Bechthold, D.A., Emerson, C.P. and Valeri, C.R. (1981) *In vitro* interactions of ^{51}Cr in human red blood cells and hemolysates. *Vox Sang.* **40**, 260–272.

Kuijpers, R.W.A.M., Modderman, P.W., Bleeker, Pauline M.M., Ouwehand, W.H. and von dem Borne, A.E.G.Kr. (1989) Localization of the platelet specific Ko-system antigen Ko[a]/Ko[b] in GP/1b/1x. *Blood*, **74**, Suppl. I, 226a.

Kuijpers, R.W.A.M., Faber, N.M., Cuypers, H.Th.M., Ouwehand, W.H. and von dem Borne, A.E.G.Kr. (1992a) The N-terminal globular domain of human platelet glycoprotein Ibx has a methionine[145]/threonine[145] amino-acid polymorphism, which is associated with the HPA-2 (Ko) alloantigens. *J. clin. Invest.* **89**, 381–384.

Kuijpers, R.W.A.M., von dem Borne, A.E.G.Kr., Kiefel, V., Mueller-Eckhardt, Ch., Waters, A.H., Zupanska, Barbara, Barz, Dagmar, Taaning, Ellen, Termijtelen, Annemarie and Ouwehand, W.H. (1992b) The leucine[33]/proline[33] substitution in human platelet glycoprotein IIIa determines the HLA DRW52a (DW24) association of the immune response against HPA-1a (Zw[a]/PL[A]1) and HPA-1b(Zw[b]/PL[A]2). *Hum. Immunol.* in press.

Kumpel, Belinda M., Leader, Katherine A., Merry, A.H., Hadley, A.G., Poole, G.D., Blancher, Antoine, Goossens, Dominique, Hughes-Jones, N.C. and Bradley, B.A. (1989a) Heterogeneity in the ability of IgG1 monoclonal anti-D to promote lymphocyte-mediated red cell lysis. *Eur. J. Immunol.* **19**, 2283–2288.

Kumpel, B.M., Wiener, E. Urbaniak, S.J. and Bradley, B.A. (1989b) Human monoclonal anti-D antibodies II. The relationship between IgG subclass, Gm allotype and Fc mediated function. *Brit. J. Haemat.* **71**, 415–420.

Kumpel, B.M. and Hadley, A.G. (1990) Functional interaction of red cells sensitized by IgG1 and IgG3 human monoclonal anti-D with enzyme modified human monocyte and FcR-bearing cell lines. *Molec. Immunol.* **27**, 247–256.

Kühnl, P., Seidl, S. and Böhm. B.O. (1989) Reduction of virus load in blood donations by screening methods, in *Virus Inactivation in Plasma Products*, ed J.J. Morgenthaler, pp. 9–12. *Current Studies in Hematology and Blood Transfusion*. S. Karger, Basel.

Kunicki, T.J., Tuccelli, M., Becker, G.A. and Aster, R.H. (1975) A study of variables af-fecting the quality of platelets stored at room temperature. *Transfusion*, **15**, 414.

Kunicki, T.J. and Aster, R.H. (1979) Isolation and immunologic characterization of the human platelet alloantigen, Pl[A1]. *Molecular Immunology*, **16**, 353–360.

Kunicki, T.J., Pidard, D., Cazenave, J.-P. Nurden, A.T. and Caen, J.P. (1981a) Inheritance of the human platelet alloantigen, Pl[A1], in Glanzmann's thrombasthenia. *J. clin. Invest.* **67**, 712–724.

Kunicki, T.J., Pidard, D., Rosa, J.P. and Nurden, A.T. (1981b) The formation of Ca^{2+}-dependent complexes of platelet membrane glycoproteins IIb and IIIa in solution, as determined by crossed immunoelectrophoresis. *Blood*, **58**, 268–278.

Kunkel, H.G. and Rockey, J.H. (1963) β_2A and other immunoglobulins in isolated anti-A antibodies. *Proc. Soc. exp. Biol.* (*N.Y.*), **113**, 278.

Kuo, G. and 19 others (1989) An assay for circulating antibodies to a major etiologic virus of human non-A, non-B hepatitis. *Science*, **244**, 362–364.

Kurata, Y. and 10 others (1989) New approach to eliminate HLA class I antigens from platelet surface without cell damage: acid treatment at pH 3.0. *Vox Sang.* **57**, 199–204.

Kurlander, R.J., Rosse, W.F. and Logue, G.L. (1978) Quantitative influence of antibody and complement coating of red cells on monocyte-mediated cell lysis. *J. clin. Invest.* **61**, 1309.

Kurtides, E.S., Salkin, M.S. and Widen, A.L. (1966) Hemolytic reaction due to anti-Jk[b]. *J. Amer. med. Assoc.* **197**, 816.

Kusnierz-Alejska, Grazyna and Bochenek, Stanislawa (1992) Haemolytic disease of the newborn due to anti-Di[a] and incidence of the Di[a] antigen in Poland. *Vox Sang.* **62**, 124–126.

Kutt, S.M., Larison, P.J., Lewis, C.A. (1988) Evaluation of a microplate test system for blood banks. *Amer. clin. Prod. Rev.* **7**, 8–11.

Kuwakhara S.S. (1980) Prekallikrein activator (Hageman factor fragment) in human plasma fractions. *Transfusion*, **20**, 433–439.

Kuypers, F.A., van Linde-Sibenius-Trip, Margreet, Roelofsen, B., Op den Kamp, J.A.F., Tanner, M.J.A. and Anstee, D.J. (1985) The phospholipid organisation in the membranes of McLeod and Leach phenotype erythrocytes. *FEBS Letters*, **184**, 20–24.

Kwok, S. Lipka, J.J., McKinney, N., Kellogg, D.E., Poiesz, B., Foung, S.K.H. and Sninsky, J.J. (1990) Low incidence of HTLV infections in random blood donors with indeterminate Western blot patterns. *Transfusion*, **30**, 491–494.

Lacey, P. (1978) An unexpected case of severe

hemolytic disease of the newborn due to anti-D (Abstract). *Transfusion*, **18**, 642.

Lachman, E., Hingley, Susan M., Bates, Gillian, Ward, A.M., Stewart, C.R. and Duncan, Sheila L.B. (1977) Detection and measurement of fetomaternal haemorrhage: serum alpha-fetoprotein and the Kleihauer technique. *Brit. med. J.* **1**, 1377.

Lachmann, P.J. (1979) An evolutionary view of the complement system. *Behring Inst. Mitteil.* **63**, 25–37.

Lachmann, P.J., Pangburn, M.K. and Oldroyd, R.G. (1982) Breakdown of C3bi to C3c, C3d and a new fragment-C3g. *J. exp. Med.* **156**, 205–216.

Lachmann, P.J., Voak, D., Oldroyd, R.C., Downie, D.M. and Bevan, P.C. (1983) Use of monoclonal anti-C3 antibodies to characterise the fragments of C3 that are found on erythrocytes. *Vox Sang.* **45**, 367–372.

Ladipo, O.A. (1972) Management of third stage of labour, with particular reference to reduction of feto-maternal transfusion. *Brit. med. J.* **i**, 721.

Lagaaij, Emma and 9 others (1989) Effect of one-HLA-DR-matched and completely HLA-DR-mismatched blood transfusions on survival of heart and kidney allografts. *New Engl. J. Med.* **321**, 701–705.

Lahav, M., Rosenberg, I. and Wysenbeek, A.J. (1989) Steroid-responsive idiopathic cold agglutinin disease: a case report. *Acta haemat.* **81**, 166–168.

Laine, M.L. and Beattie, K.M. (1985) Frequency of alloantibodies accompanying autoantibodies. *Transfusion*, **25**, 545–546.

Lalezari, P., Nussbaum, M., Gelman, S. and Spaet, T.H. (1960) Neonatal neutropenia due to maternal isoimmunization. *Blood*, **15**, 236.

Lalezari, P. and Bernard, G.E. (1966) A new neutrophile-specific antigen. Its role in the pathogenesis of neonatal neutropenia. *Fed. Proc.* **25**, 371.

Lalezari, P. and Murphy, G.B. (1967) Cold reacting leukocyte agglutinins and their significance, in *Histocompatibility Testing*, eds E.S. Curtoni, P.L. Mattiuz and R.M. Tosi, p. 421. Munksgaard, Copenhagen.

Lalezari, P. (1968) A new method for detection of red blood cell antibodies. *Transfusion*, **8**, 372.

Lalezari. P., Murphy, G.B. and Allen, F.H. (1971) NB1, a new neutrophil antigen involved in the pathogenesis of neonatal neutropenia. *J. clin. Invest.* **50**, 1108.

Lalezari, P., Malamut, Dorothy C., Dreisiger, Martha E. and Sanders, C. (1973) Anti-s and anti-U cold-reacting antibodies. *Vox Sang.* **25**, 390.

Lalezari, P. and Radel, Eva (1974) Neutrophil-specific antigens: immunology and clinical significance. *Semin. Hemat.* **11**, 281.

Lalezari, P., Talleyrand, N.P., Wenz, B., Schoenfeld, M.E. and Tippett, P. (1975a) Development of direct antiglobulin reaction accompanying alloimmunization in a patient with Rh^d (D, category III) phenotype. *Vox Sang.* **28**, 19.

Lalezari, P., Jiang, An-Fu, Yegen, Lonna and Santorineou, Maria (1975b) Chronic autoimmune neutropenia due to anti-NA2 antibody. *New Engl. J. Med.* **293**, 744.

Lalezari, P. (1977) Neutrophil antigens: immunology and clinical implications, in *The Granulocyte: Function and Clinical Utilization, Progress in Clinical and Biological Research*, eds T.J. Greenwalt and G.A. Jamieson, p. 209. Alan R. Liss, New York.

Lalezari, P. and Jiang. A.F. (1980) The manual polybrene test: a simple and rapid procedure for detection of red cell antibodies. *Transfusion*, **20**, 206–211.

Lalezari, P. and Driscoll, Ann M. (1982) Ability of thrombocytes to acquire HLA specificity from plasma. *Blood*, **59**, 167–170.

Lalezari, P., Louie, J.E. and Fadlallah, N. (1982) Serologic profile of alphamethyldopa-induced hemolytic anemia: correlation between cell-bound IgM and hemolysis. *Blood*, **59**, 61–68.

Lamberson, H., McMillan, J., Weiner, L., Williams, M., Clark, D., McMahon, C., Bousman, E. and Patti, A. (1984) Nursery acquired CMV infection in transfused neonates (Abstract). *Transfusion*, **24**, 430.

Lamberson, H.V. (1985) Cytomegalovirus (CMV): the agent, its pathogenesis and its epidemiology, in *Infection, Immunity and Blood Transfusion*, eds. R.Y. Dodd and L.F. Baker, pp. 149–173. Alan R. Liss, New York.

Lambert, S.W. (1908) Melaena neonatorum with report of a case cured by transfusion. *Med. Rec., N.Y.* **73**, 885.

Lambert, R., Edwards, Jacqueline and Anstee, D.J. (1978) A simple method for the standardization of proteolytic enzymes used in blood group serology. *Med. Lab. Sciences*, **35**, 233.

Lampe, T.L., Moore, S.B. and Pineda, A.A. (1979) Survival studies of Lan-positive red blood cells in a patient with anti-Lan (Abstract). *Transfusion*, **19**, 640.

Landois, L. (1875) *Die Transfusion des Blutes*. F.C.W. Vogel, Leipzig.

Landsteiner, K. (1900) Zur Kenntnis der anti-fermentativen, lytischen und agglutinierenden Wirkungen des Blutserums und der Lymphe. *Zbl. Bakt.* **27**, 357.

Landsteiner, K. (1901) Über Agglutinationserscheinungen normalen menschlichen Blutes. *Klin. Wschr.* **14**, 1132.

Landsteiner, K. (1903) Über Beziehungen zwischen dem Blutserum und den Körperzellen. *Münch. med. Wschr.* **50**, 1812.

Landsteiner, K. and Miller, C.P. (1925) Serological studies on the blood of the primates. II. The blood groups in anthropoid apes. *J. exp. Med.* **42**, 853.

Landsteiner, K. and Levine, P. (1926) On the cold agglutinins in human serum. *J. Immunol.* **12**, 441.

Landsteiner, K. and Witt, D.H. (1926) Observations on the human blood groups. Irregular reactions. Iso-agglutinin in sera of group 4. The factor A_1. *J. Immunol.* **11**, 221.

Landsteiner, K. and Levine, P. (1927) Further observations on individual differences of human blood. *Proc. Soc. exp. Biol.* (*N.Y.*), **24**, 941.

Landsteiner, K., Levine, P. and Janes, M.L. (1928) On the development of isoagglutinins following transfusions. *Proc. Soc. exp. Biol.* (*N.Y.*), **25**, 672.

Landsteiner, K. and Levine, P. (1929) On isoagglutinin reactions of human blood other than those defining the blood groups. *J. Immunol.* **17**, 1.

Landsteiner, K. (1931) Individual differences in human blood. *Science*, **73**, 405.

Landsteiner, K. and Wiener, A.S. (1940) An agglutinable factor in human blood recognizable by immune sera for Rhesus blood. *Proc. Soc. exp. Biol.* (*N.Y.*), **43**, 223.

Landsteiner, K. and Wiener, A.S. (1941) Studies on an agglutinogen (Rh) in human blood reacting with anti-Rhesus sera and with human iso-antibodies. *J. exp. Med.* **74**, 309.

Landsteiner, E.K. and Finch, C.A. (1947) Hemoglobinemia accompanying transurethral resection of the prostate. *New Engl. J. Med.* **237**, 310.

Lane, T.A. and Windle, B.E. (1979) Granulocyte concentrate preservation: effect of temperature on granulocyte preservation. *Blood*, **54**, 216–255.

Lane, T.A. and Lamkin, G.E. (1984) Hydrogen ion maintenance improves the chemotaxis of stored granulocytes. *Transfusion*, **24**, 231–237.

Lane, T.A. (1990) Granulocyte storage. *Transfus. Med. Rev.* **IV**, 23–35.

Langdell, R.D., Adelson, E., Furth, F.W. and Crosby, W.H. (1958) Dextran and prolonged bleeding time: results of a sixty-gram, one-liter infusion given to one hundred and sixty-three normal human subjects. *J. Amer. med. Assoc.* **162**, 346.

Langenscheidt, F., Kiefel, V., Santoso, S., Nau, A. and Mueller-Eckhardt, Ch. (1989) Quantitation of platelet antigens after chloroquine treatment. *Eur. J. Haemat.* **42**, 186–192.

Langer, R., Linhardt, R.J., Hoffberg, S., Larsen, A.K., Cooney, C.L., Tapper, D. and Klein, M. (1982) An enzymatic system for removing heparin in extracorporeal therapy. *Science*, **217**, 261–263.

Langkilde, N.C., Wolf, H. and Orntoft, T.F. (1990) Lewis negative phenotype and bladder cancer (Letter). *Lancet*, **i**, 926.

Langlois, R.G., Bigbee, W.L. and Jensen, R.H. (1985) Flow cytometric characterization of normal and variant cells with monoclonal antibodies specific for glycophorin A. *J. Immunol.* **134**, 4009–4017.

Lanore, J.J., Quarre, M.C., Audibert, J.D., Chiche, J.D., Woimant, G., Dreyfus, F., Brunet, F., Dhainaut, J.F. and Varet, B. (1989) Acute renal failure following transfusion of accidentally frozen autologous red blood cells. *Vox Sang.* **56**, 293.

Lapierre, Y., Rigal, D., Adam, J., Josef, D., Meyer, F., Greber, S. and Drot, C. (1990) The gel test: a new way to detect red cell antigen-antibody reactions. *Transfusion*, **30**, 109–113.

Lapinid, I.M., Steib, M.D. and Noto, T.A. (1984) Positive direct antiglobulin tests with anti-lymphocyte globulin. *Amer. J. clin. Path.* **81**, 514–17.

Larsen, G.L., McCarthy, K., Webster, R.V., Henson, J. and Henson, P.M. (1980) A differential effect of $C5^a$ and $C5^a$ des Arg. in induction of pulmonary inflammation. *Amer. J. Path.* **100**, 179–192.

Lasky, L.C. (1986) The blood bank as a source of hematopoietic stem cells, in *Transfusion Medicine: Recent Technological Advances*, eds K. Munawski and F. Peetoom, pp. 199–225. Alan R. Liss, New York.

Lathem, W. (1959) The renal excretion of hemoglobin. Regulatory mechanisms and the differential excretion of free and protein-bound hemoglobin. *J. clin. Invest.* **38**, 652.

Lathem, W., Davis, B.B. Zweig, P.H. and Dew, R. (1960) The demonstration and localization of renal tubular reabsorption of hemoglobin by stop flow analysis. *J. clin. Invest.* **39**, 840.

Lattes, L. and Cavazutti, A. (1924) Sur l'existence d'un troisième élément d'isogglutination. *J. Immunol.* **9**, 407.

Lau, P., Sholtis, Carol M. and Aster, R.H. (1980) Post-transfusion purpura: an enigma of alloimmunization. *Amer. J. Hemat.* **9**, 331–336.

Lau, P., Sererat, S., Moore, Vicky, McLeish, K. and Alousi, M. (1983) Paroxysmal cold haemoglobinuria in a patient with klebsiella pneumonia. *Vox Sang.* **44**, 167–172.

Lauer, A. (1941) Zur Konstanz der Blutgruppen. *Z. Immun.-Forsch.* **99**, 433.

Lauf, P.K. and Joiner, C.H. (1976) Increased potassium transport and ouabain binding in human Rh_{null} red blood cells. *Blood*, **48**, 457.

Laurell, C.-B. and Nyman, Margareta (1957) Studies on the serum haptoglobin level in hemoglobinemia and its influence on renal excretion of hemoglobin. *Blood*, **12**, 493.

Laurent, J.C., Noel, P. and Fancon, M. (1978) Expression of a cryptic cell surface antigen in primary cultures from human breast cancer. *Biomedicine*, **29**, 260.

Laurenti, F., Ferro, R., Isacchi, G., Panero, A., Savignoni, P.G., Malagnino, F., Palermo, D., Mandelli, F. and Bucci, G. (1981) Polymorphonuclear leukocyte transfusion in the treatment of sepsis in the newborn infant. *J. Pediat.* **98**, 118–123.

Lauterburg, B.H., Pineda, A.A., Dickson, E.R, Baldus, W.P. and Taswell, H.F. (1978) Plasmaperfusion for the treatment of intractable pruritus and cholestasis. *Mayo Clin. Proc.* **53**, 403.

Law, S.K., Lichtenberg, N.A. and Levine, R.P. (1980) Covalent binding and hemolytic activity of complement proteins. *Proc. nat. Acad. Sci. USA*, **77**, 7194–7198.

Lawler, Sylvia D. and van Loghem, J.J. (1947) The Rhesus antigen C^w causing haemolytic disease of the newborn. *Lancet*, **ii**, 545.

Lawler, Sylvia D. and Shatwell, H.S. (1967) A study of anti-5b-leuco-agglutinins. *Vox Sang.* **13**, 187.

Layrisse, M., Arends, T. and Sisco, R.D. (1955) Nuevo grupo sanguineo encontrado en descendientes de Indios. *Acta med. venez.* **3**, 132.

Layrisse, M. and Arends, T. (1956) The Diego blood factor in Chinese and Japanese. *Nature (Lond.)*, **177**, 1083.

Lazarus, H.M., Kaniecki-Green, Eve A., Warm, Sarah E., Aikawa, M. and Herzig, R.H. (1981) Therapeutic effectiveness of frozen platelet concentrates for transfusion. *Blood*, **57**, 243–249.

Lazarus, H.M. and 9 others (1991) Selective *in vivo* removal of rheumatoid factor by an extracorporeal treatment device in rheumatoid arthritis patients. *Transfusion*, **31**, 122–128.

Leader, K.A., Kumpel, B.M., Poole, G.D., Kirkwood, J.D., Merry, A.H. and Bradley, B.A. (1990) Human monoclonal anti-D with reactivity against category D^VI cells used in blood grouping and determination of the incidence of the category D^VI phenotype in the D^u population. *Vox Sang.* **58**, 106–111.

Leading Article (1980) Haemodynamic monitoring in the intensive care unit. *Brit. med. J.* **280**, 1035–1036.

Leak, M., Poole, J., Kaye, T., Garner, S., Chatfield, C., Milkins, C., Banks, J. and Reid, M. (1990) The rare M^kM^k phenotype in a Turkish antenatal patient and evidence for clinical significance of anti-En^a (Abstract). *Transfusion Med.* **1**, Suppl. 1, 26.

Lechler, R.J. and Batchelor, J.R. (1982) Restoration of immunogenicity to passenger cell depleted kidney allografts by the addition of donor strain dentritic cells. *J. exp. Med.* **155**, 31–41.

Lechner, K., Thaler, E. and Niessner, H. (1983) Ursache, klinische Bedeutung und Therapie von Antithrombin III-Mangelzustanden. *Acta med. Austriaca*, **10**, 129–135.

Leddy, J.P. and Bakemeier, R.F. (1967) A relationship of direct Coombs test pattern to autoantibody specificity in acquired hemolytic anemia. *Proc. Soc. exp. Biol. (N.Y.)*, **125**, 808.

Lederman, M.M., Ratnoff, O.D., Scillian, J.J., Jones, P.K. and Schachter, B. (1983) Impaired cell-mediated immunity in patients with classic haemophilia. *New Engl. J. Med.* **308**, 79–83.

Lee, D., Flowerday, M.H.E. and Tomlinson, J. (1977) The use of IgM anti-D coated cells in the deliberate immunization of Rh-negative male volunteers. *Vox Sang.* **32**, 189.

Lee, D., Remnant, M. and Stratton, F. (1984) 'Naturally occurring' anti-Rh in Rh(D) negative volunteers for immunization. *Clin. lab. Haemat.* **6**, 33–38.

Lee, E.J. and Schiffer, C.A. (1985) Management of platelet alloimmunization, in *Immunological Aspects of Platelet Transfusion*, eds L.F. McCarthy and J.E. Menitove. Amer. Assoc. Blood Banks, Arlington, VA.

Lee, T.H., Kanki, P., McLane, M.F., Tachibana, N. and Essex, M. (1985) Pathobiology of human T-cell leukemia virus, in *Infection, Immunity and Blood Transfusion.* eds R.Y. Dodd and L.F. Barker, pp. 213–221. Alan R. Liss, New York.

Lee, S.I., Heiner, D.C. and Wara, Diane (1986) Development of serum IgG subclass levels in children. *Monograph. Allergy*, **19**, 108–121.

Lee, E.J. and Schiffer, C.A. (1987) Serial measurement of lymphocytotoxic antibody and response to nonmatched platelet transfusion in alloimmunized patients. *Blood*, **70**, 1727–1729.

Lee, E.J. and Schiffer, C.A. (1989) ABO compatibility can influence the results of platelet transfusion. Results of a randomized trial. *Transfusion*, **29**, 384–389.

Lee, H., Swanson, P., Shorty, V.S., Zack, J.A, Rosenblatt, J.D. and Onen, I.S.Y. (1989) High rate of HTLV-II infection in seropositive IV drug abusers in New Orleans. *Science*, **244**, 471–75.

Lee, S., Zambas, Eleni, D., Marsh, W.L. and Redman, C.M. (1991) Molecular cloning and primary structure of Kell blood group protein. *Proc. nat. Acad. Sci. USA*, **88**, 6353–6357.

Leeksma, O.C., Giltay, J.C., Zandbergen-Spaargaren, J., Modderman, P.W., van Mourik, J.A. and von dem Borne, A.E.G.Kr.

(1987) The platelet alloantigen Zwᵃ or Pl^{A1} is expressed on cultured endothelial cells. *Brit. J. Haemat.* **66**, 369–373.

Leen, C.L.S., Yap, P.L., Neill, G., McClelland, D.B.L. and Westwood, A. (1986) Serum ALT levels in patients with primary hypogamma-globulinaemia receiving replacement therapy with intravenous immunoglobulin or fresh frozen plasma. *Vox Sang.* **50**, 26–32.

Leffler, H. and Svanborg-Edén, Catharina (1981) Glycolipid receptors for uropathogenic *Escherichia coli* on human erythrocytes and uro-epithelial cells. *Infection and Immunity*, **34**, 920–929.

Lefrère, J-J., Courouçé, A.M., Bertrand, Y. and Soulier, J.P. (1986) Infections à parvovirus B 19. *Rev. franç. Transfus. Immunohémat.* **29**, 149–162.

Lefrère, J-J., Elghouzzi, Marie-Helene, Paquez, F., N'Dalla, J. and Nubel, L. (1992) Interviews with anti-HIV-positive individuals detected through the systematic screening of blood donations: consequences on predonation medical interview. *Vox Sang.* **62**, 25–28.

Lehane, D. (1967) Production of plasma for making anti-D γ-globulin (Abstract). *Brit. J. Haemat.* **13**, 800.

Lehman, H.A., Lehman, Leorosa O., Rustagi, P.K., Rustgi, R.N., Plunkett, R.W., Farolino, Deborah L., Conway, J. and Logne, G.L. (1987) Complement-mediated autoimmune thrombocytopenia. Monoclonal IgM antiplatelet antibody associated with lymphoreticular malignant disease. *New Engl. J. Med.* **316**, 194–198.

Lehner, P., Hutchings, Patricia, Lydyard, P.M. and Cooke, Anne (1983) Regulation of the immune response by antibody: II. IgM mediated enhancement; dependency on antigen dose. T cell requirement and lack of evidence for an idiotype related mechanism. *Immunology*, **50**, 503–509.

Leikola, J. and Pasanen, V.J. (1970) Influence of antigen receptor density on agglutination of red blood cells. *Int. Arch. Allergy*, **39**, 352.

Leikola, J., Fudenberg, H.H., Vyas, G.N. and Perkins, H.A. (1971) Isoantibodies to human IgM: serologic and immunochemical investigations. *J. Immunol.* **106**, 1147.

Leikola, J., Koistinen, J. Lehtinen, Marja and Virolainen, M. (1973) IgA-induced anaphylactic transfusion reactions: a report of four cases. *Blood*, **42**, 111.

Leikola. J. and Perkins, H.A. (1980a) Enzyme-linked antiglobulin test: an accurate and simple method to quantify red cell antibodies. *Transfusion*, **20**, 138–144.

Leikola, J. and Perkins, H.A. (1980b) Red cell antibodies and low ionic strength: a study with enzyme-linked antiglobulin test. *Transfusion*, **20**, 224–228.

Leikola, J. (1987) Self-sufficiency in blood products: background and overview. *Plasma Therap. transfus. Technol.* **8**, 215–220.

Leikola, J. (1989) Plasma procurement worldwide. *Beitr. Infusionstherap.* **24**, 69–73.

Leikola, J. (1990) Formulation of a national blood programme, in *Management of Blood Transfusion*, eds S.R. Hollan, W. Wagstaff, J. Leikola and F. Lothe. World Health Organization, Geneva.

Leitman, Susan F., Boltansky, H., Alter, H.J., Pearson, F.C. and Kaliner, M.A. (1986) Allergic reactions in healthy plateletpheresis donors caused by sensitization to ethylene oxide gas. *New Engl. J. Med.* **315**, 1192–1196.

Lelie, P.N., van der Poel, C.L., Reesink, H.W. Huisman, H.G. Boucher, C.A.B. and Goudsmit, J. (1989) Efficacy of the latest generation of antibody assays for (early) detection of HIV 1 and HIV 2 infection. *Vox Sang.* **56**, 59–61.

Lemaire, J.M., Coste, J. and Habibi, B. (1991) Attitude pratique devant la découverte d'une sérologie HTLV-I/II positive chez un donneur de sang. *Rev. franç. Transfus. Hémobiol.* **34**, 305–313.

Lenes, B.A. and Sacher, R.A. (1981) Blood component therapy in neonatal medicine. *Clin. lab. Med.* **1**, 285–309.

Lenny, L.L., Hurst, Rosa, Goldstein, J., Benjamin, L.J. and Jones, R.L. (1991) Single-unit transfusion of RBC enzymatically converted from group B to group O to A and O normal volunteers. *Blood*, **77**, 1383–1388.

Leonard, G.L., Ellisor, S.S., Reid, M.E., Sanchez, P.D. and Tippett, P. (1976) An unusual Rh immunization. *Vox Sang.* **31**, 275.

Le Pendu, J., Lemieux, R.U. and Oriol, R. (1982) Purification of anti-Leᶜ antibodies with specificity for βDGal(1–3) βDGlcNAcO using a synthetic immunoadsorbent. *Vox Sang.* **43**, 188–195.

Le Pendu, J. (1983) α-2-L-fucosyltransferase activities of human serum, properties of two distinct enzymes and their relationships with the genetics of H tissue antigens, In *Red Cell Membrane Glycoconjugates and Related Genetic Markers*, eds J.P. Cartron, P. Rouger and C. Salmon, pp. 183–191.

Le Pendu, J., Lambert, F., Gerard, G., Vitrac, D., Mollicone, R. and Oriol, R. (1986) On the specificity of human anti-H antibodies. *Vox Sang.* **50**, 223–226.

Letendre, P.L., Williams, M.A. and Ferguson, D.J. (1987) Comparison of a commercial hexa-dimethrine bromide method and low-ionic-strength solution for antibody detection with special reference to anti-K. *Transfusion*, **27**, 138–141.

Levaditi (1902) État de la cytase hémolytique. *Ann. Inst. Pasteur*, **16**, 233.

Levene, C., Sela, R., Rudolphson, Y., Nathan, A., Karplus, M. and Dvilansky, A. (1977) Hemolytic disease of the newborn due to anti-PP$_1$P^k(anti-Tj^a). *Transfusion*, 17, 569.

Levene, C. (1979) Live children and abortions of p mothers (Letter). *Transfusion*, 19, 224.

Lever, A.M.L., Webster, A.D.B., Brown, D. and Thomas, H.C. (1984) Non-A, non-B hepatitis occurring in agammaglobulinaemic patients after intravenous immunoglobulin. *Lancet*, ii, 1062–1064.

Lever, A.M.L. and Webster, A.D.B. (1987) IgG antibodies in intravenous gammaglobulins. *Lancet*. i, 99.

Levine, P. and Katzin, B.M. (1938) Temporary agglutinability of red cells. *Proc. Soc. exp. Biol. (N.Y.)*, 39, 167.

Levine, P. and Stetson, R. (1939) An unusual case of intra-group agglutination. *J. Amer. med. Assoc.* 113, 126.

Levine, P. and Polayes, S.H. (1941) An atypical hemolysin in pregnancy. *Ann. intern. Med.* 14, 1903.

Levine, P., Burnham, L., Katzin, E.M. and Vogel, P. (1941) The role of iso-immunization in the pathogenesis of erythroblastosis fetalis. *Amer. J. Obstet. Gynec.* 42, 925.

Levine, P. (1943) Serological factors as possible causes in spontaneous abortions. *J. Hered.* 34, 71.

Levine, P. (1944) Landsteiner's concept of the individuality of human blood. *Exp. Med. Surg.* 11, 36.

Levine, P. and Waller, R.K. (1946) Erythroblastosis fetalis in the first-born; prevention of its most severe forms. *Blood*, 1, 143.

Levine, P., Backer, May, Wigod, M. and Ponder, Ruth (1949) A new human hereditary blood property (Cellano) present in 99.8 per cent of all bloods. *Science*, 109, 464.

Levine, P., Bobbitt, O.B., Waller R.K. and Kuhmichel, A. (1951a) Isoimmunization by a new blood factor in tumor cells. *Proc. Soc. exp. Biol. (N.Y.)*, 77, 403.

Levine, P., Kuhmichel, A.B., Wigod, M. and Koch, Elizabeth (1951b) A new blood factor, s, allelic to S. *Proc. Soc. exp. Biol. (N.Y.)*, 78, 218.

Levine, P., Ferraro, L.R. and Koch, E. (1952) Hemolytic disease of the newborn due to anti-S. *Blood*, 7, 1030.

Levine, P., Vogel, P. and Rosenfield, R.E. (1953) Hemolytic disease of the newborn. *Advanc. Pediat.* 6, 97.

Levine, P. and Koch, Elizabeth (1954) The rare human isoagglutinin anti-Tj^a and habitual abortion. *Science*, 120, 239.

Levine, P., Robinson, Elizabeth A., Herrington, L.B. and Sussman, L.N. (1955) Second example of the antibody for the high-incidence blood factor Vel. *Amer. J. clin. Path.* 25, 751.

Levine, P., Robinson, E.A, Layrisse, M., Arends, T. and Sisco, R.D. (1956) The Diego blood factor. *Nature (Lond.)*, 177, 40.

Levine, P., Celano, M. and Staveley, J.M. (1958) The antigenicity of P-substance in echinococcus cyst fluid coated onto tanned red cells. *Vox Sang.* 3, 434.

Levine, P. (1958) The influence of the ABO system on hemolytic disease. *Hum. Biol.* 30, 14.

Levine, P., Celano, M., Fenichel, R., Pollack, W. and Singher, H. (1961a) A 'D-like' antigen in rhesus monkey, human Rh positive and human Rh negative red blood cells. *J. Immunol.* 87, 6.

Levine, P., White, Jane A. and Stroup, Marjory (1961b) Seven Ve^a (Vel) negative members in three generations of a family. *Transfusion*, 1, 111.

Levine, P., Celano, M.J., Vos, G.H. and Morrison, J. (1962) The first human blood ---/---, which lacks the 'D-like' antigen. *Nature (Lond.)*, 194, 304.

Levine, P., Celano, M.J. and Falkowski, F. (1963a) The specificity of the antibody in proxysmal cold hemoglobinuria (P.C.H.). *Transfusion*, 3, 278.

Levine, P., Celano, M.J., Wallace, J. and Sanger, Ruth (1963b) A human 'D-like' antibody. *Nature (Lond.)*, 198, 596.

Levine, B.B., Ojeda, A. and Benacerraf, B. (1963c) Studies of artificial antigens. III. The genetic control of the immune response to hapten-poly-l-lysine conjugates in guinea pigs. *J. exp. Med.* 118, 953.

Levine, P., Celano, M.J., Falkowski, F., Chambers, Jane W., Hunter, O.B. jr. and English, Carol T. (1964) A second example of ---/--- blood or Rh$_{null}$. *Nature (Lond.)*, 204, 892.

Levine, P.H., Brettler, Doreen B. and Sullivan, J.L. (1985) Haemophilia and acquired immune deficiency syndrome, in *Infection, Immunity and Blood Transfusion*, eds R.Y. Dodd and L.F. Barker, pp. 287–296. Alan R. Liss, New York.

Levine, P.H. (1990) The American T-cell leukemia/lymphoma registry (ATLR): an update, in *Human Retrovirology HTLV*, ed W.A. Blattner, pp. 469–473. Raven, New York.

Levy, G.J., Shabot, M.M., Hart, M.E., Mija, W.W. and Goldfinger, D. (1986) Transfusion associated non-cardiogenic pulmonary edema. *Transfusion*, 26, 278–281.

Levy, J.A. (1989) Human immunodeficiency viruses and the pathogenesis of AIDS. *J. Amer. med. Assoc.* 261, 2997–3006.

Levy, P.C., Looney, R.J., Shen, L., Graziano, R.F., Fanger, M.W., Roberts, N.J., Ryan, D.H. and Utell, M.J. (1990) Human alveolar macrophage FcR-mediated cytotoxicity.

Heteroantibody-versus conventional antibody-mediated target cell lysis. *J. Immunol.* **144**, 3693–3700.

Lewis, S. and Clarke, T.K. (1960) A hitherto undescribed phenomenon in ABO haemolytic disease of the newborn. *Lancet*, **ii**, 456.

Lewis, S.M., Dacie, J.V. and Szur, L. (1960) Mechanism of haemolysis in the cold-haemagglutinin syndrome. *Brit. J. Haemat.* **6**, 154.

Lewis, S.M. (1962) Red-cell abnormalities and haemolysis in aplastic anaemia. *Brit. J. Haemat.* **8**, 322.

Lewis, S.M., Grammaticos, P. and Dacie, J.V. (1970) Lysis by anti-I in dyserythropoietic anaemias: role of increased uptake of antibody. *Brit. J. Haemat.* **18**, 465.

Lewis, R., Reid, Marion, Ellisor, Sandra and Avoy, D.R. (1980) A glucose-dependent pan-hemagglutinin. *Vox Sang.* **39**, 205–211.

Lewis, Marion and 27 others (1985) ISBT Working Party on Terminology for Red Cell Surface Antigens: Munich Report. *Vox Sang.* **49**, 171–175.

Lewis, M. and 32 others (1990) Blood group terminology (1990). From the ISBT Working Party on Terminology for Red Cell Surface Antigens. *Vox Sang.* **58**, 152–169.

Lewis, M. and 29 others (1991) ISBT Working Party on Terminology for Red Cell Surface Antigens: Los Angeles Report. *Vox Sang.* **61**, 158–160.

Lewisohn, R. (1915) Blood transfusion by the citrate method. *Surg. Gynec. Obstet.* **21**, 37.

Ley, A.B., Harris, J.P., Brinkley, M., Liles, B., Lack, J.A. and Cahan, A. (1958a) Circulating antibody directed against penicillin. *Science*, **127**, 1118.

Ley, A.B., Mayer, K. and Harris, J.P. (1958b) Observations on a 'specific autoantibody'. *Proc. 6th Congr. Int. Soc. Blood Transfus.*, Boston, 1956.

Ley, T.J., Griffith, Patricia and Nienhuis, A.W. (1982) Transfusion haemosiderosis and chelation therapy. *Clinics in Haematology*, **11**, 437–464.

Li, T.C., Bromham, D.R. and Balmer, B.M. (1988) Fetomaternal macrotransfusion in the Yorkshire region. 1. Prevalence and obstetric factors. *Brit. J. Obstet. Gynaec.* **95**, 1144–1151.

Lian, E.C.Y., Harkness, D.R., Byrnes, J.J., Wallach, H. and Nunez, R. (1979) Presence of a platelet aggregating factor in the plasma of patients with thrombotic thrombocytopenic purpura (TTP) and its inhibition by normal plasma. *Blood*, **53**, 333–338.

Liang, T.J., Hasegawa, K., Rimon, N., Wands, J.R. and Ben-Porath, E. (1991) A hepatitis-B virus mutant associated with an epidemic of fulminant hepatitis. *New Engl. J. Med.* **324**, 1705–1709.

Lichtiger, B. and Hester, J.P. (1986) Transfusion of Rh-incompatible blood components to cancer patients. *Haematologia*, **19**, 81–88.

Lichtman, H.C., Watson, R. Janet, Feldman, F., Ginsburg, V. and Robinson, Jean (1953) Studies on thalassemia. Part I. An extracorpuscular defect in thalassemia major. Part II. The effects of splenectomy in thalassemia major with an associated acquired hemolytic anemia. *J. clin. Invest.* **32**, 1229.

Lieberman, H.M., La Brecque, D.R., Kew, M.C., Hadziyannis, S.J. and Shafritz, D.A. (1983) Detection of hepatitis B virus DNA directly in human serum by a simplified molecular hybridisation test: comparison to HBeAg/anti-HBe status in HBsAg carriers. *Hepatology*, **3**, 285–291.

Liedén, Gudrun (1973) Iron state in regular blood donors. *Scand. J. Haemat.* **11**, 342.

Liedén, Gudrun (1975) Iron supplement to blood donors. I. Trials with intermittent iron supply. *Acta med. scand.* **197**, 31.

Liedén, Gudrun, Höglund, S. and Ehn, L. (1975) Iron supplement to blood donors. II. Effect of continuous iron supply. *Acta med. scand.* **197**, 37.

Liedholm, P. (1971) Feto maternal haemorrhage in ectopic pregnancy. *Acta obstet. gynecol. scand.* **50**, 367.

Liew, Y.W., Bird, G.W.G. and King, M.J. (1982) The human erythrocyte cryptantigen Tk: exposure by an endo-beta galactosidase from *Flavobacterium keratolyticus*. *Rev. franç. Transfus. Immunohémat.* **25**, 639–641.

Liley, A.W. (1961) Liquor amnii analysis in management of pregnancy complicated by rhesus sensitization. *Amer. J. Obstet. Gynec.* **82**, 1359.

Liley, A.W. (1963) Intrauterine transfusion of foetus in haemolytic disease. *Brit. med. J.* **ii**, 1107.

Lillehoj, E.P., Alexander, S.S., Dubrule, C.J., Wiktor, S., Adams, R., Tai, C-C., Manns, Angela, and Blattner, W.A. (1990) Development and evaluation of a human T-cell leukaemia virus type 1 serologic confirmatory assay incorporating a recombinant envelope polypeptide. *J. clin. Microbiol.* **28**, 2653–2658.

Lim, V.S., de Gowin, R.L., Lavola, D., Kirchner, P.T., Abels, R., Perry, P. and Faughan, J. (1989) Recombinant human erythropoietin treatment in pre-dialysis patients. *Ann. intern. Med.* **110**, 108–114.

Lin-Chu, Marie and Broadberry, R. (1990) The Lewis phenotypes among Chinese in Taiwan, in *Second International Workshop on Monoclonal Antibodies against Human Red Cells and Related Antigens*, eds M.A. Chester, U. Johnson, A. Lundblad, B. Low, L. Messeter and B. Samuelson, p. 79. Lund, Sweden.

Lin-Chu, M., Broadberry, R.E., Chang, F.C. and Ting, F. (1991) Hemolytic disease of the newborn (HDN) due to maternal anti-Di[b] in a Chinese infant. *Abstracts, 2nd Congr. W. Pacific Region Int. Soc. Blood Transfus.*, Hong Kong.

Lind, Patricia E. and McArthur, Norma R. (1947) The distribution of 'T' agglutinins in human sera. *Aust. J. exp. Biol. med. Sci.* **25**, 247.

Lindahl-Kiessling, K. and Safwenberg, J. (1971) Inability of UV-irradiated lymphocytes to stimulate allogeneic cells in mixed lymphocyte culture. *Int. Arch. Allergy appl. Immunol.* **41**, 670–678.

Lisowska, E. (1987) MN monoclonal antibodies as blood group reagents, in *Monoclonal Antibodies Against Human Red Blood Cell and Related Antigens*, eds P. Rouger and C. Salmon. Paris.

Lionetti, F.J., Valeri, C.R., Bond, J.C. and Fortier, N.L. (1964) Measurement of hemoglobin binding capacity of human serum or plasma by means of dextran gels. *J. Lab. clin. Med.* **64**, 519.

Litwin, S.D. (1973) Allotype preference in human Rh antibodies. *J. Immunol.* **110**, 717.

Ljungstrom, K-G., Renck, H., Hedin, H., Richter, W. and Wiholm, B.E. (1988) Hapten inhibition and dextran anaphylaxis. *Anaesthesia*, **43**, 729–732.

Lo, K.J. and 10 others (1985) Combined passive and active immunization for interruption of perinatal transmission of hepatitis B virus in Taiwan. *Hepatogastroenterology*, **32**, 65–68.

Lobo, P.I., Westervelt, F.B., White, Clarence and Rudolf, L.E. (1980) Cold lymphocytotoxins: an important cause of acute tubular necrosis occurring immediately after transplantation. *Lancet*, **ii**, 879–881.

Lo Buglio, A.F., Court, W.S., Vincour, L., Maglott, G. and Shaw, G.M. (1983) Immune thrombocytopenic purpura. Use of [121]I-labeled anti-human IgG monoclonal antibody to quantify platelet-bound IgG. *New Engl. J. Med.* **309**, 459–463.

Locasciulli, Anna and 9 others (1991) Hepatitis C virus infection and chronic liver disease in children with leukemia in long-term remission. *Blood*, **78**, 1619–1622.

Loeb, V. jr, Moore, C.V. and Dubach, R. (1953) The physiological evaluation and management of chronic bone marrow failure. *Amer. J. Med.* **15**, 499.

Lomas, Christine G. and Tippett, Patricia (1985) Use of enzymes in distinguishing anti-LW[a] and anti-LW[ab] from anti-D. *Med. Lab. Sciences*, **42**, 88–89.

Lomas, Christine, Bruce, M., Watt, A., Gabra, G.S., Muller, S. and Tippett, Patricia (1986) TAR + individuals with anti-D, a new category D[VII] (Abstract). *Transfusion*, **26**, 560.

Lomas, C., Tippett, P., Thompson, K.M., Melamed, M.D. and Hughes-Jones, N.C. (1989) Demonstration of seven epitopes on the Rh antigen D using human monoclonal anti-D antibodies and red cells from D categories. *Vox Sang.* **57**, 261–264.

Lomberg, Helena, Cedergren, B., Leffler, H., Nilsson, B., Carlström, Ann-Sofie and Svanborg-Edén, Catharina (1986) Influence of blood group on the availability of receptors for attachment of uropathogenic *Escherichia coli. Infection and Immunity*, **51**, 919–926.

London, I.M., Shemin. D., West, R. and Rittenberg, D. (1949) Heme synthesis and red blood cell dynamics in normal humans and in subjects with polycythemia vera, sickle cell anemia and pernicious anemia. *J. biol. Chem.* **179**, 463.

London, I.M. (1961) The metabolism of the erythrocyte. *Harvey Lect.* **56**, 151.

Longster, G.H. and Major, K.E. (1975) Anti-Kell (K1) in ascitic fluid. *Vox Sang.* **28**, 253.

Longster, G. and Giles, C.M. (1976) A new antibody specificity, anti-Rg[a], reacting with a red cell and serum antigen, *Vox Sang.* **30**, 175.

Longster, G.H., North, D.I. and Robinson, E.A.E. (1981) Further examples of anti-In[b] detected during pregnancy. *Clin. lab. Haemat.* **3**, 351–356.

Longster, G.H. and Johnson, E. (1988) IgM anti-D as auto-antibody in a case of cold autoimmune haemolytic anaemia. *Vox Sang.* **54**, 174–176.

Loomes, L.M. and 9 others (1984) Erythrocyte receptors for *Mycoplasma pneumoniae* are sialylated oligosaccharides of Ii antigen type. *Nature (Lond.)*, **307**, 560–562.

Lopas, H. and Birndorf, N.I. (1971) Haemolysis and intravascular coagulation due to incompatible red cell transfusion in isoimmunized monkeys. *Brit. J. Haemat.* **21**, 399.

Lopas, H., Birndorf, N.I. and Robboy, S.J. (1971) Experimental transfusion reactions and disseminated intravascular coagulation produced by incompatible plasma in monkeys. *Transfusion*, **11**, 196.

Lopez, M., Benali, J., Cartron, J.P. and Salmon, C. (1980) Some notes on the specificity of anti-A$_1$ reagents. *Vox Sang.* **39**, 271–276.

Lopez, M., Cartron, J., Cartron, J.P., Mariotti, M., Bony, V., Salmon, C. and Levene, C. (1983) Cytotoxicity of Anti-PP$_1$P[k] antibodies and possible relationship with early abortions of p mothers. *Clin. Immunol. Immunopath.* **28**, 296–303.

Loutit, J.F., Mollison, Margaret D. and van der Walt, E.D. (1942) Venous pressure during venesection and blood transfusion. *Brit. med. J.* **ii**, 658.

Loutit, J.F. and Mollison, P.L. (1943) Advantages

of a disodium-citrate-glucose mixture as a blood preservative. *Brit. med. J.* **ii**, 744.

Loutit, J.F., Mollison, P.L. and Young, I. Maureen (1943) Citric acid-sodium-citrate-glucose mixtures for blood storage. *Quart. J. exp. Physiol.* **32**, 183.

Loutit. J.F. and Mollison, P.L. (1946) Haemolytic icterus (acholuric jaundice) congenital and acquired. *J. Path. Bact.* **58**, 711.

Loutit, J.F. and Morgan, W.T.J. (1946) Unpublished observations.

Lovelock, J.E. (1952) Resuspension in plasma of human red blood cells frozen in glycerol. *Lancet*, **i**, 1238.

Lovelock, J.E. (1953a) The haemolysis of human red blood cells by freezing and thawing. *Biochim. biophys. Acta*, **10**, 414.

Lovelock, J.E. (1953b) The mechanism of the protective action of glycerol against haemolysis by freezing and thawing. *Biochim. biophys. Acta.* **11**, 28.

Lovric, V.A. and Klarkowski, D.B. (1989) Donor blood frozen and stored between −20°C and −25°C with 35-day post-thaw shelf life. *Lancet*, **i**, 71–73.

Löw, B. (1955) A practical method using papain and incomplete Rh-antibodies in routine Rh blood-grouping. *Vox Sang. (O.S.)*, **5**, 94.

Löw, B. and Messeter, L. (1974) Antiglobulin test in low-ionic strength salt solution for rapid antibody screening and cross-matching. *Vox Sang.* **26**, 53.

Low, P.S. (1986) Structure and function of the cytoplasmic domain of band 3: center of erythrocyte membrane-peripheral protein interactions. *Biochim biophys Acta*, **864**, 145–167.

Lowenstein, J., Faulstick, D.A., Yiengst, M.J. and Shock, N.W. (1961) The glomerular clearance and renal transport of hemoglobin in adult males. *J. clin. Invest.* **40**, 1172.

Lowenthal, R.M. (1977) Chronic leukaemias—treatment by leucapheresis. *Exp. Haemat.* **5**, Suppl. 1, 73.

Lown, J.A.G., Holland, P.A.T. and Barr A.L. (1984) Inhibition of serological reactions with enzyme-treated red cells by complement binding alloantibodies. *Vox Sang.* **46**, 300–305.

Lown, J.A.G. and Ivy, J.G. (1988) Laboratory techniques. Polybrene technique for red cell antibody screening using microplates. *J. clin. Path.* **41**, 556–557.

Lozman, J., Powers, S.R. jr, Older, T., Dutton, R.E., Roy, R.J., English, M., Marco, D. and Eckert, C. (1974) Correlation of pulmonary wedge and left atrial pressures. *Arch. Surg.* **109**, 270.

Lubenko, A. (1985) Analysis of the binding site specificity of hyperimmune human anti-A and -A,B sera using monoclonal antibodies

Abstracts 3rd Annual Meeting, Brit. Blood Transfus. Soc., Oxford, p. 61.

Lubenko, A. and Ivanyi, Y. (1986) Epitope specificity of blood-group-A-reactive murine monoclonal antibodies. *Vox Sang.* **51**, 136–142.

Lubenko, A. and Contreras, M. (1989) A review: low-frequency red cell antigens. *Immunohematology*, **5**, 7–14.

Lubenko, A. and Savage, Julia (1989) Analysis of the heterogeneity of the binding site specificities of hyperimmune human anti-A and -A,B sera: the application of competition assays using murine monoclonal antibodies. *Vox Sang.* **57**, 254–260.

Lubenko, A., Savage, J., Forsi, L., Garner, S. and Contreras, M. (1990) Functional and serological analysis of monoclonal anti-D reagents, in *Proceedings of the Second International Workshop and Symposium on Monoclonal antibodies against Human Red Blood Cell Antigens and Related Antigens*, eds M.A. Chester, U. Johnson. A. Lundblad, B. Low, L. Messeter and B. Samuelsson, p. 161. Lund, Sweden.

Lubenko, A. and Contreras, Marcela (1992) The incidence of HDN attributable to anti-Wr^a (Letter). *Transfusion*, **32**, 87–88.

Luce, J.M., Montgomery, A.B., Marks, J.D., Turner, J., Metz, C.A. and Murray, J.F. (1988) Ineffectiveness of high dose methylprednisolone in preventing parenchymal lung injury and improving mortality in patients with septic shock. *Amer. Rev. resp. Dis.* **138**, 62–68.

Ludbrook, J. and Wynn, V. (1958) Citrate intoxication. A clinical and experimental study. *Brit. med. J.* **ii**, 523.

Ludlum, C.A., Chapman, D., Cohen, B. and Litton, P.A. (1989) Antibodies to hepatitis C virus in haemophilia. *Lancet*, **ii**, 560–561.

Ludorf, M., Wolfmeyer, K., Collins, J., Aster, R.H. and McFarland, J.G. (1988) Posttransfusion purpura (PTP) associated with both Pl^{A2} and Bak^a platelet-specific alloantibodies (Abstract) *Blood*, **72**, Suppl., 267a.

Ludvigsen, C.W. jr, Swanson, Jane L., Thompson, T.R. and McCullough, J. (1987) The failure of neonates to form red cell alloantibodies in response to multiple transfusions. *Amer. J. clin. Path.* **87**, 250–251.

Lundberg, W.B. and McGinniss, M.H. (1975) Hemolytic transfusion reaction due to anti-A$_1$. *Transfusion*, **15**, 1.

Lundgren, G. and 11 others (1986) HLA-matching and pretransplant blood transfusions in cadaveric renal transplantation—a changing picture with cyclosporin. *Lancet*, **ii**, 66–69.

Lundsgaard-Hansen, P. (1977a) Volume limitations of plasmapheresis. *Vox Sang.* **32**, 20.

Lundsgaard-Hansen, P. (1977b) Intensive plasmapheresis as a risk factor for arteriosclerotic cardiovascular disease? *Vox Sang.* **33**, 1–4.

Lundsgaard-Hansen, P. and Tschirren, B. (1978) Modified fluid gelatin as a plasma substitute, in *Blood Substitutes and Plasma Expanders*, eds G.A. Jamieson and T.J. Greenwalt. Alan R. Liss, New York.

Lundsgaard-Hansen, P., Bucher, U., Tschirren, B., Haase, S., Kuske, B., Lüdi, H., Stankiewicz, L.A. and Hässig. A. (1978) Red cells and gelatin as the core of a unified program for the national procurement of blood components and derivatives: prediction, performance, and impact on supply of albumin and Factor VIII. *Vox Sang.* **34**, 261.

Lundsgaard-Hansen, P. (1981) Donor safety in plasmapheresis, in joint WHO/IABS Symposium on the Standardization of Albumin, Plasma Substitutes and Plasmapheresis, Geneva, 1980. *Develop. biol. Standard.* **48**, 287–295. S. Karger, Basel.

Lundsgaard-Hansen, P., Ehrengruter, E., Frei, E., Papp, E., Seun, A. and Tschirren, B. (1983) Antithrombin III and related parameters in surgical patients receiving blood components. *Vox Sang.* **46**, 19–28.

Lundsgaard-Hansen, P., Doran, J.E., Rubli, E., Papp, E., Morgenthaler, J. and Spath, P. (1985) Purified fibronectin administration to patients with severe abdominal infections. *Ann. Surg.* **202**, 745–758.

Luner, S.J., Sturgeon, P., Azklarek, D., and McQuiston, D.T. (1975) Effects of proteases and neuraminidase on RBC surface charge and agglutination. A kinetic study. *Vox Sang.* **28**, 184.

Lung, J.A. and Wilson, S.D. (1971) Development of arterio-venous fistula following blood donation. *Transfusion*, **11**, 145.

Lusher, Jeanne M., Shapiro, S.S., Palascak, J.E., Rao, A.V., Levine, P.H., Blatt, P.M. and The Hemophilia Study Group (1980) Efficacy of prothrombin-complex concentrates in hemophiliacs with antibodies to Factor VIII. *New Engl. J. Med.* **303**, 421–425.

Lusher, Jeanne M., Arkin, S., Abilgaard, C.F., Hilgartner, Margaret H. and The Kogenate$_T$ ^{M} Study Group (1991) Observations in previously untreated hemophiliacs receiving (R) F VIII (Abstract). *Thrombos. Haemostas.* Abstract 182.

Luthra, M.G., Friedman, J.M. and Sears, D.A. (1979) Studies of density fractions of normal human erythrocytes labelled with iron-59 in vivo. *J. Lab. clin. Med.* **94**, 879–896.

Lutz, H.U. (1978) Vesicles isolated from ATP-depleted erythrocytes and out of thrombocyte-rich plasma. *J. supramolec. Structure*, **8**, 375–389.

Luyet, B.J. and Gehenio, P.M. (1940) Life and death at low temperature. *Biodynamica*, Normady, Mo., U.S.A.

Lyman, Suzanne, Aster, R.H., Visentin, G.P. and Newman, P. (1990) Polymorphism of human platelet membrane glycoprotein IIb associated with the Bak^a/Bak^b alloantigen system. *Blood*, **75**, 2343–2348.

Lynn, R.I., Honig, Christine L., Jatlow, P.I. and Kliger, A.S. (1979) Resin hemoperfusion for treatment of ethchlorvynol overdose. *Ann. intern. Med.* **91**, 549–553.

Lyon, Mary, F. (1972) X-chromosome inactivation and developmental patterns in mammals. *Biol. Rev.* **47**, 1–35.

MacAfee, C.A.J., Fortune, D.W. and Beischer, N.A. (1970) Non-immunological hydrops fetalis. *J. Obstet. Gynaec. Brit. Cwlth.* **77**, 226.

McAlpine, Lindsay, Parry, J.V. and Tosswill, Jennifer, H.C. (1992) An evaluation of an enzyme immunoassay for the combined detection of antibodies to HIV-1, HIV-2, HTLV-I and HTLV-II. *AIDS*, **6**, 387–391.

McCafferty, J., Griffiths, A.D., Winter, G. and Chiswell, D.J. (1990) Phage antibodies: filamentous phage displaying antibody variable domains. *Nature (Lond.)*, **348**, 552–554.

McCarthy, D.M. and Goldman, J.M. (1984) Transfusion of circulating stem cells. *CRC Crit. Rev. clin. lab. Sci.*, **20**, 1–24.

McCarthy, P.M., Popovsky, M.A., Schaff, H.V., Orszulak, T.A., Williamson, K.R., Taswell, H.F. and Ilstrup, D.M. (1988) Effect of blood conservation efforts in cardiac operations at the Mayo Clinic. *Mayo Clin. Proc.* **63**, 225–229.

McCluskey, D.R. and Boyd, N.A.M. (1990) Anaphylaxis with intravenous gamma-globulin. *Lancet*, **i**, 874.

McCullough, J., Weiblen, Barbara J. and Quie, P.G. (1974) Chemotactic activity of human granulocytes preserved in various anticoagulants. *J. Lab. clin. Med.* **84**, 902–906.

McCullough, J., Weiblen, Barbara J., Peterson, P.K. and Quie, P.G. (1978) Effect of temperature on granulocyte preservation. *Blood*, **52**, 301–310.

McCullough, J., Weiblen, B.J., Clay, M.E. and Forstrom, L. (1981) Effect of leukocyte antibodies on the fate *in vivo* of indium-111-labeled granulocytes. *Blood*, **58**, 164–170.

McCullough, J., Clay, M.E., Richards, K. Forstrom, L. and Loken, M. (1982) Leukocyte antibodies: their effect on the fate *in vivo* of indium-111 labeled granulocytes (Abstract). *Blood*, **60**, 80a.

McCullough, J., Weiblen, Barbara J. and Fine, O. (1983) Effects of storage of granulocytes on their fate *in vivo*. *Transfusion*, **23**, 20–24.

McCullough, J., Clay, M.E., Press, C. and Kline, W. (1988a) *Granulocyte Serology: A Clinical and*

Laboratory Guide. A.S.C.P. Press, American Society of Clinical Pathologists, Chicago.

McCullough, J., Steeper, T.A., Connelly, D.P., Jackson, B., Huntington, Sally and Scott, E.P. (1988b) Platelet utilization in a university hospital. *J. Amer. med. Assoc.* **259**, 2414–2418.

McCurdy, P.R. (1969) ^{32}DFP and ^{51}Cr for measurement of red cell life span in abnormal hemoglobin syndromes. *Blood,* **33**, 214.

MacDonald, K.A. and Marsh, W.L. (1958) Frozen red cells. A modified recovery technique. *J. med. lab. Technol.* **15**, 22.

Macdonald, W.B. and Berg, R.B. (1959) Hemolysis of transfused cells during use of the injection (push) technique for blood transfusion. *Pediatrics,* **23**, 8.

MacDonald, S., Webster, A.D.B. and Platts-Mills, T.A.E. (1982) An analysis of the lymphocytotoxic activity found in sera from patients with hypogammaglobulinaemia. *Scand. J. Immunol.* **15**, 379–382.

MacDonald, E.B. and Gerns, L.M. (1986) The use of murine monoclonal antibodies in blood grouping. *Abstracts, 19th Congr. Int. Soc. Blood Transfus.,* Sydney.

McDougal, J.S., Martin, L.S., Cort, S.P., Mozen, M., Heldebrant, C.M. and Evatt, B.L. (1985) Thermal inactivation of the acquired immunodeficiency syndrome virus, human T-lymphotrophic virus III/lymphadenopathy-associated virus, with special reference to antihemophilic factor. *J. clin. Invest.* **76**, 875–877.

McDowell, M.A., Stocker, I., Nance, S. and Garratty, G. (1986) Auto anti-Sc1 associated with autoimmune hemolytic anemia (Abstract). *Transfusion,* **26**, 578.

McFadzean, A.J.S. and Tsang, K.C. (1956) Antibody formation in cryptogenetic splenomegaly. I. The response to particulate antigen injected intravenously. *Trans. roy. Soc. trop. Med. Hyg.* **50**, 433.

McFadzean, A.J.S., Todd, D. and Tsang, K.C. (1958) Observations on the anemia of cryptogenetic splenomegaly. I. Hemolysis. *Blood,* **13**, 513.

McGinniss, M.H., Schmidt, P.J. and Carbone, P.P. (1964) Close association of I blood group and disease. *Nature (Lond.),* **202**, 606.

McGinniss, Mary H. and Goldfinger, D. (1971) Drug reactions due to passively transfused penicillin antibody. *Commun. Amer. Assoc. Blood Banks,* Chicago.

McGinniss, M.H., Leiberman, R. and Holland, P.V. (1979) The Jk^b red cell antigen and gram-negative organisms. *Transfusion,* **19**, 663.

McGinniss. J.D., MacLowry, J.D. and Holland P.V. (1984) Acquisition of K : 1-like antigen during terminal sepsis. *Transfusion,* **24**, 28–30.

McGrath, K., Wolf, M., Bishop, J., Veale, M.,

Ayberk, H., Szer, J., Cooper, I. and Whiteside, M. (1988) Transient platelet and HLA antibody formation in multitransfused patients with malignancy. *Brit. J. Haemat.* **68**, 345–350.

McGrath, K., Minchinton, R., Cunningham, I. and Ayberk, H. (1989) Platelet anti Bak^b antibody associated with neonatal alloimmune thrombocytopenia. *Vox Sang.* **57**, 182–184.

Machin, S.J., Defreyn, G., Chamone, D.A.F. and Vermylen, J. (1980) Plasma 6-keto PGF$_{ix}$ levels after plasma exchange in thrombotic thrombocytopenic purpura. *Lancet,* **i**, 661.

Machin, S.J., McVerry, B.A., Cheingsong-Popov, R. and Tedder, R.S. (1985) Seroconversion for HTLV-III since 1980 in British haemophiliacs. *Lancet,* **i**, 336.

McHugh, T.M., Reid, Marion E., Stites, D.P., Chase E.S. and Casavant, C.H. (1987) Detection of the human erythrocyte surface antigen Gerbich by flow cytometry using human antibodies and phycoerythrin for extreme immunofluorescence sensitivity. *Vox Sang.* **53**, 231–234.

McIntosh, Sue, O'Brien, R., Schwartz, A. and Pearson, H. (1973) Neonatal isoimmune purpura. Response to platelet infusions. *J. Pediat.* **82**, 1020.

McIntosh, R.V., Docherty, N., Fleming, D. and Foster, P.R. (1987) A high yield Factor VIII concentrate suitable for advanced heat-treatment (Abstract). *Thromb. Haemostas.* **58**, 306.

McIntyre, C., Finigan, L. and Larsen, A.L. (1976) Anti-Co^a implicated in hemolytic disease of the newborn. *Transfusion,* **16**, 76.

MacIntyre, E.A., Linch, D.C., Macey, M.G. and Newland, A.C. (1985) Successful response to intravenous immunoglobulin in autoimmune haemolytic anaemia. *Brit. J. Haemat.* **60**, 387–388.

McKay, D.C. (1965) *Disseminated Intravascular Coagulation. An Intermediary Mechanism of Disease.* Harper & Row, New York.

McKelvey, Jo K. and Edwards, Joann M. (1984) Cold acid elution: another look at a useful technique. *Lab. Med.* **15**, 44 46.

MacKenzie, F.A.F., Elliot, D.H., Eastcott, H.H.G., Hughes-Jones, N.C., Barkhan, P. and Mollison, P.L. (1962) Relapse in hereditary spherocytosis with proven splenunculus. *Lancet,* **i**, 1102.

MacKenzie, M.R., MacKey, Gail and Fudenberg, H.H. (1967) Antibodies to IgM in normal human sera. *Nature (Lond.),* **216**, 690.

MacKenzie, M.R., Brown, Ellen, Fudenberg, H.H. and Goodenday, Lucy (1970a) Waldenström's macroglobulinemia: correlation between expanded plasma volume and increased serum viscosity. *Blood,* **35**, 394.

MacKenzie, M.R., Fudenberg, H.H. and O'Reilly, R.A. (1970b) The hyperviscosity syndrome. I. In IgG myeloma. The role of protein concentration and molecular shape. *J. clin. Invest.* **49**, 15.

MacLean, L.D. and van Tyn, R.A. (1961) Ventricular defibrillation. *J. Amer. med. Assoc.* **175**, 471.

McLean, F.C. and Hastings, A.B. (1934) A biological method for the estimation of calcium ion concentration. *J. biol. Chem.* **107**, 337.

MacLennan, Sheila, Barbara, J.A., Hewitt, Patricia, Moore, Christine and Contreras, Marcela (1992) Screening blood donations for HCV. *Lancet*, **i**, 131–132.

McLeod, B.C. and Sassetti, R.J. (1980) Plasmapheresis with return of cryoglobulin-depleted autologous plasma (cryoglobulin-pheresis) in cryoglobulinemia. *Blood*, **55**, 866–870.

MacLeod, A., Catto, G., Mather, A., Mason, R., Stewart, K., Power, D., Shewan, G. and Urbaniak, S. (1985) Beneficial antibodies in renal transplantation developing after blood transfusion: evidence for HLA linkage. *Transplant. Proc.* **27**, 1057–1058.

McLeod, B.C., Sassetti, R.J., Cole, E.R. and Scott, J.P. (1988) Long-term frequent plasma exchange donation of cryoprecipitate. *Transfusion*, **28**, 307–310.

McLoughlin, K. and Rogers, J. (1970) Anti-Ge^a in an untransfused New Zealand male. *Vox Sang.* **19**, 94.

McManus, T.F. and Borgese, T.A. (1961) Effect of pyruvate on metabolism of inosine by erythrocytes. *Fed. Proc.* **20**, 65.

McMaster Conference (1977) Prevention of Rh immunization. *Vox Sang.* **36**, 50.

McMillan, R., Tani, P., Milland, F., Berchthold, L., Renshaw, L. and Woods, V.L. (1987) Platelet-associated and plasma anti-glycoprotein autoantibodies in chronic ITP. *Blood*, **70**, 1040–145.

McMonigal, K., Horwitz, C.A., Henle, W., Henle, G., Lawton, J., Polesky, H. and Peterson, L. (1983) Post-perfusion syndrome due to Epstein-Barr virus. Report of two cases and review of the literature. *Transfusion*, **23**, 331–335.

McNabb, Trudy, Koh, T-Y, Dorrington, K.J. and Painter, R.H. (1976) Structure and function of immunoglobulin domains. V. Binding of immunoglobulin G and fragments to placental membrane preparations. *J. Immunol.* **117**, 882.

McNair, T.J. and Dudley, H.A.F. (1959) The local complications of intravenous therapy. *Lancet*, **ii**, 365.

McNamara, J.J., Molot, M.D. and Stremple, J.F. (1970) Screen filtration pressure in combat casualties. *Ann. Surg.* **172**, 334.

McNeil, C., Helmick, W.M. and Ferrari, A. (1963) A preliminary investigation into automatic blood grouping. *Vox Sang.* **8**, 235.

MacQuaide, D.H.G. and Mollison, P.L. (1940) Treatment of anaemia with concentrated red cell suspensions. *Brit. med. J.* **ii**, 555.

McShine, R.L. and Kunst, V.A.J.M. (1970) The stimulation of immune antibodies anti-A and anti-B in patients after treatment with cryoprecipitate and factor IX concentrate (P.P.S.B. according to Soulier). *Vox Sang.* **18**, 435.

McSwain, Byrdie and Robins, C. (1988) A clinically significant anti-Cr^a (Letter). *Transfusion*, **28**, 289–290.

McVay, P.A., Hoag, R.W., Hoag, M.S. and Toy, P.T. (1989) Safety and use of autologous blood donation during the third trimester of pregnancy. *Amer. J. Obstet. Gynec.* **160**, 1479–1488.

McVay, P.A., Andrews, A., Kaplan, E.B., Black, D.B., Stehling, L.C., Strauss, R.G. and Toy, P.T.C.Y. (1990) Donation reactions among autologous donors. *Transfusion*, **30**, 249–252.

McVerry, B.A., O'Connor. M.C., Price, A., Tylden, E. and Gorman, A. (1977) Isoimmunisation after narcotic addiction. *Brit. med. J.* **i**, 1324.

Madhok, R. and Forbes, C.D., (1990) HIV-1 infection in haemophilia. The treatment of haemophilia: a double-edged sword, in *Haematology in HIV Disease*, ed Christine Costello. *Baillière's Clinical Haematology*, **3**, 79–101.

Maeda, Y. and 9 others (1984) Prevalence of possible adult T-cell leukemia virus-carriers among volunteer blood donors in Japan: a nation-wide study. *Int. J. Cancer*, **33**, 717–720.

Maffei, L.M. and Thurer, R.L. (1988) Foreword, in *Autologous Blood Transfusion. Current issues.* eds L.M. Maffei and R.L. Thurer, pp. xi–xii. Amer. Assoc. Blood Banks, Arlington, VA.

Magee, J.M. (1985) A study of the effects of treating platelets with paraformaldehyde for use in the platelet suspension immunofluorescence test. *Brit. J. Haemat.* **61**, 513–516.

Magnaval, J.F., Brochier, B., Charlet, J.P., Gonzaga dos Santos, L. and Larrouy, G. (1985) Dépistage de la maladie de Chagas par immunoenzymologie. Comparaison de l'ELISA avec l'immunofluoresence et l'hémagglutination indirecte chez 976 donneurs de sang. *Rev. franç. Transfus. Immunohémat.* **28**, 201–212.

Mahnovski, V., Cheung, Mary H., Lipsey, A.I. and Keyomarsi, K. (1987) Drugs in blood donors. *Clin. Chem.* **33**, 189.

Mainwaring, U.R. and Pickles, Margaret M. (1948) A further case of anti-Lutheran immunization, with some studies on its capacity for human sensitization. *J. clin. Path.* **1**, 292.

Maizels, M. and Paterson, J.H. (1940) Survival of stored blood after transfusion. *Lancet*, **ii**, 417.

Maizels, M. and Whittaker, N. (1940) Diluents for stored blood. *Lancet*, **i**, 590.

Maizels, M. (1941a) Preservation of organic phosphorous compounds in stored blood by glucose. *Lancet*, **i**, 722.

Maizels, M. (1941b) Unpublished report to the Blood Transfusion Research Committee of the Medical Research Council.

Majer, R.V. and Hyde, R.D. (1988) High-dose intravenous immunoglobulin in the treatment of autoimmune haemolytic anaemia. *Clin. lab. Haemat.* **10**, 391–395.

Mäkelä, O. and Mäkelä, P. (1956) Le[b] antigen: studies on its occurrence in red cells, plasma and saliva. *Ann. Med. exp. fenn.* **34**, 157.

Mäkelä, O., Mäkelä, Pirjo and Krüppe, M. (1959) Zur Spezifizität der anti-B Phythämagglutinine. *Z. Immun.-Forsch.* **117**, 220.

Malchesky, P.S., Asanuma, Y., Zawicki, I., Blumenstein, M., Calabrese, L., Kyo, A., Krakauer, R. and Nose, Y. (1980) On-line separation of macromolecules by membrane filtration with cryogelation, in *Plasma Exchange: Plasmapheresis-Plasma-Separation*, ed H.G. Sieberth, pp. 133–139. Schattaver Verlag.

Malde, Ranjan, Kelsall, Gail and Knight, R.C. (1986) The manual low-ionic strength polybrene technique for the detection of red cell antibodies. *Med. lab. Sciences*, **43**, 360–363.

Mallinson, G., Martin, P.G., Anstee, D.J., Tanner, M.J.A., Merry, A.H., Tills, D. and Sonneborn, H.H. (1986) Identification and partial characterization of the human erythrocyte membrane component(s) which express the antigens of the LW blood group system. *Biochem. J.* **234**, 649–652.

Malyska, H., Kleeman, Jeanine E., Masouredis, S.P. and Victoria, E.J. (1983) Effects on blood group antigens from storage at low ionic stength in the presence of neomycin. *Vox Sang.* **44**, 375–384.

Mammen, E.F., Koets, M.N. and Washington, B.C. (1985) Hemostasis during cardiopulmonary bypass surgery. *Semin. Thrombos. Hemostas.* **11**, 281–292.

Mangal, A.K., Growe, G.H., Sinclair, M., Stillwell, G.F., Reeve, C.E. and Naiman, S.C. (1984) Acquired hemolytic anemia due to 'auto'-anti-A or 'auto'-anti-B induced by group O homograft in renal transplant recipients. *Transfusion*, **24**, 201–205.

Mann, J.D., Cahan, A., Gelb, A.G., Fisher, Nathalie, Hamper, Jean, Tippett, Patricia, Sanger, Ruth and Race, R.R. (1962) A sex-linked blood group. *Lancet*, **i**, 8.

Mann, M., Sacks, H.J. and Goldfinger, D. (1983) Safety of autologous blood donation prior to elective surgery for a variety of potentially

"high-risk" patients. *Transfusion*, **23**, 229–232.

Mannarino, A.D. and MacPherson, C.R. (1963) Copper sulfate screening of blood donors: report of a donor passing the test with less than eight grams of hemoglobin. *Transfusion*, **3**, 398.

Mannessier, Lucienne, Rouger, P., Johnson, C.L., Mueller, Kathleen A. and Marsh, W. (1986) Acquired loss of red-cell Wj antigen in a patient with Hodgkin's disease. *Vox Sang.* **50**, 240–244.

Mannoni, P., Bracq, Christine, Yvart, J. and Salmon, Ch. (1970) Anomalie de fonctionnement du locus Rh au cours d'une myélofibrose. *Nouv. Rev. franç. Hémat.* **10**, 381.

Manns, A. and Blattner, W.A. (1991) The epidemiology of the human T-cell lymphotrophic virus type I and type II: etiologic role in human disease. *Transfusion*, **31**, 67–75.

Mannucci, P.M., Lobina, G.F., Caocci, L. and Dioguardi, N. (1969) Effect on blood coagulation of massive intravascular haemolysis. *Blood*, **33**, 207.

Mannucci, P.M., Federici, A.B. and Sirchia, G. (1982) Hemostasis testing during massive blood replacement. *Vox Sang.* **42**, 113–123.

Mannucci, P.M., Colombo, M. and Rodeghiero, F. (1985a) Non-A, non-B hepatitis after factor VIII concentrate treated by heating and chloroform. *Lancet*, **ii**, 1013.

Mannucci, P.M., Amnassari, M., Gringeri, A., Geroldi, D., and Zanetti, A.R. (1985b) Anti-LAV and concentrate consumption in Italian haemophiliacs. *Thrombos. Haemostas.* **54**, 556.

Mannucci, P.M. (1986) Desmopressin (DDAVP) for treatment of disorders of hemostasis. *Prog. Hemostas. Thrombos.* **8**, 19–45.

Mannucci, P.M., Colombo, M., Gatti, L., Rafanelli, D., Colombo, M., Geroldi, D., Einarsson, M. and Zanetti, A.R. (1988) Virucidal treatment of clotting factor concentrates. *Lancet*, **ii**, 782–785.

Mannucci, P.M. (1992) Outbreak of hepatitis A among Italian patients with haemophilia. *Lancet*, **i**, 819.

Manny, W., Levene, C., Sela, R., Johnson, C.L., Mueller, K.A. and Marsh, W.L. (1983) Autoimmunity and the Kell blood groups: autoanti-Kp[b] in a Kp(a + b −) patient. *Vox Sang.* **45**, 252–256.

Mansberger, A.R., Doran, J.E., Treat, R., Hawkins, M., May, J.R., Callaway, B.D., Horowitz, B. and Shulman, R. (1989) The influence of fibronectin administration on the incidence of sepsis and septic mortality in severely injured patients. *Ann. Surg.* **210**, 297.

Manuelidis, E .G. Kim, J.H. Mericangas, J.R. and Manuelidis, L. (1985) Transmission to animals of Jakob–Creutzfeld disease from human blood. *Lancet*, ii, 896–897.

Marcel, Y.L. and Noel, S.P. (1970) Contamination of blood stored in plastic packs. *Lancet*, i, 35.

Marcellin, P., Martinot, M., Boyer, N., Pouteau, M., Aumont, P., Erlinger, S. and Benhamou J-P. (1991) Second generation (RIBA) test in diagnosis of chronic hepatitis C (Letter). *Lancet*, i, 551–552.

Marchal, G., Dausset, J. and Colombani, J. (1960) Fréquence des anticorps anti-plaquettaires chez les malades polytransfusés. *Commun. 8th Congr. Int. Soc. Blood Transfus.*, Tokyo.

Marcus, D.M., and Cass, Louise (1969) Glycosphingolipids with Lewis blood group activity: uptake by human erythrocytes. *Science*, **164**, 553.

Marcus, D.M., Naiki, M. and Kundu, S.K. (1976) Abnormalities in the glycosphingolipid content of human P^k and p erythrocytes. *Proc. nat. Acad. Sci. USA*, **73**, 3263.

Marcus, D.M., Kundu, S.K. and Suzuki. A. (1981) The P blood group system: recent progress in immunochemistry and genetics. *Semin. Haemat.* **18**, 63–71.

Marcus, R.E. and Adams, J. (1983) Leukapheresis in the Sézary syndrome. A case report and review of the literature. *Apheresis Bull.* **1**, 46–50.

Marcus, R.E. and Huehns, E.R. (1985) Transfusional iron overload. *Clin. lab. Haemat.* **7**, 195–212.

Marcus, R.E., Wonke, B., Bantock, H.M., Thomas, M.J.G., Parry, E.S., Taite, H. and Huehns, E.R. (1985) A prospective trial of young red cells in 48 patients with transfusion-dependent thalassaemia. *Brit. J. Haemat.* **60**, 153–159.

Marcus, C.S., Myhre, B.A., Angulo, M.C., Salk, R.D. Essex, C.E. and Demianew, S.H. (1987) Radiolabelled red cell viability I. Comparison of ^{51}Cr, ^{99m}Tc, and ^{111}In for measuring the viability of autologous stored red cells. *Transfusion*, **27**, 415–419.

Margolis, J. (1976) Improvements in production of antihaemophilic factor (Factor VIII) concentrates. *Proc. 11th Congr. Wld. Fed. Haemophilia*, p. 233.

Marker, S.C., Asher, N.L., Kalis, J.M., Simmons, R.L., Najarian, J.S. and Balfour, H.H. jr (1979) Epstein-Barr virus antibody responses and clinical illness in renal transplant recipients. *Surgery*, **85**, 433–440.

Marley, P.B. and Gilbo, C.M. (1981) Temperature sensitivity within the pasteurization temperature range of prekallikrein activator in stable plasma protein solution (SPPS). *Transfusion*, **21**, 320–324.

Marquet, R.L. and Heystek, G.A. (1981) Induction of suppressor cells by donor-specific

blood transfusion and heart transplantation in rats. *Transplantation*, **31**, 272–274.

Marquet, R.L., de Bruin, R.W.F., Dallinga, R.J., Singh, S.K. and Jeekel, J. (1986) Modulation of human growth by allogeneic blood transfusion. *J. Cancer Res. clin. Oncol.* **3**, 50–53.

Marriott, H.L. and Kekwick, A. (1940) Volume and rate in blood transfusion for the relief of anaemia. *Brit. med. J.* i, 1043.

Marsh, W.L. (1972) Scoring of hemagglutination reaction. *Transfusion*, **12**, 352.

Marsh, S.G.E. and Bodmer, J.G. (1989) HLA-DR and -DQ epitopes and monoclonal antibody specificity. *Immunology Today*, **10**, 305–312.

Marsh, W.L. and Redman, C.M.(1990) The Kell blood group system: a review. *Transfusion*, **30**, 158–167.

Marsden, P.D. (1984) Chagas' disease: clinical aspects, in *Recent Advances in Tropical Medicine*, ed H.M. Gilles. pp. 63–87. Churchill Livingstone, Edinburgh.

Marsh, W.L. and Jenkins, W.J. (1960) Anti-i: a new cold antibody. *Nature (Lond.)*, **188**, 753.

Marsh, W.L. (1960) The pseudo B antigen. A study of its development. *Vox Sang.* **5**, 387.

Marsh, W.L. (1961) Anti-i: a cold antibody defining the iI relationship in human red cells. *Brit. J. Haemat.* **7**, 200.

Marsh, W.L. and Jenkins, W.J. (1968) Anti-Sp_1: the recognition of a new cold auto-antibody. *Vox Sang.* **15**, 177.

Marsh, W.L., Nichols, Margaret E. and Jenkins, W.J. (1968) Automated detection of blood group antibodies. *J. med. lab. Technol.* **25**, 335.

Marsh, G.W., Stirling, Yvonne and Mollison, P.L. (1970) Accidental injection of anti-D immunoglobulin to an infant. *Vox Sang.* **19**, 468.

Marsh, W.L., Reid, Marion E. and Scott, Patricia (1972) Autoantibodies of U blood group specificity in autoimmune haemolytic anaemia. *Brit. J. Haemat.* **22**, 625.

Marsh, W.L., Øyen, Ragnhild, Nichols, Margaret E. and Allen, F.H. jr (1975) Chronic granulomatous disease and the Kell blood groups. *Brit. J. Haemat.* **29**, 247.

Marsh, W.L. and Øyen, R. (1978) A study of soluble Lewis and P_1 substances produced for use in immunohematology. *Transfusion*, **18**, 743.

Marsh, W.L., Nichols, M.E., Øyen, R., Thayer, R.S., Deere. W.L. Freed, P.J. and Schmelter, S.E. (1978) Naturally-occurring anti-Kell stimulated by *E. coli* enterocolitis in a 20-day-old child. *Transfusion*, **18**, 149.

Marsh, W.L., Øyen, R., Alicea, Edith, Linter, M. and Horton, Susan (1979) Autoimmune hemolytic anemia and the Kell blood groups. *Amer. J. Hemat.* **7**, 155–162.

Marsh, W.L., Johnson, C.L., DiNapoli, J., Øyen, R., Alicea, E., Rao, A.H. and Chandrasekaran, V. (1980b) Immune hemolytic anemia caused by auto anti-Sd^x: a report on 6 cases (Abstract). *Transfusion*, **20**, 647.

Marsh, W.L., Marsh, N.J., Moore, A., Symmans, W.A., Johnson, C.L. and Redman, C.M. (1981) Elevated serum creatine phosphokinase in subjects with McLeod syndrome. *Vox Sang.* **40**, 403–411.

Marsh, W.L. and Johnson, C.L. (1985) Possible identity of Wj and Anton antigens (Letter). *Transfusion*, **25**, 443–444.

Marshall, Joan V. (1973) The Bg antigens and antibodies. *Canad. J. med. Technol.* **35**, 26.

Marshall, B.E., Ellison, N., Wurzel, H.A., Neufeld, G.R. and Soma, L.R. (1975a) Microaggregate formation in stored blood. II. Influence of anticoagulants and blood components. *Circulatory Shock*, **2**, 185.

Marshall, B.E., Wurzel, H.A., Ellison, N., Neufeld, G.R. and Soma, L.R. (1975b) Microaggregate formation in stored blood. III. Comparison of Bentley, Fenwal, Pall and Swank micropore filtration. *Circulatory Shock*, **2**, 249.

Mårtensson, L. and Fudenberg, H.H. (1965) Gm genes and γG-globulin synthesis in the human fetus. *J. Immunol.* **94**, 514.

Martin, D.J., Lucas, C.E., Ledgerwood, Anna M., Hoschner, Judith, McGonigal, M.D. and Crabon, D. (1985) Fresh frozen plasma supplement to massive red blood cell transfusion. *Ann. Surg.* **202**, 505–511.

Martinez-Letona J., Barbolla, L., Frieyro, E., Bouza, E., Gilsanz, F. and Fernandez, M.N. (1977) Immune haemolytic anaemia and renal failure induced by streptomycin. *Brit. J. Haemat.* **35**, 561.

Martinelli, G.P., Horowitz, Cheryl, Chiang Konan, Racelis, D. and Schauzer, H. (1987) Pretransplant conditioning with donor-specific transfusions using heated blood and cyclosporine. *Transplantation*, **43**, 140–145.

Martlew, Vanessa, J. (1986) Immune haemolytic anaemia and nomifensine treatment in north-west England 1984–85: report of six cases. *J. clin. Path.* **39**, 1147–1150.

Mason. S.J., Muller, L.H., Shiroishi, T., Dvorak, J.A. and McGinniss, M.N. (1977) The Duffy blood group determinants: their role in the susceptibility of human and animal erythrocytes to *Plasmodium knowlesi* malaria. *Brit. J. Haemat.* **36**, 327.

Mason, E.C. (1978) Thaw-syphon technique for the production of cryoprecipitate concentrate of factor VIII. *Lancet*, **ii**, 15.

Masouredis, S.P. (1959) Reaction of I^{131} trace labeled human anti-Rh$_0$ (D) with red cells. *J. clin. Invest.* **38**, 279.

Masouredis, S.P. (1960) Relationship between Rh$_0$ (D) genotype and quantity of ^{131}I anti-Rh$_0$ (D) bound to red cells. *J. clin. Invest.* **39**, 1450.

Masouredis, S.P., Dupuy, Mary E. and Elliot, Margaret (1967) Relationship between Rh$_0$ (D) zygosity and red cell Rh$_0$ (D) antigen content in family members. *J. clin. Invest.* **46**, 681.

Masouredis, S.P., Sudora, E.J., Mahan, L. and Victoria, E.J. (1976) Antigen site densities and ultrastructural distribution patterns of red cell Rh antigens. *Transfusion*, **16**, 94.

Masouredis, S.P., Sudora, E., Mahan, L.C. and Victoria, E.J. (1980a) Immunoelectron microscopy of Kell and Cellano antigens on red cell ghosts. *Haematologia*, **13**, 59–64.

Masouredis, S.P., Sudora, E., Mahan, L. and Victoria, E.J. (1980b) Quantitative immunoferritin microassay of Fy^a, Fy^b, Jk^a, U and Di^b antigen site numbers on human red cells. *Blood*, **56**, 969–977.

Massey, G.V., McWilliams, N.B. and Mueller, D.G. (1987) Intravenous immunoglobulin in neonatal isoimmune thrombocytopenia. *J. Pediat.* **111**, 133–135.

Matsumoto, H., Tamaki, Y., Sato, S. and Shibata, K. (1981) A case of hemolytic disease of the newborn caused by anti-M: serological study of maternal blood. *Acta Obstet. Gynaec. Japan*, **33**, 525–528.

Matté, C. (1971) Le Groupamatic, appareil pour la détermination automatique des groupes sanguins. *Proc. 12th Congr. Int. Soc. Blood Transfus*, Moscow.

Matthew, A.H. (1912) *Life and Times of Rodrigo Borgia*, p. 66.

Matthews, C.D. and Matthews, A.E.B. (1969) Transplacental haemorrhage: spontaneous and induced abortion. *Lancet*, **i**, 694.

Mattingly, J.A. and Waksman, B. (1978) Immunologic suppression after oral administration of antigen. I. Specific suppressor cells formed in rat's Peyer's patches after oral administration of sheep erythrocytes and their systemic migration. *J. Immunol.* **121**, 1878.

Mattox, K.L., Walker, L.E., Beall, A.C. and Jordan, G.L. (1975) Blood availability for the trauma patient—autotransfusion. *J. Trauma*, **15**, 633.

Matuhasi, T. (1959) Plasma protein and antibody fractions observed from the serological point of view. *Proc. 15th Gen. Assembly Jap. Med. Congr.*, Tokyo, **4**, 80.

Matuhasi, T., Kumazawa, H. and Usui, M. (1960) Question of the presence of so-called cross-reacting antibody. *J. Jap. Soc. Blood Transfus.* **6**, 295.

Maunsell, Kate (1944) Urticarial reactions and desensitization in allergic recipients after serum transfusions. *Brit. med. J.* **ii**, 236.

Mawle, Alison, C. and McDougal, J.S. (1992)

Immunologic aspects of human immuno-deficiency virus infection, in *AIDS Testing. Methodology and Management Issues*, eds G. Schochetman and J.R. George, pp. 30–47. Springer-Verlag, New York.

Mayer, K. and D'Amaro, J. (1964) Improvement of methods of differential haemolysis by haemoglobinometry. *Scand. J. Haemat.* **1**, 331.

Mayer, K., Ley, A.B. and D'Amaro, J. (1966) Impairment of red cell viability by exposure to 'excess' acid-citrate dextrose. *Blood*, **28**, 513.

Mayer, K., Dwyer, Andrea and Laughlin, J.S. (1970) Spleen scanning using ACD-damaged red cells tagged with ^{51}Cr. *J. nuclear med.* **11**, 455.

Mayer, K. (1982) A different view of transfusion safety—type and screen, transfusion of Coombs incompatible cells, fatal transfusion induced graft versus host disease, in *Safety in Transfusion Practices*, eds H.F. Polesky and R.H. Walker. College of American Pathologists, Skokie, Illinois.

Mayne, K.M., Bowell, P.J. and Pratt, G.A. (1990a) The significance of anti-Kell sensitization in pregnancy. *Clin. lab. Haemat.* **12**, 379–385.

Mayne, K., Bowell, P., Woodward, T., Sibley, C., Lomas, C. and Tippett, P. (1990b) Rh immunization by the partial D antigen of category D^{Va}. *Brit. J. Haemat.* **76**, 537–539.

Mayr, W.R., Kemkes, Astrid, Kowalkski, Rita, Goertz-Kaiser, Birgit and Mayr Dorotea (1990) Lymphocytotoxic activity in ABH and Lewis monoclonal antibodies, in *the Second International Workshop on Monoclonal Antibodies against Human Red Cells and Related Antigens*, eds M.A. Chester, U. Johnson, A. Lundblad, B. Low, L. Messeter and B. Samuelson, p. 52. Lund, Sweden.

Mazur, P., Leibo, S.P. and Chu, E.H.Y. (1972) A two-factor hypothesis of freezing. *Exp. Cell Res.* **71**, 345.

Means, R.T., Olsen, Nancy J., Krantz, S.B., Dessypris, E.N., Graber, S.E., Stone, W.J., O'Neill, Vicky L. and Pincus, T. (1989) Treatment of the anemia of rheumatoid arthritis with recombinant human erythropoietin: clinical and *in vitro* studies. *Arthritis and Rheumatism*, **32**, 638.

Medearis, A.L., Hensleigh, P.A., Parks, D.R. and Herzenberg, L.A. (1984) Detection of fetal erythrocytes in maternal blood postpartum with the fluorescence-activated cell sorter *Amer. J. Obstet. Gynec.* **148**, 290–295.

Medical Research Council (1944) Report prepared by a Sub-committee of the Blood Transfusion Research Committee. Fainting in blood donors. *Brit. med. J.* **i**, 279.

Medical Research Council (1954) The Rh blood groups and their clinical effects. *Memor. Med. Res. Coun. (Lond.)*, **27**.

Medical Research Council (1957) Thrombophlebitis following intravenous infusions: trial of plastic and red rubber giving-sets. Report of a Sub-committee. *Lancet*, **i**, 595.

Medical Research Council (1969) Hypogamma-globulinaemia in the United Kingdom (Report of a Medical Research Council Working Party). *Lancet*, **i**, 163.

Medical Research Council (1974a) Report of a Working Party on the use of anti-D immunoglobulin for the prevention of isoimmunization of Rh-negative women during pregnancy. *Brit. med. J.* **ii**, 75.

Medical Research Council (1974b) Post-transfusion hepatitis in a London hospital: results of a two-year prospective study. *J. (Camb.)*, **73**, 173.

Medical Research Council (1978) An assessment of the hazards of amniocentesis (Report of a Working Party). *Brit. J. Obstet. Gynaec.* **85**, Suppl. 2, 1.

Meijler, F.L. and Durrer, D. (1959) The influence of polyvinyl-chloride tubing on the isolated perfused rat's heart. *Vox Sang.* **4**, 239.

Melamed, M.D., Gordon, J., Ley, S.J., Edgar, D. and Hughes-Jones, N.C. (1985) Senescence of a human lymphoblastoid clone producing anti-Rhesus(D). *Eur. J. Immunol.* **15**, 742–746.

Melamed, M.D., Thompson, K.M., Gibson, T. and Hughes-Jones, N.C. (1987) Requirements for the establishment of heterohybridomas secreting monoclonal human antibody to rhesus (D) blood group antigen. *J. immunol. Methods*, **104**, 245–251.

Melbye, M. (1986) The natural history of human T-lymphotropic virus-III infection: the cause of AIDS. *Brit. med. J.* **292**, 5–12.

Melbye, M. and 11 others (1986) Evidence for heterosexual transmission and clinical manifestations of human immunodeficiency virus infection and related conditions in Lusaka, Zambia. *Lancet*, **ii**, 1113–1115.

Melbye, M., Biggar, R.J., Wantzin, P., Krogsgaard, K., Ebbesen, P. and Becker, N.G. (1990) Sexual transmission of hepatitis C virus: cohort study (1981–1989) among European homosexual men. *Brit. med. J.* **301**, 210–212.

Mellander, S. and Lewis, D.H. (1963) Effect of hemorrhagic shock on the reactivity of resistance and capacitance vessels and on capillary filtration transfer in cat skeletal muscle. *Circulat. Res.* **11**, 105.

Mellbye, O.J. (1966) Reversible agglutination of trypsinised red cells by a γM globulin synthesized by the human foetus. *Scand. J. Haemat.* **3**, 310.

Mellbye, O.J. (1967) Reversible agglutination of trypsinised red cells by normal human sera. *Scand. J. Haemat.* **4**, 135.

Mellbye, O.J. (1969a) Properties of the trypsinised red cell receptor reacting in reversible agglutination by normal sera. *Scand. J. Haemat.* **6**, 139.

Mellbye, O.J. (1969b) Specificity of natural human agglutinins against red cells modified by trypsin and other agents. *Scand. J. Haemat.* **6**, 166.

Meltz, D.J., Bertles. J.F., David, D.S. and DeCiutiis, A.C. (1971) Delayed haemolytic transfusion reaction with renal failure. *Lancet*, **ii**, 1348.

Menache, D. and 17 others (1990) Evaluation of the safety, recovery, half-life, and clinical efficacy of antithrombin III (human) in patients with hereditary antithrombin III deficiency. *Blood*, **75**, 33–39.

Menitove, J.E. and 10 others (1983) T-lymphocyte subpopulations in patients with classic hemophilia treated with cryoprecipitate and lyophilized concentrates. *New Engl. J. Med.* **308**, 83–86.

Menolasino, N.J., Davidsohn, I. and Lynch, Dorothy E. (1954) A simplified method for the preparation of anti-M and anti-N typing sera. *J. Lab. clin. Med.* **44**, 495.

Menticoglou, S.M., Harman, C.R., Manning, F.A. and Bowman, J.M. (1987) Intraperitoneal fetal transfusion: paralysis inhibits red cell absorption. *Fetal Therapy*, **2**, 154.

Meredith, L.C. (1985) Anti-Fy5 does not react with e variants (Abstract). *Transfusion*, **25**, 482.

Merrill, B.S., Mills, D.L., Rogers, W. and Weinberg, P.C. (1980) Autotransfusion: intraoperative use in ruptured ectopic pregnancy. *J. reprod. Med.* **24**, 14–16.

Merritt, M. and Hardy, J. (1955) Notes on a serum containing anti-P in high titre. *J. clin. Path.* **8**, 329.

Merry, A.H., Thomson, Eileen E., Anstee, D.J and Stratton, F. (1984a) The quantification of erythrocyte antigen sites with monoclonal antibodies. *Immunology*, **51**, 793–800.

Merry, A.H., Thomson, Eileen E., Rawlinson, Violet I. and Stratton, F. (1984b) Quantitation of IgG on erythrocytes: correlation of number of IgG molecules per cell with the strength of the direct and indirect antiglobulin tests. *Vox Sang.* **47**, 73–81.

Merry, A.H., Gardner, B., Parsons, S.F. and Anstee, D.J. (1987) Estimation of the number of binding sites for a murine monoclonal anti-Lu^b on human erythrocytes. *Vox Sang.* **53**, 57–60.

Merry, A.H., Brojer, Eva, Zupanska, Barbara, Hadley, A.G., Kumpel, Belinda, M. and Hughes-Jones, N.C. (1988) Comparison of the ability of monoclonal and polyclonal anti-D antibodies to promote the binding of erythrocytes to lymphocytes, granulocytes and monocytes. *Biochem. Soc. Transact.* **16**, 727–728.

Merry, A.H., Brojer, E., Zupanska, B., Hadley, A.G., Kumpel, B.M. and Hughes-Jones, N.C. (1989) Ability of monoclonal anti-D antibodies to promote the binding of red cells to lymphocytes, granulocytes and monocytes. *Vox Sang.* **56**, 48–53.

Merskey, C. (1949) Red cell fragility, endogenous uric acid and red cell survival in polycythaemia vera. *S. Afr. J. med. Sci.* **14**, 1.

Meryman. H.T. (1956) Mechanics of freezing in living cells and tissues. *Science*, **124**, 515.

Meryman, H.T. (1971) Osmotic stress as a mechanism of freezing injury. *Cryobiology*, **8**, 489–000.

Meryman, H.T. and Hornblower, M. (1972) A method for freezing and washing red blood cells using a high glycerol concentration. *Transfusion*, **12**, 145.

Meryman, H.T. and Hornblower, M. (1976) Freezing and deglycerolizing sickle-trait red blood cells. *Transfusion*, **16**, 627–632.

Meryman, H.T. and Hornblower, M. (1978) Advances in red cell freezing (Abstract). *Transfusion*, **18**, 632.

Meryman, H.T. (1989) Cryopreservation of blood cells and tissues, in *Clinical Practice of Transfusion Medicine*, eds L.D. Petz and S.N. Swisher, 2nd edn, pp. 297–314. Churchill Livingstone, Edinburgh.

Messeter, L. and Johnson, U. (1990) Preface to the proceedings on monoclonal antibodies against human red blood cells and related antigens. *J. Immunogenet.* **17**, 213–215.

Messmer, K., Lewis, D.H., Sunder-Plassman, L., Klovekorn, W.P., Mendler, N. and Holper, K. (1972) Acute normovolemic hemodilution. *Europ. surg. Res.* **4**, 55.

Messmer, K. (1975) Hemodilution. *Surg. Clin. Amer.* **55**, 659.

Messmer, K. (1988) Characteristics, effects and side-effects of plasma substitutes, in *Blood Substitutes. Preparation, Physiology and Medical Applications*, ed K.C. Lowe, pp. 51–70. Ellis Horwood, Chichester.

Messmer, K., Ljungstrom, K-G., Gruber, U-F, Richter, W. and Hedin, H. (1980) Prevention of dextran-induced anaphylactoid reactions by hapten inhibition (Letter). *Lancet*, **i**, 975.

Messmer, K.F.W. (1987) Acceptable haematocrit levels in surgical patients. *World J. Surg.* **11**, 41–46.

Metaxas, M.N. and Metaxas-Bühler, M. (1970) An agglutinating example of anti-Xg^a and Xg^a frequencies in 559 Swiss blood donors. *Vox Sang.* **19**, 527.

Metaxas, M.J., Metaxas-Buehler, M. and Tippett, P. (1975) A 'new' antibody in the P blood group system. *Commun. 14th Congr. Int. Soc. Blood Transfus.*, Helsinki.

Metzger, H. (1970) Structure and function of γM macroglobulin. *Adv. Immunol.* **12**, 57.

Meyer, C.J.L.M., Cnossen, Jetske, Lafeber, Geertruida J.M., Damsteeg, Mieke J.M. and Cats, A. (1982) Autoantibodies against Tμ and B lymphocytes in patients with rheumatoid arthritis. *Clin. exp. Immunol.* **47**, 368–380.

Meyers, J.D., Flournoy, N. and Thomas, E.D. (1986) Risk factors for cytomegalovirus infection after allogeneic marrow transplantation. *J. infect. Dis.* **153**, 478–488.

Meyrick, B.O., Ryan, U.S. and Brigham, K.L. (1986) Direct effects of *E. coli* endotoxin on stucture and permeability of pulmonary endothelial layer of internal implants. *Amer. J. Path.* **122**, 140–151.

Michaelsen, T.E. and Kornstad, L. (1987) IgG subclass distribution of anti-Rh, anti-Kell and anti-Duffy antibodies measured by sensitive haemagglutination assays. *Clin. exp. Immunol* **67**, 637–645.

Michel, F.W. (1964) The occurrence of bloodgroup specific material in the plasma and serum of stored blood. *Vox Sang.* **9**, 471.

Michel, J. and Sharon, R. (1980) Non-haemolytic adverse reaction after transfusion of a blood unit containing penicillin. *Brit. med. J.* **i**, 152–153.

Michlmayr, G., Pathouli, Christina, Huber, C. and Huber, H. (1976) Antibodies for T lymphocytes in systemic lupus erythematosus. *Clin. exp. Immunol.* **24**, 18.

Middleton, Janice and Crookston, Marie (1972) Chido-substance in plasma. *Vox Sang.* **23**, 256.

Middleton, Janice and 13 others (1974) Linkage of Chido and HL-A. *Tissue Antigens.* **4**, 366.

Mielke, C.H. jr, Kaneshiro, M.M., Maher, I.A., Weiner, J.M. and Rapaport, S.I. (1969) The standardized normal Ivy bleeding time and its prolongation by aspirin. *Blood*, **34**, 204.

Miescher, P. and Fauconnet, M. (1954) Mise en évidence de différents groupes leucocytaires chez l'homme. *Schweiz. med. Wschr.* **84**, 597.

Miescher, P. (1956a) Hypersplenie. *Helv. med. Acta*, **23**, 457.

Miescher, P. (1956b) Le mécanisme de l'erythroclasie a l'état normal. *Rev. Hémat.* **11**, 248.

Miescher, P., Burger, H., Gilardi, A. and Hegglin, O. (1958) Die Lebensdauer von ⁵¹Crmarkierten Erythrocyten in verschiedenen Lebensaltern. *Strahlentherapie*, **38**, Suppl. 3, p. 236.

Miescher, P.A. and Muller-Eberhard, H.J. (eds) (1978) *Seminars in Immunopathology* vol 1: *Immunodeficiency Diseases*. Springer-Verlag, Berlin.

Mikaelson, M., Nilsson, I.M., Vilhardt, H. and Wiechel, B. (1982) Factor VIII concentrate prepared from blood donors stimulated with intranasal DDAVP. *Transfusion*, **22**, 229–233.

Miles, R.M., Maurer, H.M. and Valdes, O.S. (1971) Iron-deficiency anaemia at birth. Two examples secondary to chronic fetal-maternal hemorrhage. *Clin. Pediat.* **10**, 223.

Millar, D.S., Davis, L.R., Rodeck, C.H., Nicolaides, K.H. and Mibashan, R.S. (1985) Normal blood cell values in the early midtrimester fetus. *Prenatal Diagnosis*, **5**, 367–373.

Miller, G., McCoord, Augusta B., Joos, H.A. and Clausen, S.W. (1954a) Studies of serum electrolyte changes during exchange transfusion. *Pediatrics*, **13**, 412.

Miller, E.B., Rosenfield, R.E., Vogel, P., Haber, Gladys and Gibbel, Natalie (1954b) The Lewis blood factors in American Negroes. *Amer. J. phys. Anthrop.* **12**, 427.

Miller, W.V., Holland, P.V., Sugarboker, E., Strober, W. and Waldmann, T.A. (1970) Anaphylactic reactions to IgA: a difficult transfusion problem. *Amer. J. clin. Path.* **54**, 618.

Miller, R.D., Robbins, T.O., Tong, M.J. and Barton, S.L. (1971) Coagulation defects associated with massive blood transfusions. *Ann. Surg.* **174**, 794.

Miller, L.H. (1975) Transfusion malaria, in *Transmissible Disease and Blood Transfusion*, eds T.J. Greenwalt and G.A. Jamieson. Grune & Stratton, New York.

Miller, L.H., Mason, S.J., Clyde, D.F. and McGinniss, Mary H. (1976) The resistance factor to *Plasmodium vivax* in blacks. The Duffy blood group genotype, *FyFy*. *New Engl. J. Med.* **295**, 302.

Miller, R.H. and Purcell, R.H. (1990) Hepatitis C virus shares amino acid sequence similarity with pestiviruses and flaviviruses as well as members of two plant virus supergroups. *Proc. nat. Acad. Sci. USA*, **87**, 2057–2061.

Miller, W.J., McCullough, J., Balfour, H.H. jr, Haake, R.J., Ramsay, N.K.C., Goldman, A., Bowman, R. and Kersey, J. (1991) Prevention of cytomegalovirus infection following bone marrow transplantation: a randomized trial of blood product screening. *Bone Marrow Transplantation*, **7**, 227–234.

Mills, J.N. (1946) The life-span of the erythrocyte. *J. Physiol. (Lond.)*, **105**, 16(P).

Milne, R.W. and Dawes, C. (1973) The relative contributions of different salivary glands to the blood group activity of whole saliva in humans. *Vox Sang.* **25**, 298.

Milner, P.F. (1982) Chronic transfusion regimens for sickle cell disease, in *Advances in the*

Pathophysiology, Diagnosis and Treatment of Sickle Cell Disease, ed R.B. Scott. *Progress in Clinical and Biological Research*, **98**, 97–107. Alan R. Liss, New York.

Milstein, C. (1980) Monoclonal antibodies. *Scientific American*, **243**, 56–64.

Milstein, C. (1981) Monoclonal antibodies from hybrid myelomas. *Proc. roy. Soc. Lond. B.* **211**, 393–412.

Mimms, L., Vallari, D., Ducharme, L., Holland, P., Kuramoto, I.K. and Zeldis, J. (1990) Specificity of anti-HCV ELISA assessed by reactivity to three immunodominant HCV regions (Letter). *Lancet*, **ii**, 1590–1591.

Minev, M. (1975) Differences in the immunogenicity of the HL-A antigens. *Vox Sang.* **29**, 433.

Mintz, P.D. and Sullivan, M.F. (1985) Preoperative crossmatch ordering and blood use in elective hysterectomy. *Obstet. Gynec.* **65**, 389–392.

Mir, N., Samson, D., House, M.H. and Kovar, I.Z. (1988) Failure of antenatal high-dose immunoglobulin to improve fetal platelet count in neonatal alloimmune thrombocytopenia. *Vox Sang.* **55**, 188–189.

Mishler, J.M., Higby, D.J., Rhomberg, W., Nicora, R.W. and Holland, J.F. (1975) Leucapheresis: increased efficiency of collection by the use of hydroxyethyl starch and dexamethasone, in *Leucocytes: Separation, Collection and Transfusion*, eds J.M. Goldman and R.M. Lowenthal. Academic Press, New York.

Mishler, J.M., Janes, A.W., Lowes, B., Farfan, Carol and Emerson, Pauline M. (1976) The utilization of a new strength citrate anticoagulant during centrifugal plateletpheresis. 1. Assessment of donor effects. *Brit. J. Haemat.* **34**, 387.

Mishler. J.M. (1977) The effects of corticosteroids on mobilization and function of neutrophils. *Exper. Hemat.* **5**, Suppl. 1. p. 15.

Mishler, J.M., Borberg, H., Reuter, J. and Gross. R. (1977) The utilization of a new strength citrate anticoagulant during centrifugal plateletpheresis. II. Assessment of *in vitro* platelet function. *Blut*, **34**, 237.

Mishler, J.M., Darley, J.H., Cederholm-Williams, S. and Wright, G. (1978) Whole blood storage in citrate and phosphate solutions containing half-strength trisodium citrate: cellular and biochemical studies. *J. Path.* **124**, 125.

Mishler, J.M., Darley, J.H., Haworth, Catherine and Mollison, P.L. (1979) Viability of red cells stored in diminished concentration of citrate. *Brit. J. Haemat.* **43**, 63–67.

Mishler, J.M. (1982) *Pharmacology of Hydroxyethyl Starch*. Oxford University Press, Oxford.

Mishler, J.M., Hester, J.P., Huestis, D.W., Rock, G.A. and Strauss, R.G. (1983) Panel II: dosage

and scheduling regimens for erythrocyte sedimenting macromolecules. *J. clin. Apheresis*, **1**, 130–143.

Mitsuno, T., Ohyanagi, H. and Naito, R. (1982) Clinical studies of a perfluorochemical whole blood substitute (Fluosol-DA). *Ann. Surg.* **195**, 60–69.

Mittal, K.M., Ruder, E.A. and Green, D. (1976) Matching of histocompatibility (HL-A) antigens for platelet transfusion. *Blood*, **47**, 31.

Miyamoto, M. and Sasakawa, S. (1987) Studies on granulocyte preservation: III. Effect of agitation on granulocyte concentrates. *Transfusion*, **27**, 165–166.

Miyamoto, M., Sasakawa, S., Ishikawa, Y., Ogawa, A., Nishimura, T. and Kuroda, T. (1989) Leukocyte-poor platelet concentrates at the bedside by filtration through Sepacell-PL. *Vox Sang.* **57**, 164–167.

Miyoshi, K., Kaneto, Y., Lawai, H., Ochi, H., Hasegawa, K., Shirakami, A. and Yamamo, T. (1988) X-linked dominant control of F-cells in normal adult life: characterization of the Swiss type as hereditary persistence of fetal hemoglobin regulated dominantly by gene(s) on X chromosome. *Blood*, **72**, 1854–1860.

Modell, C.B. (1975) Transfusion and haemochromatosis, in *Iron Metabolism and its Disorders*, ed H. Kiel. Excerpta Medica, Amsterdam.

Modell, Bernadette (1985) Chorionic villus sampling. Evaluating safety and efficacy. *Lancet*, **i**, 737–740.

Moe, P.J. (1970) Hemoglobin, hematocrit and red blood cell count in 'capillary' (skin-prick) blood compared to venous blood in children. *Acta paediat. scand.* **59**, 49.

Moeschlin, S. and Wagner, K. (1952) Agranulocytosis due to the occurrence of leucocyte agglutinins (pyramidon and cold agglutinins). *Acta haemat.* **8**, 29.

Moffat, Elisabeth H., Gerrish, P., Mir, M.A. and Darke, C. (1982) Remission of posttransfusion thrombocytopenic purpura with high dose intravenous corticosteroids. *Clin. lab. Haemat.* **4**, 333–336.

Mohandas, N., Greenquist, A.C. and Shohet, S.B. (1978) Effects of heat and metabolic depletion on erythrocyte deformability, spectrin extractability and phosphorylation, in *The Red Cell*, ed G.J. Brewer. Alan R. Liss, New York.

Moheng, M.C., McCarthy. P. and Pierce, S.R. (1985) Anti-Do[b] implicated as the cause of a delayed hemolytic transfusion reaction. *Transfusion*, **25**, 44–46.

Mohini, R. (1989) Clinical efficacy of recombinant human erythropoietin in hemodialysis patients. *Semin. Nephrol.* **9**, Suppl. 1, 16–21.

Mohn, J.F., Lambert, R.M., Bowman, H.S. and Brason, F.W. (1961) Experimental transfusion of donor plasma containing blood-group antibodies into incompatible normal human recipients. I. Absence of destruction of red-cell mass with anti-Rh, anti-Kell and anti-M. *Brit. J. Haemat.* **7**, 112.

Mohn, J.F., Bowman, H.S., Lambert, R.M. and Brason. F.W. (1964) The formation of Rh specific autoantibodies in experimental isoimmune hemolytic anemia in man. *Commun. 10th Congr. Int. Soc. Blood Transfus.*, Stockholm.

Moise, K.J. jr, Cano, Lorraine, E. and Sala, Debra J. (1990) Resolution of severe thrombocytopenia in a pregnant patient with rhesus-negative blood with autoimmune thrombocytopenic purpura after intravenous rhesus immune globulin. *Amer. J. Obstet. gynec.* **162**, 1237–1238.

Möller, G. (1964) Isoantibody-induced cellular resistance of immune haemolysis *in vivo* and *in vitro. Nature (Lond.)*, **20 2**, 357.

Möller, G. (1965) Survival of H-2 incompatible mouse erythrocytes in untreated and isoimmune recipients. *Immunology*, **8**, 360.

Mollison, P.L. and Young, I. Maureen (1941a) Failure of *in vitro* tests as a guide to the value of stored blood. *Brit. med. J.* **ii**, 797.

Mollison, P.L. and Young, I. Maureen (1941b) Iso-agglutinin changes after transfusion of incompatible blood and serum. *Lancet*, **ii**, 635.

Mollison, P.L. and Young, I. Maureen (1942) *In vivo* survival in the human subject of transfused erythrocytes after storage in various preservative solutions. *Quart. J. exp. Physiol.* **31**, 359.

Mollison, P.L. (1943a) The investigation of haemolytic transfusion reactions. *Brit. med. J.* **i**, 529, 559.

Mollison, P.L. (1943b) The survival of transfused red cells in haemolytic disease of the newborn. *Arch. Dis. Childh.* **18**, 161.

Mollison, P.L. (1947) The survival of transfused erythrocytes, with special reference to cases of acquired haemolytic anaemia. *Clin. Sci.* **6**, 137.

Mollison, P.L. and Cutbush, Marie (1949a) Haemolytic disease of the newborn: criteria of severity. *Brit. med. J.* **i**, 123.

Mollison, P.L. and Cutbush, Marie (1949b) Haemolytic disease of the newborn due to anti-A antibodies. *Lancet*, **ii**, 173.

Mollison, P.L. and Cutbush, Marie (1949c) La maladie hémolytique chez un enfant D^u. *Rev. Hémat.* **4**, 608.

Mollison, P.L., Veall, N. and Cutbush, Marie (1950) Red cell volume and plasma volume in newborn infants. *Arch. Dis. Childh.* **25**, 242.

Mollison, P.L. (1951) *Blood Transfusion in Clinical Medicine*, Blackwell Scientific Publications, Oxford.

Mollison, P.L. and Cutbush, Marie (1951) A method of measuring the severity of a series of cases of hemolytic disease of the newborn. *Blood*, **6**, 777.

Mollison, P.L. and Sloviter, H.A. (1951) Successful transfusion of previously frozen human red cells. *Lancet*, **ii**, 862.

Mollison, P.L. and Walker, W. (1952) Controlled trials of the treatment of haemolytic disease of the newborn. *Lancet*, **i**, 429.

Mollison, P.L., Sloviter, H.A. and Chaplin, H. jr (1952) Survival of transfused red cells previously stored for long periods in the frozen state. *Lancet*, **ii**, 501.

Mollison, P.L. (1954) The life-span of red blood cells. *Lectures on the Scientific Basis of Medicine*, **2**, 269.

Mollison, P.L. and Cutbush Marie (1954) Haemolytic disease of the newborn, in *Recent Advances in Paediatrics*, ed D. Gairdner. J. & A. Churchill, London.

Mollison, P.L. and Cutbush, Marie (1955) The use of isotope-labelled red cells to demonstrate incompatibility *in vivo. Lancet* i, 1290.

Mollison, P.L. and Veall, N. (1955) The use of the isotope ^51Cr as a label for red cells. *Brit. J. Haemat.* **1**, 62.

Mollison, P.L. (1956) *Blood Transfusion in Clinical Medicine*, 2nd edn. Blackwell Scientific Publications, Oxford.

Mollison, P.L. and Hughes-Jones, N.C. (1958) Sites of removal of incompatible red cells from the circulation. *Vox Sang.* **3**, 243.

Mollison, P.L., Robinson, Margaret A. and Hunter, Denise A. (1958) Improved method of labelling red cells with radioactive phosphorus. *Lancet*, **i**, 766.

Mollison, P.L. (1959a) Measurement of survival and destruction of red cells in haemolytic syndromes. *Brit. med. Bull.* **15**, 59.

Mollison, P.L. (1959b) Factors determining the relative clinical importance of different blood group antibodies. *Brit. med. Bull.* **15**, 92.

Mollison, P.L. (1959c) Further studies on the removal of incompatible red cells from the circulation. *Acta haemat.* (Basel), Fasc. **10**, 495.

Mollison, P.L. (1959d) Blood group antibodies and red cell destruction. *Brit. med. J.* **ii**, 1035 and 1123.

Mollison, P.L. and Robinson, Margaret A. (1959) Observations on the effects of purine nucleosides on red-cell preservation. *Brit. J. Haemat.* **5**, 331.

Mollison, P.L. and Thomas, Ann R. (1959) Haemolytic potentialities of human blood group antibodies revealed by the use of animal complement. *Vox Sang.* **4**, 185.

Mollison, P.L. (1961a) Further observations on

the normal survival curve of ^{51}Cr-labelled red cells. *Clin. Sci.* **21**, 21.

Mollison, P.L. (1961b) *Blood Transfusion in Clinical Medicine.* 3rd edn. Blackwell Scientific Publications, Oxford.

Mollison, P.L. (1962) Destruction of incompatible red cells *in vivo* in relation to antibody characteristics, in *Mechanism of Cell and Tissue Damage Produced by Immune Reactions,* 2nd International Symposium on Immunopathology, Brook Lodge (Mich., U.S.A.), 1961, p. 267. Schwabe, Basel.

Mollison, P.L., Polley, Margaret J. and Crome, Patricia (1963) Temporary suppression of Lewis blood-group antibodies to permit incompatible transfusion. *Lancet,* **i**, 909.

Mollison, P.L., Crome, Patricia, Hughes-Jones, N.C. and Rochna, Erna (1965) Rate of removal from the circulation of red cells sensitized with different amounts of antibody. *Brit. J. Haemat.* **11**, 461.

Mollison, P.L. (1965) The role of complement in haemolytic processes *in vivo,* in *Ciba Foundation Symposium, Complement,* eds G.E.W. Wolstenholme and J. Knight, p. 323. J. & A. Churchill, London.

Mollison, P.L. (1967) *Blood Transfusion in Clinical Medicine,* 4th edn. Blackwell Scientific Publications, Oxford.

Mollison, P.L. and Hughes-Jones, N.C. (1967) Clearance of Rh positive cells by low concentration of Rh antibody. *Immunology,* **12**, 63.

Mollison, P.L., Hughes-Jones, N.C., Lindsay, Margaret and Wessely, Jane (1969) Suppression of primary Rh immunization by passively-administered antibody. Experiments in volunteers. *Vox Sang.* **16**, 421.

Mollison, P.L. (1970) The effect of isoantibodies on red-cell survival. *Ann. N.Y. Acad. Sci.* **169**, 199.

Mollison, P.L., Frame, Marion and Ross, Margaret E. (1970) Differences between Rh(D) negative subjects in response to Rh(D) antigen. *Brit. J. Haemat.* **19**, 257.

Mollison, P.L. (1972a) *Blood Transfusion in Clinical Medicine,* 5th edn. Blackwell Scientific Publications, Oxford.

Mollison, P.L. (1972b) Quantitation of transplacental haemorrhage. *Brit. med. J.* **iii**, 31 and 115.

Mollison, P.L. and Newlands, Marion (1976) Unusual delayed haemolytic transfusion reaction characterised by the slow destruction of red cells. *Vox Sang.* **31**, 54.

Mollison, P.L., Johnson, Carole A. and Prior. Dilys M. (1978) Dose-dependent destruction of A_1 cells by anti-A_1. *Vox Sang.* **35**, 149.

Mollison, P.L. (1979) *Blood Transfusion in Clinical Medicine,* 6th edn. Blackwell Scientific Publications, Oxford.

Mollison, P.L. (1981) Determination of red cell survival using ^{51}Cr, in *A Seminar on Immune-Mediated Cell Destruction,* Amer. Assoc. Blood Banks, Chicago.

Mollison, P.L. (1982) The clinical significance of red cell alloantibodies (and autoantibodies) in blood transfusion, in *Safety in Transfusion Practices,* eds H.F. Polesky and R.H. Walker, pp. 131–149. College of American Pathologists, Stokie, Illinois.

Mollison, P.L. (1983) *Blood Transfusion in Clinical Medicine,* 7th edn. Blackwell Scientific Publications, Oxford.

Mollison, P.L. (1984a) Methods of determining the post-transfusion survival of stored red cells. *Transfusion,* **24**, 93–96.

Mollison, P.L. (1984b) Some aspects of Rh hemolytic disease and its prevention, in *Hemolytic Disease of the Newborn,* ed G. Garratty. Amer. Assoc. Blood Banks, Arlington, VA.

Mollison, P.L. (1985) Antibody-mediated destruction of foreign red cells, in *Antibodies; Protective, Destructive and Regulatory Role,* eds F. Milgrom, C.J. Abeyounis and B. Albini, pp. 65–74, Karger, Basel.

Mollison, P.L. (1986) Survival curves of incompatible red cells. An analytical review. *Transfusion,* **26**, 43–50.

Mollison, P.L., Engelfriet, C.P. and Contreras, Marcela (1987) *Blood Transfusion in Clinical Medicine,* 8th edn. Blackwell Scientific Publications, Oxford.

Mollison, P.L. (1989) Further observations on the patterns of clearance of incompatible red cells. *Transfusion,* **29**, 347–354.

Moloney, M.D., Bulmer, J.N., Scott, J.S., Need J.A. and Pattison, N.S. (1989) Maternal immune responses and recurrent miscarriage (Letter). *Lancet,* **i**, 46.

Molthan, L., Crawford, Mary N. and Tippett, Patricia (1973) Enlargement of the Dombrock blood group system: the finding of anti-Do^b. *Vox Sang.* **24**, 382.

Molthan, L. and Crawford, M.N. (1978) Anti-Fy^a. Second example in a black (Abstract). *Transfusion,* **18**, 386.

Molthan, L. and Strohm, Patricia L. (1981) Hemolytic transfusion reaction due to anti-Kell undetectable in low-ionic-strength solution. *Amer. J. clin. Path.* **75**, 629–631.

Monafo, W.W., Chuntrasakul, C. and Ayvazian, V.H. (1973) Hypertonic sodium solutions in the treatment of burn shock. *Amer. J. Surg.* **126**, 778–783.

Moncharmont, P., Juron-Dupraz, F., Rigal, M., Vignal, M. and Meyer, F. (1990) Haemolytic disease of two newborns in a rhesus anti-e alloimmunised woman. Review of literature. *Haematologia,* **23**, 97–100.

Moncrieff, R.E. and Thompson, W.P. (1975)

Delayed hemolytic transfusion reaction with four antibodies detected by pretransfusion tests. *Amer. J. clin. Path.* **64**, 251.

Monjardino, J.P. and Saldanha, J.A. (1990) Delta hepatitis. The disease and the virus. *Brit. med. Bull.* **46**, 399–407.

Monsen, E.R., Critchlow, C.W., Finch, C.A. and Donohue, D.M. (1983) Iron balance in super-donors. *Transfusion*, **23**, 221–225.

Montoro, J.B., Rodriguez, S., Altisent, C. and Tussell, J.M. (1991) Transient Factor VIII inhibitor and treatment with monoclonal-antibody-purified Factor VIII. *Lancet*, **ii**, 1222.

Moore, C.V. (1948) Iron metabolism and hypochromic anemia, in *Nutritional Anemia*. Robert Gould Research Foundation, Cincinnati, USA.

Moore, J.M. (1958) Uncontrollable post-operative haemorrhage after incompatible blood transfusion. *Brit. med. J.* **ii**, 1201.

Moore, B.P.L. and Hughes-Jones, N.C. (1970) Automated assay of anti-D concentration in plasmapheresis donors, in *Advances in Automated Analysis*. Technicon Int. Congr. Chicago.

Moore, J.A. and Chaplin, H. jr (1973) Autoimmune hemolytic anemia associated with an IgG cold incomplete antibody. *Vox Sang.* **24**, 236.

Moore, H.C., Issitt, P.D. and Pavone, B.G. (1975) Successful transfusion of Chido-positive blood to two patients with anti-Chido. *Transfusion*, **15**, 266.

Moore, B.F.L. (1976) Biological and clinical significance of differences between RBC membrane (Rh) and non-membrane (ABH, MN, P) antigenic sites. *Rev. franç. Transfus. Immunohémat.* **19**, 629.

Moore, H.C. and Mollison, P.L. (1976) Use of a low-ionic-strength medium in manual tests for antibody detection. *Transfusion*, **16**, 291.

Moore, S.B., Taswell, H.F., Pineda, A.A. and Sonnenberg, Cheryl L. (1980) Delayed hemolytic transfusion reactions. Evidence of the need for an improved pretransfusion compatibility test. *Amer. J. clin. Path.* **74**, 94–97.

Moore, G.L., Peck. C.C., Sohmer, P.R. and Zuck, T.F. (1981) Some properties of blood stored in anticoagulant CPDA-1 solution. A brief summary. *Transfusion*, **21**, 135–137.

Moore, S., Woodrow, Christina F. and McClelland, B.L. (1982) Isolation of membrane components associated with human red cell antigens Rh(D), ($\bar{c}$), (E) and Fy^a. *Nature (Lond.)*, **295**, 529–531.

Moore, S. (1983) Identification of red cell membrane components associated with rhesus blood group antigen expression, in *Red Cell Membrane Glycoconjugates and Related Genetic Markers*, eds J.P. Cartron, P. Rouger and C. Salmon, pp. 97–106. Lib. Arnette, Paris.

Moore, H.H. (1984) Automated reading of red cell antibody identification tests by a solid phase antiglobulin technique. *Transfusion*, **24**, 218–221.

Moore, G.L. and Ledford, M.E. (1985) Effect of 4000 rad irradiation on the *in vitro* storage properties of packed red cells. *Transfusion*, **25**, 583–585.

Moore, S. and Green, C. (1987) The identification of specific Rhesus polypeptide blood group ABH active glycoprotein complexes in the human red cell membrane. *Biochem. J.* **244**, 735–741.

Moores, P., Botha, M.C. and Brink, S. (1970) Anti-N in the serum of a healthy type MN person—a further example. *Amer. J. clin. Path.* **54**, 90.

Moores, P. (1972) The 'Bombay' blood-type in Natal. *Commun. 13th Congr. Int. Soc. Blood Transfus.*, Washington, D.C.

Moores. P., Pudifin, D. and Patel, P.L. (1975) Severe hemolytic anemia in an adult associated with anti-T. *Transfusion*, **15**, 329.

Moraes, J.R. and Stastny, P. (1977) Human endothelial cell antigens: molecular independence from HLA and expression in blood monocytes. *Transplant Proc.* **9**, 605.

Morehead, R.T., Anderson, K., Grunewald, S., Casey, D. and McCullough, J. (1974) A comparison of AutoAnalyzer and manual methods for red cell antibody screening. *Transfusion*, **14**, 586.

Morel, P., Hill, V., Bergren, M. and Garratty, G. (1975) Sera exhibiting hemagglutination of N red blood cells stored in media containing glucose (Abstract). *Transfusion*, **15**, 522.

Morel, Phyllis A., Garratty, G. and Perkins, H.A. (1978) Clinically significant and insignificant antibodies in blood transfusion. *Amer. J. med. Technol.* **44**, 122.

Morel, P. and Tyler, V. (1979) LISS autoagglutinins of no apparent clinical significance (Abstract). *Transfusion*, **19**, 647.

Morel, P.A. and Hamilton, H.B. (1979) Ok^a: an erythrocytic antigen of high frequency. *Vox Sang.* **36**, 182–185.

Morel, P.A., Bergren, M.O., Hill, V., Garratty, G. and Perkins, H.A. (1981) M and N specific hemagglutinins of human erythrocytes stored in glucose solutions. *Transfusion*, **21**, 652–662.

Morell, A., Terry, W.D. and Waldmann, T.A. (1970) Metabolic properties of IgG subclasses in man. *J. clin. Invest.* **49**, 673.

Morell, A., Skvaril, F., van Loghem, Erna and Kleemola, Marjaana (1971) Human IgG subclasses in maternal and fetal serum. *Vox Sang.* **21**, 481.

Morell, A., Skvaril, F. and Rufener, J..L. (1973)

Characterization of Rh antibodies formed after incompatible pregnancies and after repeated booster injections. *Vox Sang.* **24**, 323.

Morell, A., Schurch, Beatrice, Ryser, D., Hofer, F., Skvaril, F. and Barandun, S. (1980) In vivo behaviour of gamma globulin preparations. *Vox Sang.* **38**, 272–283.

Moreno, C. and Kabat, E.A. (1969) Studies on human antibodies. VIII. Properties and association constant of human antibodies to blood group A substance purified with insoluble specific adsorbants and fractionally-eluted with mono- and oligosaccharides. *J. exp. Med.* **129**, 871.

Moreschi, C. (1908) Neue Tatsachen über die Blutkörperchen Agglutinationen. *Zbl. Bakt.* **46**, 49 and 456.

Morgan, W.T.J. and Watkins, Winifred M. (1948) The detection of a product of the blood group O gene and the relationship of the so-called O-substance to the agglutinogens A and B. *Brit. J. exp. Path.* **29**, 159.

Morgan, P., Wheeler, C.B. and Bossom, E.L. (1967) Delayed transfusion reaction attributed to Jk^b. *Transfusion*, **7**, 307.

Morgan, W.T.J. and Watkins, Winifred M. (1969) Genetic and biochemical aspects of human blood-group A-, B-, H-, Le^a- and Le^b- specificity. *Brit. med. Bull.* **25**, 30.

Morgan, G., Linch, D.C., Knott. L.T., Davies, E.G., Sieff, C., Chessels, J.M., Hale, G., Waldmann, H. and Levinsky, R.J. (1986) Successful haploidentical mismatched bone marrow transplantation in severe combined immunodeficiency: T cell removal using CAMPATH-I monoclonal antibody and E-rosetting. *Brit. J. Haemat.* **62**, 421–430.

Morgan, C., Hyland, C. and Young, I.F. (1990) Hepatitis C antibody and transaminase activities in blood donors (Letter). *Lancet*, i, 921.

Morgan, C.L., Cannell, G.R., Addison, R.S. and Minchinton, R.M. (1991) The effect of intravenous immunoglobulin on placental transfer of a platelet-specific antibody: anti-Pl^A1 *Transfus. Med.* **1**, 209–216.

Morgenthaler, J-J. (1989) Effect of ethanol on viruses, in *Virus Inactivation in Plasma Products*, ed J.J. Morgenthaler, pp. 109–121. *Current Studies in Hematology and Blood Transfusion*. S. Karger, Basel.

Moriau, M. and 10 others (1977) Haemostasis disorders in open heart surgery with extracorporeal circulation. Importance of the platelet function and the heparin neutralization. *Vox Sang.* **32**, 41.

Moroff, G. (1981) Aggregation: release response of platelets stored at 22°C. *Vox Sang.* **40**, 110–114.

Moroff, G. and 10 others (1984) Platelet viability following storage for 5 days. Influence of holding whole blood for 8 hours at 20 to 24°C before concentrate preparation. *Transfusion*, **24**, 382–385.

Moroff, G. and George, V.M. (1990) The maintenance of platelet properties upon limited discontinuation of agitation during storage. *Transfusion*, **30**, 427–430.

Moroff, G., Holme, S., Heaton, W.A.L., Kevy, S., Jacobson, M. and Popovsky, M. (1990) Effect of an 8-hour holding period on in vivo and in vitro properties of red cells and Factor VIII content of plasma after collection in a red cell additive system. *Transfusion*, **30**, 828–830.

Moroff, G. and Holme, S. (1991) Concepts about current conditions for the preparation and storage of platelets. *Transfus. Med. Rev*, **5**, 48–59.

Morrison, F.S. (1966) The effect of filters on the efficiency of platelet transfusion. *Transfusion*, **6**, 493.

Morrison, F.S., Mollison, P.L. and Robson, D.C. (1968) Post-transfusion survival of red cells stored in liquid nitrogen. *Brit. J. Haemat.* **14**, 215.

Morrison, J.C., Whybrew, W.D. and Bucovaz, E.T. (1978) Use of partial exchange transfusion preoperatively in patients with sickle cell hemoglobinopathies. *Amer. J. Obstet. Gynec.* **132**, 59–63.

Morrison, J.C., Schneider, J.M., Whybrew, W.D., Bucovaz, E.T. and Menzel, D.M. (1980) Prophylactic transfusions in pregnant patients with sickle hemoglobinopathies: benefit versus risk. *Obstet. Gynec.* **56**, 274–280.

Morse, E.E., Freireich, E.J., Carbone, P.P., Bronson, W. and Frei, Emil III (1966) The transfusion of leukocytes from donors with chronic myelocytic leukemia to patients with leukopenia. *Transfusion*, **8**, 183.

Morse, E.E. (1978) Interdonor incompatibility as a cause of reaction during granulocyte transfusion. *Vox Sang.* **35**, 215.

Mortimer, P.P., Luban, N.L.C., Kelleher, J.F. and Cohen, B.J. (1983) Transmission of serum parvovirus-like virus by clotting-factor concentrates. *Lancet*, ii, 482–484.

Mortimer, P.P., Parry, J.V. and Mortimer, J.V. (1985) Which anti-HTLV-III/LAV assays for screening and confirmatory testing? *Lancet*, ii, 877–878.

Morton, J.A. and Pickles, M.M. (1947) Use of trypsin in the detection of incomplete anti-Rh antibodies. *Nature (Lond.)*, **159**, 779.

Morton, J.A. (1962) Some observations on the action of blood-group antibodies on red cells treated with proteolytic enzymes. *Brit. J. Haemat.* **8**, 134.

Morton, J.A., Pickles, M.M. and Sutton, L. (1969) The correlation of the Bg^a blood group with the HL-A7 leucocyte group: demonstration of antigenic sites on red cells and leucocytes. *Vox Sang.* **17**, 536.

Morton, J.A., Pickles, M.M. and Terry, A.M. (1970) The Sd^a blood group antigen in tissues and body fluids. *Vox Sang.* **19**, 472.

Morton, J.A., Pickles, M.M., Sutton, L. and Skov, F. (1971) Identification of further antigens on red cells and lymphocytes. Association of Bg^b with W17 (Te57) and Bg^c with W28 (Da15, Ba*). *Vox Sang.* **21**, 141.

Morton, J.A., Pickles, M.M. and Darley, J.H. (1977) Increase in strength of red cell Bg^a antigen following infectious mononucleosis. *Vox Sang.* **32**, 26.

Morton, J.A., Pickles, M.M., Turner, J.E. and Cullen, P.R. (1980) Changes in red cell Bg antigens in haematological disease. *Immunol. Commun.* **9**, 173–190.

Morville, P. (1929) Investigation on isohaemagglutination in mothers and newborn children. *Acta path. microbiol. scand.* **6**, 39.

Mosher, D.F. (1975) Cross-linking of cold-insoluble globulin by fibrin-stabilizing factor. *J. biol. Chem.* **250**, 6614.

Mosmann, T.R., Gallatin, M. and Longenecker, B.M. (1980) Alteration of apparent specificity of monoclonal (hybridoma) antibodies recognizing polymorphic histocompatibility and blood group determinants. *J. Immunol.* **125**, 1152–1156.

Moss, W.L. (1910) Studies on isoagglutinins and isohemolysins. *Bull. Johns Hopk. Hosp.* **21**, 63.

Moss, G.S., Lowe, R.J., Jilek, J. and Levine, H.D. (1981) Colloid or crystalloid in the resuscitation of hemorrhagic shock; a controlled clinical trial. *Surgery*, **89**, 434–438.

Moss, G.S., Gould, S.A., Rosen, A.L., Sehgal, L.R. and Sehgal, Hansa L. (1989) Results of the first clinical trial with a polymerised hemoglobin solution (Abstract). *Biomat. artif. Cells artif. Organs*, **17**, 633.

Most, A.S., Ruocco, N.A. and Gewirtz, H. (1986) Effect of a reduction in blood viscosity on maximal oxygen delivery distal to a moderate coronary stenosis. *Circulation*, **74**, 1085–1092.

Motschman, T.L., Reisner, R.K. and Taswell, H.F. (1985) Evaluation of the antibody screen and crossmatch (Abstract). *Transfusion*, **25**, 451.

Motulsky, A.G., Casserd, F., Giblett, Eloise R., Broun, G.O. and Finch, C.A. (1958) Anemia and the spleen. *New Engl. J. Med.* **259**, 1164 and 1215.

Moulds, J.J., Polesky, H.F., Reid, M. and Ellisor, S.S. (1975) Observations on the Gy^a and Hy antigens and the antibodies that define them. *Transfusion*, **15**, 270.

Moulinier, J. (1957) Iso-immunisation maternelle antiplaquettaire et purpura néo-natal. Le système de groupe plaquettaire 'Duzo'. *Proc. 6th* *Congr. Europe. Soc. Haemat.* Copenhagen, p. 817.

Moullec, J. (1947) Substance A des hématies humaines et anatoxine diphtérique. *C.R. Soc. Biol. (Paris)*, **141**, 20.

Moullec, J., Sutton, E. and Burgada, M. (1955) Une variante faible de l'agglutinogène de groupe B. *Rev. Hémat.* **10**, 574.

Mourant, A.E. (1949) Rh phenotypes and Fisher's CDE notation. *Nature (Lond.)*, **163**, 913.

Mourant, A.E., Kopéc, Ada C. and Domaniewska-Sobczak, Kazimiera (1976) *The Distribution of the Human Blood Groups and Other Biochemical Polymorphisms*, 2nd edn. Oxford University Press.

Mourant, A.E. (1977) Disease associations with polymorphisms other than HLA, in *HLA and Disease*, eds J. Dausset and A. Svejgaard, pp. 12–19. Munksgaard, Copenhagen.

Moureau, F. (1945) Les réactions post-transfusionnelles. *Rev. belge Sci. méd.* **16**, 258.

Mowbray, J.F., Underwood, J.C., Michel, M., Forbes, P.R. and Beard, R.W. (1987) Immunization with paternal lymphocytes in women with recurrent spontaneous abortion. *Lancet*, **ii**, 679–680.

MRC. *See* Medical Research Council.

Mueller-Eckhardt, C., Mueller-Eckhardt, G., Willen-Ohff, H., Norz, A., Küenzlen, E., O'Neill, G.J. and Schendel, D.J. (1985b) Immunogenicity of and immune response to the human platelet antigen Zw^a is strongly associated with HLA-B8 and -DR3. *Tissue Antigens*, **26**, 71–76.

Mueller-Eckhardt, C., Becker, T., Weisheit, M., Witz, C. and Santoso, S. (1986) Neonatal alloimmune thrombocytopenia due to feto-maternal Zw^b incompatibility. *Vox Sang.* **50**, 94–96.

Mueller-Eckhardt, C. and Kiefel, V. (1988) High-dose IgG for post-transfusion purpura-revisited. *Blut*, **57**, 163–167.

Mueller-Eckhardt, Ch., Kiefel, V. and Grubert, A. (1989a) High-dose IgG treatment for neonatal alloimmune thrombocytopenia. *Blut*, **59**, 145–146.

Mueller-Eckhardt, Ch., Kiefel, V., Kroll, H. and Mueller-Eckhardt, Gertrud (1989b) HLA-Drw6, a new immune response marker for immunization against the platelet alloantigen Br^a. *Vox Sang.* **57**, 90–91.

Mueller-Eckhardt, Ch. (1991) Platelet allo- and autoantigens and their clinical implications, in *Transfusion Medicine in the 1990s*, ed Sandra T. Nance. American Association of Blood Banks, Arlington, Virginia.

Mulet, C., Cartron, J.-P., Schenkel-Brunner, H., Duchet, D., Sinay, P. and Salmon, C. (1979) Probable biosynthetic pathway for the synthesis of the B antigen from B_h variants. *Vox Sang.* **37**, 272–280.

Mullard, G.W., Haworth, Clare and Lee, D. (1978) A case of atypical polyagglutinability due to Tk transformation. *Brit. J. Haemat.* **40**, 571.

Müller, H.E. and Gramlich, F. (1965) Über den Plasmaproteinfilm an der Oberfläche menschlicher Erythrocyten. *Acta haemat.* **34**, 239.

Müller-Eberhard, U., Liem, H.H., Hanstein, A. and Saarinen, P.A. (1969) Studies on the disposal of intravascular heme in the rabbit. *J. Lab. clin. Med.* **73**, 210.

Müller-Eberhard, Ursula, Bosman, C. and Liem, H.H. (1970) Tissue localization of the hemehemopexin complex in the rabbit and the rat as studied by light microscopy with the use of radioisotopes. *J. Lab. clin. Med.* **76**, 426.

Mullis, K.B. and Faloona, F.A. (1987) Specific synthesis of DNA *in vitro* via a polymerase-catalyzed chain reaction. *Methods Enzymol.* **155**, 335–350.

Munk-Andersen, G. (1956) Demonstration of incomplete ABO-antibody with special reference to its passage through the placenta. I. The content of complete ABO-antibody in umbilical cord serum. *Acta path. microbiol. scand.* **39**, 407.

Munk-Andersen, G. (1958) Excess of group O-mothers in ABO-haemolytic disease. *Acta path. microbiol. scand.* **42**, 43.

Munn, L.R. and Chaplin, H. jr. (1977) Rosette formation by sensitized red cells — effects of source of peripheral leukocyte monolayers. *Vox Sang.* **33**, 129.

Munro, J.R. and Schachter, H. (1973) The presence of two GPD-L-fucose: glycoprotein fucosyltransferases in human serum. *Arch. Biochem. Biophys.* **156**, 534.

Murphy, S., Sayar, S.N. and Gardner, F.H. (1970) Storage of platelet concentrates at 22°C. *Blood*, **35**, 549.

Murphy, J.R. (1973) Influence of temperature and method of centrifugation on the separation of erythrocytes. *J. Lab. clin. Med.* **82**, 334.

Murphy, S., Sayar, S.N., Abdou, N.L. and Gardner, F.H. (1974) Platelet preservation by freezing. Use of dimethylsulfoxide as cryoprotective agent. *Transfusion*, **14**, 139.

Murphy, S. and Gardner, F.H. (1976) Room temperature storage of platelets. *Transfusion*, **16**, 2.

Murphy, S., Kahn, R.A., Holme, S., Phillips, G.L., Sherwood, W., Davisson, W. and Buchholz, D.H. (1982) Improved storage of platelets for transfusion in a new container. *Blood*, **60**, 194–200.

Murphy, S. (1985) Platelet storage for transfusion. *Semin. Hemat.* **22**, 165–177.

Murphy, S. (1986) Evolution, current state of the art, and further trends of platelet preservation. *Abstracts, 19th Congr. Int. Soc. Blood Tranfus.*, Sydney, p. 78.

Murphy, M.E., Metcalf, P., Thomas, H., Eve, J., Ord, J., Lister, T.A. and Waters. A.H. (1986) Use of leucocyte-poor blood components and HLA-matched platelet donors to prevent HLA-alloimmunization. *Brit. J. Haemat.* **62**, 529–534.

Murphy, E.L., Hanchard, B., Figueroa, J.P., Gibbs, W.N., Lofters, W.S., Campbell, M., Goedert, J.J. and Blattner, W.A. (1989) Modelling the risk of adult T-cell leukemia/lymphoma in persons infected with human T-lymphotopic virus type I. *Int. J. Cancer*, **43**, 250–253.

Murray, J. and Clark, E.C. (1952) Production of anti-Rh in guinea pigs from human erythrocyte extracts. *Nature (Lond.)*, **169**, 886.

Murray, S. (1957) The effect of Rh genotypes on severity in haemolytic disease of the newborn. *Brit. J. Haemat.* **3**, 143.

Murray, R.K., Connell, G.E. and Pert, J.M. (1961) The role of haptoglobin in the clearance and distribution of extracorpuscular hemoglobulin. *Blood*, **17**, 45.

Murray, Sheilagh, Knox, E.G. and Walker, W. (1965) Rhesus haemolytic disease of the newborn and the ABO groups. *Vox Sang.* **10**, 6.

Murray, J.F., Matthay, M.A., Luce, J.M. and Flick, M.R. (1988) An expanded definition of the adult respiratory distress syndrome. *Amer. Rev. resp. Dis.* **136**, 720–723.

Musial, J., Niewiarowski, S., Hershock, D., Morinelli, T.A., Colman, R.W. and Edmunds, L.H. jr (1985) Loss of fibrinogen receptors from the platelet surface during simulated extracorporeal circulation. *J. Lab. clin. Med.* **105**, 514–522.

Mygind, K. and Ahrons, S. (1973) IgG cold agglutinins and first trimester abortion. *Vox Sang.* **23**, 552.

Myhre, B.A. (1972) Antibody screening with the AutoAnalyzer using donors' plasma in place of serum. *Amer. J. clin. Path.* **58**, 698.

Myhre, B.A., Koepke, J.A., Polesky, H.F., Walker, R. and van Schoonhoven, P. (1977) The CAP blood bank comprehensive survey program—1975. *Amer. J. clin. Path.* **68**, *Suppl.*, 175.

Myhre, B.A., Demaniew, S. and Nelson. E.J. (1984) Preservation of red cell antigens during storage of blood with different anticoagulants. *Transfusion*, **24**, 499–501.

Myhre, B.A., Marcus, C.S. and Wheeler, N.C. (1990) The prediction of autologous red cell survival. *Ann. clin. lab. Sci.* **20**, 258–262.

Myllylä, G. (1991) Whole blood and plasma procurement and the impact of plasmapheresis, in *Blood Separation and Plasma Fractionation*, ed J.R. Harris, pp. 15–42. Wiley-Liss, New York.

Myllylä, G., Furuhjelm, U., Nordling, S., Pirkola, Anna, Tippett, Patricia, Gavin, June and Sanger, Ruth (1971) Persistent mixed field polyagglutinability. Electrokinetic and serological aspects. *Vox Sang.* **20**, 7.

Nadler, S.B., Hidalgo, J.U. and Bloch, T. (1962) Prediction of blood volume in normal human adults. *Surgery*, **51**, 224.

Nagashima, H., Wiedermann, G., Hermann, G. and Miescher, P.A. (1965) Influence of 2-mercaptoethanol treatment on opsonizing activity of human and rabbit 7S antibodies. *Vox Sang.* **10**, 333.

Nagashima, M., Matsushima, M., Massuoko, H., Ogawa, A. and Okumura, N. (1987) High-dose gammaglobulin therapy for Kawasaki disease. *J. Pediat.* **110**, 710–712.

Nagel, R.L. (1990) Red-cell cytoskeletal abnormalities—implications for malaria (Editorial). *New Engl. J. Med.* **323**, 1558–1560.

Nagington, J., Cossart, Y.E. and Cohen. B.J. (1977) Reactivation of hepatitis B after transplantation operations. *Lancet*, **i**, 558–560.

Naidu, S. (1983) Central nervous system lesions in neonatal isoimmune thrombocytopenia. *Arch. Neurol.* **40**, 552–554.

Naiki, M. and Marcus, D.M. (1975) An immunochemical study of the human blood group P_1, P and P^k glycosphingolipid antigens. *Biochemistry*, **14**, 4837.

Naiki, M., Fong, J.. Ledeen, R. and Marcus, D.M. (1975) Structure of the human erythrocyte blood group P_1. *Biochemistry*, **14**, 4831.

Nakada, K., Kohakura, M., Komoda, H. and Hinum, Y. (1984) High incidence of HTLV antibody in carriers of *Strongyloides stercoralis* (Letter). *Lancet*, **i**, 633.

Nakajima, H. and Ito, K. (1978) An example of anti-Jr^a causing haemolytic disease of the newborn and frequency of Jr^a antigen in the Japanese population. *Vox Sang.* **35**, 265–267.

Nakao, M., Nakao, T., Arimatsu, Y. and Yoshikawa, H. (1960) A new preservative medium maintaining the level of adenosine triphosphate and the osmotic resistance of erythrocytes. *Proc. Jap. Acad.* **36**, 43.

Nakao, K., Wada, T. and Kamiyama, T. (1962) A direct relationship between adenosine triphosphate-level and *in vivo* viability of erythrocytes. *Nature (Lond.)*, **194**, 877.

Nakasone, N., Watkins, E. jr, Janeway, C.A. and Gross, R.E. (1954) Experimental studies of circulatory derangement following the massive transfusion of citrated blood. Comparison of blood treated with ACD solution and blood decalcified by ion exchange resin. *J. Lab. clin. Med.* **43**, 184.

Nance, S. and Garratty, G. (1984) Correlates between *in vivo* hemolysis and the amount of rbc bound IgG measured by flow cytometry (Abstract). *Blood*, **64**, Suppl. **1**, 88a.

Nance, S., Nelson, J., Horenstein, J., O'Neill, P. and Garratty, G. (1986) Predictive value of amniocentesis versus monocyte monolayer assays in pregnant women with Rh antibodies (Abstract). *Transfusion*, **26**, 570.

Nance, S.J. and Garratty, G. (1987) A new potentiator of red blood antigen–antibody reactions. *Amer. J. clin. Path*, **87**, 633–635.

Nance, S.J., Arndt, P. and Garratty, G. (1987) Predicting the clinical significance of red cell alloantibodies using a monocyte monolayer assay. *Transfusion*, **27**, 449–452.

Nance, Sandra J., Arndt, Patricia and Garratty, G. (1988) The effect of fresh normal serum on monocyte monolayer assay reactivity (Letter). *Transfusion*, **28**, 398–399.

Nance, Sandra J., Nelson, Janice M., Horenstein, Janet, Arndt, Patricia A., Platt, L.D. and Garratty, G. (1989) Monocyte monolayer assay: an efficient noninvasive technique for predicting the severity of haemolytic disease of the newborn. *Amer. J. clin. Path.* **92**, 89–92.

Nason, S.G., Vengelen-Tyler, V., Cohen, N., Best, M. and Quirk, J. (1980) A high incidence antibody (anti-Sc3) in the serum of a Sc: –1, –2 patient. *Transfusion*, **20**, 531–535.

Natvig, J.B. (1965) Incomplete anti-D antibody with changed Gm specificity. *Acta path. microbiol. scand.* **65**, 467.

Natvig, J.B. and Kunkel, H.G. (1968) Genetic markers of human immunoglobulins: the Gm and Inv systems. *Ser. Haemat.* **1**, 66.

Neefjes, J.J., Breur-Vriesendorp, Birgitta S., van Seventer, G.A., Ivany, P. and Ploegh, H.G. (1986) An improved biochemical method for the analysis of poly-morphism of HLA class-I antigens. Definition of new HLA class-I subtypes. *Hum. Immunol.* **16**, 169–181.

Negrin, R.S., Haeber, D.H., Nagler, A., Kobayashi, Y. Sklar, J., Donlon, T., Vincent, Martha and Greenberg, P.L. (1990) Maintenance treatment of patients with myelodysplastic syndromes using recombinant human granulocyte colony-stimulating factor. *Blood*, **76**, 36–43.

Neimann-Sørensen, A., Rendel, J. and Stone, W.H. (1954) The J substance of cattle. II. A comparison of normal antibodies and antigens in sheep, cattle and man. *J. Immunol.* **73**, 407.

Nelken, D. (1961) False positive anti human globulin tests caused by reticulocytes. *Vox Sang.* **6**, 348.

Nemunaitis, J., Singer, J.W., Buckner, C.D., Hill, R., Storb, R., Thomas, E.D. and Appelbaum,

F.R. (1988) Use of recombinant human granulocyte-macrophage colony-stimulating factor in autologous marrow transplantation for lymphoid malignancies. *Blood*, **72**, 834–836.

Ness, P.M. and Salamon, J.L. (1986) The failure of postinjection Rh immune globulin titers to detect large fetal–maternal hemorrhages. *Amer. J. clin. Path.* **85**, 604–606.

Ness, P.M., Baldwin, M.L. and Walsh, P.C. (1987) Pre-deposit autologous transfusion in radical retropubic prostatectomy (Abstract). *Transfusion*, **27**, 518.

Ness, P.M., Shirey, R.S., Thoman, S.K. and Buck, S.A. (1990) The differentiation of delayed serologic and delayed hemolytic transfusion reactions: incidence, long-term serologic findings, and clinical significance. *Transfusion*, **30**, 688–693.

Neter, E. (1936) Observations of abnormal isoantibodies following transfusions. *J. Immunol.* **30**, 255.

Neuberger, A. and Niven, Janet S.E. (1951) Haemoglobin formation in rabbits. *J. Physiol.* **112**, 292.

Nevanlinna, H.R. (1953) Factors affecting maternal Rh immunization. *Ann. Med. exp. fenn.* **31**, Suppl. 2.

Nevanlinna, H.R. and Vainio, T. (1956) The influence of mother-child ABO incompatibility on Rh immunization. *Vox Sang.* **1**, 26.

Nevanlinna, H.R. (1965) ABO protection in Rh immunization. *Commun. 10th Congr. Europ. Soc. Haemat.*, Strasbourg.

Newland, A.C., Treleaven, J.G., Minchinton, R.M. and Waters, A.H. (1983) High-dose intravenous IgG in adults with autoimmune thrombocytopenia. *Lancet*, **i**, 84–87.

Newland, A.C., Macey, A.C., Macintyre, E.A. and Linch, D.C. (1986) The role of intravenous IgG in autoimmune haemolytic anaemia, in *Abstracts, 21st Congr. Int. Soc. Blood Transfus.*, Sydney.

Newman, P.J., Derbes, R.S. and Aster, R.H. (1989) The human platelet alloantigens Pl^A1 and Pl^A2 are associated with a leucine[33]/proline[33] amino acid polymorphism in membrane glycoprotein IIIa and are distinguishable by DNA typing. *J. clin. Invest.* **83**, 1778–1781.

Newsom-Davis, J., Pinching, A.J., Vincent, Angela and Wilson, S.G. (1978) Function of circulating antibody to acetylcholine receptors in myasthenia gravis: investigation by plasma exchange. *Neurology*, **28**, 266.

Ng, P.K., Fournel, M.H. and Lundblad, J.L. (1981) PPF: product improvement studies. *Transfusion*, **21**, 682–685.

Nicholls, R.J., Davies, P. and Kenwright, Marga-

ret G. (1970) Thrombocytopenic purpura after blood transfusion. *Brit. med. J.* **ii**, 581.

Nicholls, A. (1986) Ethylene oxide and anaphylaxis during haemodialysis. *Brit. med. J.* **292**, 1221–1222.

Nichols, Margaret E., Rosenfield, R.E. and Rubinstein, P. (1985) Two blood group M epitopes disclosed by monoclonal antibodies. *Vox Sang.* **49**, 138–148.

Nichols, Margaret E., Rosenfield, R.E. and Rubinstein, P. (1987a) Monoclonal anti-K14 and anti-K2. *Vox Sang.* **52**, 231–235.

Nichols, Margaret E., Rubinstein, P., Barnwell, J., De Cordoba, S.R. and Rosenfield, R.E. (1987b) A new human Duffy blood group specificity defined by a murine monoclonal antibody. *J. exp. Med.* **166**, 776–785.

Nicholson-Weller, A., Burge, J., Fearon, D.T., Weller, P.F. and Austen, K.F. (1982) Isolation of a human erythrocyte membrane glycoprotein with decay accelerating activity for C3 convertases of the human complement system. *J. Immunol.* **129**, 184–189.

Nicholson-Weller, A., March, J.P., Rosenfield, S.I. and Austen, K.F. (1983) Affected erythrocytes of patients with paroxysmal nocturnal hemoglobinuria are deficient in the complement regulatory protein, decay accelerating factor. *Proc. nat. Acad. Sci. USA*, **80**, 5066–5070.

Nicolaides, K.H. and Rodeck, C.H. (1985) Rhesus disease: the model for fetal therapy. *Brit. J. hosp. Med.* **34**, 141–148.

Nicolaides, K.H., Rodeck, C.H., Millar, D.S. and Mibashan, R.S. (1985a) Fetal haematology in rhesus isoimmunization. *Brit. med. J.* **290**, 661–663.

Nicolaides, K.H., Warenski, J.C. and Rodeck, C.H. (1985b) The relationship of fetal plasma protein concentration and hemoglobin level to the development of hydrops in rhesus isoimmunization. *Amer. J. Obstet. Gynaec.* **152**, 341–344.

Nicolaides, K.H., Rodeck, C.H., Mibashan, R.S. and Kemp, J.R. (1986) Have Liley charts outlived their usefulness? *Amer. J. Obstet. Gynec.* **155**, 90–94.

Nicolaides, K.H., Soothill, P.W., Clewell, W.H., Rodeck, C.H., Mibashan, R.S. and Campbell, S. (1988) Fetal haemoglobin measurement in the assessment of red cell immunisation. *Lancet*, **i**, 1073–1075.

Nicolini, U. and Rodeck, C.H. (1988) A proposed scheme for planning intrauterine transfusion in patient with severe Rh-immunisation. *J. Obstet. Gynec.* **9**, 162–163.

Nicolini, U., Kochenour, N.K., Greco, P., Letsky, Elizabeth A., Johnson, R.D., Contreras, Marcela and Rodeck, C.H. (1988a) Consequences of fetomaternal haemorrhage after intra-uterine transfusion. *Brit. Med. J.* **297**, 1379–1381.

Nicolini, V., Rodeck, C.H., Kochenowe, N.K., Greco, P., Fisk, N.M., Letsky, E. and Lubenko, A. (1988b) *In utero* platelet transfusion for alloimmune thrombocytopenia. *Lancet*, **ii**, 506.

Nicolson, G.L., Masouredis, S.P. and Singer, S.J. (1971) Quantitative two-dimensional ultrastructural distribution of $Rh_0(D)$ antigenic sites on human erythrocyte membranes. *Proc. nat. Acad. Sci. USA*, **68**, 1416.

NIH (National Institutes of Health) (1985) Fresh frozen plasma. Indications and risks. *J. Amer. med. Assoc.* **253**, 551–553.

NIH (1986) *The Impact of Routine HTLV-III Antibody Testing on Public Health*. National Institutes of Health Consensus Development Conference Statement, **6**, pp. 1–9.

NIH (1987) Consensus Development Conference. Platelet transfusion. *J. Amer. med. Assoc.* **257**, 1777–1780.

Nijenhuis, L.E. and Bratlie, K. (1962) ABO antibodies in twins. *Vox Sang.* **7**, 236.

Nilsson, I.M., Walter, H., Mikaelsson, M. and Vilhardt, H. (1979) Factor VIII concentrate prepared from DDAVP stimulated blood donor plasma. *Scand. J. Haemat.* **22**, 42–46.

Nilsson, T., Rudolphi, O. and Cedergren, B. (1983) Effects of intensive plasmapheresis on the haemostatic system. *Scand. J. Haemat.* **30**, 201–206.

Nishida, T., Nakagawa, S., Awata, T., Tani, Y. and Manabe, R. (1983) Fibronectin eyedrops for traumatic recurrent corneal erosion. *Lancet*, **ii**, 521.

Nishimura, Y., Yamaguchi, K., Kiyokawa, T., Takatsuki, K., Imamura, Y. and Fujiwara, H. (1989) Prevention of transmission of human T-cell lymphotropic virus type-I by blood transfusion by screening of donors (Letter). *Transfusion*, **29**, 372.

Nishioka, K. (1990) Hepatitis C virus: hepatocellular carcinoma and mode of infection. *Transfusion Today*, **6**, 3–4.

Nisonoff, A. and Pressman, D. (1957) Closeness of fit and forces involved in the reactions of antibody homologous to the p-(p-azophenylazo)-benzoate ion group. *J. Amer. chem. Soc.* **79**, 1616.

Nissen, Catherine, Tichelli, A., Gratwohl, A., Speck, B., Miene, Alison, Gordon-Smith, E.C. and Schaedelin, J. (1988) Failure of recombinant human granulocyte-macrophage colony-stimulating factor therapy in aplastic anemia with severe neutropenia. *Blood*, **72**, 2045–2047.

Noble, R.P. and Gregersen, M.I. (1946) Blood volume in clinical shock. II. The extent and cause of blood volume reduction in trau-matic, hemorrhagic, and burn shock. *J. clin. Invest.* **25**, 172.

Noble, T.C. and Abbott, J. (1959) Haemolysis of stored blood mixed with isotonic dextrose-containing solutions in transfusion apparatus. *Brit. med. J.* **ii**, 865.

Noble, R.C., Kane, M.A., Reeves, Sally A. and Roeckel, Irene (1984) Post-transfusion hepatitis A in a neonatal intensive care unit. *J. Amer. med. Assoc.* **252**, 2711–2715.

Noël, A. (1981) Anti-A isoagglutinins and pneumococcal vaccine. *Lancet*, **ii**, 687–688.

Nordhagen, R. and Ørjasaeter, H. (1974) Association between HL-A and red cell antigens. An AutoAnalyzer study. *Vox Sang.* **26**, 97.

Nordhagen, R. (1977) Association between HLA and red cell antigens. IV. Further studies of haemagglutinins in cytotoxic HLA antisera. *Vox Sang.* **32**, 82.

Nordhagen, R. (1978) Association between HLA and red cell antigens. V. A further study of the nature and behaviour of the HLA antigens on red blood cells and their corresponding haemagglutinins. *Vox Sang.* **35**, 49.

Nordhagen, R. and Aas, M. (1978) Association between HLA and red cell antigens. VII. Survival studies of incompatible red cells in a patient with HLA-associated haemagglutinins. *Vox Sang.* **35**, 319.

Nordhagen, R. (1979) HLA antigens on red blood cells. Two donors with extraordinarily strong reactivity. *Vox Sang.* **37**, 209–215.

Nordhagen. R. and Aas, M. (1979) Survival studies of ^{51}Cr Ch(a+) red blood cells in a patient with anti-Ch^a, and massive transfusion of incompatible blood. *Vox Sang.* **37**, 179–181.

Nordhagen, Rannveig, Olaisen, B., Teisberg, B. and Gedde-Dahl, T. jr (1980) Association between the electrophoretically determined C4M haplotype product and partial inhibition of anti-Ch^a. *J. Immunogenet.* 301–306.

Nordhagen, R. (1983) Cross-reactions in the HLA system revealed by red blood cells expressing HLA determinants, with particular reference to cross-reactions between HLA-A2 and B17. *Vox Sang.* **44**, 218–224.

Nordhagen, R. and Kornstad, L. (1984) The manual polybrene test in relation to low concentration red cell antibodies. *Abstracts, 18th Congr. Int. Soc. Blood Transfus.*, Munich, p. 218.

Nordhagen, R., Conradi, M. and Dromtorp, S.M. (1986) Pulmonary reaction associated with transfusion of plasma containing anti-5b. *Vox Sang.* **51**, 102–108.

Norfolk, D.R., Bowen, M., Cooper, E.H. and Robinson. A.E. (1985) Changes in plasma fibronectin during donor apheresis and therapeutic plasma exchange. *Brit. J. Haemat.* **61**, 641–647.

Northoff, H., Martin, A. and Roelcke, D. (1987) An IgG κ-monotypic anti-Pr$_{ih}$ associated with fresh varicella infection. *Eur. J. Haemat.* **38**, 85–88.

Nossaman, Janis K. (1981) Laboratory evaluation of the immunized patient, in *Prenatal and Perinatal Immunohematology*, eds W.M. Tregellas and C.H. Wallas. Amer. Assoc. Blood Banks, Arlington, VA.

Notes on Epidemiology (1977) Human immunoglobulin by the intravenous route. *Brit. med. J.* **i**, 521.

Nouri, A., Macfarlane, T.W., Mackenzie, D. and McGowan, D.A. (1989) Should recent dental treatment exclude potential blood donors? *Brit. med. J.* **298**, 295.

Noyes, W.D., Bothwell, T.H. and Finch, C.A. (1960) The role of the reticulo-endothelial cell in iron metabolism. *Brit. J. Haemat.* **6**, 43.

Noyes, W.D. and Garby, L. (1967) Rate of haptoglobin synthesis in normal man. Determination by the return to normal levels following hemoglobin infusion. *Scand. J. clin. Lab. Invest.* **20**, 33.

Nsongkla, M., Hummert, J. and Chaplin, H. jr (1982) Weak "false positive" DAT reactions with polyspecific antiglobulin reagents—lack of correlation with rbc-bound C3d. *Transfusion*, **22**, 273–278.

Nunn, J.F. and Freeman, J. (1964a) Problems of oxygenation and oxygen transport during anaesthesia. *Anaesthesia*, **19**, 120.

Nunn, J.F. and Freeman, J. (1964b) Problems of oxygenation and oxygen transport during-haemorrhage. *Anaesthesia*, **19**, 206.

Nurden, A.T., Dupuis, D., Pidard, D., Kieffer, Nelly, Kunicki, T.J. and Cartron, J.-P. (1982) Surface modifications in the platelets of a patient with alpha-N-acetyl-D-galactosamine residues, the Tn-syndrome. *J. clin. Invest.* **70**, 1281–1291.

Nusbacher, J. and Naiman, R. (1989) Longitudinal follow-up of blood donors found to be reactive for antibody to human immunodeficiency virus (anti-HIV) by enzyme-linked immunoassay (EIA) but negative by western blot (WB). *Transfusion*, **29**, 365–367.

Nyman, Margareta, Gydell, K. and Nosslin, B. (1959) Haptoglobin und Erythrokinetik. *Clin. chim. Acta*, **4**, 82.

Nymand, G. (1974) Complement-fixing and lymphocytotoxic antibodies in serum of pregnant women at delivery. *Vox Sang.* **27**, 322.

Oakes, J., Taylor, D., Johnson, C. and Marsh, W.L. (1978) Fy^3 antigenicity of blood of newborns (Letter). *Transfusion*, **18**, 127.

Oberdorfer, C.E., Kahn, B., Moore, V., Zelenski, K., Øyen, R. and Marsh, W.L. (1974) A second example of anti-Fy^3 in the Duffy blood group system. *Transfusion*, **14**, 608.

Oberman, H.A. (1974) Transfusion of the neonatal patient. *Transfusion*, **14**, 183.

Oberman, H.A., Barnes, B.A. and Friedman, B.A. (1978) The risk of abbreviating the major crossmatch in urgent or massive transfusion. *Transfusion*, **18**, 137.

Oberman, H.A. (1984) In International Forum: How much plasma, relative to his body weight, can a donor give over a certain period without a continuous deviation of his plasma protein metabolism in the direction of plasma protein deficiency? *Vox Sang.* **47**, 442–443.

Oberman, H.A. (1985) Uses and abuses of fresh frozen plasma, in *Current Concepts in Transfusion Therapy*, ed G. Garratty. Amer. Assoc. Blood Banks, Arlington, VA.

Oberman, H.A. (1990) Appropriate use of plasma and plasma derivatives, in *Transfusion Therapy: Guidelines for Practice*, eds S.H. Summers, D.M. Smith and D.M. Agranenko. Amer. Assoc. Blood Banks, Arlington, VA.

Obregon, E. and McKeever, B.G. (1980) Studies in offspring of pp mothers (Abstract). *Transfusion*, **20**, 621–622.

Ochs, H.D., Fischer, S.H., Virant, F.S., Lee, M.L., Kingdon, H.S. and Wedgwood, R.J. (1986) Non-A, Non-B hepatitis and intravenous immunoglobulin. *Lancet*, **i**, 404–405.

Ochs, H.D., Fischer, S.H., Virant F.S., Lee, M.L., Mankarious, S., Kingdon. H.S. and Wedgwood, R.J. (1986) Non-A, Non-B hepatitis after intravenous gamma-globulin (Letter). *Lancet*, **i**, 322–323.

O'Connel, B.A. and Schiffer, C.A. (1990) Donor selection for alloimmunized patients by platelet crossmatching of random donor platelet concentrates. *Transfusion*, **30**, 314–317.

O'Connor, B., Clifford, Jacqueline S., Lawrence, W.D. and Logue, G.L. (1989) Alpha-interferon for severe cold agglutinin disease. *Ann. intern. Med.* **111**, 255.

Oda, H., Honda, A., Sugita, K., Nakamura, A. and Nakajima, H. (1985) High-dose intravenous intact IgG infusion in refractory auto immune hemolytic anemia (Evans syndrome). *J. Pediat.* **107**, 744–746.

O'Day, T. (1987) A second example of autoanti-Jk3. *Transfusion*, **27**, 442.

Oehlecker, F. (1928) Hämolyse trotz Blutgruppenbestimmung. Anhang: experimentelle Studien über den Eintritt der Hämolyse. *Arch. für klin. Chir.* **152**, 477.

Officer, R. (1945) Experimental transfusion with malaria infected blood. *Med. J. Aust.* **i**, 271.

Ogasawara, K. and Mazda, T. (1989) Differences in substrate specificities for cysteine proteinases used in blood group serology, and the use of bromelain in a two-phase inhibitor technique. *Vox Sang.* **57**, 72–76.

Ogata, T. and Matuhasi, T. (1962) Problems of specificity and cross reactivity of blood group antibodies. *Proc. 8th Congr. Int. Soc. Blood Transfus*, Tokyo, 1960, p. 208.

Ogata, T. and Matuhasi, T. (1964) Further observations on the problems of specific and cross reactivity of blood group antibodies. *Proc. 9th Congr. Int. Soc. Blood Transfus.*, Mexico, 1962, p. 528.

Ogata, N., Alter, H.J., Miller, R.H. and Purcell, R.H. (1991) Nucleotide sequence and mutation rate of the H strain of hepatitis C virus. *Proc. nat. Acad. Sci. USA*, **88**, 3392–3396.

Ogden, J.E., Woodrow, J., Perks, K., Harris, R., Coghlan, D., Chan, B., Jones, G. and Wilson, M.T. (1991) Expression and assembly of functional human haemoglobin in *Saccharomyces cerevisiae* (Abstract). *Transfus. Med.* Suppl. 2, 14.

Ogle, J.W. (1881) *The Harveian Oration, 1880.* Burt & Co. (Printers), London.

Ohnishi, Y. and Kitazawa, M. (1980) Application of perfluorochemicals in human beings. *Acta Path. Japan.* **30**, 489–504.

Oien, L., Nance, S. and Garratty, G. (1985) Zygosity determinations using flow cytometry—a superior method (Abstract). *Transfusion*, **25**, 474.

Oikawa, T., Hosokawa, M., Iwamura, M., Sendo, F., Nakayama, Gotodha, E., Kodama, T. and Kobayshi, H. (1977) Anti-tumour immunity by normal allogenic blood transfusion in rat. *Clin. exp. Immunol.* **27**, 549–554.

Okochi, K. and Sato, H. (1985) Adult T-cell leukemia virus, blood donors and transfusion: experience in Japan, in *Infection, Immunity and Blood Transfusion*, eds R.Y. Dodd and L.F. Barker, pp. 245–256. A.R. Liss, New York.

Okochi, K. and Sato, H. (1989) Blood transfusion and HTLV-I in Japan, in *HTLV-I and the Nervous System*, eds C.G. Román, J.C. Vernant and M. Osame, pp. 527–532. Alan R. Liss, New York.

Okubo, Y., Yamaguchi, H., Nagao, N., Tomita, T., Seno, T. and Tanaka, M. (1986) Heterogeneity of the phenotype Jk(a–b–) found in Japanese. *Transfusion*, **26**, 237–239.

Olesen, H. (1966) Thermodynamics of the cold agglutinin reaction. *Scand. J. clin. Lab. Invest.* **18**, 1.

Olivares-Lopez, F., Cruz-Carranza, G., Peterz-Rodriguez, G.E. and Camacho-Gutierrez, M.G.R. (1985) Malaria inducida por transfusión de sangre. Análisis de 44 casos. *Rev. med. Inst. Mex. Seg. Soc.* **23**, 153–157.

Olson, P.R., Cox, C. and McCullough, J. (1977) Laboratory and clinical effects of the infusion of ACD solution during plateletpheresis. *Vox Sang.* **33**, 79.

O'Neill, G.J., Yang, S.Y., Tegoli, J., Berger, R. and Dupont, B. (1978) Chido and Rodgers blood groups are distinct antigenic components of human complement C4. *Nature (Lond.)*, **273**, 668.

O'Neill, Patricia, Shulman, Ira A., Simpson, R.B., Halima, Diana and Garratty, G. (1986) Two examples of low ionic strength-dependent autoagglutinins with anti-Pr_a specificity. *Vox Sang.* **50**, 107–111.

Onkelinx, E., Meuldermans, W., Joniau, M. and Lontie, R. (1969) Glutaraldehyde as a coupling reagent in passive haemagglutination. *Immunology*, **16**, 35.

Opelz, G., Sengar, D.P.S., Mickey, M.R. and Terasaki, P.I. (1973) Effect of blood transfusions on subsequent kidney transplants. *Transplant Proc.* **5**, 253.

Opelz, G. (1984) Ninth international histocompatibility workshop renal transplant study, in *Histocompatibility Testing* 1984, eds E.D. Albert, M.P. Baur and W.R. Mayr. Springer-Verlag.

Opelz, G. (1985) Effect of HLA matching, blood transfusion and presensitization in cyclosporine-treated kidney transplant recipients. *Transplant. Proc.* **12**, 2179–2183.

Opelz, G. (1987) Improved kidney graft survival in non-transfused recipients. *Transplant. Proc.* **19**, 149–153.

Opelz, G. (1988) Importance of HLA antigen splits for kidney transplant matching. *Lancet*, **ii**, 61–64.

Oral, A., Nusbacker, J., Hill, J.B. and Lewis, J.H. (1984) Intravenous gammaglobulin in the treatment of chronic idiopathic thrombocytopenic purpura in adults. *Amer. J. Med.* **76** (3a), 187–192.

Ordman, C.W., Jennings, C.G. and Janeway, C.A. (1944) Chemical, clinical and immunological studies on the products of human plasma fractionation. XII. The use of concentrated normal human serum gamma globulin (human immune serum globulin) in the prevention and attenuation of measles. *J. clin. Invest.* **23**, 541.

O'Reilly, R.A., Lombard, C.M. and Azzi, R.L. (1985) Delayed hemolytic transfusion reaction associated with Rh antibody anti-f: first reported case. *Vox Sang.* **49**, 336–339.

Oriol, R., Cartron, J., Yvart, J., Bedrossian, J., Duboust, A., Bariety, J., Gluckman, J.C. and Gagnadoux, M.F. (1978) The Lewis system: new histocompatibility antigens in renal transplantation. *Lancet*, **i**, 574.

Oriol, R., Baur, M.P., Danilovs, J., Pollock, C. and Mayr, W. (1980a) Combined ABH-Lewis-secretor antigens, in *Histocompatibility Testing, 1980*, ed P.I. Terasaki, p. 585. UCLA Tissue Typing, Los Angeles.

Oriol, R., Danilovs, J., Lemieux, R., Terasaki, P. and Bernoco, D. (1980b) Lymphocytoxic definition of combined ABH and Lewis antigens and their transfer from sera to lymphocytes. *Human Immunol.* **3**, 195–205.

Oriol, R. (1990) Genetic control of the fucosylation of ABH precursor chains. Evidence for new epistatic interactions in different cells and tissues. *J. Immunogenet.* **17**, 235–245.

Oriol, R., Samuelsson, B.E. and Messeter. L. (1990) ABO antibodies — serological behaviour and immuno-chemical characterization. *J. Immunogenet.* **17**, 279–299.

Orlin, J.B. and Berkman, E.M. (1980) Partial exchange using albumin replacement: removal and recovery of normal plasma constituents. *Blood*, **56**, 1055–1059.

Orlina, A. and Josephson, A. (1969) Comparative viability of blood stored in ACD and CPD. *Transfusion*, **9**, 62.

Orlina, A.R., Josephson, A.M. and McDonald, Barbara J. (1970) The poststorage viability of glucose-6-phosphate dehydrogenase-deficient erthrocytes. *J. Lab. clin. Med.* **75**, 930.

Orlina, A.R., Brim, L.H., Gilbert, R. jr, McDonald, B.J. and Josephson, A.M. (1972) Preliminary evaluation of an automated disposable continuous centrifugal washing system for frozen-stored blood. *Transfusion*, **12**, 227.

Orlina, A.R., Unger, Phyllis J. and Koshy, Mabel (1978) Post-transfusion alloimmunization in patients with sickle cell disease. *Amer. J. Hemat.* **5**, 101.

Ørntoft, T.F., Holmes, E.H., Johnson, P., Hakomori, S-I. and Clausen H. (1991) Differential tissue expression of the Lewis blood group antigens: enzymatic, immunohistologic, and immunochemical evidence for Lewis a and b antigen expression in Le(a–b–) individuals. *Blood*, **77**, 1389–1396.

Osame, M., Usuku, K. and Izumo, S. (1986) HTLV-I associated myelopathy. A new clinical entity (Letter). *Lancet*, **ii**, 1031–1032.

Osame, M., Igata, A., Matsumoto, M., Kohka, M., Usuku, K. and Izumo, S. (1990) HTLV-I associated myelopathy (HAM) treatment trials, retrospective survey and clinical and laboratory findings. *Haematol. Rev.* **3**, 271–284.

Osband, M.E., Lavin, P.T., Babayan, R.K., Graham, S., Lamm, D.L., Parker, Barbara, Sawczuk, I., Ross, Susan, Crane, R. J. (1990). Effect of autolymphocyte therapy on survival and quality of life in patients with metastatic renal-cell carcinoma. *Lancet*, **i**, 994–998.

Osborn, L.M., Lenarsky, C., Oakes, R.C. and Reiff, M.I. (1984) Phototherapy in full-term infants with hemolytic disease secondary to ABO incompatibility. *Pediatrics*, **74**, 371–374.

Oski, F.A., Marshall, B.E., Cohen, P.J., Sugerman, H.J. and Miller, L.D. (1971a) Exercise with anemia. The role of the left-shifted or right-shifted oxygen—hemoglobin equilibrium curve. *Ann. intern. Med.* **74**, 44–46.

Oski, F.A., Travis, Susan F., Miller, L.D., Delivoria-Papadopoulos, Maria and Cannon, Elizabeth (1971b) The *in vitro* restoration of red cell 2,3-diphosphoglycerate levels in banked blood. *Blood*, **37**, 52.

Ostrow, J.D., Jandl, J.H. and Schmid, R. (1962) The formation of bilirubin from hemoglobin *in vivo. J. clin. Invest*, **41**, 1628.

Otsuka, S. and 10 others (1989) Fatal erythroderma (suspected graft-versus-host disease) after cholecystectomy. *Transfusion*, **29**, 544.

Otsuka, S., Kunieda, K., Kitamura, F., Misawa, K., Sasaoka, I., Hirose, M., Kasuya, S., Saji, S. and Noma, A. (1991) The critical role of blood from HLA-homozygous donors in fatal transfusion-associated graft-versus-host disease in immunocompetent patients. *Transfusion*, **31**, 260–264.

Ottenberg, R. (1908) Transfusion and arterial anastomosis. Some experiments in arterial anastomosis and a study of transfusion with presentation of two clinical cases. *Ann. Surg.* **47**, 486.

Ottenberg, R. (1911) Studies in isoagglutination. I. Transfusion and the question of intravascular agglutination. *J. exp. Med.* **13**, 425.

Ottenberg, R. and Kaliski, D.J. (1913) Accidents in transfusion. Their prevention by preliminary blood examination: based on experience of one hundred and twenty-eight transfusions. *J. Amer. med. Assoc.* **61**, 2138.

Ottenberg, R. and Thalheimer, W. (1915) Studies in experimental transfusion. *J. med. Res.* **33**, 213.

Ottenberg, R. (1937) Reminiscences of the history of blood transfusion. *J. Mt. Sinai Hosp.* **4**, 264.

Ottenberg, R. and Fox, C.L. (1938) Rate of removal of hemoglobin from the circulation and its renal threshold in human beings. *Amer. J. Physiol.* **123**, 516.

Ottensooser, F. and Willenegger, H. (1938) Ueber die gruppen spezifischen A-reaktionen von Impfstoffen. Pepton- und Pepsin-präparaten. *Schweiz. Z. allg. Path.* **1**, 421.

Ottensooser, F. and Silberschmidt, K. (1953) Haemagglutinin anti-N in plant seeds. *Nature* (*Lond.*), **172**, 914.

Ovary, Z. and Spiegelman, J. (1965) The production of cold 'autohemagglutinins' in the rabbit as a consequence of immunization with isologous erythrocytes. *Ann. N.Y. Acad. Sci.* **124**, 147.

Overweg, J. and Engelfriet, C.P. (1969) Cytotoxic leucocyte iso-antibodies formed during the first pregnancy. *Vox Sang.* **16**, 97.

Owen, R.D. (1954) Heterogeneity of antibodies to

the human blood groups in normal and immune sera. *J. Immunol.* **73**, 29.

Owen, R.D., Woon, H.R., Foord, A.G., Sturgeon, P. and Baldwin, L.G. (1954) Evidence for actively acquired tolerance to Rh antigens. *Proc. nat. Acad. Sci. USA*, **40**, 420.

Owens, M., Cimino, C. and Donnelly, J. (1991) Cryopreserved platelets have decreased adhesive capacity. *Transfusion*, **31**, 160–163.

Owings, Debra V., Kruskall, Margot S., Thurer, R.L. and Donovan, Lillian M. (1989) Autologous blood donations prior to elective cardiac surgery: safety and effect on subsequent blood use. *J. Amer. med. Assoc.* **262**, 1963–1968.

Ozawa, N., Shimiza, M., Imai, M., Miyakawa, Y. and Maynini, M. (1985) Selective absence of immunoglobulin A1 or A2 among blood donors and hospital patients. *Transfusion*, **26**, 73–76.

Ozer, F.L. and Chaplin, H. (1963) Agglutination of stored erythrocytes by a human serum. Characterization of the serum factor and erythrocyte changes. *J. clin. Invest.* **42**, 1735.

Pace, N., Lozner, E.L., Consolazio, W.V., Pitts, G.C. and Pecora, L.J. (1947) The increase in hypoxia tolerance of normal men accompanying the polycythemia induced by transfusion of erythrocytes. *Amer. J. Physiol.* **148**, 152.

Page, P.L., Langevin, S., Petersen, R.A. and Kruskall, Margot S. (1987) Reduced association between the Ii blood group and congenital cataracts in White patients. *Amer. J. clin. Path.* **87**, 101–102.

Pahwa, S., Kaplan, M., Firkig, S., Pahwa, R., Sarngadharan, M.G., Popovic, M. and Gallo, R.C. (1986) Spectrum of human T-cell lymphotropic virus type III infection in children. Recognition of symptomatic, asymptomatic, and seronegative patients. *J. Amer. med. Assoc.* **255/17**, 2299–2305.

Pai, M.K.R., Bedritis, I. and Zipursky, A. (1977) Massive transplacental hemorrhage: clinical manifestations in the newborn. *Canad. med. Assoc. J.* **112**, 585.

Painter, R.H. and Minta, J.O. (1969) Stability of immune serum globulin during storage: effects of modifications in the fractionation scheme. *Vox Sang.* **17**, 434.

Palek, J., Mirćevová, L., Brabec, V., Friedmann, B. and Májský, A. (1968) The effect of anti-A antibody on red cell organic phosphates and adenosine triphosphatase activity *in vitro*. *Scand. J. Haemat.* **5**, 191.

Palek, J. and Lambert, S. (1990) Genetics of the red cell membrane skeleton. *Semin. Hemat.* **27**, 290–332.

Palosuo, T. and Milgrom, F. (1980) Appearance of dextrans and anti-dextran antibodies in human sera. *Int. Arch. Allergy appl. Immunol.* **57**, 153–161.

Pamphilon, D.H., Carbin, S.A., Saunders, J. and Tandy, N.P. (1989) Applications of ultraviolet light in the preparation of platelet concentrates. *Transfusion*, **29**, 379–383.

Pamphilon, D.H., Potter, M., Cutts, M., Meenaghan, M., Rogers, W., Slade, R.R., Saunders, J., Tandy, N.P. and Fraser, I.D. (1990) Platelet concentrates irradiated with ultraviolet light retain satisfactory *in vitro* storage characteristics and *in vivo* survival. *Brit. J. Haemat.* **75**, 240–244.

Pangburn, M.K. and Muller-Eberhard, H.J. (1984) The alternative pathway of complement, in *Springer Seminars in Immunopathology*, eds P.A. Miescher and H.J. Muller-Eberhard, **7**, 163–192. Springer Verlag.

Pannacciulli, I., Tizianello, A., Ajmar, F. and Salvidio, E. (1965) The course of experimentally induced hemolytic anemia in a primaquine-sensitive caucasian. *Blood*, **25**, 92.

Panzer, S., Salama, A., Bodeker, R.H. and Mueller-Eckhardt, C. (1984a) Quantitative evaluation of elution methods for red cell antibodies. *Vox Sang.* **46**, 330–335.

Panzer, S., Mueller-Eckhardt, G., Salama, A., Strauss, B.-E., Kietel, V. and Mueller-Eckhardt, C. (1984b) The clinical significance of HLA antigens on red cells. Survival studies in HLA-sensitized individuals. *Transfusion*, **24**, 486–489.

Pao, C.C., Yao, D-S., Lin, C-Y., Kao, S-M., Tsao, K-C., Sun, C-F. and Liaw, Y-F. (1991) Serum hepatitis B virus DNA in hepatitis B virus seropositive and seronegative patients with normal liver function. *Amer. J. clin. Path.* **95**, 591–596.

Pappenheimer, A.M. (1940) Anti-egg albumin antibody in the horse. *J. exp. Med.* **71**, 263.

Pareira, M.D., Serkes, K.D. and Lang, S. (1964) Enhanced efficacy of plasma after ageing in treatment of tourniquet shock. *Proc. Soc. exp. Biol. (N.Y.)*, **115**, 660.

Parinaud, J., Blanc, M., Grandjean, H., Fournie, A., Bierme, S. and Pontonnier, G. (1985) IgG subclasses and Gm allotypes of anti-D antibodies during pregnancy: correlation with the gravity of the fetal disease. *Amer. J. Obstet. Gynec.* **151**, 1111–1115.

Parish, H.J. and Macfarlane, R.G. (1941) Effect of calcium in a case of autohaemagglutination. *Lancet*, **ii**, 447.

Park, B.H., Goon, R.A., Gate, J. and Burke, B. (1974) Fatal graft-versus-host reaction following transfusion of allogeneic blood and plasma in infants with combined immunodeficiency disease. *Transplant. Proc.* **6**, 385.

Parker, A.C., Willis, G., Urbarniak, S.J. and

Innes, E.M. (1978) Autoimmune haemolytic anaemia with anti-A autoantibody. *Brit. med. J.* i, 26.

Parkes, A.S. (1985) *Off-beat Biologist; the Autobiography of A.S. Parkes*, p. 439. The Galton Foundation, Cambridge.

Parkman, R., Mosier, D., Umansky, I., Cochran, W., Carpenter, C.B. and Rosen, F.S. (1974) Graft-versus-host disease after intrauterine and exchange transfusions for hemolytic disease of the newborn. *New Engl. J. Med.* 290, 359.

Parr, L.W. and Krischner, H. (1932) Hemolytic transfusion fatality with donor and recipient in the same blood group. *J. Amer. med. Assoc.* 98, 47.

Parsons, S.F., Judson, P.A. and Anstee, D.J. (1982) A monoclonal antibody with a specificity related to the Kell blood group system. *J. Immunogenet.* 9, 377–380.

Parsons, S.F., Mallinson, G., Judson, P.A., Anstee, D.J. Tanner, M.J.A. and Daniels, G.L. (1987) Evidence that the Lu^b blood group antigen is located on red cell membrane glycoproteins of 85 and 78 kd. *Transfusion*, 27, 61–63.

Parsons, Polly E., Worthen, G.S., Moore, E.R. Tate, R.M. and Hensen, P.M. (1989) The association of circulating endotoxin with the development of the adult respiratory distress syndrome. *Amer. Rev. resp. Dis.* 240, 249–310.

Parsons, S.F., Gardner, B. and Anstee, D.J. (1991) Monoclonal antibodies to epitopes on Kell protein; serology, immunochemistry and quantitation of antigen sites (Abstract). *Transfus. Med.* 1, Suppl. 2, 48.

Pasternack, A. and Furuhjelm, U. (1964) Heavy agglutination of leucocytes complicating haemodialysis. *Lancet*, ii, 1095.

Pasvol, G., Anstee, D. and Tanner, M.J.A. (1984) Glycophorin C and the invasion of red cells by *Plasmodium falciparum. Lancet*, i, 907–908.

Patten, E., Beck, C.E., Scholl, C., Stroope, R.A. and Wukasch, C. (1977) Autoimmune hemolytic anemia with anti-Jk^a specificity in a patient taking aldomet. *Transfusion*, 17, 517.

Patten, R., Reddi, C.R., Riglin, H. and Edwards, J. (1982) Delayed hemolytic transfusion reaction caused by a primary immune response. *Transfusion*, 22, 248–250.

Patten, Ethel and Patel, S. (1989) Preparation of leukocyte-poor platelet concentrates. *Transfusion*, 29, 562–563.

Pattison, J.R., Jones, S.E., Hogdson, J., Davis, L.R., White, J.M., Stroud, C.E. and Murtaza, L. (1981) Parvovirus infections and hypoplastic crisis in sickle-cell anaemia. *Lancet*, i, 664.

Pattison, J.R., (1987) B19 virus—a pathogenic human parvovirus. *Blood Reviews*, 1, 58–64.

Paul, L.C., Baldwin, W.M., Claas, H.J., van Es, L.A. and van Rood, J.J. (1984) Monocyte alloantigens in man: genetics and expression on the renal endothelium, in *Mononuclear Phagocyte Biology*, ed A. Volkmann. M. Dekker Inc., New York.

Paul, Deborah, Falk, L., Knigge, M., Landay, A., Bice, M. and Blaaw, B. (1986) Potential use of serum assays for HTLV III Ag and Ab in following disease progression in Ab+ individuals. *Abstracts, International Conference on AIDS*, Paris, p. 146.

Paulson, O.B., Parring, H-H., Olsen. J. and Skinhoj, E. (1973) Influence of carbon monoxide and of hemodilution on cerebral blood flow and blood gases in man. *J. appl. Physiol.* 35, 111.

Pavone, Beverly G. and Issitt, P.D. (1974) Anti-Bg antibodies in sera used for red cell typing. *Brit. J. Haemat.* 27, 607.

Pavone, B.G., Pirkola, A., Nevanlinna, H.R. and Issitt, P.D. (1978) Demonstration of anti-Wr^b in a second serum containing anti-En^a. *Transfusion*, 18, 155.

Pavone, B.G., Billman, R., Bryani, J., Sniecinski, I. and Issitt, P.D. (1981) An auto-anti-En^a, inhibitable by MN sialoglycoprotein. *Transfusion*, 21, 25–31.

Pawlak, Z. and Lopez, M. (1979) Développement des antigènes ABH et Ii chez les enfants de O à 16 ans. *Rev. franç. Transfus. Immunohémat.* 22, 253–263.

Payne, Rose (1957) The association of febrile transfusion reactions with leukoagglutinins. *Vox Sang.* 2, 233.

Payne, R. and Rolfs, M.R. (1958) Fetomaternal leucocyte incompatibility. *J. clin. Invest.* 37, 1756.

Pearce, R.M. (1904) The experimental production of liver necroses by intravenous injection of haemagglutinins. *J. med. Res.* 12, 329.

Pearl, R.G., Halperin, B.D., Mihm, F.G. and Rosenthal, M.H. (1988) Pulmonary effects of crystalloid and colloid resuscitation from hemorrhagic shock in the presence of oleic acid-induced pulmonary capillary injury in the dog. *Anesthesiology*, 68, 12 20.

Pearson, E.S. and Hartley, H.O. (eds) (1954) *Biometrika Tables for Statisticians*, 2nd edn, vol. I, p. 203. Cambridge University Press (for the Biometrika Trustees).

Pearson, H.A. and Diamond, L.K. (1959) Fetomaternal transfusion. *Amer. J. Dis. Childh.* 97, 267.

Pearson, H.A. and Vertrees, K.M. (1961) Site of binding of chromium 51 to haemoglobin. *Nature (Lond.)*, 189, 1019.

Peevy, K.J. and Wiseman, H.J. (1978) ABO hemolytic disease of the newborn: evaluation of management and identification of racial and antigenic factors. *Pediatrics*, 61, 475.

Pegels, J.G., von dem Borne, A.E.G.Kr., Thomas, L.L.M., Tytgat, G.N. and Engelfriet, C.P. (1980) Auto-immune granulocytopenia, possibly associated with levamisole therapy. *Clin. lab. Haemat.* **2**, 339–346.

Pegels, J.G., Bruynes, E.C.E., Engelfriet, C.P. and von dem Borne, A.E.G.Kr. (1981) Post-transfusion purpura: a serological and immunochemical study. *Brit. J. Haemat.* **49**, 521–530.

Pegels, J.G., von dem Borne, A.E.G.Kr., Bruynes, E.C.E. and Engelfriet, C.P. (1982) Pseudo-thrombocytopenia: an immunological study on platelet antibodies dependent on ethylene diamine tetra-acetate. *Blood*, **59**, 157.

Pejandier, L., Kickenin-Martin, V. Boffa, M.C. and Stembuch, M. (1987) Appraisal of the protein composition of prothrombin complex concentrates of different origins. *Vox Sang.* **52**, 1–9.

Pellegrino, M.A., Ferrone, S. and Theofilopoulos, A.N. (1976) Isolation of human T and B lymphocytes by rosette formation with 2-aminoethyliso thiouronium bromide (AET)-treated sheep red blood cells and with monkey red blood cells. *J. immunol. Methods*, **11**, 273.

Pelosi, M.A., Bauer, J.L., Langer, A. and Hung, C.T. (1974) Transfusion of incompatible blood after neutralization of Lewis antibodies. *Obstet. Gynec.* **4**, 590.

Pembrey, M.E., Weatherall, D.J. and Clegg, J.B. (1973) Maternal synthesis of haemoglobin F in pregnancy. *Lancet*, **i**, 1350.

Penny, R., Rozenberg, M.C. and Firkin, B.G. (1966) The splenic platelet pool. *Blood*, **27**, 1.

Penny, A.F., Townley, Alison, Robinson, Angela, E., Warrington, R., Learoy, D.P., Gilkes, L. and Tovey, L.A.D. (1984) Pilot study of an automated dual component plasmapheresis collection system. *Apheresis Bull.* **2**, 3–12.

Pepper, D.S. (1983) A review of column technology as applied to apheresis. *Apheresis Bull.* **1**, 114–124.

Pepperell, R.J., Barrie, J.U. and Fliegner, J.R. (1977) Significance of red-cell irregular antibodies in the obstetric patient. *Med. J. Aust.* **ii**, 453.

Pereira, A., Monteagudo, J., Rovira, M., Mazzara, R., Reverter, J.C. and Castillo R. (1989) Anti-K1 of the IgA class associated with *Morganella morganii* infection. *Transfusion*, **29**, 549–551.

Pereira, A., Mazzara, R. and Castillo, R. (1990) Transfusion of racially unmatched blood (Letter). *New Engl. J. Med.* **323**, 1421.

Perine, P.L. (1983) Non-venereal treponemes: yaws, endemic syphilis and pinta, in *Oxford Textbook of Medicine*, eds, D.J. Weatherall, J.G.G. Ledingham and D.A. Warrell, pp. 5.301–5.303. Oxford University Press, Oxford.

Perkins, H.A., Day, Dorothy and Hill, Elaine (1964) An immunologic basis for massive loss of red blood cells after open heart surgery. *Proc. 9th Congr. Int. Soc. Blood Transfus.*, Mexico, 1962, p. 97.

Perkins, H.A., Payne, Rose, Ferguson, Joyce and Wood, Mildred (1966) Nonhemolytic febrile transfusion reactions. Quantitative effects of blood components with emphasis on isoantigenic incompatibility of leukocytes. *Vox Sang.* **11**, 578.

Perkins, H.A. (1975) In *Transfusion and Immunology*, eds Ikkala and Nykanon, *Plenary Session Lectures, 14th Congr. Int. Soc. Blood Transfus.*, Helsinki.

Perkins, H.A., McIlroy, M., Swanson, J. and Kadin, M. (1977) Transient LW-negative red blood cells and anti-LW in a patient with Hodgkin's disease. *Vox Sang.* **33**, 299.

Perkins, S.J., Nealis, A.S., Sutton, B.J. and Feinstein, A. (1991) Solution structure of human and mouse immunoglobulin M by synchroton X-ray scattering and molecular graphics modelling. *J. mol. Biol.* **221**, 1345–1366.

Perrault, R. and Högman, C. (1971) Automated red cell antibody analysis. A parallel study. II. Identification of serological specificity. *Vox Sang.* **20**, 356.

Perrault, R.A. and Högman, C.F. (1972) Low concentration red cell antibodies. III. 'Cold' IgG anti-D in pregnancy: incidence and significance. *Acta Universitatis uppsaliensis*, No. 120.

Perrault, R. (1973a) 'Cold' IgG autologous anti-LW. *Vox Sang.* **24**, 150.

Perrault, R. (1973b) Naturally-occuring anti-M and anti-N with special case: IgG anti-N in a NN donor. *Vox Sang.* **24**, 134.

Persijn, G.G., Hendriks, G.F.J. and van Rood, J.J. (1984) HLA matching, blood transfusion and renal transplantation, in *Clinical Immunology and Allergy*, eds J.J. van Rood and R.R.P. de Vries. W.B. Saunders, London.

Pert, J.H., Schork, P.K. and Moore, R. (1963) A new method of low-temperature blood preservation using liquid nitrogen and a glycerol sucrose additive. *Clin. Res.* **11**, 197.

Peterman, T.A., Jaffe, H.W., Feorino, P.M., Getchell, Jane, P., Warfield, Donna, T., Haverkos, H.W., Stoneburner, R.L. and Curran, J.W. (1985) Transfusion-associated acquired immunodeficiency syndrome in the United States. *J. Amer. med. Assoc.* **254**, 2913–2917.

Peterman, T.A. (1987) Transfusion-associated acquired immunodeficiency syndrome. *World J. Surg.* **11**, 36–40.

Petermans, M.E. and Cole-Dergent, J. (1970) Haemolytic transfusion reaction due to anti-Sd^a. *Vox Sang.* **18**, 67.

Peters, B., Reid, M.E., Ellisor, S.S. and Avoy, D.R. (1978) Red cell survival studies of Lu^b incompatible blood in a patient with anti-Lu^b (Abstract). *Transfusion*, **18**, 623.

Peters, A.M., Klonizakis, I., Lavender, J.P. and Lewis, S.M. (1980) Use of ^{111}Indium-labelled platelets to measure spleen function. *Brit. J. Haemat.* **46**, 587–593.

Peters, A.M., Saverymuttu, S.H., Wonke, B., Lewis, S.M. and Lavender, J.P. (1984) The interpretation of sites of abnormal platelet destruction. *Brit. J. Haemat.* **57**, 637–649.

Peters, A.M., Saverymuttu, S.H., Bell, R.N. and Lavender, J.P. (1985) Quantification of the distribution of the marginating granulocyte pool in man. *Scand. J. Haemat.* **34**, 111–120.

Petit, A., Duong, T.H., Brémond, J.L., Barrabes, A., Binet, Ch., Combescot, Ch. and Leroux, M.E. (1981) Allo-anticorps irréguliers anti-P$_1$ et Clonorchiase à clonorchis sinensis. *Rev. franç. Transfus. Immunohémat.* **24**, 197–210.

Petranyi, C.C., Padanyi, A., Horuzsko, A., Rethy, M., Gyodi, E. and Perner, F. (1988) Mixed lymphocyte culture evidence that pretransplant transfusion with platelets induces FcR and blocking antibody production similar to that induced by leucocyte transfusion. *Transplantation*, **45**, 823–824.

Petricciani, J.C., McDougal, J.S. and Evatt, B.L. (1985) Case for concluding that heat treated licensed anti-hemophilic factor is free from HTLV-III. *Lancet*, **ii**, 803–804.

Pettenkofer, H.J. and Hoffbauer, H. (1954) Über die Bedeutung des Lewis-Blutgruppensystems für die Entstehung eines Morbus haemolyticus neonatorum. *Zbl. Gynäk.* **76**, 576.

Petty, T. and Ashburgh, D.G. (1971) The adult respiratory distress syndrome: clinical features, factors influencing prognosis and principles of management. *Chest*, **60**, 223–239.

Petz, L.D. and Fudenberg, H.H. (1966) Coombs-positive hemolytic anemia caused by penicillin administration. *New Engl. J. Med.* **274**, 171.

Petz, L.D. and Garratty, G. (1975) Laboratory correlations in immune hemolytic anemias, in *Laboratory Diagnosis of Immunologic Disorders*, eds G.N. Vyas, D.P. Sites and G. Brecher. Grune & Stratton, New York.

Petz, L.D. and Garratty, G (1980) *Acquired Immune Hemolytic Anemias*. Churchill Livingstone, New York.

Petz, L.D. and Branch, D.R. (1983) Serological tests for the diagnosis of immune haemolytic anaemias, in *Methods in Haematology: Immune Cytopenias*, ed R. McMillan, pp. 9–48. Churchill Livingstone, New York.

Petz, L.D. and Branch, D.R. (1985) Drug-induced hemolytic anemia in *Immune Hemolytic Anemias*, ed H. Chaplin, pp. 47–94. Churchill-Livingstone, New York.

Petz, L.D. and Swisher, S.N. (1989) Blood transfusion in acquired hemolytic anemias, in *Clinical Practice of Transfusion Medicine*, eds L.D. Petz and S.N. Swisher, pp. 549–582. Churchill Livingstone, New York.

Petz, L.D., Saxton, E., Lee, H., Chen, I.S.Y., Chin, E., Delamarter, R., Rosenblatt, J.D., Harper, M. and Ness, P.M. (1989) A case of transfusion transmitted HTLV-I associated myelopathy (Abstract). *Transfusion*, **29**, 55S.

Petz, L.R. (1991) The expanding boundaries of transfusion medicine, in *Clinical and Basic Science Aspects of Immunohematology*, ed Sandra T. Nance. American Association of Blood Banks, Arlington, VA.

Phan, T.M., Foster, C.S., Bornchoff, S.A., Zagachin, L.M. and Colvin, R.B. (1987) Topical fibronectin in the treatment of persistent corneal epithelial defects and trophic ulcers. *Amer. J. Ophthalmol.* **104**, 494.

Phibbs, R.H., Johnson, P. and Tooley, W.H. (1974) Cardiorespiratory status of erythroblastic newborn infants. II. Blood volume, hematocrit, and serum albumin concentration in relation to hydrops fetalis. *Pediatrics*, **53**, 13.

Phillips, P.K., Prior, Dilys and Dawes, B. (1984) A modified azo-albumin technique for the assay of proteolytic enzymes for use in blood group serology. *J. clin. Path.* **37**, 329–331.

Phillips, P.K. (1987) A preparation for calibrating the assay of the blood group antibody anti-c. *Brit. J. Haemat.* **65**, 57–59.

PHLS Malaria Reference Laboratory (1983) Malaria prophylaxis. *Brit. med. J.* **286**, 787–789.

Pichlmayer, R., Ringe, B., Laanchart, W. and Wonigeit, K. (1987) Liver transplantation. *Transplant. Proc.* **29**, 103–112.

Pickles, M.M. (1946) Effect of cholera filtrate on red cells as demonstrated by incomplete Rh antibodies. *Nature (Lond.)*, **158**, 880.

Pickles, Margaret M. (1949) *Haemolytic Disease of the Newborn*. Blackwell Scientific Publications, Oxford.

Pickles, Margaret M. and Morton, J.A. (1977) The Sd^a blood group, in *Human Blood Groups*, eds J.F. Mohn, R.W. Plunkett, R.K. Cunningham and R.M. Lambert, pp. 277–286. S. Karger, Basel.

Pickles, M.M., Jones, M.N., Egan, J., Dodsworth, H. and Mollison, P.L. (1978) Delayed haemolytic transfusion reactions due to anti-C. *Vox Sang.* **35**, 32.

Pien, F.D., Smith, T.F., Taswell, H.F. and Hable, Kathleen A. (1974) Cold reactive antibodies in a case of congenital cytomegalo-virus infection. *Amer. J. clin. Path.* **61**, 352.

Pierce, S.R., Hardman, J.T., Hunt, J.S. and Beck, M.L. (1980) Anti-Yt^a: characterization by IgG subclass composition and macrophage assay (Abstract). *Transfusion*, **20**, 627–628.

Pietersz, Ruby N.I., Reesink, H.W., Dekker, W.J.A. and Fyen, F.J. (1987) Preparation of leukocyte-poor platelet concentrates from buffy coats. I. Special inserts for centrifuge cups. *Vox Sang.* **53**, 203–208.

Pietersz, Ruby N.I., Dekker, W.J.A. and Reesink, H.W. (1989a) A new cellulose acetate filter to remove leucocytes from buffy-coat-poor red cell concentrates. *Vox Sang.* **56**, 37–40.

Pietersz, R.N.I., de Korte, D., Reesink, H.W., Dekker, W.J.A., van den Ende, A. and Loos, J.A. (1989b) Storage of whole blood for up to 24 hours at ambient temperature prior to component preparation. *Vox Sang.* **56**, 145–150.

Pikul, F.J., Farrar, R.P., Boris, M.B., Estok, L., Marlo, D., Wildgen, M. and Chaplin, H. (1989) Effectiveness of two synthetic fiber filters for removing white cells from AS-I red cells. *Transfusion*, **29**, 590–595.

Piller, F. and Cartron, J.P. (1983) Biosynthesis of antigenic structures, in *Red Cell Membrane Glycoconjugates and Related Genetic Markers*, eds J.P. Cartron, P. Rouger and C. Salmon, pp. 175–181. Lib. Arnette, Paris.

Pindyck, J., Waldman, A., Zang, E., Olesko, W., Lowy, M. and Bianco, C. (1985) Measures to decrease the risk of acquired immune deficiency transmission by blood transfusion. *Transfusion*, **25**, 3–9.

Pineda, A.A. and Taswell, H.F. (1975) Transfusion reactions associated with anti-IgA antibodies: report of four cases and review of the literature. *Transfusion*, **15**, 10.

Pineda, A.A., Brzica, S.M. jr and Taswell, H.F. (1977) Continuous semicontinuous-flow blood centrifugation systems; therapeutic applications with plasma, platelet and eosinapheresis. *Transfusion*, **17**, 407–416.

Pineda, A.A., Taswell, H.F. and Brzica, S.M. jr (1978a) Delayed hemolytic transfusion reaction. An immunologic hazard of blood transfusion. *Transfusion*, **18**, 1.

Pineda, A.A., Brzica, S.M. and Taswell, H.F. (1978b) Hemolytic transfusion reaction. Recent experience in a large blood bank. *Mayo Clin. Proc.* **53**, 378.

Pineda, A.A., Chase, C.J. and Taswell, H.F. (1987) Red cell antibodies: clinical and laboratory relevance in multitransfused patients, in *Thalassemia Today. The Mediterranean Experience, Proc. 2nd Mediterranean Meeting on Thalassemia*, eds G. Sirchia and A. Zanella, Milano, 1985. Centro Trasfusionale Ospedale Maggiore Policlinico di Milano Editore.

Pineda, A.A. and Valbonesi, M. (1990) Intra-operative blood salvage, in *Blood Transfusion: the Impact of New Technologies*, ed Marcela Contreras. *Baillière's Clinical Haematology*, **3**, 385–403.

Pingleton, M.D., Coalson, Jacqueline, J., Hinshaw, L.B. and Guenter, C.A. (1972) Effects of steroid pretreatment on development of shock lung. *Lab. Invest.* **27**, 445.

Pinkerton, F.J., Mermod, L.E., Liles, B.A., Jack, J. jr and Noades, J. (1959) The phenotype Jk(a–b–) in the Kidd blood group system. *Vox Sang.* **4**, 155.

Pinkerton, P.H., Tilley, C.A. and Crookston, M.C. (1977) cited by Bird and Wingham (1977a).

Pinkerton, P.H. and nine others (1979) Proficiency testing in immunohematology in Ontario, Canada, 1975–1977. *Amer. J. clin. Path.* **72**, 559–563.

Pinkerton, P.H. and nine others (1981) Proficiency testing in immunohaematology in Ontario, Canada 1977–1979. *Clin. lab. Haemat.* **3**, 155–164.

Pinkerton, P.H., Zuber, Edna D., Barr, R.M., Croucher, Betsy, E.E., Quantz, Marie, C., Rapson, Dilys, A., Wood, D.E., Crockford, Joan and Moore, B.P.L. (1984) Sensitivity of routine blood bank methods for the detection of anti-D as determined during proficiency testing. *Amer. J. clin. Path.* **82**, 326–329.

Pinkerton, P.H., Zuber, E.D., Wood, D.E., Holburn, A.M. and Prior, D. (1985) Proficiency testing in immunohaematology in Ontario, Canada, and in the United Kingdom: a comparative study. *J. clin. Path.* **38**, 570–574.

Piomelli, S., Lurinsky, Gertrude and Wasserman, L.R. (1967) The mechanism of red cell aging. 1. Relationship between cell age and specific gravity evaluated by ultracentrifugation in a discontinuous density gradient. *J. Lab. clin. Med.* **69**, 659.

Piomelli, S., Seaman, Carol, Reibman, Joan, Tytun, A., Graziano, J., Tabachnik, Nina and Corash, L. (1978) Separation of younger red cells with improved survival *in vivo*; an approach to chronic transfusion therapy. *Proc. nat. Acad. Sci. USA*, **75**, 3474.

Pirofsky, B. and Cordova, Maria de la S. (1963) Bivalent nature of incomplete anti-D (Rho). *Nature (Lond.)*, **197**, 392.

Pirofsky, B. and Nelson, Helen M. (1964) The determination of hemoglobin in blood banks. *Transfusion* **4**, 45.

Pischel, K.D., Bluestein, H.G. and Woods W.L. (1988) Platelet glycoprotein Ia, Ic and IIa are physicochemically indistinguishable from the very late activation adhesion-related proteins of lymphocytes and other cell types. *J. clin. Invest.* **81**, 585–513.

Pitney, W.R., Thomas, H.N. and Wells, J.V. (1968) Cold haemagglutinins associated with splenomegaly in New Guinea. *Vox Sang.* **14**, 438.

Pittman, Margaret (1953) A study of bacteria implicated in transfusion reactions and of bacteria isolated from blood products. *J. Lab. clin. Med.* **42**, 273.

Plapp, F. V., Sinor, L.T., Rachel, G.M., Beck, M.L., Coenen, W.M. and Bayer, W.L. (1984) A solid phase antibody screen. *Amer. J. clin. Path.* **82**, 719–721.

Plapp, F.V., Rachel, J.M., Beck, M.L. *et al.* (1984) Blood antigens and antibodies: solid-phase adherence assays. *Lab. Manag.* **22**, 39–47.

Plapp, F.V., Rachel, J.M. and Simor, C.T. (1986) Dipsticks for determining ABO blood groups. *Lancet* i, 1465–1466.

Plischka, H. and Schäfer, E. (1972) A study on the immunoglobulin class of the anti-A_1 iso-agglutinin. *J. Immunol.* **108**, 782.

Plow, E.F., Birdwell, C. and Grinsberg, M.N. (1979) Identification and quantification of platelet-associated fibronectin antigen. *J. clin. Invest.* **63**, 540–543.

Podack, E.R. (1986) Assembly and functions of the terminal components, in *Immunobiology of the Complement System*, ed. G.D. Ross, pp. 115–137 Academic Press.

Poiesz, B.J., Ruscetti, F.W., Gazdar, A.F., Bunn, P.A., Minna, J.D. and Gallo, R.C. (1980) Detection and isolation of type C retrovirus particles from fresh and cultured lymphocytes of a patient with cutaneous T-cell lymphoma. *Proc. nat. Acad. Sci. USA*, **77**, 7415–7419.

Poles, F.C. and Boycott, M. (1942) Syncope in blood donors. *Lancet*, ii, 531.

Polesky, H.F. and Bove, J.R. (1964) A fatal hemolytic transfusion reaction with acute autohemolysis. *Transfusion*, **4**, 285.

Polesky, H.F. and Swanson, J.L. (1966) Studies on the distribution of the blood group antigen Do^a (Dombrock) and the characteristics of anti-Do^a. *Transfusion*, **11**, 162.

Polge, C., Smith, Audrey U. and Parkes, A.S. (1949) Revival of spermatozoa after vitrification and dehydration at low temperatures. *Nature (Lond.)*, **164**, 666.

Pollack, W., Hager, H.J. and Hollenberger, L.L. jr (1962) The specificity of anti-human gamma globulin reagents. *Transfusion*, **2**, 17.

Pollack, W. (1965) Some physicochemical aspects of hemagglutination. *Ann. N.Y. Acad. Sci.* **127**, 892.

Pollack, W., Hager, H.J., Reckel, R., Toren, D.A. and Singher, H.O. (1965) A study of the forces involved in the second stage of the hemagglutination. *Transfusion*, **5**, 158.

Pollack, W., Gorman, J.G., Hager, H.J., Freda, V.J. and Tripodi, D. (1968a) Antibody-mediated immune suppression to the Rh factor; animal models suggesting mechanism of action. *Transfusion*, **8**, 134.

Pollack, W., Gorman, J.G., Freda, V.J., Ascari, W.Q., Allen, A.E. and Baker, W.J. (1968b) Results of clinical trials of RhoGAM in women. *Transfusion*, **8**, 151.

Pollack, W., Ascari, W.Q., Kochesky, R.J., O'Connor, R.R., Ho, T.Y. and Tripodi, D. (1971a) Studies on Rh prophylaxis. I. Relationship between doses of anti-Rh and size of antigenic stimulus. *Transfusion*, **11**, 333.

Pollack, W., Ascari, W.Q., Crispen, J.F., O'Connor, R.R. and Ho, T.Y. (1971b) Studies on Rh prophylaxis. II. Rh immune prophylaxis after transfusion with Rh-positive blood. *Transfusion*, **11**, 340.

Pollack, W. (1980) Preparation of a broad-spectrum antiglobulin reagent using monoclonal antibodies against human complement components. *Abstracts, 18th Congr. Int. Soc. Hemat.*, Montreal.

Pollack, S., Cunningham-Rundles, C., Smithwick, E.M., Barandun, S. and Good, R.A. (1982) High dose intravenous gamma globulin in autoimmune neutropenia. *New Engl. J. Med.* **307**, 253.

Polley, Margaret J. and Mollison, P.L. (1961) The role of complement in the detection of blood group antibodies. Special reference to the antiglobulin test. *Transfusion*, **1**, 9.

Polley, Margaret J., Mollison, P.L. and Soothill, J.F. (1962) The role of 19S gamma globulin blood group antibodies in the antiglobulin reaction. *Brit. J. Haemat.* **8**, 149.

Polley, Margaret J., Adinolfi, M. and Mollison, P.L. (1963) Serological characteristics of anti-A related to type of antibody protein ($7S\gamma$ or $19S\gamma$). *Vox Sang.* **8**, 385.

Polley, Margaret J. (1964) The development and use of the antiglobulin sensitization test for the study of the serological characteristics of blood-group antibodies and for the quantitive estimation of certain serum proteins. Ph.D. Thesis, University of London.

Polley, Margaret J., Mollison, P.L., Rose, Jane and Walker, W. (1965) A simple serological test for antibodies causing ABO-haemolytic disease of the newborn. *Lancet*, i, 291.

Pollock, A. (1968) Transplacental haemorrhage after external cephalic version. *Lancet*, i, 612.

Pollock, T.M. and Reid, D. (1969) Immunoglobulin for the prevention of infectious hepatitis in persons working overseas. *Lancet*, i, 281.

Pollock, Janet M. and Bowman, J.M. (1990) Anti-Rh(D) subclasses and severity of Rh hemolytic disease of the newborn. *Vox Sang.* **59**, 176–179.

Pondman, K.W., Rosenfield, R.E., Tallal, L. and Wasserman, L.R. (1960) The specificity of the complement antiglobulin test. *Vox Sang.* **5**, 297.

Ponfick, Prof. (1875) Experimentelle Beiträge zur Lehre von der Transfusion. *Virchows Arch. path. Anat.* **62**, 273.

Pool, Judith G. (1970) Cryoprecipitated Factor VIII concentrate. *Bibl. haemat. (Basel)*, **34**, 23.

Poole, Joyce and Giles, Carolyn M. (1982) Observations on the Anton antigen and antibody. *Vox Sang.* **43**, 220–222.

Poon, Annette and Wilson, S. (1980) Simple manual method for harvesting granulocytes. *Transfusion*, **20**, 71–74.

Popat, N., Wood, W.G. and Weatherall, D.J. (1977) Pattern of maternal F-cell production during pregnancy. *Lancet*, **ii**, 377.

Popovic, M., Sarngadharan, M.G., Read, I. and Gallo, R.C. (1984) Detection, isolation and continuous production of cytopathic retrovirus HTLV-III from patients with AIDS and pre-AIDS. *Science*, **224**, 497–500.

Popovsky, M.A., Abel, M.D. and Moore, S.B. (1983) Transfusion-related acute lung injury associated with passive transfer of antileukocyte antibodies. *Amer. Rev. resp. Dis.* **128**, 185–189.

Popovsky, M.A. and Moore, S.B. (1985) Diagnostic and pathogenetic considerations in transfusion-related acute lung injury. *Transfusion*, **25**, 573–577.

Popovsky, M.A. (1987) The role of autologous transfusion in surgery and the emergency room, in *Autologous and Directed Blood Programs*, eds R. J. Garner and A. J. Silvergleid. pp. 47–63. Amer. Assoc. Blood Banks, Arlington, VA.

Popovsky, M.A. (1990) Babesiosis and lyme disease: a transfusion medicine perspective, in *Emerging Global Patterns in Transfusion Transmitted Infections*, eds R.G. Westphal, K.B. Carlson and J.M. Ture, pp. 45–64. Amer. Assoc. Blood Banks, Arlington, VA.

Popper, H. (1988) Pathobiology of hepatocellular carcinoma, in *Viral Hepatitis and Liver Disease*, ed A.J. Zuckerman, pp. 719–722, Alan R. Liss, New York.

Portugal, C.L., Pinho, M.O., Barbosa, M., Mettrau, M.C., de Azevedo, J.G., Contreras, M., Cervi, P. and Lubenko, A. (1990) The first example of severe haemolytic disease in an infant born to an Rh null proposita. *Abstracts, Joint Congress of Int. Soc. Blood Transfus. and Amer. Assoc. Blood Banks*, Los Angeles.

Posner, M.P., McGeorge, M.B., Mendez-Picon, G., Mohanakumar, T. and Lee, H.M. (1986) The importance of the Lewis system in cadaver renal transplantation. *Transplantation*, **41**, 474–477.

Postoway, N., Nance, S., O'Neill, P. and Garratty, G. (1985) Comparison of a practical differen-tial agglutination procedure to flow cytometry in following the survival of transfused red cells (Abstract). *Transfusion*, **25**, 453.

Potapov, M.I. (1970) Detection of the antigen of the Lewis system, characteristic of the erythrocytes of the secretory group Le(a – b –). *Probl. Hemat. Blood Transfus.* **15**, 45.

Potter, M.L. and Moore, M. (1977) Human mixed lymphocyte culture using separated lymphocyte preparations. *Immunol.* **32**, 359.

Poulain, M. and Huchet, J. (1971) Appréciation de l'hémorragie foeto-maternelle après l'accouchement en vue de la prévention de l'immunisation anti-D. (Bilan de 5.488 tests de Kleihauer.) *Rev. franç. Transfus.* **14**, 219.

Poulsen, Anne-Grethe, Kvinesdal, Birgit, Aaby, P., Molbak, Kåre, Frederiksen, Kirsten, Dias, F. and Lauritzen, E. (1989) Prevalence of and mortality from human immunodeficiency virus type 2 in Bissau, West Africa. *Lancet*, **i**, 827–831.

Powell, F.S. and Doran, J.E. (1991) Current status of fibronectin in transfusion medicine: focus on clinical studies. *Vox Sang.* **60**, 193–202.

Pratt, G.A., Bowell, P.J., MacKenzie, I.Z., Ferguson, Jane and Selinger, M. (1989) Production of additional atypical antibodies in Rh(D)-sensitised pregnancies managed by intrauterine investigation method. *Clin. lab. Haemat.* **11**, 241–248.

Prchal, J.T., Huang, S.T., Court, W.S. and Poon, M.C. (1985) Immune hemolytic anemia following administration of antithymocyte globulin. *Amer. J. Haemat.* **19**, 95–98.

Preiksaitis, J.K., Rosno, S., Grumet, C. and Merigan, T.C. (1983) Infections due to herpes viruses in cardiac transplant recipients: role of the donor heart and immunosuppressive therapy. *J. infect. Dis.* **147**, 974–981.

Preiksaitis, J. (1991) Indications for the use of cytomegalovirus-seronegative blood products. *Transfus. Med. Rev.* **5**, no. 1, 1–17.

Prentice, T.C., Olney, J.M. jr, Artz, C.P. and Howard, J.M. (1954) Studies of blood volume and transfusion therapy in the Korean battle casualty. *Surg. Gynec. Obstet.* **99**, 542.

Prentice, C.R.M. (1985) Acquired coagulation disorders, in *Coagulation Disorders*, ed A.N. Ruggeri. *Clinics in Haemat.* **14**, 413–442.

Preston, A.E. and Barr, A. (1964) The plasma concentration of Factor VIII in the normal population. II. The effects of age, sex and blood group. *Brit. J. Haemat.* **10**, 238.

Preston, F.E., Hay, C.R.M., Dewar, M.S., Greaves, M. and Triger, D.R. (1985) Non-A, non-B hepatitis and heat-treated Factor VIII concentrates (Letter). *Lancet*, **ii**, 213.

Prince, A.M. (1968) An antigen detected in the blood during the incubation period of serum hepatitis. *Proc. nat. Acad. Sci. USA*, **60**, 814.

Prince, A.M. (1975) Post-transfusion hepatitis: etiology and prevention, in *Transfusion and Immunology, Plenary Session Lectures of the 14th Congr. Int. Soc. Blood Transfus.*, Helsinki.

Prince, A.M., Horowitz, B., Horowitz, M.S. and Zang, E. (1987) The development of virus-free labile blood derivatives. A review. *Eur. J. Epidemiol*, **3**, 103–118.

Prins, H.K. and Loos, J.A. (1970) Studies on biochemical properties and viability of stored packed cells, in *Modern Problems of Blood Preservation*, eds W. Spielmann and S. Seidl. Gustav Fischer, Stuttgart.

Prins, H.K., De Bruyn, J.C.G.H., Henrichs, H.P.J. and Loos, J.A. (1980) Prevention of micro-aggregate formation by removal of "buffy-coats". *Vox Sang.* **39**, 48–51.

Pritchard, J.A. and Weisman, R. jr (1957) The absorption of labelled erythrocytes from the peritoneal cavity of humans. *J. Lab. clin. Med.* **49**, 756.

Prokop, O., Uhlenbruck, G. and Kohler, W. (1968) A new source of antibody-like substances having anti-blood group specificity. A discussion on the specificity of helix agglutinins. *Vox Sang.* **14**, 321.

Propper, R.D., Cooper, B., Rufo, R.R., Nienhuis, A.W., Anderson, W.F., Bunn, H.F., Rosenthal, A. and Nathan, D.G. (1977) Continuous subcutaneous administration of deferoxamine in patients with iron overload. *New Engl. J. Med.* **297**, 418.

Propper, R.D., Button, L.N. and Nathan, D.G. (1980) New approaches to the transfusion management of thalassaemia. *Blood*, **55**, 55–60.

Pross, H.F. and Eidinger, D. (1974) Antigenic competition: a review of nonspecific antigen-induced suppression, in *Advances in Immunology*, eds F.J. Dixon and H. G. Kunkel, Vol. 18. Academic Press, London.

Prou, O. (1985) Mise en evidence de *Plasmodium falciparum* par immunofluorescence indirecte a l'aide d'anticorps monoclonaux murins specifiques. *Rev. franç. Transfus. Immunohémat.* **28**, 659–670.

Pruitt, B.A., Moncrief, J.A. and Mason, A.D. (1965) Effect of buffered saline solution upon the blood volume of man after acute measured hemorrhage. *Annual Research Progress Report U.S. Army Surgical Research Unit, Texas.*

Pruitt, B.A. jr (1978) Advances in fluid therapy and the early care of the burn patient. *World J. Surg.* **2**, 139–150.

Pruzanski, W., Cowan, D.H. and Parr, D.M. (1974) Clinical and immunochemical studies of IgM cold agglutinins with lambda type

light chains. *Clin. Immunol. Immunopath.* **2**, 234.

Pruzanski, W., Farid, N., Keystone, E., Armstrong, M. and Greaves, M.F. (1975) The influence of homogeneous cold agglutinins on human B and T lymphocytes. *Clin. Immunol. Immunopath.* **4**, 248.

Pruzanski, W., Roelcke, D., Donnelly, E. and Lui, L-C. (1986) Persistent cold agglutinins in AIDS and related disorders. *Acta haemat.* **75**, 171–173.

Przestwor, E. (1964) Distribution of ABH group substances in amniotic fluid. *Poznanski Towarzystwo Przjaciol Nauk.* **29**, 197.

Puckett, A. (1986a) A sterility testing method for blood products. *Med. Lab. Sciences*, **43**, 249–251.

Puckett, A. (1986b) Bacterial contamination of blood for transfusion: a study of the growth characteristics of four implicated organisms. *Med. Lab. Sciences*, **43**, 252–257.

Puckett, A., Davison, G., Entwistle, C.C. and Barbara, J.A.J. (1992) Post transfusion septicaemia 1980–1989: importance of donor arm cleansing. *J. clin. Pathol.* **45**, 155–157.

Puig, N., Carbonell, F. and Marty, M.L. (1986) Another example of mimicking Anti-Kp[b] in a Kp(a + b –) patient. *Vox Sang.* **51**, 57–59.

Purcell, R.H., London, W.T., Newman, J., Gerin, J.L., Cicmance, J., Mindrea, M.E.H., Poppen, H. and Eigberg, J.W. (1985) Hepatitis B virus, hepatitis non-A, non-B virus and hepatitis delta virus in lyophilized anti-hemophilic factor; relative sensitivity to heat. *Hepatology*, **5**, 1091–1099.

Purcell, R.H. and Ticehurst, J.R. (1988) Enterically transmitted non-A, non-B hepatitis: epidemiology and clinical characteristics, in *Viral Hepatitis and Liver Disease*, ed A.J. Zuckerman, pp. 131–137. Alan R. Liss, New York.

Pusey, C.D. (1983) Vascular access for plasma exchange. *Apheresis Bull.* **1**, 87–91.

Quaranta, V., Imai, K., Molinaro, G.A. and Ferrone, S. (1980) Manufacture of monoclonal antibodies to human melanoma associated and histocompatibility antigens, in *Immunology, Clinical Laboratory Techniques for the 1980s*, eds R.M. Nakamura, W.R. Dito and E.S. Tucjer. Alan R. Liss, New York.

Quick, A.J., Georgatsos, J.G. and Hussey, Clara V. (1954) The clotting activity of human erythrocytes: theoretical and clinical implications. *Amer. J. Med. Sci.* **228**, 207.

Quigley, R.L., Wood, K.J. and Morris, P.J. (1989) Transfusion induces blood donor-specific suppressor cells. *J. Immunol.* **142**, 463–470.

Quintiliami, L. and 9 others (1991) Effects of blood transfusion on the immune responsiveness and survival of cancer patients: a prospective study. *Transfusion*, **31**, 713–718.

Rabiner, S.F. and Friedman, L.H. (1968) The role of intravascular haemolysis and the reticulo-endothelial system in the production of a hypercoagulable state. *Brit. J. Haemat.* **14**, 105.

Rabiner, S.F., O'Brien, K., Peskin, G.W. and Friedman, Lila H. (1970) Further studies with stroma-free hemoglobin solution. *Ann. Surg.* **171**, 615.

Race, R.R. (1944) An 'incomplete' antibody in human serum. *Nature (Lond.)*, **153**, 771.

Race, R.R., Mourant, A.E., Lawler, Sylvia, D. and Sanger, Ruth (1948a) The Rh chromosome frequencies in England. *Blood*, **3**, 689.

Race, R.R., Sanger, Ruth and Lawler, Sylvia, D. (1948b) The Rh antigen D^u. *Ann. Eugen. (Camb.)*, **14**, 171.

Race, R.R. and Sanger, Ruth (1950) *Blood Groups in Man*. Blackwell Scientific Publications, Oxford.

Race, R.R., Sanger, Ruth and Selwyn, J.G. (1951) A possible deletion in a human Rh chromosome: a serological and genetical study. *Brit. J. exp. Path.* **32**, 124.

Race, R.R. (1952) An unsuccessful attempt to discover some more blood groups. *Vox Sang. (O.S.)*, **3**, 191.

Race, R.R., Sanger, Ruth and Lehane, D. (1953) Quantitative aspects of the blood-group antigen Fy^a. *Ann. Eugen. (Camb.)*, **17**, 255.

Race, R.R. and Sanger, Ruth (1954) *Blood Groups in Man*, 2nd edn. Blackwell Scientific Publications, Oxford.

Race, R.R. and Sanger, Ruth (1962) *Blood Groups in Man*, 4th edn. Blackwell Scientific Publications, Oxford.

Race, R.R. and Sanger, Ruth (1968) *Blood Groups in Man*, 5th edn. Blackwell Scientific Publications, Oxford.

Race, Caroline and Watkins, Winifred M. (1972a) The enzymic products of the human A and B blood group genes in the serum of 'Bombay' O_h donors. *FEBS Letters*, **27**, 125.

Race, Caroline and Watkins, Winifred M. (1972b) The action of the blood group B gene-specified α-galactosyltransferase from human serum and stomach mucosal extracts on group O and 'Bombay' O_h erythrocytes. *Vox Sang.* **23**, 385.

Race, R.R. and Sanger, Ruth (1975) *Blood Groups in Man*, 6th edn. Blackwell Scientific Publications, Oxford.

Rachel, J.M., Sinor, L.T., Beck, M.L. and Plapp, F.V. (1985a) A solid-phase antiglobulin test. *Transfusion*, **25**, 24–26.

Rachel, Jane M., Sinor, L.T., Tawfik, D.W., Summers, T., Beck, M.L., Bayer, W.L. and Plapp, F.V. (1985b) A solid-phase red cell adherence test for platelet cross-matching. *Med. Lab. Sciences*, **42**, 194–195.

Rachel, Jane M., Summers, T.C., Sinor, L.T. and Plapp, F.V. (1988) Use of a solid phase red blood cell adherence method for pretransfusion platelet compatibility testing. *Amer. J. clin. Path.* **90**, 63–68.

Rachkewich, R.A., Crookston, M.C., Tilley, C.A. and Wherrett, J.R. (1978) Evidence that blood-group A antigen on lymphocytes is derived from the plasma. *J. Immunogenet.* **5**, 25.

Rackow, E.C., Falk, J.L., Fein, A., Siegel, J.S., Packman, M.I., Haupt, Marilyn T., Kaufman, B.S. and Putnam, D. (1983) Fluid resuscitation in circulatory shock: a comparison of the cardiorespiratory effects of albumin, hetastarch and saline solutions in patients with hypovolemic and septic shock. *Critical Care Medicine*, **11**, 839–850.

Radermecker, M., Bruwier, M., François, C., Brocteur, J., Salmon, J., André, A. and van Cauwenberger, H. (1975) Anti-P_1 activity in pigeon breeders' serum. *Clin. exp. Immunol.* **22**, 546.

Radovic, M., Balint, B., Milenkovic, L., Tiska-Rudman, L. and Taseski, J. (1991) Therapeutic leukapheresis. *Transfus. Sci.* **12**, 193–196.

Raevsky, C.A., Cohn, D.L., Wolf, F.C. and Judson, F.N. (1986) Transfusion-associated human T-lymphotropic virus type III/lymphadeno-pathy-associated virus infection from a sero-negative donor-Colorado. *MMWR.* **35**, 389–391.

Ragni, Margaret V. and 10 others (1986) AIDS retrovirus antibodies in hemophiliacs treated with factor VIII or factor IX concentrates, cryoprecipitate, or fresh frozen plasma: prevalence, seroconversion rate, and clinical correlations. *Blood*, **67**, 592–595.

Rajan, V.P., Larsen, R.D., Ajmera, S., Ernst, Linda K. and Lowe, J.B. (1989) A cloned human DNA restriction fragment determines expression of a GDP-L-fucose: β-D-galactoside 2-α-L-fucosyltransferase in transfected cells. *J. biol. Chem.* **264**, 11158–11167.

Ramirez, M.A. (1919) Horse asthma following blood transfusion: report of a case. *J. Amer. med. Assoc.* **73**, 985.

Ramirez, A.M., Woodfield, D.G., Scott, R. and McLachan, J. (1987) High potassium levels in stored irradiated blood (Letter). *Transfusion*, **27**, 444–445.

Ramsey, G., Nusbacher, J., Starzl, T.E. and Lindsay, Gwenn D. (1984) Isohemagglutinins of graft origin after ABO-unmatched liver transplantation. *New Engl. J. Med.* **311**, 1167–1170.

Ramsey, G., Israel, Linda, Lindsay, Gwenn D., Mayer, T.K. and Nusbacher, J. (1986) Anti-Rh_o(D) in two Rh-positive patients receiving kidney grafts from an Rh-immunized donor. *Transplantation*, **41**, 67–69.

Ramsey, G. and Larson, P. (1988) Loss of red cell antibodies over time. *Transfusion*, **28**, 162–165.

Ramsey, G., Cornell, F.W., Hahn, L.F., Issitt, L.B. and Starzl, T.E. (1989a) Red cell antibody problems in 1000 liver transplants. *Transfusion*, **29**, 396–400.

Ramsey, C., Hahn, Linda F., Cornell, F.W., Boczkowski, D.J., Staschak, Sandee, Clark, Roxann, Hardesty, R.L., Griffith, B.P. and Starzl, T.E. (1989b) Low rate of rhesus immunization from Rh-incompatible blood transfusions during liver and heart transplant surgery. *Transplantation*, **47**, 993–995.

Rand, B.P., Olson, J.D. and Garratty, G. (1978) Coombs negative immune hemolytic anemia with anti-E occurring in the red blood cell eluate of an E-negative patient. *Transfusion*, **18**, 174.

Randazzo, Paula, Streeter, B. and Nusbacher, J. (1973) A common agglutinin reactive only against bromelin-treated red cells (Abstract). *Transfusion*, **13**, 345.

Ranki, Annamari, Valle, S-L., Krohn, M., Antonen, J., Allain, J-P., Leuther, M., Franchini, G. and Krohn, K. (1987) Long latency precedes overt seroconversion in sexually transmitted human immunodeficiency-virus infection. *Lancet*, **ii**, 589–593.

Rao, Neeraja, Ferguson, D.J., Lee, S-F. and Telen, Marilyn J. (1991) Identification of human erythrocyte blood group antigens on the C3b/C4b receptor. *J. Immunol.* **146**, 3502–3507.

Rapoport, M. and Stokes, J. (1937) Reactions following the intramuscular injection of whole blood. *Amer. J. Dis. Childh.* **53**, 471.

Rapoport, S. (1947) Dimensional, osmotic and chemical changes of erythrocytes in stored blood. I. Blood preserved in sodium citrate, neutral and acid citrate-glucose (ACD) mixtures. *J. clin. Invest.* **26**, 591.

Ratcliff, A.P. and Hardwicke, J. (1964) Estimation of serum haemoglobin-binding capacity (haptoglobin) on Sephadex G 100. *J. clin. Path.* **17**, 676.

Ratkin, G.A., Osterland, C.K. and Chaplin, H. jr (1973) IgG, IgA and IgM cold-reactive immunoglobulin in 19 patients with elevated cold agglutinins. *J. Lab. clin. Med.* **82**, 67.

Rathbun, E.J., Nelson, E.J. and Davey, E.J. (1989) Posttransfusion survival of red cells frozen for 8 weeks after 42-day liquid storage in AS-3. *Transfusion*, **29**, 213–217.

Rauner, R.A. and Tanaka, K.R. (1967) Hemolytic transfusion reactions associated with the Kidd antibody (Jk^a). *New Engl. J. Med.* **276**, 1486.

Rausen, A.R., LeVine, R., Hsu, R.C.S. and Rosenfield, R.E. (1975) Compatible transfusion therapy for paroxysmal cold hemoglobinuria. *Pediatrics*, **55**, 275.

Ravitch, M.M., Farmer, T.W. and Davis, B. (1949) Use of blood donors with positive serologic tests for syphilis—with a note on the disappearance of passively transferred reagin. *J. clin. Invest.* **28**, 18.

Rawson, A.J. and Abelson, Neva M. (1960a) Studies of blood group antibodies. III. Observations on the physicochemical properties of isohemagglutinins and isohemolysins. *J. Immunol.* **85**, 636.

Rawson, A.J. and Abelson, Neva M. (1960b) Studies of blood group antibodies. IV. Physico-chemical differences between iso-anti-A,B and iso-anti-A or iso-anti-B. *J. Immunol.* **85**, 640.

Rawson, A.J. and Abelson, Neva M. (1964) Studies of blood group antibodies. VI. The blood group isoantibody activity of γ_{1A} globulin. *J. Immunol.* **93**, 192.

Ray, R.N., Cassell, Mona and Chaplin, H. jr (1959) *In vitro* and *in vivo* observations on stored sickle trait red blood cells. *Amer. J. clin. Path.* **32**, 430.

Ray, P.K., and Raychaudhuri, S. (1982) Differential binding affinity of immobilized concanavalin-A-Sepharose-4B for normal and myelomatous immunoglobulins. *Biomed. Pharmacol.* **36**, 206–210.

Read, E.J., Crabill, H.E. and Davey, R.J. (1985) Flow cytometric determination of transfused red blood cell (rbc) survival in a patient with autoimmune hemolytic anemia (AIHA) (Abstract). *Transfusion*, **25**, 451.

Read, E.J., Cardine, L.L. and Yu, M.Y. (1991) Flow cytometric detection of human red cells labeled with a fluorescent membrane label: potential application to *in vivo* survival studies. *Transfusion*, **31**, 502–508.

Rearden, A. and Masouredis, S.P. (1977) Blood group D antigen content of nucleated red cell precursors. *Blood*, **50**, 981.

Reckel, R.P. and Harris, J. (1978) The unique characteristics of covalently polymerized bovine serum albumin solutions when used as antibody detection media. *Transfusion*, **18**, 397.

Redman, M., Malde, Ranjan and Contreras, Marcela (1990) Comparison of IgM and IgG anti-A and anti-B levels in Asian, Caucasian and Negro donors in the north-west Thames region. *Vox Sang.* **59**, 89–91.

Reed, T.E. and Moore, B.P.L. (1964) A new variant of blood group A. *Vox Sang.* **9**, 363.

Reed, R.L., Heimbach, D.M., Counts, R.B., Ciaverella, D., Baron, Lois, Carrico, C.J. and Pavlin, E. (1986) Prophylactic platelet administration during massive transfusion. *Ann. Surg.* **203**, 40–48.

Reepmaker, J. (1952) Relation between polyagglutinability of erythrocytes *in vivo* and the

Hübener-Thomsen-Friedenreich phenomenon. *J. clin. Path.* **5**, 266.

Reesink, H.W., van der Hart, Mia and van Loghem. J.J. (1972) Evaluation of a simple method for the determination of the IgG titre of anti-A or -B in cases of possible ABO blood group incompatibility. *Vox Sang.* **22**, 397.

Reesink, H.W., Wesdorp, I.C.E., Grijm, R., Hengeveld, P., Jöbsis, A.C., Aay, C. and Reerink-Brongers, E.E. (1980) Follow-up of blood donors positive for hepatitis B surface antigen. *Vox Sang.* **38**, 138.

Reesink, H.W. and van der Poel, C.L. (1989) Blood transfusion and hepatitis: still a threat? *Blut*, **58**, 1–6.

Regan, L. (1991) Recurrent miscarriage. *Brit. med. J.* **302**, 543–544.

Reich, M.L., Heilweil, L. and Fischel, E.E. (1970) Complement preservation in citrated human blood. *Transfusion*, **10**, 14.

Reid, W.O., Lucas, O.N., Francisco, J., Geisler, P.H. and Erslev, A.J. (1964) The use of epsilon-aminocaproic acid in the management of dental extractions in the hemophiliac. *Amer. J. med. Sci.* **248**, 184.

Reid, M.E., Ellisor, S.S. and Frank, B.A. (1975) Another potential source of error in Rh-hr typing. *Transfusion*, **15**, 485.

Reid, M.E., Ellisor, S.S., Barker, J.M., Lewis, T. and Avoy, D.R. (1981) Characteristics of an antibody causing agglutination of M-positive non-enzymatically glycosylated human red cells. *Vox Sang.* **41**, 85–90.

Reid, Marion, E., Vengelen-Tyler, Virginia, Shulman, Ira, and Reynolds, Marilyn, V. (1988) Immunochemical specificity of autoanti-Gerbich from two patients with autoimmune haemolytic anaemia and concomitant alteration in the red cell membrane sialoglycoprotein beta. *Brit. J. Haemat.* **69**, 61–66.

Reid, Marion E. (1989) Biochemistry and molecular cloning analysis of human red cell sialoglycoproteins that carry Gerbich blood group antigens, in *Blood Group Systems: MN and Gerbich*, eds Phyllis J. Unger and Barbara Laird-Fryer. Amer. Assoc. Blood Banks, Arlington, VA.

Reisner, E.G., Kostyu, D.D., Phillips, G., Walker, C. and Dawson, D.V. (1987) Alloantibody responses in multiply transfused sickle cell patients. *Tissue Antigens*, **30**, 161–166.

Rekvig, O.P. and Hannestad, K. (1977) Acid elution of blood group antibodies from intact erythrocytes. *Vox Sang.* **33**, 280.

Remenchik, A.P., Schuckmell, Natalie, Dyniewicz, J.M. and Best, W.R. (1958) The survival of Cr^{51}-labelled autogenous erythrocytes in children. *J. Lab. clin. Med.* **51**, 753.

Remington, J.W. and Baker, C.H. (1959) Plasma volume changes accompanying reactions to infusions of blood or plasma. *Amer. J. Physiol.* **197**, 193.

Remuzzi, G., Rossi, E.C., Misiani, R., Marchesi, D., Mecca, G., de Gaetano, G. and Donati, M.B. (1980) Prostacyclin and thrombotic microangiopathy. *Semin. Thrombos. Haemostas.* **6**, 391–394.

Renaer, M., van de Putte, I. and Vermylen, C. (1976) Massive feto-maternal hemorrhage as a cause of perinatal mortality and morbidity. *Europ. J. Obstet. Gynec. reprod. Biol.* **6**, 125.

Rendel, J., Neimann-Sørensen, A. and Irwin, M.R. (1954) Evidence for epistatic action of genes for antigenic substances in sheep. *Genetics*, **39**, 396.

Renkonen, K.O. (1948) Studies on hemagglutinins in seeds of some representatives of the family of *Leguminosae. Ann. Med. exp. fenn.* **26**, 66.

Renkonen, K.O. and Seppälä, M. (1962) The sex of the sensitizing Rh-positive child. *Ann. Med. exp. fenn.* **40**, 108.

Renkonen, K.O. and Timonen, S. (1967) Factors influencing the immunization of Rh-negative mothers. *J. med. Genet.* **4**, 166.

Rent, Rosemarie, Ertel, Nancy, Eisenstein, R. and Gewurz, H. (1975) Complement activation by interaction of polyanions and polycations. I. Heparin-protamine induced consumption of complement. *J. Immunol.* **114**, 120.

Renton, P.H. and Hancock, Jeanne A. (1962) Uptake of A and B antigens by transfused group O erythrocytes. *Vox Sang.* **7**, 33.

Renton, P.H. and Hancock, Jeanne A. (1964) A simple method of separating erythrocytes of different ages. *Vox Sang.* **9**, 183.

Renton, P.H., Howell, P., Ikin, Elizabeth W., Giles, Carolyn M. and Goldsmith, K.L.G. (1967) Anti-Sd^a, a new blood group antibody. *Vox Sang.* **13**, 493.

Report from 9 Collaborating Laboratories (1991) Results of tests with different cellular bioassays in relation to severity of Rh D haemolytic disease. *Vox Sang.* **60**, 225–229.

Report of National Academy of Sciences—National Research Council (1974) Chemical specifications for adenine for medical use. *Transfusion*, **14**, 185.

Report of NHS (National Health Service) Advisory Group (1975) *Second Report of the Advisory Group on Testing for the Presence of Hepatitis B Surface Antigen and its Antibody.* Her Majesty's Stationery Office, London.

Restrepo, F.A. and Chaplin, H. (1962) Measurement of *in vivo* survival of red blood cells by means of starch block hemoglobin electrophoresis. *Amer. J. clin. Path.* **6**, 557.

Reul, G.J. jr, Beall, A.C. jr and Greenberg, S.D. (1974) Protection of the pulmonary microvasculature by fine screen blood filtration. *Chest,* **66**, 4.

Reverberi, R. and Menini, C. (1990) Clinical efficacy of five filters specific for leukocyte removal. *Vox Sang.* **58**, 188–191.

Revill, J.A., Emblin, K.F. and Hutchinson, R.M. (1979) Failure of anti-D immunoglobulin to remove fetal red cells from maternal circulation. *Vox Sang.* **36**, 93–96.

Reviron, M., Janvier, D., Reviron, J. and Lagabrielle, J.F. (1984) An anti-I cold autoagglutinin enhanced in the presence of sodium azide. *Vox Sang.* **46**, 211–216.

Reyes, F., Lejonc, J.L., Gourdin, M.F., Tonthat, H. and Breton Gorius, J. (1974) Human normoblast A antigen seen by immunoelectron microscopy. *Nature (Lond.),* **247**, 461.

Reyes, F., Gourdin, M.F., Lejonc, J.L., Cartron, J.P., Breton Gorius, J. and Dreyfus, B. (1976) The heterogeneity of erythrocyte antigen distribution on human normal phenotypes: an immunoelectron microscopy study. *Brit. J. Haemat.* **34**, 613.

Reyes, G.R., Purdy, M.A., Kim, J.P., Luk, K-C., Young LaVonne, M., Fry, K.B. and Bradley, D.W. (1990) Isolation of a cDNA from the virus responsible for enterically transmitted non-A, non-B hepatitis. *Science,* **247**, 1335–1339.

Reynes, M., Zignego, L., Samuel, D., Fabiani, B., Gugenheim, J., Tricottet, V., Brechot, C. and Bismuth, H. (1989) Graft hepatitis delta virus infection after orthotopic liver transplantation in HDV cirrhosis. *Transplant Proc.* **21**, 2424–2425.

Reynolds, Marilyn V., Vengelen-Tyler, Virginia and Morel, Phyllis A. (1981) Autoimmune haemolytic anaemia associated with auto-anti-Ge. *Vox Sang.* **41**, 61–67.

Reznikoff-Etiévant, M.F., Dangu, C. and Lobet, R. (1981) HLA-B8 antigen and anti-P1A1 alloimmunization. *Tissue Antigens,* **18**, 66–68.

Reznikoff-Etiévant, M.F., Muller, J-Y., Lulien, F. and Patereau, C. (1983) An immune response gene linked to MHC in man. *Tissue Antigens,* **22**, 312–314.

Reznikoff-Etiévant, M.F. (1988) Management of alloimmune neonatal and antenatal thrombocytopenia. *Vox Sang.* **55**, 193–201.

Rhame, F.S., Root, R.K., Maclowry, J.D., Dadisman, T.A. and Bennett, J.V. (1973) *Salmonella* septicemia from platelet transfusions: study of an outbreak traced to a hematogenous carrier of *Salmonella cholera suis. Ann. intern. Med.* **78**, 633–641.

Richert, N.D., Willingham, M.C. and Pastan, I.H. (1983) Epidermal growth factor receptor: characterization of a monoclonal antibody specific for the receptor of A431 cells. *J. biol. Chem.* **258**, 8902–8907.

Rickard, K.A., Robinson, R.J. and Worlledge,

Sheila M. (1969) Acute acquired haemolytic anaemia associated with polyagglutination. *Arch. Dis. Childh.* **44**, 102.

Riddell, V. (1939) *Blood Transfusion.* Oxford University Press, Oxford.

Ridgwell, K., Tanner, M.J.A. and Anstee, D.J. (1984) The Rhesus (D) polypeptide is linked to the human erythrocyte cytoskeleton. *FEBS Letters,* **174**, 7–10.

Ridgwell, Kay, Tanner, M.J.A. and Anstee, D.J. (1983) The Wr[b] antigen, a receptor for *Plasmodium falciparum* malaria, is located on a helical region of the major membrane sialoglycoprotein of human red blood cells. *Biochem. J.* **209**, 273–276.

Ries, C.A., Garratty, G., Petz, L.D. and Fudenberg, H.H. (1971) Paroxysmal cold hemoglobinuria: report of a case with an exceptionally high thermal range Donath-Landsteiner antibody. *Blood,* 38, 491.

Riley, J.Z., Ness, P.M., Taddie, S.J., Barrasso, C. and Baldwin, M.L. (1982) Detection and quantitation of fetal maternal hemorrhage utilizing an enzyme-linked antiglobulin test. *Transfusion,* **22**, 472–474.

Rinaldo, Jean E. and Rogers, R.N. (1986) Adult respiratory distress syndrome (Editorial). *New Engl. J. Med.* **315**, 578–580.

Rinaldo, Jean E. and Christman, J.W. (1990) Mechanisms and mediators of the adult respiratory distress syndrome. *Clinics Chest Med.* **11**, 621–632.

Ring, J. and Messmer, K. (1977) Incidence and severity of anaphylactoid reactions to colloid volume substitutes. *Lancet,* **i**, 466.

Ring, J., Sharkoff, D. and Richter, W. (1980) Using HES in man. *Vox Sang.* **39**, 181–185.

Rinker, Judy and Galambos, J.T. (1981) Prospective study of hepatitis B in thirty-two inadvertently infected people. *Gastroenterology,* **81**, 686–691.

Risseeuw-Appel, I.M. and Kothe, F.C. (1983) Transfusion syphilis: a case report. *Sex. transmitted Dis.* **10**, 200–201.

Ritch, P.S. and Anderson, T. (1987) Reversal of autoimmune hemolytic anemia associated with chronic lymphocytic leukemia following high-dose immunoglobulin. *Cancer,* **60**, 2637–2640.

Rivera, R. and Scornik, J.C. (1986) HLA antigens on red cells. Implications for achieving low HLA antigen content in blood transfusion. *Transfusion,* **26**, 375–381.

Rivet, C., Baxter, A. and Rock, C. (1989) Potassium levels in irradiated blood (Letter). *Transfusion,* **29**, 185.

Rizza, C.R. (1961) Effect of exercise on the level of antihaemophilic globulin in human blood. *J. Physiol. (Lond.),* **156**, 128.

Rizza, C.R. and Biggs, Rosemary (1969) Blood

products in the management of haemophilia and Christmas disease, in *Recent Advances in Blood Coagulation*, ed L. Poller. J. & A. Churchill, London.

Rizzetto, M. (1983) The delta agent. *Hepatology*, **3**, 729–737.

Rø, J. (1937) Über gruppenspezifische Reaktionen nach Bluttransfusionen. Ein Fall von hämolytischer Reaktion. *Acta chir. scand.* **80**, 283.

Robbins, G., Petersen, C.V. and Brozović, B. (1985) Lymphocytopenia in donors undergoing regular platelet apheresis with cell separators. *Clin. lab. Haemat.* **7**, 225–230.

Robert-Guroff, M., Goedert, J.J., Naugle, C.J. Jennings, A.M., Blattner, W.A. and Gallo, R.C. (1988) Spectrum of HIV-1 neutralizing antibodies in a cohort of homosexual men: results of a 6 year prospective study. *AIDS Research and Human Retroviruses*, **4**, 343–350.

Roberts, J.A. (1957) Blood groups and susceptibility to disease. *Brit. J. prev. soc. Med.* **11**, 107.

Roberts, S.C. (1989) Quality control for computers in blood banks. *Transfus. Sci.* **10**, 233–240.

Robertson, O.H. (1917) The effects of experimental plethora on blood production. *J. exp. Med.* **26**, 221.

Robertson, O.H. (1918) Transfusion with preserved red blood cells. *Brit. med. J.* i, 691.

Robertson, O.H. and Bock, A.V. (1919) Memorandum on blood volume after haemorrhage. *Spec. Rep. Ser. med. Res. Cttee. (Lond.)*, No. 25.

Robertson, L.B. (1924) Exsanguination-transfusion. A new therapeutic measure in the treatment of severe toxemias. *Arch. Surg.* **9**, 1–15.

Robertson, M., Boulton, F.E., Doughty, R., Machennan, J.R., Collins, A., McLelland, D.B.L. and Prowse, C.V. (1985) Macroaggregate formation in optimal addition red cells. *Vox Sang.* **49**, 259–266.

Robinson, Angela E. and Tovey, L.A.D. (1980) Intensive plasma exchange in the management of severe Rh disease. *Brit. J. Haemat.* **45**, 621–631.

Robinson, Angela E. (1981) Unsuccessful use of absorbed autologous plasma in Rh-incompatible pregnancy (Letter). *New Engl. J. Med.* **305**, 1346.

Robinson, Angela E. (1984) Principles and practice of plasma exchange in the management of Rh hemolytic disease of the newborn. *Plasma Therapy*, **5**, 7–14.

Robinson, A. (1990a) Hazards of apheresis and the U.K. approach to guidelines. *Transfus. Sci.* **11**, 305–308.

Robinson, A. (1990b) Analysis of European Society for Haemapheresis questionnaire on apheresis guidelines. *Transfus. Sci.* **11**, 333–336.

Rocchi, G., deFelici, A., Ragona, G. and Heinz, A. (1977) Quantitative evaluation of Epstein-Barr virus-infected mononuclear peripheral blood leukocytes in infectious mononucleosis. *New Engl. J. Med.* **296**, 131–134.

Rochant, N., Tonthat, H., Eitevant, Marie Françoise, Intrator, Lilian, Sylvestre, R. and Dreyfus, B. (1972) Lambda cold agglutinin with anti-A_1 specificity in a patient with reticulosarcoma. *Vox Sang.* **22**, 45.

Roche, M., Perez–Gimenez, M.E., Layrisse, M. and di Prisco, E. (1957) Study of urinary and fecal excretion of radioactive chromium Cr^{51} in man. Its use in the measurement of intestinal blood loss associated with hookworm infection. *J. clin. Invest.* **36**, 1183.

Rochna, Erna and Hughes–Jones, N.C. (1965) The use of purified ^{125}I-labelled anti-γ globulin in the determination of the number of D antigen sites on red cells of different phenotypes. *Vox Sang.* **10**, 675.

Rock, R.C., Bove, J.R. and Nemerson, Y. (1969) Heparin treatment of intravascular coagulation accompanying hemolytic transfusion reactions. *Transfusion*, **9**, 57.

Rock, G. and Wise, P. (1979) Plasma expansion during granulocyte procurement: cumulative effects of hydroxyethyl starch. *Blood*, **53**, 1156–1163.

Rock, G.A., Cruikshanks, W.H., Tackaberry, E.S. and Palmer, D.S. (1979) Improved yields of factor VIII from heparinized plasma. *Vox Sang.* **36**, 294–300.

Rock, G.A. and Palmer, D.S. (1980) Intermediate purity factor VIII production utilizing a cold-insoluble globulin technique. *Thrombos. Res.* **18**, 551–556.

Rock, G., McCombie, N. and Tittley, P. (1981) A new technique for the collection of plasma: machine plasmapheresis. *Transfusion*, **21**, 241–246.

Rock, G.A., Blanchette, V.S., McKendry, R.J. and Kardish, R. (1982) Plasmapheresis and cryoglobulinemia: an evaluation of cold precipitation as a method of removing abnormal protein (Abstract). *Blood*, **60**, Suppl. 1, 181 A.

Rock, Gail, Herzig, R., McCombie, N., Lazarus, H.M. and Tittley, P. (1983a) Automated platelet production during plasmapheresis. *Transfusion*, **23**, 290-293.

Rock, G., Tocch, M. and Tackaberry, E. (1983b) Plasticized red blood cells: good or bad? (Abstract). *Transfusion*, **23**, 426.

Rock, G., Sherring, V.A. and Tittley, P. (1984a) Five-day storage of platelet concentrates. *Transfusion*, **24**, 147–152.

Rock, G., Zurakowski, S., Baxter, A. and Adams, G. (1984b) Simple and rapid preparation of granulocytes for the treatment of neonatal septicemia. *Transfusion*, **24**, 511–512.

Rock, G., Wise, P., Kardish, R. and Huestis, D.W. (1984c) Modified fluid gelatin in leukapheresis; accumulation and persistence in the body. *Transfusion,* **24,** 68–73.

Rock, Gail and McCombie, N. (1985) Alternate dosage regimens for high-molecular-weight hydroxyethyl starch. *Transfusion,* **25,** 417–419.

Rock, C. and Tittley, P. (1990) A comparison of results obtained by two different chromium-51 methods of determining platelet survival and recovery. *Transfusion,* **30,** 407–410.

Rock, C., White, J. and Labow, R. (1991a) Storage of platelets in balanced salt solution: a simple platelet storage medium. *Transfusion,* **31,** 21–25.

Rock, Gail A., Shumak, K.H., Buskard, N.A., Blanchette, V.S., Kelton, J.G., Nair, R.C., Spasoff, R.A. and the Canadian Apheresis Study Group (1991b) Comparison of plasma exchange with plasma infusion in the treatment of thrombotic thrombocytopenic purpura. *New Engl. J. Med.* **325,** 393–397.

Rodeck, C.H., Nicolaides, K.H., Warshof, S.L., Fysh, W.J., Gamsu, H.R. and Kemp, J.R. (1984) The management of severe rhesus isoimmunization by fetoscopic intravascular transfusions. *Amer. J. Obstet. Gynec.* **150,** 769–774.

Rodeck, C.H. and Letsky, Elizabeth (1989) How the management of erythroblastosis fetalis has changed (Commentary). *Brit. J. Obstet. Gynaec.* **96,** 759–763.

Rodeghiero, F., Castaman, G., Meijer, D. and Manucci, M. (1992) Replacement therapy with virus-inactivated plasma concentrate in Von Willebrand's disease. *Vox Sang.* **62,** 193–200.

Roelcke, D. and Uhlenbruck, G. (1970) Letter to the Editor. *Vox Sang.* **18,** 478.

Roelcke, D. (1973) Specificity of IgA cold agglutinins: anti-Pr1. *Eur. J. Immunol.* **3,** 206–212.

Roelcke, D., Ebert, W. and Feizi, Ten (1974) Studies on the specificities of two IgM lambda cold agglutinins. *Immunology.* **27,** 879.

Roelcke, D., Ebert, W. and Geisen, H.P. (1976) Anti-Pr₃: serological and immunochemical identification of a new anti-Pr subspecificity. *Vox Sang.* **30,** 122.

Roelcke, D., Riesen, W., Geisen, H.P. and Ebert, W. (1977) Serological identification of the new cold agglutinin specificity anti-Gd. *Vox Sang.* **33,** 304.

Roelcke, D., Pruzanski, W., Ebert, W., Römer, W., Fischer, Elisabeth, Lenhard, V. and Rutenberg, E. (1980) A new human monoclonal cold agglutinin Sa recognizing terminal N-acetylneuraminyl groups on the cell surface. *Blood,* **55,** 677–681.

Roelcke, D. (1981a) The Lud cold agglutinin: a further antibody recognizing N-acetylneuraminic acid-determined antigens not fully expressed at birth. *Vox Sang.* **41,** 316–318.

Roelcke, D. (1981b) A further cold agglutinin. F1, recognizing a N-acetylneuraminic acid-determined antigen. *Vox Sang.* **41,** 98–101.

Roelcke, D. and Kreft, H. (1984) Characterization of various anti-Pr cold agglutinins. *Transfusion,* **24,** 210–213.

Roelcke, D., Kreft, Heidi and Pfister, Anne-Marie (1984) Cold agglutinins Vo. An IgM lambda monoclonal human antibody recognizing a sialic acid determined antigen fully expressed on newborn erythrocytes. *Vox Sang.* **47,** 236–241.

Roelcke, P., Dahr, W. and Kalden, J.R. (1986) A human monoclonal IgM κ cold agglutinin recognizing oligosaccharides with immunodominant sialyl groups preferentially at the blood group M-specific peptide backbone of glycophorins: anti-Prᴹ. *Vox Sang.* **51,** 207–211.

Rogers, Margaret J., Stiles, Patricia A. and Wright, J. (1974) A new minus-minus phenotype: three Co(a − b −) individuals in one family (Abstract). *Transfusion,* **14,** 508.

Rogers, Martha, F. and Schochetman, G. (1992) Human immunodeficiency virus infection in children, in *AIDS Testing. Methodology and Management Issues,* eds G. Schochetman and J.R. George, pp. 152–167. Springer-Verlag, New York

Roggen, G., Bertschmann, M., Berchtold, H. and Mühlemann, H. (1964) A contribution to the comparative chemical and biological assay procedures for plastic containers used for blood preservation. *Vox Sang.* **9,** 546.

Rohr, T.E., Smith, D.F., Zopf, D.A. and Ginsburg, V. (1980) Leᵇ-active glycolipid in human plasma: measurement by radioimmunoassay. *Arch. Biochem. Biophys.* **199,** 265–269.

Roitt, I. (1988) *Essential Immunology,* 6th edn. Blackwell Scientific Publications, Oxford.

Roitt, I., Brostoff, J. and Male, D. (1989) *Immunology,* 2nd edn. Gower Medical Publications, London.

Rolih, S.D. and Issitt, P.D. (1978) Effects of trypsin on the *Vicia graminea* receptors of glycophorin A and B (Abstract). *Transfusion,* **18,** 637.

Roman, G.C. and Osame, M. (1988) Identity of HTLV-I associated tropical spastic paraparesis and HTLV-I-associated myelopathy (Letter). *Lancet,* **i,** 651.

Romano, E.L., Hughes-Jones, N.C. and Mollison, P.L. (1973) Direct antiglobulin reaction in ABO-haemolytic disease of the newborn. *Brit. med. J.* **i,** 524.

Romano, E.L., Stolinski, C. and Hughes-Jones, N.C. (1974) An antiglobulin reagent labelled with colloidal gold for use in electron microscopy. *Immunochemistry*, **11**, 521.

Romano, E.L., and Mollison, P.L. (1975) Red cell destruction *in vivo* by low concentrations of IgG anti-A. *Brit. J. Haemat.* **29**, 121.

Romano, E.L., Stolinski, C. and Hughes-Jones, N.C. (1975) Distribution and mobility of the A, D and c antigens on human red cell membranes: studies with a gold-labelled antiglobulin reagent. *Brit. J. Haemat.* **30**, 507.

Romano, E.L., Mollison, P.L. and Linares, J. (1978) Number of B sites generated on group O red cells from adults and newborn infants. *Vox Sang.* **34**, 14.

Romano, E.L., Linares, J. and Suarez, G. (1982) Plasma fibrinogen concentration in ABO-hemolytic disease of the newborn. *Int. Arch. Allergy appl. Immunol.* **67**, 74–77.

Romano, E.L., Soyano, A. and Linares, J. (1987) Preliminary human study of synthetic trisaccharide representing blood group substance A. *Transplant. Proc.* **19**, 4475–4478.

Romans, D.G., Tilley, C.A., Crookston, M.C., Falk, R.E. and Dorrington, K.J. (1977) Conversion of incomplete antibodies to direct agglutinins by mild reduction: evidence for segmental flexibility within the Fc fragment of immunoglobulin G. *Proc. nat. Acad. Sci. USA*, **74**, 2531.

Romans, D.G., Tilley, C.A. and Dorrington, K.J. (1979) Interactions between Fab and Fc regions in liganded immunoglobulin G. *Molec. Immunol.* **16**, 859–879.

Romans, D.G., Tilley, C.A. and Dorrington, K.J. (1980) Monogamous bivalency of IgG antibodies. I. Deficiency of branched ABHI-active oligosaccharide chains on red cells of infants causes the weak antiglobulin reactions in hemolytic disease of the newborn due to ABO incompatibility. *J. Immunol.* **124**, 2807–2811.

Ronalds, C.J., Grint, P.C.A., Hardiman, A.E. and Heath R.B. (1989) Testing for hepatitis B surface antigen — a critical review. *Serodiagnosis and Immunotherapy in Infectious Disease*, **3**, 293–297.

Rook, A.H. and Quinnan, G.V. jr (1982) Cytomegalovirus infections following blood transfusion, in *Infectious Complications of Blood Transfusion*, ed E. Tabor, pp. 45–63. Academic Press, New York.

Roord, J.J., van der Meer, J.W.M., Kuis, Wietske, de Windt, G.E., Zegers, B.J.M., van Furth, R. and Stoop, J.W. (1982) Home treatment in patients with antibody deficiency by slow subcutaneous infusion of gammaglobulin. *Lancet*, i, 689–690.

Ropars, C., Gerbal, A., Poncey, C., Cartron, J., Doinel, Ch. and Salmon, Ch. (1971) Accident transfusionnel de type anaphylactique en rapport avec un anticorps anti-IgA. *Rev. franç. Transfus.* **14**, 401.

Ropars, C., Whylie, S., Cartron, J.P., Doinel, C., Gerbal, A. and Salmon, C. (1973) Anticorps chez les polytransfusés dirigés contres certaines immunoglobulines IgM. *Nouv. Rev franç Hémat.* **13**, 459.

Ropars, C., Caldera, L.H., Griscelli, C., Homberg, J.C. and Salmon, C. (1974) Anti-immunoglobulin antibodies in immunodeficiencies: their influence on intolerance reactions to γ-globulin administration. *Vox Sang.* **27**, 294.

Ropars, C., Geay-Chicot, D., Cartron, J.P., Doinel, C. and Salmon, C. (1979) Human IgE response to the administration of blood components. II. Repeated gammaglobulin injections. *Vox Sang.* **37**, 149–157.

Rørth, M. (1969) 2,3-DPG as regulator of T_{50}. *Försvarsmedicin*, **5**, 167.

Rosa, Raymonde, Audit, Isabella and Rosa, J. (1975) Evidence for three enzymatic activities in one electrophoretic band of 3-phosphoglycerate mutase from red cells. *Biochimie*, **57**, 1059.

Rosati, L.A., Barnes, B., Oberman, H.A. and Penner, J.A. (1970) Hemolytic anemia due to anti-A in concentrated antihemophilic factor preparations. *Transfusion*, **10**, 139.

Rosen, H. and Sears, D.A. (1969) Spectral properties of hemopexin-heme: the Schumm test. *J. Lab. clin. Med.* **74**, 941.

Rosenblatt, J.D., Cann, A.J., Golde, D.W. and Chen, I.S.Y. (1986) Structure and function of the human T-cell leukemia virus genome. *Cancer Rev.* **1**, 115.

Rosenblatt, J.D. and 9 others (1990) A clinical, haematologic, and immunologic analysis of 21 HTLV-II infected intravenous drug users. *Blood*, **76**, 409–417.

Rosenfield, R.E., Vogel, P. and Race, R.R. (1950) A further example of the human blood group antibody anti-Fy[a]. *Rev. Hémat.* **5**, 315.

Rosenfield, R.E. and Vogel, P. (1951) The identification of hemagglutinins with red cells altered with trypsin. *Trans. N.Y. Acad. Sci.* **13**, 213.

Rosenfield, R.E., Vogel, P. Gibbel, Natalie, Sanger, Ruth and Race, R.R. (1953) A 'new' Rh antibody, anti-f. *Brit. med. J.* i, 975.

Rosenfield, R.E. and Ohno, Grace (1955) A-B hemolytic disease of the new-born. *Rev. Hémat.* **10**, 231.

Rosenfield, R.E. (1955) A-B hemolytic disease of the newborn. Analysis of 1480 cord blood specimens, with special reference to the direct anti-globulin test and to the group O mother. *Blood*, **10**, 17.

Rosenfield, R.E. and Haber, Gladys V. (1958) An Rh blood factor, rh_i (Ce), and its relationship to hr (ce). *Amer. J. hum. Genet.* **10**, 474.

Rosenfield, R.E., Haber, Gladys V., Kissmeyer-Nielsen, F., Jack, J.A., Sanger, Ruth and Race, R.R. (1960) Ge, a very common red-cell antigen. *Brit. J. Haemat.* **6**, 344.

Rosenfield, R.E., Allen F.H. jr, Swisher, S.N. and Kochwa, S. (1962) A review of Rh serology and presentation of a new terminology. *Transfusion*, **2**, 287.

Rosenfield, R.E., Schroeder, Ruth, Ballard, Rachel, van der Hart, Mia, Moes, Mieke and van Loghem, J.J. (1964a) Erythrocyte antigenic determinants characteristic of H, I in the presence of H[IH], or H in the absence of i [H(−i)]. *Vox Sang.* **9**, 415.

Rosenfield, R.E., Szymanski, Irma, O. and Kochwa, S. (1964b) Immunochemical studies of the Rh system: III. Quantitative hemagglutination that is relatively independent of source of Rh antigens and antibodies. *Cold Spr. Harb. Symp. quant. Biol.* **29**, 427.

Rosenfield, R.E., Schmidt, P.J., Calvo, R.C. and McGinniss, Mary H. (1965) Anti-i, a frequent cold agglutinin in infectious mononucleosis. *Vox Sang.* **10**, 631.

Rosenfield, R.E., Rubinstein, P., Lalezari, P., Dausset, J. and van Rood J.J. (1967a) Hemagglutination by human anti-leukocyte serums. *Vox Sang.* **13**, 461.

Rosenfield, R.E., Vitale, B. and Kochwa, S. (1967b) Immune mechanisms for destruction of erythrocytes *in vivo*. II. Heparinization for protection of lysin-sensitized erythrocytes. *Transfusion*, **7**, 261.

Rosenfield, R.E., Berkman, E.M., Nusbacher, J., Hyams, L., Dabinsky, C., Stux, S., Hirsch, A. and Kochwa, S. (1971) Specific agglutinability of erythrocytes from whole blood stored at 4 °C. *Transfusion*, **11**, 177.

Rosenfield, R.E. (1974) Early twentieth century origins of modern blood transfusion therapy. *The Mnt. Sinai J. Med.* **41**, 626.

Rosenfield, R.E. and Jagathambal (1976) Transfusion therapy for autoimmune hemolytic anemia. *Semin. Hemat.* **13**, 311.

Rosenfield, R.E., Kochwa, S. and Kaczera, Z. (1976) Solid-phase serology for the study of human erythrocytic antigen-antibody reactions. *Abstracts, 15th Congr. Int. Soc. Blood Transfus.*, Paris. pp. 27–33.

Rosenfield, R.E. (1977) In memoriam Alexander S. Wiener. *Haematologia*, **11**, 5.

Rosenfield, R.E. and Jagathambal (1978) Antigenic determinants of C3 and C4 complement components on washed erythrocytes from normal persons. *Transfusion*, **18**, 517.

Rosenfield, R.E., Shaikh, Shirin H., Innella, Filomena, Kaczera, Z. and Kochwa, S. (1979) Augmentation of hemagglutination by low ionic conditions. *Transfusion*, **19**, 499–510.

Rosenfield, R.E. (1989) Who discovered Rh? A personal glimpse of the Levine–Wiener argument. *Transfusion*, **29**, 355–357.

Rosenthal, M.C. and Schwartz, L. (1951) Reversible agglutination of trypsin-treated erythrocytes by normal human sera. *Proc. Soc. exp. Biol.* (*N.Y.*), **76**, 635.

Rosina, F., Saracco, G. and Rizzetto, M. (1985) Risk of post-transfusion infection with the hepatitis delta virus. A Multicenter Study. *New Engl. J. Med.* **312**, 1488–1491.

Ross, J.F., Finch, C.A., Peacock, W.C. and Sammons, M.E. (1947) The *in vitro* preservation and post-transfusion survival of stored blood. *J. clin. Invest.* **26**, 687.

Ross, C.R., Yount, W.J., Walport, M.J., Winfield, J.B., Parker, C.J., Fuller, C.R., Taylor, R.P., Myones, B.L. and Lachmann, P.J. (1985) Disease-associated loss of erythrocyte complement receptors (CR_1, C3b receptors) in patients with systemic lupus erythematosus and other diseases involving autoantibodies and/or complement activation. *J. Immunol.* **1235**, 2005–2014.

Ross, G.D. (1986) Opsonization and membrane complement receptors, in *Immunobiology of the Complement System*, ed G.D. Ross. Academic Press, New York.

Ross, G.D. (1989) Complement and complement receptors. *Current Opinion in Immunology.* **2**, 50–62.

Ross, D.G., Heaton, W.A.L. and Holme, S. (1989) Additive solution for the suspension and storage of deglycerolized red blood cells. *Vox Sang.* **56**, 75–79.

Rosse, W.F., Dourmashkin, R. and Humphrey, J.H. (1966) Immune lysis of normal human and paroxysmal nocturnal haemoglobinuria (PNH) red blood cells. III. The membrane defects caused by complement lysis. *J. exp. Med.* **123**, 969.

Rosse, W.F., Borsos, T. and Rapp, H.J. (1968) Cold-reacting antibodies: the enhancement of antibody fixation by the first component of complement (C'1a). *J. Immunol.* **100**, 259.

Rosse, W.F. (1968) Fixation of the first component of complement (C'1a) by human antibodies. *J. clin. Invest.* **47**, 2430.

Rosse, W.F. (1986) The control of complement activation by the blood cells in paroxysmal nocturnal haemoglobinuria. *Blood*, **67**, 268–269.

Rosse, W.F. (1989) Paroxysmal nocturnal hemoglobinuria: the biochemical defects and the clinical syndrome. *Blood Reviews*, **3**, 192–200.

Rosse, W.F., Gallagher, Diane, Kinney, T.R., Castro, O., Dosik, H., Moohr, J., Wang, Winfred, Levy, P.S. and the Cooperative Study of Sickle Cell Disease (1990) Transfusion and alloimmunization in sickle cell disease. *Blood*, **76**, 1431–1437.

Rothman, I.K., Alter, H.J. and Strewler, G.J. (1976) Delayed overt hemolytic transfusion reaction due to anti-U antibody. *Transfusion*, **16**, 357.

Rouger, P., Riveau, D. and Salmon, C. (1979) Detection of the H and I blood group antigens in normal plasma. A comparison with A and i antigens. *Vox Sang.* **37**, 78–83.

Rouger, P.H., Dosda, F., Girard, M., Fouillade, M.T. and Salmon, C. (1982a) Étude de la sensibilité de l'antigène Yt^a aux enzymes protéolytiques. *Rev. franç. Transfus. Immunohémat.* **25**, 45–47.

Rouger, P., Goossens, D., Gane, P. and Salmon, C. (1982b) Antigens common to blood cells and tissues: from red cell antigens to tissue antigens, in *Blood Groups and Other Red Cell Surface Markers in Health and Disease*, ed C. Salmon, pp. 101–109. Masson Inc., USA.

Rouger, P., Lee, H. and Juszczak, G. (1983) Murine monoclonal antibodies against Gerbich antigens. *J. Immunogenet.* **10**, 333–335.

Rouger, P., Goossens, D., Champomier, F., Tsikas, G., Liberge, G., Leblanc, J., Richard, C., Bailleul, C. and Salmon, C. (1985) Utilisation diagnostique et therapeutique d' anticorps monoclonaux humains anti-D (Rho). Bilans et perspectives. *Rev. franç. Transfus. Immunohemat.* **28**, 671–679.

Rouger, P. and Anstee, B. (1987) First International Workshop on Monoclonal Antibodies Against Human Red Blood Cell and Related antigens (Final report). *Vox Sang.* **55**, 57–61.

Rous, P. and Turner, J.R. (1916) Preservation of living red blood corpuscles *in vitro*. II. The transfusion of kept cells. *J. exp. Med.* **23**, 219.

Rous, P. and Robertson, O.H. (1918) Free antigen and antibody circulating together in large amounts (hemagglutinin and agglutinogen in the blood of transfused rabbits). *J. exp. Med.* **27**, 509.

Rowley, D.A. (1950) The formation of circulating antibody in the splenectomized human being following intravenous injection of heterologous erythrocytes. *J. Immunol.* **65**, 515.

Roy, R.B. and Lotto, W.N. (1962) Delayed hemolytic reaction caused by anti-c not detectable before transfusion. *Transfusion*, **2**, 342.

Roy, A.J., Jaffe, N. and Djerassi, I. (1973) Prophylactic platelet transfusions in children with acute leukemia: a dose response study. *Transfusion*, **13**, 283.

Royal, J.E. and Seeler, R.A. (1978) Hypertension, convulsions, and cerebral haemorrhage in sickle-cell anaemia patients after blood-transfusion. *Lancet*, **ii**, 1207.

Royston, D., Bidstrup, B.P., Taylor, K.M. and Sapsford, R.N. (1987) Effect of aprotinin on need for blood transfusion after repeat open heart surgery. *Lancet*, **ii**, 1289–1290.

Rubin, H. (1963) Antibody elution from red blood cells. *J. clin. Path.* **16**, 70.

Rubin, H. and Solomon, A. (1967) Cold agglutinins of anti-i specificity in alcoholic cirrhosis. *Vox Sang.* **12**, 227.

Rubin, R.H. and 10 others (1985) Multicenter seroepidemiologic study of the impact of cytomegalo-virus infection on renal transplantation. *Transplantation*, **40**, 243–249.

Rubinstein, D., Kashket, S., Blostein, R. and Denstedt, O.F. (1959) Studies on the preservation of blood. VII. The influence of inosine on the metabolic behaviour of the erythrocyte during the preservation of blood in the cold. *Canad. J. Biochem.* **37**, 69.

Rubinstein, P. (1972) Cyclical variations in anti-Rh titer detected by automatic quantitative hemagglutination. *Vox Sang.* **23**, 508.

Rubinstein, A., Sicklick, M., Mehra, V., Rosen, F.S. and Levey, R.H. (1981) Anti-helper T cell autoantibody in acquired agammaglobulinemia. *J. clin. Invest.* **67**, 42–50.

Rubinstein, P. (1982) Repeated small volume plasmapheresis in the management of hemolytic disease of the newborn, in *Rh Hemolytic Disease: New Strategy for Eradication*, eds F.D. Frigoletto, J.F. Jewett and Angelyn A. Konugres. G.K. Hall, Boston.

Rubli, E., Buessard, S., Frei, E., Lundsgaard-Hansen, P. and Pappova, E. (1983) Plasma fibronectin and associated variables in surgical intensive care patients. *Ann. Surg.* **197**, 310.

Rubo, J. and Wahn, V. (1991) High-dose intravenous gammaglobulin in rhesus-haemolytic disease (Letter). *Lancet*, **337**, 914.

Rudowski, W. and Kostrzewska, Ewa (1976) Aspects of treatment. Blood substitutes. *Ann. roy. Coll. Surg. England*, **58**, 115.

Ruffie, J. and Carriere, M. (1951) Production of a blocking anti-D antibody by injection of D^u red cells. *Brit. med. J.* **ii**, 1564.

Rush, B.F. (1974) Volume replacement: when, what and how much?, in *Treatment of Shock: Principles and Practice*, eds W. Schumer and L.M. Nyhus. Lea & Febiger, Philadelphia.

Ryden, S.E. and Oberman, H.A. (1975) Compatibility of common intravenous solutions with CPD blood. *Transfusion*, **15**, 250.

Rzad, L., Murphy, S., Buchholz, D.H., Davisson, W., Gajewski, M. and Aster, R.H. (1982) Storage of platelet concentrate for seven days in PL-732 plastic. *Transfusion*, **22**, 417.

Saarinen, Ulla M., Kekomaki, R., Siimes, M.A. and Myllyla, G. (1990) Effective prophylaxis against platelet refractoriness in multitransfused patients by use of leucocyte-free blood components. *Blood*, **75**, 512–517.

Saba, T.M., Blumenstock, F.A., Scovill, W.A. and Bernard, H. (1978) Cryoprecipitate reversal of opsonic alpha 2 surface binding glycoprotein deficiency in septic surgical and trauma patients. *Science*, **201**, 622.

Saba, T.M. and Jaffe, E. (1980) Plasma fibronectin (opsonic glycoprotein), its synthesis by vascular endothelial cells and role in cardiopulmonary integrity after trauma is related to reticulo-endothelial function. *Amer. J. Med.* **68**, 577–594.

Saba, T.M. and 9 others (1986) Reversal of opsonic deficiency in surgical, trauma and burn patients by infusion of purified human plasma fibronectin. *Amer. J. Med.* **80**, 229.

Sabo, B., Moulds, J.J. and McCreary, J. (1978) Anti-JMH: another high titer-low avidity antibody against a high frequency antigen (Abstract). *Transfusion*, **18**, 387.

Sacher, R.A., Abbondanzo, S.L., Miller, D.K. and Womack, B. (1989) Clinical and serologic findings of seven patients from one hospital and review of the literature. *Amer. J. clin. Path.* **91**, 304–309.

Sachs, H.W., Reuter, W., Tippett, Patricia and Gavin, June (1978) An Rh gene complex producing both C^w and c antigen. *Vox Sang.* **35**, 272.

Sack, E.S. and Nefa, O.M. (1970) Fibrinogen and fibrin degradation products in hemolytic transfusion reactions. *Transfusion*, **10**, 317.

Sacks, M.S., Wiener, A.S., Jahn, Elsa F., Spurling, C.L. and Unger, L.J. (1959) Isosensitization to a new blood factor, Rh^D, with special reference to its clinical importance. *Ann. intern. Med.* **51**, 740.

Sacks, D.A., Johnson, C.S. and Platt, L.D. (1985) Isoimmunization in pregnancy to Gerbich antigen. *Amer. J. Perinatology*, **2**, 208–210.

Sadler, J.E., Paulson, J.C. and Hill, R.L. (1979) The role of sialic acid in the expansion of human MN blood group antigens. *J. biol. Chem.* **254**, 2112–2119.

Sahota, A., Simmonds, H.A., Potter, C.F., Watson, J.G., Hugh-Jones, K. and Perrett, D. (1980) Adenosine and deoxyadenosine metabolism in the erythrocytes of a patient with adenosine deaminase deficiency. *Adv. exp. Med. Biol.* **122A**, 397–401.

Saiki, R.K., Bugawan, Teodirica, L., Horn, G.T., Mullis, Kary, B., and Erlich, H.A. (1986) Analysis of enzymatically amplified beta-globin and HLA-DQ alpha DNA with allele-specific oligonucleotide probes. *Nature (Lond.)*, **324**, 163–166.

Saiki, R.K., Gelfand, D.H., Stoffel, S., Scharf, S.J., Higuchi, R., Horn, G.T., Mullis, K.B., and Erlich, H.A. (1988) Primer-directed enzymatic amplification of DNA with a thermostable DNA polymerase. *Science*, **239**, 487–491.

Saji, H., Maruya, E., Fujii, H. Moekawa, T., Akiyema, Y., Matsoura, T. and Hosoi, T. (1989) New platelet antigen, Sib^a involved in platelet transfusion refractoriness in a Japanese man. *Vox Sang.* **56**, 283.

Sakatibara, T. and Juji, T. (1986) Post-transfusion graft-versus-host disease after open heart surgery. *Lancet*, **ii**, 1099.

Salahuddin, S.Z., Groopman, J.E., Markahm, P.D., Sarngadharan, M.G., Redfield, R.R., McLane, M.F., Essex, M., Sliski, A. and Gallo, R.C. (1984) HTLV-III in symptom-free sero-negative persons. *Lancet*, **ii**, 1418–1420.

Salahuddin, S.Z. and 10 others (1986) Isolation of a new virus, HBLV, in patients with lymphoproliferative disorders. *Science*, **234**, 596–601.

Salama, A. and Mueller-Eckhardt, C. (1982) Elimination of the prozone effect in the anti-globulin reaction by a simple modification. *Vox Sang.* **42**, 157–160.

Salama, A. and Mueller-Eckhardt, C. (1984) Delayed hemolytic transfusion reactions. Evidence for complement activation involving allogeneic and autologous red cells. *Transfusion*, **24**, 188–193.

Salama, A., Mahn, I., Neuzner, J., Granbuer, M. and Mueller-Eckhardt, C. (1984) IgG therapy in autoimmune haemolytic anaemia of warm type. *Blut*, **48**, 391–392.

Salama, A. and Mueller-Eckhardt, C. (1985) The role of metabolite specific antibodies in nomifensine-dependent immune hemolytic anemia. *New Engl. J. Med.* **313**, 469–474.

Salama, A., Mueller-Eckhardt, C. and Bhakdi, S. (1985) A two-stage immunoradiometric assay with ^{125}I-staphylococcal protein A for the detection of antibodies and complement on human blood cells. *Vox Sang.* **48**, 239–245.

Salama, A., Kiefel, V. and Mueller-Eckhardt, C. (1986) Effect of IgG anti-Rh°(D) in adult patients with chronic autoimmune thrombocytopenia. *Amer. J. Haemat.* **22**, 241–250.

Salama, A. and Mueller-Eckhardt, C. (1987a) Cianidanol and its metabolites bind tightly to red cells and are responsible for the production of auto- and/or drug-dependent antibodies against these cells. *Brit. J. Haemat.* **66**, 263–266.

Salama, A. and Mueller-Eckhardt, C. (1987b) On the mechanisms of sensitization and attachment of antibodies to RBC in drug-induced immune hemolytic anemia. *Blood*, **69**, 1006–1010.

Salama, A., Gottsche, B., Vaidya, V., Santoso, S. and Mueller-Eckhardt, C. (1988) Complement-independent lysis of human red blood cells by cold hemagglutinins. *Vox Sang.* **55**, 21–25.

Salama, A., Schutz, B., Kiefel, V., Breithaupt, H.

and Mueller-Eckhardt, C. (1989) Immune-mediated agranulocytosis related to drugs and heterogeneity of antibodies. *Brit. J. Haemat.* **72**, 127–132.

Salmon, C., Dreyfus, B. and André, R. (1958) Double population de globules, différant seulement par l'antigène de groupe ABO, observée chez un malade leucémique. *Rev. Hémat.* **13**, 148.

Salmon, C., André, R. and Dreyfus, B. (1959a) Existe-t-il des mutations somatiques du gène de groupe sanguin A au cours de certaines leucemies aiguës? *Rev. franç. Étud. clin. biol.* **4**, 468.

Salmon, C., Schwartzenberg, L. and André, R. (1959b) Anémie hémolytique post-transfusionelle chez un sujet A_3 à la suite d'un injection massive de sang A_1. *Sang.* **30**, 223.

Salmon, C., Schwartzenberg, L. and André, R. (1959c) Observations sérologiques et génétiques sur le groupe sanguin A. *Sang.* **30**, 227.

Salmon, C. and Homberg, J.C. (1971) Les anticorps associés au cours des anémies hémolytiques acquises avec auto-anticorps, in *Les anémies hémolytiques. Rapports présentés au 38e Congrès de Medécine, Beyrouth*, p. 83. Masson, Paris.

Salmon, Ch., Ropars, C., Gerbal, A., Habibi, B., Andreu, G. and Salmon, D. (1973) Quelques aspects des anti-immunoglobulines chez les polytransfusés. *Rev. franç. Transfus.* **16**, 373.

Salmon, Ch. (1976) Les phénotypes B faibles B_3, B_x, B_{el}. Classification pratique proposée. *Rev. franç. Transfus. Immunohémat.* **19**, 89.

Salmon, Ch. and Cartron, J.P. (1977) ABO phenotypes, in *CRC Handbook Series in Clinical Laboratory Science, Section D: Blood Banking*, eds T.J. Greenwalt and E.A. Steane, vol. 1, pp. 71–105. CRC Press Inc., Cleveland, USA.

Salmon, C., Cartron, J.P. and Rouger, P. (1984) *The Human Blood Groups*. Masson Publishing, USA.

Salsbury, A.J. and Clarke, J.A. (1967) Surface changes, in red blood cells undergoing agglutination. *Rev. franç. Étud. clin. biol.* **12**, 981.

Salvatierra, O. and 11 others (1980) Deliberate donor-specific blood transfusions prior to living related renal transplantation. *Ann. Surg.* **192**, 543–552.

Salvatierra, O. jr and 9 others (1981a) Incidence, characteristics and outcome of recipients sensitized after donor-specific blood transfusions. *Transplantation*, **32**, 528–531.

Salvatierra, O. jr and 11 others (1981b) Pretreatment with donor-specific blood transfusion in related recipients with high MLC. *Transplant. Proc.* **13**, 142–149.

Salvatierra, O., Melzer, Juliet, Potter, D., Garovoy, M., Vincenti, F., Amend, W.J.C., Husing,

R., Hopper, Susan and Feduska, N.J. (1986) A seven-year experience with donor-specific blood transfusions. Results and considerations for maximum efficacy. *Transplantation*, **40**, 654–659.

Salzman, E.W. and 11 others (1986) Treatment with desmopressin acetate to reduce blood loss after cardiac surgery. *New Engl. J. Med.* **314**, 1402–1406.

Samet, S. and Bowman, H.S. (1961) Feto-maternal ABO incompatibility: intravascular hemolysis, fetal hemoglobinemia and fibrinogenopenia in maternal circulation. *Amer. J. Obstet. Gynec.* **81**, 49.

Sampietro, M., Thein, Swee, L., Contreras, Marcela and Pazmany, L. (1992) Variation of HbF and F-cell number with the G-gamma Xmn l (C-T) polymorphism in normal individuals (Letter). *Blood*, **79**, 832–833.

Sampliner, R.E., Hamilton, F.A., Iseri, O.A., Tabor, E. and Boitnot, J. (1979) The liver histology and frequency of clearance of the hepatitis B surface antigen (HBsAg) in chronic carriers. *Amer. J. med. Sci.* **277**, 17–22.

Samson, Diana and Mollison, P.L. (1975) Effect on primary Rh immunization of delayed administration of anti-Rh. *Immunology*, **28**, 349.

Sander, R.P. Hardy, N.M. and van Meter, S. (1987) Anti-Jk^a autoimmune hemolytic anemia in an infant. *Transfusion*, **27**, 58–60.

Sandiford, F.M., Chiariello, L., Hallman, G.L. and Cooley, D.A. (1974) Aorto-coronary bypass in Jehovah's witnesses. Report of 36 patients. *J. thorac. cardiovasc. Surg.* **68**, 1.

Sandler, S.G. and Nusbacher, J. (1982) Health risks of leukapheresis donors. *Haematologia*, **15**, 57–69.

Sandler, S.G. (1983) Overview, in *Autologous Transfusion*, eds S.G. Sandler and A. Silvergleid. Amer. Assoc. Blood Banks, Arlington, VA.

Sandler, S.G., Fang, C.T. and Williams, A.E. (1991) Human T-cell lymphotropic virus type I and II in transfusion medicine. *Transfus. Med. Rev.* **5**, 93–107.

Sandor, M. and Langone, J.J. (1982) Demonstration of high and low affinity complexes between protein A and rabbit immunoglobulin-G antibodies depending on hapten density. *Biochem. biophys. Res. Commun.* **106**, 761–767.

Sanger, Ruth, Race, R.R., Walsh, R.J. and Montgomery, Carmel (1948) An antibody which subdivides the human MN blood groups. *Heredity*, **2**, 131.

Sanger, Ruth, Gavin, June, Tippett, Patricia, Teesdale, Phyllis and Eldon, K. (1971) Plant agglutinin for another human blood-group (Letter). *Lancet*, **i**, 1130.

Sanger, Ruth and Tippett, Patricia (1979) Live

children and abortions of p mothers (Letter). *Transfusion*, **19**, 222.

Sangster, J.M., Kenwright, M.G., Walker, M.P. and Pembroke, A.C. (1979) Anti-blood group M autoantibodies with livedo reticularis, Raynaud's phenomenon and anaemia. *J. clin. Path.* **32**, 154–157.

Sansby, J.M. (1925) Intraperitoneal transfusion of citrated blood. The effect of an intraperitoneally produced plethora on the hemopoietic activity of the bone marrow. *Amer. J. Dis. Child.* **30**, 659.

Santoso, S., Shibata, Y., Kiefel, V. and Mueller-Eckhardt, Ch. (1987) Identification of the Yuk^b alloantigen on platelet glycoprotein IIIa. *Vox Sang.* **53**, 48–51.

Santoso, S., Kiefel, V. and Mueller-Eckhardt, Ch. (1989) Human platelet alloantigens Br^a/Br^b are expressed on the very late activation antigen 2 (VLA-2) of T lymphocytes. *Hum. Immunol.* **25**, 237–246.

Sarnaik, S., Soorya, D., Kim, J., Ravindranath, Y. and Lusher, J. (1979) Periodic transfusions for sickle cell anaemia and CNS infarction. *Amer. J. Dis. Child.* **133**, 1254–1257.

Sarnaik, S., Schornak, J. and Lusher, J.M. (1986) The incidence of development of irregular red cell antibodies in patients with sickle cell anemia. *Transfusion*, **26**, 249–252.

Sato, H. and Okochi, K. (1986) Transmission of human T cell leukaemia virus (HTLV-I) by blood transfusion: demonstration of proviral DNA in recipients' blood lymphocytes. *Int. J. Cancer*, **37**, 397–400.

Satow, Y-I., Hashido, M., Ishikawa, K-I., Honda, H., Mizuno, M., Kawana, T. and Hayami, M. (1991) Detection of HTLV-I antigen in peripheral and cord blood lymphocytes from carrier mothers. *Lancet*, **ii**, 915–916.

Sausais, Laima, Krevans, J.R. and Townes, A.S. (1964) Characteristics of a third example of anti-Xg^a (Abstract). *Transfusion*, **4**, 312.

Savage, C.O.S., Pusey, C.D., Bowman, C., Rees, A.J. and Lockwood, C.M. (1986) Antiglomerular basement membrane antibody mediated disease in the British Isles 1980–4. *Brit. med. J.* **292**, 301–304.

Saverymuttu, S.H., Peters, A.M., Keshavarzian, A., Reavy, H.J. and Lavender, J.P. (1985) The kinetics of 111 Indium distribution following injection of 111 Indium labelled autologous granulocytes in man. *Brit. J. Haemat.* **61**, 675–685.

Savitsky, J.P., Doczi, J., Black, J. and Arnold, J. D. (1978) A clinical safety trial of stroma-free hemoglobin. *Clin. Pharmacol. Therap.* **23**, 73–80.

Saxinger, C., Polesky, H., Eby, N., Grufferman, S., Murphy, R., Tegtmeir, G., Parekh, V., Memon, S. and Hung, C. (1988) Antibody reactivity with HBLV (HHV-6) in U.S. populations. *J. virol. Methods*, **21**, 199–208.

Sayers, M.H., Anderson, K.C. Goodnough, L.T., Kurtz, S.R., Lane, T.A., Pisciotto, Patricia and Silberstein, L.E. (1992) Reducing the risk for transfusion-transmitted cytomegalovirus infection. *Ann. intern. Med.* **116**, 55–62.

Sazama, K. (1990) Reports of 355 transfusion-associated deaths: 1976 through 1985. *Transfusion*, **30**, 583–590.

Schachter, H., Michaels, M.A., Crookston, Marie C., Tilley, Christine A. and Crookston, J.H. (1971) A quantitative difference in the activity of blood group A-specific N-acetylgalactosaminyl-transferase in serum from A$_1$ and A$_2$ human subjects. *Biochem. biophys. Res. Commun.* **45**, 1011.

Schachter, H., Michaels, M.A., Tilley, Christine A., Crookston, Marie C. and Crookston, J.H. (1973) Qualitative differences in the N-acetyl-D-galactosaminyltransferases produced by human A^1 and A^2 genes. *Proc. nat. Acad. Sci. USA*, **70**, 220.

Schanfield, M.S., Stevens, J.O. and Bauman, D. (1981) The detection of clinically significant erythrocyte alloantibodies using a human mononuclear phagocyte assay. *Transfusion*, **21**, 571–576.

Schanfield, M.S. and van Loghem, Erna (1986) Human immunoglobulin allotypes, in *Handbook of Experimental Immunology. Vol 3: Genetics and Molecular Immunology*, ed D.M. Weir, pp. 94.1–94.18. Blackwell Scientific Publications, Oxford.

Schechter, Geraldine P., Soehlen, Frances and McFarland, W. (1972) Lymphocyte response to blood transfusion in man. *New Engl. J. Med.* **28**, 1169.

Schedel, L. (1986) Application of immunoglobulin preparations in multiple myeloma, in *Clinical Uses of Intravenous Immunoglobulins*, eds A. Morell and U.E. Nydegger, pp. 123–132. Academic Press, London.

Schellong, G. (1964) Über den Einfluss mütterlicher Antikörper des ABO-systems auf Reticulocyten-zahl und Serumbilirubin bei Frühgeborenen. *Commun. 10th Congr. Int. Soc. Blood Transfus.*, Stockholm.

Schenkel-Brunner, H. and Tuppy, H. (1969) Enzymatic conversion of human O into A erythrocytes and of B into AB erythrocytes. *Nature (Lond.)*, **223**, 1272.

Schenkel-Brunner, H., Chester, M.A. and Watkins, Winifred M. (1972) α-L-fucosyltransferases in human serum from donors of different ABO, secretor and Lewis blood-group phenotypes. *Eur. J. Biochem.* **30**, 269.

Schenkel-Brunner, H. (1980a) Blood-group-ABH antigens of human erythrocytes. Quantitative studies on the distribution of H antigenic sites among different classes of membrane components. *Eur. J. Biochem.* **104**, 529–534.

Schenkel-Brunner, H. (1980b) Blood group ABH antigens on human cord red cells. Number of *A* antigenic sites and their distribution among different classes of membrane constituents. *Vox Sang.* **38**, 310–314.

Schenkel-Brunner, H. and Hanfland, P. (1981) Immunochemistry of the Lewis blood-group system. III. Studies on the molecular basis of the Le^x property. *Vox Sang.* **40**, 358–366.

Scherer, R., Morarescu, A. and Ruhenstroth-Bauer, G. (1975) Die spezifische Wirkung der Plasmaproteine bei der Blutkörperchensenkung. *Klin. Wschr.* **53**, 265.

Schierman, L.W. and McBride, R.A. (1967) Adjuvant activity of erythrocyte isoantigens. *Science*, **156**, 658.

Schierman, L.W., Leckband, E. and McBride, R.A. (1969) Immunological interaction of erythrocyte isoantigens: effect of passive antibody. *Proc. Soc. exp. Biol. (N.Y.)*, **130**, 744.

Schiff, F. (1924) Über gruppenspezifische Serumpräcipitine. *Klin. Wschr.* **3**, 679.

Schiff, F. (1934) Zur Kenntnis der Blutantigene des Shigabazillus. *Z. Immun.-Forsch.* **82**, 46.

Schiff, P. and Kemp, A. (1991) Safety of IVIG made from HCV-antibody-screened plasma (Letter). *Lancet*, **ii**, 1076.

Schiffer, L.M., Atkins, H.L., Chanana, A.D., Cronkite, E.P., Greenberg, M.L., Johnson, H.A., Robertson, J.S. and Stryckmans, P.A. (1966) Extracorporeal irradiation of the blood in humans: effects upon erythrocyte survival. *Blood*, **27**, 831.

Schiffer, C.A., Lichtenfeld, J.L., Wiernik, P.H., Mardiney, M. and Mehsen Joseph, J. (1976) Antibody response in patients with acute nonlymphocytic leukemia. *Cancer*, **37**, 2177.

Schiffer, C.A. (1981) In International Forum: Which are the parameters to be controlled in platelet concentrates in order that they may be offered to the medical profession as a standardised product with specific properties? *Vox Sang.* **40**, 122–124.

Schiffer, C.A., Aisner, J., Dutcher, J.P., Daly, P.A. and Wiernik, P.H. (1982) A clinical program of platelet cryopreservation, in *Progress in Pheresis*, ed W.R. Vogler. Alan R. Liss, New York.

Schiffer, C.A. (1987) Management of patients refractory to platelet transfusion. An evaluation of methods of donor selection. *Prog. Hemat.* **15**, 91.

Schiffer, C.A. (1990) Granulocyte transfusions: an overlooked therapeutic modality. *Transfus. Med. Rev.* **4**, 2–7.

Schimpf, K. and 13 others (1987) Absence of hepatitis after treatment with a pasteurised Factor VIII concentrate in patients with hae-

mophilia and no previous transfusion. *New Engl. J. Med.* **316**, 918–922.

Schmidt, P.J. and Kevy, S.V. (1958) Air embolism. *New Engl. J. Med.* **258**, 424.

Schmidt, P.J., Nancarrow, J.F., Morrison, Eleanor G. and Chase, G. (1959) A hemolytic reaction due to the transfusion of A$_x$ blood. *J. Lab. clin. Med.* **54**, 38.

Schmidt, R. Pauline, Griffitts, J.J. and Northman, F.F. (1962a) A new antibody anti-Sm, reacting with a high incidence antigen. Cited by Race, R.R. and Sanger, Ruth (1962).

Schmidt, P.J., Morrison, E.G. and Shohl, Jane (1962b) The antigenicity of the Rh$_0$(D^u) blood factor. *Blood*, **20**, 196.

Schmidt, P.J., Barile, M.F. and McGinniss, Mary H. (1965) Mycoplasma (pleuropneumonia-like organism) and blood group I; associations with neoplastic disease. *Nature (Lond.)*, **205**, 371.

Schmidt, P.J. and Holland, P.V. (1967) Pathogenesis of the acute renal failure associated with incompatible transfusion. *Lancet*, **ii**, 1169.

Schmidt, P.J. and Vos, G.H. (1967) Multiple phenotypic abnormalities associated with Rh$_{null}$ (.../...). *Vox Sang.* **13**, 18–20.

Schmidt, P.J. (1968) Transfusion in America in the eighteenth and nineteenth centuries. *New Engl. J. Med.* **279**, 1319.

Schmidt, A.P. and Taswell, H.F. (1969) Co-existence of MN erythrocytes and apparent anti-M antibody. *Transfusion*, **9**, 203.

Schmidt, A.P., Taswell, F. and Gleich, G.J. (1969) Anaphylactic transfusion reactions associated with anti-IgA antibody. *New Engl. J. Med.* **280**, 188.

Schmidt, P.J. (1978) Red cells for transfusion. *New Engl. J. Med.* **299**, 1411.

Schmidt, P.J. (1980a) The mortality from incompatible transfusion, in *Immunobiology of the Erythrocyte*, eds S.G. Sandler, J. Nussbacher and M.S. Schanfeld. Alan R. Liss Inc., New York.

Schmidt, P.J. (1980b) Transfusion mortality; with special reference to surgical and intensive care facilities. *J. Fla. med. Assoc.* **67**, 151–153.

Schmitz, N., Djibey, I., Kretschmer, V., Mahn, I. and Mueller-Eckhardt, C. (1981) Assessment of red cell autoantibodies in autoimmune haemolytic anaemia of warm type by a radioactive anti-IgG test. *Vox Sang.* **41**, 224–230.

Schmuñis, G.A. (1991) *Trypanosoma cruzi*, the etiologic agent of Chagas' disease: status in the blood supply in endemic and nonendemic countries. *Transfusion*, **31**, 547–557.

Schneider, C.L. (1956) Mechanisms of production of acute fibrinogen deficiencies. *Progr. Hemat.* **1**, 202.

Schneider, J. and Preisler, O. (1966) Untersuchungen zur serologischen Prophylaxe der Rh-Sensibilisierung. *Blut*, **12**, 1.

Schneider, J. (1969) Prophylaxe der Rh-Sensibiliserung durch Anti-D-Applikation, in Ergebnissc der Bluttransfusionsforschung. *Bibl. haemat. (Basel)*, **32**, 113.

Schochetman, G. (1992) Biology of human immunodeficiency viruses in *AIDS Testing*, eds G. Schochetman and J.R. George, pp. 18–29. Springer-Verlag, New York.

Schochetman, G. and George, J.R. (1992) *AIDS Testing. Methodology and Management Issues.* Springer-Verlag, New York.

Schonermark, Sabine, Rauterberg, E.W., Shin, M.L., Loke, S., Roelcke, D. and Hansch, Gertrud M. (1986) Homologous species restriction in lysis of human erythrocytes: a membrane-derived protein with C8-binding capacity functions as an inhibitor. *J. Immunol.* **136**, 1772–1776.

Schorr, J.B., Schorr, Phyllis T., Francis, Rose, Spierer, G. and Dugan, Evelyn (1971) The antigenicity of C and E antigens when transfused into Rh-negative (rr) and Rh-positive recipients. *Commun. Amer. Assoc. Blood Banks*, Chicago.

Schreiber, A.D. and Frank, M.M. (1972) Role of antibody and complement in the immune clearance and destruction of erythrocytes. I. *In vivo* effects of IgG and IgM complement-fixing sites. *J. clin. Invest.* **51**, 575.

Schreiber, A.D., Herskovitz, B.S. and Goldwein, M. (1977) Low-titer cold-hemagglutinin disease. Mechanism of hemolysis and response to corticosteroids. *New Engl. J. Med.* **296**, 1490.

Schrier, S.L., Moore, L.D. and Chiapella, A.P. (1968) Inhibition of human erythrocyte membrane mediated ATP synthesis by anti-D antibody. *Amer. J. med. Sci.* **256**, 340.

Schultze, H.E. and Heremans, J.F. (1966) *Molecular Biology of Human Proteins with Special Reference to Plasma Proteins*, vol. 1. Elsevier, Amsterdam.

Schumer, W. and Nyhus, L.M. (1974) Preface to *Treatment of Shock: Principles and Practice*, eds W. Schumer and L.W. Nyhus. Lea & Febiger, Philadelphia.

Schupbach, J., Haler, O., Vogt, M., Luthy, R., Joller, Helen, Oelz, O., Popovic, M., Sarngadharan, M.G. and Gallo, R.C. (1985) Antibodies to HTLV-III in Swiss patients with AIDS and pre-AIDS and in groups at risk for AIDS. *New Engl. J. Med.* **312**, 265–270.

Schur, P.H. and Christian, G.D. (1964) The role of disulfide bonds in the complement-fixing and precipitating properties of 7S rabbit and sheep antibodies. *J. exp. Med.* **120**, 531.

Schur, P.H., Alpert, E. and Alper, C. (1973) Gamma G subgroups in human fetal, cord,

and maternal sera. *Clin. Immunol. Immunopath.* **2**, 62.

Schwarting, G.A., Marcus, D.M. and Metaxas, M. (1977) Identification of sialosylparagloboside as the erythrocyte receptor for an 'anti-p' antibody. *Vox Sang.* **32**, 257.

Schwarting, G.A., Kundu, S.K. and Marcus, D.M. (1979) Reaction of antibodies that cause paroxysmal cold hemoglobinuria (PCH) with globoside and Forssman glycosphingolipids. *Blood*, **53**, 186–192.

Schwartz, B.S., Williams, E.C., Conlan, M.C. and Mosher, D.F. (1986) Epsilon-aminocaproic acid in the treatment of patients with acute promyelocytic leukemia and acquired alpha-2-plasmin inhibitor deficiency. *Ann. intern. Med.* **105**, 873–877.

Scott, J.R. (1976) Immunologic risks to fetuses from maternal to fetal transfer of erythrocytes, in *Proceedings of Symposium on Rh antibody Mediated Immunosuppression.* Ortho Research Institute, Raritan, New Jersey.

Scott, E.P. and Slichter, S.J. (1980) Viability and function of platelet concentrates stored in CPD-adenine (CPDA-1). *Transfusion*, **20**, 489–497.

Scott, J.R., Rote, N.S. and Cruickshank, D.P. (1983) Antiplatelet antibodies and platelet counts in pregnancies complicated by autoimmune thrombocytopenia. *Amer. J. Obstet. Gynec.* **145**, 932–939.

Scott, Marion L. (1991) The principles and applications of solid-phase blood group serology. *Transfus. Med. Rev.* **5**, 60–72.

Scott, Marion L. and Phillips, P.K. (1987) Sensitive two-stage papain technique without cell washing. *Vox Sang.* **52**, 67–70.

Scott, M.L., Johnson, C.A. and Phillips, P.K. (1987a) The pH optima for papain and bromelain treatment of red cells. *Vox Sang.* **52**, 223–227.

Scott, J.R., Rote, N.S. and Branch, D.W. (1987b) Immunologic aspects of recurrent abortion and fetal death. *Obstet. Gynec.* **70**, 645–656.

Scott, M.L., Voak, D. and Downie, D.M. (1988a) Optimum enzyme activity in blood grouping, and a ncw technique for antibody detection: an explanation for the poor performance on the one-stage mix technique. *Med. Lab. Sciences*, **45**, 7–18.

Scott, E.P., Moilan-Bergeland, J. and Dalmasso, A.P. (1988b) Posttransfusion thrombocytopenia associated with passive transfusion of a platelet-specific antibody. *Transfusion*, **28**, 73–76.

Scott, M.L., Guest, A.R. and Anstee, D.J. (1989) Subclass dependence of reduction and alkylation of incomplete IgG monoclonal anti-D to complete anti-D (Abstract). *Transfusion*, **29**, Suppl. 57S.

Seaman, M.J., Benson, R., Jones, M.N., Morton, J.A. and Pickles, M.M. (1967) The reactions of the Bennett-Goodspeed group of antibodies tested with the AutoAnalyzer. *Brit. J. Haemat.* **13**, 464.

Seaman, Muriel J., Chalmers, D.G. and Franks, D. (1968) Siedler: an antibody which reacts with A_1 Le(a−b+) red cells. *Vox Sang.* **15**, 25.

Searle, J.F. (1973) Anaesthesia in sickle cell states. A review. *Anaesthesia*, **28**, 48.

Sebring, Elizabeth S. (1984) Fetomaternal hemorrhage-incidence and methods of detection and quantitation, in *Hemolytic Disease of the Newborn*, ed G. Garratty, pp. 87–117. Amer. Assoc. Blood Banks, Arlington, VA.

Sebring, E.S. and Polesky, H.F. (1990) Fetomaternal hemorrhage: incidence, risk factors, time of occurrence, and clinical effects. *Transfusion*, **30**, 344–357.

Second International Workshop on Red Cell Monoclonal Antibodies (1990) *Proceedings of the Second International Workshop and Symposium on Monoclonal Antibodies against Human Red Blood Cells and Related Antigens*, eds M.A. Chester., U. Johnson, A. Lundblad, B. Low, L. Messeter and B. Samuelsson, Lund, Sweden.

Seeberg, S., Brandberg, Å., Hermodsson, S., Larsson, P. and Lundgren, S. (1981) Hospital outbreak of hepatitis A secondary to blood exchange in a baby (Letter). *Lancet*, **i**, 1155–1156.

Seeff, L.B. and 13 others (1977) A randomized, double blind controlled trial of the efficacy of immune serum globulin for the prevention of posttransfusion hepatitis. *Gastroenterology*, **72**, 111.

Seeger, W. Schneider, U., Kreusler, B., von Witzleben, E., Walmrath, D., Grimminger, F. and Neppert, J. (1990) Reproduction of transfusion-related acute lung injury in an *ex-vivo* lung model. *Blood*, **76**, 1438–1444.

Seemayer, T.A. and Bolande, R.P. (1980) Thymic involution mimicking thymic dysplasia. A consequence of transfusion induced graft versus-host disease in a premature infant. *Arch. Path. lab. Med.* **104**, 141–144.

Seger, R., Joller, P., Bird, G.W.G., Wingham, J., Wuest, J., Kenny, A., Rapp, A., Garzoni, D., Hitzig, W.H. and Duc, G. (1980) Necrotising enterocolitis and neuraminidase-producing bacteria. *Helv. paediat. Acta*, **35**, 121–128.

Seghatchian, M.J., Vickers, M., Ip, A.H.L., Cutts, M. Tandy, N., Gasgoine, M.E. and Booker, W. (1990) Changes in the mean platelet volume and the quality control of platelet concentrates (Abstract). *Joint Congr. Int. Soc. Blood Transfus. AABB*, Los Angeles.

Segre, D. and Kaeberle, M.L. (1962) The immunologic behavior of baby pigs. I. Production of antibodies in three-week-old pigs. *J. Immunol.* **89**, 782.

Sehgal, L.R., Rosen, A.L., Gould, S.A., Sehgal, H., Dalton, L., Mayoral, J. and Moss, G.S. (1980) *In vitro* and *in vivo* characteristics of poly-merized-pyridoxylated hemoglobin solution. *Fed. Proc.* **39**, 718.

Seidl, S. and Spielmann, W. (1970) Comparative studies on the effect of different nucleosides in red cell preservation, in *Modern Problems of Blood Preservation*, eds W. Spielmann and S. Seidl. Gustav Fischer, Stuttgart.

Sela, M. and Mozes, Edna (1966) Dependence of the chemical nature of antibodies on the net electrical charge of antigens. *Proc. nat. Acad. Sci. USA*, **55**, 445.

Selbie, F.R. (1943) Viability of *Treponema pallidum* in stored plasma. *Brit. J. exp. Path.* **24**, 150.

Seligmann, M. (1990) Immunological features of human immunodeficiency virus disease, in *Haematology in HIV Disease*, ed Christine Costello. Baillière Tindall, London, **3**, 37–63.

Selwyn, J.G., Seright, W., Donald, J. and Wallace, J. (1968) Matching blood for recipients of dextrans. *Lancet*, **ii**, 1032.

Sender, A., Maigret, P., Poulain, M., Boeswill-wald, M. and Lepage, F. (1971) La règle de compatibilité transfusionnelle A.B.C. à la période néo-natale. *Bull. Fed. Soc. Gynec. Obstet.* **23**, 560.

Senhauser, D.A., Westphal, R.G., Bohman, J.E. and Neff, J.C. (1982) Immune system changes in cytapheresis donors. *Transfusion*, **22**, 302–304.

Seppälä, M. and Ruoslahti, E. (1972) Radio-immunoassay of maternal serum alpha feto-protein during pregnancy and delivery. *Amer. J. Obstet. Gynec.* **112**, 208.

Sererat, M.N., Schifano, J.V., Lau, P., Beikert, Earla, Bhumbra, A. and Nankervis, G.A. (1986) Evaluation of cytomegalovirus (CMV) antibody screening tests for blood donors. *Amer. J. clin. Path.* **86**, 523–526.

Settle, J.A.D. (1982) Fluid therapy in burns. *J. Roy. Soc. Med.* **75**, Suppl. 1, 6–11.

Severns, M.L., Kline, L.M. and Epley, K.M. (1989) Computerized threshold determination for automated ABO/Rh tests. *Vox Sang.* **56**, 87–92.

Sevitt, S. (1958–9) Hepatic jaundice after blood transfusion in injured and burned subjects. *Brit. J. Surg.* **46**, 68.

Seyfried, Halina, Frankowska, Krystyna and Giles, Carolyn M. (1966) Further examples of anti-Bu^a found in immunized donors. *Vox Sang.* **11**, 512.

Seyfried, Halina, Gorska, Barbara, Maj, S., Sylwestrowicz, T., Giles, Carolyn M. and Goldsmith, K.L.G. (1972) Apparent depression of antigens of the Kell blood group system associated with autoimmune acquired haemolytic anaemia. *Vox Sang.* **23**, 528.

Shackelford, D.A. and Strominger, J.L. (1980) Demonstration of structural polymorphism among HLA-DR light chains by two-dimensional gel electrophoresis. *J. exp. Med.* **151**, 144–165.

Shackelford, D.A., Kaufman, A.J., Korman, A.J. and Strominger, J.L. (1982) HLA-DR antigens: structure, separation, of subpopulations, gene cloning and function. *Immunol. Rev.* **66**, 133–188.

Shanwell, H., Sallander, S., Olsson, I., Gullikson, H., Pedagas, I. and Lerner, R. (1991) An allo-immunised, thrombocytopenic patient successfully transfused with acid-treated random donor platelets. *Brit. J. Haemat.* **79**, 462–465.

Sharon, B.I. and Honig, G. (1991) Management of congenital hemolytic anemias, in *Principles of Transfusion Medicine*, eds E.C. Rossi, T.L. Simon and G.S. Moss, pp. 131–149. Williams and Wilkins Baltimore, Maryland, USA.

Sharpey-Schafer, E.P. and Wallace, J. (1942a) Retention of injected serum in the circulation. *Lancet*, **i**, 699.

Sharpey-Schafer, E.P. and Wallace, J. (1942b) Circulatory overloading following rapid intravenous injections. *Lancet*, **ii**, 304.

Sharpey-Schafer, E.P. (1945) Transfusion and the anaemic heart. *Lancet*, **ii**, 296.

Shattock, A.G., Irwin, Fiona M., Morgan, Bridget M., Hillary, Irene B., Kelly, M.G., Fielding, J.F., Kelly, Deirdre A. and Weir, D.G. (1985) Increased severity and morbidity of acute hepatitis in drug abusers with simultaneously acquired hepatitis B and hepatitis D virus infections. *Brit. med. J.* **290**, 1377–1380.

Sheetz, M.P. (1983) Membrane skeletal dynamics: role in modulation of red cell deformability, mobility of transmembrane proteins, and shape. *Semin. Haemat.* **20**, 175–188.

Shemin, D. and Rittenberg, D. (1946) The life-span of the human red blood cell. *J. biol. Chem.* **166**, 627.

Shen, S.C., Ham, T.H. and Fleming, E.M. (1943) Studies in destruction of red blood cells. III. Mechanism and complications of hemoglobinuria in patients with thermal burns: spherocytosis and increased osmotic fragility of red blood cells. *New Engl. J. Med.* **229**, 701.

Shepherd, L.P., Feingold, E. and Shanbrom, E. (1969) An unusual occurrence of anti-Xg[a]. *Vox Sang.* **16**, 157.

Sherertz, R.J., Russell, B.A. and Reuman, P.D. (1984) Transmission of hepatitis A by transfusion of blood products. *Arch. intern. Med.* **144**, 1579–1580.

Sheridan, W.P. and 9 others (1989) Granulocyte colony-stimulating factor and neutrophil re-

covery after high-dose chemotherapy and autologous bone marrow transplantation. *Lancet*, **ii**, 891–895.

Sherman, S.P. and Taswell, H.F. (1977) The need for transfusion of saline-washed red blood cells to patients with paroxysmal nocturnal haemoglobinuria: a myth (Abstract). *Transfusion*, **17**, 683.

Sherwood, R.A., Brent, L. and Rayfield, L.S. (1986) Presentation of alloantigens by host cells. *Eur. J. Immunol.* **16**, 596–574.

Shibata, Y., Baba, M. and Kaniyoki, M. (1983) Studies on the retention of passively transferred antibodies in man II. Antibody activity in the blood after intravenous or intramuscular administration of anti-HBs human immunoglobulin. *Vox Sang.* **45**, 77–82.

Shibata, Y., Miyaji, T., Ischikawa, Y. and Matsuda, I. (1986a) Yuk[a], a new platelet antigen involved in two cases of neonatal alloimmune thrombocytopenia. *Vox Sang.* **50**, 177–181.

Shibata, Y., Miyaji, T., Ischikawa, Y. and Matsuda, I. (1986b) A new platelet antigen system, Yuk[a]/Yuk[b]. *Vox Sang.* **51**, 334–337.

Shields, C.E. (1968) Comparison studies of whole blood stored in ACD and CPD and with adenine. *Transfusion*, **8**, 1.

Shields, C.E. (1969a) Studies on stored whole blood. II. Use of packed red blood cells. *Transfusion*, **9**, 1.

Shields, C.E. (1969b) Effect of adenine on stored erythrocytes evaluated by autologous and homologous transfusion. *Transfusion*, **9**, 115.

Shields, C.E. (1970) Studies on stored whole blood: IV. Effects of temperature and mechanical agitation on blood with and without plasma. *Transfusion*, **10**, 155.

Shields, C.E. (1971) Effect of plasma removal on blood stored in ACD with adenine. *Transfusion*, **11**, 134.

Shih, W.K., Esteban, M.J.I. and Alter, H.J. (1986) Non-A, non-B hepatitis: advances and unfulfilled expectations of the first decade. *Prog. Liver Dis.* **8**, 433–452.

Shih, J.W.K., Lee, H.H., Falchek, M., Canavaggio, M., Jett, B.W., Allain, J-P. and Alter, H.J. (1990) Transfusion-transmitted HTLV-I/II infection in patients undergoing open-heart surgery. *Blood*, **75**, 546–549.

Shinowawa, G.Y. (1951) Enzyme studies on human blood. XI. The isolation and characterisation of thromboplastic cell and plasma components. *J. Lab. clin. Med.* **38**, 11.

Shirey, R.S., Smith, B., Sensenbrenner, L., Bauer, T.W., Ness, P.M., Kickler, T.S. and Gibble, J.W. (1983) Red cell sensitization due to anti-D in an anti-lymphocyte globulin. *Transfusion*, **23**, 396–397.

Shirey, R.S., Oyen, R., Heeb, K.N., Kickler, T.S. and Ness, P.M. (1988) ^{51}Cr radiolabelled survival studies in a patient with anti-Lu12. *Transfusion*, **28**, 375.

Shore, G.M. and Steane, E.A. (1977) Survival of incompatible red cells in a patient with anti-Cs[a] and three other patients with antibodies to high-frequency red cell antigens. *Commun. Amer. Assoc. Blood Banks*, Atlanta.

Shrand, J. (1964) Visceral larva migrans: *Toxacara canis* infection. *Lancet*, **i**, 1357.

Shulman, N.R., Aster, R.H., Leitner, A. and Hiller, Merilyn C. (1961) Immunoreactions involving platelets. V. Post-transfusion purpura due to a complement-fixing antibody against a genetically controlled platelet antigen. A proposed mechanism for thrombocytopenia and its relevance in 'autoimmunity'. *J. clin. Invest.* **40**, 1597.

Shulman, N.R., Marder, V.J., Hiller, Merilyn C. and Collier, Ellen M. (1964) Platelet and leukocyte isoantigens and their antibodies: serologic, physiologic and clinical studies. *Progr. Hemat.* **4**, 222.

Shulman, N.R. (1966) Immunological considerations attending platelet transfusion. *Transfusion*, **6**, 39.

Shulman, N.R., Leissinger, C.A., Hotchkiss, A.J. and Kantz, C.A. (1982) The non-specific nature of platelet-associated IgG. *Trans. Assoc. Amer. Phycns.* **14**, 213–220.

Shulman, I.A., Saxena, S., Nelson, Janice M. and Furmanski, M. (1984) Neonatal exchange transfusions complicated by transfusion-induced malaria. *Pediatrics*, **73**, 330–332.

Shulman, Ira A., Branch, D.R., Nelson, Janice M., Thompson, J.C., Saxena, S. and Petz, L.D. (1985) Autoimmune hemolytic anemia with both cold and warm autoantibodies. *J. Amer. med. Assoc.* **253**, 1746–1748.

Shulman, N.R. and Jordan, J.V. (1987) Platelet immunobiology, in *Haemostasis and Thrombosis*, eds R.W. Colman, J. Hirsch, V.G. Marder and E.W. Salzmann, 2nd edn, pp. 452–529. Lippincott, Philadelphia.

Shulman, Ira A., Meyer, E.A., Lam, H.T. and Nelson, J.M. (1987) Additional limitations of the immediate spin crossmatch to detect ABO incompatibility (Letter). *Amer. J. clin. Path.* **87**, 667.

Shulman, I.A. and Appleman, Maria, D. (1990) An overview of unusual diseases transmitted by blood transfusion within the United States, in *Emerging Global Patterns in Transfusion Transmitted Infections*, eds R.G. Westphal, K.B. Carlson and J.M. Turc, p.1. Amer. Assoc. Blood Banks, Arlington, VA.

Shulman, Ira A., Vengelen-Tyler, Virginia, Thompson, J.C., Nelson, Janice M. and Chen, D.C.T. (1990) Autoanti-Ge associated with severe autoimmune hemolytic anemia. *Vox Sang.* **59**, 232–234.

Shulman, N.R. (1991) Posttransfusion purpura: clinical features and the mechanism of platelet destruction, in *Clinical and Basic Science Aspects of Immunohematology*, ed Sandra T. Nance. Amer. Assoc. of Blood Banks, Arlington, VA.

Shulman, Ira A. and Calderon, C. (1991) Effect of delayed centrifugation or reading on the detection of ABO incompatibility by the immediate-spin crossmatch. *Transfusion*, **31**, 197–200.

Shumak, K.H., Rachkewich, Rose A., Crookston, Marie C. and Crookston, J.H. (1971) Antigens of the Ii system on lymphocytes. *Nature, New Biol.* **231**, 148.

Shumak, K.H., Beldotti, Lorraine E. and Rachkewich, Rose A. (1979) Diagnosis of haematological disease with anti-i. *Brit. J. Haemat.* **41**, 399–405.

Shumak, K.H. and Rock, Gail A. (1984) Therapeutic plasma exchange. *New Engl. J. Med.* **310**, 762–771.

Shwe, K.H., Love, E.M., Lieberman, B.A. and Newland, A.C. (1991) High-dose intravenous immunoglobulin in the prenatal management of neonatal alloimmune thrombocytopenia. *Clin. lab. Haemat.* **13**, 75–79.

Siber, G.R., Ambrosino, Donna M. and Gorgone, Barbara C. (1982) Blood group A-like substance in a preparation of pneumococcal vaccine. *Ann. intern. Med.* **96**, 580–586.

Sickles, Gretchen R. and Murdick, P.P. (1953) Isoagglutinin responses to injections of specific substances A and B. *Amer. J. clin. Path.* **23**, 322.

Siddiqui, B. and Hakomori, S. (1971) A revised structure for the Forssman glycolipid hapten. *J. biol. Chem.* **246**, 5766.

Sideman, S., Mor, L., Brandes, J.M., Thaler, I., Mordohovich, D. and Lupovich, L. (1981) *In vitro* and *in vivo* bilirubin removal by hemoperfusion on ion exchange column. *Israel J. med. Sci.* **17**, 1207.

Sidiropoulos, D., Bohme, U., von Muralt, H., Morell, A. and Barandun, S. (1981) Immunoglobulin Substitution bei der Behandlung der neonatalen Sepsis. *Schweiz. med. Wschr.* **111**, 1649–1655.

Sidiropoulos, D. and Straume, B. (1984) Treatment of neonatal isoimmune thrombocytopenia with intravenous immunoglobulin (IgG i.v.). *Blut*, **48**, 383–386.

Sieg, von W., Borner, P., Pixberg, H.J. and Deicher, H. (1970) Die Elimination Rh-positiver fetaler Erythrozyten aus der Blutbahn Rh-negativer Erwachsener durch körpereigene Isoagglutinine. *Blut*, **21**, 69.

Siegel, S.E., Lunde, M.N., Gelderman, A.H., Halterman, R.H., Brown, J.A., Levine, A.S. and Graw, R.G. jr (1971) Transmission of toxoplasmosis by leukocyte transfusion. *Blood*, **37**, 388.

Siena, S. and 9 others (1991) Flow cytometry for clinical estimation of circulating hematopoietic progenitors for autologous transplantation in cancer patients. *Blood*, **77**, 400–409.

Silbert, J.A., Bove, J.R., Dubin, S. and Bush, W.S. (1981) Patterns of fresh frozen plasma use. *Connecticut Medicine*, **45**, 507–511.

Silvergleid, A.J., Hafleigh, E.B., Harabin, M.A., Wolf, R.M. and Grumet, F.C. (1977) Clinical value of washed-platelet concentrates in patients with non-hemolytic transfusion reactions. *Transfusion*, **17**, 33.

Silvergleid, A.J., Wells, R.F., Hafleigh, E.B., Korn, G., Kellner, R.T. and Grumet, F.C. (1978) Compatibility test using ^{51}chromium-labelled red blood cells in crossmatch positive patients. *Transfusion*, **18**, 8.

Silvergleid, A.J. (1987) Safety and effectiveness of predeposit autologous transfusion in preteen and adolescent children. *J. Amer. med. Assoc.* **257**, 3403–3404.

Silvergleid, A.J. (1991) Preoperative autologous donation: what have we learned? (Editorial). *Transfusion* **31**, 99–101.

Silvestre, D., Kourilsky, F.M., Niccolai, M.G. and Levy, J.P. (1970) Presence of HLA antigens on human reticulocytes as demonstrated by electron microscopy. *Nature (Lond.)*, **228**, 67.

Sim, R.B., Twose, T.W., Paterson, D.S. and Sim, E. (1981) The covalent-binding reaction of complement component C3. *Biochem. J.* **193**, 115–127.

Simmonds, P. and 9 others (1990) Hepatitis C quantification and sequencing in blood products, haemophiliacs, and drug users. *Lancet*, **ii**, 1469–1472.

Simmons, R.T. and Woods, E.F. (1946) Anti-Rh human sera preserved with merthiolate. *Aust. J. Sci.* **8**, 108.

Simon, E.R. (1962) Red cell preservation: further studies with adenine. *Blood*, **20**, 485.

Simon, E.R., Chapman, R.G. and Finch, C.A. (1962) Adenine in red cell preservation. *J. clin. Invest.* **41**, 351.

Simon, I.C., Nelson, E.J., Carmen, R. and Murphy, S. (1983) Extension of platelet concentrate storage. *Transfusion*, **23**, 207–212.

Simon, T.L., Collins, Janice, Kunicki, T.J., Furihata, K., Smith, K.J. and Aster, R.H. (1988) Posttransfusion purpura associated with alloantibody specific for the platelet antigen, Pen^a. *Amer. J. Hemat.* **29**, 38–40.

Simon, T.L., Sohmer, P. and Nelson, E.J. (1989) Extended survival of neocytes produced by a new system. *Transfusion*, **29**, 221–225.

Simonovits, I., Timár, Irma and Bajtai, G. (1980) Rate of Rh immunization after induced abortion. *Vox Sang.* **38**, 161–164.

Simpson, M.B., Dunstan, R.A., Rosse, W.F., Munro, A.C., Fraser, R. and Nichols, M.E. (1987) Status of the MNSs antigens on human platelets. *Transfusion*, **27**, 15–18.

Sims, D.G., Barron, S.L., Wadehra, V. and Ellis, H.A. (1976) Massive chronic feto-maternal bleeding associated with placental chorioangiomas. *Acta paediat. scand.* **65**, 271.

Singer, K., Robin, S., King, J.C. and Jefferson, R.N. (1948) The life-span of the sickle cell in the pathogenesis of sickle-cell anemia. *J. Lab. clin. Med.* **33**, 975.

Singer, S.J. and Nicolson, G.L. (1972) The fluid mosaic model of the structure of cell membranes. *Science*, **175**, 720.

Sinor, L.T., Rachel, J.M., Beck, M.L., Bayer, W.L., Coenen, W.M. and Plapp, F.V. (1985) Solid-phase ABO grouping and Rh typing. *Transfusion*, **25**, 21–23.

Sintnicolaas, K., Sizoo, W., Haye, W.G., Abels, J., Vriesendorp, H.M., Stenfert-Kroeze, W.F., Hop, W.C.J. and Löwenberg, B. (1981) Delayed immunization by random single donor platelet transfusions. *Lancet*, **i**, 750.

Sintnicolaas, K., van der Steuijt, K.J.B., van Putten, W.L.J. and Bolhuis, R.L.H. (1987) A microplate ELISA for the detection of platelet alloantibodies: comparison with the platelet immunofluorescence test. *Brit. J. Haemat.* **66**, 363–367.

Sioufi, H.A., Button, L.N., Jacobson, M.S. and Kevy, S.V. (1990) Nonradioactive chromium technique for red cell labeling. *Vox Sang.* **58**, 204–206.

Sirchia, G., Ferrone, S. and Mercuriali, F. (1970) Leukocyte antigen-antibody reaction and lysis of paroxysmal nocturnal hemoglobinuria erythrocytes. *Blood*, **36**, 334.

Sirchia, G., Parravicini, P., Rebulla, N., Fattori, I. and Milani, S. (1980) Evaluation of three procedures for the preparation of leukocyte-poor and leukocyte-free red blood cells for transfusion. *Vox Sang.* **38**, 197–204.

Sirchia, G., Parravicini, A., Rebulla, P., Greppi, N., Scalamogna, A. and Morelati, F. (1982) Effectiveness of red blood cells filtered through cotton wool to prevent anti-leukocyte antibody production in multitransfused patients. *Vox Sang.* **42**, 190–197.

Sirchia, G., Parravicini, A., Rebulla, P., Bertolini, F., Morelati, F. and Marconi, M. (1983) Preparation of leucocyte-free platelets for transfusion by filtration through cotton wool. *Vox Sang.* **44**, 115–120.

Sirchia, G., Zanella, A., Parrovincini, A., Morelati, F., Rebulla, P. and Masera, C. (1985) Red cell alloantibodies in thalassaemia major. *Transfusion*, **25**, 110–112.

Sistonen, P., Nevanlinna, H.R., Virtaranta-Knowles, K., Pirkola, A., Leikola, J., Kekomäki, R., Gavin, June and Tippett, Patricia (1981) Ne^a, a new blood group antigen in Finland. *Vox Sang.* **40**, 352–357.

Sistonen, P. and Tippett, Patricia (1982) A 'new' allele giving further insight into the LW blood group system. *Vox Sang.* **42**, 252–255.

Sistonen, P. (1984) The Jk (a–b–) phenotype in a Finnish family (Abstract). *18th Congr. Internat. Soc. Blood Transfus.* p. 164, Munich, Karger, Basel.

Skidmore, S.J., Pasi, K.J., Mawson, S.J., Williams, M.D. and Hill, F.G.H. (1990) Serological evidence that dry heating of clotting factor concentrates prevents transmission of non-A, non-B hepatitis. *J. med. Virol.* **30**, 50–52.

Skikne, B., Lynch, S., Borek, D. and Cook, J. (1984) Iron and blood donation, in *Blood Transfusion and Blood Banking*, ed. W.L. Bayer, *Clinics in Haemat.* **13**. W.B. Saunders Co., London.

Skogen, B., Rossebo Hansen, B., Husebekk, A., Havnes, T. and Hannestad, K. (1988) Minimal expression of blood group A antigen on thrombocytes from A$_2$ individuals. *Transfusion*, **28**, 456–459.

Skov, F. (1976) Observations of the number of available G (rh^G, Rh 12) antigen sites on red cells. *Vox Sang.* **31**, 124.

Skov, F. and Hughes-Jones, N.C. (1977) Observations on the number of available C antigen sites on red cells. *Vox Sang.* **33**, 170.

Slaastad, R.A. and Eika, C. (1973) Failure to trigger intravascular coagulation by water-induced haemolysis in rabbits. *Scand. J. Haemat.* **11**, 217.

Slater, J.L., Griswold, D.J., Wojtyniak, L.S. and Reisling, M.J. (1989) Evaluation of the polyethylene glycol-indirect antiglobulin test for routine compatibility testing. *Transfusion*, **29**, 686–688.

Slichter, S.J. and Harker, L.A. (1976a) Preparation and storage of platelet concentrates. I. Factors influencing the harvest of viable platelets from whole blood. *Brit. J. Haemat.* **34**, 395.

Slichter, S.J. and Harker, L.A. (1976b) Preparation and storage of platelet concentrates. II. Storage variables influencing platelet viability and function. *Brit. J. Haemat.* **34**, 403.

Slichter, Sherrill J. (1978) Efficacy of platelets collected by semi-continuous flow centrifugation (Haemonetics Model 30). *Brit. J. Haemat.* **38**, 131.

Slichter, S.J. (1980) Controversies in platelet transfusion therapy. *Amer. Rev. Med.* **31**, 509–540.

Slichter, Sherrill J. (1982) Post-transfusion purpura: response to steroids and association with red blood cell and lymphocytotoxic antibodies. *Brit. J. Haemat.* **50**, 599–605.

Slichter, S.J. (1985) Optimum platelet concentrate preparation and storage, in *Current Concepts in Transfusion Therapy*, ed G. Garratty. Amer. Assoc. Blood Banks, Arlington, VA.

Slichter, Sherrill J., O'Dormell, Margaret R., Weiden, F.L., Storb, R. and Schroeder, Maria-Louise (1986) Canine platelet alloimmunization: the role of donor selection. *Brit. J. Haemat.* **63**, 713–727.

Slichter, Sherrill J., Deeg, H.J. and Kennedy, M.S. (1987) Prevention of platelet alloimmunization in dogs with systemic cyclosporine and by UV-irradiation of cyclosporine-loading of donor platelets. *Blood*, **69**, 414–418.

Sloand, E.M. and Klein, H.G. (1990) Effect of white cells on platelets during storage. *Transfusion*, **30**, 333–338.

Slocombe, G.W., Newland, A.C. and Colvin, B.T. (1981) The role of intensive plasma exchange in the management of haemorrhage in patients with inhibitors to factor VIII. *Brit. J. Haemat.* **47**, 577–585.

Slotki, I.N., MacIver, J.E., Mallick, N.P. and Palmer, H.M. (1976) Acute intravascular hemolysis with minimal renal impairment in clostridium perfringens infection. *Clin. Nephrol.* **6**, 451.

Sloviter, H.A. (1951) *In vivo* survival of rabbit's red cells recovered after freezing. *Lancet*, i, 1350.

Sloviter, H.A., Petkovic, M., Ogoshi, S. and Yamada, H. (1969) Dispersed fluorochemicals as substitutes for erythrocytes in intact animals. *J. appl. Physiol.* **27**, 666.

Sloviter, H.A. (1976) Physiological and metabolic aspects of freezing erythrocytes with historical notes, in *Clinical Uses of Frozen-thawed Red Blood Cells*. Alan R. Liss, New York.

Smalley, C.E. and Tucker, E.M. (1983) Blood group A antigen site distribution and immunoglobulin binding in relation to red cell age. *Brit. J. Haemat.* **54**, 209–219.

Smedile, A. and 12 others (1982) Influence of delta infection on severity of hepatitis B. *Lancet*, ii, 945–947.

Smilovici, W., Ducos, J. and Mariniere, A. (1984) Anti-HBc testing is reliable for blood donor screening. *Lancet*, i, 1024.

Smit Sibinga, C.Th., Welbergen, H., Das, P.C. and Griffin, B. (1981) High-yield method of production of freeze-dried purified factor VIII by blood banks. *Lancet*, ii, 449–450.

Smit Sibinga, C.Th. (1989) Factor VIII in regional blood banking practice, in *Factor VIII — von Willebrand Factor*, eds M.J. Seghatchian and G.F. Savidge, Vol. I, pp. 280–288. CRC Press, Boca Raton, Florida.

Smit Sibinga, C.Th. (1990) Application of computers in blood transfusion, in *Blood Transfusion: the Impact of New Technologies*, ed Marcela Contreras, *Baillière's Clinical Haematology*, **3**, 405–422.

Smith, T. (1909) Active immunity produced by so-called balanced or neutral mixtures of diphtheria toxin and antitoxin. *J. exp. Med.* **11**, 241.

Smith, H.W. (1940) The physiology of the renal circulation. *Harvey Lect.* **35**, 166.

Smith, G.H. (1945) Isoagglutinin titres in heterospecific pregnancy. *J. Path. Bact.* **57**, 113.

Smith, Audrey U. (1950) Prevention of haemolysis during freezing and thawing of red blood-cells. *Lancet,* ii, 910.

Smith, G.N., Griffiths, Birgit, Mollison, D.P. and Mollison, P.L. (1972) Uptake of IgG following intramuscular and subcutaneous injection. *Lancet,* i, 1208.

Smith, G.N. and Mollison, P.L. (1974) Responses in rabbits to the red cell alloantigen Hg^A. *Immunology,* **26**, 865.

Smith, T.D. and Richards, P. (1976) A simple kit for the preparation of ^{99m}Tc-labeled red blood cells. *J. nucl. Med.* **17**, 126.

Smith, G.N. and Mollison, D.P. (1977) Unpublished observations.

Smith, M.L. and Beck, M.L. (1977) *The Immunoglobulin Class of Antibodies with M Specificity.* Commun. Amer. Assoc. Blood Banks, Atlanta.

Smith, T.R., Sherman, S., Nelson, C. and Taswell, H.F. (1977) *Formation of Anti-G by the Transfusion of D-Negative Blood.* Commun. Amer. Assoc. Blood Banks, Atlanta.

Smith, J.W., Wysenbeek, A.J. and Krakauer, R.S. (1981) Plasmapheresis 1: Membrane filtration methods. *Plasma Therapy,* **2**, 53–60.

Smith, D., Wright, P., Estes, W., Krueger, L., Wallas, C., Moldovan, R. and Tanley, P. (1984) Posttransfusion cytomegalovirus infection in neonates weighing less than 1,250 grams (Abstract). *Transfusion,* **24**, 430.

Smith, R.P., Evans, A.T., Popovsky, M., Mills, Letha and Spielman, A. (1986) Transfusion-acquired babesiosis and failure of antibiotic treatment. *J. Amer. med. Assoc.* **256**, 2726–2727.

Smith, D.S., Stratton, F., Johnson, T., Brown, R., Howell, P. and Riches, R. (1969) Haemolytic disease of the newborn caused by anti-Lan antibody. *Brit. med. J.* **3**, 90.

Smith, K.J., Coonce, L.S., South, S.F. and Troup, G.M. (1983) Anti-Cr^a: family study and survival of chromium-labeled incompatible red cells in a Spanish-American patient. *Transfusion,* **23**, 167–169.

Smith, J.W., Kelton, J.G., Horsewood, P., Brown, C., Giles, A., Meyer, R., Woods, V. and Burrows, R. (1989) Platelet specific alloantigens on the platelet glycoprotein Ia/IIa complex. *Brit. J. Haemat.* **72**, 534–538.

Smith, J.K. (1990) Trends in the production and use of coagulation factor concentrates, in *Developments in Hematology and Immunology,*

Vol. 26. Kluwer Academic Publishers, Dordrecht, Boston, London.

Smith, D.M. (1991) Transfusion-transmitted human immunodeficiency virus infection, in *Transfusion Transmitted Infections,* eds D.M. Smith and R.Y. Dodd, pp. 73–79. ASCP Press, Chicago.

Smoller, B.R. and Kruskall, Margot S. (1986) Phlebotomy for diagnostic laboratory tests in adults. Pattern of use and effect on transfusion requirements. *New Engl. J. Med.* **314**, 1233–1235.

Snary, D., Barnstable, C.J., Bodmer, W.F. and Crumpton, M.J. (1977a) Molecular structure of human histocompatibility antigens: the HLA-C series. *Eur. J. Immunol.* **8**, 580.

Snary, D., Barnstable, C., Bodmer, W.F., Goodfellow, P. and Crumpton, M.J. (1977b) Human Ia antigens — purification and molecular structure. *Cold Spr. Harb. Symp. quant. Biol.* **41**, 379.

Sneath, Joan S. and Sneath, P.H.A. (1955) Transformation of the Lewis groups of human red cells. *Nature (Lond.),* **176**, 172.

Sneath, Joan S. and Sneath, P.H.A. (1959) Adsorption of blood-group substances from serum on to red cells. *Brit. med. Bull.* **15**, 154.

Sniecinski, I.J., Petz, L.D., Orien, L. and Blume, K.G. (1987) Immunohematologic problems arising from ABO incompatible bone marrow transplantation. *Transplant. Proc.* **19**, 4609–4611.

Sniecinski, I., O'Donnel, M.R., Nowicki, B. and Hill, L.R. (1988) Prevention of refractoriness and HLA-alloimmunization using filtered blood products. *Blood,* **71**, 1402–1407.

Sniecinski, I.J., Orien, L., Petz, L.P. and Blume, K.G. (1988) Immunohematologic consequences of major ABO-mismatched bone marrow transplantation. *Transplantation,* **45**, 530–534.

Sniecinski, Iren, Margolin, Kim, Shulman, Ira, Oien, Linda, Meyer, Elisabeth and Branch, D.R. (1988) High titer, high thermal amplitude cold agglutinin not associated with hemolytic anemia. *Vox Sang.* **55**, 26–29.

Snyder, E.L., Grum, B.S., Cooper–Smith, M. and James, R. (1979) Transfusion of platelets through microaggregate filters. *Anaesthesiology,* **51**, Suppl., S 205.

Snyder, E.L., Hezzey, A., Joyner, R., Davisson, W. and Buchholz, D.H. (1983) Stability of red cell antigens during prolonged storage in citrate-phosphate-dextrose and a new preservative solution. *Transfusion,* **23**, 165–166.

Snyder, E.L., Ferri, Patricia, Brown, R., Gallup, Peggy and Roberts, S. (1985) Evaluation of flatbed reciprocal motion agitators for resuspension of stored platelet concentrates. *Vox Sang.* **48**, 269–275.

Snyder, E.L., Pope, C., Ferri, P.M., Smith, E.D., Walter, S.D. and Ezekowitz, M.D. (1986a) The effect of mode of agitation and type of plastic bag on storage characteristics and *in vivo* kinetics of platelet concentrates. *Transfusion*, **26**, 125–130.

Snyder, E.L., Moroff, T., Simon, A., Heaton, A. and Members of the *ad hoc* Platelet Radio Labelling Study Group (1986b) Recommended methods for conducting radiolabelled platelet survival studies. *Transfusion*, **26**, 37–42.

Snyder, E.L., Depalma, L. and Napychank, P. (1988) Use of polyester filters for the preparation of leukocyte-poor platelet concentrates. *Vox Sang.* **54**, 21–23.

Sobeslavsky, O. (1978) HBV as a global problem, in *Viral Hepatitis, Proceedings of 2nd Symposium on Viral Hepatitis,* San Francisco, March 1978, eds G.N. Vyas, S.N. Cohen and R. Schmid. Franklin Institute Press, Philadelphia.

Söderström, T., Enskog, A., Samuelsson, B.E. and Cedergren, B. (1985) Immunoglobulin subclass (IgG3) restriction of anti-P and anti-P^k antibodies in patients of the rare p blood group. *J. Immunol.* **134**, 1–3.

Soendjojo, A., Boedisantoso, M., Ilias, M.I. and Rahardjo, D. (1982) Syphilis d'emblée due to blood transfusion. Case report. *Brit. J. vener. Dis.* **58**, 149–150.

Soh, Cecilia P.C., Morgan, W.T.J., Watkins, W.M. and Donald, A.S.R. (1980) The relationship between the N-acetylgalactosamine content and the blood group Sd^a activity of Tamm and Horsfall urinary glycoprotein. *Biochem. biophys. Res. Commun.* **93**, 1132–1139.

Sohmer, P.R., Beutler, E. and Moore, G.L. (1981) Clinical trials with CPD-A2 (Abstract). *Transfusion*, **21**, 600.

Sokol, R.J., Hewit, S. and Stamps, Barbara K. (1981) Autoimmune haemolysis: an 18-year study of 865 cases referred to a regional transfusion centre. *Brit. med. J.* **i**, 2023–2027.

Sokol, R.J., Hewitt, S. and Stamps, Barbara K. (1982) Autoimmune haemolysis associated with Donath–Landsteiner antibodies. *Acta haemat.* **68**, 268–277.

Sokol, R.J., Hewitt, S. and Stamps, Barbara K. (1983) Autoimmune haemolysis: mixed warm and cold type antibody. *Acta haemat.* **69**, 266–274.

Sokol, R.J., Hewitt, S., Stamps, Barbara K. and Hitchen, Patricia A. (1984) Autoimmune haemolysis in childhood and adolescence. *Acta haemat.* **72**, 245–257.

Sokol, R.J., Hewitt, S., Booker, P.J. and Stamps, R. (1985) Enzyme linked direct antiglobulin tests in patients with autoimmune haemolysis. *J. clin. Path.* **38**, 912–914.

Sokol, R.J., Hewitt, S., Booker, D.J. and Stamps,

R. (1987) Small quantities of erythrocyte bound immunoglobulins and autoimmune haemolysis. *J. clin. Path.* **40**, 254–257.

Sokol, R.J., Hewitt, S., Booker, D.J., Stamps, R. and Booth, J.R. (1988) An enzyme-linked direct antiglobulin test for assessing erythrocyte bound immunoglobulins. *J. immunol. Methods*, **106**, 31–35.

Solem, J.H. and Jörgensen, W. (1969) Accidentally transmitted infectious mononucleosis. *Acta med. scand.* **186**, 433.

Solis, R.T., Goldfinger, D., Gibbs, M.B. and Zeller, J.A. (1974) Physical characteristics of microaggregates in stored blood. *Transfusion*, **14**, 538.

Solomon, J.M. (1964) Behavior of incomplete antibodies in quantitative hemagglutination reactions. *Transfusion*, **4**, 101.

Somers, H. and Kuhns, W.J. (1972) Blood group antibodies in old age. *Proc. Soc. exp. Biol. Med. (N.Y.)*, **141**, 1104.

Sonneborn, H.H., Uthemann, H. and Pfeffer, A. (1983) Monoclonal antibody specific for human blood group k (cellano). *Biotest Bulletin*, **4**, 328–330.

Sosler, S.D., Behzad, O., Garratty, G., Lee, C.L., Postoway, Nina and Khomo, O. (1984) Acute hemolytic anemia associated with a chlorpropamide-induced apparent auto-anti-Jk^a. *Transfusion*, **24**, 206–209.

Soulier, J.P. (1958) Les modifications du Ca^{++} dans les transfusions massives et la circulation extracorporéale utilisant du sang citraté. *Rev. Hémat.* **13**, 437.

Soulier, J.-P., Patereau, C., Gobert, N., Achach, P. and Muller, J.-Y. (1979) Post-transfusional immunologic thrombocytopenia. A case report. *Vox Sang.* **37**, 21–29.

Soulier, J.P. (1984) Diseases transmissible by blood transfusion. *Vox Sang.* **47**, 1–6.

Spaet, T.H. and Ostrom, Betty W. (1952) Studies on the normal serum panagglutinin active against trypsinated human erythrocytes. I. The mechanism of agglutination reversal. *J. clin. Path.* **5**, 332.

Spear, P.W., Sass, M. and Cincotti, J.J. (1956) Ammonia levels in transfused blood. *J. Lab. clin. Med.* **48**, 702.

Spanos, T., Karageorga, M., Lapis, V., Peristeri, J., Hatziliami, A. and Kattamis, C. (1990) Red cell alloantibodies in patients with thalassemia. *Vox Sang.* **58**, 50–55.

Speiser, P., Schwarz, J. and Lewkin, D. (1951) Statistische Ergebnisse von 10,000 Blutgruppen- und Blutfaktorenbestimmungen in der Wiener Bevölkerung 1948 bis 1950. *Klin. Med. (Wien)*, **6**, 105.

Speiser, P. (1956) Zur Frage der Vererbbarkeit des irregulaeren Agglutinins Anti-A$_1$ (α_1). *Acta Genet. med. (Roma)*, **3**, 192.

Speiser, P. (1964) Anti-Körperbildung von Kindern gegen die Gm-Gruppe ihrer Mutter (Weitere Beobachtungen). *Commun. 10th Congr. Int. Soc. Blood Transfus.*, Stockholm.

Speiser, P., Kühböck, J., Mickerts, D., Pausch, V., Reichel, G., Lauer, D., Poremba, I., Doering, I. and Hamacher, H. (1966) 'Kamhuber' a new human blood group antigen of familial occurrence, revealed by a severe transfusion reaction. *Vox Sang.* **11**, 113.

Spensieri, S. Carnevale, Arella E. and Caldana, P.L. (1968) Iso-immunizzazione Rh e passagio transplacentare di eritrociti fetali. *Monit. ostet.-ginec.* **39**, Suppl., 889.

Sprague, C.C., Harrington, W.J., Lange, R.D. and Shapleigh, J.B. (1952) Platelet transfusions and the pathogenesis of idiopathic thrombocytopenic purpura. *J. Amer. med. Assoc.* **150**, 1193.

Sprat, T. (1667) *The History of the Royal Society of London, for the Improving of Natural Knowledge.* Printed by T.R. for J. Martyn at the Bell without Temple-bar and J. Allestry at the Rose and Crown in Duck-lane, Printers to the Royal Society.

Spring, F.A. and Anstee, D.J. (1991) Evidence that the Yt blood group antigens are located on human erythrocyte acetylcholinesterase (AChE). *Transfusion Medicine*, **1**, Suppl. 2, 42.

Springer, G.F. and Ansell, Norma J. (1958) Inactivation of human erythrocyte agglutinogens M and N by influenza viruses and receptor-destroying enzyme. *Proc. nat. Acad. Sci. USA*, **44**, 182.

Springer, G.F., Horton, R.E. and Forbes, M. (1959) Origin of anti-human blood group B agglutinins in white leghorn chicks. *J. exp. Med.* **110**, 221.

Springer, G.F. and Tritel, H. (1962) Influenza virus vaccine and blood group A-like substances. *J. Amer. med. Assoc.* **182**, 1341.

Springer, G.F., Williamson, P. and Readler, B.L. (1962) Blood group active gram-negative bacteria and higher plants. *Ann. N.Y. Acad. Sci.* **97**, 104.

Springer, G.F. and Schuster, R. (1964) Stimulation of isohemolysins and isohemagglutinins by influenza virus preparations. *Vox Sang.* **9**, 589.

Springer, G.F. and Horton, R.E. (1969) Blood group isoantibody stimulation in man by feeding blood group-active bacteria. *J. clin. Invest.* **48**, 1280.

Springer, G.F., Desai, P.R. and Banatwala, I. (1974) Blood group MN specific substances and precursors in normal and malignant human breast tissue. *Naturwissenschaften*, **61**, 457.

Springer, G.F. and Tegtmeyer, Herta (1981) Origin of anti-Thomsen-Friedenreich (T) and Tn agglutinins in man and in white leghorn chicks. *Brit. J. Haemat.* **47**, 453–460.

Springer, G.F., Desai, P.R., Fry, W.A., Goodale, R.L., Shearen, J.G. and Scanlon, E.F. (1983) Patients immune response to CA-associated T antigen, in *Cellular Oncology*, Vol. 1, eds P.J. Moloy and G.L. Nicolson. pp. 99–130. Praeger, New York.

Springer, G.F., Taylor, C.R., Howard, D.R., Tegtmeyer, Herta, Desai, P.R., Murthy, S.M., Felder, Barbara and Scanlon, E.F. (1985) Tn, a carcinoma associated antigen, reacts with anti-Tn of normal human sera. *Cancer*, **55**, 561–569.

Squires, J.E., Larison, P.J., Charles, W.T. and Milner, P.F. (1985) A delayed hemolytic transfusion reaction due to anti-Co^b. *Transfusion*, **25**, 137–139.

Stagno, S., Pass, R.F., Cloud, Gretchen, Britt, W.J., Henderson, R.E., Walton, P.D., Veren, D.A., Page, F. and Alford, C.A. (1986) Primary cytomegalovirus infection in pregnancy. Incidence, transmission to fetus and clinical outcome. *J. Amer. med. Assoc.* **256**, 1904–1908.

Stalker, A.L. (1964) Intravascular erythrocyte aggregation. *Bibl. anat. (Basel)*, **4**, 108.

Stapleton, R.R. and Moore, B.P.L. (1959) A tube test for Rh typing using papain and incomplete anti-D. *J. Lab. clin. Med.* **64**, 640.

Starkey, J.M., MacPherson, J.L., Bolgiano, D.C., Simon, E.R., Zuck, T. and Sayers, M.H. (1989) Markers for transfusion-transmitted disease in different groups of blood donors. *J. Amer. med. Assoc.* **262**, 3452–3454.

Stastny, P. and Nunez, G. (1981) The role of endothelial and monocyte antigens in kidney transplantation. *Transplant. clin. Immunol.* **13**, 133–139.

Staub, N.C. (1974) Pulmonary edema. *Physiol Rev.* **54**, 678–811.

Stats, D. (1954) Cold hemagglutination and cold hemolysis. The hemolysis produced by shaking cold agglutinated erythrocytes. *J. clin. Invest.* **24**, 33.

Steane, E.A., Sheehan, R.G., Brooks, B.A. and Frenkel, E.P. (1982a) Therapeutic plasmapheresis in patients with antibodies to high frequency red cell antigens, in *Therapeutic Apheresis and Plasma Perfusion*, ed R.S.A. Tindall, *Progress in Clinical and Biological Research*, **106**, 347–353. Alan R. Liss, New York.

Steane, S.M., Steane, E.A. and Reyes, V.G. (1982b) Limitations of digitonin-acid elution procedure (Abstract). *Transfusion*, **22**, 430.

Steel, C.M., Ludlam, C.A., Beatson, Dianne, Peutherer, J.F., Cuthbert, R.J.G., Simmonds, P., Morrison, H. and Jones, M. (1988) HLA haplotype A1B8 DR3 as a risk factor for HIV disease. *Lancet*, **i**, 1185–1188.

Stefanini, M. (1950) Studies on the role of calcium in the coagulation of blood. *Acta med. scand.* **136**, 250.

Stefanini, M., Dameshek, W. and Adelson, E. (1952) Platelets. VII. Shortened platelet survival time and development of platelet agglutinins following multiple platelet transfusions. *Proc. Soc. exp. Biol.* (*N.Y.*), **80**, 230.

Stefanini, M., Mednicoff, Irma B., Salomon, Lucy and Campbell, E.W. (1954) Thrombocytopenia of replacement transfusion: a cause of surgical bleeding. *Clin. Res. Proc.* **2**, 61.

Steffey, Nancy B. (1983) Investigation of a probable non-red cell stimulated anti-Di^a. *Red Cell Free Press*, **8**, 24.

Stegmayr, B., Berseus, O., Björsell-Östling, Elisabet and Wirell, Marianne. (1990) Plasma exchange in patients with severe consumption coagulopathy and acute renal failure. *Transfus. Sci.* **11**, 271–277.

Stehling, L.C., Ellison, N., Faust, R.J., Grotta, A.W. and Moyers, J.R. (1987) A survey of transfusion practices among anaesthesiologists. *Vox Sang.* **52**, 60–62.

Stehling, Linda (1990) Trends in transfusion therapy. *Anesthesiol. Clin. N. Amer.* **8**, 519–531.

Stehr-Green, Jeanette K., Evatt, B.L. and Lawrence, D.N. (1991) Preventing transfusion-transmitted infections in persons with hemophilia, in *Transfusion Transmitted Infections*, eds D.M. Smith and R.Y. Dodd, pp. 271–281. ASCP Press, Chicago.

Steinberg, A.G. and Wilson, Janet (1963) Hereditary globulin factors and immune tolerance in man. *Science*, **140**, 303.

Steiner, Lisa A. and Eisen, H.M. (1967) The relative affinity of antibodies synthesised in the secondary response. *J. exp. Med.* **126**, 1185.

Stellon, A.J. and Moorhead, P.J. (1981) Polygeline compared with plasma protein fraction as the sole replacement fluid in plasma exchange. *Brit. med. J.* **i**, 696–697.

Stephan, W. (1989) Inactivation of hepatitis viruses and HIV in plasma and plasma derivatives by treatment with beta-propiolactone/UV irradiation, in *Virus Inactivation in Plasma Products*, ed J.J. Morgenthaler, pp. 122–127. S. Karger, Basel.

Stephen, C.R., Martin, Ruth C. and Bourgeois-Gavardin, M. (1955) Antihistaminic drugs in treatment of nonhemolytic transfusion reactions. *J. Amer. med. Assoc.* **158**, 525.

Stephens, J.G. (1940) Surface and fragility differences between mature and immature red cells. *J. Physiol.* (*Lond.*), **99**, 30.

Sterling, K. (1951) The turnover rate of serum albumin in man as measured by ^{131}I-tagged albumin. *J. clin. Invest.* **30**, 1228.

Stern, K., Davidsohn, I. and Masaitis, Lillian (1956) Experimental studies on Rh immunization. *Amer. J. clin. Path.* **26**, 833.

Stern, K., Davidsohn, I., Jensen, F.G. and Muratore, R. (1958) Immunologic studies on the Be^a factor. *Vox Sang.* **3**, 425.

Stern, K. (1960) Hemolytic disease of the newborn associated with type D^u. *Bull. Amer. Assoc. Blood Banks*, December.

Stern, K., Goodman, H.S. and Berger, Maya (1961) Experimental isoimmunization to hemo-antigens in man. *J. Immunol.* **87**, 189.

Stern, K. (1975) Multiple differences in red cell antigens and isoimmunization. *Transfusion*, **15**, 179.

Stevens, A.R. jr and Finch, C.A. (1954) A dangerous universal donor. Acute renal failure following transfusion of group O blood. *Amer. J. clin. Path.* **24**, 612.

Stevens, C.E., Aach, R.D., Hollinger, F.B., Mosley, J.W., Szmuness, W., Kahn, R., Werch, Jochewed and Edwards, Virginia (1984) Hepatitis B virus antibody in blood donors and the occurrence of non-A, non-B hepatitis in transfusion recipients. An analysis of the transfusion-transmitted viruses study. *Ann. intern. Med.* **101**, 733–737.

Stevens, C.E., Taylor, P.E., Pindyck, J., Choo, Q-L., Bradley, D.W., Kuo, G. and Houghton, M. (1990) Epidemiology of hepatitis C virus. A preliminary study in volunteer blood donors. *J. Amer. Med. Assoc.* **263**, 49–53.

Stewart, H.J., Shepard, E.M. and Horger, E.L. (1948) Electrocardiograph manifestations of potassium intoxication. *Amer. J. med.* **5**, 821.

Stewart, J.W. and Mollison, P.L. (1959) Rapid destruction of apparently compatible red cells. *Brit. med. J.* **i**, 1274.

Stiehm, E.R. and Fudenberg, H.H. (1965) Antibodies to gamma globulin in infants and children exposed to isologous gamma-globulin. *Pediatrics*, **35**, 229.

Stiller, R.J., Lardas, Olga and Haynes de Regt, Roberta (1990) Vel isoimmunisation in pregnancy. *Amer. J. Obstet. Gynec.* **162**, 1071–1072.

Stockwell, M.A., Soni, N. and Riley, B. (1992a) Colloid solutions in the critically ill. A randomised comparison of albumin and polygeline. 1. Outcome and duration of stay in the intensive care unit. *Anaesthesia*, **47**, 3–6.

Stockwell, M.A., Scott, A., Day, A., Riley, B. and Soni, N.A. (1992b) Colloid solutions in the critically ill. A randomised comparison of albumin and polygeline. Serum albumin concentration and incidences of pulmonary oedema and renal failure. *Anaesthesia*, **47**, 7–9.

Stoddart, J.C. (1960) Nickel sensitivity as a cause of infusion reactions. *Lancet*, **ii**, 741.

Stoffel, W. and Demant, T. (1981) Selective removal of apolipoprotein B-containing serum lipoproteins from blood plasma. *Proc. nat. Acad. Sci. USA*, **78**, 611–615.

Stohlman, F. jr and Schneiderman, M.A. (1956) Application of the ^{51}Cr technique to the study of experimental hemolysis in the dog. *J. Lab. clin. Med.* **47**, 72.

Stone, B. and Marsh, W.L. (1959) Haemolytic disease of the newborn caused by anti-M. *Brit. J. Haemat.* **5**, 344.

Stormont, C. (1949) Acquisition of the J-substance by bovine erythrocytes. *Proc. nat. Acad. Sci. USA*, **35**, 232.

Stout, T.D., Moore, B.P.L., Allen, F.H. jr and Corcoran, Patricia (1963) A new phenotype D + G – (Rh: 1, –12). *Vox Sang.* **8**, 262.

Strahl, M., Pettenkofer, H.J. and Hasse, W. (1955) A haemolytic transfusion reaction due to anti-M. *Vox Sang. (O.S.)*, **5**, 34.

Stramer, Susan L., Heller, J.S., Coombs, R.W. Parry, J.V., Ho, D.D. and Allain, J-P. (1989) Markers of HIV infection prior to IgG antibody seropositivity. *J. Amer. Med. Assoc.* **262**, 64–69.

Strange, C.A. and Cross, J. (1981) An anti-A agglutinin active only in the presence of borate. *Vox Sang.* **41**, 235–238.

Stratton, F. (1946) A new Rh allelomorph. *Nature (Lond.)*, **158**, 25.

Stratton, F. (1954) Polyagglutinability of red cells. *Vox Sang. (O.S.)*, **4**, 58.

Stratton, F. (1955a) Iso-immunization to blood group antigens, in *Modern Trends in Blood Diseases*, ed J.F. Wilkinson. Butterworth, London.

Stratton, F. (1955b) Rapid Rh-typing: a sandwich technique. *Brit. med. J.* **i**, 201.

Stratton, F. and Dimond, E.R. (1955) The value of a serum and albumin mixture for use in the detection of blood group antigen-antibody reactions. *J. clin. Path.* **8**, 218.

Stratton, F. and Jones, A.R. (1955) The reactions between normal human red cells and antiglobulin (Coombs) serum. *J. Immunol.* **75**, 423.

Stratton, F. and Renton, P.H. (1958) *Practical Blood Grouping*, p. 87. Blackwell Scientific Publications, Oxford.

Stratton, F., Renton, P.H. and Rawlinson, V.I. (1960) Serological difference between old and young cells. *Lancet*, **ii**, 1388.

Stratton, F. (1963) Erythrocyte antibodies and autoimmunity. *Lancet*, **ii**, 626.

Stratton, F., Rawlinson, V.I., Chapman, S.A., Pengelly, C.D.R. and Jennings, R.C. (1972) Acquired hemolytic anemia associated with IgA anti-e. *Transfusion*, **12**, 157.

Stratton, F., Rawlinson, Violet I., Gunson, H.H. and Phillips, P.K. (1973) The role of zeta potential in Rh agglutination. *Vox Sang.* **24**, 273.

Stratton, F. and Rawlinson, Violet I. (1976) C3 components on red cells under various conditions, in *The Nature and Significance of Complement Activation*. Ortho Research Institute, Raritan, New Jersey.

Stratton, F., Rawlinson, Violet I., Merry, A.H. and Thomson, Eileen E. (1983) Positive direct antiglobulin test in normal individuals. II. *Clin. lab. Haemat.* **5**, 17–21.

Strauss, Dorothea, Roigas, H., Raderecht, H.J. and Gülke, L. (1969) Sechswöchige Lagerung von Erythrozytenresuspensionen und Erythrozytenkonzentrat. *Z. ges. inn. Med.* **24**, 891.

Strauss, Dorothea and Raderecht, H.J. (1974) Zum Einfluss von Adenin und Guanosin auf die Überlebensrate von Erythrozyten nach Lagerung bei Temperaturen zwischen 4°C und 25°C. *Folia Haematol. (Leipzig)*, **101**, 232.

Strauss, R.G., Spitzer, R.E., Stitzel, A.E., Urmson, J.R., Maguire, L.C., Koepke, J.A. and Thompson, J.S. (1980) Complement changes during leukapheresis. *Transfusion*, **20**, 32–38.

Strauss, R.G. and Crouch, J. (1981) Preservation of neutrophils in CPD-adenine. *Transfusion*, **21**, 354–356.

Strauss, R.A., Gloster, Elizabeth, Shanfield, M.S., Kittinger, Sandra P. and Morgan, B.B. (1983a) Anaphylactic transfusion reaction associated with a possible anti-A2m(1). *Clin. lab. Haemat.* **5**, 371–377.

Strauss, R.G., Huestis, D.W., Wright, D.G. and Hester, Jeane P. (1983b) Cellular depletion by apheresis (Panel V). *J. clin. Apheresis*, **1**, 158–165.

Strauss, R.G. (1986) Current issues in neonatal transfusions. *Vox Sang.* **51**, 1–9.

Strauss, R.G. (1989) Directed and limited-exposure donor programmes for children, in *Contemporary Issues in Pediatric Transfusion Medicine*, eds R.A. Sacher and R. Strauss, pp. 1–11. Amer. Assoc. Blood Banks, Arlington, VA.

Strauss, R.G. and 9 others (1990) Commentary on small-volume red cell transfusions for neonates. *Transfusion*, **30**, 565–570.

Stricker, R.B., Lewis, B.H., Corark, L. and Shumar, M.A. (1987) Posttransfusion purpura associated with an autoantibody directed against a previously undefined platelet antigen. *Blood*, **69**, 1458–1463.

String, T., Robinson, A.J. and Blaisdell, F.W. (1971) Massive trauma. Effect of intravascular coagulation on prognosis. *Arch. Surg.* **102**, 406.

Stroncek, D.F., K.M. Skubitz and McCullough, J.J. (1990) Biochemical characterization of the neutrophil-specific antigen NB1. *Blood*, **75**, 744–755.

Stroup, Marjory MacIlroy, Mija (1965) Evaluation of the albumin antiglobulin technic in antibody detection. *Transfusion*, **5**, 184.

Strumia, M.M. (1954a) Analytical review: the preservation of blood for transfusion. *Blood*, **9**, 1105.

Strumia, M.M. (1954b) Methods of blood preservation in general and preparation, preservation and use of red cell suspensions. *Amer. J. clin. Path.* **24**, 260.

Strumia, M.M., Colwell, Louise S. and Ellenberger, Katherine (1955) The preservation of blood for transfusion. I. The effect of plastic containers on red cells. *J. Lab. clin. Med.* **46**, 225.

Strumia, M.M., Colwell, L.S. and Dugan, Ann (1958) The measure of erythropoiesis in anemias. I. The mixing time and the immediate post-transfusion disappearance of T-1824 dye and of Cr^{51}-tagged erythrocytes in relation to blood volume determination. *Blood*, **8**, 128.

Strumia, M.M., Colwell, Louise S. and Dugan, Ann (1959) The preservation of blood for transfusion. III. Mechanism of action of containers on red blood cells. *J. Lab. clin. Med.* **53**, 106.

Strumia, M.M., Dugan, A., Taylor, L., Strumia, P.V. and Basster, D. (1962) Splenectomy in leukemia and myelofibrosis: changes in the erythrocytic values. *Amer. J. clin. Path.* **37**, 491.

Strumia, M.M., Strumia, P.V. and Dugan, A. (1968) Significance of measurement of plasma volume and of indirect estimation of red cell volume. *Transfusion*, **8**, 197.

Strumia, M.M., Strumia, P.V. and Eusebi, A.J. (1970) The preservation of blood for transfusion. VII. Effect of adenine and inosine on the adenosine triphosphate and viability of red cells when added to blood stored from zero to seventy days at 1°C. *J. Lab. clin. Med.* **75**, 244.

Strunk, R. and Colten, H.R. (1976) Inhibition of the enzymatic activity of the first component of complement (C1) by heparin. *Clin. Immunol. Immunopath.* **6**, 248.

Stuckey, M.A., Osoba, D. and Thomas, J.W. (1964) Haemolytic transfusion reactions. *Canad. med. Assoc. J.* **90**, 739.

Sturgeon, P., Moore, B.P.L. and Weiner, W. (1964) Notations for two weak A variants: A_{end} and A_{el}. *Vox Sang.* **9**, 214.

Sturgeon, P. and Jennings, E.R. (1968) Anti-γ-globulins in women treated with anti-Rh γ-globulin. *Transfusion*, **8**, 343.

Sturgeon, P. (1970) Hematological observations on the anemia associated with blood type Rh_{null}. *Blood*, **36**, 310.

Sturgeon, P. and Arcillia, M.B. (1970) Studies on the secretion of blood group substances—1. Observations on the red cell phenotype Le(a+b+x+). *Vox Sang.* **18**, 301.

Sturgeon, P., Smith, L.E., Chun, H.M.T., Hurvitz, C.H., Garratty, G., Morel, P. and Goldfinger, D. (1979) Autoimmune hemolytic anemia associated exclusively with IgA of Rh specificity. *Transfusion*, **19**, 324–328.

Suarez, C.R. and Anderson, C. (1987) High-dose intravenous gammaglobulin (IVG) in neonatal immune thrombocytopenia. *Amer. J. Hemat.* **26**, 247–253.

Sugg, U., Schenzle, D. and Hess, G. (1988) Antibodies to hepatitis B core antigen in blood donors screened for alanine aminotransferase level and hepatitis non-A, non-B in recipients. *Transfusion*, **28**, 386–388.

Sugita, Y. and Simon, E.R. (1965) The mechanism of action of adenine in red cell preservation. *J. clin. Invest.* **44**, 629.

Sullivan, C.M., Kline, W.E., Rabin, B.I., Johnson, C.L. and Marsh, W.L. (1987) The first example of auto-anti-Kx. *Transfusion*, **27**, 322–324.

Sullivan, K.M. and 13 others (1989) Graft versus host disease as adoptive immunotherapy in patients with advanced hematologic neoplasms. *New Engl. J. Med.* **320**, 828–834.

Sullivan, Marian, Williams, A.E., Fang, C.T., Grandinetti, Teresa, Poiesz, B.J., Ehrlich, G.D. and The American Red Cross HTLV-IIII Collaborative Study Group (1991) Transmission of human T-lymphotrophic virus types I and II by blood transfusion. *Arch. intern. Med.* **151**, 2043–2048.

Sultan, Y., Bussel, A., Maisonneuve, P., Poupeney, M., Sitty, X. and Gajdos, P. (1979) Potential danger of thrombosis after plasma exchange in the treatment of patients with immune disease. *Transfusion*, **19**, 588–593.

Sultan, J., Kazatchkine, M.D., Maisonneuve, P. and Nydegger, U.E. (1984) Anti-idiotype suppression of autoantibodies to factor VIII (anti-haemophilic factor) by high-dose intravenous gammaglobulin. *Lancet*, **ii**, 765–768.

Sundsmo, J.S. and Fair, D.S. (1983) Relationships among the complement, kinin, coagulation and fibrinolytic systems. *Springer Seminars in Immunopathology*, **9**, 231–238.

Surgenor, D.M., Wallace, E.L., Hao, S.H.S. and Chapman, R.H. (1990) Collection and transfusion of blood in the United States, 1982–1988. *New Engl. J. Med.* **322**, 1646–1651.

Susal, C., Terness, P. and Opelz, G. (1990) An experimental model for preventing alloimmunization against platelet transfusions by pretreatment with antibody-coated cells. *Vox Sang.* **59**, 209–215.

Sussman, L.N. and Miller, E.B. (1952) Un nouveau facteur sanguin 'Vel'. *Rev. Hémat.* **7**, 368.

Sutherland, D.A., Eisentraut, Anna M. and Mc-Call, Mary Sue (1963) The direct Coombs test and reticulocytes. *Brit. J. Haemat.* **9**, 68.

Sutton, D.M.C., Cardella, C.J., Uldall, P.R. and Deveber, G.A. (1981) Complications of intensive plasma exchange. *Plasma Therapy*, **2**, 19–23.

Suyama, K. and Goldstein, J. (1990) Enzymatic evidence for differences in the placement of Rh antigens within the red cell membrane. *Blood*, **75**, 255–260.

Suzuki, T. and Dale, G.L. (1987) Biotinylated erythrocytes: *in vivo* survival and *in vitro* recovery. *Blood*, **70**, 791–795.

Svejgaard, A., Platz, P. and Ryder, L.P. (1983) Associations between HLA and some diseases. *Immunol. Rev.* **70**, 193–218.

Swan, H.J.C., Ganz, W., Forester, J., Marcus, H., Diamond, G. and Chonette, D. (1970) Catheterisation of the heart in man with use of a flow-directed balloon-tipped catheter. *New Engl. J. Med.* **283**, 447.

Swank, R.L. (1961) Alteration of blood on storage: measurement of adhesiveness of 'aging' platelets and leucocytes and their removal by filtration. *New Engl. J. Med.* **265**, 728.

Swanson, Jane and Matson, G.A. (1964) Third example of a human 'D-like' antibody or anti-LW. *Transfusion*, **4**, 257.

Swanson, Jane, Polesky, H.F., Tippett, Patricia and Sanger, Ruth (1965) A 'new' blood group antigen Do^a. *Nature (Lond.)*, **206**, 313.

Swanson, Jane, Zweber, Mary and Polesky, H.F. (1967) A new public antigenic determinant Gy^a (Gregory). *Transfusion*, **7**, 304.

Swanson, Jane, Crookston, Marie C., Yunis, E., Azar, M., Gatti, R.A. and Good, R.A. (1971a) Lewis substances in a human marrow-transplantation chimæra (Letter). *Lancet*, **i**, 396.

Swanson, Jane, Olsen, Jeanne and Azar, M.M. (1971b) Serological evidence that antibodies of Chido-York-Cs^a specificity are leukocyte antibodies (Abstract). *Fed. proc.* **30**, 248.

Swanson, Jane L., Issitt, C.H., Mann, E.W., Condie, R.M., Simmons, R.L. and McCullough, J. (1984) Resolution of red cell compatibility testing problems in patients receiving anti-lymphoblast or anti-thymocyte globulin. *Transfusion*, **24**, 141–143.

Swanson, Jane L. and Sastamoinen, R. (1985) Chloroquine stripping of HLA A,B antigens from red cells. *Transfusion*, **25**, 439–440.

Swanson, J., Sastamoinen, R., Sebring, E. and Chopek, M. (1985) Rh and Kell antibodies of probable donor origin produced after solid organ transplantation (Abstract). *Transfusion*, **25**, 467.

Swanson, Jane, Sebring, Elizabeth, Sastamoinen, R. and Chopek, M. (1987) Gm allotyping to determine the origin of the anti-D causing hemolytic anemia in a kidney transplant recipient. *Vox Sang.* **52**, 228–230.

Sweeley, C.C. and Dawson, G. (1969) Lipids of the erythrocyte, in *Red Cell Membrane: Structure and Function*, eds G.A. Jamieson and T.J. Greenwalt. J.B. Lippincott, Philadelphia.

Swisher, S.N. and Young, L.E. (1954) Studies of the mechanisms of erythrocyte destruction initiated by antibodies. *Trans. Assoc. Amer. Phycns.* **67**, 124.

Sykes, M.K. (1963) Venous pressure as a clinical indication of adequacy of transfusion. *Ann. roy. Coll. Surg.* **33**, 185.

Symmans, W.A., Shepherd, C.S., Marsh, W.L., Øyen, R., Shohet, S.B. and Linehan, B.J. (1979) Hereditary acanthocytosis associated with the McLeod phenotype of the Kell blood group system. *Brit. J. Haemat.* **42**, 575–583.

Szalóky, A. and van der Hart, M. (1971) An auto-antibody anti-Vel. *Vox Sang.* **20**, 376.

Szatkowski, N.S., Kunicki, T.J. and Aster, R.H. (1986) Identification of glycoprotein Ib as a target of autoantibody in idiopathic (auto-immune) thrombocytopenic purpura. *Blood*, **67**, 310–315.

Szulman, A.E. (1965) The ABH antigens in human tissues and secretions during embryonal development. *J. Histochem. Cytochem.* **13**, 752.

Szulman, A.E. (1980) The ABH blood groups and development, in *Current Topics in Developmental Biology*, ed M. Friedlander, pp. 127–145. Academic Press, New York.

Szumness, W., Stevens, C.E., Harley, E.J., Zang, Edith A., Oleszko, W.R., William, D.C., Sadovsky, R., Morrison, J.M. and Kellner, A. (1980) Hepatitis B vaccine: demonstration of efficacy in a controlled clinical trial in a high-risk population in the United States. *New Engl. J. Med.* **303**, 833–841.

Szymanski, I.O. and Valeri, C.R. (1968) Automated differential agglutination technic to measure red cell survival. II. Survival *in vivo* of preserved red cells. *Transfusion*, **8**, 74.

Szymanski, I.O., Valeri, C.R., McCallum, L.E., Emerson, C.P. and Rosenfield, R.E. (1968) Automated differential agglutination technic to measure red cell survival. I. Methodology. *Transfusion*, **8**, 65.

Szymanski, I.O. and Valeri, C.R. (1969) Clinical evaluation of concentrated red cells. *New Engl. J. Med.* **280**, 281.

Szymanski, I.O. and Valeri, C.R. (1970) Factors influencing chromium elution from tagged red cells *in vivo* and the effect of elution on red cell survival measurements. *Brit. J. Haemat.* **19**, 397.

Szymanski, I.O. and Valeri, C.R. (1971) Lifespan of preserved red cells. *Vox Sang.* **21**, 97.

Szymanski, Irma O., Roberts, P.L. and Rosenfield, R.E. (1976) Anti-A autoantibody with severe intravascular hemolysis. *New Engl. J. Med.* **294**, 995.

Szymanski, Irma O., Tilley, Christine A., Crookston, Marie C., Greenwalt, T.J. and Moore, Susan (1977) A further example of human blood group chimaerism. *J. med. Genet.* **14**, 279.

Szymanski, I.O. and Odgren, P.R. (1979) Studies on the preservation of red blood cells. Attachment of the third component of human complement to erythrocytes during storage at 4°C. *Vox Sang.* **36**, 213–224.

Szymanski, I.O., Huff, S.R. and Delsignore, R. (1982) An autoanalyzer test to determine immunoglobulin class and IgG subclass of blood group antibodies. *Transfusion*, **22**, 90–95.

Szymanski, I.O. and Gandhi, J.G. (1983) A new low ionic strength test for assessment of pre-transfusion compatibility. Studies *in vitro* and *in vivo*. *Amer. J. clin. Path.* **80**, 37–42.

Szymanski, I.O. and Odgren, P.R. (1984) Measurement of fragments of the third component of human complement on erythrocytes by a new immunochemical method. *Vox Sang.* **46**, 92–102.

Szymanski, I.O., Swanton, R.E. and Odgren, P.R. (1984) Quantitation of the third component of complement on stored red cells. *Transfusion*, **24**, 194–197.

Taaning, Ellen, Antonsen, H., Peterson, S., Svejgaard, A. and Thomson, M. (1983) HLA antigens and maternal antibodies in allo-immune neonatal thrombocytopenia. *Tissue Antigens*, **21**, 351–360.

Taaning, E., Morling, N., Ovesen, H. and Svejgaard, A. (1985) Post transfusion purpura and anti-Zw^b(–Pl^{A2}). *Tissue Antigens*, **26**, 143–146.

Taaning, Ellen and Skov, F. (1991) Elution of anti-Zw^a (–Pl^{A}1) from autologous platelets after normalization of platelet count in post-transfusion purpura. *Vox Sang.* **60**, 40–44.

Tabb, P.A., Inglis, J., Savage, D.C.L. and Walker, C.H.M. (1972) Controlled trial of phototherapy of limited duration in the treatment of physiological hyperbilirubinaemia in low-birth-weight infants. *Lancet*, **2**, 1211.

Tabor, E. (1982) *Infectious Complications of Blood Transfusion*. Academic Press, New York.

Taddie, S.J., Barrasso, C. and Ness, P.M. (1982) A delayed transfusion reaction caused by anti-K6. *Transfusion*, **22**, 68–69.

Taft, E.G. (1981) Apheresis in platelet disorders. *Plasma Therapy*, **2**, 181–209.

Taguchi, H., Kobayashi, M. and Miyoshi, I. (1991) Immunosuppression by HTLV-I infection (Letter). *Lancet*, **i**, 308.

Takahashi, K., Imai, M., Nomura, M., Oinuma, A., Machida, A., Funatsu, G., Miyakawa, Y. and Mayumi, M. (1981) Demonstration of the immunogenicity of hepatitis B core antigen in a hepatitis B e antigen polypeptide (P19). *J. gen. Virol.* **57**, 325–330.

Takamizawa, A. and 9 others (1991) Structure and organization of the hepatitis C virus genome isolated from human carriers. *J. Virol.* **65**, 1105–1113.

Takeda, A., Tuazon, C.U. and Ennis, F.A. (1988) Antibody-enhanced infection by HIV-1 via Fc receptor-mediated entry. *Science*, **242**, 580–583.

Takeuchi, K. and 9 others (1990) The putative nucleocapsid and envelope protein genes of hepatitis C virus determined by comparison of the nucleotide sequences of two isolates derived from an experimentally infected chimpanzee and healthy human carriers. *J. gen. Virol.* **71**, 3027–3033.

Taliano, V., Guévin, R.-M., Hébert, Diane, Daniels, G.L., Tippett, Patricia, Anstee, D.J., Mawby, W.J. and Tanner, M.J.A. (1980) The rare phenotype En(a–) in a French-Canadian family. *Vox Sang.* **38**, 87–93.

Talmage, D.W. (1959) Immunological specificity. *Science*, **129**, 1463.

Tanaka, H. and Okubo, Y. (1977) Acute acquired hemolytic anemia with T-polyagglutination. *Annales paediatrici Japonici*, **23**, 49.

Tanner, M.J.A., Anstee, D.J., Mallinson, G., Ridgwell, K., Martin, P.G., Avent, N.D. and Parsons, S.F. (1988) Effect of endoglycosidase F preparations on the surface components of the human erythrocyte. *Carbohydrate Research*, **178**, 203–212.

Tannirandorn, Y. and Rodeck, C.H. (1990) New approaches in the treatment of haemolytic disease of the fetus, in *Blood Transfusion: the Impact of New Technologies*, ed Marcela Contreras. *Baillière's Clinical Haematology*, **3**, 289–320.

Tassopoulos, N.C., Papaevangelou, G.J. and Roumeliotou-Karayannis, Anastasia (1986) Heterosexual transmission of hepatitis B virus from symptomless HBsAg carriers positive for anti-HBe. *Lancet*, **ii**, 972.

Taswell, H.G., Pineda, A.A. and Brzica, S.M. (1976) Chronic granulomatous disease: successful treatment of infection with granulocyte transfusions resulting in subsequent hemolytic transfusion reaction. *Commun. Amer. Assoc. Blood Banks*, San Francisco.

Taswell, H.F., Pineda, A.A. and Moore, S.B. (1981) Hemolytic transfusion reactions: frequency and clinical and laboratory aspects, in *A Seminar on Immune-mediated Cell Destruction* Amer. Assoc. Blood Banks, Chicago.

Tate, Hermine, Cunningham, C., McDade, Mary G., Tippett, Patricia A. and Sanger, Ruth

(1960) An Rh gene complex Dc – . *Vox Sang.* **5**, 398.

Tate, Y., Sorensen, R.L., Gerrard, J.M., White, J.G. and Krivit, W. (1977) An immunoenzyme histochemical technique for the detection of platelet antibodies from the serum of patients with idiopathic (autoimmune) thrombocytopenic purpura. *Brit. J. Haemat.* **37**, 265.

Tateishi, J. (1985) Transmission of Jakob–Creuzfeld disease from human blood and urine into mice. *Lancet*, **ii**, 1074.

Taylor, G.L., Race, R.R., Prior, Aileen M. and Ikin, Elizabeth W. (1942) Frequency of the isoagglutinin α_1 in the serum of the subgroups A_2 and A_2B. *J. Path. Bact.* **54**, 514.

Taylor, W.C., Gillis, C.N., Nash, C.W. and Kullman, G.L. (1961) Experimental observations on cardiac arrhythmia during exchange transfusion in rabbits. *J. Pediat.* **58**, 470.

Taylor, I.W. and Rutherford, C.E. (1963) Accidental loss of plastic tube into venous system. *Arch. Surg.* **86**, 177.

Taylor, Patricia A., Rachkewich, Rose A., Gare, D.J., Falk, Judith A., Shumak, K.H. and Crookston, Marie C. (1974) Effect of pregnancy on the reactions of lymphocytes with cytotoxic antisera. *Transplantation*, **17**, 142.

Taylor, C. and Falk, W.P. (1981) Prevention of recurrent abortion with leucocyte transfusions. *Lancet*, **ii**, 68–70.

Tedder, R.S., Cameron, C.H., Wilson-Croome, Ruth, Howell, D.R., Colgrove, Anne and Barbara, J.A.J. (1980a) Contrasting patterns and frequency of antibodies to the surface, core, and e antigens of hepatitis B virus in blood donors and in homosexual patients. *J. med. Virol.* **6**, 323–332.

Tedder, R.S., Cameron, C.H., Barbara, J.A.J. and Howell, D. (1980b) Viral hepatitis markers in blood donors with history of jaundice (Letter). *Lancet*, **i**, 595–596.

Tedder, R.S., Briggs, Moya and Howell, D.R. (1982) U.K. prevalence of delta infection. *Lancet*, **ii**, 764–765.

Tedder, R.S. and Weiss, R.A. (1990) Retrovirus infections of humans, in Topley and Wilson's *Principles of Bacteriology, Virology and Immunity*, 8th edn, eds L.H. Collier and Morag C. Timbury, ch. 4, 32, Vol. 4, pp. 631–655. Edward Arnold, London.

Teesdale, P.W., de Silva, P.M., Fleetwood, P., Smithers, S., Gee, S., Schwarz, G. and Contreras, M. (1988) Responsiveness to Rh(D) and its association with HLA, red cell and serum markers. *Abstracts, 20th Congr. Int. Soc. Blood Transfus.*, London.

Teesdale, Phyllis, de Silva, Mahes and Contreras, Marcela (1991) Development of non-Rh antibodies in volunteers stimulated for the pro-

duction of hyperimmune anti-D. *Vox Sang.* **61**, 37–39.

Tegoli, J., Sausais, L. and Issitt, P.D. (1967a) Another example of a 'naturally-occurring' anti-K1. *Vox Sang.* **12**, 305.

Tegoli, J., Harris, Jean P., Issitt, P.D. and Sanders, C.W. (1967b) Anti-IB, an expected 'new' antibody detecting a joint product of the *I* and *B* genes. *Vox Sang.* **13**, 144.

Tegoli, J., Harris, J.P., Nichols, M.F., Marsh, W.L. and Reid, M.E. (1970) Autologous anti-I and anti-M following liver transplant. *Transfusion*, **10**, 133.

Tegoli, J., Cortez, Myrna, Jensen, Leila and Marsh, W.L. (1971) A new antibody, anti-ILe^{bH}, reacting with an apparent interaction product of the *I*, *Le*, *Se* and *H* genes. *Vox Sang.* **21**, 397.

Tegtmeier, G.E., Buckley, S.E., Jenkins, D.C., Hall, R.T., Kurth, C.G., Luetkemeyer, R.B., Sheehan, M.B. and Bayer, W.L. (1984) Acquired cytomegalovirus infections in transfused, premature neonates. *Abstracts, 18th Congr. Int. Soc. Blood Transfusion*, Münich, p. 180.

Tegtmeier, G.E. (1986) Transfusion-transmitted cytomegalovirus infections: significance and control. *Vox Sang.* **51**, suppl. 1, 22–30.

Tegtmeier, G.E. (1989) Posttransfusion cytomegalovirus infections. *Arch. Path. lab. Med.* **113**, 236–245.

Telen, M.J., Eisenbarth, G.S. and Haynes, B.F. (1983) Human erythrocyte antigens. Regulation of expression of a novel erythrocyte surface antigen by the inhibitor Lutheran *In (Lu)* gene. *J. clin. Invest.* **71**, 1878–1886.

Telen, Marilyn J. and Chasis, J.A. (1990) Relationship of the human erythrocyte Wr^b antigen to an interaction between glycophorin A and Band 3. *Blood*, **76**, 842–848.

Telischi, M., Behzad, O., Issitt, P.D. and Pavone, B.G. (1976) Hemolytic disease of the newborn due to anti-N. *Vox Sang.* **31**, 109.

Terasaki, P.I., McClelland, J.C., Park, M.S. and McCurdy, B. (1973) Microdroplet lymphocyte cytotoxicity test, in *Manual of Tissue Typing Techniques*. DHEW publ. (NIH) 74–545. Government Printing Office, Washington, D.C.

Terasaki, P. (1984) The beneficial transfusion effect on kidney graft survival attributed to clonal deletion. *Transplantation*, **37**, 119–125.

Terman, D.S., Tavel, T., Petty, D., Racic, M.R. and Buffaloe, G. (1977) Specific removal of antibody by extracorporeal circulation over antigen immobilized in collodion-charcoal. *Clin. exp. Immunol.* **29**, 180.

Terres, G. and Wolins, W. (1959) Enhanced sensitization in mice by simultaneous injection of antigen and specific rabbit antiserum. *Proc. Soc. exp. Biol. Med.* **102**, 632.

Terres, G. and Wolins, W. (1961) Enhanced immunological sensitization of mice by the simultaneous injection of antigen and specific antiserum. I. Effect of varying the amount of antigen used relative to the antiserum. *J. Immunol.* **86**, 361.

Terry, M.F. (1970) A management of the third stage to reduce feto-maternal transfusion. *J. Obstet. Gynaec. Brit. Cwlth.* **77**, 129.

Testa, U., Rochant, H., Henri, A., Titeux, M., Ton That, H. and Vainchenker, W. (1981) Change in i-antigen expression of erythrocytes during *in vivo* aging. *Rev. franç. Transfus. Immunohémat.* **24**, 299–305.

Thakur, M.L., Welch, M.J., Joist, J.H. and Colewan, R.A. (1976) Indium-111 labelled platelets: studies on preparation and evaluation of *in vitro* and *in vivo* functions. *Thrombos. Res.* **9**, 345–357.

Thakur, M.L., Lavender, J.P., Arnot, Rosemary N., Silvester, D.J. and Segal, A.W. (1977a) Indium-111-labeled autologous leukocytes in man. *J. nucl. Med.* **18**, 1014.

Thakur, M.L., Coleman, R.E. and Welch, M.J. (1977b) Indium-111-labeled leukocytes for the localization of abscesses: preparation, analysis, tissue distribution, and comparison with gallium-67 citrate in dogs. *J. Lab. clin. Med.* **89**, 217.

Thaler, M., Shamis, A., Orgad, S., Huszar, Monica, Nussinovitch, N., Meisel, S., Gazit, E., Lavee, J. and Smolinsky, A. (1989) The role of blood from HLA-homozygous donors in fatal transfusion-associated graft-versus-host disease after open-heart surgery. *New Engl. J. Med.* **321**, 25–28.

Thalheimer, W. (1921) Hemoglobinuria after a second transfusion with the same donor. *J. Amer. med. Assoc.* **76**, 1345.

Tharakan, J., Strickland, D., Burgess, W., Drohan, W.N., Clark, D.B. (1990) Development of an immunoaffinity process for Factor IX purification. *Vox Sang.* **58**, 21–29.

The, T.H. (1984) In International Forum: Transfusion-transmitted CMV infections. *Vox Sang.* **46**, 387–414.

Thiers, V. and 10 others (1988) Transmission of hepatitis B from hepatitis-B-seronegative subjects. *Lancet*, **ii**, 1273–1276.

Thomaidis, T., Fouskaris, G. and Matsaniotis, N. (1967) Isohemagglutinin activity in the first day of life. *Amer. J. Dis. Child.* **113**, 654.

Thompson, P.R., Childers, D.M. and Hatcher, D.E. (1967) Anti-Di[b]—first and second examples. *Vox Sang.* **13**, 314.

Thompson, J.S. and Severson, C.D. (1980) *Granulocyte Antigens in Blood Cells and Body Fluids.* Amer. Assoc. Blood Banks, Washington, D.C. pp. 151–187.

Thompson, J.S., Overlin, V., Severson, C.D.,

Parsons, T.J., Herbick, J., Strauss, R.G., Burns, C.P. and Claas, F.H.J. (1980a) Demonstration of granulocyte, monocyte, and endothelial cell antigens by double fluorochromatic microcytotoxicity testing. *Transplant. Proc.* **12**, Suppl. 1, 26–31.

Thompson, J.S., Herbick, J.M., Klassen, L.W., Severson, C.D., Overlin, V.L., Blaschke, J.W., Silverman, M.A. and Vogel, C.L. (1980b) Studies on levamisole-induced agranulocytosis. *Blood*, **56**, 388–396.

Thompson, G.R. (1981) Plasma exchange for hypercholesterolaemia. *Lancet*, **i**, 1246–1248.

Thompson, K.M. and Hughes-Jones, N.C. (1990) Production and characterization of monoclonal anti-Rh, in *Blood Transfusion; the Impact of New Technologies*, ed Marcela Contreras. *Baillière Clinical Haematology*, **3**, 243–253.

Thompson, K., Barden, G., Sutherland, J., Beldon, I. and Melamed, M. (1991) Human monoclonal antibodies to human blood group antigens Kidd Jk[a] and Jk[b]. *Transfus. Med.* **1**, 91–96.

Thomsen, O. (1927) Ein vermehrungsfähiges Agens als Veränderer des isoagglutinatorischen Verhaltens der roten Blutkörperchen, eine bisher unbekannte Quelle der Fehlbestimmung. *Z. Immun.-Forsch.* **52**, 85.

Thomsen, O. and Thisted, A. (1928a) Untersuchungen über Isohämolysin in Menschenserum. I. Reaktivierung. *Z. Immun.-Forsch.* **59**, 479.

Thomsen, O. and Thisted, A. (1928b) Untersuchungen über Isohämolysin in Menschenserum. II. Die relative Stärke des α und β-lysins. *Z. Immun.-Forsch.* **59**, 491.

Thomsen, O. and Kettel, K. (1929) Die Stärke der menschlichen Iso-agglutinine und entsprechenden Blutkörperchenrezeptoren in verschiedenen Lebansaltern. *Z. Immun.-Forsch.* **63**, 67.

Thomsen, O. (1930) Immunisierung von Menschen mit Antigenem Gruppenfremden Blute. *Z. Rassenphysiol.* **2**, 105.

Thomson, Amanda, Contreras, Marcela, Gorick, Barbara, Kumpel, Belinda, Chapman, G., Lane, R.S., Teesdale, Phyllis, Hughes-Jones, N.C. and Mollison, P.L. (1990) Human monoclonal IgG3 and IgG1 anti-Rh D mediate clearance of D positive red cells. *Lancet*, **ii**, 1147–1150.

Thorogood, J., Persijn, G.G., Schreuder, G.M.TH., D'Amaro, J., Zantvoort, F.A., Van Houwelingen, J.C. and van Rood, J.J. (1990) The effect of HLA-matching on kidney graft survival, in separate post-transplantation time intervals. *Transplantation*, **58**, 146–150.

Thorpe, Susan J. (1989) Detection of Rh D-associated epitopes in human and animal tissues using human monoclonal anti-D anti-bodies. *Brit. J. Haemat.* **73**, 527–536.

Thorpe, Susan J. (1990) Reactivity of human monoclonal antibody against Rh D with the intermediate filament protein vimentin. *Brit. J. Haemat.* **76**, 116–120.

Thorsby, E. (1984) The role of HLA in T-cell activation. *Hum. Immunol.* **9**, 1–9.

Thorsen, G. and Hint, H. (1950) Aggregation, sedimentation and intravascular sludging of erythrocytes. *Acta chir. scand.* Suppl. 154.

Thurer, R.L., Lytle, B.W., Cosgrove, D.M. and Loop. F.D. (1979) Autotransfusion following cardiac operations: a randomized prospective study. *Ann. thorac. Surg.* **27**, 500–507.

Tijhuis, G.J., Klaassen, R.J.L., Modderman, P.W., Ouwehand, W.H. and von dem Borne, A.E.G.Kr. (1991) Quantification of platelet-bound immunoglobulins of different class and subclass using radiolabelled monoclonal antibodies: assay conditions and clinical application. *Brit. J. Haemat.* **77**, 93–101.

Tilley, C.A., Crookston, M.C., Brown, B.L. and Wherrett, J.R. (1975) A and B and A_1Le^b substances in glycosphingolipid fractions of human serum. *Vox Sang.* **28**, 25.

Tilley, C.A., Crookston, M.C., Haddad, S.A. and Shumak, K.H. (1977) Red blood cell survival studies in patients with anti-Ch[a], anti-Yk[a], anti-Ge and anti-Vel. *Transfusion*, **17**, 169.

Tilley, C.A., Crookston, M.C., Crookston, J.H., Shindman, J. and Schachter, H. (1978a) Human blood group A- and H-specified glycosyl-transferase levels in the sera of newborn infants and their mothers. *Vox Sang.* **34**, 8.

Tilley, C.A., Romans, D.G. and Crookston, Marie C. (1978b) Localisation of Chido and Rodgers determinants to the C4d fragment of human C4. *Nature (Lond.)*, **276**, 713.

Ting, A. (1983) The lymphocytotoxic crossmatch test in clinical renal transplantation. *Transplantation*, **35**, 403–407.

Tinsley, J.C., Moore, C.V., Dubach, R., Minnich, V. and Grinstein, M. (1949) The role of oxygen in the regulation of erythropoiesis. Depression of the rate of delivery of new red cells to the blood by high concentrations of inspired oxygen. *J. clin. Invest.* **28**, 1544.

Tiollais, P., Charnay, P. and Vyas, G.N. (1981) Biology of hepatitis B virus. *Science*, **213**, 406–411.

Tiollais, P., Buendia, Marie-Annick, Bréchot, C., Dejean, Anne, Michel, Marie-Louise and Pourcel, Christine (1988) Structure, genetic organization, and transcription of Hepadna viruses, in *Viral Hepatitis and Liver Disease*, ed A.J. Zuckerman, pp. 295–300. Alan R. Liss, New York.

Tippett, Patricia, Noades, Jean, Sanger, Ruth, Race, R.R., Sausais, Laima, Holman, C.A. and

Buttimer, R.J. (1960) Further studies of the I antigen and antibody. *Vox Sang.* **5**, 107.

Tippett, Patricia and Sanger, Ruth (1962) Observations on subdivisions of the Rh antigen D. *Vox Sang.* **7**, 9.

Tippett, Patricia (1963) Serological Study of the Inheritance of Unusual Rh and Other Blood Group Phenotypes. Ph.D. Thesis, University of London.

Tippett, Patricia, Sanger, Ruth, Race, R.R., Swanson, Jane and Busch, Shirley (1965) An agglutinin associated with the P and the ABO blood group systems. *Vox Sang.* **10**, 269–280.

Tippett, Patricia (1972) A present view of Rh. *Pathologica*, **64**, 29.

Tippett, Patricia (1975) Antibodies in the sera of p and P[k] people. *Abstracts, 14th Congr. Int. Soc. Blood Transfus.*, Helsinki, p. 94.

Tippett, Patricia and Sanger, Ruth (1977) Further observations on subdivisions of the Rh antigen D. *Arztl. Lab.* **23**, 476–480.

Tippett, Patricia (1986) Contributions of monoclonal antibodies to understanding one new and some old blood group systems in *Red Cell Antigens and Antibodies*, ed G. Garratty, pp. 83–98. Amer. Assoc. of Blood Banks, Arlington, VA.

Tippett, Patricia and Moore, A. (1990) Monoclonal antibodies against Rh and Rh related antigens. *J. Immunogenet.* **17**, 309–319.

Tippett, Patricia and Lomas, Christine (1992) Partial D antigens: definition in terms of D epitopes, to be published.

Tisdall, L.H., Garland, D.M. and Wiener, A.S. (1946a) A critical analysis of the value of the addition of A and B group-specific substances to group O blood for use as universal donor blood. *J. Lab. clin. Med.* **31**, 437.

Tisdall, L.H., Garland, D.M., Szanto, P.B., Hand, A.M. and Bonnett, J. (1946b) The effects of the transfusion of group O blood of high iso-agglutinin titer into recipients of other blood groups. *Amer. J. clin. Path.* **16**, 193.

Tobey, R.E., Kopriva, C.J., Homer, L.D., Solis, R.T., Dickson, L.G. and Herman, C.M. (1974) Pulmonary gas exchange following hemorrhagic shock and massive transfusion in the baboon. *Ann. Surg.* **179**, 316.

Todd, C. and White, R.G. (1911) On the fate of red blood corpuscles when injected into the circulation of an animal of the same species: with a new method for the determination of the total volume of blood. *Proc. roy. Soc. Lond. B*, **84**, 255.

Toivanen, P. and Hirvonen, T. (1969) Iso- and heteroagglutinins in human fetal and neonatal sera. *Scand. J. Haemat.* **6**, 42.

Tokunaga, E. and 9 others (1979) Two apparently healthy Japanese individuals of type M^kM^k have erythrocytes which lack both the blood group MN and Ss-active sialoglyco-proteins. *J. Immunogenet.* **6**, 383–390.

Tomar, R.H., John, Patricia, Hennig, Anne, K. and Kloster, B. (1985) Cellular target anti-lymphocyte antibodies in AIDS and LAS. *Clin. Immunol. Immunopath.* **37**, 37–47.

Tomasi, T.B. jr, Tan, E.M., Solomon, A. and Prendergast, R.A. (1965) Characteristics of an immune system common to certain external secretions. *J. exp. Med.* **121**, 101.

Tomasi, T.B. (1980) Oral tolerance. *Transplantation*, **29**, 353–356.

Tomasulo, P.A., Anderson, A.J., Paluso, M.B., Gutschenritter, M.A. and Aster R.H. (1980) A study of criteria for blood donor deferral. *Transfusion*, **20**, 511–518.

Tomita, M. and Marchesi, V.T. (1975) Amino-acid sequence and oligosaccharide attach-ment sites of human erythrocyte glycophorin. *Proc. nat. Acad. Sci. USA*, **72**, 2964–2968.

Tong, S., Li J., Vitvitski, Ludmila, and Trépo, C. (1990) Active hepatitis B virus replication in the presence of anti-HBe is associated with viral variants containing an inactive pre-C region. *Virology*, **176**, 596–603.

Tongio, M.M., Berrebi, A. and Mayer, S. (1972) A study of lymphocytotoxic antibodies in multi-parous women having had at least four preg-nancies. *Tissue Antigens*, **2**, 378.

Tongio, M.M., Falkenrodt, A., Mitsuishi, Y., Urlacher, A., Bergerat, J.P., North, M.L. and Mayer, S. (1985) Natural HLA antibodies. *Tissue Antigens*, **26**, 271–285.

Tonthat, H., Rochant, H., Henry, A., Leporrier, M. and Dreyfus, B. (1976) A new case of monoclonal IgA kappa cold agglutinin with anti-Pr$_1$d specificity in a patient with persis-tent HB antigen cirrhosis. *Vox Sang.* **30**, 464.

Topley, Elizabeth, Jackson, D.MacG., Cason, J.S. and Davies, J.W.L. (1962) Assessment of red cell loss in the first two days after severe burns. *Ann. Surg.* **155**, 581.

Topley, Elizabeth, Bull, J.P., Maycock, W.d'A., Mourant, A.E. and Parkin, Dorothy (1963) The relation of the isoagglutinins in pooled plasma to the haemolytic anaemia of burns. *J. clin. Path.* **16**, 79.

Topley, E., Knight, R. and Woodruff, A.W. (1973) The direct antiglobulin test and immu-noconglutinin titres in patients with malaria. *Trans. roy. Soc. Trop. Med. Hyg.* **67**, 51.

Topping, M.D. and Watkins, Winifred M. (1975) Isoelectric points of the human blood group A^1, A^2, and B gene-associated glycosyltrans-ferases in ovarian cyst fluids and serum. *Bio-chem. biophys. Res. Commun.* **64**, 89.

Tosswill, Jennifer, H.C., Parry, J.V. and Weber, J.A.J. (1992) Application of screening and confirmatory assays for anti-HTLV I/II in UK populations. *J. med. Virol.* **36**, 167–171.

Tovey, G.H. (1945) A study of the protective factors in heterospecific group pregnancy and their role in the prevention of haemolytic disease of the newborn. *J. Path. Bact.* **57**, 295.

Tovey, A.D. (1958) The incidence, distribution and life history of the anti-A and anti-B haemolysins in the general population. *Vox Sang.* **3**, 363.

Tovey, G.H. and Lennon, G.G. (1962) Blood vol-ume studies in accidental haemorrhage. *J. Obstet. Gynaec. Brit. Cwlth.* **5**, 749.

Tovey, G.H., Nelson, S.D. and Moore, Barbara (1973) Response in pregnancy to LA and Four series antigens. *Series Immunobiol. Standard*, **18**, 53.

Tovey, G.H. (1974) Preventing the incompatible blood transfusion. *Haematologia*, **8**, 389.

Tovey, L.A.D., Murray, Jane, Stevenson, Beryll J. and Taverner, J.M. (1978) The prevention of Rhesus haemolytic disease. *Brit. med. J.* **2**, 106.

Tovey, L.A.D., Townley, A., Stevenson, B.J. and Taverner, J. (1983) The Yorkshire antenatal anti-D immunoglobulin trial in primi-gravidae. *Lancet*, **2**, 244–246.

Tovey, L.A.D. (1986) Haemolytic disease of the newborn—the changing scene. *Brit. J. Obstet. Gynaec.* **93**, 960–966.

Toy, P.T., Reid, M., Lewis, T., Ellisor, S. and Avoy, D.R. (1981) Does anti-Jr^a cause haemolytic disease of the newborn? *Vox Sang.* **41**, 40–44.

Travis, G.H. and Salvesen, G.S. (1983) Human plasma proteinase inhibitors. *Ann. Rev. Bio-chem.* **52**, 655–709.

Tregellas, W.M., Moulds, J.J. and South, S.F. (1978) Successful transfusion of a patient with anti-LW and LW positive blood (Ab-stract). *Transfusion*, **18**, 384.

Tremper, K.K., Friedman, A.E., Levine, E.M., Lapin, R. and Camarillo, Debra (1982) The preoperative treatment of severely anemic patients with a perfluorochemical oxygen-transport fluid, Fluosol-DA. *New Engl. J. Med.* **307**, 277–283.

Trepo, C., Hantz, O., Jacquier, M.F., Nemoz, G., Cappel, R. and Trepo, D. (1978) Different fates of hepatitis B virus markers during plasma fractionation. A clue to the infectivity of blood derivatives. *Vox Sang.* **35**, 143.

Triger, D.R. and Preston, F.E. (1990) Chronic liver disease in haemophiliacs. *Brit. J. Hae-mat.* **74**, 241–245.

Trudeau, L.R., Judd, W.J., Oberman, H.A. and Butch, S.H. (1981) Is a room temperature crossmatch necessary for the detection of ABO errors? (Abstract). *Transfusion*, **21**, 625.

Tsai, C.M., Zopf, D.A. and Ginsburg, V. (1978) The molecular basis for cold agglutination: effect of receptor density upon thermal am-plitude of a cold agglutinin. *Biochem. biophys. Res. Commun.* **80**, 905.

Tschirren, B., Affolter, U., Elsässer, R., Freihofer, U.A., Grawehr, R., Müller, P.H. and Lundsgaard-Hansen, P. (1973/74) Der klinsche Plasmaersatz mit Gelatine: zwölf Jahre Erfahrungen mit 39320 Einheiten Physiogel. *Infusionstherapie*, 1, 651–662.

Tsubakio, T., Tani, P., Curd, J.R. and McMillan, R. (1986) Complement activation *in vitro* by anti platelet antibodies in chronic immune thromboyctopenic purpura. *Brit. J. Haemat.* 63, 293–300.

Tubbs, R.R., Hoffman, G.C., Deodhar, S.D. and Hewlett, J.S. (1976) IgM monoclonal gammography. Histopathologic and clinical spectrum. *Cleveland Clin. Quart.* 43, 21.

Tucker, Elizabeth M. and Ellory, J.C. (1970) The M-L blood group system and its influence on red cell potassium levels in sheep. *Anim. Blood Grps. biochem. Genet.* 1, 101.

Tucker, J., Murphy, M.F., Gregory, W.M., Lim, J., Rohatinez, A.Z.S., Waters, A.H. and Lister, T.A. (1989) Apparent removal of graft-versus-leukaemia effect by the use of leucocyte-poor blood components in patients with acute myeloblastic leukaemia. *Brit. J. Haemat.* 73, 584–785.

Tuddenham, E.G.D., Takase, T., Thomas, A.E., Awidi, A.S., Mandanat, F.F., Hajir, M.M.A. and Kernoff, P.B.A. (1989) Homozygous protein C deficiency with delayed onset of symptoms at 7 to 10 months. *Thrombos. Res.* 53, 475–484.

Tui, C. and Schrift, M.N. (1942) Production of pyrogen by some bacteria. *J. Lab. clin. Med.* 27, 569.

Turner, T.B. and Diseker, T.K. (1941) Duration of infectivity of *Treponema pallidum* in citrated blood stored under conditions obtaining in blood banks. *Bull. Johns Hopk. Hosp.* 68, 269.

Turner, A.R., MacDonald, R.N. and Cooper, B.A. (1972) Transmission of infectious mononucleosis by transfusion of pre-illness plasma. *Ann. intern. Med.* 77, 751.

Tursz, T., Preud'Homme, J-L., Labanne, Sylvaine, Matuchansky, C. and Seligmann, M. (1977) Autoantibodies to B lymphocytes in a patient with hypoimmunoglobulinemia. Characterization and pathogenic role. *J. clin. Invest.* 60, 405–410.

Twigley, Alison J. and Hillman, K.M. (1985) The end of the crystalloid era? *Anaesthesia*, 40, 860–871.

Uchikawa, H and Tohyama, H. (1986) A potent cold autoagglutinin that recognizes type 2H determinant on red cells. *Transfusion*, 26, 240–242.

Ueda, E., Kinoshita, T., Terasawa, T., Shischiscima, T., Yawata, Y. Inoue, K. and Kitani, T. (1990) Acetylcholinesterase and lymphocyte function-associated antigen 3 found on decay-accelerating factor-negative erythrocytes from some patients with paroxysmal nocturnal haemoglobinuria are lost during erythrocyte aging. *Blood*, 75, 762–769.

Uhlenbruck, G., Dahr, W., Schmalisch, R. and Janssen, E. (1976) Studies on the receptors of the MNSs blood group system. *Blut*, 32, 163.

U.K. BTS/NIBSC (1990) *Guidelines for the Blood Transfusion Services in the United Kingdom 1989.* HMSO, London.

U.K. Haemophilia Centre Directors (1986) Prevalence of antibody to HTLV-III in haemophiliacs in the United Kingdom. *Brit. med. J.* 293, 175–176.

Umlas, J. (1979) Coagulation and component therapy in trauma and surgery, in *Hemotherapy in Trauma and Surgery*, eds A. Barnes and J. Umlas, pp. 31–41. Amer. Assoc. Blood Banks, Arlington, V.A.

Unger, L.J. (1921) Precautions necessary in selection of a donor for blood transfusion. *J. Amer. med. Assoc.* 76, 9.

Unger, L.J. (1951) A method for detecting Rh_0 antibodies in extremely low titer. *J. Lab. clin. Med.* 37, 825.

Unger, L.J. and Wiener, A.S. (1959) Observations on blood factors Rh^A, Rh^α, Rh^B and Rh^C. *Amer. J. clin. Path.* 31, 95.

Urbaniak, S.J. (1979a) ADCC(K-cell) lysis of human erythrocytes with Rhesus alloantibodies. I. Investigation of *in vitro* culture variables. *Brit. J. Haemat.* 42, 303–314.

Urbaniak, S.J. (1979b) ADCC(K-cell) lysis of human erythrocytes sensitized with alloantibodies. II. Investigation into the mechanism of lysis. *Brit. J. Haemat.* 42, 315–328.

Urbaniak, S.J. and Robertson, A.E. (1981) A successful program of immunizing Rh-negative male volunteers for anti-D production using frozen/thawed blood. *Transfusion*, 21, 64–69.

Urbaniak, S.J. (1983) Replacement fluids in plasma exchange. *Apheresis Bull.* 1, 104–113.

Urbaniak, S.J. (1984) Therapeutic plasma exchange and cellular apheresis, in *Blood Transfusion and Blood Banking*, ed W.L. Bayer, *Clinics in Haematology*, 13, 217 251.

Urbaniak, S.J., Greiss, M.A., Crawford, R.J. and Fergusson, M.J.C. (1984) Prediction of the outcome of rhesus haemolytic disease of the newborn: additional information using an ADCC assay. *Vox Sang.* 46, 323–329.

Usher, R., Shepard, M. and Lind, J. (1963) The blood volume of the newborn infant and placental transfusion. *Acta paediat. (Uppsala)*, 52, 497.

Vadhan-Raj, S., Keating, M.D., Le Maistre, A., Hittelman, W.N., McGredie, K. Trujillo, J.M., Broxmeijer, H.E., Henney, Ch. and Gutterman, J.U. (1987) Effects of recombinant human granulocyte-macrophage colony stimulating factor in patients with myeloplastic syndromes. *New Engl. J. Med.* **317**, 1545–1552.

Vadhan-Raj, S. and 11 others (1988) Stimulation of myelopoiesis in patients with aplastic anemia by recombinant human granulocyte-macrophage colony-stimulating factor. *New Engl. Med.* **319**, 1628–1634.

Vainchenker, W., Testa, V., Deschamps, Jeanne, Henri, Annie, Titeux, Monique, Breton-Gorius, Janine, Rochant, H., Lee, D. and Cartron, J-P. (1982) Clonal expression of the Tn antigen in erythroid and granulocyte colonies and its application to determination of the clonality of the human megakaryocyte colony assay. *J. clin. Invest.* **69**, 1081–1091.

Vainchenker, W., Vinci, G., Testa, U., Henri, Annie, Tabillo, A., Fache, M-P., Rochaert, H. and Cartron, J-P. (1985) Presence of the Tn antigen on hematopoietic progenitors from patients with the Tn syndrome. *J. clin. Invest.* **75**, 541–546.

Väisänen, V., Korhonen, T.K., Jokinen, M., Gahmberg, C.G. and Ehnholm, C. (1982) Blood group M specific haemagglutinin in pyelonephritogenic *Escherichia coli* (Letter). *Lancet*, **i**, 1192.

Vakkila, J. and Myllyla, G. (1987) Amount and type of leukocytes in 'leukocyte-free' red cell and platelet concentrates. *Vox Sang.* **53**, 76–82.

Valentine, G.H. (1958) ABO incompatibility and haemolytic disease of the newborn. *Arch. Dis. Childh.* **33**, 185.

Valentin, N., Vergracht, A., Bignon, J.D., Cheneau, M.L., Blanchard, D., Kaplan, C., Reznikoff-Etiévant, M.F. and Muller, J.Y. (1990) HLA-DRw52a is involved in alloimmunization against Pl-A[1] antigen. *Hum. Immunol.* **27**, 73–80.

Valeri, C.R. (1965a) Effect of resuspension medium on *in vivo* survival and supernatant hemoglobin of erythrocytes preserved with glycerol. *Transfusion*, **5**, 25.

Valeri, C.R. (1965b) The *in vivo* survival, mode of removal of the non-viable cells, and the total amount of supernatant hemoglobin in deglycerolized, resuspended erythrocytes. I. The effect of the period of storage in ACD at 4°C prior to glycerolization. II. The effect of washing deglycerolized, resuspended erythrocytes after a period of storage at 4°C. *Transfusion*, **5**, 273.

Valeri, C.R. and McCallum, Linda (1965) The age of human erythrocytes lost during freezing and thawing with glycerol using the Cohn Fractionator. *Transfusion*, **5**, 421.

Valeri, C.R., Mercado-Lugo, R. and Danon, D. (1965) Relationship between osmotic fragility and *in vivo* survival of autologous deglycerolized resuspended red blood cells. *Transfusion*, **5**, 267.

Valeri, C.R., Booth, W., Gildea, S. and McCallum, L. (1968) Observations on the chromium labelling of ACD-stored and previously frozen red cells. *Transfusion*, **8**, 210.

Valeri, C.R. and Hirsch, N.M. (1969) Restoration *in vivo* of erythrocyte adenosine triphosphate, 2,3-diphosphoglycerate, potassium ion, and sodium ion concentrations following the transfusion of acid-citrate-dextrose-stored human red blood cells. *J. Lab. clin. Med.* **73**, 722.

Valeri, C.R. and Runck, A.H. (1969) Long term frozen storage of human red blood cells: studies *in vivo* and *in vitro* of autologous red blood cells preserved up to six years with high concentrations of glycerol. *Transfusion*, **9**, 5.

Valeri, C.R., Szymanski, I.O. and Runck, A.H. (1970) Therapeutic effectiveness of homologous erythrocyte transfusions following frozen storage at −80°C for up to seven years. *Transfusion*, **10**, 102.

Valeri, C.R. and Zaroulis, C.G. (1972) Rejuvenation and freezing of outdated stored human red cells. *New Engl. J. med.* **287**, 1307.

Valeri, C.R., Cooper, A.G. and Pivacek, L.E. (1973) Limitations of measuring blood volume with iodinated I^{125} serum albumin. *Arch. intern. Med.* **132**, 534.

Valeri, C.R. (1974) Factors influencing the 24-hour post-transfusion survival and the oxygen transport function of previously frozen red cells preserved with 40 per cent w/v glycerol and frozen at −80°C. *Transfusion*, **14**, 1.

Valeri, C.R. (1975) Simplification of the methods for adding and removing glycerol during freeze-preservation of human red blood cells with the high or low glycerol methods: biochemical modification prior to freezing. *Transfusion*, **15**, 195.

Valeri, C.R., Kuehl, G.V., Skrabut, E.M., Bechthold, D.A., Vecchione, J.J., Harkness, D.R. and Emerson, C.P. (1981a) Studies on the *in vivo* elution of ^{51}Cr from baboon red blood cells. *Vox Sang.* **40**, 338–345.

Valeri, C.R., Valeri, D.A., Anastasi, J., Vecchione, J.J., Dennis, R.C. and Emerson, C.P. (1981b) Freezing in the primary polyvinylchloride plastic collection bag: a new system for preparing and freezing nonrejuvenated and rejuvenated red blood cells. *Transfusion*, **21**, 138–149.

Valeri, C.R. (1985) Measurement of viable ADSOL-preserved human red cells. *New Engl. J. Med.* **312**, 377–378.

Valeri, C.R., Landrock, R.D., Pivacek, L.E., Gray, A.D., Fink, J.G. and Szymanski, I.O. (1985) Quantitative differential agglutination method using the Coulter counter to measure survival of compatible but identifiable red blood cells. *Vox Sang.* **49**, 195–205.

Valeri, C.R., Feingold, H., Cassidy, G., Ragno, Gina, Khuri, S. and Altschule, M.D. (1987) Hypothermia-induced reversible platelet dysfunction. *Ann. Surg.* **205**, 175–181.

Valeri, C.R. and 10 others (1989) The safety and therapeutic effectiveness of human red cells stored at –80°C for as long as 21 years. *Transfusion*, **29**, 429–437.

Valko, Denise A. (1988) The Duffy blood group system: biochemistry and role in malaria, in *Blood Group Systems: Duffy, Kidd and Lutheran*, eds S.R. Pierce and C.R. MacPherson. Amer. Assoc. Blood Banks, Arlington VA.

Valtis, D.J. and Kennedy, A.C. (1954) Defective gas-transport function of stored red blood cells. *Lancet*, **i**, 119.

van Aken, W.G. (1989) Does perioperative blood transfusion promote tumor growth? *Transfus. Med. Rev.* **3**, 243–252.

van Alphen, L., Poole, Joyce and Overbeeke, Marijke (1986) The Anton blood group antigen is the erythrocyte receptor for *Haemophilus influenzae*. *FEMS Microbiol. Letters*, **37**, 69–71.

van Buren, N.L., Stroncek, D.F., Clay, M.E., McCullough, J. and Dalmasso, A.P. (1990) Transfusion-related acute lung injury caused by an NB2 granulocyte-specific antibody in a patient with thrombotic thrombocytopenic purpura. *Transfusion*, **30**, 42–45.

van der Giessen, M., van der Hart, Mia and van der Weerdt, Ch.M. (1964) Fractionation of sera containing antibodies against red cells or platelets with special reference to anti-D sera. *Vox Sang.* **9**, 25.

van der Hart, Mia and van Loghem, J.J. (1953) A further example of anti-Jk^a. *Vox Sang.* (*O.S.*), **3**, 72.

van der Hart, Mia, Engelfriet, C.P., Prins, H.K. and van Loghem, J.J. (1963) A haemolytic transfusion reaction without demonstrable antibodies *in vitro*. *Vox Sang.* **8**, 363.

van der Hart, M., Szaloky, A., van der Berg-Loonen, E.M., Engelfriet, C.P. and van Loghem, J.J. (1974) Présence d'antigènes HL-A sur les hématies d'un donneur normal. *Nouv. Rev. franç. Hémat.* **14**, 555.

van der Meer, J., Daenen, S., van Imhoff, G.W., de Wolf, J.T.M. and Halie, M.R. (1986) Absence of seroconversion for HTLV-III in haemophiliacs intensively treated with heat treated factor VIII concentrate. *Brit. med. J.* **292**, 1049.

van der Meulen, F.W., de Bruin, H.G., Goosen, P.C.M., Bruynes, E.C.E., Joustra-Maas, C.J., Telkamp, H.G., von dem Borne, A.E.G.Kr. and Engelfriet, C.P. (1980a) Quantitative aspects of the destruction of red cells sensitized

with IgG1 autoantibodies: an application of flow cytofluorometry. *Brit. J. Haemat.* **46**, 47–56.

van der Meulen, J.A., McNabb, Trudy C., Haeffner-Cavaillon, Nicole, Klein, M. and Dorrington, K.J. (1980b) The Fc receptor on human placental plasma membrane. I. Studies on the binding of homologous and heterologous immunoglobulin G. *J. Immunol.* **124**, 500–507.

van der Poel, C.L., Reesink, H.W., Lelie, P.N., Leentvaar-Kuypers, A., Choo, Q-L., Kuo, G. and Houghton, M. (1989a) Anti-hepatitis C antibodies and non-A, non-B posttransfusion hepatitis in The Netherlands. *Lancet*, **ii**, 297–298.

van der Poel, C., Lelie, N., Reesink, H., Ehlers, P., Bakker, E. and Huisman, H. (1989b) Prevalence of HTLV-I antibodies in blood donors in The Netherlands (Abstract). *5th Int. Conf. AIDS*, Montreal, p. 248.

van der Poel, C.L., Reesink, H.W., Lelie, P.N., Exel-Oehlers, P., Winkel, I., Schaasberg, W., Polito, A. and Houghton, H. (1990) Anti-HCV and transaminase testing of blood donors. *Lancet*, **ii**, 187–188.

van der Poel, C.L. (1991) Hepatitis C Virus: Studies on Transmission and Epidemiology. Academic Thesis, University of Amsterdam.

van der Poel, C.L. and 14 others (1991) Confirmation of hepatitis C virus infection by new four-antigen recombinant immunoblot assay. *Lancet*, **i**, 317–319.

van der Poel, C.L. and 12 others (1992) Early anti-HCV response with second generation C200/C22 ELISA. *Vox Sang.* **62**, 208–213.

van der Salm, T.J., Ansell, J.E., Okike, O.N., Marsciano, T.H., Lew, R., Stephenson, Wendy P. and Rooney, Kathy (1988) The role of epsilon-aminocaproic acid in reducing bleeding after cardiac operation; a double-blind randomised study. *J. Thorac. cardiovasc. Surg.* **95**, 538–540.

van der Schoot, C. Ellen, Webster, M. Mieke, von dem Borne, A.E.G.Kr. and Huisman, H.G. (1986) Characterization of platelet-specific alloantigens by immunoblotting: localization of Zw and Bak antigens. *Brit. J. Haemat.* **64**, 715–723.

van der Schoot, C. Ellen, Daams, Marjolein, Huiskes, Elly, Clay, Mary, McCullough, J., van Dalen, Carla M. and von dem Borne, A.E.G.Kr. (1992) Antigenic polymorphism of the Leu-CAM family recognized by human leukocyte alloantisera. *Brit. J. Haemat.* in press.

van der Sluis, J.J., Ten Kate, F.J.W., Vuzevski, V.D., Kothe, F.C., Aelbers, G.M.N. and Van Eijk, R.V.W. (1985) Transfusion syphilis, survival of *Treponema pallidum* in stored donor blood. II-Dose dependence of experimentally determined survival times. *Vox Sang.* **49**, 390–399.

van der Vegt, S.G.L., Ruben, A.M.Th., Werre, J.M., Palsma, D.M.H., Verhoef, C.W., de Gier, J. and Staal, G.E.J. (1985a) Counterflow centrifugation of red cell populations: a cell age related separation technique. *Brit. J. Haemat.* **61**, 393–403.

van der Vegt, S.G.L., Ruben, A.M.Th., Werre, J.M., de Gier, J. and Stall, G.E.J. (1985b) Membrane characteristics and osmotic fragility of red cells, fractionated with anglehead centrifugation and counter flow centrifugation. *Brit. J. Haemat.* **61**, 405–413.

van der Weerdt, C.M., van de Wiel-Dorfmeyer, Hanny, Engelfriet, C.P. and van Loghem, J.J. (1962) A new platelet antigen. *Proc. 8th Congr. Europ. Soc. Haemat.*, Vienna, 1961, p. 379.

van der Weerdt, C.M., Veenhoven-von Riesz, L.E., Nijenhuis, L.E. and van Loghem, J.J. (1963) The Zw blood group system in platelets. *Vox Sang.* **8**, 513.

van der Woude, F.J., Rasmussen, N., Lobatto, S, Wiik, A., Permin, H., van Es, L.A., van der Giessen, M., van der Hem, G.K. and The, T.H. (1985) Autoantibodies against neutrophils and monocytes: tool for diagnosis and marker for disease activity in Wegener's granulomatosis. *Lancet*, **i**, 425–429.

van de Winkel, J.G.J., Tax, W.J.M., Groeneveld, A., Tamboer, W.P.M., de Mulder, P.H.M. and Capel, P.J.A. (1988) A new radiometric assay for the quantitation of surface-bound IgG on sensitized erythrocytes. *J. immunol. Methods*, **108**, 95–103.

van Dijk, B.A., Barrera Rico, P., Hoitsma, A. and Kunst, V.A.J.M. (1989) Immune hemolytic anemia associated with tolmetin and suprofen. *Transfusion*, **29**, 638–641.

Vandongen, R. and Gordon, R.D. (1969) Generation and survival of angiotensin in nonrefrigerated plasma: an explanation for presence of pressor material in human plasma protein solutions used clinically. *Transfusion*, **9**, 205.

van Hooff, J.P., Kalff, M.W., van Poelgeest, A.E., Persijn, G.G. and van Rood, J.J. (1976) Blood transfusions and kidney transplantation. *Transplantation*, **22**, 306.

van Kessel, A.H.M.G., Stoker, K., Claas, F.H.J., van Agothoren, A.J. and Hagemeier, A. (1983) Assignment of the leucocyte group five surface antigens to human chromosome 4. *Tissue Antigens*, **21**, 213–218.

van Leeuwen, A. (1979) Alloantibodies that react with subsets of human T cells. *Tissue Antigens*, **14**, 437–443.

van Leeuwen, A., Festenstein, H. and van Rood, J.J. (1980) Human alloimmune sera against T cell subsets. Detection and influence on pokeweed mitogen-stimulated Ig production in vitro. *J. exp. Med.* **152**, 235–242.

van Leeuwen, E.F., von dem Borne, A.E.G.Kr., von Riesz, L.E., Nijenhuis, L.E. and Engelfriet, C.P. (1981) Absence of platelet-specific alloantigens in Glanzmann's thrombasthenia. *Blood*, **57**, 49–54.

van Leeuwen, A., Festenstein, H. and van Rood, J.J. (1982a) Di-allelic alloantigenic systems on subsets of T-cells. *Hum. Immunol.* **4**, 109–121.

van Leeuwen, Eleonoor F., van der Ven, J.Th.M., Engelfriet, C.P. and von dem Borne, A.E.G.Kr. (1982b) Specificity of autoantibodies in autoimmune thrombocytopenia. *Blood*, **59**, 23–26.

van Loghem, J.J. (1947) Production of Rh agglutinins anti-C and anti-E by artificial immunization of volunteer donors. *Brit. med. J.* **ii**, 958.

van Loghem, J.J., Bartels, H.L.J.M. and van der Hart, Mia (1949) La production d'un anticorps anti-C^w par immunization artificielle d'un donneur bénévole. *Rev. Hémat.* **4**, 173.

van Loghem, J.J., Kresner, M., Coombs, R.R.A. and Fulton Roberts, G. (1950) Observations on a prozone phenomenon encountered in using the anti-globulin sensitization test. *Lancet*, **ii**, 729.

van Loghem, J.J., Harkink, H. and van der Hart, Mia (1953a) Production of the antibody anti-e by artificial immunization. *Vox Sang.* (O.S.), **3**, 22.

van Loghem, J.J. and van der Hart, Mia (1954) Varieties of specific auto-antibodies in acquired haemolytic anaemia. *Vox Sang.* (O.S.) **4**, 2.

van Loghem, J.J., van der Hart, Mia and Land, Madeleine E. (1955) Polyagglutinability of red cells as a cause of severe haemolytic transfusion reaction. *Vox Sang.* (O.S.), **5**, 125.

van Loghem, J.J., Dorfmeier, Hanny and van der Hart, Mia (1957) Two A antigens with abnormal serologic properties. *Vox Sang.* **2**, 16.

van Loghem, J.J., van der Hart, Mia, Hijmans, W. and Schutt, H.R.E. (1958) The incidence and significance of complete and incomplete white cell antibodies with special reference to the use of the Coombs consumption test. *Vox Sang.* **3**, 203.

van Loghem, J.J., Dorfmeier, Hanny and van der Hart, Mia (1959) Serological and genetical studies on a platelet antigen (Zw). *Vox Sang.* **4**, 161.

van Loghem, J.J., Peetoom, F., van der Hart, Mia, van der Veer, Marga, van der Giessen, Marijke, Prins, H.K., Zurcher, C. and Engelfriet, C.P. (1963) Serological and immunochemical studies in haemolytic anaemia with high-titre cold agglutinins. *Vox Sang.* **8**, 33.

van Loghem, J.J. (1965) Some comments on autoantibody induced red cell destruction. *Ann. N.Y. Acad. Sci.* **124**, 465.

van Loghem, J.J., van der Hart, Mia, Moes, Mieke and von dem Borne, A.E.G.Kr. (1965) Increased red cell destruction in the absence of demonstrable antibodies *in vitro*. *Transfusion*, **5**, 525.

van Loghem, Erna (1974) Familial occurrence of isolated IgA deficiency associated with antibodies to IgA. Evidence against a structural gene defect. *Europ. J. Immunol.* **4**, 56.

van Loghem, Erna and de Lange, Gerda (1975) Transfusion reactions caused by antibodies against immunoglobulins, in *Dr. Karl Landsteiner Foundation Annual Report*, Central Laboratory of the Netherlands Red Cross Blood Transfusion Service.

van Loghem, Erna, Zegers, B.J.M., Bast, E.J.E.G. and Kater, L. (1983) Selective deficiency of IgA2. *J. clin. Invest.* **72**, 1918–1923.

van Marwijk Kooy, M., van Prooyen, H.C., Borghuis, L. and Akkerman, J.W.N. (1989) The use of iloprost for leukocyte depletion of platelet concentrates by filtration. *Vox Sang.* **56**, 291–292.

van Marwijk Kooy, M., van Prooijen, H.C., Moes, M., Bosma-Stants,, Ineke, Akkerman, J.W.N. (1991) The use of leukocyte-depleted platelet concentrates for the prevention of refractoriness and primary HLA alloimmunization; a prospective, randomized trial. *Blood*, **77**, 201.

van Oss, C.J., Edberg, S.C. and Bronson, P.M. (1973) Valency of IgM, in *Specific Receptors of Antibodies, Antigens and Cells*, eds D. Pressman, T.B. Tomasi jr, A.L. Grossberg and N.R. Rose. S. Karger, Basel.

van Oss, C.J., Mohn, J.F. and Cunningham, R.K. (1978) Influence of various physicochemical factors on hemagglutination. *Vox Sang.* **34**, 351.

van Oss, C.J., Absolom, D.R., Grossberg, A.L. and Neumann, A.W. (1979) Repulsive van der Waals forces. I. Complete dissociation of antigen-antibody complexes by means of negative van der Waals forces. *Immunol. Commun.* **8**, 11–29.

van Oss, C.J., Beckers, D., Engelfriet, C.P., Absolom, D.R. and Neumann, A.W. (1981) Elution of blood group antibodies from red cells. *Vox Sang.* **40**, 367–371.

van Oss, C.J. and Absolom, D.R. (1983) Hemagglutination and the closest distance approach of normal, neuraminidase and papain-treated erythrocytes. *Vox Sang.* **47**, 250–256.

van Prooyen, H.C., van Marwijk Kooy, M., van Wilden, H.C., Aarts-Riemers, M.J., Borghuis, L. and Akkerman, J.W.N. (1990) Evaluation of a new source for irradiation of platelet concentrates. *Brit. J. Haemat.* **75**, 573–577.

van Rhenen, D.J., Thijssen, P.M.H.J. and Overbeeke, Marijke A.M. (1989) Testing efficacy of anti-D sera by a panel of donor red cells with weak reacting D antigen and with partial D antigens. *Vox Sang.* **56**, 274–277.

van Rood, J.J. (1958) Leucocyte antibodies in sera from pregnant women. *Nature (Lond.)*, **181**, 1735.

van Rood, J.J. and van Leeuwen, A. (1963) Leukocyte grouping. A method and its application. *J. clin. Invest.* **42**, 1382.

van Rood, J.J. and Ernisse, J.G. (1968) The detection of transplantation antigens in leukocytes. *Semin. Hemat.* **5**, 2.

van Rood, J.J., van Leeuwen, A. and van Santen, M.C.T. (1970) Anti-HL-A2 inhibitor in normal serum. *Nature (Lond.)*, **226**, 366.

van Rood, J.J., van Leeuwen, A., Keuning, J.J. and Blussé van Oud Alblas, A. (1975) The serological recognition of the human MLC determinants using a modified cytotoxicity technique. *Tissue Antigens*, **5**, 73,

van Rood, J.J., van Leeuwen, A., Termijtelen, A. and Keuning, J.J. (1976a) B-cell antibodies, Ia-like determinants, and their relation to MLC-determinants in man. *Transplant. Rev.* **30**, 122.

van Rood, J.J., van Leeuwen, A. and Ploem, J.S. (1976b) Simultaneous detection of two cell populations by two-colour fluorescence and application to the recognition of B-cell determinants. *Nature (Lond.)*, **262**, 795.

van Rood, J.J., van Leeuwen, A., Jonker, M., Termijtelen, A. and Keuning, J.J. (1976c) The HLA linkage group. *Exp. Hemat.* **4**, 237–242.

van't Veer, M.B., van Wieringen, P.M.V., van Leeuwen, I., Overbeeke, M.A.M., von dem Borne, A.E.G.Kr. and Engelfriet, C.P. (1981) A negative direct antiglobulin test with strong IgG red cell auto-antibodies present in the serum of a patient with autoimmune haemolytic anaemia. *Brit. J. Haemat.* **49**, 383–386.

van't Veer, M.B., van Leeuwen, I., Haas, F.J.L.M., Smelt, M., Overbeeke, M.A.M. and Engelfriet, C.P. (1984) Red-cell autoantibodies mimicking anti-Fy^b specificity. *Vox Sang.* **47**, 88–91.

van't Veer-Korthof, E.T., Niterink, J.S.G., van Nieuwkoop, J.A. and Eernisse, J.G. (1981) IgG subclasses in Rhesus-D immunization. Effects of weekly small volume plasmapheresis. *Vox Sang.* **41**, 207–211.

van Twuyver, Esther, Kast, W.M., Mooijaart, R.J.D., Wilmink, J.M., Melief, C.J.M. and de Waal, L.P. (1989) Allograft tolerance induction in adult mice associated with functional deletion of specific CTL precursors. *Transplantation*, **48**, 844–847.

van Twuyver, Esther, Kast, W.M., Mooijaart, R.J.D., Melief, C.J.M. and de Waal, L.P. (1990)

Induction of transplantation tolerance by intravenous injection of allogeneic lymphocytes across an H-2 class II mismatch. Different mechanisms operate in tolerization across an H-2 class I vs. H-2 class II disparity. *Eur. J. Immunol.* **20**, 441–444.

van Twuyver, Esther, Mooijaart, R.J.D., Ten Berge, Ineke, van der Horst, Anneke R., Wilmink, J.M., Kast, M., Melief, C.J.M. and de Waal, L.P. (1991) Pretransplantation blood transfusion revisited. *New Engl. J. Med.* **325**, 1210–1213.

Vartdal, F., Gaudernack, G., Funderud, S., Bratlie, Anne, Tor, Lea, Ugelstad, J. and Thorsby, E. (1986) HLA class I and II typing using cells positively selected from blood by immunomagnetic isolation—a fast and reliable technique. *Tissue Antigens*, **28**, 301–312.

Vaudin, M., Wolstenholme, A.J., Tsiquaye, K.N., Zuckerman, A.J. and Harrison, T.J. (1988) The complete nucleotide sequence of the genome of a hepatitis B virus isolated from a naturally infected chimpanzee. *J. gen Virol.* **69**, 1383–1389.

Vaughan, Janet M. (1942) Pigment metabolism following transfusion of fresh and stored blood. *Brit. med. J.* **i**, 548.

Vaughan-Neil, E.F., Ardeman, S., Bevan, G., Blakeman, A.C. and Jenkins, W.J. (1975) Post-transfusion purpura associated with unusual platelet antibody (anti-Pl^{B1}). *Brit. med. J.* **i**, 436.

Veall, N. and Mollison, P.L. (1950) The rate of red cell exchange in replacement transfusion. *Lancet*, **ii**, 792.

Vengelen-Tyler, V. and Morel, P. (1979) Serological and IgG subclass characterization of multiple examples of Cartwright^a (Yt^a) and Gerbich antibodies (Abstract). *Transfusion*, **19**, 650.

Vengelen-Tyler, V., Anstee, D.J., Issitt, P.D., Pavone, B.G., Ferguson, S.J., Mawby, W.J., Tanner, M.J.A., Blajchman, M.A. and Lorque, P. (1981) Studies on the blood of an Mi^v homozygote. *Transfusion*, **21**, 1–14.

Vengelen-Tyler, Virginia (1983) Letter to the Editor. *Red Cell Free Press*, **8**, 14.

Vengelen-Tyler, Virginia, Goya, K., Mogck, W., Kleinman, S., Wells, D.C. and Ridolfi, R.L. (1983) Autoantibody-hr^B appearing as an alloantibody: report of two cases (Abstract). *Transfusion*, **23**, 408.

Vengelen-Tyler, Virginia and Morel, P.A. (1983) Serologic and IgG subclass characterization of Cartwright (Yt) and Gerbich (Ge) antibodies. *Transfusion*, **23**, 114–116.

Vengelen-Tyler, Virginia (1984) The serological investigation of hemolytic disease of the newborn caused by antibodies other than anti-D, in *Hemolytic Disease of the Newborn*, ed G.

Garratty. Amer. Assoc. Blood Banks, Arlington, VA.

Vengelen-Tyler, Virginia (1985) Anti-Fy^a preceding anti-Fy3 or -Fy5: a study of five cases (Abstract). *Transfusion*, **25**, 482.

Vengelen-Tyler, Virginia, Gonzalez, B., Garratty, G., Kruppe, C., Johnson, C.L., Mueller, K.A. and Marsh, W.L. (1987) Acquired loss of red cell Kell antigens. *Brit. J. Haemat.* **65**, 231–234.

Vercellotti, G.M., Hammerschmidt, D.E., Craddock, P.R. and Jacob, H.S. (1982) Activation of plasma complement by perfluorocarbon artificial blood: probable mechanism of adverse pulmonary reactions in treated patients and rationale for corticosteroid prophylaxis. *Blood*, **59**, 1299–1304.

Verheugt, F.W.A., von dem Borne, A.E.G.Kr., Decary, F. and Engelfriet, C.P. (1977) The detection of granulocyte alloantibodies with an indirect immunofluorescence test. *Brit. J. Haemat.* **36**, 533.

Verheugt, F.W.A., von dem Borne, A.E.G.Kr., van Noord-Bokhorst, J.C., Nijenhuis, L.E. and Engelfriet, C.P. (1978) ND$_1$, a new neutrophil granulocyte antigen. *Vox Sang.* **35**, 13.

Verheugt, F.W.A., van Noord-Bokhorst, J.C., von dem Borne, A.E.G.Kr. and Engelfriet, C.P. (1979) A family with allo-immune neonatal neutropenia: group-specific pathogenicity of maternal antibodies. *Vox Sang.* **36**, 1–8.

Vernant, J.C., Maurs, L., Gessain, A., Barin, F., Gout, O., Delaporte, J.M., Sanhadji, K., Buisson, G. and de The, G. (1987) Endemic tropical spastic paraparesis associated with T-lymphotropic virus type I: a clinical and seroepidemiological study of 25 cases. *Ann. Neurol.* **21**, 123–130.

Veronese, F.D., Copeland, T.D., Oroszlan, S, Gallo, R.C. and Sarngadharan, M.G. (1988) Biochemical and immunological analysis of human immunodeficiency virus *gag* gene products p17 and p24. *J. Virol.* **62**, 795–801.

Verrier Jones, J. (1990) Staphylococeal protein A as an extracorporeal immunosorbent: theoretical and practical considerations. *Transfus. Sci.* **11**, 153–159.

Vessman, J. and Rietz, Gunilla (1978) Formation of mono(ethylhexyl)phthalate from di(ethylhexyl)phthalate in human plasma stored in PVC bags and its presence in fractionated plasma proteins. *Vox Sang.* **35**, 75.

Vest, M., Strebel, L. and Hauenstein, D. (1965) The extent of 'shunt' bilirubin and erythrocyte survival in the newborn infant measured by the administration of (^{15}N) glycine. *Biochem. J.* **95**, 11c.

Vettore, L., de Matteis, Maria C. and Zampini, Patrizia (1980) A new density gradient system for the separation of human red blood cells. *Amer. J. Hemat.* **8**, 291–297.

Vicariot, M., Abgroll, J.F., Dutel, J.L., Leglise, M.C. and Brieze, J. (1984) Alloimmunization anti-leuco-plaquettaire en reanimation hematologique. Les transfusions de plaquettes de donneurs uniques presentent-elles un avantage sur les plaquettes de donneurs multiples. *Rev. franç. Transfus. Immunohémat.* **27**, 35–43.

Vichinsky, E.P., Earles, Ann, Johnson, R.A., Hoag, Silvija M., Williams, A. and Lubin, B. (1990) Alloimmunization in sickle cell anaemia and transfusion of racially unmatched blood. *New Engl. J. Med.* **322**, 1617–1622.

Victoria, E.J., Muchmore, E.A., Sudora, E.J. and Masouredis, S.P. (1975) The role of antigen mobility in anti-Rh_0 (D)-induced agglutination. *J. clin. Invest.* **56**, 292.

Viggiano, E., Clary, N.L. and Ballas, S.K. (1982) Autoanti-K antibody mimicking an alloantibody. *Transfusion*, **22**, 329–332.

Vilaseca, J.A., Cerisola, J.A., Olarte, J.A. and Zothner, A. (1966) The use of crystal violet in the prevention of the transmission of Chagas-Mazza disease (South American trypansomiasis). *Vox Sang.* **11**, 711.

Vilmer, E. and 10 others (1984) Isolation of a new lymphotropic retrovirus from two siblings with haemophilia B, one with AIDS. *Lancet*, **i**, 753–757.

Vincenzi, F.F. and Hinds, T.R. (1988) Decreased Ca pump ATPase activity associated with increased density in human red blood cells. *Blood Cells*, **14**, 139–148.

Vinci, G. and 10 others (1984) Immunologic study of *in vivo* maturation of human megakaryocytes. *Brit. J. Haemat.* **56**, 589–605.

Virgilio, R.W., Smith, D.E., Rice, C.L., Hobelmann, C.F. and Peters, R.M. (1977) To filter or not to filter? (Abstract). *Intensive Care Medicine*, **3**, 144.

Virgilio, R.W., Rice, C.L., Smith, D.E., James, D.R., Zarins, C.K., Hobelmann, C.F. and Peters, R.M. (1979) Crystalloid vs. colloid resuscitation: is one better? *Surgery*, **85**, 129–139.

Virmani, R., Warren, D., Rees, R., Fink, L.M. and English, D. (1983) Effects of perfluorochemical on phagocytic function of leukocytes. *Transfusion*, **23**, 512–515.

Vlahakes, G.J., Lee, R., Jacobs, E.E. jr, Laraia, P.J. and Austen, W.G. (1990) Hemodynamic effects and oxygen transport properties of a new blood substitute in a model of massive blood replacement. *J. thoracic cardiovasc. Surg.* **100**, 379–388.

Voak, D. and Lodge, T.W. (1968) The role of H in the development of A. *Vox Sang.* **15**, 345.

Voak, D., Lodge, T.W., Hopkins, J. and Bowley, C.C. (1968) A study of the antibodies of the H'O'I-B complex with special reference to their occurrence and notation. *Vox Sang.* **15**, 353.

Voak, D. (1969) The pathogenesis of ABO haemolytic disease of the newborn. *Vox Sang.* **17**, 481.

Voak, D. and Bowley, C.C. (1969) A detailed serological study on the prediction and diagnosis of ABO haemolytic disease of the newborn (ABO HD). *Vox Sang.* **17**, 321.

Voak, D., Lodge, T.W. and Reed, J.V. (1969) The enhancement of *Ulex europaeus* anti-H activity by human serum. *Vox Sang.* **17**, 134.

Voak, D., Lodge, T.W., Stapleton, R.R., Fogg, H. and Roberts, H.E. (1970) The incidence of H-deficient A_2 and A_2B bloods and family studies on the AH/ABH status of an A_{int} and some new variant blood types. *Vox Sang.* **19**, 73–84.

Voak, D. and Williams, M.A. (1971) An explanation of the failure of the direct antiglobulin test to detect erythrocyte sensitization in ABO haemolytic disease of the newborn and observations on pinocytosis of IgG anti-A antibodies in infant (cord) red cells. *Brit. J. Haemat.* **20**, 9.

Voak, D. (1972) Observations on the rare phenomenon of anti-A prozone and the non-specific blocking of haemagglutination due to C1 complement fixation by IgG anti-A antibodies. *Vox Sang.* **22**, 408.

Voak, D., Abu-Sin, A.Y. and Downie, D.M. (1973) Observations on the thermal optimum, saline agglutinating activity and partial neutralization characteristics of IgG anti-A antibodies. *Vox Sang.* **24**, 246.

Voak, D., Downie, D.M., Haigh, T. and Cook, N. (1982) Improved antiglobulin tests to detect difficult antibodies: detection of anti-Kell by LISS. *Med. Lab. Sciences*, **39**, 363–370.

Voak, D., Lachmann, P.J., Downie, D.M., Oldroyd, R.G. and Bevas, P.C. (1983) Monoclonal antibodies—C3 serology. *Biotest Bulletin*, **4**, 339–347.

Voak, D., Downie, D.M., Moore, B.P.L. and Engelfriet, C.P. (1986a) Anti-human globulin reagent specification. The European and ISBT/ICSH view. *Biotest Bulletin*, **1**, 7–22.

Voak, D., Downie, D.M., Moore, B.P.L., Ford, D.S., Engelfriet, C.P. and Case, J. (1986b) Quality control of anti-human globulin tests: use of replicate tests to improve performance. *Biotest Bulletin*, **1**, 41–52.

Voak, D. (1990) Monoclonal antibodies as blood grouping reagents, in *Blood Transfusion, the Impact of New Technologies*, ed Marcela Contreras. *Baillière's Clinical Haematology*, **3**, 219–242.

Vogel, P., Rosenthal, N. and Levine, P. (1943) Hemolytic reactions as a result of isoimmunization following repeated transfusions of homologous blood. *Amer. J. clin. Path.* **13**, 1.

Vogelsang, Georgina B., Kickler, T.S. and Bell, W.R. (1986) Post-transfusion purpura: a report of five patients and a review of the pathogenesis and management. *Amer. J. Hemat.* **21**, 259–267.

Vogelsang, Georgina B. (1990) Transfusion-associated graft-versus-host disease in non-immunocompromised hosts. *Transfusion*, **30**, 101–103.

Vogler, W.R. and Winton, E.F. (1977) A controlled study of the efficacy of granulocyte transfusions in patients with neutropenia. *Amer. J. Med.* **63**, 548.

Vogt, Else, Krystad, Elly, Heistö, Helge and Myhere, Käre (1958) A second example of a strong anti-E reacting *in vitro* almost exclusively with enzyme-treated E-positive cells. *Vox Sang.* **3**, 118.

Voller, A. and Draper, C.C. (1982). Immunodiagnosis and seroepidemiology of malaria. *Brit. med. Bull.* **38**, 173–177.

von dem Borne, A.E.G.Kr., Engelfriet, C.P., Beckers, Do. van der Kort-Henkes, Gerda, van der Giessen, Marijke and van Loghem, J.J. (1969) Autoimmune haemolytic anaemias. II. Warm haemolysins—serological and immunochemical investigations and ^{51}Cr studies. *Clin. exp. Immunol.* **4**, 333.

von dem Borne, A.E.G.Kr., Beckers, Do., van der Meulen, F.W. and Engelfriet, C.P. (1977) IgG4 autoantibodies against erythrocytes, without increased haemolysis. *Brit. J. Haemat.* **37**, 137.

von dem Borne, A.E.G.Kr., Verheught, F.W.A., Oosterhof, F., von Riesz, E., de la Riviere, A.B. and Engelfriet, C.P. (1978) A simple immunofluorescence test for the detection of platelet antibodies. *Brit. J. Haemat.* **39**, 195.

von dem Borne, A.E.G.Kr., von Riesz, E., Verheught, F.W.A., Ten Cate, J.W., Koppe, J.G., Engelfriet, C.P. and Nijenhuis, L.E. (1980) Bak^a, a new platelet-specific antigen involved in neonatal alloimmune thrombocytopenia. *Vox Sang.* **39**, 113–120.

von dem Borne, A.E.G.Kr., van Leeuwen, Eleonore F., von Riesz, L. Elly, van Boxtel, C.J. and Engelfriet, C.P. (1981) Neonatal alloimmune thrombocytopenia: detection and characterization of the responsible antibodies by the platelet immunofluorescence test. *Blood*, **57**, 649–656.

von dem Borne, A.E.G.Kr., Mol, J.J., Joustra-Maas, N., Pegels, J.G., Langenhuijsen, M.M.A.C. and Engelfriet, C.P. (1982) Autoimmune haemolytic anaemia with monoclonal IgM (K) anti-P cold autohaemolysins. *Brit. J. Haemat.* **50**, 345–350.

von dem Borne, A.E.C.Kr. and van der Plas-van Dalen, C.M. (1985) Further observations on posttransfusion purpura (Letter). *Brit. J. Haemat.* **61**, 374–375.

von dem Borne, A.E.G.Kr. and van der Plas-van Dalen, C.M. (1986) Bak^a and Lek^a are identical antigens. *Brit. J. Haemat.* **62**, 404–405.

von dem Borne, A.E.G.Kr., Pegels, J.G., van der Stadt, R.J., van der Plas-van Dalen, C.M. and Helmerhorst, F.M. (1986a) Thrombocytopenia associated with gold therapy: a drug-induced autoimmune disease? *Brit. J. Haemat.* **63**, 509–516.

von dem Borne, A.E.G.Kr., van der Lelie, J., Vox, J.J.E., van der Plas-van Dalen, C.M., Risseeuw-Bogaert, J., Ticheler, M.D.A. and Pegels, J.G. (1986b) Antibodies against crypt-antigens of platelets. Characterization and significance for the serologist, in *Platelet Serology, Research Progress and Clinical Implications*, eds F. Décary and G.A. Rock. S.A. Karger, Basel.

von dem Borne, A.E.G.Kr., Vos, J.J.E., van de Lelie, J., Bossers, B. and van Dalen, C.M. (1986c) Clinical significance of a positive immunofluorescence test in thrombocytopenia, in *Brit. J. Haemat.*, **64**, 767–776.

von dem Borne, A.E.G.Kr, Bos, M.J.E., Joustra-Maas, N., Tromp, J.F., Van Wijngaarden-du Bois and Tetteroo P.A.T. (1986d) A murine monoclonal IgM antibody specific for blood group P antigen (globoside). *Brit. J. Haemat.* **63**, 35–46.

von dem Borne, A.E.G.Kr. and Décary, Francine (1990) ICSH/ISBT Working Party on Platelet Serology Nomenclature of Platelet-Specific Antigens. *Vox Sang.* **55**, 176.

von Dungern (1900) Beitrage zur Immunitätslehre. *Munch. med. Wschr.* **47**, 677.

von Fliedner, V., Higby, D.J. and Kim, U. (1982) Graft-versus-host reaction following blood product transfusion. *Amer. J. Med.* **72**, 951–961.

von Restorff, W., Höfling, B., Holtz, J. and Bassenge, E. (1975) Effect of increased blood fluidity through hemodilution on coronary circulation at rest and during exercise in dogs. *Pflügers Arch.* **357**, 15–34.

Vontver, L.A. (1973) Rh sensitization associated with drug use. *J. Amer. med. Assoc.* **226**, 469.

Vos, G.H., Vos, Dell, Kirk, R.L. and Sanger, Ruth (1961) A sample of blood with no detectable Rh antigens. *Lancet*, **i**, 14.

Vos, G.H., Celano, M.J., Falkowski, F. and Levine, P. (1964) Relationship of a hemolysin resembling anti-Tj^a to threatened abortion in Western Australia. *Transfusion*, **4**, 87.

Vos, G.H. (1965) A comparative observation of the presence of anti-Tj^a-like hemolysins in relation to obstetric history, distribution of the various blood groups and the occurrence of immune anti-A or anti-B hemolysins among aborters and nonaborters. *Transfusion*, 5, 327.

Vos, G.H. (1966) The serology of anti-Tjᵃ-like hemolysins observed in the serum of threatened aborters in Western Australia. *Acta haemat.* (*Basel*), 35, 272.

Vos, G.H., Petz, L.D. and Fudenberg, H.H. (1970) Specificity of acquired haemolytic anaemia autoantibodies and their serological characteristics. *Brit J. Haemat.* 19, 57.

Vroclans-Deiminas, M. and Boivin, P. (1980) Analyse des resultats observés au cours de la recherche d'une auto-sensibilisation anti-erythrocytaire chez 2400 malades. *Rev. franç. Transfus. Immuno-hémat.* 23, 105–117.

Vullo, C. and Tunioli, Anna Maria (1961) The selective destruction of 'compatible' red cells transfused in a patient suffering from thalassaemia major. *Vox Sang.* 6, 583.

Vyas, G.N., Perkins, H.A. and Fudenberg, H.H. (1968) Anaphylactoid transfusion reactions associated with anti-IgA. *Lancet*, ii, 312.

Vyas, G.N., Holmdahl, L., Perkins, H.A. and Fudenberg, H.H. (1969) Serological specificity of human anti-IgA and its significance in transfusion. *Blood*, 34, 573.

Vyas, G.N. (1970) Antibodies to IgA causing anaphylactic reactions to small transfusions. *Amer. Assoc. Blood Banks Workshop on Transfusion Problems*, 2, 21.

Vyas, G.N. and Fudenberg, H.H. (1970) Immunobiology of human anti-IgA: a serologic and immunogenetic study of immunization to IgA in transfusion and pregnancy. *Clin. Genet.* 1, 45.

Vyas, G.N., Levin, A.S. and Fudenberg, H.H. (1970) Intrauterine isoimmunization caused by maternal IgA crossing the placenta. *Nature* (*Lond.*), 225, 275.

Vyas, G.N., Perkins, H.A., Yang, Y.M. and Basantani, G.K. (1975) Healthy blood donors with selective absence of immunoglobulin A: prevention of anaphylactic transfusion reactions caused by antibodies to IgA. *J. Lab. clin. Med.* 85, 838.

Vyas, G.N. and Perkins, H.A. (1976) Anti-IgA in blood donors (Letter). *Transfusion*, 16, 289.

Wadenvik, H. and Kutti, J. (1991) The *in vivo* kinetics of ¹¹¹In- and ⁵¹Cr-labelled platelets: a comparative study using both stored and fresh platelets. *Brit. J. Haemat.* 78, 523–528.

Wadsworth, G.R. (1955) Recovery from acute haemorrhage in normal men and women. *J. Physiol.* (*Lond.*), 129, 583.

Wagner, S.J., Friedman, L.I. and Dodd, R.Y. (1991) Approaches to the reduction of viral infectivity in cellular blood components and single donor plasma. *Transfus. Med. Rev.* 5, no. 1, 18–32.

Wagstaff, W. (1984) Use of plasma, plasma proteins and plasma substitutes. *Vox Sang.* 46, Suppl. 1, 10–11.

Wahl, C.M., Herman, J.H., Shirey, R.S., Kickler, T.S. and Ness, P.M. (1989) The activation of maternal and cord blood. *Transfusion*, 29, 635–637.

Wain-Hobson, S., Sonigo, P., Danos, O., Cole, S. and Alizon, M. (1985) Nucleotide sequence of the AIDS virus, LAV. *Cell*, 40, 9–17.

Wake, C.T., Long, E.O. and March, B. (1982) Allelic polymorphism and complexity of the genes for HLA-DR*β* chains—direct analysis by DNA–DNA hybridization. *Nature* (*Lond.*), 300, 372–374.

Waldman, A.A. and Shander, C. (1980) Human blood components I. Preparation and characteristics of leukocyte concentrates from single units of human blood. *Transfusion*, 20, 384–392.

Walker, W., Murray, Sheilagh and Russell, J.K. (1957) Stillbirth due to haemolytic disease of the newborn. *J. Obstet. Gynaec. Brit. Emp.* 44, 573.

Walker, W. (1958) The changing pattern of haemolytic disease of the newborn (1948–1957). *Vox Sang.* 3, 225 and 336.

Walker, L.G. (1973) Carrel's direct transfusion of a five day old infant. *Surg. Gynec. Obstet.* 137, 494.

Walker, R.H. (1982) Is a crossmatch using the indirect antiglobulin test necessary for patients with a negative antibody screen, in *Safety in Transfusion Practices*, eds H.F. Polesky and R.H. Walker. College of American Pathologists, Skokie, Illinois.

Walker, R.H. (1984) Relevance in the selection of serologic tests for the obstetric patient, in *Hemolytic Disease of the Newborn*, ed G. Garratty, pp. 173–200. Amer. Assoc. Blood Banks, Arlington, VA.

Walker, W.S., Yap, P.L., Kilpatrick, D.C., Bolton, F.E., Crawford, R.J. and Sang, C.T.M. (1988) Post transfusion purpura following open heart surgery: management by high dose intravenous immunoglobulin transfusion. *Blut*, 57, 323–325.

Walker, R.H., Dong-Tsamn, Lin and Hartrick, Mary B. (1989) Alloimmunization following blood transfusion. *Arch. Path. lab. Med.* 113, 254–261.

Walker, R.H. and Hartrick, M.B. (1991) Non-ABO clinically significant erythrocyte alloantibodies in Caucasian obstetric patients (Abstract). *Transfusion*, 31, Suppl. 52S.

Wallace, J. and Sharpey-Schafer, E.P. (1941) Blood changes following controlled haemorrhage in man. *Lancet*, ii, 393.

Wallace, J., Milne, G.R. and Barr, A. (1972) Total screening of blood donations for Australia (hepatitis associated) antigen and its antibody. *Brit. med. J.* **i**, 663.

Wallace, J. (1977) *Blood Transfusion for Clinicians.* Churchill Livingstone, Edinburgh.

Wallace, Margaret E. and Green, Trudell S. (1983) Special techniques, in *Selection of Procedures for Problem Solving*, p. 103. Amer. Assoc. Blood Banks, Arlington, VA.

Waller, Marion and Lawler, Sylvia D. (1962) A study of the properties of the Rhesus antibody (Ri) diagnostic for the rheumatoid factor and its application to Gm grouping. *Vox Sang.* **7**, 591.

Wallerstein, H. and Brodie, S.S. (1948) The efficiency of blood substitution. *Amer. J. clin. Path.* **18**, 857.

Wallhermfechtel, M.A., Pohl, B. and Chaplin, H. (1984) Alloimmunization in patients with warm autoantibodies: a retrospective study employing 3 donor alloabsorptions to aid in antibody detection. *Transfusion*, **24**, 482–485.

Wallvik, J. and Åkerblom, O. (1990) The platelet storage capability of different plastic containers. *Vox Sang.* **58**, 40–44.

Wallvik, J., Stenke, L. and Åkerblom, O. (1990) The effect of different agitation modes on platelet metabolism, tromboxane formation, and alpha-granular release during platelet storage. *Transfusion*, **30**, 639–643.

Walsh, R.J., Thomas, E.D., Chow, S.K., Fluharty, R.G. and Finch, C.A. (1949) Iron metabolism. Heme synthesis *in vitro* by immature erythrocytes. *Science*, **110**, 396.

Walsh, J.H., Purcell, R.H., Morrow, A.G., Chanock, R.H. and Schmidt, P.J. (1970) Posttransfusion hepatitis after open-heart operations. *J. Amer. med. Assoc.* **211**, 261.

Walter, C.W. and Murphy, W.P. (1952) A closed gravity technique for the preservation of whole blood in ACD solution utilizing plastic equipment. *Surg. Gynec. Obstet.* **94**, 687.

Walter, C.W., Kundsin, Ruth B. and Button, L.N. (1957) New technic for detection of bacterial contamination in a blood bank using plastic equipment. *New Engl. J. Med.* **257**, 364.

Walter, H., Biermann, L. and Sass, M.D. (1962) Preferential labelling of young erythrocytes by chromium *in vitro*. *Exp. Cell Res.* **27**, 193.

Wands, J.R., Fujita, Y.K., Isselbacher, K.J., Degott, C., Schellekens, H., Dazza, Marie-Christine, Thiers, Valerie, Tiollais, P. and Brechot, C. (1986) Identification and transmission of hepatitis B virus-related variants. *Proc. Nat. Acad. Sci. USA*, **83**, 6608–6612.

Wang, A.C., Faulk, W.P., Stuckey, M.A. and Fudenberg, H.H. (1970) Chemical differences of adult, fetal and hypogammaglobulinemic IgG immunoglobulins. *Immunochemistry*, **7**, 703.

Wang, L., Juji, T., Shibata, Y., Kuwata, S. and Tokunaga, K. (1991) Sequence variation of human platelet membrane glycoprotein IIIa associated with the Yuk[a]/Yuk[b] alloantigen system. *Proc. Jap. Acad.* **67**, 102–106.

Ward, H.K. (1957) The persistence of antibodies in the absence of antigenic stimulus. *Aust. J. exp. Biol. med. Sci.* **35**, 499.

Ward, H.K., Walsh, R.J. and Kooptzoff, Olga (1957) Rh antigens and immunological tolerance. *Nature (Lond.)*, **179**, 1352.

Ward, H.N. (1970) Pulmonary infiltrates associated with leukoagglutinin transfusion reactions. *Ann. intern. Med.* **73**, 689.

Ward, J.W. and 9 others (1987) Risk of human immunodeficiency virus infection from blood donors who later developed the acquired immunodeficiency syndrome. *Ann. intern. Med.* **106**, 61–62.

Ward, J.W. and 10 others (1988) Transmission of human immunodeficiency virus (HIV) by blood transfusions screened as negative for HIV antibody. *New Engl. J. Med.* **318**, 473–478.

Ward, J.W. and 14 others (1989) The natural history of transfusion-associated infection with human immunodeficiency virus. *New Engl. J. Med.* **321**, 947–952.

Warkentin, Phyllis I., Yomtovian, Roslyn, Hurd, D., Brunning, R., Swanson, Jane, Kersey, J.H. and McCullough, J. (1983) Severe delayed hemolytic transfusion reaction complicating an ABO-incompatible bone marrow transplantation. *Vox Sang.* **45**, 40–47.

Warkentin, Phyllis I., Hilden, Joanne M., Kersey, J.H., Ramsay, Norma K.C. and McCullough, J. (1985) Transplantation of major ABO-incompatible bone marrow depleted of red cells by hydroxyethyl starch. *Vox Sang.* **48**, 89–104.

Warner, W.L. (1970) Red cell preservation and survival determinations in anticoagulant systems, in *Modern Problems of Blood Preservation*, eds W. Spielmann and S. Seidl. Gustav Fischer, Stuttgart.

Warren, R.C., Butler, Joan, Morsman, J.M., McKenzie, Christine and Rodeck, C.H. (1985) Does chorionic villus sampling cause fetomaternal haemorrhage? *Lancet*, **i**, 691.

Wasi, P., Na-Nakorn, S., Pootrakul, P., Sonakul, D., Piankijagum, A. and Pacharee, P. (1978) A syndrome of hypertension, convulsion, and cerebral haemorrhage in thalassaemic patients after multiple blood-transfusions. *Lancet*, **ii**, 602.

Waśniowska, Kazimiera, Drzeniek, Zofia and Lisowska, Elwira (1977) The amino acids of M and N blood group glycopeptides are different. *Biochem. biophys. Res. Comm.* **76**, 385.

Watanabe, K. and Hakomori, S. (1976) Status of blood group carbohydrate chains in ontogenesis and oncogenesis. *J. exp. Med.* **144**, 644–653.

Watanabe, K., Hakomori, S., Childs, R.A. and Feizi, T. (1979) Characterization of a blood group I-active ganglioside. Structural requirements for I and i specificities. *J. biol. Chem.* **254**, 3221–3228.

Watanabe, T., Seiki, M. and Yoshida, M. (1984) HTLV type I (U.S. isolate) and ATLV (Japanese isolate) are the same species of human retrovirus. *Virology*, **133**, 238–241.

Waters, A.H. and 9 others (1987) Fetal platelet transfusions in the management of alloimmune thrombocytopenia (Abstract). *Thrombos. Haemostas.* **58**, 323.

Watkins, Winifred M. and Morgan, W.T.J. (1959) Possible genetical pathways for the biosynthesis of blood group mucopolysaccharides. *Vox Sang.* **4**, 97.

Watkins, Winifred M. (1966) Blood-group substances. *Science*, **152**, 172.

Watkins, Winifred M. and Morgan, W.T.J. (1976) Immunochemical observations on the human blood group P system. *J. Immunogenet.* **3**, 15.

Watkins, Winifred M. (1980) Biochemistry and genetics of the ABO, Lewis, and P blood group systems, in *Advances in Human Genetics*, eds H. Harris and K. Hirschhorn. Plenum Publishing Corporation, New York.

Watkins, M. Winifred, Greenwell, Pamela and Yates, A.D. (1980) Blood group A and B transferase levels in serum and red cells of human chimaeras. *Rev. franç. Transfus. Immunohémat.* **23**, 531–544.

Watkins, W.M., Greenwell, P. and Yates, A.D. (1981) The genetic and enzymic regulation of the synthesis of the A and B determinants in the ABO blood group system. *Immunol. Commun.* **10**, 83–100.

Watkins, Winifred, M. (1990) Monoclonal antibodies as tools in genetic studies on carbohydrate blood group antigens. *J. Immunogenet.* **17**, 259–276.

Watson, K.C. and Joubert, S.M. (1960) Haemagglutination of cells treated with antibiotics. *Nature (Lond.),* **188**, 505.

Weatherall, D.J. and Clegg, J.B. (1981) *The Thalassaemia Syndromes*. Blackwell Scientific Publications, Oxford.

Weatherall, D.J. (1991) *The New Genetics and Clinical Practice*. 3rd edn. Oxford University Press, Oxford.

Weber, J.N. and 10 others (1987) Human immunodeficiency virus infection in two cohorts of homosexual men: neutralising sera and association of anti-gag antibody with prognosis. *Lancet*, **i**, 119–122.

Webster, A.D.B. and Lever, A.M.L. (1986) Non-A, non-B hepatitis after intravenous gammaglobulin. *Lancet*, **i**, 322.

Wedzicha, J.A., Rudd, R.M., Apps, M.C.P., Cotter, F.E., Newland, A.C. and Empey, D.W. (1983) Erythrapheresis in patients with polycythaemia secondary to hypoxic lung disease. *Brit. med. J.* **i**, 511–514.

Weech, A.A., Vann, Dorothea and Grillo, Rose A. (1941) The clearance of bilirubin from the plasma. A measure of the excretory power of the liver. *J. clin. Invest.* **20**, 323.

Weed, R.I. and LaCelle, P.L. (1969) ATP dependence of erythrocyte membrane deformability, in *Red Cell Membrane Structure and Function*, eds G.A. Jamieson and T.J. Greenwalt. Lippincott, Philadelphia.

Weeden, Ann R., Datta, Naomi and Mollison, P.L. (1960) Adsorption of bacteria on to red cells leading to positive antiglobulin reactions. *Vox Sang.* **5**, 523.

Wegmann, T.G. and Smithies, O. (1966) A simple hemagglutination system requiring small amounts of red cells and antibodies. *Transfusion*, **6**, 67.

Weiden, P.L., Flournoy, N., Thomas, E.D.,Prentice, R., Fefer, A., Buckner, C.D. and Sturb, R. (1979) Anti-leukemic effect of graft-versus-host disease in human recipients of allogenic marrow grafts. *New Engl. J. Med.* **300**, 1068.

Weigelt, J.A., Norcross, J.F., Borman, Karen R. and Snyder III, W.H. (1985) Early steroid therapy for respiratory failure. *Arch. Surg.* **120**, 536–540.

Weil, R. (1915) Sodium citrate in the transfusion of blood. *J. Amer. med. Assoc.* **64**, 425.

Weiland, D., Mattsson, L. and Glaumann, H. (1986) Non-A, non-B hepatitis after intravenous gammaglobulin. *Lancet*, **i**, 976–977.

Weiner, W., Battey, D.A., Cleghorn, T.E., Marson, F.G.W. and Meynell, M.J. (1953) Serological findings in a case of haemolytic anaemia; with some general observations on the pathogenesis of the syndrome. *Brit. med. J.* **ii**, 125.

Weiner, W., Tovey, G.H., Gillespie, E.M., Lewis, H.B.M. and Holliday, T.D.S. (1956) Albumin auto-agglutinating property in three sera. A pitfall for the unwary. *Vox Sang.* **1**, 279.

Weiner, W. (1961) Reconstitution of frozen red cells. *Lancet*, **i**, 1264.

Weiner, W. and Vos, G.H. (1963) Serology of acquired hemolytic anemias. *Blood*, **22**, 606.

Weiner, W., Gordon, E.G. and Rowe, D. (1964) A Donath-Landsteiner antibody (non-syphilitic type). *Vox Sang.* **9**, 684.

Weiner, Amy J. and 11 others (1990a) HCV testing in low-risk populations (Letter). *Lancet*, **ii**, 695.

Weiner, Amy J., Kuo, G., Bradley, D.W., Bonino F., Saracco, G., Lee, Cindy, Rosenblatt, Jody, Choo, Q-L. and Houghton, M. (1990b) Detection of hepatitis C viral sequences in non-A, non-B hepatitis. *Lancet*, **i**, 1–3.

Weiner, Amy J. and 10 others (1991) Variable and hypervariable domains are found in the regions of HCV corresponding to the flavivirus envelope and NS1 proteins and the pestivirus envelope glycoproteins. *Virology*, 180, 842–848.

Weinstein, L. and Taylor, E.S. (1975) Hemolytic disease of the neonate secondary to anti-Fy[a]. *Amer. J. Obstet. Gynec.* 121, 643.

Weisberg, L.J. and Linker, C.A. (1984) Prednisone therapy of post-transfusion purpura. *Ann. intern. Med.* 100, 76–77.

Weisel, R.D., Dennis, R.C., Manny, J., Mannick, J.A., Valeri, C.R. and Hechtmann, H.B. (1978) Adverse effects of transfusion therapy during abdominal aortic aneurysmectomy. *Surgery*, 83, 682.

Weisert, O. and Marstrander, J. (1960) Severe anemia in a newborn caused by protracted feto-maternal "transfusion". *Acta Paediat.* 49, 426.

Weiss, R.A. (1990) Human immunodeficiency viruses, in *Haematology in HIV Disease*, ed. Christine Costello. *Baillière's Clinical Haematology*, 3, 207–214.

Weitzel, H., Hunermann, B., Stolp, W., Dennhardt, Angelika and Schneider, J. (1974) Immunclearance D-positiver Erythrozyten nach Anwendung unterschiedlicher anti-D-Präparate, in *Prophylaxe der Rhesus-Sensibilisierung*, eds J. Schneider and H. Weitzel. Medizinische Verlagsgesellschaft, Frankfurt.

Wells, J.V., Bleumers, J.F. and Fudenberg, H.H. (1973) Immunobiology of human anti-IgM iso-antibodies. I. Clinical and serological studies. *Clin. Immunol. Immunopath.* 1, 257.

Wells, G.M., Woodward, T.E., Fiset, P. and Hornick, R.B. (1978) Rocky mountain spotted fever caused by blood transfusion. *J. Amer. med. Assoc.* 239, 2763–2765.

Wells, J.V. (1980) Immunoglobulins: biosynthesis and metabolism, in *Basic and Clinical Immunology*, 3rd edn, eds H.H. Fudenberg, D.P. Sites, J.L. Caldwell and J.V. Wells pp. 64–78. Lange Med. Publications, Los Altos, California.

Wells, Linda and Ala, F.A. (1985) Malaria and blood transfusion *Lancet*, i, 1317–1319.

Welsh, K.J., Burgoss, H. and Batchelor, R. (1977) Immune response to allogeneic rat platelets: Ag-B antigens in matrix lacking Ia. *Eur. J. Immunol.* 7, 267–272.

Wendel, S. and Gonzaga, A.L. (1992) Chagas disease and blood transfusion: a new world problem? *Vox Sang.* in press.

Wenk, R.E., Goldstein, P. and Felix, J.K. (1985) Kell alloimmunization, hemolytic disease of the newborn, and perinatal management. *Obstet. Gynec.* 66, 473–476.

Wensley, R.T. and Snape, T.J. (1980) Preparation of improved cryoprecipitated Factor VIII concentrate: a controlled study of three variables affecting the yield. *Vox Sang.* 38, 222–228.

Wenz, B. and Apuzzo, J. (1989) Polyethylene glycol improves the indirect antiglobulin test. *Transfusion*, 29, 218–220.

Wenz, B., Apuzzo, J. and Shah, D.P. (1990) Evaluation of the polyethylene glycol-potentiated indirect antiglobulin test. *Transfusion*, 30, 318–321.

Wernet, Ch., Klouda, P.T., Carrea, M.C., Vassali, P. and Jeannet, M. (1977) Isolation of B and T lymphocytes by nylon filter columns. *Tissue Antigens*, 9, 227.

Wessler, S. and Gitel, S.N. (1979) Heparin: new concepts relevant to clinical use. *Blood*, 53, 525–544.

West, C.D., Hong, R. and Holland, Nancy H. (1962) Immunoglobulin levels from the newborn period to adulthood and in immunoglobulin deficiency states. *J. clin. Invest.* 41, 2054.

West, N.C., Jenkins, J.A., Johnston, B.R. and Modi, N. (1986) Interdonor incompatibility due to anti-Kell antibody undetectable by automated antibody screening. *Vox Sang.* 50, 174–176.

Westman, B.J.M. (1972) Serum creatinine and creatinine clearance after transfusion and ACD-adenine blood and ACD blood. *Transfusion*, 12, 371.

Westman, M. (1974) Studies for evaluation of blood preservation procedures with special regard to the oxygen release function and the toxicity of adenine. Doctoral Thesis, University of Uppsala.

Westphal, O. (1957) Pyrogens, in *Polysaccharides in Biology*. Transactions 2nd Conf., 1956, p. 115. Josiah Macy jr Foundation, New York.

Westphal, R.G. (1984) Health risks to cytapheresis donors, in *Blood Transfusion and Blood Banking, Clinics in Haemat.* 13, 289–301.

Westphal, R. (1991a) Transfusion-transmitted malarial infections in *Transfusion-Transmitted Infections*, ed D.M. Smith and R.Y. Dodd, pp. 167–180. ASCP Press, Chicago.

Westphal, R. (1991b) Other parasitic organisms transmitted by transfusion in *Transfusion-Transmitted Infections*, eds D.M. Smith and R.Y. Dodd, pp. 181–193. ASCP Press, Chicago.

Wewers, M.D., Casolaro, M.A. and Sellers, B.E. (1987) Replacement therapy for alpha$_1$-antitrypsine deficiency associated with emphysema. *New Engl. J. Med.* 316, 1055–1062.

Wexler, L.B., Pincus, J.B., Matelson, S. and Lugovoy, J. (1949) The fate of citrate in erythroblastic infants treated with exchange transfusion. *J. clin. Invest.* **28**, 474.

White, W.D., Issitt, C.H. and McGuire, D. (1974) Evaluation of the use of albumin controls in Rh phenotyping. *Transfusion*, **14**, 67.

White, J.V. (1981) Complement activation during cardiopulmonary bypass (Letter). *New Engl. J. Med.* **305**, 51.

White, N.J. (1987) Chloroquine for donated blood? *Lancet*, 100–101.

White, P.M.B. (1988) Comparison of assays for antibody to HTLV-I. *J. clin. Path.* **41**, 700–702.

White, G., Gomperts, E., Lin-Maruya, S. and the Recombinate$_T^M$ Collaborative Study Group (1991) Long-term safety and efficiency clinical trial with recombinant Factor VIII. *Thrombos. Haemostas. Abstracts XIIIth Congress of the International Society on Thrombosis and Haemostasis*, Abstract, 180.

Whitrow, W. and Ross, D.W. (1990) Automation in blood grouping: impact of microplate technology, in *Blood Transfusion: the Impact of New Technologies*, ed Marcela Contreras. *Baillière's Clinical Haematology*, **3**, pp. 255–266.

WHO (1971) Prevention of Rh sensitization. *Technical Report Series*, **468**.

WHO (1975) Meeting on the utilization and supply of human blood and blood products, Bern, Switzerland, in *Resolutions, Recommendations and Decisions on Blood Transfusion*. League of Red Cross and Red Crescent Societies, Geneva.

WHO (1976) Review of the notation for the allotypic and related markers of human immunoglobulins. Amended report of WHO meeting. 1974. *J. Immunol.* **117**, 1056.

WHO (1977) Twenty-eighth Report of WHO Expert Committee on Biological Standardization. *Technical Report Series*, **610**.

WHO (1983) Viral hepatitis. The use of normal and specific immunoglobulin. *Weekly epid. Record*, **58**, 237.

WHO (1985) Immunodiagnosis of malaria. *WHO/ Malaria document*, pp. 10–18.

WHO (1986) Severe and complicated malaria. *Transact. Roy. Soc. trop. Med. Hyg.* **80**, 1–50.

WHO (1987) Recommendations following the meeting and consultation on the safety of blood and blood products, in *AIDS: The Safety of Blood and Blood Products*, eds J.C. Petricciani, I.D. Gust, P.A. Hoppe and H.W. Krijnen. pp. 355–359. John Wiley & Sons Ltd., U.K.

WHO (1989) Requirements for the collection, processing and quality control of blood, blood components and plasma derivatives, in *WHO Technical Series Report*, **786**, pp. 94–176.

WHO (1990) Acquired immunodeficiency syndrome (AIDS). Proposed criteria for interpreting results from Western blot assays for HIV-1, HIV-2 and HTLV-I/HTLV-II. *Weekly Epidemiol. Record*, **65**, 281–288.

WHO (1992) Global programme on AIDS. Current and future dimensions of the HIV/AIDS pandemic, a capsule summary.

Wickerhauser, M. and Williams, C. (1984) A single-step method for the isolation of antithrombin III. *Vox Sang.* **47**, 397–405.

Wiener, A.S. (1934) Longevity of the erythrocyte. Letter to the Editor. *J. Amer. med. Assoc.* **102**, 1779.

Wiener, A.S. and Peters, H.R. (1940) Hemolytic reactions following transfusions of blood of the homologous group, with three cases in which the same agglutinogen was responsible. *Ann. intern. Med.* **13**, 2306.

Wiener, A.S. (1941a) Subdivisions of group A and group AB. II. Isoimmunization of A_2 individuals against A_1 blood; with special reference to the role of the subgroups in transfusion reactions. *J. immunol.* **41**, 181.

Wiener, A.S. (1941b) Hemolytic reactions following transfusions of blood of the homologous group. II. Further observations on the role of property Rh, particularly in cases without demonstrable iso-antibodies. *Arch. Path.* **32**, 227.

Wiener, A.S. (1942a) Hemolytic transfusion reactions. I. Diagnosis, with special reference to the method of differential agglutination. *Amer. J. clin. Path.* **12**, 189.

Wiener, A.S. (1942b) Hemolytic transfusion reactions. III. Prevention, with special reference to the Rh and cross-match tests. *Amer. J. clin. Path.* **12**, 302.

Wiener, A.S. (1943) *Blood Groups and Transfusion.* C.C. Thomas, Springfield, Illinois, U.S.A.

Wiener, A.S. and Moloney, W.C. (1943) Hemolytic transfusion reactions. IV. Differential diagnosis. 'Dangerous universal donor' or intragroup incompatibility. *Amer. J. clin. Path.* **13**, 74.

Wiener, A.S. and Unger, L.J. (1944) Isoimmunization to factor P by blood transfusion. *Amer. J. clin. path.* **14**, 616.

Wiener, A.S. (1944) A new test (blocking test) for Rh sensitization. *Proc. Soc. exp. Biol. (N.Y.)*, **56**, 173.

Wiener, A.S., Hurst, Jane G. and Sonn-Gordon, Eve B. (1947) Studies on the conglutination reaction, with special reference to the nature of conglutinin. *J. exp. Med.* **86**, 267.

Wiener, A.S. (1949) Further observations on isosensitization to the Rh factor. *Proc. Soc. exp. Biol. (N.Y.)*, **70**, 576.

Wiener, A.S., Wexler, L.B. and Hurst, Jane G. (1949) The use of exchange transfusion for the treatment of severe erythroblastosis due to A-B sensitization with observations on the pathogenesis of the disease. *Blood*, **4**, 1014.

Wiener, A.S. (1950) Reaction transfusionnelle hémolytique due à une sensibiliation anti-M. *Rev. Hémat.* **5**, 3,

Wiener, A.S. (1951a) The Rh-Hr blood types: serology, genetics and nomenclature. *Trans. N.Y. Acad. Sci.* **13**, 198.

Wiener, A.S. (1951b) Origin of naturally occurring hemagglutinins and hemolysins: a review. *J. Immunol.* **66**, 287.

Wiener, A.S., Samwick, A.A., Morrison, H. and Cohen, L. (1953a) Studies on immunization in man. I. The blood group substances A and B. *Exp. Med. Surg.* **11**, 267.

Wiener, A.S., Samwick, A.A., Morrison, H. and Cohen, L. (1953b) Studies on immunization in man. II. The blood factor C. *Exp. Med. Surg.* **11**, 276.

Wiener, A.S., Unger, L.J. and Gordon, Eve B. (1953c) Fatal hemolytic transfusion reaction caused by sensitization to a new blood factor U. *J. Amer. med. Assoc.* **153**, 1444.

Wiener, A.S. (1954) Newer blood factors and their clinical significance. *N.Y. State J. Med.* **54**, 3071.

Wiener, A.S., Samwick, A.A., Morrison, H. and Cohen, L. (1955) Studies on immunization in man. III. Immunization experiments with pooled human blood cells. *Exp. Med. Surg.* **13**, 347.

Wiener, A.S., Unger, L.J., Cohen, L. and Feldman, J. (1956) Type-specific cold autoantibodies as a cause of acquired hemolytic anemia and hemolytic transfusion reactions: biologic test with bovine red cells. *Ann. intern. Med.* **44**, 221.

Wiener, A.S. (1958) Blood group nomenclature. *Science*, **128**, 849.

Wiener, E. and Garner, S.F. (1985) The use of cultured macrophages and anti-human globulin reagents to detect complement-fixing red cell antibodies. *Abstracts, 3rd annual meeting Brit. Blood Transfus. Soc.*, Oxford.

Wiener, E. and Garner, S.F. (1987) The use of macrophages stimulated by immune interferon as indicator cells in the mononuclear phagocyte assay. *Clin. lab. Haemat.* **9**, 397–408.

Wiener, E., Atwal, A., Thompson, K.M., Melamed, M.D., Gorick, B. and Hughes-Jones, N.C. (1987) Differences between the activities of human monoclonal IgG1 and IgG3 subclasses of anti-Rh(D) antibodies in their ability to mediate red cell binding to macrophages. *Immunology*, **62**, 401–404.

Wiener, E., Jolliffe, V.M., Scott, H.C.F., Kumpel, B.M., Thompson, K.M., Melamed, D. and Hughes-Jones, N.C. (1988) Differences between the activities of human monoclonal IgG1 and IgG3 anti-D antibodies of the Rh blood group system in their abilities to mediate effector functions of monocytes. *Immunology*, **65**, 159–163.

Wiklander, O. (1956) Blood volume determinations in surgical practice. A comparative analysis of the Evans blue dye method, the radioactive phosphorus method and the alveolar CO method, with special reference to determinations under pre- and post-operative conditions. *Acta chir. scand.* Suppl. 208.

Wikström, U., Backman, B.G., Danielson, B.G., Fellström, B., Sjöberg, O. and Wahlberg, J. (1990) Plasmapheresis of HLA-immunized uremic patients before renal transplantation. *Transfus. Sci.* **11**, 341.

Wiktor, S.Z., Pate, E.J., Weiss, S.H., Gohd, R.S., Correa, P., Fontham, Elizabeth, Hanchard, B., Biggar, R.J. and Blattner, W.A. (1991) Sensitivity of HTLV-I antibody assays for HTLV-II (Letter). *Lancet*, **ii**, 512–513.

Wilczynska, Z., Miller-Podraza, H. and Koscielak, J. (1980) The contribution of different glycoconjugates to the total ABH blood group activity of human erythrocytes. *FEBS Letters*, **112**, 277–279.

Wilhelm, R.E., Nutting, H.M., Devlin, H.B., Jennings, E.R. and Brines, O.A. (1955) Antihistaminics for allergic and pyrogenic transfusion reactions. *J. Amer. med. Assoc.* **158**, 529.

Wilkerson, D.K., Rosen, A.L., Gould, S.A., Sehgal, L.R., Sehgal, H.L. and Moss, G.S. (1987) Oxygen extraction ratio: a valid indicator of myocardial metabolism in anemia. *J. surg. Res.* **42**, 629–634.

Williams, R.J. (1976) A proposed mechanism for PVP cryoprotection (Abstract). *Cryobiology*, **13**, 653.

Williams, J., Goff, J.R. and Anderson, H.R. (1980) Efficacy of transfusion therapy for one to two years in patients with sickle cell disease and cerebrovascular accidents. *J. Pediat.* **96**, 205–208.

Williams, D., Johnson, C.L. and Marsh, W.L. (1981) Duffy antigen changes on red blood cells stored at low temperature. *Transfusion*, **21**, 357–359.

Williams, J.G., Riley, T.R.D. and Moody, R.A. (1983) Resuscitation experience in the Falkland Islands campaign. *Brit. med. J.* **286**, 775–777.

Williams, B.D., O'Sullivan, Margaret M. and Ratanckaiyovong, Suvina (1985) Reticuloendothelial Fc function in normal individuals and its relationship to the HLA antigen DR3. *Clin. exp. Immunol.* **60**, 532–538.

Williams, P.E., Yap, P.L., Gillon, J., Crawford, R.J., Urbaniak, S.J. and Galea, G. (1989) Transmission of non-A, non-B hepatitis by pH4-treated intravenous immunoglobulin. *Vox Sang.* **57**, 15–18.

Williams, S.F., Bitran, J.D., Richards, J.M., de-Christopher, P.J., Barker, E., Conant, J., Golomb, H.M. and Orlina, A.R. (1990) Peripheral blood-derived stem cell collections for use in autologous transplantation after high dose chemotherapy: an alternative approach. *Bone Marrow Transplantation*, **5**, 129–133.

Williams, A.E. and Sullivan Marian, T. (1991) Other retroviruses transmitted by blood transfusion, in *Transfusion Transmitted Infections*, eds D.M. Smith and R.Y. Dodd, pp. 81–114. ASCP Press, Chicago.

Williamson, K.R. and Taswell, H.F. (1988) Intraoperative autologous transfusion (IAT): experience in over 8,000 surgical procedures (Abstract). *Transfusion*, **28**, 11S.

Williamson, K.R., Taswell, H.F., Rettke, S.R. and Crumb, R.A.F. (1989) Intraoperative autologous transfusion: its role in orthotopic liver transplantation. *Mayo Clin. Proc.* **64**, 340–345.

Wimer, B.M., Marsh, W.L., Taswell, H.F. and Galey, W.R. (1977) Haematological changes associated with the McLeod phenotype of the Kell blood group system. *Brit. J. Haemat.* **36**, 219.

Winchester, R.J. and Kunkel, H.G. (1979) The human Ia system. *Advances in Immunology*, **28**, 221–293.

Winearls, C.G., Oliver, D.O., Pippard, M.J., Reid, C., Downing, M.R. and Cotes, P. Mary (1986) Effect of human erythropoietin derived from recombinant DNA on the anaemia of patients maintained by chronic haemodialysis. *Lancet*, **ii**, 1175–1178.

Winkelstein, J.A. and Mollison, P.L. (1965) The antigen content of 'inagglutinable' group B erythrocytes. *Vox Sang.* **10**, 614.

Winkler, A.W. and Hoff, H.E. (1943) Potassium and the cause of death in traumatic shock. *Amer. J. Physiol.* **139**, 686.

Winston, D.J., Ho, W.G., Howell, C.L., Miller, M.J., Mickey, R., Martin, W.J., Lin, C.H. and Gale, R.P. (1980) Cytomegalovirus infections associated with leukocyte transfusions. *Ann. intern. Med.* **93**, 671–675.

Winston, D.J., Ho, W.G. and Gale, R.P. (1982) Therapeutic granulocyte transfusions for documented infections. A controlled trial in ninety-five infectious granulocytopenic episodes. *Ann. intern. Med.* **97**, 509–515.

Witebsky, E. (1946) Isolation and purification of blood group A and B substances; their use in conditioning universal donor blood, in neutralizing anti-Rh sera, and in the production of potent grouping sera. *Ann. N.Y. Acad. Sci.* **46**, 887.

Witebsky, E. (1948) Interrelationship between the Rh system and the ABO system. *Blood*, **3**, 66.

Witebsky, E. and Engasser, Lillian M. (1949) Blood groups and subgroups of the newborn. I. The A factor of the newborn. *J. Immunol.* **61**, 171.

With, T.K. (1949) On jaundice. *Acta med. scand.* Suppl. **234**.

Wolach, B., Heddle, Nancy, Barr, R.D., Zipursky, A., Pai, K.R.M. and Blajchman, M.A. (1981) Transient Donath-Landsteiner haemolytic anaemia. *Brit. J. Haemat.* **48**, 425–434.

Wolf, P.L., McCarthy, L.J. and Hafleigh, Betsy (1970) Extreme hypercalcemia following blood transfusion combined with intravenous calcium. *Vox Sang.* **19**, 544.

Wolf, C.F.W and Canale, V.C. (1976) Fatal pulmonary hypersensitivity reaction to HLA in compatible blood transfusion: report of a case and review of the literature. *Transfusion*, **16**, 135–140.

Wolf, M.W. and Roelcke, D. (1989) Incomplete warm hemolysins. II. Corresponding antigens and pathogenetic mechanisms in autoimmune hemolytic anemias induced by incomplete warm hemolysins. *Clin. Immunol. Immunopath.* **51**, 68–76.

Wolfe, M.S. (1975) Parasites, other than malaria, transmissible by blood transfusion, in *Transmissible Disease and Blood Transfusion*, eds T.J. Greenwalt and G.A. Jamieson. Grune & Stratton, New York.

Woll, Judith E., Smith, C.M. and Nusbacher, J. (1974) Treatment of acute cold agglutinin hemolytic anemia with transfusion of adult i RBCs. *J. Amer. med. Assoc.* **229**, 1779.

Wollman, E.E., Guilherme, L., Lepage, V. and Dausset, J. (1984) Non HLA antigenic determinants expressed on activated T and B human lymphocytes. *Tissue Antigens*, **23**, 1–11.

Wong, K.H., Skelton, S.K. and Feeley, J.C. (1985) Interaction of *Campylobacter jejuni* and *Campylobacter coli* with lectins and blood group antibodies. *J. clin. Microbiol.* **22**, 134–135.

Wong-Staal, Flossie and Gallo, R.C. (1985) Human T-lymphotropic retroviruses. *Nature (Lond.)*, **317**, 395–403.

Wong-Staal, Flossie, Shaw, G.M., Hahn, B.H., Salahuddin, S.Z., Popovic, M., Markham, P., Redfield, R. and Gallo, R.C. (1985) Genomic diversity of human T-lymphotrophic virus type III (HTLV-III). *Science*, **229**, 759–762.

Wong-Staal, F., Chanda, P.K. and Ghrayeb, J. (1987) Human immunodeficiency virus: the eighth gene. *AIDS Res. Hum. Retrov.* **3**, 33–39.

Wood, E.E. (1955) Brucellosis as a hazard of blood transfusion. *Brit. med. J.* **i**, 27.

Wood, L. and Beutler, E. (1967) The viability of

human blood stored in phosphate adenine media. *Transfusion*, **7**, 401.

Wood, L. and Beutler, E. (1971) Storage of erythrocytes in artificial media. *Transfusion*, **11**, 123.

Wood, L.A. and Beutler, E. (1973) The effect of ascorbate on the maintenance of 2,3-disphosphoglycerate (2,3-DPG) in stored red cells. *Brit. J. Haemat.* **25**, 611.

Wood, L. and Beutler, E. (1974) The effect of ascorbate and dihydroxyacetone on the 2,3-diphosphoglycerate and ATP levels of stored human red cells. *Transfusion*, **14**, 272.

Wood, W.I. and 13 others (1984) Expression of active human factor VIII from recombinant DNA clones. *Nature (Lond.)*, **312**, 330–337.

Wood, G.M., Levy, Lesley J., Losowsky, M.S., Cooke, D.I., Read, A.E., Hambling, M.H., Clarke, Suzanne, K.R., Waight, Pauline and Polakoff, Sheila. (1989) Chronic liver disease. A case control study of the effect of previous blood transfusion. *Public Health*, **103**, 105–112.

Woodfield, G., Giles, C., Poole, J., Oraka, R. and Tolanu, T. (1986) A further null phenotype (Sc-1-2) in Papua New Guinea. *Proc. 19th Congr. Int. Soc. Blood Transfus.*, Sydney, p. 651.

Woodford-Williams, E., Webster, D., Dixon, M.P. and Mackenzie, W. (1962) Red cell longevity in old age. *Geront. clin. (Basel)*, **4**, 183.

Woodrow, J.C., and 9 others (1965) Prevention of Rh-haemolytic disease: a third report. *Brit. med. J.* **i**, 279.

Woodrow, J.C. and Finn, R. (1966) Transplacental haemorrhage. *Brit. J. Haemat.* **12**, 297.

Woodrow, J.C. and Donohoe, W.T.A. (1968) Rh-immunization by pregnancy: results of a survey and their relevance to prophylactic therapy. *Brit. med. J.* **iv**, 139.

Woodrow, J.C., Bowley, C.C., Gilliver, B.E. and Strong, S.J. (1968) Prevention of Rh immunization due to large volumes of Rh-positive blood. *Brit. med. J.* **i**, 148.

Woodrow, J.C., Finn, R. and Krevans, J.R. (1969) Rapid clearance of Rh positive blood during experimental Rh immunization. *Vox Sang.* **17**, 349.

Woodrow, J.C. (1970) Rh immunization and its prevention. *Ser. Haemat.* **3**, No. 3.

Woodrow, J.C., Clarke, C.A., Donohoe, W.T.A., Finn, R., McConnell, R.B., Sheppard, P.M., Lehane, D., Roberts, Freda M. and Gimlette, T.M.D. (1975) Mechanism of Rh prophylaxis: an experimental study on specificity of immunosuppression. *Brit. med. J.* **2**, 57.

Woodruff, A.W., Topley, Elizabeth, Knight, R. and Downie, C.G.B. (1972) The anaemia of kala azar. *Brit. J. Haemat.* **22**, 319.

Woodruff, M.F.A. and van Rood, J.J. (1983) Possible implication of the effect of blood transfusion on allograft survival. *Lancet*, **i**, 1201–1202.

Woods, V.L., Oh, Esther H., Mason, Donna and McMillan, R. (1984a) Autoantibodies against the glycoprotein IIb/IIIa complex in patients with chronic ITP. *Blood*, **63**, 368–375.

Woods, V.L., Kurata, Y., Montgomery, R.R., Tani, Patricia, Mason, Donna, Oh, Esther H. and McMillan, R. (1984b) Autoantibodies against platelet glycoprotein Ib in patients with chronic ITP. *Blood*, **64**, 156–160.

Woods, V.L., Pischel, E.D., Avery, E.D. and Bluestein, H.G. (1989) Antigenic polymorphism of human very late activation protein-2 (platelet glycoprotein Ia-IIa): platelet alloantigen Hc^a. *J. clin. Invest.* **83**, 978–985.

Woof, J.M., Partridge, L.J., Jefferis, R. and Burton, D.R. (1986) Localization of the monocyte-binding region on human immunoglobulin G. *Molec. Immunol.* **23**, 319–330.

Worlledge, Sheila M. and Rousso, C. (1965) Studies on the serology of paroxysmal cold haemoglobinuria (P.C.H.), with special reference to its relationship with the P blood group system. *Vox Sang.* **10**, 293.

Worlledge, Sheila M., Carstairs, K.C. and Dacie, J.V. (1966) Autoimmune haemolytic anaemia associated with α-methyldopa therapy. *Lancet*, **ii**, 135.

Worlledge, Sheila, M. (1969) Immune drug-induced haemolytic anaemias. *Semin. Haemat.* **6**, 181.

Worlledge, Sheila M. and Dacie, J.V. (1969) Haemolytic and other anaemias in infectious mononucleosis, in *Infectious Mononucleosis*, eds R.L. Carter and H.G. Penman. Blackwell Scientific Publications, Oxford.

Worlledge, Sheila, Ogiemudia, S.E., Thomas, C.O., Ikoku, B.N. and Luzzatto, L. (1974) Blood group antigens and antibodies in Nigeria. *Ann. trop. Med. Parasit.* **68**, 249.

Worlledge, S.M. (1977) Red cell antigens in dyserythropoiesis, in *Dyserythropoiesis*, eds S.M. Lewis and R.A.L. Verwilghen. Academic Press, New York.

Worlledge, Sheila (1978) Results published in the 6th edition of this book, p. 397.

Worsley, A., Cuttner, J., Gordon, R., Reilly, M., Ambinder, E.P. and Conjalka, M. (1982) Therapeutic leukapheresis in a patient with hairy cell leukemia presenting with a white cell count greater than 500,000/μl. *Transfusion*, **22**, 308–310.

Worwood, M. (1980) Serum ferritin, in *Iron in Biochemistry and Medicine* 2, ed A. Jacobs, Academic Press, New York.

Worwood, M. (1987) The diagnostic value of serum ferritin determinations for assessing iron status. *Haematologia*, **20**, 229–235.

Wren, M.R. and Issitt, P.D. (1988) Evidence that Wr[a] and Wr[b] are antithetical. *Transfusion*, **28**, 113–118.

Wright, G. and Sanderson, J.M. (1974) A.C.D. and C.P.D. blood preservation. *Lancet*, **ii**, 173.

Wright, J., Freedman, J., Lim, F.C. and Garvey, M.B. (1979) Crossmatch difficulties following the prophylactic use of Rh immune globulin. *Canad. med. Assoc. J.* **120**, 1235–1238.

Wright, D.G., Karsh, J., Fauci, A.S., Kippel, J.H., Decker, J.L., O'Donnel, J. and Deisseroth, A.B. (1981) Lymphocyte depletion and immuno-suppression with repeated leukapheresis by continuous flow centrifugation. *Blood*, **58**, 451–458.

Wright, A., Hecke, J.F. and Lewis, G.B.H. (1985) Use of transdermal glyceryl trinitrate to reduce failure of intravenous infusion due to phlebitis and extravasation. *Lancet*, **ii**, 1148–1150.

Wrobel, Damiana M., McDonald, Ione, Race, Caroline and Watkins, Winifred M. (1974) 'True' genotype of chimeric twins revealed by blood-group gene products in plasma. *Vox Sang.* **27**, 395.

Wurmser, R., Filitti-Wurmser, S. and Briault, R. (1942) Sur la conservation du sang. *Rev. Canad. Biol.* **1**, 372.

Wurzel, H.A., Gottlieb, A.J. and Abelson, Neva M. (1971) Immunoglobulin characterization of anti-Tj[a] antibodies. *Commun. Amer. Assoc. Blood Banks*, Chicago.

Wyke, R.J., Tsiquaye, K.N., Thornton, A., White, Y., Portmann, B., Das, P.K., Zuckerman, A.J. and Williams, R. (1979) Transmission of non-A non-B hepatitis to chimpanzees by factor-IX concentrates after fatal complications in patients with chronic liver disease. *Lancet*, **i**, 520–524.

Wyler, D.J. (1983) Resurgence, resistance and research. *New Engl. J. Med.* **308**, 875–878, 934–940.

Yamada, K.M. and Olden, K. (1978) Fibronectin-adhesive glycoproteins of cell surface and blood. *Nature (Lond.)*, **275**, 179.

Yamada, A., Cohen, P.L. and Winfield, J.B. (1985) Subset specificity of anti-lymphocyte antibodies on systemic lupus erythematosus. Preferential reactivity with cells bearing the T4 and autologous erythrocyte receptor phenotypes. *Arthr. Rheumat.* **28**, 262–270.

Yamato, K., Taguchi, H., Yoshimoto, S., Fujishita, M., Yameshita, M., Ohtsuki, Y., Hoshino, H. and Miyoshi, I. (1986) Inactivation of lymphocyte-transforming activity of human T-cell leukemia virus type I by heat. *Jap. J. Cancer. Res.* (Gann) **77**, 13–15.

Yamamoto, F., Marken, J., Tsuji, T., White, T., Clausen, H. and Hakomori, S. (1990a) Cloning and characterization of DNA complemen-

tary to human UDP-GalNAc: Fuc $\alpha 1 \rightarrow 2$Gal $\alpha 1 \rightarrow 3$ GalNAc transferase (histo-blood group A transferase) mRNA. *J. biol. Chem.* **265**, 1146–1151.

Yamamoto, F., Clausen, H., White, T., Marken, J. and Hakomori, S. (1990b) Molecular genetic basis of the histo-blood group ABO system. *Nature (Lond.)*, **345**, 229–233.

Yamamoto, N. and 9 others (1990c) A platelet membrane glycoprotein (GP) deficiency in healthy blood donors: Nak[a]-platelets lack detectable GPIV (CD36). *Blood*, **76**, 1698–1703.

Yamamoto, F. (1991) Molecular genetic basis of histo-blood group ABO system (A[1] and A[2] subtypes). *Crime Lab. Digest*. **18**, 206.

Yang, S.Y. (1989) Population analysis of class I HLA antigens by one-dimensional isoelectric focusing gel electrophoresis. Workshop Summary report, in *Immunobiology of HLA*, ed B. Dupont, pp. 309–331. Springer-Verlag, New York, Berlin, Heidelberg.

Yankee, R.A., Graff, K.S., Dowling, Regina and Henderson, E.S. (1973) Selection of unrelated compatible platelet donors by lymphocyte HL-A matching. *New Engl. J. Med.* **288**, 760.

Yao, Alice C., Moinian, M. and Lind, J. (1969) Distribution of blood between infant and placenta after birth. *Lancet*, **ii**, 871.

Yap, P.L. and Williams, P.E. (1990) Novel intravenous immunoglobulins and their applications, in *Blood Transfusion: the Impact of New Technologies*, ed Marcela Contreras. *Ballière's Clinical Haematology*, **3**, 423–449.

Yarrish, R.L., Janas, J.A.S., Nosanchuk, J.S., Steigbigel, R.T. and Nusbacher, J. (1982) Transfusion malaria. Treatment with exchange transfusion after delayed diagnosis. *Arch. intern. Med.* **142**, 187–188.

Yates, A.D. and Watkins, W.M. (1982) Biosynthesis of blood group B determinants by the blood group A gene-specified anti-3-N-acetyl-D-galactosaminyl-transferase. *Biochem. biophys. Res. Commun.* **109**, 958–965.

Yates, A.D., Greenwell, P. and Watkins, W.M. (1983) Overlapping specification of the glycosyl-transferases specified by the blood-group A and B genes: a possible explanation for aberrant blood-group expression in malignant tissues. *Biochem. Soc. Transact.* **11**, 300–301.

Yates, A.D., Feeney, J., Donald, A.S.R. and Watkins, W.M. (1984) Characterisation of a blood-group A-active tetrasaccharide synthesized by a blood group B gene-specified glycosyltransferase. *Carbohydrate Res.* **130**, 251–260.

Yeager, Anne S., Grumet, F.C., Hafleigh, Elizabeth B., Arvin, Ann M., Bradley, J.S. and Prober, C.G. (1981) Prevention of transfusion-acquired cytomegalovirus infections in new-born infants. *J. Pediat.* **98**, 281–287.

Yeung, C.Y. and Hobbs, J.R. (1968) Serum-γG-globulin levels in normal, premature, post-mature, and 'small-for-dates' newborn babies. *Lancet*, **ii**, 1167.

Yliruokanen, A. (1948) Blood transfusions in premature infants. *Ann. Med. exp. Biol. fenn.* **26**, Suppl. 6.

Yoell, J.H. (1966) Immune anti-N agglutinin in human serum. Report of apparent associated hemolytic reaction. *Transfusion*, **6**, 592.

Yokoyama, M. and Fudenberg, H.H. (1964) Studies on 'cross-reacting' isoagglutinins. *J. Immunol.* **92**, 966.

Yokoyama, M. and McCoy, J.E. jr (1967) Further studies on auto-anti-Xg^e antibody. *Vox Sang.* **13**, 15.

Yomtovian, R., Abramson, J., Quie, P. and McCullogh, J. (1981) Granulocyte transfusion therapy in chronic granulomatous disease. *Transfusion*, **21**, 739–743.

Yomtovian, R., Kline, W., Press, C., Clay, M., Engman, H., Hammerschmidt, D. and McCullough, J. (1984) Severe pulmonary hypersensitivity associated with passive transfusion of a neutrophil-specific antibody. *Lancet*, **i**, 244–246.

Yoshida, A., Yamaguchi, H. and Okubo, Y. (1980a) Genetic mechanism of *cis* AB inheritance. I. A case associated with unequal chromosomal crossing over. *Amer. J. hum. Genet.* **32**, 332–338.

Yoshida, A., Yamaguchi, H. and Okubo, Y. (1980b) Genetic mechanism of *cis* AB inheritance. II. Cases associated with structural mutation of blood group glycosyltransferases. *Amer. J. hum. Genet.* **32**, 645–650.

Yoshida, Y., Yoshida, H., Tatsumi, K., Asoh, T., Hoshino, T. and Matsumoto, H. (1981a) Successful antibody elimination in severe M-incompatible pregnancy. *New Engl. J. Med.* **305**, 460–461.

Yoshida, A., Dave, V., Tregellas, W.M., McCormick, S. and Babcock, L. (1981b) Abnormal blood group galactosyltransferase in blood type B subjects whose serum contains anti-B agglutinin (Abstract). *Blood*, **58**, Suppl. 1, 92a.

Yoshida, M., Miyoshi, I. and Hinuma, Y. (1982) Isolation and characterization of retrovirus from cell lines of human adult T-cell leukemia and its implications in the disease. *Proc. nat. Acad. Sci. USA*, **79**, 2031–2035.

Yoshida, H., Ito, K., Emi, N., Kanzaki, H. and Matsuura, S. (1984) A new therapeutic antibody removal method using antigen-positive red cells. II. Application to a P-incompatible pregnant woman. *Vox Sang.* **47**, 216–223.

Young, L.E., Platzer, R.F., Yuile, C.L. and Woodruff, R.L. (1947) Recovery of group O recipient after transfusion of two litres of group A blood. *Amer. J. clin. Path.* **17**, 777.

Young, L.E., Ervin, D.M. and Yuile, C.L. (1949) Hemolytic reactions produced in dogs by transfusion of incompatible dog blood and plasma. I. Serologic and hematologic aspects. *Blood*, **4**, 1218.

Young, L.E., Christian, R.M., Ervin, D.M., Swisher, S.N., O'Brien, W.A., Stewart, W.B. and Yuile, C.L. (1950) Erythrocyte-iso-antibody reactions in dogs. *Commun. 3rd Int. Congr. Haemat.*, Cambridge. See also (1951) *Blood*, **6**, 291.

Young, L.E. (1954) Blood groups and transfusion reactions. *Amer. J. Med.* **16**, 885.

Young, W.W. jr, Portoukalian, J. and Hakomori, S. (1981) Two monoclonal anticarbohydrate antibodies directed to glycosphingolipids with a lacto-N-glycosyl type II chain. *J. biol. Chem.* **256**, 10967–10972.

Young, W.W. jr and 10 others (1983) Characterization of monoclonal antibodies specific for the Lewis human blood group determinant. *J. biol. Chem.* **258**, 4890–4894.

Young, N. and Mortimer, P. (1984) Viruses and bone marrow failure. *Blood*, **63**, 729–737.

Young, H., Moyes, A., McMillan, A. and Patterson, J. (1992) Enzyme immunoassay for anti-treponemal IgG: screening or confirmatory test? *J. clin. Path.* **45**, 37–41.

Yuile, C.L., van Zandt, T.F., Ervin, D.M. and Young, L.E. (1949) Hemolytic reactions produced in dogs by transfusion of incompatible dog blood and plasma. II. Renal aspects following whole blood transfusions. *Blood*, **4**, 1232.

Yunis, J.J. and Yunis, E.J. (1963) Cell antigens and cell specialization. I. A study of blood group antigens on normoblasts. *Blood*, **22**, 53.

Yunis, J.J. and Yunis, E.J. (1964) Cell antigens and cell specialization. II. Demonstration of some red cell antigens of human normoblasts. *Blood*, **24**, 522.

Zack, J.A. and Chen, I.S.Y. (1991) The biology of retroviruses, in *Transfusion Transmitted Infections*, eds. D.M. Smith and R.Y. Dodd, pp. 53–72. ASCP Press, Chicago.

Zade-Oppen, A.M.M. (1968) The effect of mannitol, sucrose, raffinose and dextran on post-hypertonic hemolysis. *Acta physiol. scand.* **74**, 195.

Zak, S.J. and Good, R.A. (1959) Immunochemical studies of human serum gamma globulins. *J. clin. invest.* **38**, 579.

Zanetti, A.R., Tanzi, E., Zehender, G., Magni, E., Incarbone, C., Zonaro, A., Primi, D. and Cariani, E. (1990) Hepatitis C virus RNA in symptomless donors implicated in post-transfusion non-A, non-B hepatitis (Letter). *Lancet*, **ii**, 448.

Zaroulis, C.G., Spector, J.I., Emerson, C.P. and Valeri, C.R. (1979) Therapeutic transfusions of previously frozen washed human platelets. *Transfusion*, **19**, 371–378.

Zeitlin, R.A., Sanger, Ruth and Race, R.R. (1958) Unpublished data cited by Race and Sanger (1975), p. 240.

Zelenski, K.R. (1986) Serologic characterization of monoclonal anti-A and anti-B blood group antibodies. *Abstracts, 19th Congr. Int. Soc. Blood Transfus.*, Sydney, p. 502.

Zeller, W.J., Scholler, P., Rossler, W., Lenhard, K., Dreikorn, E., Weber, E. and Schmahl, D. (1986) Allogenic blood transfusion and experimental tumor growth. *Transplant. Proc.* **18**, 1448–1449.

Zettner, A. and Bove, J.R. (1963) Hemolytic transfusion reaction due to interdonor incompatibility. *Transfusion*, **3**, 48.

Zimmerman, L.M. and Howell, Katharine M. (1932) History of blood transfusion. *Ann. med. Hist. (N.S.)*, **4**, 415.

Zimmerman, T.S. and Müller-Eberhard, H.J. (1971) Blood coagulation initiation by a complement-mediated pathway. *J. exp. med.* **134**, 1601.

Zinkernagel, R.M. and Doherty, P.C. (1974) Restriction of *in vitro* T cell mediated cytotoxicity in lymphocyte choriomeningitis within a syngeneic or semi-allogeneic system. *Nature (Lond.)*, **248**, 701.

Zipursky, A., Pollock, Janet, Neelands, P., Chown, B. and Israels, L.G. (1963a) The transplacental passage of foetal red blood-cells and the pathogenesis of Rh immunization during pregnancy. *Lancet*, **ii**, 489.

Zipursky, A., Pollock, Janet, Chown, B. and Israels, L.G. (1963b) Transplacental foetal hemorrhage after placental injury during delivery or amniocentesis. *Lancet*, **ii**, 493.

Zipursky, A., Pollock, J., Chown, B. and Israels, L.G. (1965) Transplacental isoimmunization by foetal red blood cells. *Birth Defects, Original Article Series*, **1**, 84.

Zipursky, A. (1971) The universal prevention of Rh immunization. *Clin. Obstet. Gynec.* **14**, 869.

Zuckerman, A.J. and Taylor, P.E. (1969) Persistence of the serum hepatitis (SH-Australia) antigen for many years. *Nature (Lond.)*, **223**, 81.

Zuckerman, A.J. (1990) Viral hepatitis. *Brit. med. Bull.* **46**, 1–564.

Zuckerman, Jane, N., Cockcroft, Anne and Griffiths, P. (1991) Hepatitis A immunisation. *Brit. med. J.* **303**, 247.

Zuelzer, W.W. and Kaplan, E. (1954) ABO heterospecific pregnancy and hemolytic disease. IV. Pathologic variants. *Amer. J. Dis. Child.* **88**, 319.

Zupańska, B., Lawkowicz, W., Górska, B., Kozlowska, J., Ochocka, M., Rokicka-Milewska, R., Derulska, D. and Ciepielewska, D. (1976) Autoimmune haemolytic anaemia in children. *Brit. J. Haemat.* **34**, 511.

Zupańska, Barbara, Thomson, Eileen E. and Merry, A.H. (1986) Fc receptors for IgG1 and IgG3 on human mononuclear cells—an evaluation with known levels of erythrocyte-bound IgG. *Vox Sang.* **50**, 97–103.

INDEX

Antibodies are not listed unless they are of substantial clinical importance (e.g anti-K, anti-HPA-1a) or unless their name is different from that of the system to which they belong (e.g. anti-U of the MNSs system). Those not listed can be found by looking up the entry for the corresponding antigen.

A, B and H antigens *see also* A_1, etc.; B_3, etc.
    and Anti-A and -B
  A reacting with anti-B   154
  A weakening B   153
  acquired B   156–7, 315
  amniotic fluid   159
  animal tissues   173–4
  B converted to O   157
  B reacting with anti-A   154
  B weakening A   153
  B_3, B_x, B_{el} 152
  on bacteria   101, 157, 160
  biosynthesis   191–203
  Blacks and Whites compared   150
  carcinoma, changes   88, 202–3
  chemistry   194–203
  cis AB   153, 199
  cloning of *A, B* and *H* 203
  cryoprecipitates   172
  development   89, 155–6, 160
  on epidermis   160
  on fetal red cells   155–6, 160
  gene frequencies   85
  h (Bombay and para-Bombay)
      phenotypes   154–5, 159, 169, 199
  H, type I and II chains   159, 195–7
  H as structural gene   195, 198, 200
  Hh   150
  immune responses to A and B   170–5, 530
  inhibiting anti-A, etc.   158–9, 165, 322, 370, 583
  leukaemia, changes   88, 156
  in liver, etc.   160
  on lymphocytes and platelets   159–60
  numbers of antigen sites   154
  O converted to A or B   157, 199
  pig A substance   173–5
  in plasma (and serum) 158–9, 322
  purified human A substance   165, 172, 174
  on red cells of newborn   588–9
  on reticulocytes   89
  in saliva   157–8, 175
  secretors and non-secretors
    H with A or B or both in body fluids of
      secretors   157–8

  infections more frequent in non-
      secretors   200
  Se a regulator or structural gene 194–5, 198, 200
  Se and *se* influencing Lewis
      phenotype   175–8
  only secretor fetuses stimulate maternal
      anti-A and -B   172
  specific oligosaccharides   370, 590–1
  on spermatozoa   160
  subgroups of A *see* A_1, A_2, etc.
  subgroups of B   152–3
  transferases in serum   198–9
  transferases weakened in pregnancy   199
  uptake onto red cells from plasma   159
  in urine   158
  in vaccines   173–4
  in various secretions   158
A_1 and A_2 (also A_1B and A_2B)
  chemistry   200–1
  difference between A^1 and A^2 genes   203
  distinction *in vitro*   150–1, 156, 167–8, 200–1
  distinction *in vivo*   168, 463–4, 506
  frequencies   150
  in haemolytic disease (ABO) of the newborn 588–9
  in newborn infants   150–1
A_3, A_{el}, A_{end}, A_m, A_x 151–2, 154, 330
A_h and B_h 154–5
ABO system (including Hh)
  antibodies *see* Anti-A, B; Anti-A_1 *and* Anti-H
      and -HI
  antigens *see* A, B and H
  carcinoma of stomach   87
  discovery   78
  Factor VIII levels   662
  gene frequencies in Britain   85
  genotypes and phenotypes   85
  phenotype frequencies in selected
      populations   85–6, 150
  routine grouping   358–9
ABO-incompatibility *see also* Haemolytic disease
      (ABO) of newborn *and* Incompatible
      transfusions

973

MNSs system (*cont'd*)
  anti-V   264–5, 534, 583
  anti-Vw   101, 260, 264–5, 279
  Bauhinea purpurea, B. varieagata   84, 263
  chemistry of antigens   258–60
  DAT positive in subject with weak MN
    antigens   258
  differences between MM and MN   256, 259,
    359, 449–50
  effect of enzymes on antigens   83, 259–60,
    327–8
  En(a –)   257
  Iberis amara 262
  Ig class of antibodies   261–4
  Miltenberger (Mi.I, etc.)   257
  Mit   545
  M^k 257
  Moluccella laevis   263–4
  monoclonal antibodies   108, 262
  'N'   256, 260
  naming of M antigen   78
  Nf (formaldehyde N)   263
  N_{vg} 263
  rare genetic variants   257
  trypsin-sensitive low-frequency antigens on
    MN sialoglycoprotein   328
  Vicia graminea   84, 124, 263–4
Mo^a 279
Molucella laevis   263–4
Monoclonal antibodies
  advantages as reagents   329
  constructing new antibodies   110
  disadvantages as reagents   109–10, 329–30
  effect of pH   109
  human monoclonals   109
  hybridomas   108
  murine monoclonals   108–9
  reacting with
    A, B and H   108, 154, 163, 201, 330
    band 3   108
    complement components   108–9, 272
    D   109, 214, 330, 469
    En^a TS   108
    endotoxin   54
    Fy6   253
    Ge (related)   108, 273
    glycophorins A, B and C   108
    H type I, H type II   108
    HLA   603
    I   108
    IgG, IgG1, etc.   108–9
    Jk^a, Jk^b 109, 256
    k   108, 250
    K (related)   251
    Le^a, Le^b 108, 181–2
    Le^y 108
    LKE   193
    Lu^b 108, 266
    M,N,S   108, 262
    P, P_1, P^k 108
    Rh (c, E, etc.)   109
    Rh (D)   109, 214, 330,
    Rh-related polypeptides   208
    s (related)   108

    T, Tn   108
    Y (Le^y)   108
Monocyte monolayer assay (MMA)   136,
  462–3, 562
Monocyte phagocyte system (MPS) *see also*
  Extravascular destruction of red cells
  capacity for removing red cells   473–5
  competition between
    antibody-coated red cells and
     platelets   674
    bacteria and red cells   524
  corticosteroids   485
  overloading as cause of intravascular
    lysis   519–20
  survival of stored red cells affected by MPS
    function   404
Monocytes and macrophages
  ADCC assays *see* Bioassays
  antigens   607, 611
  chemiluminescence assays   137
  erythrophagocytosis   132–6, 463
  lysing IgG-coated red cells *in vitro*   132,
    136–7
  macrophage and monocyte assays *see*
    Bioassays
  receptors for
    fragments of C3 and C4   134
    IgG1 and IgG3   132
  rosetting   135 *see also* Bioassays
Monogamous bivalency   125, 166
Mosaics   89, 119, 134
MPT *see* Manual polybrene test
Mt^a *see* MNSs system
Mur   258
Mycobacterium leprae   773
Mycoplasma   292

N, *see* MNSs system
N-acetylneuraminic acid (NeuNAc) *see* Sialic
  acid
NA1, etc.   608
NANA (*N*-acetylneuraminic acid) *see* Sialic acid
NANB hepatitis *see* Non-A, non-B hepatitis
NATP *see* Neonatal alloimmune
  thrombocytopenia
Naturally occurring red cell alloantibodies *see*
  also Anti-A and -B; MNSs system; Rh
  antibodies, etc.
  characteristics (including Ig class)   102, 160
  definition   80, 100, 102
  effect of antigenic stimulus   101, 168,
    170–5, 183, 189
  prevalence   100
  relation to heteroagglutinins   80, 101
  response to specific stimulus
    A_1 168
    Le   183, 484
    P_1 189
  specificities
    A, B   102, 162–3
    A_1 67
    Cs, etc.   102, 218, 275, 458
    Di^a 101E   102, 458